Pitfalls in Musculoskeletal Radiology

Wilfred C.G. Peh

Editor

Pitfalls in Musculoskeletal Radiology

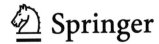 Springer

Editor
Wilfred C.G. Peh, MD, FRCP (Edin), FRCP (Glasg), FRCR
Department of Diagnostic Radiology
Khoo Teck Puat Hospital
Singapore
Republic of Singapore

ISBN 978-3-319-53494-7   ISBN 978-3-319-53496-1   (eBook)
DOI 10.1007/978-3-319-53496-1

Library of Congress Control Number: 2017941712

Printed on acid-free paper

This Springer imprint is published by Springer Nature
The registered company is Springer International Publishing AG
The registered company address is: Gewerbestrasse 11, 6330 Cham, Switzerland

Foreword

I am honored to be able to write a foreword for this new and timely book *Pitfalls in Musculoskeletal Radiology*, edited by my good friend, Wilfred Peh, with a contributing cast that includes many of the distinguished members of the International Skeletal Society. I am very familiar with the time commitment and hard work that the preparation of such books involves, having myself been involved with the publication of books in the past. Although Wilfred suggests that his task was simple, merely "conceptualizing the contents of this book and then approaching these friends to contribute their considerable expertise," I know for fact that it takes a motivated and knowledgeable editor to determine what subjects need to be addressed and who specifically would be the correct person or persons to complete the work. Clearly, it helps if that editor has a worldwide reputation as an educator with the ability to identify the right people and obtain their approval as contributors. The result is a book that is desperately needed and will become an instant success.

There are countless texts currently available that cover the spectrum of musculoskeletal imaging in a variety of disorders, but there is none that emphasizes those pitfalls that cause confusion in image interpretation and misdiagnosis. Such pitfalls include many anatomic variants and technique-specific artifacts, and they are encountered every day in clinical practice. I myself have struggled with these throughout my career and, until now, had no single place to go to figure out with what I was dealing. Now I do. Indeed, in the pages of this book can be found reference to pitfalls in conventional radiography, ultrasonography, computed tomography, magnetic resonance, nuclear medicine, arthrography, and interventional procedures, with information collected and detailed by experts in each one of these modalities and techniques. General, disease-specific, and regional-specific artifacts and variants are covered, with succinct and clear writing, vivid illustrations, and pertinent references for further reading. Each chapter is well organized and a pleasure to read, providing useful information that will allow the reader to avoid mistakes in interpretation that otherwise would occur daily.

Wilfred Peh is not new to book-writing. His impressive resume confirms a lifelong commitment to education. His previous texts have all been well received. But *Pitfalls in Musculoskeletal Radiology* will likely turn out to be the most successful of the lot, because this book addresses a subject that has been largely ignored and one that has a great clinical impact. Purchase this book, place it at an easily accessible spot on your desk or shelf, and refer to it often and I can guarantee that you will become better in the interpretation of imaging studies related to the musculoskeletal system. Congratulations Wilfred and contributors (many of whom are friends of mine), this is a job well done! I am privileged to be able to write this foreword.

San Diego, USA   Donald Resnick, MD
30 July 2016

Preface

The growing applications of advanced imaging modalities such as high-resolution ultrasound (US) imaging, dual-energy computed tomography, and magnetic resonance imaging (MRI) have made the daily clinical practice of musculoskeletal radiology progressively complex. While these modalities can show a larger number of musculoskeletal structures in greater detail, with more sensitivity and higher resolution, they may also result in the production of technique-specific artifacts and the detection of unsuspected anatomical variants. Failure to recognize these imaging artifacts and variants may lead to diagnostic error and misinterpretation, with resultant medicolegal implications.

Potentially correctable pitfalls may also result from inadequate imaging technique, lack of training/inexperience, and failure to correlate with other imaging findings, in particular radiographs. Pitfalls in imaging interpretation also occur during imaging of trauma to structures such as bones, joints, tendons, ligaments, and muscles, in different regions of the musculoskeletal system at different ages, as well as various diseases affecting these structures, such as inflammatory arthritides, infections, metabolic bone lesions, congenital skeletal dysplasias, tumors, and tumorlike conditions. Recognition of these pitfalls is crucial in helping the practicing radiologist achieve a more accurate diagnosis. However, it is increasingly difficult for musculoskeletal radiologists, let alone general radiologists and residents, to know all of these pitfalls. This textbook aims at highlighting the spectrum of pitfalls that may occur in musculoskeletal radiology and, where possible, provides suggestions for overcoming or avoiding these pitfalls.

This book came about as I was nearing the tail end of completing the well-received *Pitfalls in Diagnostic Radiology*, published by Springer-Verlag (Berlin/Heidelberg) in 2015. As with the previous book project, I sounded out the idea for *Pitfalls in Musculoskeletal Radiology* to my good friend, Dr. Ute Heilmann, editorial director of clinical medicine at Springer-Verlag, who replied within days saying "Again a very promising project from you!....I am confident that under your leadership, a sound project, worthwhile to be published and of value to the community." I once again thank Ute, for her decisive and complete support, and her staff, for competently managing this project.

This book addresses a topic very close to my heart and also to the hearts of many of my musculoskeletal radiologist friends, the majority of whom are distinguished members of the International Skeletal Society. Hence, I was left with the relatively simple task of conceptualizing the contents of this book and then approaching these friends to contribute their considerable expertise. The resultant *Pitfalls in Musculoskeletal Radiology* highlights musculoskeletal imaging pitfalls in a comprehensive and systematic manner and draws on the vast collective experiences of an international group of 97 radiologists from 51 reputable centers in 18 countries located in different parts of the world – as far as I know, the only such book available. To my willing author friends, I give my sincere thanks.

The resultant book consists of 43 chapters, well illustrated with 892 figures and 1,585 individual images. As with *Pitfalls in Diagnostic Radiology*, I have tried to edit the contributions of these experts with a light touch so as to retain, as much as possible, the original flow of each chapter according to the diverse experiences and perspectives of each author. Some overlap among chapters will be inevitable but not necessarily a bad thing. For example, the magic angle phenomenon is first explained in Chap. 4 on MRI artifacts but is also highlighted in chapters on MRI pitfalls of shoulder injury (Chap. 15), elbow injury (Chap. 17), wrist and hand injuries (Chap. 19), and cartilage imaging (Chap. 40), among others. In a similar vein, the anisotropy artifact appears in Chap. 2 on US imaging artifacts, as well as in chapters dealing with US pitfalls of injuries to the shoulder (Chap. 16), elbow (Chap. 18), and hip (Chap. 22). Discussion of diagnostic pitfalls in these individual chapters would not have been complete without a mention of these two artifacts. Similarly, marrow reconversion is relevant in topics as diverse as elbow injury (Chap. 17), knee injury (Chap. 23), treated musculoskeletal tumors (Chap. 32), multifocal and multisystemic bone lesions (Chap. 36), hematological and circulatory bone conditions (Chap. 37), and pediatric lesions (Chap. 38).

My grateful thanks go to my good friend and role model Professor Donald Resnick, who graciously wrote the foreword for this book.

Pitfalls in Musculoskeletal Radiology is dedicated to my dearest mother, Libby Tin Peh. She is the best mother that any son can wish for and is the most wonderful human being.

Singapore   Wilfred C.G. Peh
31 December 2016

Contents

Part I   Imaging Modality and Technique Pitfalls Related to the Musculoskeletal System

1   **Radiography Limitations and Pitfalls**   3
    Keynes T.A. Low and Wilfred C.G. Peh

2   **Ultrasound Imaging Artifacts**   33
    Lana Hiraj Gimber and Mihra S. Taljanovic

3   **Computed Tomography Artifacts**   45
    Derik L. Davis and Prasann Vachhani

4   **Magnetic Resonance Imaging Artifacts**   61
    Dinesh R. Singh, Helmut Rumpel, Michael S.M. Chin,
    and Wilfred C.G. Peh

5   **Nuclear Medicine Imaging Artifacts**   83
    Anbalagan Kannivelu, Kelvin S.H. Loke, Sean X.X. Yan,
    Hoi Yin Loi, and David C.E. Ng

6   **Arthrographic Technique Pitfalls**   99
    Teck Yew Chin and Robert S.D. Campbell

7   **Ultrasound-Guided Musculoskeletal Interventional
    Techniques Pitfalls** 121
    Gajan Rajeswaran and Jeremiah C. Healy

8   **Musculoskeletal Interventional Techniques Pitfalls** 139
    Paul I. Mallinson and Peter L. Munk

9   **Musculoskeletal Biopsy Pitfalls** 149
    Mark J. Kransdorf and James S. Jelinek

10 **Errors in Radiology** 165
    Andoni P. Toms

Part II   Regional and Disease-Based Imaging Pitfalls

11 **Radiographic Normal Variants** 181
    Mark W. Anderson

12 Long Bone Trauma: Radiographic Pitfalls................ 207
Robert B. Uzor, Johnny U.V. Monu,
and Thomas L. Pope

13 Spine Trauma: Radiographic and CT Pitfalls............ 257
Prudencia N.M. Tyrrell and Naomi Winn

14 Spine Trauma: MRI Pitfalls.......................... 277
Sri Andreani Utomo, Paulus Rahardjo, Swee Tian Quek,
and Wilfred C.G. Peh

15 Shoulder Injury: MRI Pitfalls........................ 293
Josephina A. Vossen and William E. Palmer

16 Shoulder Injury: US Pitfalls......................... 307
Richard W. Fawcett, Emma L. Rowbotham,
and Andrew J. Grainger

17 Elbow Injury: MRI Pitfalls.......................... 321
Mark Harmon, Elaine NiMhurchu, Gordon Andrews,
and Bruce B. Forster

18 Elbow Injury: US Pitfalls............................ 339
Graham Buirski and Javier Arnaiz

19 Wrist and Hand Injuries: MRI Pitfalls................. 355
Mingqian Huang and Mark E. Schweitzer

20 Wrist and Hand Injuries: US Pitfalls.................. 381
Graham Buirski and Javier Arnaiz

21 Hip Injury: MRI Pitfalls............................ 391
Lauren M. Ladd, Donna G. Blankenbaker,
and Michael J. Tuite

22 Hip Injury: US Pitfalls............................. 415
James Teh and David McKean

23 Knee Injury: MRI Pitfalls........................... 425
Redouane Kadi and Maryam Shahabpour

24 Knee Injury: US Pitfalls............................ 471
David McKean and James Teh

25 Ankle and Foot Injuries: MRI Pitfalls.................. 479
Yuko Kobashi, Yohei Munetomo, Akira Baba, Shinji Yamazoe,
and Takuji Mogami

26 Ankle and Foot Injuries: US Pitfalls................... 511
Philip Yoong and James Teh

27 Pediatric Trauma: Imaging Pitfalls.................... 525
Timothy Cain and John Fitzgerald

**28 Musculoskeletal Soft Tissue Tumors:
CT and MRI Pitfalls**................................. 547
Richard W. Whitehouse and Anand Kirwadi

29 Musculoskeletal Soft Tissue Tumors: US Pitfalls 581
Esther H.Y. Hung and James F. Griffith

30 Bone Tumors: Radiographic Pitfalls 597
Sumer N. Shikhare, Niraj Dubey, and Wilfred C.G. Peh

31 Bone Tumors: MRI Pitfalls 621
Remide Arkun and Mehmet Argin

**32 Musculoskeletal Tumors Following Treatment:
Imaging Pitfalls** 647
Wouter C.J. Huysse, Lennart B. Jans, and Filip M. Vanhoenacker

33 Musculoskeletal Infection: Imaging Pitfalls 671
Nuttaya Pattamapaspong

34 Inflammatory Arthritides: Imaging Pitfalls 697
Paul Felloni, Neal Larkman, Rares Dunca,
and Anne Cotten

35 Metabolic Bone Lesions: Imaging Pitfalls 713
Eric A. Walker, Jonelle M. Petscavage-Thomas,
Agustinus Suhardja, and Mark D. Murphey

**36 Multifocal and Multisystemic Bone Lesions:
Imaging Pitfalls** 743
Michael E. Mulligan

**37 Hematological and Circulatory Bone Lesions:
Imaging Pitfalls** 767
Suphaneewan Jaovisidha, Khalid Al-Ismail,
Niyata Chitrapazt, and Praman Fuengfa

**38 Pediatric Nontraumatic Musculoskeletal Lesions:
Imaging Pitfalls** 819
Eu Leong Harvey James Teo

39 Spine Nontraumatic Lesions: Imaging Pitfalls 853
Shigeru Ehara

40 Cartilage Imaging Pitfalls 881
Klaus Bohndorf

41 Bone Mineral Densitometry Pitfalls 893
Giuseppe Guglielmi, Federico Ponti, Sara Guerri,
and Alberto Bazzocchi

42 Congenital Skeletal Dysplasias: Imaging Pitfalls 925
Richa Arora and Kakarla Subbarao

**43 Musculoskeletal Lesions: Nuclear Medicine
Imaging Pitfalls** 951
Yun Young Choi, Jae Sung Lee, and Seoung-Oh Yang

Part I

Imaging Modality and Technique Pitfalls Related to the Musculoskeletal System

Radiography Limitations and Pitfalls

Keynes T.A. Low and Wilfred C.G. Peh

Contents

1.1 **Introduction** 3

1.2 **Pitfalls Related to Radiographic Image
    Acquisition** 4
1.2.1 Adequacy of Coverage and Views 4
1.2.2 Radiographic Technique and Positioning 6
1.2.3 Radiographic Artifacts 9

1.3 **Limitations of Radiographic Imaging of
    Non-osseous Structures** 12
1.3.1 Intra- and Periarticular Structures 12
1.3.2 Other Soft Tissues and Foreign Bodies 19

1.4 **Radiographically Occult Osseous
    Abnormalities** 24
1.4.1 Destructive Osseous Lesions 24
1.4.2 Trauma-Related Osseous Injuries 25
1.4.3 Osteoporosis 28

Conclusion 29

References 31

Abbreviations

ALARA As low as reasonably achievable
CT   Computed tomography
MRI   Magnetic resonance imaging
US   Ultrasound

1.1 Introduction

It is widely acknowledged that radiography should be the initial imaging modality in the evaluation of most suspected musculoskeletal lesions. They are often adequate for diagnosis, although advanced imaging modalities such as computed tomography (CT) and magnetic resonance imaging (MRI) are still often required for more detailed assessment of structures such as bone marrow and various soft tissues. Nevertheless, radiographs play an important complementary role to these newer cross-sectional imaging techniques. For example, they can provide a big picture view of bony or joint abnormalities, which allows better assessment of conditions such as the inflammatory arthritides (e.g., by showing distribution and pattern of joint involvement). Radiographs can also demonstrate calcifications and ossifications, which might not be convincingly seen on MRI. In fact, radiography still remains the most specific imaging modality for the diagnosis of bone tumors.

Radiographs are commonly obtained for acute musculoskeletal trauma, infection, chronic arthropathies, and bone or soft tissue tumors. They are also performed for follow-up imaging after treatment such as fracture fixation and joint replacement. Radiographs are widely available, inexpensive, and well tolerated and can be rapidly and easily obtained. As with any imaging modality, radiography has advantages and disadvantages. Radiographs are of limited value in the evaluation of soft tissue injuries, for example, musculotendinous, cartilaginous, or ligamentous injuries. These soft tissue structures are not clearly seen on the radiograph and are better assessed on MRI or ultrasound (US) imaging, both of which have superior soft tissue resolution. Radiography is also limited in the assessment of conditions such as osteomyelitis and non-displaced acute fractures, both of which can be radiographically occult. Certain scenarios make it challenging or impossible to accurately interpret radiographs, for example, when an external cast obscures bone or when a background of osteopenia results in a paucity of osseous detail. Apart from the aforementioned intrinsic limitations of the radiographic modality, other potential pitfalls in relation to radiographic technique can be encountered. Proper positioning of the patient is crucial in obtaining a radiograph of diagnostic quality. An adequate coverage of the area of interest and an adequate number of views are also necessary for proper evaluation.

1.2 Pitfalls Related to Radiographic Image Acquisition

Radiography is often the initial modality used in the imaging workup of patients with musculoskeletal complaints. It is the workhorse in the emergency department, where it is able to support the high patient throughput. Despite the time pressure, the radiographer has to be meticulous during the acquisition of radiographs as a multitude of potential pitfalls may occur, limiting the accuracy of the evaluation and ultimately negatively impacting upon the clinical management of patients.

1.2.1 Adequacy of Coverage and Views

When radiographic imaging is requested, one of the fundamental responsibilities of the radiolo-

gist is to ensure adequate coverage and sufficient views of the anatomical region of interest. For example, a full radiographic series of the cervical spine should include an anteroposterior view, a lateral view, and an open-mouth odontoid view. On the lateral view, the entire cervical spine should be visualized with the base of the skull seen superiorly and the cervicothoracic junction (C7-T1 level) seen inferiorly. If the routine lateral view is insufficient, attempts should be made to better visualize the cervicothoracic junction (e.g., performing a swimmer's view) (Fig. 1.1). Missing a significant injury as a result of inadequate coverage on imaging evaluation is virtually indefensible in the court of law. The example of the cervical spine radiograph is particularly pertinent due to the medicolegal implications of a missed unstable cervical spine injury, which can result in devastating neurological sequelae. CT has been shown to have superior sensitivity and has largely superseded radiography in the detection of cervical spine injuries in patients who have high risk of injury (Holmes and Akkinepalli 2005). Obtaining high-quality radiographs with adequate coverage tends to be challenging in these patients due to difficulties in positioning. However, radiography is still used for screening low-risk patients with an indication for imaging, and adequate coverage of anatomy remains crucial.

Another potential pitfall is the failure to cover separate associated anatomical regions which may be involved while imaging the primary area of interest. For example, in a patient with injury to the medial ankle structures, a Maisonneuve injury may be missed if imaging does not include the proximal fibula (Pankovich 1976) (Fig. 1.2). Associated injuries should be suspected based on the injury mechanism and the imaging of the relevant area obtained, if indicated. In another example, a calcaneal fracture is usually due to an axial loading force and should raise the suspicion of spinal injury, especially at the thoracolumbar junction.

In general, orthogonal views are sufficient in the radiographic imaging of the axial and appendicular skeleton (Fig. 1.3). However, additional views may be required based on the complexity of the anatomy, especially if the structure of

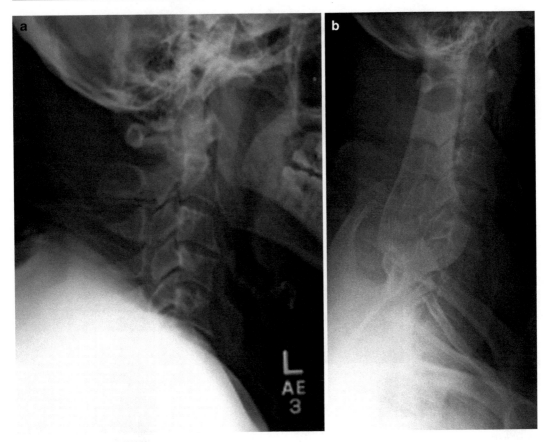

Fig. 1.1 A 47-year-old man who presented with neck pain following a motor vehicle accident. (**a**) Lateral radiograph of the cervical spine shows inadequate coverage of anatomy. The cervical spine inferior to the C5 level, as well as the cervicothoracic junction, is obscured by the shoulder girdle. (**b**) A swimmer's view was performed as a complementary study and ensured complete coverage of the region of interest

interest has a complex shape. Recognition that there are insufficient views can help to identify this pitfall and prevent potential missed diagnoses. In the knee, for example, a skyline view may demonstrate an avulsion fracture of the medial aspect of the patella in relation to transient patellar dislocation (Fig. 1.4). This finding would have been missed on routine anteroposterior and lateral views of the knee. In the case of the scaphoid bone, the standard posteroanterior and lateral radiographs of the wrist are usually insufficient for this complex-shaped bone, with additional views needed for adequate evaluation. Although previous studies show varying recommendations on the number and specific views required in the scaphoid series, a posteroanterior view of the wrist with ulnar deviation and slight tube angulation is usually part of the imaging series (Malik et al. 2004; Shenoy et al. 2007; Toth et al. 2007) (Fig. 1.5).

Sometimes, stress views are warranted for evaluation of ligamentous injuries. Examples include the clenched-fist view for assessment of scapholunate ligament integrity and the weight-bearing view for assessment of the coracoclavicular ligament. These views may demonstrate widening of the scapholunate interval and coracoclavicular distance, respectively, which indicate significant injury (Lee et al. 2011; Eschler et al. 2014). Without stress views, these injuries would likely be radiographically occult and hence be difficult to detect.

Fig. 1.2 An 87-year-old woman who presented with right ankle pain after a fall. (**a**) Frontal radiograph of the right ankle shows a spiral fracture of the distal tibia. (**b**) Frontal radiograph of the right leg shows a proximal fibular fracture (*arrow*). This Maisonneuve injury would have been missed if imaging coverage of the proximal leg was not performed

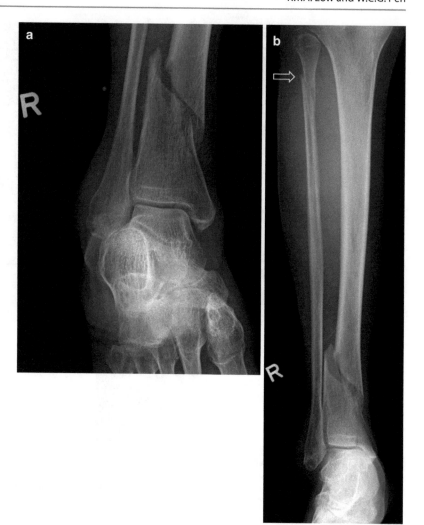

1.2.2 Radiographic Technique and Positioning

Radiographic technique refers to the selection of exposure factors, the kilovolt peak (kVp), and the milliampere-second (mAs), which determine the properties of the X-ray beam. The kVp influences the penetrative ability of the X-ray beam, while the mAs influences the quantity of radiation delivered. Good radiographic technique requires the proper selection of exposure factors such that there is optimal beam penetration of the anatomy, as well as optimal quantity of radiation reaching the detector at a radiation dose which is as low as reasonably achievable (ALARA).

In recent years, the field of diagnostic radiology has seen the transition from film/screen radiographic systems to digital imaging. For the film/screen systems, whether a film was under- or overexposed was easily appreciated, since the image would either be too white or too dark, respectively. In digital systems, however, the wide dynamic range of the detector and the ability to automatically post-process images to achieve optimal brightness allow images of acceptable quality to be produced over a larger range of exposures as compared to the film/screen systems (Murphey et al. 1992). Digital radiography is thus more forgiving with suboptimal exposures and has significantly reduced

Fig. 1.3 A 31-year-old woman who presented with left lateral ankle pain. Frontal and lateral radiographs of the left ankle were obtained. A minimally displaced distal fibular fracture is seen as a lucent line only on the lateral radiograph (*arrow*). It is occult on the frontal radiograph. This common injury illustrates the importance of having sufficient radiographic views for proper evaluation

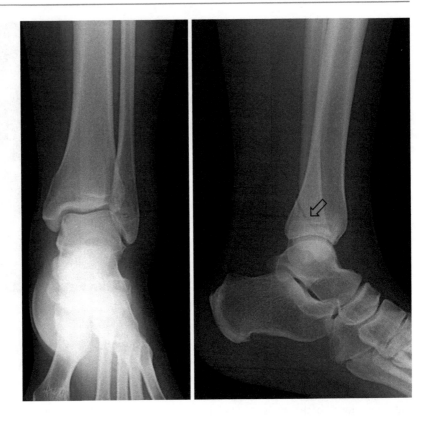

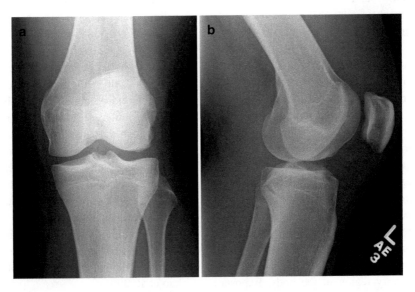

Fig. 1.4 An 18-year-old man who presented with left knee pain after a collision with another player during a football match. (**a**) Frontal and (**b**) lateral radiographs of the left knee show no fracture or dislocation. (**c**) Skyline view of the knee, however, shows a bony fragment at the medial aspect of the patella (*arrow*), suggestive of an avulsion fracture. (**d**) Axial fat-suppressed T2-W MR image of the left knee shows marrow edema at the site of the avulsion fracture (*arrow*) and disruption of the medial patellofemoral ligamentous structures (*arrowheads*), which are typical features of a transient patellar dislocation. Associated kissing bone contusion was present at the lateral femoral condyle (not shown)

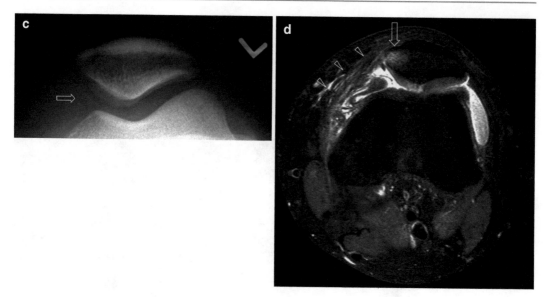

Fig. 1.4 (continued)

the number of rejected films. Even with the advantages of digital radiography, radiographic technique still affects the image quality and the radiation dose to the patient. Underexposure results in a reduction of the signal-to-noise ratio and manifests as increased quantum mottle, which might render the image unsuitable for diagnostic interpretation (Fig. 1.6). Conversely, overexposure in the digital system does not affect image quality but delivers a larger quantity of radiation than is necessary, resulting in excessive radiation dose to the patient. An optimum exposure should be given with each radiographic study, in line with the ALARA principle and producing an image of sufficient quality.

Each digital radiographic system is unique, due to differences in design and detector type. The optimal exposure settings are thus unique to each system. A technique chart should be available for each radiographic system, containing specific optimal exposure settings for each radiographic position in every region of the body. Exposure adjustment systems should then be applied to fine-tune the exposure settings based on the patient's weight and thickness of the body part to be imaged, the methods of which are beyond the scope of this chapter (Ching et al. 2014).

Standardized positioning of the patient results in radiographic views which are reproducible and optimal for interpretation. If proper positioning is not achieved during image acquisition, alignment of bones might not be accurately evaluated. For example, the posteroanterior view of the wrist should be obtained with the wrist in a neutral position, as only with proper positioning can the ulnar variance be accurately demonstrated. Supination of the forearm decreases ulnar variance, while pronation increases ulnar variance (Epner et al. 1982) (Fig. 1.7). Another example is in the radiographic evaluation of the ankle mortise. Accurate assessment of the alignment of the ankle mortise requires internal rotation of the leg and is not accurately assessed on standard anteroposterior views of the ankle (Takao et al. 2001).

Fig. 1.5 A 40-year-old
man who presented with
left wrist pain after
falling onto his
outstretched left hand.
(**a**) Frontal and (**b**)
lateral radiographs of
the left wrist show no
fracture or dislocation.
(**c**) Posteroanterior view
of the left wrist taken in
ulnar deviation and
slight tube angulation,
usually part of the
scaphoid imaging series,
shows an undisplaced
fracture of the waist of
the scaphoid (*arrow*)

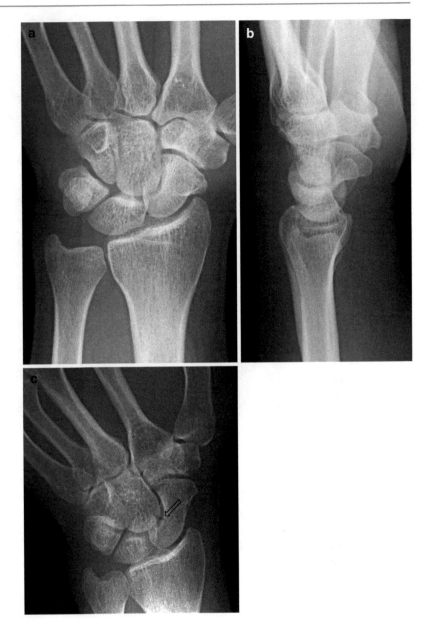

1.2.3   Radiographic Artifacts

Various technical artifacts can be produced
during the acquisition and processing of radiographs (Shetty et al. 2011; Walz-Flannigan et al.
2012). Detailed discussion of this subject is
beyond the scope of this chapter, but these artifacts are generally obvious and do not pose
clinical diagnostic problems. Occasionally

Fig. 1.6 A 29-year-old man who presented with low back pain following a motor vehicle accident. (**a**) Frontal and (**b**) lateral radiographs of the lumbar spine were obtained. Underexposure is evident, as a result of suboptimal radiographic technique. There is increase in quantum mottle especially on the lateral view, causing loss of radiographic detail and affecting the diagnostic quality of the study. This case illustrates how inappropriate selection of exposure factors can result in a poor-quality radiograph

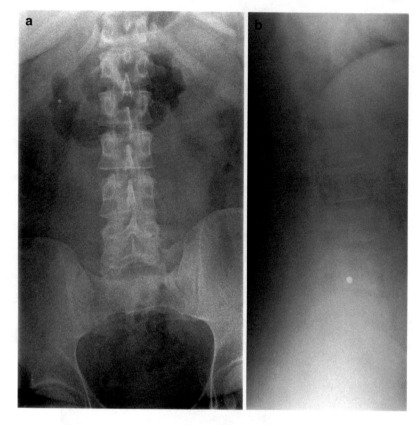

though, with relevance to musculoskeletal imaging, technical artifacts secondary to dirt or dust may mimic foreign bodies. Encountering any of these technical artifacts would usually trigger a repeat of the radiographic examination. Nevertheless, a properly trained radiographer will be able to prevent many of these technical artifacts. Artifacts which are external to the patient may cause the underlying anatomical structures to be obscured. An external cast on a postreduction radiograph is a frequently encountered example. X-rays have difficulty penetrating the cast, resulting in reduced radiographic detail of the underlying bones (Fig. 1.8). Alignment of fractures and assessment of fracture healing can therefore be difficult to assess on these limited postreduction radiographs.

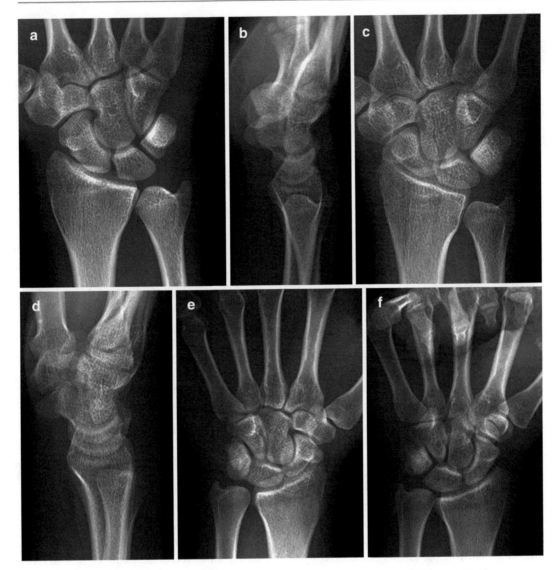

Fig. 1.7 Poor positioning affects the radiographic orthogonal views of the wrist in a 24-year-old man. (**a**) Posteroanterior and (**b**) lateral radiographs of the right wrist show inappropriate positioning of the wrist on the lateral view. After acquisition of the standard posteroanterior view, the wrist was left on the imaging plate with forearm supination performed for acquisition of the lateral view. Note the resultant identical appearances of the ulna on both images, making this a suboptimal radiographic study due to the lack of proper orthogonal views. (**c**) Posteroanterior and (**d**) lateral radiographs of the right wrist in another patient show appropriate positioning of the wrist, which remains in neutral position on both views. The ulnar variance is also influenced by the position of the wrist, increasing on pronation and decreasing on supination. Ulnar variance is therefore only accurately assessed on the standardized posteroanterior view of the wrist in the neutral position. It is noteworthy that dynamic stress maneuvers can also alter bony alignment. For example, the (**e**) frontal and (**f**) clenched-fist stress radiographs of the left wrist of a 40-year-old woman show an increase in ulnar variance on the stress view, which is a normal finding

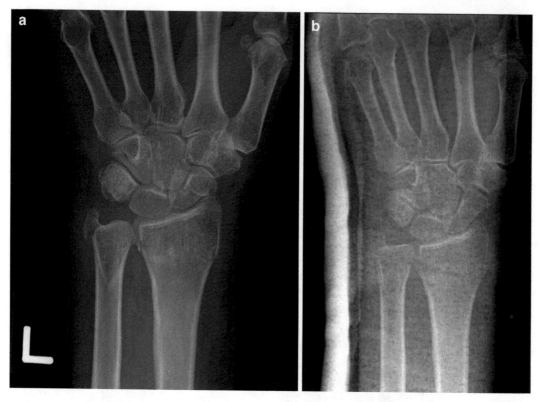

Fig. 1.8 A 66-year-old woman who presented after falling onto her outstretched left hand. (**a**) Frontal radiograph of the left wrist shows fractures of the distal radius and ulnar styloid process. (**b**) Postreduction frontal radiograph shows the presence of a backslab, which obscures the bony details

1.3   Limitations of Radiographic Imaging of Non-osseous Structures

One of the intrinsic limitations of radiography is its poor soft tissue contrast. Delineation of soft tissue structures on the radiograph may be difficult or impossible, making radiography a generally unreliable imaging modality for the assessment of soft tissue lesions. Unless there is gross morphological alteration (e.g., tendon rupture) (Fig. 1.9) or typical pattern of calcification or ossification (e.g., myositis ossificans) (Fig. 1.10), soft tissue abnormalities invariably go unnoticed on the radiograph. Radiography is generally an insensitive imaging modality compared to other cross-sectional imaging modalities, such as MRI and US imaging, in the early stages of disease processes involving the soft tissues. Early radiographic signs tend to be subtle and easily overlooked, whereas in advanced disease, osseous changes are usually readily observed. However, at the stage when such typically irreversible advanced osseous changes take place, the optimal time for therapeutic intervention might have been missed.

1.3.1   Intra- and Periarticular Structures

1.3.1.1 Articular Cartilage

The articular cartilage is essentially radiolucent and invisible on the radiograph. This makes its radiographic assessment particularly challenging. Radiographs are insensitive in the direct detection

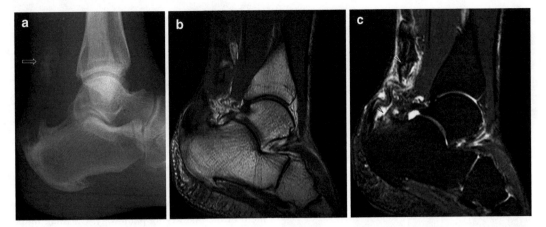

Fig. 1.9 A 41-year-old woman who presented after a fall with left ankle pain and had significant limited range of motion. (**a**) Lateral radiograph of the ankle shows background calcaneal enthesopathy, with an avulsed fragment off the dorsal aspect of the calcaneus (*arrow*). This finding, together with concordant clinical examination findings, allowed the diagnosis of a high-grade Achilles tendon tear to be made. (**b**) Sagittal T1-W MR image of the left ankle shows disruption of the fibers of the Achilles tendon in keeping with a complete tear. The associated avulsion fracture of the dorsal aspect of the calcaneus is seen, and on the (**c**) sagittal fat-suppressed T2-W MR image, there is corresponding marrow edema (*arrowheads*)

of chondral lesions, whether degenerative or traumatic in etiology. A purely chondral lesion caused by acute trauma, without involvement of the subchondral bone, cannot be appreciated on the radiograph (Fig. 1.11). The radiographic diagnosis of osteoarthritis is based on the observation of indirect features, such as the presence of marginal osteophytes, narrowing of joint space, as well as subchondral sclerosis and cyst formation. Radiographs have high specificity in the detection of advanced osteoarthritis, with the combination of indirect features allowing an easy diagnosis to be made. However, in early osteoarthritis, radiographs have low sensitivity and tend to underestimate the extent of cartilage degeneration (Blackburn et al. 1994). Despite the absence of radiographic signs of osteoarthritis, many symptomatic patients have been shown on arthroscopic evaluation to have significant degeneration of articular cartilage (Kijowski et al. 2006). In addition, the degree of joint space narrowing in patients with known osteoarthritis is a poor predictor of the actual state of the articular cartilage (Fife et al. 1991) (Fig. 1.12).

Currently, radiography is still widely used in the imaging follow-up of patients with established osteoarthritis. Nevertheless, with advances in pharmacological and surgical therapies, a more precise imaging modality is required for articular cartilage evaluation. MRI is currently the gold standard in the imaging evaluation of articular cartilage. It has the ability to assess both the morphology and the biochemical integrity of the articular cartilage and will play an increasingly important role in the noninvasive evaluation of articular cartilage both before and after therapeutic intervention (Gold et al. 2009; Crema et al. 2011).

1.3.1.2 Synovium and Joint Fluid
The synovium is normally not visible on the radiograph. When synovitis occurs, whether inflammatory such as in the inflammatory arthritides or infective in the case of septic arthritis, the radiographic appearance is usually normal early in the course of the disease. However, at this early stage, some changes may already be appreciated on MRI or US imaging. Synovial hypertrophy, hypervascularity and enhancement, and

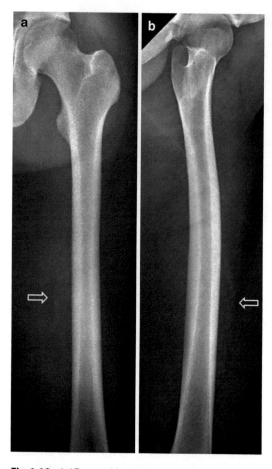

Fig. 1.10 A 17-year-old man who had a history of trauma to the left thigh 2 weeks before presentation. (a) Frontal and (b) lateral radiographs of the left femur show faint curvilinear sheet-like calcifications (*arrows*) adjacent to the mid-shaft of the femur. In the context of recent trauma, this appearance is highly suggestive of myositis ossificans. Note the external artifacts due to the patient's clothing

possible adjacent soft tissue and bone marrow signal changes are features which are usually radiographically occult (Fig. 1.13).

Small joint effusions may not be appreciated on radiography. Even if seen radiographically, without information on the state of the synovium, periarticular soft tissues, and bone marrow, this finding may not be useful in narrowing the differential diagnoses (Fig. 1.14). On the other hand, MRI, with or without intravenous contrast administration, is able to show the state of the surrounding structures, allowing better assessment of the underlying pathology. US imaging is highly sensitive in the detection of joint effusions and is able to provide real-time imaging guidance for diagnostic joint aspiration.

Radiographs have been used for more than a century in the imaging evaluation of the inflammatory arthritides, and they are able to demonstrate the osseous changes which indicate advanced disease. Currently, however, when modern therapy allows prevention or delay of irreversible joint destruction, imaging modalities with higher sensitivity for inflammatory changes (i.e., MRI and US imaging) are superior to radiographs in guiding treatment decisions (Szkudlarek et al. 2006; Weiner et al. 2008; Sankowski et al. 2013) (Fig. 1.15). Similarly, in the case of septic arthritis, irreversible joint destruction would have occurred by the time osseous changes are seen on the radiograph. Clinical judgment is of paramount importance in the management of patients with septic arthritis.

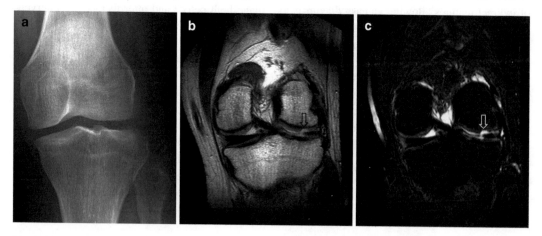

Fig. 1.11 A 42-year-old man who presented with left knee pain. (a) Frontal radiograph of the left knee shows minimal degenerative changes with preservation of the joint spaces. Coronal (b) PD-W and (c) fat-suppressed T2-W MR images of the left knee show a focal chondral defect (*arrows*) at the articular surface of the lateral femoral condyle. This finding cannot be appreciated radiographically since cartilage is essentially radiolucent

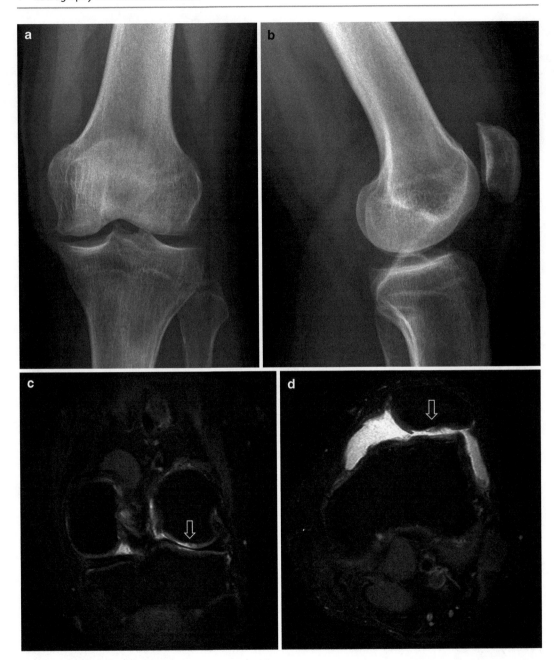

Fig. 1.12 A 44-year-old man who presented with chronic left knee pain. (**a**) Frontal and (**b**) lateral radiographs of the left knee show mild osteoarthritis with small marginal osteophytes and relative preservation of the joint spaces. A joint effusion is also noted. (**c**) Coronal and (**d**) axial fat-suppressed PD-W MR images of the left knee show partial- to full-thickness articular cartilage loss (*arrows*) involving the lateral tibiofemoral and patellofemoral joint compartments and confirm the presence of a joint effusion. As illustrated, the degree of joint space narrowing is not a sensitive method for predicting the actual state of the articular cartilage

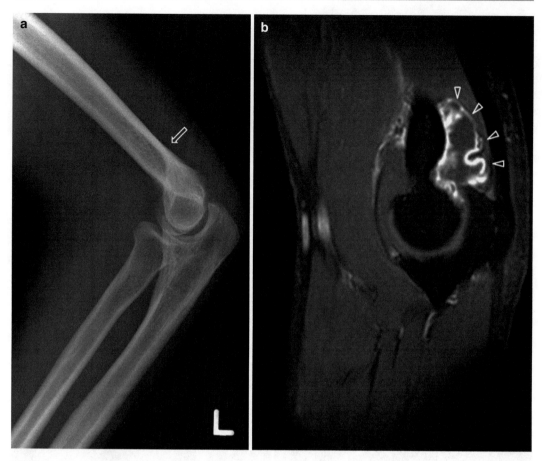

Fig. 1.13 A 36-year-old man who presented with left elbow pain after a traumatic injury. Initial radiographic evaluation of the left elbow was negative for fracture or dislocation. (**a**) Lateral radiograph shows that the posterior fat pad is just visible (*arrow*), raising suspicion of a joint effusion. (**b**) Sagittal contrast-enhanced fat-suppressed T1-W MR image of the left elbow confirms the presence of a joint effusion and shows enhancement of the synovium (*arrowheads*), consistent with synovitis. No fracture was identified. In the absence of other clinical features of infection, transient inflammatory synovitis of traumatic etiology was the primary diagnosis. The patient made a full recovery with conservative management

Joint aspiration has to be performed for the diagnosis to be established, and treatment has to be instituted without delay, as rapid progression to permanent joint destruction may otherwise ensue.

1.3.1.3 Ligaments, Tendons, and Other Fibrocartilaginous Structures

Radiographic assessment of ligaments, tendons, and fibrocartilaginous structures relies upon the observation of indirect features which indicate possible underlying pathology involving these structures. These indirect features include joint malalignment, hemarthrosis, calcific deposits, and secondary osseous changes. The latter two are seen in relation to chronic degenerative processes. In acute trauma, injuries to these structures tend to be occult on the radiograph, especially when sprains, strains, or partial tears occur. Extensive ligamentous disruption with joint dislocation is usually visible

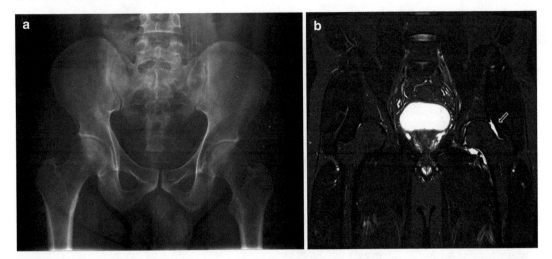

Fig. 1.14 A 38-year-old man who presented with left groin pain after a period of intense physical activity. (**a**) Frontal radiograph of the pelvis is essentially normal. (**b**) Coronal turbo inversion recovery magnitude (TIRM) MR image of the pelvis shows a left hip joint effusion (*arrow*), which was radiographically occult. This represented a reactive effusion secondary to a left groin muscular strain (not shown), and the patient subsequently made a full recovery with conservative management

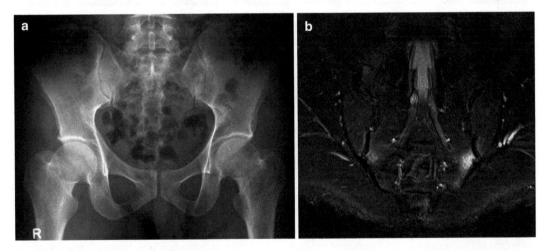

Fig. 1.15 A 35-year-old man who presented with worsening back pain, on a background of chronic back and polyarticular pain. (**a**) Frontal radiograph of the pelvis shows no significant abnormality. (**b**) Coronal TIRM MR image of the sacrum shows periarticular marrow edema involving the inferior aspect of both sacroiliac joints (worse on the left), seen as conspicuous hyperintense fluid signal which has high contrast compared with the surrounding fat-suppressed normal marrow. This case highlights the high sensitivity of MRI to the early changes of sacroiliitis, when it is radiographically occult

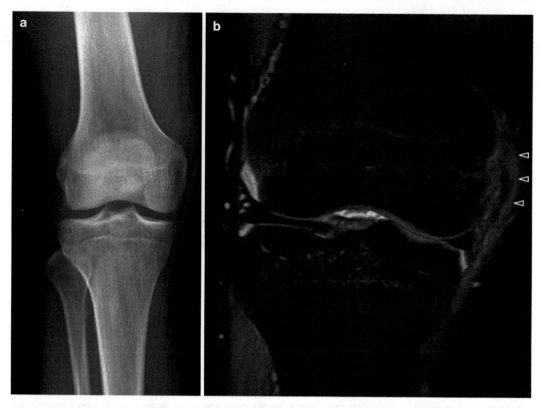

Fig. 1.16 A 25-year-old man who presented with right knee pain after sustaining an injury from a tackle during a football match. (**a**) Frontal radiograph of the right knee shows no fracture or dislocation. (**b**) Coronal fat-suppressed PD-W MR image of the right knee shows a grade 2 injury of the medial collateral ligament, evident as a partial disruption of the ligament with surrounding edema (*arrowheads*). This injury is usually not appreciable on radiography, but may be suggested if bony avulsion occurs at the attachment sites of the ligament

on the radiograph. Complete tendon rupture with tendon retraction may also be visible radiographically. However, these injuries tend to be obvious on clinical examination.

Gross disruption of the supporting ligaments of a joint, with the presence of dislocation, represents one end of the spectrum of ligamentous injuries and manifests in radiographs as a disruption of the bony alignment. Less severe ligamentous injuries range from sprains to high-grade partial tears and even complete tears of individual ligaments. These injuries are largely not appreciated on radiographs, especially in the acute setting when joint instability might not be accurately assessed on clinical examination, and the bony alignment often remains normal on imaging (Figs. 1.16 and 1.17). Sometimes, the same traumatic mechanism causing ligamentous injury may result in bone abnormalities, which

again are indirect features on the radiograph. These bone abnormalities can often be seen on the radiograph but are usually subtle and easily missed, if not suspected. In the example of an injury involving the anterior cruciate ligament of the knee, possible bony abnormalities include avulsion fractures at the femoral or tibial attachment sites, the Segond fracture, and an osteochondral impaction fracture of the lateral femoral condyle (Ng et al. 2011). Detection of any of these bony abnormalities without appreciating the underlying soft tissue injuries is a potential pitfall in the interpretation of the radiograph.

A complete tendon rupture with tendon retraction, involving a superficial large tendon such as the Achilles tendon, does not usually pose a diagnostic problem. However, in other locations, for example, the rotator cuff tendons in the shoulder, accurate assessment of tendon

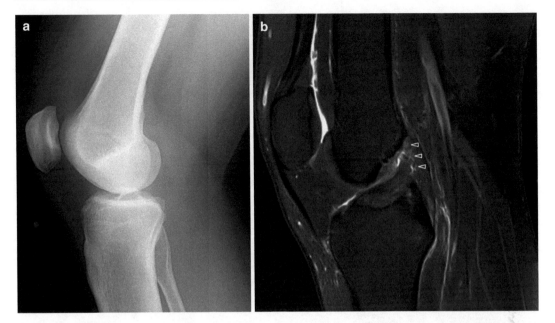

Fig. 1.17 A 35-year-old man who presented with right knee pain after a twisting injury sustained during a game of basketball. (**a**) Lateral radiograph of the right knee shows no significant bony injury or joint malalignment. A small suprapatellar joint effusion is noted. (**b**) Sagittal fat-suppressed PD-W MR image of the right knee shows a high-grade injury of the anterior cruciate ligament, evident as a disruption of the fibers at the femoral attachment (*arrowheads*). This injury is not usually discernable on radiography, although indirect osseous findings (such as Segond fracture) may suggest this injury

tears is impossible on radiographs. The rotator cuff is the archetype of a tendon which is highly susceptible to chronic degeneration. Significant chronic tendinosis and tendon tears of the rotator cuff are typically not visualized on radiographs (Fig. 1.18), though indirect findings such as osseous changes (signifying advanced disease), calcific tendinous deposits, and features of subacromial impingement may be seen. Nevertheless, other imaging modalities such as MRI and US imaging would be necessary for proper evaluation, as radiographic findings alone will not be sufficient to guide clinical management (Seibold et al. 1999). Other examples of fibrocartilaginous structures which are usually not directly visualized on radiography include intervertebral disks, menisci of the knee, glenoid labrum, and triangular fibrocartilage complex of the wrist (Figs. 1.19, 1.20, 1.21, and 1.22). Radiography plays a limited but usually complementary role in the evaluation of these structures.

1.3.2   Other Soft Tissues and Foreign Bodies

Various soft tissues, such as muscle and subcutaneous soft tissue, are usually included in the views obtained on radiography of the musculoskeletal system. Radiographs are largely limited in the assessment of muscle abnormalities, with rare exceptions such as myositis ossificans which shows typical radiographic appearances but may be diagnostically confusing on MRI early in its course (McCarthy and Sundaram 2005). Otherwise, muscle lesions are best assessed on MRI, which can demonstrate alterations in muscle signal intensity characteristics (Theodorou et al. 2012).

However, much information can still be gleaned from the radiographic appearance of the subcutaneous soft tissue. Diffuse processes such as edema and cellulitis may be appreciated by the presence of increased reticular markings and thickening of the overlying skin. However, this appearance is nonspecific, based on radiography

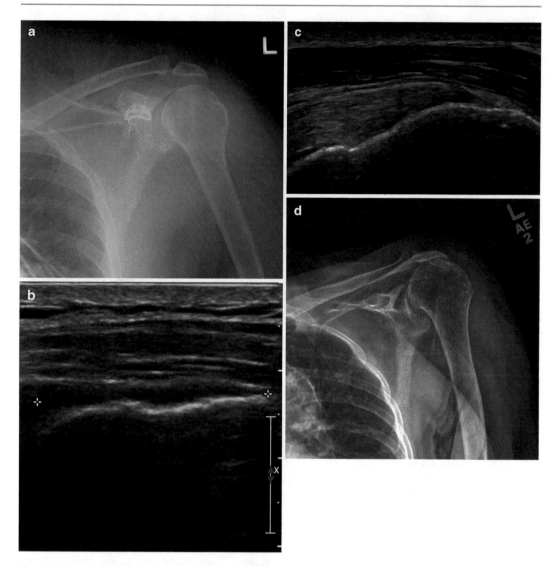

Fig. 1.18 A 46-year-old man who presented with left shoulder pain and decreased range of motion after a motor vehicle accident. (**a**) Frontal radiograph of the left shoulder shows no significant abnormality. The humerus is in an internally rotated position. (**b**) Longitudinal US image of the supraspinatus shows a complete tear of the supraspinatus tendon, with a tendon gap at its attachment to the greater tuberosity (as indicated by the crosshairs). This finding was not apparent on the radiographs.

(**c**) Longitudinal US image of another patient shows a normal fibrillar pattern of the distal supraspinatus tendon (shown for comparison). (**d**) Frontal radiograph of the left shoulder of a 70-year-old woman with advanced rotator cuff disease shows an obliterated acromiohumeral interval and secondary degenerative osseous changes, features which are radiographically discernible. At this late stage of disease, surgical intervention will not be useful

alone. Likewise, for focal pathologies such as superficial hematoma, abscess, and a myriad of other soft tissue masses (including intramuscular masses), the radiographic appearance alone is usually nonspecific. Certain radiographic

characteristics such as lesion density, the presence of calcification or ossification, and effect on adjacent osseous structures may shed some light on the nature of the soft tissue mass. Thus, although limited on its own, radiography plays a

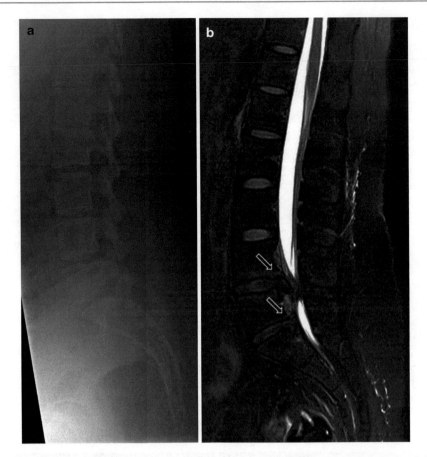

Fig. 1.19 A 25-year-old woman who presented with low back pain and bilateral lower limb numbness after lifting some heavy loads. (**a**) Lateral radiograph of the lumbar spine is essentially normal. (**b**) Sagittal fat-suppressed T2-W MR image of the lumbar spine shows posterior intervertebral disk extrusions at L4–L5 and L5-S1 levels (*arrows*), worse at the L4–L5 level where there is significant spinal canal stenosis with likely impingement of the cauda equina nerve roots. Note the reduced signal of the desiccated disks at the affected levels, as well as increased marrow signal at the endplates of L4–L5 level consistent with Modic type 1 degenerative signal changes. The other intervertebral disks have a normal appearance. Example of fibrocartilaginous structure (disk) not directly visualized on radiography

complementary role in the imaging evaluation of soft tissue masses (Gartner et al. 2009).

Radiographs are useful for the detection of suspected radiopaque foreign bodies, as well as soft tissue gas pockets. On the radiograph, gas pockets are visible on a background of soft tissue densities as their hyperlucency provides imaging contrast. Similarly, radiopaque foreign bodies can be seen, as the differences in densities provide good contrast. The higher the radiodensity of a foreign body, the greater its visibility. A limi-tation of radiography is in the detection of foreign bodies which are weakly radiopaque, especially if the material of the foreign body has a density close to that of the surrounding soft tissue (e.g., wood). These weakly radiopaque foreign bodies will not be appreciated on the radiograph. This potential pitfall should be recognized by the clinician requesting the radiograph, and if necessary, an alternative imaging modality such as US imaging should be considered (Aras et al. 2010) (Fig. 1.23).

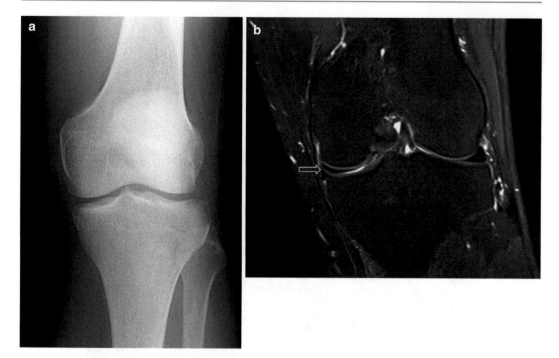

Fig. 1.20 A 37-year-old man who presented with left knee pain. (**a**) Frontal radiograph of the left knee shows no significant abnormality. (**b**) Coronal fat-suppressed PD-W MR image of the left knee shows a horizontal tear of the medial meniscus involving its inferior surface, evident as a linear area of hyperintensity (*arrow*). The lateral meniscus has a normal appearance. Example of fibrocartilaginous structure (meniscus) not directly visualized on radiography

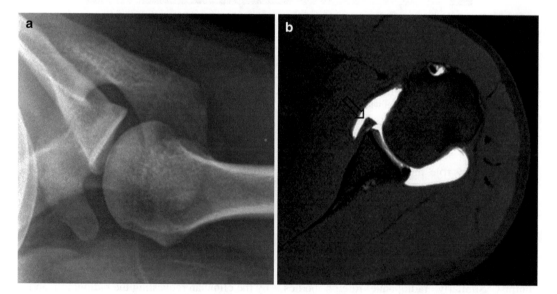

Fig. 1.21 A 22-year-old man who had recurrent episodes of anterior shoulder dislocation. (**a**) Axillary radiographic view of the left shoulder shows normal joint alignment and no significant osseous abnormality. (**b**) Axial fat-suppressed T1-W MR arthrographic image of the left shoulder shows a Perthes lesion (a variant of the Bankart lesion), manifesting as detachment of the anteroinferior glenoid labrum which remains attached to an intact but lifted periosteum of the anterior glenoid (*arrow*). The posterior glenoid labrum shows a normal appearance. Example of fibrocartilaginous structure (glenoid labrum) not directly visualized on radiography

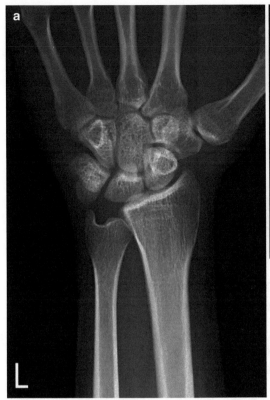

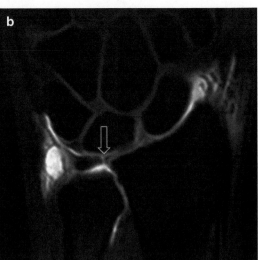

Fig. 1.22 A 28-year-old motorcyclist who had persistent ulnar-sided left wrist pain 4 months after being involved in a minor motor vehicle accident. (**a**) Frontal radiograph of his left wrist is essentially normal, with no fracture or dislocation seen. Negative ulnar variance is noted. (**b**) Coronal fat-suppressed T1-W MR arthrographic image of the left wrist shows a tear of the radial attachment site of the triangular fibrocartilage complex (TFCC), seen as linear high signal (*arrow*). Hyperintense contrast agent is seen extending into the distal radioulnar joint, a result of the TFCC tear. Example of fibrocartilaginous structure (TFCC) not directly visualized on radiography

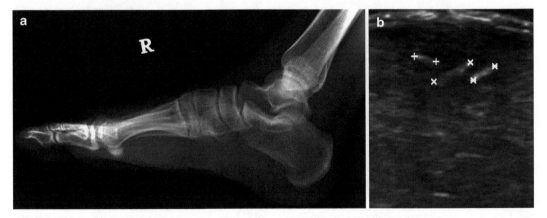

Fig. 1.23 A 34-year-old construction worker who presented with pain in the right foot after stepping barefoot onto unknown material at his work site. (**a**) Lateral radiograph of the right foot does not show any radiopaque foreign body. (**b**) US image shows a few small foreign bodies within the plantar subcutaneous layer of the right foot, seen as linear echogenic structures (as indicated by the *crosshairs*). The patient underwent removal of the foreign bodies, which turned out to be wooden splinters. Wood is weakly radiopaque and may be invisible on radiography

1.4   Radiographically Occult Osseous Abnormalities

One of the strengths of the radiograph is its ability to demonstrate the osseous structures. This gives it relatively good specificity in the evaluation of osseous abnormalities. In most cases of discrete osseous lesions, the radiographic appearance allows categorization into aggressive and nonaggressive entities and so

helps narrow the differential diagnoses. In many cases, the radiographic appearance is so characteristic as to allow a diagnosis to be made.

1.4.1   Destructive Osseous Lesions

Although radiographs display osseous anatomy well, before a destructive osseous lesion is even

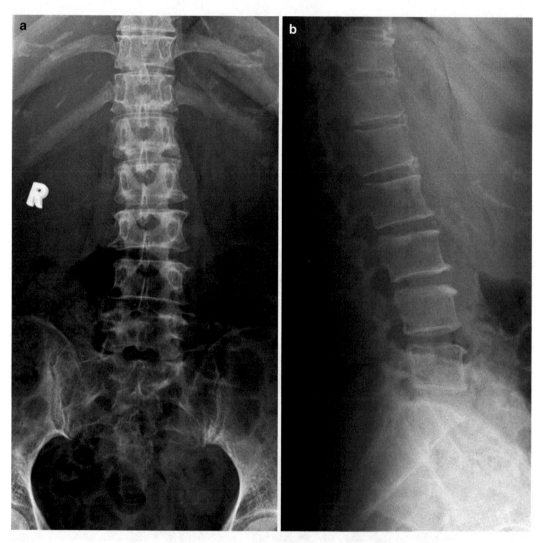

Fig. 1.24 A 53-year-old woman who was recently diagnosed with adenocarcinoma of the right lung and presented with diffuse back pain. (**a**) Frontal and (**b**) lateral radiographs of the lumbar spine show spondylotic changes. Bone density is preserved and there is no evidence of osseous destruction. (**c**) Whole-body Tc-99 m

MDP bone scintiscan shows extensive osseous metastases, evident as increased tracer uptake at multiple sites, especially in the axial skeleton including the lumbar spine. This case demonstrates the superior sensitivity of bone scintigraphy compared to radiographs in the detection of metastatic bone disease

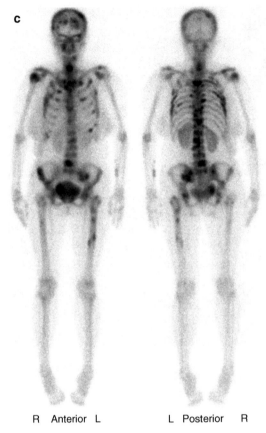

c

R   Anterior   L   L   Posterior   R

Fig. 1.24 (continued)

visible radiographically, there has to be loss of about 50% of the cortical bone mass (Osmond et al. 1975; Taoka et al. 2001). Radiography is thus significantly limited in the detection of lesions early in the course of osseous metastatic disease, since the pathology is predominantly confined to the medullary cavity of the bone at this early stage (Gold et al. 1990). In contrast to radiography, bone scintigraphy is sensitive enough to demonstrate metastatic involvement of cortical bone with a threshold of about 5–10% lesion-to-normal bone ratio (Algra et al. 1991) (Fig. 1.24).

Similarly, in osteomyelitis, before thresholds of about 50% of bone mineral content involvement and 1 cm of lesion size are reached, the lesion remains radiographically occult (Pineda et al. 2009). Thus, the radiographic features of osteomyelitis are typically delayed by about 10–14 days from the onset of infection. In the early stages of osteomyelitis, the radiograph can be normal in appearance and so is significantly limited as a diagnostic modality. However, radiographs can still be useful for demonstrating associated findings such as foreign bodies and soft tissue gas in this setting. MRI is exquisitely sensitive to bone marrow changes, making it the imaging modality of choice in the evaluation of vertebral metastases as well as osteomyelitis, both of which mainly involve the bone marrow (Algra et al. 1991; Pineda et al. 2009) (Figs. 1.25 and 1.26).

1.4.2 Trauma-Related Osseous Injuries

1.4.2.1 Undisplaced Fractures

An important limitation of radiographs is in the evaluation of acute undisplaced fractures, especially hairline ones. For an acute fracture to be visualized on the radiograph, at least a small amount of displacement or separation is usually necessary for the fracture to manifest as a radiolucent line, sclerotic line, or cortical step. Hence, even with adequate views and proper technique, an acute undisplaced fracture can be radiographically occult. It is important to be aware of this potential pitfall when interpreting radiographs of the acute trauma patient, especially if there are associated soft tissue findings in a seemingly negative radiograph. For example, elevated fat pads in the elbow joint indicate the presence of a hemarthrosis, which could be secondary to an occult undisplaced fracture. If the clinical suspicion for a fracture is high despite a negative initial radiograph, follow-up radiographs can be obtained 10–14 days later. If present, these fractures typically become increasingly visible with time as bone resorption and callus formation occur at the fracture site (Fig. 1.27).

In certain clinical scenarios, confirmation of the presence of a fracture may need to be done rapidly, as an unnecessary delay in the diagnosis would result in significant morbidity. In such cases, follow-up radiographs should not be advocated and advanced imaging evaluation should instead be performed. For example, in the elderly

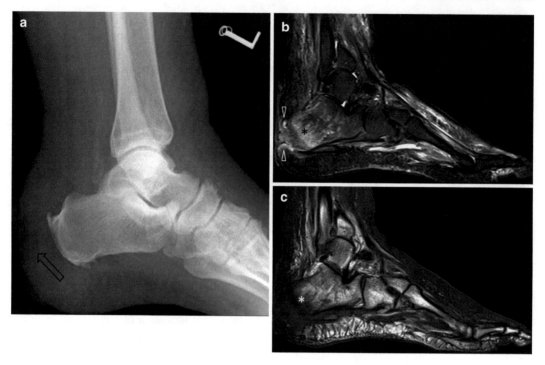

Fig. 1.25 A 62-year-old man with type 2 diabetes mellitus who presented with an infected ulcer at the left hindfoot. (**a**) Lateral radiograph of the left ankle shows a radiolucent area posterior to the calcaneum (*arrow*), corresponding to the known ulcer. No obvious radiographic sign of osteomyelitis (e.g., periosteal reaction and bone destruction) is discerned. (**b**) Sagittal TIRM MR image of the left foot shows subcutaneous inflammatory signal alteration deep to the ulcer (*arrowheads*), extending down to the calcaneum which shows abnormal marrow edema (*asterisk*). (**c**) Sagittal T1-W MR image shows the characteristic T1-hypointense marrow signal of osteomyelitis involving the calcaneum (*asterisk*)

adult with hip pain after a fall, where there is inability to weight-bear and no fracture is seen on radiographs, further advanced imaging such as MRI and CT should be arranged early to establish the presence of an undisplaced femoral neck fracture, which usually requires to be treated surgically (Oka and Monu 2004; Gill et al. 2013; Ward et al. 2013) (Fig. 1.28).

1.4.2.2 Stress Injuries

Stress injuries range in a continuum from stress reactions to established stress fractures. They develop as a result of chronic repetitive microtrauma causing fatigue of normal bone and essentially comprise microtrabecular fractures which are not visible on the radiograph. If the inciting activity causing repetitive stress is not stopped to allow bone to heal, these microtrabecular fractures accumulate and eventually result in a full cortical fracture. Formation of periosteal new bone is the earliest radiographic feature of stress fractures, and its appearance may be delayed up to 3 months from the initial injurious stimulus (Jarraya et al. 2013) (Fig. 1.29).

The earliest stage of stress injuries, termed stress reaction, is radiographically occult but may manifest on MRI as bone marrow edema without a fracture line. Due to nonspecificity of isolated bone marrow edema, CT may also be useful in distinguishing stress reaction from other entities such as osteoid osteoma (Liong and Whitehouse 2012). Since only timely management can interrupt the cycle of repetitive stress, early detection of stress injuries is crucial. An understanding of the limitation of radiography in this respect and the use of more appropriate imaging modalities is vital in establishing the diagnosis of stress injury in the early stages.

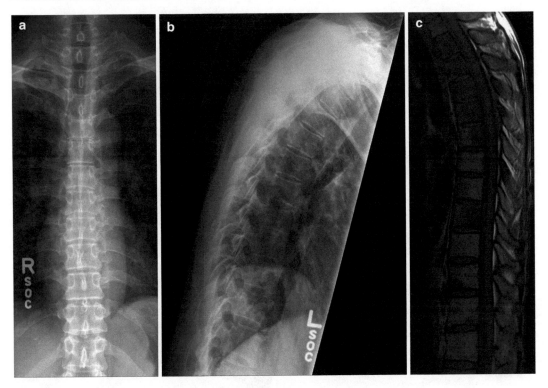

Fig. 1.26 A 51-year-old man who presented with back pain of insidious onset. (**a**) Frontal and (**b**) lateral radiographs of the thoracic spine appear essentially normal. There is no radiographic evidence of osseous metastasis. (**c**) Sagittal T1-W MR image of the thoracic spine shows abnormal hypointense marrow signal involving multiple vertebral levels. The patient had extensive osseous metastases secondary to a primary malignancy in the right lung apex, which was incidentally imaged on the frontal radiograph (**a**) and seen as right lung apical opacities

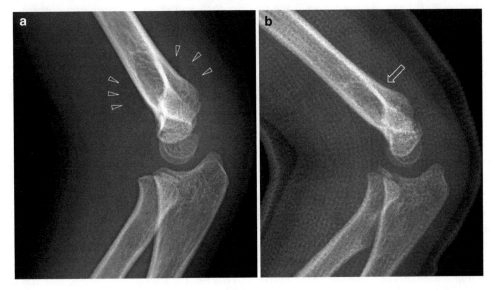

Fig. 1.27 A 6-year-old boy who presented with pain in the left elbow after a fall onto his outstretched left hand. (**a**) Lateral radiograph of the left elbow shows no displaced fracture. The joint alignment is maintained. There is however a joint effusion, as indicated by elevated anterior and posterior fat pads (*arrowheads*). This finding should raise the suspicion of an occult undisplaced fracture in the setting of trauma. (**b**) Follow-up lateral radiograph of the left elbow was performed 10 days after the initial presentation. Despite the presence of an overlying cast, periosteal reaction can be seen along the posterior aspect of the distal shaft of the humerus (*arrow*), indicating a healing undisplaced fracture

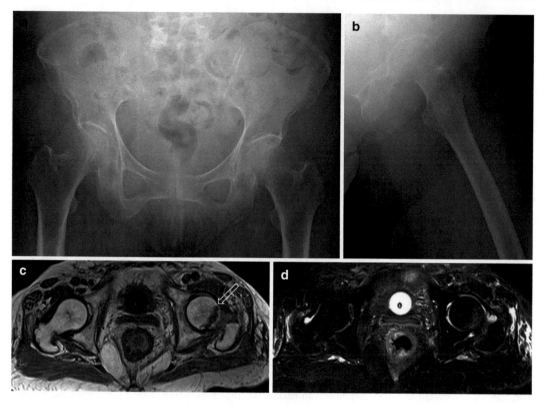

Fig. 1.28 An 83-year-old woman who presented with left hip pain after a fall. (**a**) Frontal radiograph of the pelvis and (**b**) lateral radiograph of the left hip show no appreciable fracture or dislocation. There is diffuse reduction in bone density, which limits radiographic sensitivity for minimally displaced fractures. (**c**) Axial T1-W MR image of the pelvis shows an undisplaced fracture of the neck of the left femur, seen as a hypointense fracture line (*arrow*). This fracture was radiographically occult. (**d**) Axial fat-suppressed T2-W MR image of the pelvis at the corresponding level shows associated marrow edema around the fracture site

1.4.3 Osteoporosis

Osteoporosis is defined as a reduction in bone mass, with a bone density of less than 2.5 standard deviations below that of a healthy young adult (World Health Organization 2003). It has many different causes, but its appearance on radiography is the same regardless of etiology. The diagnosis is most confidently made on a quantitative technique such as dual-energy X-ray absorptiometry (DXA). However, most cases of osteoporosis are still diagnosed on radiography (Guglielmi et al. 2011). Radiographs are inherently limited in the detection of reduced bone mass, which is only appreciable when about 30% of bone loss has occurred

(Harris and Heaney 1969). Radiographic technique may also be a confounding factor, for example, causing bones to appear more radiolucent than usual and giving a false impression of osteoporosis. This is a potential pitfall when radiographs are used in the diagnosis of osteoporosis. A combination of features such as cortical thinning, trabecular changes, and insufficiency fractures is usually needed to provide a higher degree of confidence in the diagnosis of osteoporosis on radiography (Fan and Peh 2016). Another radiographic pitfall in relation to osteoporosis is the limitation in the detection of destructive lesions and fractures. On a background of reduced bone mass, these conditions can be difficult or impossible to

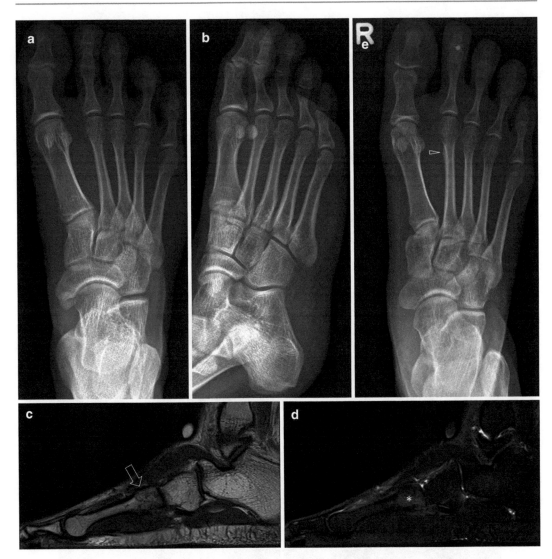

Fig. 1.29 A 24-year-old avid runner who presented with right foot pain. (**a**) Frontal and (**b**) oblique radiographs of the right foot show no significant abnormality. Incidental note is made of a type 2 os navicularis. (**c**) Sagittal T1-W MR image of the right foot shows curvilinear hypointense trabecular fracture lines in the base of the fourth metatarsal (*arrow*). (**d**) Sagittal fat-suppressed T2-W MR image of the right foot shows associated marrow edema (*aster-*

isk). With the presence of a concordant history, the findings were consistent with a stress injury. (**e**) Frontal radiograph of the right foot in another patient at a later stage in the natural progression of a stress injury shows typical periosteal reaction adjacent to the neck of the second metatarsal (*arrowhead*), indicating a healing stress fracture. This is the earliest radiographic feature of stress injury

appreciate. This is especially so early in the course of destructive processes (e.g., osteomyelitis or osseous metastasis) or when fractures are undisplaced (e.g., hip fracture in the elderly adult) (Figs. 1.28 and 1.30).

Conclusion

Radiography as an imaging modality has inherent limitations in the demonstration of lesions involving soft tissues, as well as early in the course of abnormalities involving bone. Pitfalls

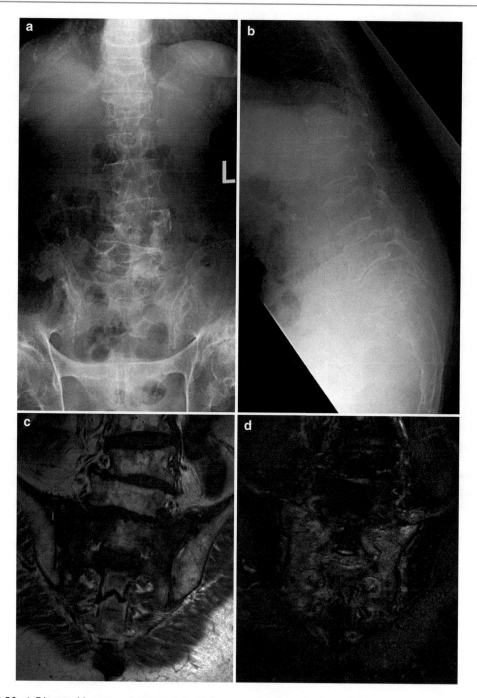

Fig. 1.30 A 74-year-old woman who presented with low back pain and tenderness in the upper gluteal region after a fall. (**a**) Frontal and (**b**) lateral radiographs of the lumbar spine show diffuse reduction in bone density consistent with osteoporosis. Known chronic osteoporotic compression fractures are seen at the thoracolumbar junction levels. Background spinal degenerative changes are evident, especially at the lower lumbar spine. (**c**) Coronal T1-W and (**d**) coronal fat-suppressed T2-W MR images of the sacrum show sacral insufficiency fractures, evident as a typical "H" pattern of T1-hypointense and T2-hyperintense marrow edema involving the bilateral sacral ala and the body of the second sacral segment. This finding is radiographically occult

are also encountered in radiographic acquisition, and if the clinician or radiologist is not cognizant of them, suboptimal diagnosis and patient management can ensue. Nevertheless, the humble radiograph remains a mainstay of diagnostic imaging in the modern day, frequently being the first-line imaging modality or assuming a complementary role to other more advanced imaging modalities.

References

Algra PR, Bloem JL, Tissing H et al (1991) Detection of vertebral metastases: comparison between MR imaging and bone scintigraphy. Radiographics 11:219–232

Aras MH, Miloglu O, Barutcugil C et al (2010) Comparison of the sensitivity for detecting foreign bodies among conventional plain radiography, computed tomography and ultrasonography. Dentomaxillofac Radiol 3:72–78

Blackburn WD, Bernreuter WK, Rominger M et al (1994) Arthroscopic evaluation of knee articular cartilage: a comparison with plain radiographs and magnetic resonance imaging. J Rheumatol 21:675–679

Ching W, Robinson J, McEntee M (2014) Patient-based radiographic exposure factor selection: a systematic review. J Med Radiat Sci 61:176–190

Crema MD, Roemer FW, Marra MD et al (2011) Articular cartilage in the knee: current MR imaging techniques and applications in clinical practice and research. Radiographics 31:37–61

Epner RA, Bowers WH, Guilford WB (1982) Ulnar variance – the effect of wrist positioning and roentgen filming technique. J Hand Surg Am 7:298–305

Eschler A, Rosler K, Rotter R et al (2014) Acromioclavicular joint dislocations: radiological correlation between Rockwood classification system and injury patterns in human cadaver species. Arch Orthop Trauma Surg 134:1193–1198

Fan YL, Peh WCG (2016) Radiology of osteoporosis: old and new findings. Semin Musculoskelet Radiol 20:235–245

Fife RS, Brandt KD, Braunstein EM et al (1991) Relationship between arthroscopic evidence of cartilage damage and radiographic evidence of joint space narrowing in early osteoarthritis of the knee. Arthritis Rheum 34:377–382

Gartner L, Pearce CJ, Saifuddin A (2009) The role of the plain radiograph in the characterisation of soft tissue tumours. Skelet Radiol 38:549–558

Gill SK, Smith J, Fox R, Chesser TJS et al (2013) Investigation of occult hip fractures: the use of CT and MRI. Sci World J 2013:830319

Gold RI, Seeger LL, Bassett LW, Steckel RJ et al (1990) An integrated approach to the evaluation of metastatic bone disease. Radiol Clin N Am 28:471–483

Gold GE, Chen CA, Koo S et al (2009) Recent advances in MRI of articular cartilage. AJR Am J Roentgenol 193:628–638

Guglielmi G, Muscarella S, Bazzocchi A (2011) Integrated imaging approach to osteoporosis: state-of-the-art review and update. Radiographics 31:1343–1364

Harris WH, Heaney RP (1969) Skeletal renewal and metabolic bone disease. N Engl J Med 280:193–202

Holmes JF, Akkinepalli R (2005) Computed tomography versus plain radiography to screen for cervical spine injury: a meta-analysis. J Trauma 58:902–905

Jarraya M, Hayashi D, Roemer FW et al (2013) Radiographically occult and subtle fractures: a pictorial review. Radiol Res Pract 2013:370169

Kijowski R, Blankenbaker D, Stanton P et al (2006) Arthroscopic validation of radiographic grading scales of osteoarthritis of the tibiofemoral joint. AJR Am J Roentgenol 187:794–799

Lee SK, Desai H, Silver B et al (2011) Comparison of radiographic stress views for scapholunate dynamic instability in a cadaver model. J Hand Surg Am 36:1149–1157

Liong SY, Whitehouse RW (2012) Lower extremity and pelvic stress fractures in athletes. Br J Radiol 85:1148–1156

Malik AK, Shetty AA, Targett C, Compson JP (2004) Scaphoid views: a need for standardisation. Ann R Coll Surg Engl 86:165–170

McCarthy EF, Sundaram M (2005) Heterotopic ossification: a review. Skelet Radiol 34:609–619

Murphey MD, Quale JL, Martin NL et al (1992) Computed radiography in musculoskeletal imaging: state of the art. AJR Am J Roentgenol 158:19–27

Ng WHA, Griffith JF, Hung EHY et al (2011) Imaging of the anterior cruciate ligament. World J Orthop 2:75–84

Oka M, Monu JUV (2004) Prevalence and patterns of occult hip fractures and mimics revealed by MRI. AJR Am J Roentgenol 182:283–288

Osmond JD, Pendergrass HP, Potsaid MS (1975) Accuracy of 99mTC-diphosphonate bone scans and roentgenograms in the detection of prostate, breast and lung carcinoma metastases. Am J Roentgenol Radium Therapy, Nucl Med 125:972–977

Pankovich AM (1976) Maisonneuve fracture of the fibula. J Bone Joint Surg Am 58:337–342

Pineda C, Espinosa R, Pena A (2009) Radiographic imaging in osteomyelitis: the role of plain radiography, computed tomography, ultrasonography, magnetic resonance imaging, and scintigraphy. Semin Plast Surg 23:80–89

Sankowski AJ, Lebkowska UM, Cwikla J et al (2013) The comparison of efficacy of different imaging techniques (conventional radiography, ultrasonography, magnetic resonance) in assessment of wrist joints and metacarpophalangeal joints in patients with psoriatic arthritis. Pol J Radiol 78:18–29

Seibold CJ, Mallisee TA, Erickson SJ et al (1999) Rotator cuff: evaluation with US and MR imaging. Radiographics 19:685–705

Shenoy R, Pillai A, Hadidi M (2007) Scaphoid fractures: variation in radiographic views - a survey of current practice in the west of Scotland region. Eur J Emerg Med 14:2–5

Shetty CM, Barthur A, Kambadakone A et al (2011) Computed radiography image artifacts revisited. AJR Am J Roentgenol 196:37–48

Szkudlarek M, Klarlund M, Narvestad E et al (2006) Ultrasonography of the metacarpophalangeal and proximal interphalangeal joints in rheumatoid arthritis: a comparison with magnetic resonance imaging, conventional radiography and clinical examination. Arthritis Res Ther 8:R52

Takao M, Ochi M, Naito K et al (2001) Computed tomographic evaluation of the position of the leg for mortise radiographs. Foot Ankle Int 22:828–831

Taoka T, Mayr NA, Lee HJ et al (2001) Factors influencing visualization of vertebral metastases on MR imaging versus bone scintigraphy. AJR Am J Roentgenol 176:1525–1530

Theodorou DJ, Theodorou SJ, Kakitsubata Y (2012) Skeletal muscle disease: patterns of MRI appearances. Br J Radiol 85:e1298–e1308

Toth F, Sebestyen A, Balint L et al (2007) Positioning of the wrist for scaphoid radiography. Eur J Radiol 64:126–132

Walz-Flannigan A, Magnuson D, Erickson D, Schueler B (2012) Artifacts in digital radiography. AJR Am J Roentgenol 198:156–161

Ward RJ, Weissman BN, Kransdorf MJ et al (2013) ACR appropriateness criteria acute hip pain – suspected fracture. J Am Coll Radiol 11:114–120

Weiner SM, Jurenz S, Uhl M et al (2008) Ultrasonography in the assessment of peripheral joint involvement in psoriatic arthritis. Clin Rheumatol 27:983–989

World Health Organization (2003) Prevention and management of osteoporosis. World Health Organ Tech Rep Ser 921:1–164

Ultrasound Imaging Artifacts

2

Lana Hiraj Gimber and Mihra S. Taljanovic

Contents

2.1   **Introduction** 33

2.2   **Ultrasound Imaging** 33
2.2.1 Equipment 33
2.2.2 Physics 34
2.2.3 Doppler US 34
2.2.4 Normal Structures 34

2.3   **Gray-Scale Artifacts** 35
2.3.1 Beam Characteristics 35
2.3.2 Velocity Errors 36
2.3.3 Attenuation Errors 37
2.3.4 Multiple Echoes 38

2.4   **Color and Power Doppler Artifacts** 40

Conclusion 44

References 44

Abbreviation

US   Ultrasound

L.H. Gimber, MD, MPH
M.S. Taljanovic, MD, PhD, FACR (✉)
Department of Medical Imaging,
The University of Arizona College of Medicine,
Banner-University Medical Center,
1501 N. Campbell Avenue, P.O. Box 245067,
Tucson, AZ 85724, USA
e-mail: lgimber@radiology.arizona.edu;
mihrat@radiology.arizona.edu

2.1 Introduction

Ultrasound (US) imaging is an accessible imaging modality that does not employ ionizing radiation. However, while US imaging is easily employed, it is also very operator dependent. In clinical practice, the US beam often deviates from the ideal physical assumptions, and artifacts are created which can be mistaken for pathology. Artifacts can be found in both B-mode gray-scale and Doppler imaging. It is therefore important to be able to identify these artifacts and to employ techniques that can help avoid or minimize them.

2.2 Ultrasound Imaging

2.2.1 Equipment

US imaging employs the use of a small transducer, or probe, and US gel which is placed directly onto the skin. The probe transmits sound waves through the gel, which acts as a coupling medium, and into the body. Once in the body, the sound waves bounce off structures and return back to the probe. The computer then uses these collected sound waves to create an image. The US transducer contains thin piezoelectric crystals, which allow electrical signal to be converted to ultrasonic waves and the returning ultrasonic waves back into electrical signal (Smith and Finnoff 2009). There are different

© Springer International Publishing AG 2017
W.C.G. Peh (ed.), *Pitfalls in Musculoskeletal Radiology*, DOI 10.1007/978-3-319-53496-1_2

frequency transducers. A transducer that has a lower frequency is often used to assess deeper structures but will however have a lower spatial resolution (Smith and Finnoff 2009). A transducer that has a higher frequency will not penetrate into the deeper tissues but will have a higher spatial resolution. In musculoskeletal US, a small footprint high-frequency linear (hockey stick) transducer is often used. This transducer accommodates small and curved surfaces and enables excellent evaluation of the superficial soft tissues.

2.2.2 Physics

Ultrasound is based on ideal physical beam assumptions. In the ideal situation, the US beam is assumed to travel in a straight line. As the US beam travels through tissues, it is assumed that the attenuation of sound is uniform. The speed of sound is assumed to be the same in all tissues. Once the US beam reaches an object, it is assumed that each reflector produces only a single echo. The echoes that are detected by the transducer are assumed to have originated from the main US beam. The depth of an object is directly related to the amount of time it takes the US echo to return to the transducer (Nilsson 2001; Feldman et al. 2009).

In clinical practice, the US beam deviates from these assumptions quite frequently. In addition to the main US beam, secondary beams outside of the main beam called side lobes and grating lobes are also created. Maximum sound wave reflection occurs when the sound wave is directly proportional to the imaged structure, which is not always possible to obtain. In addition, some sound waves are reflected back at the skin surface, while others can be absorbed in the examined tissues. When there is deviation from the ideal physical assumptions, artifacts are produced. These artifacts occur due to inherent characteristics of the US beam, errors in velocity, errors in attenuation, and presence of multiple echo paths (Feldman et al. 2009; Taljanovic et al. 2014).

2.2.3 Doppler US

Doppler US imaging was named after Christian Johann Doppler, an Austrian mathematician and physicist who described the "Doppler effect" in 1842. He stated that the observed frequency of a wave depends on the relative speed of the source and the observer (Roguin 2002). In US imaging, the "Doppler effect" is the change of frequency in a wave when a source moves relative to the receiver (Pozniak et al. 1992; Rubens et al. 2006; Teh 2006). Color, power, and spectral Doppler imaging enhance the traditional standard brightness mode (B-mode) gray-scale imaging and allow detection of vessels or abnormal blood flow in injured or pathologic tissues.

Color Doppler US produces an image that shows the presence, direction, and velocity of blood flow (Teh 2006). The image is superimposed on the gray-scale image. The differences in color on the image designates whether the flow is headed toward or away from the transducer. In addition, the mean velocity of the blood flow is color coded. Power Doppler US does not provide flow velocity and directional information. However, it has increased flow sensitivity and better vascular delineation (Martinoli et al. 1998). Power Doppler US displays the strength or power of the signal by measuring the amount of red cells passing by the beam (Martinoli et al. 1998; Teh 2006). The intensity of the blood flow is indicated by the color on the image. Spectral Doppler US interrogates a small region of a vessel, called a sample volume, and creates a spectral Doppler waveform (Rubens et al. 2006). This gives a quantitative analysis of the velocity and direction of blood flow (Teh 2006).

2.2.4 Normal Structures

Knowledge of the appearance of normal structures on US images is a prerequisite, before being able to identify US artifacts. Normal cortical bone (Fig. 2.1a) is hyperechoic and demonstrates posterior acoustic shadowing secondary to its highly reflective surface. Normal muscle (Fig. 2.1b) is hypoechoic with fine hyperechoic

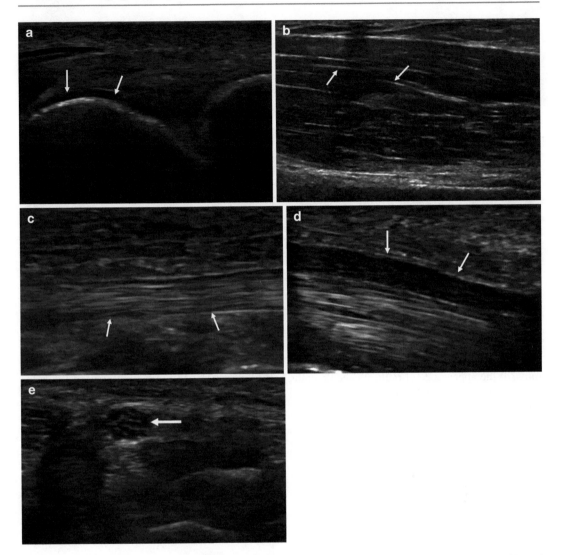

Fig. 2.1 Normal US imaging features of the musculo-skeletal tissues. (**a**) Cortical bone at the metacarpophalangeal joint – normal hyperechoic cortical bone (*arrows*) with dirty posterior acoustic shadowing. (**b**) Muscle – normal pectoralis major muscle with hypoechoic muscle bundles separated by fine hyperechoic fibroadipose septa (*arrows*). (**c**) Tendon – normal posterior tibialis tendon (*arrows*) with echogenic fibrillar echotexture. (**d**) Normal peripheral nerve in the long axis – normal median nerve (*arrows*) with a fascicular architecture and appearing hypoechoic compared to adjacent tendon. (**e**) Normal peripheral nerve in short axis – normal median nerve with a speckled or honeycomb cross-sectional appearance (*arrow*)

fibroadipose septa separating the muscle into bundles. Normal tendon (Fig. 2.1c) is hyperechoic when compared to muscle and has a fibrillar echotexture. Normal nerve (Fig. 2.1d) can be hyperechoic relative to muscle or hypoechoic relative to tendon. The cross-sectional appearance of a normal nerve demonstrates a honeycombed or speckled architecture (Fig. 2.1e).

2.3 Gray-Scale Artifacts

2.3.1 Beam Characteristics

Artifacts related to intrinsic characteristics of the US beam are side-lobe, beamwidth, and anisotropy. Side-lobe artifacts create low-level spurious

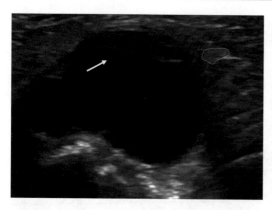

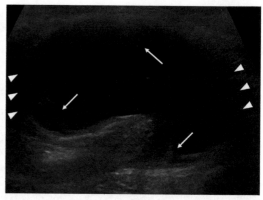

Fig. 2.2 Side-lobe artifact. Long-axis gray-scale US image taken at the dorsal aspect of the wrist shows a ganglion cyst. A spurious low-level echo (*arrow*) is seen within the cystic structure secondary to a side-lobe beam interacting with an off-axis highly reflective acoustic surface (delineated with dotted line) which is recorded as if along the main US beam path

Fig. 2.3 Beamwidth artifact. Long-axis gray-scale US image taken at the posterior aspect of the knee shows a Baker cyst which contains spurious echoes (*arrows*) generated by highly reflective objects outside of the transducer margin but inside of the widened distal beam. There is also reduced contrast at the lesion border (*arrowheads*)

echoes within cystic structures (Fig. 2.2), bright specular reflections within cystic or solid structures, or the appearance of multiple needle paths during a biopsy. Side lobes are secondary US lobes outside of the main beam (Scanlan 1991). They are much weaker than the main beam, with only 1/100 of the intensity (Laing and Kurtz 1982). Side-lobe artifact occurs when a side lobe interacts with a highly reflective acoustic surface outside of the main US path, is reflected back to the transducer, and is incorrectly recorded as if it is located in the main US beam path (Feldman et al. 2009). To distinguish if a structure is a side-lobe artifact or a true structure, an alternate plane of scanning can be used for verification.

Beamwidth artifact can cause spurious echoes to be seen within a cystic structure or reduced contrast at a lesion border (Fig. 2.3). This artifact occurs when the main US beam is too wide with respect to an imaged structure. As the main US beam travels, it normally narrows to a focal zone before fanning out and widening distally (Scanlan 1991; Feldman et al. 2009). When there is a highly reflective object outside of the margin of the transducer but inside the distal widened portion of the beam, the echo from this object is recorded at an incorrect location. Beamwidth artifact can be minimized by adjusting the focal zone to the level of the structure of interest

(Taljanovic et al. 2014). Anisotropy can mimic tears in tendons and ligaments, due to their oblique course. As mentioned previously, maximum sound wave reflection occurs when the main US beam is perpendicular to an imaged structure. This artifact occurs when the transducer is not perpendicular to an imaged structure, and therefore, many of the returning echoes are not recorded and the imaged structure may appear hypoechoic (Taljanovic et al. 2014) (Fig. 2.4). This artifact can be eliminated or minimized by heel-toe maneuvering of the transducer.

2.3.2 Velocity Errors

Artifacts related to errors in velocity are refraction and speed displacement. These artifacts occur due to the different speeds of sound through different types of tissue. For example, sound travels through bone at 4080 m/sec and travels through air at 330 m/sec, with the speeds through fat and soft tissue falling in between these values (Bushberg et al. 2012). Refraction causes widening or misplacement of structures on an US image. This artifact occurs secondary to the US beam traveling through two materials with different speeds of sound (Scanlan 1991; Nilsson 2001). As the US beam encounters the interface between these two materials, the beam

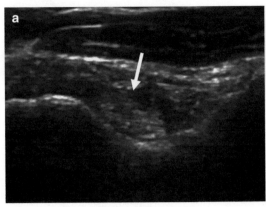

Fig. 2.4 Anisotropy. (**a**) Short-axis gray-scale US image of the long head of biceps tendon in the bicipital groove shows a normal echogenic tendon, when the transducer is properly positioned at 90 degrees to the examined struc- ture. In image (**b**), the tendon appears hypoechoic, which can mimic tendinopathy and/or tendon tear due to anisot- ropy when the US beam is not perpendicular to the exam- ined anatomical structure

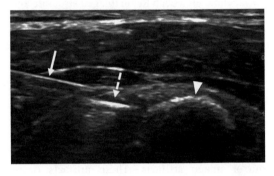

Fig. 2.5 Speed displacement. Gray-scale US image of the right supraspinatus tendon shows a biopsy needle (*solid arrow*) taken during calcium lavage for treatment of calcific tendinitis (*arrowhead*). The needle appears dis- continuous and focally displaced (*dotted arrow*) due to increased travel time of the US sound waves through the soft tissues superficial to this region

changes direction. The returning echo is then mis- placed and recorded as being in an incorrect loca- tion. This artifact can be minimized by using multiple scan planes to examine an object.

Speed displacement artifact is responsible for the discontinuous and focally displaced US appearance of biopsy needles (Fig. 2.5). The US beam in the focally displaced portion of the nee- dle travels slower in this region than the sur- rounding tissue and therefore is recorded later than the echoes in the surrounding tissue (Nilsson 2001; Feldman et al. 2009). This delay in record- ing of the returning echoes makes it appear as if this portion of the needle is focally displaced and

located farther away from the transducer, giving the needle a step-off appearance.

2.3.3 Attenuation Errors

Artifacts related to errors in attenuation are poste- rior acoustic enhancement, or increased through- transmission, and posterior acoustic shadowing. As the US beam travels through tissues, the atten- uation of sound is not uniform. Differing materi- als have different attenuation coefficients (dB/ cm). For example, at 1 MHz, water has an attenu- ation coefficient of 0.0002 dB/cm, while air has an attenuation coefficient of 40 dB/cm (Feldman et al. 2009). Increased through-transmission, or posterior acoustic enhancement, is seen as hyper- echoic soft tissues deep to a lesion (Fig. 2.6). This occurs when a weak attenuator, such as a cyst or peripheral nerve sheath tumor, is imaged. These lesions have a relatively lower attenuation of sound beam when compared to the surrounding adjacent soft tissues. Therefore, the echoes tra- versing the cystic structure or nerve sheath tumor will not be as attenuated as the echoes traversing the surrounding soft tissues (Scanlan 1991; Nilsson 2001; Taljanovic et al. 2014). The soft tis- sues deep to the lesion will appear hyperechoic compared to the surrounding soft tissues. Posterior acoustic enhancement is one way, along with lack of vascularity on Doppler interrogation, that a

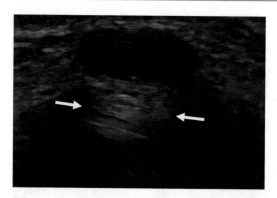

Fig. 2.6 Increased through-transmission or posterior acoustic enhancement. Gray-scale US image of a ganglion cyst at the volar aspect of the wrist shows the hyperechoic appearance of the soft tissues deep to the lesion (*arrows*) created from a relatively lower attenuation of sound beams within the lesion compared to the adjacent soft tissues

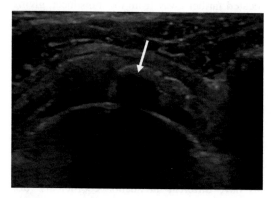

Fig. 2.7 Clean posterior acoustic shadowing. Long-axis gray-scale US image of the supraspinatus tendon shows a clean shadow with anechoic appearance deep to the calcific tendinitis (*arrow*)

cystic lesion can be differentiated from a solid one (Teh 2006).

Posterior acoustic shadowing causes an anechoic or hypoechoic area deep to an examined structure and can be seen with bone, calcification, foreign body, and gas. This artifact occurs when the US beam is reflected, absorbed, or refracted by a strongly attenuating material that causes the echoes distal to the material to be lower in intensity (Rubin et al. 1991; Feldman et al. 2009). Clean posterior acoustic shadowing manifests as an anechoic region deep to an imaged object and occurs with objects with a small radius of curvature or a rough surface (Rubin et al. 1991) (Fig. 2.7). Dirty posterior acoustic shadowing appears as a heterogeneous hypoechoic area deep to the imaged structure and occurs with objects with a large radius of curvature and smooth surface (Rubin et al. 1991) (Fig. 2.8).

2.3.4 Multiple Echoes

Artifacts related to multiple echo paths are posterior reverberation, comet-tail, ring-down, and mirror image artifacts. These artifacts occur because a reflector may produce more than a single echo. Posterior reverberation artifact causes multiple echoes at regularly spaced intervals located deep to a reflective surface, often seen when dealing with a biopsy needle (Fig. 2.9).

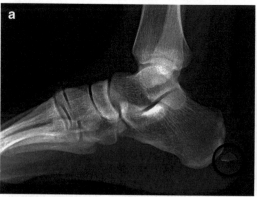
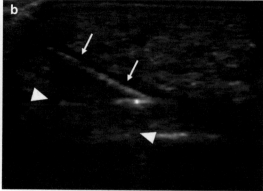

Fig. 2.8 Dirty posterior acoustic shadowing. (**a**) Lateral radiograph of the foot shows a piece of glass (*circled*) within the soft tissues posterior to the calcaneus. (**b**) Gray-scale US image in this region shows the same foreign body (*arrows*) with dirty posterior acoustic shadowing (*arrowheads*) within the soft tissues deep to this site

This artifact occurs when an echo is repeatedly reflected back and forth between two strong parallel reflectors before returning to the transducer (Scanlan 1991; Feldman et al. 2009). While the

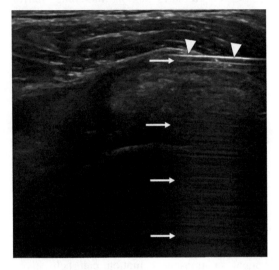

Fig. 2.9 Posterior reverberation. Gray-scale US image shows a biopsy needle (*arrowheads*) during calcium lavage of the supraspinatus tendon with numerous linear reflective echoes (*arrows*) at equally spaced distances deep to the highly reflective needle interface

first echo returns to the transducer and is displayed in the proper location, each following echo will take longer and longer to return to the transducer and will erroneously be displayed as being deeper to the echo before it.

A form of reverberation is the comet-tail artifact, which is often due to metal or calcium, where the two parallel reflectors are closely spaced together (Feldman et al. 2009; Taljanovic et al. 2014) (Fig. 2.10). The distal echoes may be attenuated with decreased amplitude. Individual echoes may be so closely spaced that they may not visually be separated from each other. Ring-down artifact can have a similar appearance to posterior reverberation and comet-tail artifacts. However, this artifact is usually seen with gas and is created through a different mechanism (Fig. 2.11). Ring-down artifact is due to fluid trapped between air bubbles, causing resonant vibrations that are recorded by the transducer (Feldman et al. 2009).

Mirror image artifact causes a duplicate image on the opposite side of a specular reflector, which is a curved highly reflective surface (Taljanovic et al. 2014) (Fig. 2.12). The duplicate image is

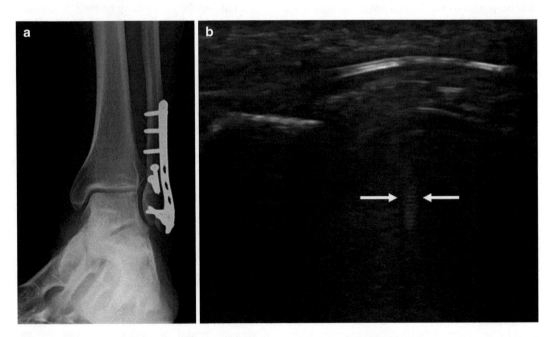

Fig. 2.10 Comet-tail artifact. (**a**) Oblique radiograph of the left ankle shows plate and screw fixation of a distal fibular diaphyseal fracture. (**b**) Gray-scale US image of this region shows a series of continuous reflective echoes (*arrows*) deep to the highly reflective metal surface related to orthopedic hardware created through a form of reverberation. It is often difficult to distinguish individual echoes

equidistant from and deep to the strongly reflective interface as the original structure (Feldman et al. 2009). This artifact occurs when an echo is reflected between the specular reflector, back of the structure of interest, back again to the specular reflector, and then back to the transducer. The delay in return of this echo causes the image to be recorded as if it is deep to the specular reflector.

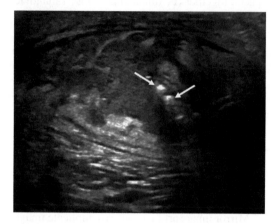

Fig. 2.11 Ring-down artifact. Long-axis gray-scale US image of the left popliteal fossa shows a heterogeneous fluid collection containing foci of air (*arrows*). Lines of parallel bands are created through resonant vibration of fluid trapped between air bubbles and extend deep to the foci of air, with a similar appearance to comet-tail artifact

2.4 Color and Power Doppler Artifacts

Artifacts related to Doppler imaging include transducer pressure, motion, blooming, mirror image, background noise, aliasing, and twinkle artifacts. Transducer pressure can cause a structure to appear to have erroneously low or no blood flow (Fig. 2.13). With this artifact, increased transducer pressure blocks vascular flow to the imaged area. Avoiding excessive transducer pressure while scanning and using copious amounts of US gel on the skin may prevent this artifact (Taljanovic et al. 2014). Contrary to transducer pressure, motion artifact can create erroneous flashes of color on Doppler US imaging, with appearance of spurious vascularity in the imaged structure (Nilsson 2001) (Fig. 2.14). This artifact occurs when there is either transducer or patient motion, creating the Doppler effect. Reducing patient or transducer motion can help avoid motion artifacts. When this is not possible, high-pass wall filters can also be used, although these will preferentially exclude slow flow moving blood (Pozniak et al. 1992; Rubens et al. 2006).

Increasing the gain setting on the US machine can create blooming artifact with artificial

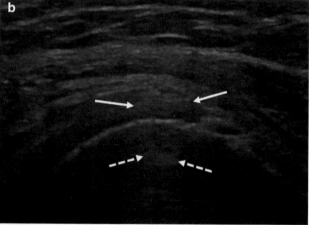

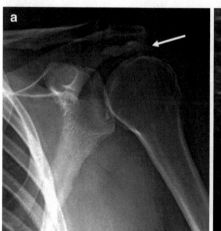

Fig. 2.12 Mirror image artifact. (**a**) Anteroposterior radiograph of the left shoulder shows calcification (*solid arrow*) in the location of the left infraspinatus tendon consistent with calcific tendonitis (calcium hydroxyapatite deposition disease). (**b**) Long-axis gray-scale US image of the same shoulder/infraspinatus tendon shows the echo-genic focus of calcium hydroxyapatite (*solid arrows*). There is a distorted mirror image (*dotted arrows*) of the infraspinatus tendon calcifications projecting into the adjacent humeral head, which acts as a highly reflective acoustic interface, creating reverberation artifact and scattering of US waves

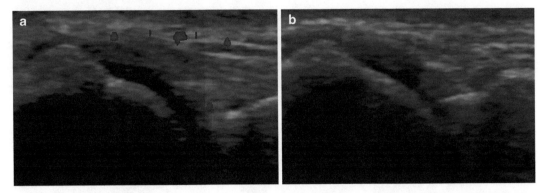

Fig. 2.13 Transducer pressure. (**a**) Long-axis power Doppler US image of the great toe metatarsophalangeal joint shows mildly increased vascularity in this region. (**b**) Power Doppler US image in the same region with increased amount of transducer pressure blocks the vascular flow to this area, and vascularity is no longer seen

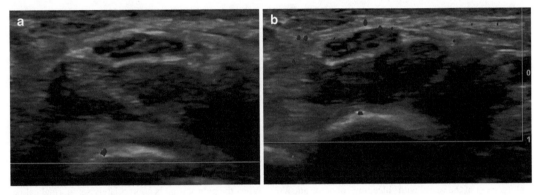

Fig. 2.14 Motion artifact. (**a**) Short-axis power Doppler US image shows a mildly enlarged median nerve without hyperemia. (**b**) Power Doppler US image in this same region shows random flashes of color in and surrounding the nerve produced by slight patient motion

enlargement of a vessel and "bleeding" of color outside of the true vessel lumen (Nilsson 2001; Rubens et al. 2006) (Fig. 2.15a). On the other hand, if the gain is set too low, there will be apparent diminished caliber of the vessel and decreased flow (Fig. 2.15b). An appropriate gain setting should be selected to accurately represent the true width of the vessel lumen (Fig. 2.15c). Background noise is also controlled with the gain setting (Pozniak et al. 1992; Teh 2006). The gain setting should be set to a level where there is almost no background noise when using color or power Doppler US imaging (Fig. 2.16a). With increased color Doppler gain setting, the background noise appears as a speckled pattern of colors, since the generated noise is a low amplitude signal containing all frequencies (Fig. 2.16b). With maximal increase of power Doppler gain, a uniformly colored background is produced, since power Doppler displays power rather than frequency (Fig. 2.16c). Mirror image artifact can also occur with Doppler imaging and is created through a similar mechanism as when dealing with gray-scale imaging (Pozniak et al. 1992; Rubens et al. 2006). Doppler mirror image artifact causes a duplicate vessel on the opposite side of a specular reflector (Fig. 2.17). As with gray-scale imaging, this duplicate image is equidistant from and deep to the strongly reflective interface as the original structure.

Aliasing occurs when the velocity range exceeds the scale available to display it and leads to inaccurate display of color Doppler velocity

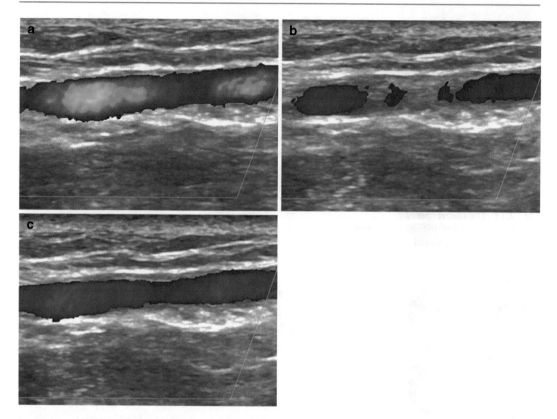

Fig. 2.15 Blooming artifact. (**a**) Long-axis power Doppler US image of the radial artery shows artificial enlargement of the vessel with "bleeding" of color outside of the artery wall secondary to increased gain setting. (**b**) When the gain setting is decreased too low, there is artificial diminishing of vessel caliber and blood flow. (**c**) When the gain setting is appropriately set, normal caliber of the radial artery is seen

(Pozniak et al. 1992; Rubens et al. 2006). The pulse repetition frequency (PRF), the number of US pulses per second that can be transmitted and received by the transducer, limits the maximum velocity scale. The maximum velocity scale must be at least twice the Nyquist limit, which is the maximum frequency shift. When this velocity scale is not at least twice the Nyquist limit, aliasing is portrayed as multiple adjacent colors within a vessel on color Doppler imaging (Nilsson 2001; Teh 2006) (Fig. 2.18a). This artifact does not occur with power Doppler (Fig. 2.18b) as this modality does not provide flow velocity information. Raising the PRF or changing the baseline can correct aliasing (Rubens et al. 2006). In addition, power Doppler imaging can be used since it does not provide flow velocity information. Twinkle artifact appears as a color signal related to a strongly reflecting interface; however, there is no associated real flow or movement (Rubens et al. 2006) (Fig. 2.19). This artifact can be seen with calcifications, calculi, bones, and foreign bodies. Twinkle is thought to be generated by intrinsic machine noise called phase (or clock) jitter (Kamaya et al. 2003). The presence of twinkle artifact can be used to help verify the presence of calcifications, stones, or foreign bodies.

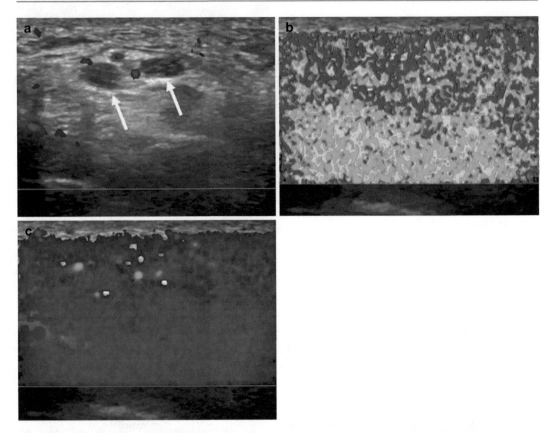

Fig. 2.16 Background noise. (**a**) Short-axis power Doppler US image shows a bifid median nerve (*arrows*) at the level of the pronator quadratus. (**b**) Color Doppler US image in the same region with the gain increased shows increased noise with random direction of flow in the Doppler box. (**c**) Power Doppler US image in the same region with the gain increased shows uniformly increased noise since power Doppler does not provide directional information of flow

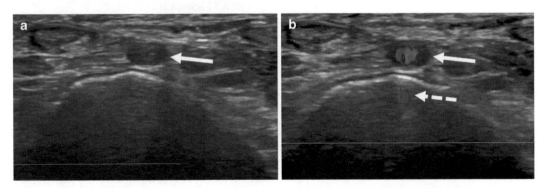

Fig. 2.17 Mirror image artifact with Doppler imaging. (**a**) Short-axis gray-scale US image shows the hypoechogenic dorsalis pedis artery (*solid arrow*). (**b**) Color Doppler US image of the same region demonstrates the red-colored dorsalis pedis artery (*solid arrow*) with mirror image artifact (*dotted arrow*) in the bone secondary to the highly reflective surface

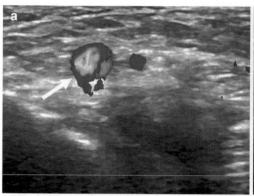

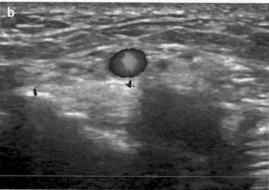

Fig. 2.18 Aliasing artifact. (**a**) Short-axis color Doppler US image of the radial artery at the distal forearm shows reversed *blue* and *green* color (aliased flow) and red color (non-aliased flow). (**b**) Power Doppler US image does not provide directional flow information, and therefore the power Doppler image in the same region shows uniform red color of the radial artery

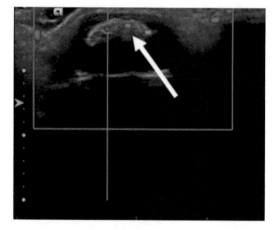

Fig. 2.19 Twinkle artifact. Power Doppler US image of the anterior scalp in a patient with familial pilomatrico-mas shows a heterogeneous solid lesion within the scalp with spurious Doppler signal (*arrow*) in the area of calcification

Conclusion

In clinical practice, US artifacts can occur quite frequently using both B-mode gray-scale and Doppler imaging. Without appropriate awareness, these artifacts can be mistaken for pathology. Radiologists should understand artifacts occurring with musculoskeletal US imaging in order to avoid erroneous interpretation and employ techniques that help avoid or minimize them.

References

Bushberg JT, Seibert JA, Leidholdt EM Jr, Boone JM (2012) The essential physics of medical imaging. Lippincott Williams and Wilkins, Philadelphia

Feldman MK, Katyal S, Blackwood MS (2009) US artifacts. Radiographics 29:1179–1189

Kamaya A, Tuthill T, Rubin JM (2003) Twinkling artifact on color Doppler sonography: dependence on machine parameters and underlying cause. AJR Am J Roentgenol 180:215–222

Laing FC, Kurtz AB (1982) The importance of ultrasonic side-lobe artifacts. Radiology 145:763–768

Martinoli C, Pretolesi F, Crespi G et al (1998) Power Doppler sonography: clinical applications. Eur J Radiol 27(Suppl 2):S133–S140

Nilsson A (2001) Artefacts in sonography and Doppler. Eur Radiol 11:1308–1315

Pozniak MA, Zagzebski JA, Scanlan KA (1992) Spectral and color Doppler artifacts. Radiographics 12:35–44

Roguin A (2002) Christian Johann Doppler: the man behind the effect. Br J Radiol 75:615–619

Rubens DJ, Bhatt S, Nedelka S, Cullinan J (2006) Doppler artifacts and pitfalls. Radiol Clin N Am 44:805–835

Rubin JM, Adler RS, Bude RO et al (1991) Clean and dirty shadowing at US: a reappraisal. Radiology 181:231–236

Scanlan KA (1991) Sonographic artifacts and their origins. AJR Am J Roentgenol 156:1267–1272

Smith J, Finnoff JT (2009) Diagnostic and interventional musculoskeletal ultrasound: part 1. Fundamentals. PM R 1:64–75

Taljanovic MS, Melville DM, Scalone LR et al (2014) Artifacts in musculoskeletal ultrasonography. Semin Musculoskelet Radiol 18:3–11

Teh J (2006) Applications of Doppler imaging in the musculoskeletal system. Curr Probl Diagn Radiol 35:22–34

Computed Tomography Artifacts

3

Derik L. Davis and Prasann Vachhani

Contents

3.1	**Introduction**	45
3.2	**Physics-Related Artifacts**	46
3.2.1	Noise	46
3.2.2	Beam Hardening	46
3.2.3	Scatter	47
3.2.4	Partial Volume Effect	47
3.2.5	Photon Starvation	48
3.2.6	Undersampling	48
3.3	**Conventional Multidetector CT Scanner Artifacts**	49
3.3.1	Ring, Windmill, and Cone Beam Artifacts	49
3.3.2	Stair Step and Zebra Artifacts	49
3.4	**Metal-Related Artifacts**	50
3.4.1	Causes of Metal-Related Artifacts	50
3.4.2	Solutions for Metal-Related Artifacts	51
3.4.3	Pitfalls of Metal Artifact Reduction	52
3.5	**Patient-Related Artifacts**	54
3.5.1	Patient Motion	54
3.5.2	Patient Positioning	54
3.5.3	Contrast-Related Artifacts	55
3.6	**Dual-Energy CT Scanner Artifacts**	55
3.6.1	Benefits of Dual-Energy CT	55
3.6.2	Pitfalls of Dual-Energy CT	56
3.7	**Dedicated Extremity Cone Beam CT Artifacts**	56
3.7.1	Benefits of Dedicated Extremity Cone Beam CT	56
3.7.2	Pitfalls of Dedicated Extremity Cone Beam CT	57
3.8	**Dynamic Four-Dimensional Musculoskeletal CT Artifacts**	57
Conclusion		58
References		58

Abbreviations

4DCT	Four-dimensional computed tomography
CBCT	Cone beam computed tomography
CT	Computed tomography
DECT	Dual-energy computed tomography
FBP	Filtered back projection
keV	Kiloelectron volts
kVp	Peak kilovoltage
mAs	Tube current
MDCT	Multidetector computed tomography

D.L. Davis, MD (✉) • P. Vachhani, MD
Department of Diagnostic Radiology &
Nuclear Medicine, University of Maryland
School of Medicine, 22 S. Greene Street,
Baltimore, MD 21201, USA
e-mail: ddavis7@umm.edu; pvacchani@umm.edu

3.1 Introduction

Computed tomography (CT) is a ubiquitous tool in modern clinical practice and is particularly useful for evaluating musculoskeletal pathology. However, CT artifacts are pitfalls which frequently

© Springer International Publishing AG 2017
W.C.G. Peh (ed.), *Pitfalls in Musculoskeletal Radiology*, DOI 10.1007/978-3-319-53496-1_3

reduce image quality. CT artifacts are manifestations of a divergence between actual attenuation coefficients and measured Hounsfield units of objects on a CT image. CT artifacts are multifactorial in origin and stem from unavoidable and avoidable causes. Unavoidable CT artifacts emanate from dense objects, while avoidable CT artifacts are outcomes of less than optimal protocol parameters affecting study acquisition and image reconstruction. This chapter reviews the cause and imaging appearance of musculoskeletal CT artifacts and also describes strategies that lessen the impact of these pitfalls.

3.2   Physics-Related Artifacts

3.2.1   Noise

Noise artifacts manifest on CT images following filtered back projection (FBP) as random dark and bright streaks (salt-and-pepper grainy appearance) in the plane of greatest attenuation (Fig. 3.1). Also known as quantum mottle, noise is a result of low photon counts (Fig. 3.2). The magnitude of noise becomes more pronounced as the photon count approaches zero (Boas and Fleischmann 2012). Noise can be decreased by increasing

mAs. Modern CT scanners with tube current modulation automatically increase or decrease mAs during image acquisition. Post-processing strategies to reduce noise include combining data from multiple scans for larger slice thickness, using soft tissue instead of bone window algorithms, or employing iterative reconstruction. Thicker slices reduce noise, but there is a trade-off with image resolution when compared to thinner slices. Iterative reconstruction techniques also allow for lower doses than FBP, but since it attempts to smooth out noise while preserving edges, it may produce images with a "plastic" appearance (Boas and Fleischmann 2012).

3.2.2   Beam Hardening

Conventional CT scanners emit polychromatic X-rays which are constituted of photons with a range of energies (Barrett and Keat 2004). Beam hardening occurs when a polychromatic X-ray passes through high-density objects that strongly absorb X-rays, preferentially those with low-energy photons, and "harden" the beam (Coupal et al. 2014). These artifacts present as dark streaks between two high-density objects (Fig. 3.3) or along the long axis of a dense object (Boas and Fleischmann 2012). Differences in beam hardening at the center versus the periphery

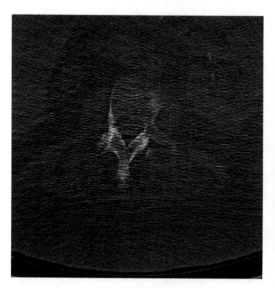

Fig. 3.1 Noise artifact. Axial CT image of the lumbar spine shows a diffuse salt-and-pepper mottled appearance

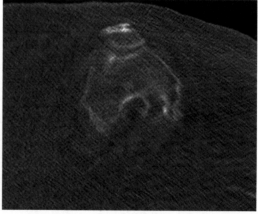

Fig. 3.2 Noise artifact in a patient with morbid obesity. Axial CT image of the knee shows poor image quality with dark and bright streaks

of an object are responsible for cupping artifacts (Barrett and Keat 2004). Adjacent bright streaks are not uncommonly produced during FBP due to inaccurate photon measurements among adjacent detectors. Increasing the kVp during image acquisition or the use of iterative reconstruction at the time of post-processing can decrease beam hardening artifacts. However, scanning at a higher kVp may result in reduced tissue contrast (Boas and Fleischmann 2012).

3.2.3 Scatter

Similar to beam hardening artifact, scatter manifests as dark streaks between two high-density objects, with associated adjacent bright streaks (Fig. 3.4). Scattered X-ray photons deflected from their original course are errantly measured by incorrect detectors, and the magnitude of this artifact increases with higher numbers of detector rows. Anti-scatter grids inherent to CT scanners are present to reduce scatter. Post-processing with scatter correction algorithms and iterative reconstruction are additional means of scatter artifact reduction. However, scatter correction may fail if all non-scatter-related photons are absorbed by a high-density object (Boas and Fleischmann 2012).

3.2.4 Partial Volume Effect

Partial volume effect is caused by an X-ray passing only partially through an off-center highly attenuating object. The resulting partial volume artifact derives from exaggeration of divergence of the X-ray along the z-axis during image reconstruction and presents as shading on the CT images. The use of thin slice acquisition can reduce partial volume artifact. Reducing slice thickness will increase noise, which can be decreased by creating thicker slices during image reconstruction (Barrett and Keat 2004).

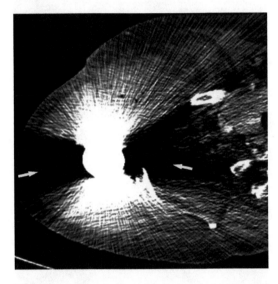

Fig. 3.3 Beam hardening artifact in a patient with a total shoulder arthroplasty. Axial CT image of the shoulder shows large dark streaks (*arrows*) as the result of beam hardening and photon starvation

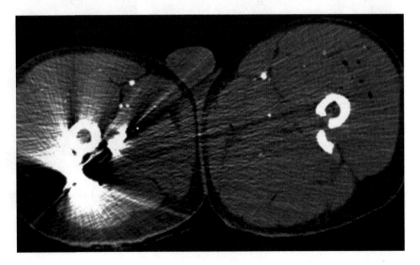

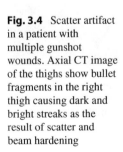

Fig. 3.4 Scatter artifact in a patient with multiple gunshot wounds. Axial CT image of the thighs show bullet fragments in the right thigh causing dark and bright streaks as the result of scatter and beam hardening

3.2.5 Photon Starvation

Photon starvation occurs if a dense object, such as metal, absorbs a large number of photons. This results in noisy images, with dark streaks on CT (Coupal et al. 2014). Photon starvation is precipitated by too few photons reaching the detector (Fig. 3.5). Increasing the mAs during scanning will reduce photon starvation artifacts. Modern scanners perform tube current modulation to increase mAs when needed while reducing the overall radiation dose (Barrett and Keat 2004).

3.2.6 Undersampling

Undersampling is an artifact related to misregistration during image reconstruction, caused by too large of a gap between projections. View aliasing artifacts manifest as fine stripes at a distance from a dense structure (Fig. 3.6). Ray aliasing artifacts appear as stripes near the edge of dense object, caused by undersampling within a projection (Fig. 3.7). Undersampling artifacts are most problematic in cases when high resolution is required. Acquiring the maximum number of projections per rotation can minimize view aliasing. CT scanner techniques utilizing flying focal spot or quarter-detector shift methods are used to decrease ray aliasing (Barrett and Keat 2004).

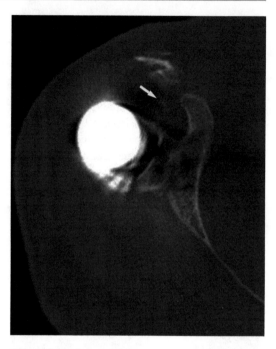

Fig. 3.6 Undersampling artifact in a patient with a total shoulder arthroplasty. Axial CT arthrographic image shows fine stripes (*arrow*) near the metallic prosthesis

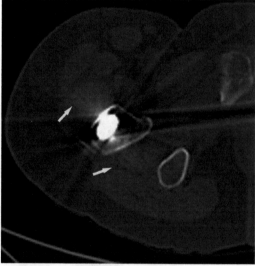

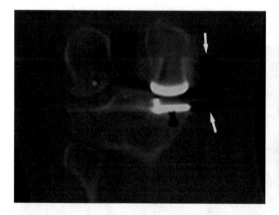

Fig. 3.5 Photon starvation artifact in a patient with a unicompartmental knee arthroplasty and acute tibial fracture. Coronal CT image of the knee shows dark streaks (*arrows*) as the result of photon starvation and beam hardening

Fig. 3.7 Undersampling artifact in a patient with a total hip arthroplasty. Axial CT image of the hip shows fine stripes (*arrows*) radiating away from the femoral stem of the hip prosthesis

3.3 Conventional Multidetector CT Scanner Artifacts

3.3.1 Ring, Windmill, and Cone Beam Artifacts

Ring artifacts are the result of detector element miscalibration. These artifacts present as concentric dark and bright rings on the CT image, along the center of rotation (Fig. 3.8). Scanners with solid-state detectors are more prone to ring artifacts than a scanner with gas detectors. Recalibration or replacement of defective detectors eliminates this artifact (Barrett and Keat 2004).

Helical multidetector row CT is prone to certain artifacts that are not seen in single-detector row CT, namely, windmill and cone beam artifacts. Windmill artifacts, also known as splay artifacts, are the result of incomplete sampling along the z-axis and are most pronounced along high-contrast boundaries, such as along the edges of metallic surgical implants (Buckwalter et al. 2011). Artifact occurs when multiple rows of detectors intersect the plane of reconstruction for every given rotation and there are inaccuracies in derived interpolated values from adjacent detectors. These artifacts appear as alternating dark and bright bands, circumferentially emanating from the edge of a dense structure (Buckwalter 2007). Reduction of pitch, or the use of a non-integer pitch value, may decrease the number of

detectors that intersect in the plane of reconstruction. Z-filter helical interpolators are also used in modern scanners to reduce windmill artifacts (Buckwalter 2007).

Cone beam artifacts are a function of the high number of parallel detector rows in modern multidetector CT (MDCT) scanners, since a wider X-ray beam in the z-axis direction must be projected to reach the entire detector array (Buckwalter 2007). These artifacts appear as shading artifacts on CT images (Barrett and Keat 2004). Software algorithms in modern scanners reduce cone beam artifact during the image reconstruction process (Defrise et al. 2001). Ensuring that collimation is less than 10 mm is also important to mitigate these artifacts (Rydberg et al. 2004).

3.3.2 Stair Step and Zebra Artifacts

Mechanisms that cause stair step and zebra artifacts are similar to ones that cause windmill artifacts mentioned previously. Stair step artifacts occur during image reconstruction as the result of a high-contrast edge between the axial plane and plane of projection. Stair step artifacts occur at the edges of structures on 2D sagittal and coronal reformatted and 3D reformatted images (Fig. 3.9). Zebra artifacts result from the non-homogenous noise distribution along the z-axis on 2D multiplanar and 3D reformatted images and are most

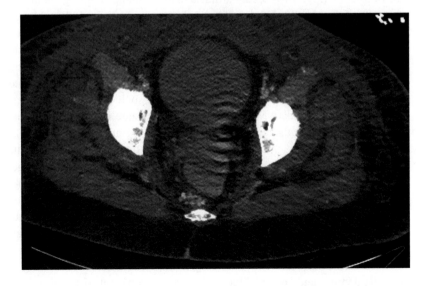

Fig. 3.8 Ring artifact. Axial CT image of the pelvis show dark and bright concentric rings at the center of the pelvis

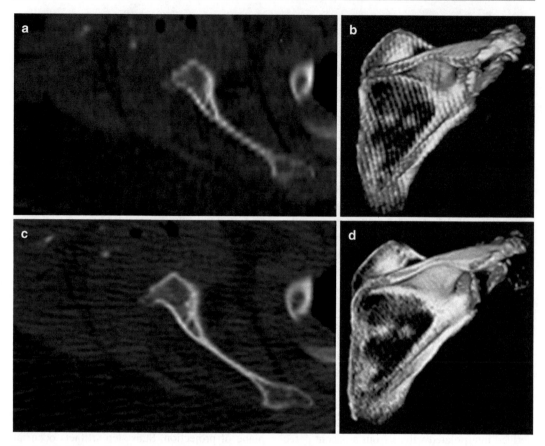

Fig. 3.9 Stair step artifact in a patient with neuropathic joint. (**a**) Axial and (**b**) coronal volume-rendered 3DCT images of the scapula reformatted from a 3 mm slice thickness show stair step artifacts. (**c**) Axial and (**d**) coronal volume-rendered 3DCT images of the scapula reformatted from a 1 mm slice thickness show elimination of the artifact

pronounced as the distance increases from the axis of rotation (Fig. 3.10). Zebra artifacts manifest as alternating bands of high and low noise on sagittal or coronal reformatted images (Boas and Fleischmann 2012). Adaptive multiple plane reconstruction and cone beam reconstruction techniques are available to mitigate stair step artifact (Flohr et al. 2005). Image reconstruction using thin slices in modern MDCT scanners also reduce stair step artifact significantly.

3.4 Metal-Related Artifacts

3.4.1 Causes of Metal-Related Artifacts

Metal creates several artifacts including noise, beam hardening, and scatter. Metal edges also create artifacts related to cone beam, windmill, undersampling, and motion. Metal artifacts present as dark and bright streaks on CT images (Boas and Fleischmann 2012). The FBP algorithm creates CT artifact from error-prone image reconstruction following attenuation of X-ray beams by metal. Bilateral metallic implants, such as bilateral hip prostheses, present on the same image will produce severe beam hardening artifacts (Fig. 3.11), usually along the left-to-right axis (Buckwalter et al. 2011). Metal alloy composition influences CT artifact intensity. Stainless steel, cobalt chrome, and nickel produce a greater amount of artifact compared to low atomic metals such as titanium on conventional MDCT. Metal artifacts are generally most severe across the long axis of a nonsymmetrical implant (Fig. 3.12). Thus, anatomy adjacent to the short axis of a nonsymmetrical

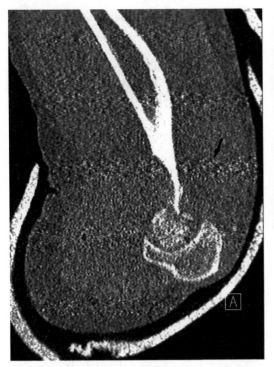

Fig. 3.10 Zebra artifact. Sagittal CT image of the elbow shows bands of alternating high noise (*arrow*) and low noise

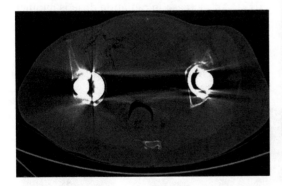

Fig. 3.11 Beam hardening artifact in a patient with bilateral total hip arthroplasty. Axial CT image of the pelvis shows dark and bright streaks extending along the left-to-right axis

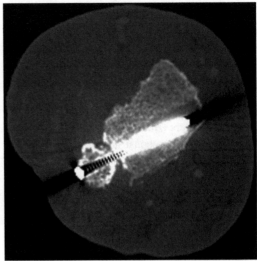

Fig. 3.12 Metallic artifact of a nonsymmetrical implant. Axial CT image of the lower leg shows that metallic artifact is most severe relative to the long axis of the syndesmotic screw

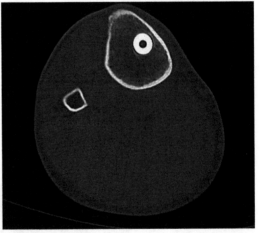

Fig. 3.13 Paucity of artifact from a symmetrical implant. Axial CT image of the lower leg shows an intramedullary rod with minimal artifact

3.4.2 Solutions for Metal-Related Artifacts

implant is less often obscured by artifact. Circular implants with a radially symmetrical shape (Fig. 3.13), such as an intramedullary rod, tend to produce fewer artifacts than a rectangular plate (Buckwalter et al. 2011). Circular intramedullary rods tend to produce streak artifacts most typically at the site of interlocking screws (Buckwalter 2007).

MDCT protocol modifications to reduce metal artifacts include scanning at 140 kVp instead of 120 kVp and increasing mAs through regions of metal (Table 3.1). Fixed mAs protocols may be necessary, since dose modulation techniques may fail in the setting of highly attenuating implants. Using a lower pitch setting can reduce windmill artifacts.

These artifacts are also significantly reduced when slice thickness is at least twice the thickness of the detector element (Buckwalter et al. 2011). Flying z spot techniques are additional methods to reduce windmill artifacts (Flohr et al. 2004).

Noise and streaking artifacts are more pronounced with high spatial resolution filters, typically bone filters (Buckwalter 2007). Soft tissue, instead of bone, reconstruction algorithms are performed to reduce metal artifacts, although there is a consequence of decreased image resolution when using FBP. Image reconstruction with thicker slices to create coronal and sagittal reformatted images (Fig. 3.14) may help reduce the amount of streaking artifact as compared to thinner slices (Buckwalter et al. 2011). However, the need to select a soft tissue reconstruction

algorithm for small and less dense implants may not be necessary (Buckwalter 2007).

Iterative reconstruction techniques are also useful for metal artifact reduction, and software is available for installation on commercially available CT scanners from several manufacturers (Figs. 3.15 and 3.16). Some methods of iterative reconstruction delete the metal data from the raw data and reconstruct the image from the nonmetal data (Boas and Fleischmann 2011). Metal deletion techniques have been shown to improve image quality more than 70% of the time for metallic implants (Boas and Fleischmann 2012).

3.4.3 Pitfalls of Metal Artifact Reduction

Best practices call for images created by iterative metal artifact reduction techniques to be compared with nonmetal artifact reduction images (Fig. 3.17), since decreased resolution or new artifacts may occur in some areas of the metal reduction images (Boas and Fleischmann 2012). An increase in radiation dose is another important parameter to consider, if an increase in kVp and mAs is used for metal artifact reduction. Lastly, the use of thicker slices for images reconstruction to decrease artifacts

Table 3.1 Strategies to reduce metal-related artifacts on conventional MDCT

Image acquisition
Increase mAs
Increase kVp
Reduce pitch
Use thin beam collimation
Post-processing
Use soft tissue reconstruction algorithm
Increase slice thickness for image reconstruction
Use iterative reconstruction
Use metal reduction software

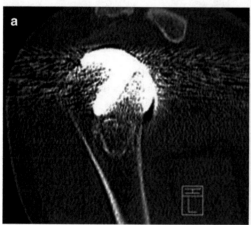 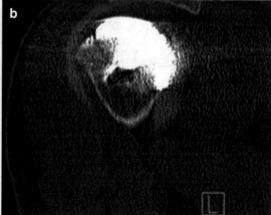

Fig. 3.14 Effect of slice thickness in a patient with a humeral head resurfacing arthroplasty. (**a**) Sagittal oblique CT arthrographic image formatted using a slice thickness of 1 mm shows extensive dark and bright streaking artifact. (**b**) Sagittal oblique CT arthrogram image formatted using a slice thickness of 2 mm shows a reduction in visible artifact

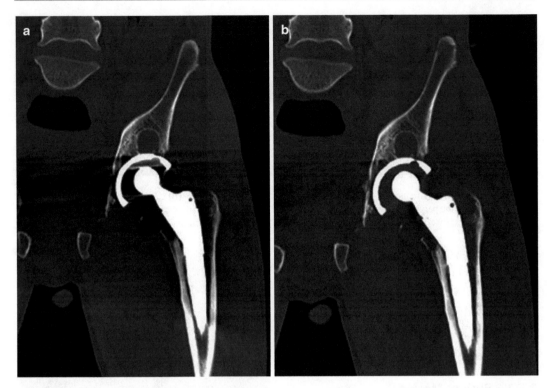

Fig. 3.15 Metal artifact reduction in a patient with a total hip arthroplasty. (**a**) Coronal CT image shows extensive dark streak artifacts obscuring the hip and pelvis. (**b**) Coronal CT image with vendor-provided metal artifact reduction software shows reduction of the metallic artifacts. The urinary bladder and medial wall of the acetabulum have improved visualization, and the osteolysis at the femoral greater trochanter is shown to greater detail

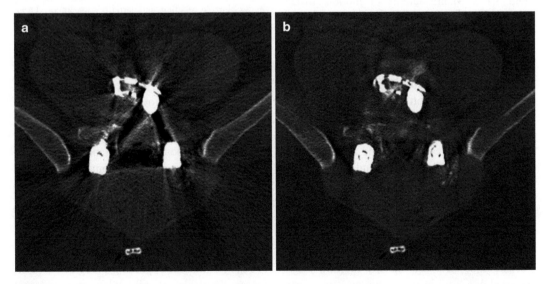

Fig. 3.16 Metal artifact reduction in a patient with posterior decompression and spinal fusion. (**a**) Axial CT image of the lumbar spine shows extensive metallic artifacts. (**b**) Axial CT image shows improved image quality following use of vendor-provided metal artifact reduction software

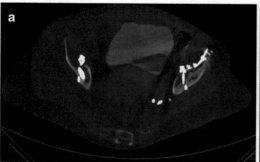 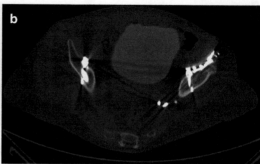

Fig. 3.17 Metal artifact reduction software pitfall. (**a**) Axial CT image of the pelvis using vendor-provided metal artifact reduction software mimics a large filling defect in the urinary bladder. (**b**) Comparison to the axial CT image without metal artifact reduction shows an absence of the urinary bladder filling defect

may not be achievable for cases requiring high resolution, such as for the wrist or ankle (Buckwalter et al. 2011).

3.5   Patient-Related Artifacts

3.5.1   Patient Motion

Patient motion artifacts are the result of misregistration during image reconstruction (Barrett and Keat 2004). Patient movement during CT scan acquisition is the major source of motion artifacts (Fig. 3.18). Manifestations of motion artifact include image blurring, shading, streaking, or partially superimposed double images (Boas and Fleischmann 2012). The use of patient restraints and positioning aids, and the alignment of the CT scan in the orientation of motion, can reduce motion artifact (Barrett and Keat 2004). Short scan time also reduces motion artifact, and this feature is more inherent in modern MDCT scanners with fast gantry rotation and a high number of detector rows (Fleischmann and Boas 2011).

3.5.2   Patient Positioning

Photon counts are reduced when X-rays must pass through the body. Raising the arm above the head can limit beam hardening, streak artifacts, and noise (Fig. 3.19), when upper extremity CT imaging is performed (Miller-Thomas

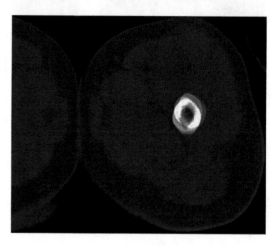

Fig. 3.18 Motion artifact. Axial CT image of the thigh shows blurring, shading, and partially superimposed double images

et al. 2005). Imaging the upper extremity in the "superman" position, in a prone position with the arms extended above the head, is an alternative method to place the arm away from the body. Subsequent securing of the upper extremity into a fixed position with tape or a restraint limits motion artifacts (Pieroni et al. 2009). Adjusting lower extremity positioning is also beneficial for reducing CT artifact. Flexing one knee and extending the opposite knee reduces beam hardening artifacts created by bilateral total knee replacements, by preventing the path of X-ray beams from passing though both prostheses. Similar positioning when only one total knee replacement is present improves image quality for evaluation of the native knee by

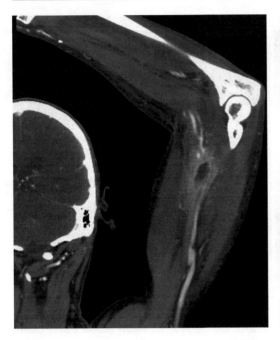

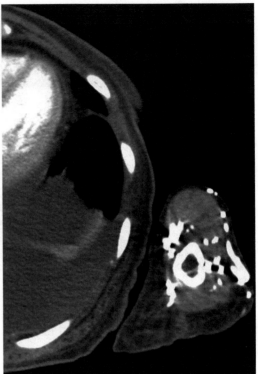

Fig. 3.19 Limb position in a patient with an arm abscess. Sagittal CT image of the upper extremity shows the arm raised above the head. No significant artifact is present

Fig. 3.20 Intravenous contrast artifact in a patient with a suspected arm mass ipsilateral to the upper extremity of contrast agent injection. Axial CT image of the upper extremity shows beam hardening and scatter artifacts reducing image quality at the arm

reducing the proximity of the knees (Buckwalter et al. 2011). Reducing the degree of knee flexion also has benefits to improve visualization of the patella in patients with a total knee arthroplasty by shifting the direction of femoral prosthesis artifact (Ho et al. 2012).

3.5.3 Contrast-Related Artifacts

Contrast agent in vessels produce beam hardening and streak artifacts on CT images (Demirpolat et al. 2011). A contrast bolus artifact (Fig. 3.20) may reduce image quality in the area of interest (Adams et al. 2012). Intravenous injection should be performed on the contralateral upper extremity, when possible (Miller-Thomas et al. 2005). Artifacts produced by contrast agent in vessels have the potential to obscure perivascular anatomy (Yun et al. 2012). Artifacts from intra-articular contrast can similarly decrease image quality of periarticular structures and may pose a challenge when coupled with metal artifact from an adjacent prosthesis.

3.6 Dual-Energy CT Scanner Artifacts

3.6.1 Benefits of Dual-Energy CT

Dual-energy CT (DECT), also known as spectral imaging, uses two different X-ray energies for simultaneous image acquisition. A common pairing includes a high-energy 140 kVp X-ray tube with a lower-energy 80 kVp X-ray tube (Nicolaou et al. 2012). As opposed to polychromatic conventional CT, DECT produces monochromatic images that are less affected by beam hardening, streak artifact, and photon starvation. DECT is useful in the setting of metallic hardware, since a range of different extrapolated energies offer a series of images of varying image quality to select for interpretation

70 keV   70 keV

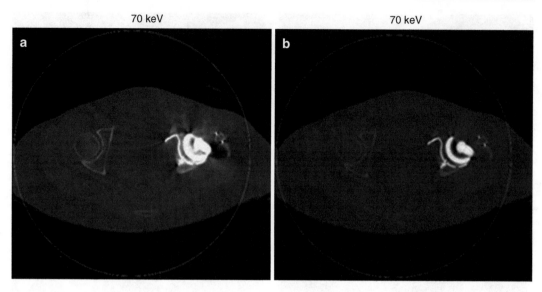

Fig. 3.21 Patient complains of pain 6 months after revision of a total left hip arthroplasty. (**a**) Axial DECT image at 70 keV shows metallic artifact emanating from the prosthesis. (**b**) Axial DECT image at 160 keV shows reduced artifact. Visualization of the acetabular prosthesis component protruding through the medial wall of the acetabulum and impinging the urinary bladder is more clearly delineated

(Fig. 3.21). Energies with the highest image quality have been reported to range from 105 to 133 keV (Coupal et al. 2014). Iterative reconstruction also can be employed with DECT to reduce noise and radiation dose (Karcaaltincaba and Aktas 2011). Furthermore, metal artifact reduction software can be used in conjunction with DECT for added benefit (Lee et al. 2012).

3.6.2   Pitfalls of Dual-Energy CT

Reconstruction of monochromatic images extrapolated from scans that omit lower-energy photon data may increase image noise. In addition, high spatial frequency detail is sacrificed, since DECT raw data are derived from soft tissue and not bone algorithm. Also, barriers exist to reconstruction of coronal and sagittal planes from DECT raw data, and a dedicated workstation for image interpretation may be required (Coupal et al. 2014). DECT does not reduce artifact from scatter and is similar to conventional MDCT in this regard (Boas and Fleischmann 2012). DECT suffers from field-of-view restrictions compared to conventional

MDCT, due to higher radiation dose and noise in patients with high body mass index (Karcaaltincaba and Aktas 2011). DECT also may be less effective for titanium prostheses as compared to stainless steel prostheses (Lee et al. 2012).

3.7   Dedicated Extremity Cone Beam CT Artifacts

3.7.1   Benefits of Dedicated Extremity Cone Beam CT

Cone beam CT (CBCT) acquires a volumetric data set in a single rotation without the patient moving through the scanner. This is accomplished through the use of >1000 detector rows with a digital flat panel detector. Dedicated musculoskeletal extremity scanners have been developed based on CBCT technology (Carrino et al. 2014). CBCT is an attractive alternative to conventional MDCT, since these systems allow for potential image acquisition under weight-bearing conditions (Choi et al. 2014).

3.7.2 Pitfalls of Dedicated Extremity Cone Beam CT

Similar to conventional MDCT, however, musculoskeletal extremity CBCT scanners are prone to beam hardening, scatter, noise, and cone beam artifacts (Carrino et al. 2014). Scatter, in particular, is a major factor limiting image quality by decreasing image contrast and spatial resolution (Sisniega et al. 2013). For musculoskeletal CBCT, image quality of periarticular soft tissues is reduced by artifacts when cortical bones near joint planes are parallel to the scanning plane. Extremity scans involving multiple joint articulations, such as the feet and hands, are the most prone to these artifacts. The flat panel detectors of CBCT are also more prone to noise compared to MDCT (Carrino et al. 2014).

Methods to address scatter include anti-scatter grids, beam blocking arrays, and software algorithms to mitigate the effects of scatter during image reconstruction (Schafer et al. 2012). The use of iterative reconstruction is an alternative to FBP techniques to reduce noise and beam hardening artifacts. Extremity positions which avoid scanning parallel to cortical bones near joint planes and the use of a noncircular detector rotation are additional measures to reduce artifacts (Carrino et al. 2014). A major drawback of CBCT is scan time, which is longer than conventional MDCT. Also, immobilization techniques may not be entirely effective in preventing patient movement (Casselman et al. 2013). Therefore, dedicated extremity CBCT scanners have a greater propensity for motion artifacts (Carrino et al. 2014).

3.8 Dynamic Four-Dimensional Musculoskeletal CT Artifacts

Four-dimensional (4D) CT imaging allows for real-time dynamic imaging of joint motion. 4DCT imaging is being performed more often for diagnostic purposes as the technology becomes more available (Tay et al. 2007). Band and motion artifacts are two artifacts encountered on 4DCT images. Banding artifacts are a manifestation of parallax errors, created by discrepancies over time as images are captured at different angular positions. Banding artifacts occur in the reconstructed coronal plane, perpendicular to the CT gantry, as a result of misalignment of the reconstructed image in the x-z-axis. The severity of banding is dependent on the velocity of motion, with slower velocities producing fewer artifacts (Neo et al. 2013). The band thickness and total number of bands are dependent on pitch and motion frequency (Tay et al. 2008).

Motion artifact is also dependent on the velocity of movement, and motion blur worsens as velocity increases (Neo et al. 2013). With 4DCT dynamic imaging, there is a linear relationship between motion velocity and image quality. The severity of motion artifacts become most pronounced when velocity exceeds 20 mm/s. However, the degree of artifact may differ between axial and reformatted coronal or sagittal images for a given motion velocity (Tay et al. 2008).

Motion and banding artifacts occur to varying degrees during different phases of motion velocity. Acceleration and deceleration phases tend to produce fewer motion and banding artifacts as compared to the mid-phase of motion, when maximum velocity occurs. Anatomical location also contributes to severity of artifact. For example, motion and banding artifacts can appear more severe for the metacarpal bones as compared to the carpal bones during wrist imaging, since the metacarpals are further from the axis of rotation and experience higher velocity of motion (Tay et al. 2007).

Image quality in 4DCT images is a function of the temporal resolution. The use of MDCT scanners with higher numbers of detector elements improves temporal resolution when compared to scanners with fewer detectors. For example, 64-slice CT scanners have better temporal resolution (165 ms) than 4-slice CT scanners (250 ms) (Tay et al. 2008). Dual source CT scanners may offer even better temporal resolution (83 ms), while 256-slice CT scanners may effectively eliminate artifacts altogether (Tay et al. 2007). Banding artifacts can be mitigated retrospectively in certain instances through adjustment of the CT gating parameters to improve the synchrony of alignment for the image acquisition with joint motion. However, motion artifacts cannot be corrected retrospectively and can only be improved prospectively through the use of faster temporal resolution or slower motion velocity (Tay et al. 2007).

Conclusion

Artifacts are commonly encountered pitfalls in musculoskeletal CT. Although unavoidable, several strategies exist to mitigate CT artifacts associated with metal. Utilizing protocol parameters specific for metal during CT acquisition and reconstruction, using metal artifact reduction software, and scanning with dual-energy CT all play a role in improving CT image quality when dense objects are present. Attention to detail for protocol optimization regarding patient-specific factors and CT acquisition and reconstruction are effective techniques to reduce the amount of avoidable CT artifacts.

References

Adams AS, Wright MJ, Johnston S et al (2012) The use of multislice CT angiography preoperative study for supraclavicular artery island flap harvesting. Ann Plast Surg 69:312–315

Barrett JF, Keat N (2004) Artifacts in CT: recognition and avoidance. Radiographics 24:1679–1691

Boas FE, Fleischmann D (2011) Evaluation of two iterative techniques for reducing metal artifacts in computed tomography. Radiology 259:894–902

Boas FE, Fleischmann D (2012) CT artifacts: causes and reduction techniques. Imaging Med 4:229–240

Buckwalter KA (2007) Optimizing imaging techniques in the postoperative patient. Semin Musculoskelet Radiol 11:261–272

Buckwalter KA, Lin C, Ford JM (2011) Managing postoperative artifacts on computed tomography and magnetic resonance imaging. Semin Musculoskelet Radiol 15:309–319

Carrino JA, Al Muhit A, Zbijewski W et al (2014) Dedicated cone-beam CT system for extremity imaging. Radiology 270:816–824

Casselman JW, Gieraerts K, Volders D et al (2013) Cone beam CT: non-dental applications. JBR-BTR 96:333–353

Choi JH, Maier A, Keil A et al (2014) Fiducial marker-based correction for involuntary motion in weight-bearing C-arm CT scanning of knees. Part II experiment. Med Phys 41:061902

Coupal TM, Mallinson PI, McLaughlin P, Nicolaou S, Munk PL, Ouellette H (2014) Peering through the glare: using dual-energy CT to overcome the problem of metal artefacts in bone radiology. Skeletal Radiol 43:567–575

Defrise M, Noo F, Kudo H (2001) Rebinning-based algorithms for helical cone-beam CT. Phys Med Biol 46:2911–2937

Demirpolat G, Yuksel M, Kavukcu G, Tuncel D (2011) Carotid CT angiography: comparison of image quality for left versus right arm injections. Diagn Interv Radiol 17:195–198

Fleischmann D, Boas FE (2011) Computed tomography – old ideas and new technology. Eur Radiol 21:510–517

Flohr T, Stierstorfer K, Raupach R, Ulzheimer S, Bruder H (2004) Performance evaluation of a 64-slice CT system with z-flying focal spot. Rofo 176:1803–1810

Flohr TG, Schaller S, Stierstorfer K, Bruder H, Ohnesorge BM, Schoepf UJ (2005) Multi-detector row CT systems and image-reconstruction techniques. Radiology 235:756–773

Ho KC, Saevarsson SK, Ramm H et al (2012) Computed tomography analysis of knee pose and geometry before and after total knee arthroplasty. J Biomech 45:2215–2221

Karcaaltincaba M, Aktas A (2011) Dual-energy CT revisited with multidetector CT: review of principles and clinical applications. Diagn Interv Radiol 17:181–194

Lee YH, Park KK, Song HT, Kim S, Suh JS (2012) Metal artefact reduction in gemstone spectral imaging dual-energy CT with and without metal artefact reduction software. Eur Radiol 22:1331–1340

Miller-Thomas MM, West OC, Cohen AM (2005) Diagnosing traumatic arterial injury in the extremities with CT angiography: pearls and pitfalls. Radiographics 25:S133–S142

Neo PY, Mat Jais IS, Panknin C et al (2013) Dynamic imaging with dual-source gated computed tomography (CT): implications of motion parameters on image quality for wrist imaging. Med Eng Phys 35:1837–1842

Nicolaou S, Liang T, Murphy DT, Korzan JR, Ouellette H, Munk P (2012) Dual-energy CT: a promising new technique for assessment of the musculoskeletal system. AJR Am J Roentgenol 199:S78–S86

Pieroni S, Foster BR, Anderson SW, Kertesz JL, Rhea JT, Soto JA (2009) Use of 64-row multidetector CT angiography in blunt and penetrating trauma of the upper and lower extremities. Radiographics 29:863–876

Rydberg J, Liang Y, Teague SD (2004) Fundamentals of multichannel CT. Semin Musculoskelet Radiol 8:137–146

Schafer S, Stayman JW, Zbijewski W et al (2012) Antiscatter grids in mobile C-arm cone-beam CT: effect on image quality and dose. Med Phys 39:153–159

Sisniega A, Zbijewski W, Badal A et al (2013) Monte Carlo study of the effects of system geometry and anti-scatter grids on cone-beam CT scatter distributions. Med Phys 40:051915

Tay SC, Primak AN, Fletcher JG et al (2007) Four-dimensional computed tomographic imaging in the wrist: proof of feasibility in a cadaveric model. Skeletal Radiol 36:1163–1169

Tay SC, Primak AN, Fletcher JG, Schmidt B, An KN, McCollough CH (2008) Understanding the relation-ship between image quality and motion velocity in gated computed tomography: preliminary work for 4-dimensional musculoskeletal imaging. J Comput Assist Tomogr 32:634–639

Yun EJ, Yoon DY, Han A, Seo YL, Lim KJ, Choi CS, Bae SH (2012) Central venous stenosis of left versus right arm: its prevalence and effects on image quality in CT of the neck. Eur J Radiol 81:e126–e131

Magnetic Resonance Imaging Artifacts

4

Dinesh R. Singh, Helmut Rumpel,
Michael S.M. Chin, and Wilfred C.G. Peh

Contents

4.1 **Introduction** 61

4.2 **MRI Artifacts** 62
4.2.1 Motion 62
4.2.2 Susceptibility and Artifacts Related to
Orthopedic Hardware 66
4.2.3 Chemical Shift 71
4.2.4 Magic Angle Phenomenon 72
4.2.5 Protocol Errors 73

4.3 **Technical Pros and Cons** 77
4.3.1 Fat-Suppression Techniques 77
4.3.2 Isotropic Imaging 77

Conclusion 79

References 80

Abbreviations

CSF   Cerebrospinal fluid
CT   Computed tomography
EPI   Echo planar imaging
FOV   Field of view
FSE   Fast spin-echo
MRI   Magnetic resonance imaging
RF   Radiofrequency
SNR   Signal-to-noise ratio

D.R. Singh, MBBS, DNB, MMed, FRCR (✉)
M.S.M. Chin, DCR • W.C.G. Peh, MD, FRCPE,
FRCPG, FRCR
Department of Diagnostic Radiology,
Khoo Teck Puat Hospital,
90 Yishun Central, Singapore 768828,
Republic of Singapore
e-mail: Rambachan.singh.dinesh@alexandrahealth.
com.sg; bluevodka99@yahoo.com;
Wilfred.peh@alexandrahealth.com.sg

H. Rumpel, PhD
Department of Diagnostic Radiology,
Singapore General Hospital, Outram Road,
Singapore 169608, Republic of Singapore
e-mail: Helmut.rumpel@sgh.com.sg

4.1 Introduction

Musculoskeletal imaging deals with pathologies of the bones, joints, and surrounding soft tissue structures. A number of imaging modalities are useful in evaluating musculoskeletal pathologies, including radiographs, ultrasound imaging, computed tomography (CT), and magnetic resonance imaging (MRI). All these modalities have a unique role in diagnosing various lesions, ranging from simple fractures to complex neoplasms. MRI is of special importance, as it involves non-ionizing radiation and has excellent soft tissue resolution. Although radiographs and CT are useful in diagnosing fractures and bone destruction, MRI is far superior for detecting lesions involving the bone marrow and in assessing adjacent soft tissue involvement. Newer high-field-strength machines have improved the image quality and have broadened the scope of imaging. Imaging is no longer limited to evaluating the

© Springer International Publishing AG 2017
W.C.G. Peh (ed.), *Pitfalls in Musculoskeletal Radiology*, DOI 10.1007/978-3-319-53496-1_4

anatomical details, and functional assessment is possible for many structures. Continuous enhancements in scanning techniques have taken MRI to a new level, making it possible to identify subtle pathologies with shorter scanning times.

MRI is, however, inherently prone to a number of artifacts; some arise from motion, while others are related to technical or external factors (Jiachen and Rao 2006). A number of these artifacts are more pronounced on high-field-strength magnets and can result in suboptimal image quality (Bernstein et al. 2006; Dietrich et al. 2008). Susceptibility artifacts have gained importance with increasing role of MRI in postoperative patients, especially after joint replacement procedures or surgical implants. Some of the artifacts can be limited by simple corrective measures, while others can be significantly reduced using various modifications to the scanning technique. Awareness of these artifacts is essential to avoid possible interpretation pitfalls. There are several other challenges to MRI on new high-field-strength machines. The advent of 3-tesla machines has greatly improved the image resolution and has reduced the scanning times. However, a number of challenges have to be overcome to allow optimal utilization of these machines. Some of these challenges include fat suppression and chemical shift artifacts (Shapiro et al. 2012).

4.2　MRI Artifacts

MRI artifacts can be broadly classified into a few subgroups. Some of the artifacts can be related to motion, which may be due to movement of the patient or even due to periodic motion. Pulsation of the cerebrospinal fluid (CSF), beating of the heart, respiration, and pulsation of the blood vessels are some causes of periodic motion artifacts. Other artifacts can be due to physical or technical factors or may be related to the machine or the scanning technique. External factors like radiofrequency (RF) interference can also cause very characteristic artifacts and can be easily reduced in most cases.

4.2.1　Motion

Motion artifacts are routinely encountered on musculoskeletal imaging. These artifacts are usually related to movement of the patient during the scan and can cause significant degradation of the quality of the MR image (Fig. 4.1). Motion artifacts can be easily recognized, and reduction measures can be applied, depending on the cause. MRI requires an absolutely stationary patient, in order to obtain the best image quality. This may, however, be difficult to achieve, as it is virtually impossible for even the most cooperative of patients to lie absolutely still for the duration of

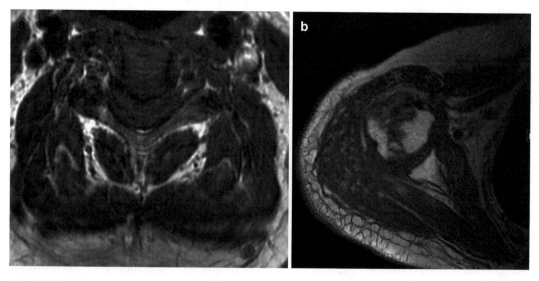

Fig. 4.1 Motion artifact. Axial T1-W MR images of the (**a**) cervical spine and (**b**) shoulder show motion artifacts resulting in poor image quality

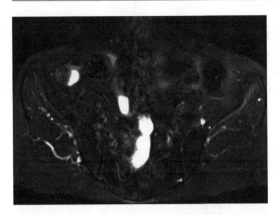

Fig. 4.2 Motion artifact arising from the bowel

the MR scan. Besides the motion related to the patient, there are many other sources of motion artifacts (Smith and Nayak 2010). These may arise from regular motion of structures, such as movement of the lungs during respiration, contraction of the heart, peristalsis of the bowel (Fig. 4.2), or even pulsation of the blood vessels. While it may be possible to restrict patient motion, it is impossible to prevent these above-mentioned causes of motion artifacts. Specific correction methods have to be applied to restrict the effect of these artifacts during the scan.

Motion artifacts are resultant of the phase-encoding gradient being unable to predictably encode the radio waves arising from the moving body structures (Peh and Chan 2001). Motion artifacts depend on factors such as speed of the moving structure and the manner in which the structure is moving. These artifacts become more prominent with increasing magnetic field strengths and are more severe on the newer MRI machines. The corrective measures depend on the cause of the motion artifact, as these can be related to voluntary or involuntary motion. Smearing and ghosting are the most typical artifacts arising from patient motion (Morelli et al. 2011). Artifacts arising from patient motion can be reduced by simple measures like restricting or limiting movement of the patient and with proper counseling before the scan. In pediatric patients, soft pads can be placed between the patient and the inner margin of the coil. Use of Velcro straps can also help in restricting the motion of the imaged body part in an uncooperative patient. In cases where the scan duration is long, simple

measures like reassuring the patient and giving the patient adequate breaks can go a long way in limiting random motion artifacts. Sedation techniques are routinely used in scanning of pediatric cases and can also be used in adult patients.

The use of PROPELLER (periodically rotated overlapping parallel lines with enhanced reconstruction) and Turboprop-MRI can help reduce these motion artifacts as well. The motion correction technique is better because retrospective motion correction can be used in addition (Tamhane and Arfanakis 2009). PROPELLER MRI technique may sometimes result in under-sampling artifacts with uneven blurring in the reconstructed image. This can be overcome by over-sampling and iterative reconstruction (Tamhane et al. 2012).

Periodic motion artifacts can result from cardiac contraction, respiratory motion, vascular pulsation, or peristalsis of the bowel. These artifacts from repetitive motion give rise to ghost images along the phase-encoding direction. The degree of brightness of these ghost images depend on factors like the speed and the amplitude of the periodic motion causing these artifacts. Many techniques have been devised to limit the effect of these artifacts, such as the use of cardiac or respiratory gating, navigator pulse, and faster MR sequences. The use of saturation bands reduces the artifacts from respiratory motion, vascular and esophageal peristalsis (Fig. 4.3). In sagittal cervical spine MRI, a saturation pulse can be applied parallel to the spine anteriorly, and this can reduce these artifacts.

CSF can cause pulsation artifacts and is typically encountered in MRI of the spine. These artifacts are more prominent as the CSF space gets bigger and are often visualized in MRI of the thoracic spine. These artifacts can easily be misinterpreted as lesions involving the spinal canal. CSF pulsation artifacts result in formation of ghost images, seen along the phase-encoding direction, and are visualized as hypointense signal areas on T2-weighted images (Singh et al. 2014). These T2-hypointense signal foci can easily mimic a flow void arising from a vascular malformation. The use of gradient-echo sequences results in reduction of these artifacts and can be used as a problem-solving tool in difficult cases (Fig. 4.4).

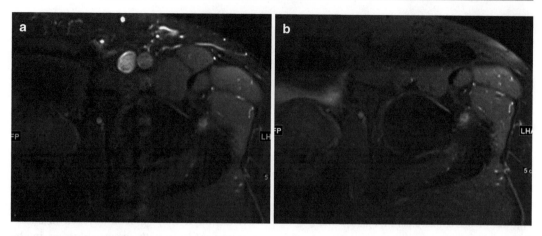

Fig. 4.3 Arterial pulsation artifact. Axial contrast-enhanced fat-suppressed T1-W MR images of the hip show (**a**) pulsation artifact from the left femoral artery, which is (**b**) reduced by using a saturation band over the vessel

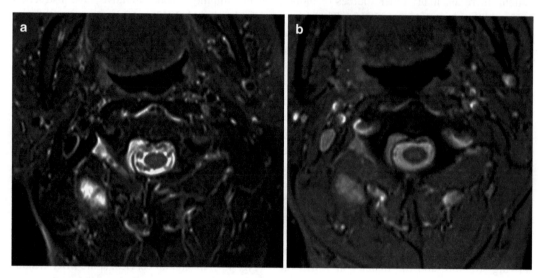

Fig. 4.4 CSF pulsation artifact. (**a**) Axial fat-suppressed T2-W MR image of the cervical spine shows CSF pulsation artifact. (**b**) The artifact is reduced on the gradient-echo image

CSF pulsation artifacts have also been found to be useful, and there is limited evidence to show that absence of these artifacts can be used as an indicator of cord compression.

Motion artifacts can also arise from flowing blood in the vascular structures and result in signal flow voids, typically seen on T2-weighted sequences. These artifacts can be useful in diagnosing vascular malformations of the spine or the soft tissue structures. The absence of these flow voids is a good indicator of an underlying vascular thrombosis. Motion artifacts arising from the blood vessels can be seen as ghost images in pulsatile flow or as high-signal areas on gradient-

echo sequences in continuous blood inflow (Peh and Chan 2001). These artifacts can be reduced by using flow compensation techniques and saturation bands or by switching the phase- and frequency-encoding directions (Singh et al. 2014). The application of additional gradient pulses minimizes the phase shifts from moving protons and rephases the signal from stationary protons. This is termed as gradient moment nulling (Morelli et al. 2011). This technique can be combined with the penalty of longer echo time (TE). The use of saturation pulse is another technique that can be used in reducing pulsation artifact. This technique uses an additional RF pulse, applied either parallel or perpendicular to the imaging plane. The most common use is in imaging of the spine, where a saturation pulse is applied anterior and parallel to the spine, to reduce pulsation-related motion artifacts. Similar to this, a saturation pulse can also be applied over a blood vessel, to reduce its pulsation artifact.

With advancement in technology, a number of newer MR scanning sequences have been devised, which have much shorter scan times without significant compromise in the image quality. MR scan time has also been significantly shortened with other advancements, such as the use of different image acquisition techniques, improvement in the coil technology (multichannel coils), higher-field-strength magnets, and improvement in the gradient strength (Morelli et al. 2011). Some of these newer image acquisition techniques include single-shot single-section imaging, multi-section imaging and parallel imaging (Singh et al. 2014). Spin-echo imaging technique is relatively insensitive to inhomogeneity in the magnetic field and has been most widely used. Fast spin-echo (FSE) techniques result in significant reduction in acquisition times; however, excessive echo train length may result in many artifacts and blurring of the image. Multi-section imaging also reduces the image acquisition time by simultaneous imaging of several interleaved sections (Morelli et al. 2011). This technique is however more susceptible to patient motion artifacts. This drawback is overcome by the use of single-shot single-section imaging techniques, which are more robust in relation to patient-motion artifacts. Techniques like HASTE (half-Fourier single-shot turbo spin echo) are excellent in reducing motion artifacts, as acquisition times are close to freezing motion. These are however more susceptible to other types of artifacts. The PROPELLER technique allows reduction of various motion artifacts encountered on MRI of the musculoskeletal system (Dietrich et al. 2011).

Fast gradient-echo sequences and steady-state sequences use shorter repetition time (TR) and result in reduced scan time. These sequences result in excellent signal-to-noise ratio (SNR) and better contrast in comparison to spoiled gradient-echo sequences (Chavhan et al. 2008).

Post-excitation refocused steady-state sequences are especially useful in evaluating menisci and the cartilage. Pre-excitation refocused steady-state sequences are useful in evaluation of the spine (Chavhan et al. 2008). Modified fully refocused steady-state sequences are useful in evaluation of the brachial plexus and the spine. The DESS (double-echo steady-state) sequence is useful in evaluation of the articular cartilage. Echo planar imaging (EPI) is a fast imaging technique that is capable of freezing motion to a large extent. It allows extremely fast image acquisition by acquiring all the spatial encoding information with a single RF excitation. Single-shot EPI acquires the entire range of phase-encoding steps in one TR. Segmented EPI in phase reduces the train length, while readout-segmented EPI reduces the inter-echo time. Any difference in susceptibility, as from local tissue to bone, leads to a magnetic field gradient and will result in substantial image distortions. Readout-segmented EPI is useful in evaluation of the vertebra and the spinal cord and can be helpful in differentiating benign from metastatic compression fractures (Rumpel et al. 2013).

Parallel imaging is a method for encoding the MR signal that allows reduction in the scan time, due to a reduced number of phase-encoding steps needed to form the image. This technique is especially useful in musculoskeletal MRI (Shapiro et al. 2012) and uses multichannel multicoil technology, where signal from different regions is received by different coils with known efficiency. Parallel imaging reduces the scanning time by reducing the number of phase-encoding steps, depending on a parallel imaging factor. Parallel imaging uses special image reconstruction algorithms, such as sensitivity encoding (SENSE), generalized autocalibrating partially parallel acquisition (GRAPPA), partially parallel imaging with localized sensitivity, and integrated parallel acquisition techniques (Singh et al. 2014). Although parallel imaging is useful in reducing scan time, there is reduction in the overall SNR with compromise in the image uniformity. Artifacts can be seen on parallel imaging, such as noise enhancement and residual aliasing (Deshmane et al. 2012). Noise enhancement makes the structures appear grainy, the severity of which varies across the image. Residual aliasing may arise due to inaccurate coil sensitivity map and can be seen if the patient moves after the initial planning scan. It can also be seen with errors in the GRAPPA weights. This can result in a bright ridge in the region of interest, especially seen when the edge of the object is bright (Deshmane et al. 2012). These artifacts can be reduced by optimization of the parallel imaging parameters and by choosing the appropriate reconstruction algorithm and the coil array.

4.2.2 Susceptibility and Artifacts Related to Orthopedic Hardware

MRI is susceptible to artifacts arising due to inhomogeneity of the magnetic field. This may be due to inhomogeneous distribution of the main magnetic field or may be due to external factors related to the patient, causing the field inhomogeneity. Magnetic susceptibility is described as the degree of magnetization of a structure or an object, when placed in an external magnetic field. When this occurs, a structure produces a magnetic field on its own, the degree and nature of which depend on its inherent properties. The magnetic field contribution may be in or opposite to the direction of the main magnetic field, depending on whether the structure is paramagnetic or diamagnetic. The degree of magnetic susceptibility is directly proportional to the strength of the external magnetic field (Dietrich et al. 2008). As a result, the magnetic susceptibility artifacts are stronger on higher-field-strength magnets. Different structures have different magnetic susceptibilities, and susceptibility artifacts typically arise at the interface of the structures, due to magnetic field inhomogeneity. This causes magnetic field distortion and results in spatial misregistration (Peh and Chan 2001).

There are various causes for susceptibility artifacts on MRI. The presence of dental prostheses can severely affect the image quality in imaging of the head and neck (Eggers et al. 2005). Susceptibility artifacts are commonly seen when imaging a joint with underlying metallic prosthesis (Hargreaves et al. 2011). They are also seen around metallic clips or fine metallic debris.

Susceptibility artifacts are known to be stronger with some metals. Titanium alloy implants are known to cause less severe susceptibility artifacts, compared to stainless steel implants (Lee et al. 2007). The severity of the magnetic susceptibility artifacts also depends on the type of sequences used for scanning. Gradient-echo sequences result in more severe metal susceptibility artifacts and in an exaggerated hypointense signal around the metallic object. This phenomenon is known as blooming and often results in a distorted image, with the soft tissues appearing smaller and the bone appearing disproportionately larger. These blooming artifacts can very easily be misinterpreted as an abnormality, thereby resulting in a misdiagnosis. Hypointense signal from the susceptibility artifacts arising from small metallic objects or debris in the spine can be misinterpreted as abnormal bone or thecal sac signal. In joint imaging, similar small foci can be misinterpreted as pseudolesions, especially the susceptibility artifacts caused by air bubbles on MR arthrography.

Susceptibility artifacts have become more important with the increasing use of MRI in the postoperative spine and in patients with metallic implants (Cha et al. 2011; Mansson et al. 2015) (Fig. 4.5). CT has a limited role in these cases, with limited assessment of the soft tissue structures and the bone marrow. The presence of metallic objects also causes beam hardening artifacts on CT, thereby causing further problems in accurate assessment (Lee et al. 2007). The severity of these artifacts depends on the field strength, and hence, these artifacts are more prominent on 3 T compared to 1 T or 1.5 T machines (Bernstein et al. 2006). There has been a progressive increase in the number of joint replacement procedures, mainly involving the hip and the knee joints. The use of metallic orthopedic hardware can result in artifacts on MRI that can be seen both in the primary imaging plane (in-plane artifacts) and in the adjacent planes (through-plane artifacts). The main artifact types are signal pileup or loss, insufficient inversion, and displacement artifacts (Sutter et al. 2012). The use of fat-suppression techniques in these cases can result in failure of fat and water suppression around, and even away, from the metallic hardware. Specific correction measures have to be

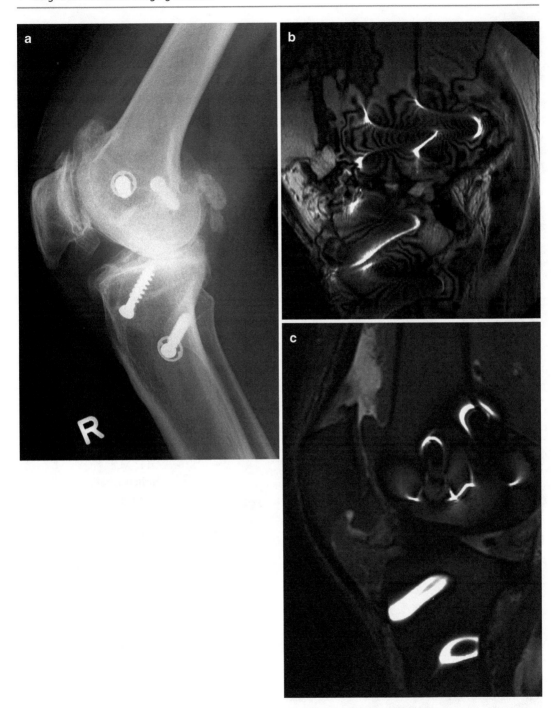

Fig. 4.5 Susceptibility artifacts. (**a**) Lateral radiograph of the knee shows reconstruction screws located in the distal femur and tibia. (**b**) Sagittal fat-suppressed PD-W MR image shows severely compromised image quality due to these screws. (**c**) There is marked improvement in the image quality on TIRM sagittal image

applied to reduce these artifacts and are discussed in the subsequent paragraphs.

One needs to first identify the source of the susceptibility artifact, before finding a way to reduce it. Sometimes, metallic objects may be located in the patient clothing and can be easily removed. In cases where the metallic object is located within the patient, e.g., postoperative spine with metal implants and joint replacement with metallic prosthesis, several other reduction strategies can be adopted (Christina et al. 2011). The use of gradient-echo sequences causes severe susceptibility artifacts and should be avoided in these situations. Spin-echo sequences cause less severe artifacts and can be preferentially used in these cases, especially FSE sequences with short echo times (Buckwalter et al. 2011) (Fig. 4.6). Other correction measures include using small field of view (FOV), increasing the receiver bandwidth, using high-resolution matrix and higher gradient strength (Lee et al. 2007). Aligning the frequency-encoding gradient along

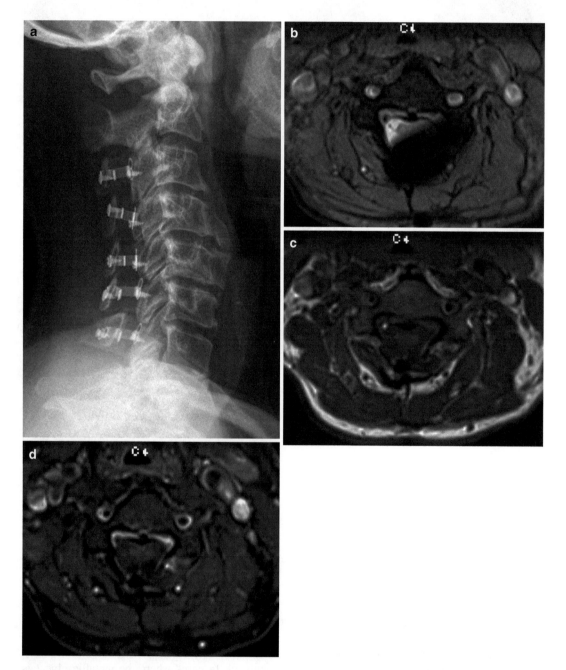

Fig. 4.6 Susceptibility artifacts. (**a**) Lateral radiograph of the cervical spine shows implants from posterior spinal fixation. (**b**) Axial gradient-echo MR image shows severe degradation of the image quality due to blooming. There is marked improvement in the image quality using (**c**) T1-W and (**d**) T2-W spin-echo sequences

the direction of the long axis of the pedicle screw can reduce susceptibility artifacts in patients with spinal instrumentation. The use of newer titanium alloy implants causes significantly less susceptibility artifacts (Rutherford et al. 2007). Metal susceptibility artifacts can also be reduced by the use of special dual-component implants which are made of a paramagnetic material and have a diamagnetic coating.

Special changes in MRI techniques have also been extremely useful in dealing with metal susceptibility artifacts, especially in cases of joint imaging after metallic implants (Fig. 4.7). Although view-angle tilting (VAT) technique can significantly

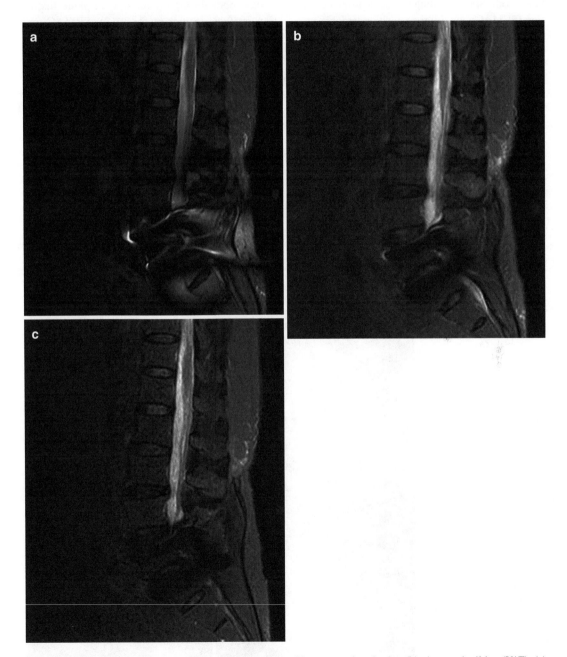

Fig. 4.7 Susceptibility artifacts. (**a**) Sagittal fat-suppressed T2-W MR image of the lumbar spine shows prominent susceptibility artifacts due to metal implants. These are reduced using (**b**) view-angle tilting (VAT). (**c**) There is however blurring and reduced SNR associated with VAT, as evident on increasing the bandwidth

reduce in-plane distortion artifacts, it does not correct the through-slice distortion. This technique adds a gradient of similar amplitude to the slice-select gradient on the slice-select axis during readout (Butts et al. 2005). The disadvantage of VAT is blurring of the image, which can be reduced by increasing the readout and reducing the excitation bandwidth. Slice encoding for metal artifact correction (SEMAC) and multi-acquisition variable-resonance image combination (MAVRIC) can be useful in imaging of patients with metallic joint implants (Koch et al. 2009; Lu et al. 2009; Lee et al. 2014). These techniques not only reduce the susceptibility artifacts but also improve the visualization of the metal-bone interface. This enables optimal evaluation, especially in cases with suspected infection. Images acquired using these techniques have been shown to be of similar quality as the conventional T1-weighted, T2-weighted, and proton density MR images (Singh et al. 2014). These techniques are superior to fast spin-echo sequences, in reduction of the susceptibility artifacts and also in measurements of the implant geometry.

MAVRIC limits the excitation bandwidth and uses several resonant frequency offset acquisi-tions, in order to cover the entire spectral range. SEMAC builds on the VAT and corrects the image distortion and metallic susceptibility artifact. It uses a 3D spin-echo acquisition with an additional slice-encoding gradient, in addition to a conventional fast spin-echo sequence (Lee et al. 2013). SEMAC in combination with VAT can reduce both through-plane and in-plane distortion artifacts (Sutter et al. 2012). SEMAC and MAVRIC have also been used in a combination technique, known as MAVRIC-SL (Choi et al. 2015). These techniques have been useful for through-plane artifact reduction, where the metal is in a plane adjacent to the image plane. Iterative decomposition of water and fat with echo asymmetry and least-squares estimation (IDEAL) is another imaging technique that has been useful in MRI in cases with metallic devices (Reeder et al. 2005; Cha et al. 2011). This technique reduces the rim of hyperintense signal around the metallic device and also achieves uniform fat suppression (Cha et al. 2011) (Fig. 4.8). The associated image distortion however shows limited improvement. IDEAL is a Dixon-based technique to separate fat-only and water-only images. This technique

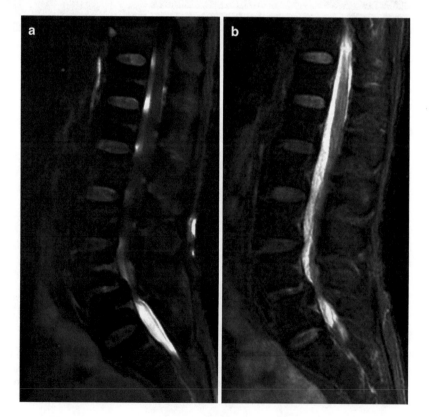

Fig. 4.8 Inhomogeneous fat suppression. (**a**) Sagittal fat-suppressed T2-W MR image of the lumbar spine shows inhomogeneous fat suppression, which is (**b**) reduced using the IDEAL technique

provides images with a high SNR and has been effectively used in T2-weighted and contrast-enhanced evaluation of the spine (Reeder et al. 2005; Shikhare et al. 2014). There is improved visualization of the spine and the adjacent structures, in addition to the reduction in metallic susceptibility artifacts and uniform fat suppression, around the metallic device.

4.2.3 Chemical Shift

Chemical shift phenomenon is also known as "misregistration" or "mismapping." Different tissues have different chemical compositions and therefore have different resonating frequencies. The resonating frequency increases with increase in the strength of the external magnetic field (Peh and Chan 2001). Chemical shift artifacts are therefore stronger on 3 T imaging, as compared to MRI on a 1.5 T magnet (Dietrich et al. 2008). This artifact is characteristically seen in the frequency-encoding direction and arises as the resonating frequency of fat is less than that of water. Chemical shift artifacts can be seen on all MR sequences and depend on the receiver bandwidth per pixel.

In MRI of the spine, chemical shift artifacts are seen as a hyperintense band on one side and as a hypointense band on the other side of a vertebral body (Fig. 4.9). The hyperintense band is typically seen at the overlapping interface of fat and water, while the hypointense band is seen at the region of the separating interface. These artifacts have been noted at several regions in spinal MRI. Chemical shift artifacts can be seen at the vertebral endplates, around the epidural fat and also around the ligamentum flavum (Fig. 4.10). These artifacts can also be seen around lipomatous and cystic lesions in the spine, such as lipoma or synovial cyst. Although chemical shift artifacts can result in loss of image quality due to superimposition of fat signal on surrounding structures, it has also been extremely useful in many ways.

Chemical shift artifacts have also been beneficial in abdominal imaging, for example, to characterize

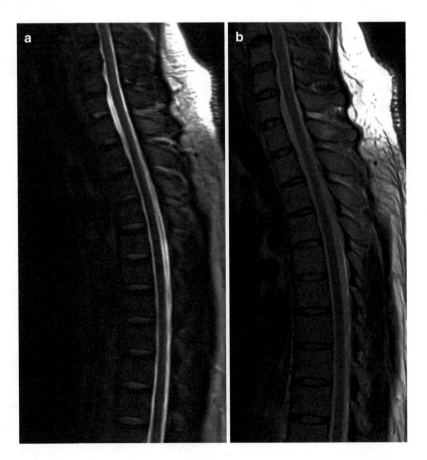

Fig. 4.9 Chemical shift artifact. (**a**) Sagittal T2-W MR image of the thoracic spine shows the chemical shift artifact as a dark band at the vertebral endplates, which (**b**) is reduced by increasing the bandwidth on the repeat MR image

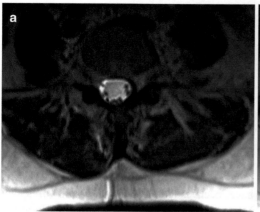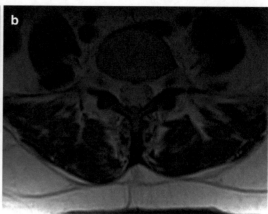

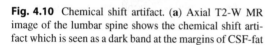

Fig. 4.10 Chemical shift artifact. (**a**) Axial T2-W MR image of the lumbar spine shows the chemical shift artifact which is seen as a dark band at the margins of CSF-fat separation and as a bright band at the margins of CSF-fat overlap. (**b**) The artifact is reduced by increasing the bandwidth on the repeat MR image

the adrenal nodules, to look for hepatic steatosis, and to identify presence of fat in lesions. These artifacts may, however, cause problems while interpreting the MR images of the spine and may need to be reduced. Chemical shift artifacts depend on the bandwidth and can be reduced by increasing the receiver bandwidth per pixel (Peh and Chan 2001). These artifacts can also be reduced by decreasing the gradient strength and are hence less prominent on lower-field-strength machines. They can also be reduced by switching the phase- and frequency-encoding directions and by using fat-suppressed sequences (Singh et al. 2014).

4.2.4 Magic Angle Phenomenon

Dipolar interaction between two nuclei has angular dependence. This is especially important for tissues with a dense molecular structure such as collagen. The term "$3\cos^2\theta-1$" modulates the dipolar interactions, where θ denotes angle of the structures with the static magnetic field (Bydder et al. 2007). The value of this equation becomes 0, when θ is approximately 54.7° (the magic angle). When the nuclei are oriented close to this magic angle, the dipolar interaction due to the static field is minimized, and the T2 value lengthens, resulting in a spurious signal on the MR image. Magic angle phenomenon is a unique artifact on MRI, seen on sequences using short echo time (TE), typically less than 36 ms. This artifact

can be seen on T1-weighted, gradient-echo, and proton density images. Magic angle artifacts occur in anisotropic structures, such as the tendons, ligaments, menisci, and hyaline cartilage (Singh et al. 2014). It can also be seen in intervertebral disks, fibrocartilage, and peripheral nerves. Magic angle phenomenon is not seen on sequences with a "critical" TE of more than 37 ms (Peh and Chan 1998).

The magic angle phenomenon involving the tendons, ligaments, or menisci produces an area of spurious hyperintense signal and hence may mimic pathology by simulating a tear, tendinopathy, or degeneration. Typical sites of this artifact include the supraspinatus tendon (Fig. 4.11), the triangular fibrocartilage complex of the wrist, the proximal posterior cruciate ligament, the infrapatellar tendon, and the Achilles tendon (Du et al. 2009) (Fig. 4.12). It can also be seen involving the peroneal tendons around the lateral malleolus (Mengiardi et al. 2006). This artifact can also cause simulation of a tear or degeneration of the articular cartilage of the knee (Disler et al. 2000; Xia 2000; Wang and Regatte 2015). Magic angle phenomenon can also cause pitfalls on MR neurography, a technique useful in the assessment of peripheral nerves and brachial plexus nerve roots (Chappell et al. 2004). Spurious hyperintense signal in the nerves can be misinterpreted as being due to an underlying disease (Kastel et al. 2011). A magic angle artifact can be reduced by using MR sequences with long TE, such as

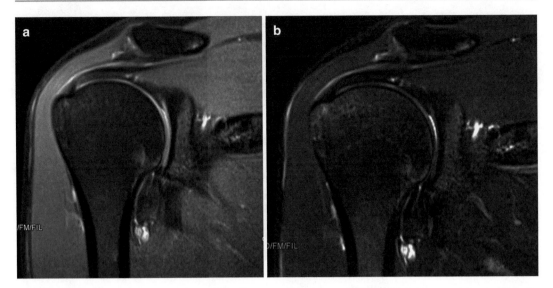

Fig. 4.11 Magic angle phenomenon. (**a**) Coronal fat-suppressed PD-W MR image of the shoulder shows an artifactual hyperintense signal in the supraspinatus tendon due to the magic angle phenomenon. TE was 33 ms. (**b**) There is reduction of the artifact on the repeat coronal MR image obtained with a TE of 76 ms

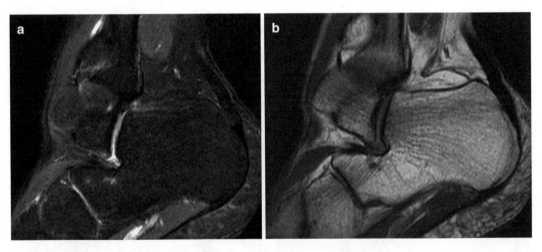

Fig. 4.12 Magic angle phenomenon. (**a**) Sagittal fat-suppressed PD-W MR image of the ankle shows spurious high signal in the Achilles tendon due to the magic angle phenomenon. TE was 33 ms. (**b**) There is reduction of the artifact on the repeat sagittal MR image obtained after increasing the TE to >36 ms

T2-weighted images. The signal abnormalities seen on sequences with short TE can be compared with corresponding T2-weighted images. Persistent signal abnormality is indicative of pathology, while correction of the signal abnormality suggests magic angle phenomenon. These artifacts can also be corrected by repositioning the patient, as this changes the orientation of the structures to the main magnetic field (Peh and Chan 2001). External rotation of the arm has been shown to reduce the magic angle artifact involving the supraspinatus tendon during MRI evaluation of the shoulder.

4.2.5 Protocol Errors

Protocol error artifacts include partial volume averaging, RF interference, saturation, shading, truncation, and wraparound and arise due to poor planning or improper parameter selection during the MR scan. Avoiding these artifacts needs proper training and knowledge of the technicalities of MRI.

4.2.5.1 Partial Volume Averaging

This artifact is dependent on the voxel size or slice thickness used during MR scanning. When the selected slice thickness or voxel size is similar to or lesser than the imaged structure, the resulting signal comes entirely from the imaged structure. However, when the slice thickness or voxel size is larger than the imaged structure, the final signal is a combination of the signal from all the structures, within the voxel. This can result in problems in assessment of small structures. One good example would be assessment of pathology in small structures such as menisci or glenoid labrum. If a larger voxel size or slice thickness is selected in imaging these structures, partial volume averaging artifact can easily mimic a radial meniscal tear or labral tear. It can also result in image distortion. These artifacts can be reduced by using thinner slices or by using a smaller FOV (Singh et al. 2014).

4.2.5.2 Radiofrequency Interference

RF interference is also known as "zipper artifact." The artifact can arise due to external electromagnetic waves leaking within the scan room. These waves can arise from various sources, such as fluorescent lights, radio stations, electronic devices, static discharge, or even hardware dysfunction (Peh and Chan 2001). RF interference artifact results in spurious bands of varying signal intensity and are seen in a direction perpendicular to the frequency-encoding direction (Peh and Chan 2001) (Fig. 4.13).

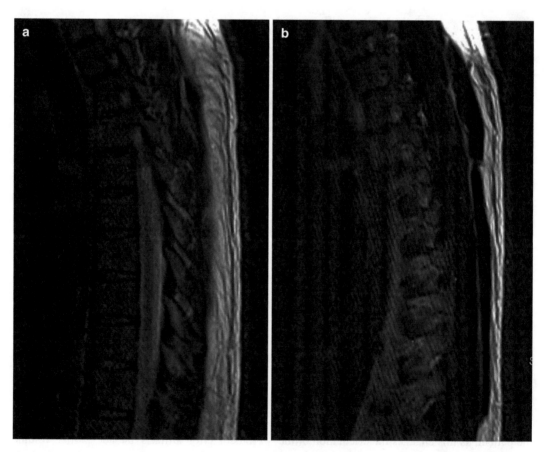

Fig. 4.13 Radiofrequency interference artifacts. (**a**, **b**) Sagittal T2-W MR images of the thoracic spine show RF interference artifacts as spurious bands of varying signal intensity

4.2.5.3 Saturation

Saturation artifact arises due to intersection of the imaging slices with different obliquities (Peh and Chan 2001). This is typically due to poor planning and results in repeated RF excitation of the tissues, in the region of overlap. Simultaneous RF excitation of the overlapping slice occurs during the excitation of the first slice and causes reduction in the signal. This is seen as a hypointense band on the MR image, typically on axial imaging of the lumbar spine (Fig. 4.14). Saturation artifacts can

also been seen in MRI of the knee and can be seen in the region of the menisci. Proper planning during the MR scan is essential to correct this artifact. The simplest way is to avoid intersecting slices. If this is difficult to avoid, one has to try placing the zone of intersection away from the point of interest. Gradient-echo imaging can also be useful in reducing these artifacts as the tissue magnetization is only flipped by a small angle on gradient-echo sequences, thereby allowing easy recovery (Singh et al. 2014).

4.2.5.4 Shading

Shading artifact is seen as nonuniform signal intensity across the MR image (Fig. 4.15). This can be due to nonuniform excitation of the protons, resulting in inhomogeneous signal intensity across the image. Another cause of shading artifact is improper placement of the coils, resulting in uneven coverage of the region of interest (Smith and Nayak 2010). The resultant image shows areas of hypointense signal, characteristically located progressively further away from the coil. Shading artifact can also arise due to improper coupling of the coils, leading to signal loss at the coupling point. Inhomogeneity of the RF field can also result in loss of signal, thereby causing this artifact. Shading artifacts are problematic, as they can result in signal loss, variable image contrast, and loss of brightness. The artifact is worse in regions further away from the coil, commonly seen with the use of surface coils.

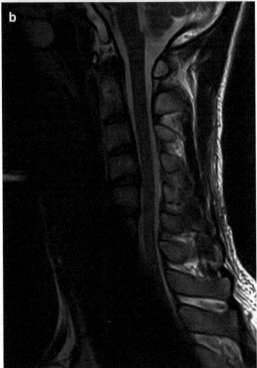

Fig. 4.14 Saturation artifact. (**a**) Axial T1-W MR image of the lumbar spine and (**b**) sagittal T2-W MR image of the cervical spine show the saturation artifact as a dark band partially obscuring the vertebral body

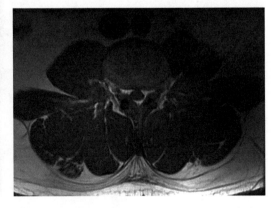

Fig. 4.15 Shading artifact. Axial T1-W MR image of the lumbar spine shows a gradual reduction in image brightness and contrast, toward the left side, due to the shading artifact

Reduction of shading artifact requires identification of its cause. In cases of improper coil placement or improper coupling, readjustment of the coils can eliminate this artifact. One needs to ensure that there is no direct contact between the patient and the coil. This can be achieved by placing water bags or foam pads separating the coil from the patient. In larger patients, the use of a larger surface coil or an enclosing coil can be useful. In cases where the artifact persists even on readjusting or checking the coil placement, changing the coil has to be considered. Surface coil intensity correction has also been found useful to limit these artifacts (Smith and Nayak 2010). Proper shimming techniques, such as active or passive shimming, can be useful to limit shading artifacts. These artifacts can also be limited by the use of RF pulses that are non-dependent on the field homogeneity.

4.2.5.5 Truncation

These artifacts are also called as "ringing" or "Gibbs phenomenon" and appear as parallel lines in region of a high-contrast interface. These artifacts can result in a false hyperintense signal involving the spinal cord, which can be misinterpreted as cord edema, syrinx, or myelomalacia (Fig. 4.16). To avoid the truncation artifacts, one needs to increase the matrix or decrease the FOV, if possible. Fat-suppression techniques can also be useful in reducing truncation artifacts.

4.2.5.6 Wraparound

Wraparound artifact is a protocol error artifact and is also known as aliasing artifact (Fig. 4.17). It is seen when the imaging FOV is smaller than the imaged body part (Peh and Chan 2001). The simplest way to correct this artifact is to increase

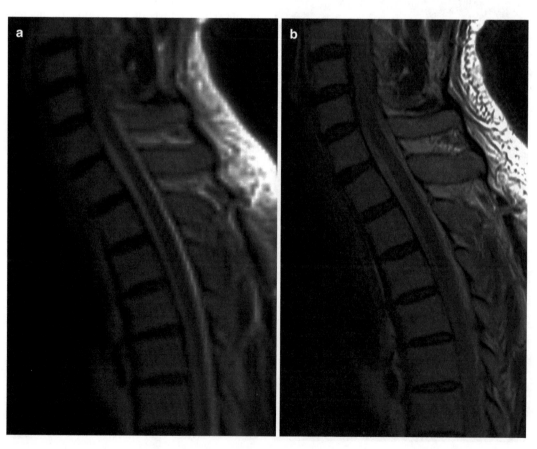

Fig. 4.16 Truncation artifact. (**a**) Sagittal T2-W MR image of the cervical spine shows linear hyperintense signal mimicking a syrinx in the spinal cord. (**b**) The trunca-tion artifact is reduced by increasing the matrix size on the repeat sagittal MR image

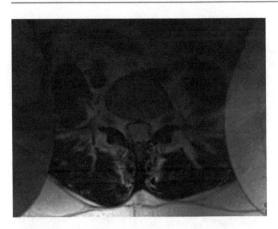

Fig. 4.17 Wraparound artifacts seen on axial T2-W MR image of the lumbar spine

the FOV. One can also switch the phase- and frequency-encoding gradients with the use of a rectangular matrix, if the geometry allows it. Saturation techniques can also be used to limit the wraparound artifacts arising from structures outside the desired FOV. These artifacts can also be overcome by the "no phase wrap" technique, without any increase in scan time or loss of spatial resolution. This may, however, result in reduced SNR. This "no phase wrap" technique doubles the FOV in the phase-encoding direction with doubling of the phase-encoding steps, thus maintaining the spatial resolution (Peh and Chan 2001).

4.3 Technical Pros and Cons

4.3.1 Fat-Suppression Techniques

The signal produced during MRI is mainly contributed by the hydrogen nuclei from water and fat. The signal from the fat molecules in adipose tissue needs to be suppressed in many situations, especially during musculoskeletal imaging. This needs good fat-suppression techniques, which also improve the image contrast. Water and fat have different resonant frequencies, and a fat-suppression module can be inserted at the beginning of an MR sequence in order to suppress the fat signal. A number of fat-suppression techniques are available, each with distinct pros and cons. Spectral fat suppression, STIR (short T1 inversion recovery), and DIXON are the main fat-suppression techniques. Spectral fat saturation is a frequency-dependent technique, and fat is suppressed by a frequency-selective saturation pulse, followed by spoiling gradients, to dephase the fat signal (the latter is not mandatory). The water signal is however not affected. The separation of water and fat is twice at 3 T compared to 1.5 T, but susceptibility artifacts partially "eat up" this advantage. The technique is susceptible to main magnetic field inhomogeneity and has a limited role in postoperative imaging in the presence of metallic implants. One advantage of this technique is that the SNR is preserved.

STIR is a relaxation-dependent technique and uses a value of the TI (inversion time) so that the fat signal is nulled. The resultant fat void image is inherently T1 weighted with inversion of the T1 contrast. This technique has a longer acquisition time and is sensitive to B1 (RF) inhomogeneity. The SNR is reduced using this technique. The advantage of this technique is that it is insensitive to the main magnetic field inhomogeneity. It can therefore be effectively used in cases with metallic implants (Fig. 4.18). It is also useful in low-field-strength and poorly shimmed magnets. DIXON is a phase-dependent technique and works on the fact that fat and water precess at different rates in the transverse plane, as they have different Larmor frequencies (Fig. 4.19). Two separate images can be acquired by adjusting the sequence timing, with water and fat protons in phase and opposed phase. Averaging the sum and the difference yields "pure water" and "pure fat" images.

4.3.2 Isotropic Imaging

Musculoskeletal MRI has conventionally been performed using two-dimensional (2D) multislice acquisitions, especially FSE sequences. Although these sequences provide excellent images for diagnosing meniscal, ligamentous, and cartilage abnormalities, there are a number of drawbacks related to this technique. The main disadvantage is anisotropic voxels with relatively thick slices, as

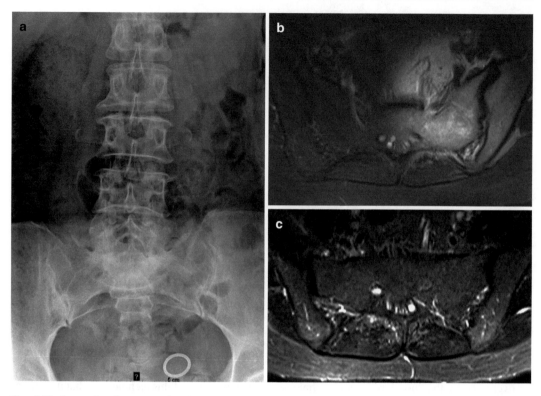

Fig. 4.18 Incomplete fat suppression due to a metallic object. (**a**) Frontal lumbar spine radiograph shows a contraceptive device projected over the pelvic cavity. (**b**) Axial fat-suppressed T2-W MR image of the pelvis shows incomplete fat suppression, resulting in artifactual signal abnormality involving the sacrum. (**c**) The artifact is reduced on repeat STIR imaging

compared to the in-plane resolution (Shapiro et al. 2012). This results in partial volume artifact. The images cannot be reformatted into different planes, and hence, separate image sets have to be acquired if visualization is needed in oblique planes. Volume calculations are also suboptimal using this method. These disadvantages are overcome with newer three-dimensional (3D) imaging techniques. Not only do these newer techniques allow multiplanar reconstructions, but they also allow accurate quantification of various important structures. The partial volume artifacts are also reduced, as thinner slices can be acquired. The overall scan time can also be reduced by reconstructing different planes from a single acquisition. 3D isotropic imaging provides thin contiguous slices, useful in MRI evaluation of the shoulder, wrist, knee, and ankle. The 3D technique also provides excellent fat suppression; however, the individual sequences have longer scan time.

Several 3D sequences are routinely used in musculoskeletal imaging. T1-weighted spoiled gradient-recalled echo (SPGR), dual-echo steady-state (DESS), steady-state free precession (SSFP), and FLASH are some of the 3D gradient-echo sequences that are especially useful in assessment of the articular cartilage (Naraghi and White 2012). These are however limited in patients with metallic implants, as these sequences are more prone to susceptibility artifacts. There is also an increase in the scan time. Magic angle phenomenon is a problem on SSFP sequences. Sampling perfection with application-optimized contrast with different flip angle evolutions (SPACE) and FSE cube acquisition are examples of 3D FSE sequences. One has to carefully plan the scanning protocols to incorporate the high-resolution 3D sequences, in addition to the 2D sequences. This will limit the overall time penalty with the added advantages that the 3D sequences offer over conventional 2D ones.

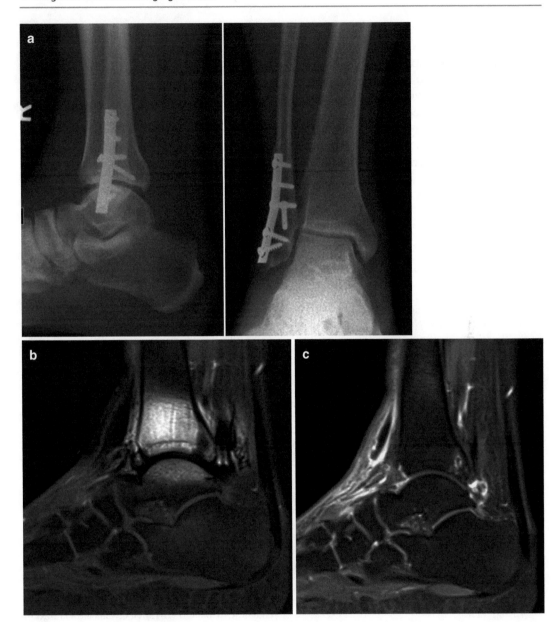

Fig. 4.19 Incomplete fat suppression due to metallic implants. (**a**) Frontal and lateral radiographs of the ankle show plating of the distal fibula. (**b**) Sagittal contrast-enhanced fat-suppressed T1-W MR image shows susceptibility artifacts from the distal fibular implants which have resulted in inhomogeneous fat suppression. (**c**) There is marked improvement in the image quality of the repeat sagittal MR image obtained using the DIXON technique of fat suppression

Conclusion

MRI is prone to a number of artifacts. Some arise due to poor scan planning, while others are related to the patient, the MRI machine, or a number of external factors. These artifacts not only affect the image quality but also can mimic pathology. Some of the artifacts can easily be mistaken for abnormal cord signal or even a meniscal or ligamentous injury. MRI artifacts related to metallic implants, especially in the joints and in the spine, can pose a significant challenge to the reporting radiologist. The radiologist needs to be aware of all these artifacts and the measures needed to correct them, in order to provide an accurate diagnosis. This chapter has described the various artifacts and discusses the individual correction measures. We have also discussed the technical pros and cons in choosing various fat-suppression techniques, in addition to the advantages and disadvantages of 2D versus 3D MR sequences, and related artifacts.

References

Bernstein MA, Huston J, Ward HA (2006) Imaging artifacts at 3.0T. J Magn Reson Imaging 24:735–746

Buckwalter KA, Lin C, Ford JM (2011) Managing postoperative artifacts on computed tomography and magnetic resonance imaging. Semin Musculoskelet Radiol 15:309–319

Butts K, Pauly JM, Gold GE (2005) Reduction of blurring in view angle tilting MRI. Magn Reson Med 53:418–424

Bydder M, Rahal A, Fullerton GD et al (2007) The magic angle effect: a source of artifact, determinant of image contrast, and technique for imaging. J Magn Reson Imaging 25:290–300

Cha JG, Jin W, Lee MH et al (2011) Reducing metallic artifacts in postoperative spinal imaging: usefulness of IDEAL contrast-enhanced T1- and T2-weighted MR imaging- phantom and clinical studies. Radiology 259:885–893

Chappell KE, Robson MD, Stonebridge-Foster A et al (2004) Magic angle effects in MR neurography. Am J Neuroradiol 25:431–440

Chavhan GB, Babyn PS, Jankharia BG et al (2008) Steady-state MR imaging sequences: physics, classification, and clinical applications. Radiographics 28:1147–1160

Choi SJ, Koch KM, Hargreaves BA et al (2015) Metal artifact reduction with MAVRIC SL at 3-T MRI in patients with hip arthroplasty. AJR Am J Roentgenol 204:140–147

Christina A, Chen BA, Chen W et al (2011) New MR imaging methods for metallic implants in the knee: artifact correction and clinical impact. J Magn Reson Imaging 33:1121–1127

Deshmane A, Gulani V, Griswold MA et al (2012) Parallel MR imaging. J Magn Reson Imaging 36:55–72

Dietrich O, Reiser MF, Schoenberg SO (2008) Artifacts in 3-tesla MRI: physical background and reduction strategies. Eur J Radiol 65:29–35

Dietrich TJ, Ulbrich EJ, Zanetti M et al (2011) PROPELLER technique to improve image quality of MRI of the shoulder. AJR Am J Roentgenol 197:93–100

Disler DG, Recht MP, McCauley TR (2000) MR imaging of the articular cartilage. Skeletal Radiol 29:367–377

Du J, Pak BC, Znamirowski R et al (2009) Magic angle effect in magnetic resonance imaging of the Achilles tendon and enthesis. Magn Reson Imaging 27:557–564

Eggers G, Rieker M, Kress B et al (2005) Artefacts in magnetic resonance imaging caused by dental material. MAGMA 18:103–111

Hargreaves BA, Worters PW, Pauly KB et al (2011) Metal-induced artifacts in MRI. AJR Am J Roentgenol 197:547–555

Jiachen Z, Rao PG (2006) MR artifacts, safety, and quality control. Radiographics 26:275–297

Kastel T, Heiland S, Baumer P et al (2011) Magic angle effect: a relevant artifact in MR neurography at 3T? Am J Neuroradiol 32:821–827

Koch KM, Lorbiecki JE, Hinks RS et al (2009) A multispectral three-dimensional acquisition technique for imaging near implants. Magn Reson Med 61:381–390

Lee MJ, Kim S, Lee SA et al (2007) Overcoming artifacts from metallic orthopedic implants at high-field-strength MR imaging and multi-detector CT. Radiographics 27:791–803

Lee YH, Lim D, Kim E et al (2013) Usefulness of slice encoding for metal artefact correction (SEMAC) for reducing metallic artifacts in 3-T MRI. Magn Reson Imaging 31:703–706

Lee YH, Lim D, Kim E et al (2014) Feasibility of fat-saturated T2-weighted magnetic resonance imaging with slice encoding for metal artefact correction (SEMAC) at 3T. Magn Reson Imaging 32:1001–1005

Lu W, Pauly KB, Gold GE et al (2009) SEMAC: slice encoding for metal artifact correction in MRI. Magn Reson Med 62:66–76

Mansson S, Muller GM, Wellman F et al (2015) Phantom-based qualitative and quantitative evaluation of artifacts in MR images of metallic hip prostheses. Phys Med 31:173–178

Mengiardi B, Pfirrmann CW, Schottle PB et al (2006) Magic angle effect in MR imaging of ankle tendons: influence of foot positioning on prevalence and site in asymptomatic patients and cadaveric tendons. Eur Radiol 16:2197–2206

Morelli JN, Runge VM, Ai F et al (2011) An image-based approach to understanding the physics of MR artifacts. Radiographics 31:849–866

Naraghi A, White LM (2012) Three-dimensional MRI of the musculoskeletal system. AJR Am J Roentgenol 199:283–293

Peh WCG, Chan JHM (1998) The magic angle phenomenon in tendons: effect of varying the MR echo time. Br J Radiol 71:31–36

Peh WCG, Chan JHM (2001) Artifacts in musculoskeletal magnetic resonance imaging: identification and correction. Skeletal Radiol 30:179–191

Reeder SB, Pineda AR, Wen Z et al (2005) Iterative decomposition of water and fat with echo asymmetry and least-squares estimation (IDEAL): application with fast spin-echo imaging. Magn Reson Med 54:636–644

Rumpel H, Chong Y, Porter DA et al (2013) Benign versus metastatic compression fractures: combined diffusion-weighted MRI and MR spectroscopy aids differentiation. Eur Radiol 23:541–550

Rutherford EE, Tarplett LJ, Davies EM (2007) Lumbar spine fusion and stabilization: hardware, techniques, and imaging appearances. Radiographics 27:1737–1749

Shapiro L, Harish M, Hargreaves B et al (2012) Advances in musculoskeletal MRI: technical considerations. J Magn Reson Imaging 36:775–787

Shikhare SN, Singh DR, Peh WCG (2014) Variants and pitfalls in MR imaging of the spine. Semin Musculoskelet Radiol 18:23–35

Singh DR, Chin MS, Peh WCG (2014) Artifacts in musculoskeletal MR imaging. Semin Musculoskelet Radiol 18:12–22

Smith TB, Nayak KS (2010) MRI artifacts and correction strategies. Imaging Med 2:445–457

Sutter R, Ulbrich EJ, Jellus V et al (2012) Reduction of metal artifacts in patients with total hip arthroplasty with slice-encoding metal artifact correction and view-angle tilting MR imaging. Radiology 265:204–214

Tamhane AA, Arfanakis K (2009) Motion correction in periodically-rotated overlapping parallel lines with enhanced reconstruction (PROPELLER) and turboprop MRI. Magn Reson Med 62:174–182

Tamhane AA, Arfanakis K, Anastasio M et al (2012) Rapid PROPELLER-MRI: a combination of iterative reconstruction and under-sampling. J Magn Reson Imaging 36:1241–1247

Wang L, Regatte RR (2015) Investigation of regional influence of magic-angle effect on t2 in human articular cartilage with osteoarthritis at 3T. Acad Radiol 22:87–92

Xia Y (2000) Magic-angle effect in magnetic resonance imaging of articular cartilage: a review. Invest Radiol 35:602–621

Nuclear Medicine Imaging Artifacts

5

Anbalagan Kannivelu, Kelvin S.H. Loke,
Sean X.X. Yan, Hoi Yin Loi, and David C.E. Ng

Contents

5.1   **Introduction** 83

5.2   **Types of Artifacts** 84
5.2.1 Radiopharmaceutical Related 84
5.2.2 Instrumentation Related 85
5.2.3 Patient Related 88

5.3   **SPECT/CT-Specific Artifacts** 90
5.3.1 SPECT Causes 90
5.3.2 CT Causes 92

5.4   **PET/CT-Specific Artifacts** 93

5.5   **DXA-Specific Artifacts** 96

Conclusion 97

References 97

A. Kannivelu, MBBS, FRCR (✉)
Department of Diagnostic Radiology, Khoo Teck
Puat Hospital, 90 Yishun Central, Singapore 768828,
Republic of Singapore
e-mail: kannivelu.anbalagan@alexandrahealth.com.sg

K.S.H. Loke, MBBS, MRCP • S.X.X. Yan, MD, ABNM
D.C.E. Ng, MBBS, FRCPE
Department of Nuclear Medicine and PET, Singapore
General Hospital, Outram Road,
Singapore 169608, Republic of Singapore
e-mail: kelvin.loke.s.h@sgh.com.sg;
sean.yan.x.x@sgh.com.sg; david.ng.c.e@sgh.com.sg

H.Y. Loi, MMed, MRCP, FRCR
Department of Diagnostic Imaging, National
University Hospital, 5 Lower Kent Ridge Road,
Singapore 119074, Republic of Singapore
e-mail: loi_hoi_yin@nuhs.edu.sg

Abbreviations

BMD   Bone mineral densitometry
CT   Computed tomography
DXA   Dual-energy X-ray absorptiometry
PET   Positron-emission tomography
SPECT   Single-photon emission computed tomography

5.1   Introduction

Nuclear medicine imaging has progressed with evolution from early rectilinear scanners to complex hybrid imaging techniques and concurrent developments of new radiopharmaceuticals (Ng et al. 2015). Typically, nuclear medicine scanners capture gamma radiation emitted from nuclear processes of gamma emitters or annihilation reactions of positron emitters and *bremsstrahlung* radiation from interactions of beta particles. But there are several problems associated with the clinical use and imaging of traditional and advanced molecular imaging radiopharmaceuticals, and the most important among them are artifacts. Artifacts may potentially interfere with the interpretation of the imaging and can effectively lead to false-positive and negative diagnoses, which in turn jeopardizes the patient management.

© Springer International Publishing AG 2017
W.C.G. Peh (ed.), *Pitfalls in Musculoskeletal Radiology*, DOI 10.1007/978-3-319-53496-1_5

5.2   Types of Artifacts

An artifact can be defined as an abnormality seen in imaging that does not represent a true physiological or pathological process. Nuclear medicine imaging artifacts can be broadly divided into three main categories, namely, (1) radiopharmaceutical related, (2) instrumentation related, and (3) patient related (Agrawal et al. 2015). Recognition and reduction of these artifacts from all these sources are necessary for the proper performance and correct interpretation of nuclear medicine studies. Nuclear medicine physicians should also be aware of the normal variants and interpretation pitfalls in order to avoid misdiagnosis. We will discuss the artifacts in the above-mentioned broad divisions in general, followed by single-photon emission computed tomography (SPECT)/computed tomography (CT), positron-emission tomography (PET)/CT, and dual-energy X-ray absorptiometry (DXA) scan-related artifacts specifically.

5.2.1   Radiopharmaceutical Related

Multiple important factors affect the biodistribution of radiopharmaceuticals, which can be described in the following major categories: (1) preparation and formulation, (2) administration techniques and procedures, (3) pathophysiological and biochemical changes, (4) medical procedures, and (5) drug therapy and interaction (Hung et al. 1996; Vallabhajosula et al. 2010).

5.2.1.1 Preparation and Formulation
The quality of the radiopharmaceuticals can be affected by radionuclide impurity or radiochemical impurity. The most common examples of radionuclide impurities are molybdenum (Mo)-99 contamination of technetium (Tc)-99m radiopharmaceuticals and iodine (I)-125 and I-124 contamination of I-123-labeled radiopharmaceuticals. They lead to more unnecessary radiation exposure to patients and also affect the quality of the scans. Many sorts of radiochemical impurities can occur during radiolabeling or decomposition, due to unwanted chemical reactions. These

impurities should be within allowed limits during regular quality checks; otherwise, they result in altered distribution of the radiotracers. For example, during Tc-99m methylene diphosphonate (MDP) bone scan, excess free pertechnetate uptake is seen in the stomach, gastrointestinal tract, thyroid, and salivary glands. If excessive stannous ion (Sn^{++}) is present in the kit, Tc-99m colloid will get formed, and it is usually phagocytized by the cells of reticuloendothelial system located in the liver, spleen, and bone marrow (Holese et al. 1994). If the Tc-99m particle sizes are more than 10 µm, they are filtered at the level of pulmonary capillaries before reaching the systemic circulation. These impurities cause nontargeted accumulation of Tc-99m, producing artifacts and degrading the quality of the bone scan (Davis 1975).

5.2.1.2 Administration Techniques and Procedures
The most common defect related to radiopharmaceutical administration is inadvertent extravascular infiltration of the radiopharmaceuticals (Hung et al. 1996). This usually leads to loss of activity and inadequate availability of tracer for imaging purpose. They can obscure nearby bone lesions, especially if the injection is done in the larger central veins. Sometimes, subcutaneous extravasation courses through local lymph vessels and localizes in the regional lymph nodes, producing artifacts (Ongseng et al. 1995). If we withdraw blood into the syringe containing radiopharmaceuticals to check the patency of intravenous cannula, the radiopharmaceutical could then bind to the formed blood clots, and these can localize in the lungs, producing focal "hot spots" (Goldberg and Lieberman 1977). The administration of Tc-99m radiopharmaceuticals via heparinized catheters may produce artifacts, because Tc-99m can bind to heparin and the Tc-99m heparin complex may avidly localize in the kidneys (Hung et al. 1996).

5.2.1.3 Pathophysiological and Biochemical Changes
Artifacts may sometimes occur as a result of unanticipated or atypical pathophysiological and

biochemical mechanisms beyond the purpose of the original indication of the study. Tc-99m MDP localizes by cationic substitution for calcium ions in bone hydroxyapatite crystals, and this uptake depends on local blood flow, osteoblastic activity, and extraction efficiency (Vallabhajosula et al. 2010). Increased muscle uptake and poor contrast due to renal failure degrade the image quality significantly. In advanced cases of renal failure, hypercalcemia can produce metabolic super scan due to altered biodistribution, producing intense skull uptake which can mask lesions (Loutfi et al. 2003; Gnanasegaran et al. 2009).

5.2.1.4 Medical Procedures

The biodistribution of radiopharmaceuticals can be affected significantly by various medical procedures such as radiotherapy, surgery, and hemodialysis (Lentle et al. 1979). In the early phase of radiation therapy, predominant inflammatory response and increased vascular permeability produce increased Tc-99m MDP activity during the bone scan. Tc-99m MDP activity is also increased in the soft tissue areas of radiation port (Morrison and Steuart 1995). After a few months, the radiation therapy leads to fibrosis; this results in significantly reduced bone tracer uptake which is often identified as a well-defined region of less tracer uptake confined to the field of radiotherapy (Vallabhajosula et al. 2010). Flare phenomenon, which is often seen immediately after chemotherapy, can make the known lesions more prominent, and follow-up bone scans are mandatory to differentiate it from progression (Tu et al. 2009). Recent surgery also increases the tracer uptake in tissues of surgical site, probably due to local edema. During hemodialysis and peritoneal dialysis, prolonged blood pool activity and increased clearance through the liver are observed due to background compromised renal function. Thus, the radiotracer can move from the bloodstream to dialysate, instead of localizing in the target organs, because of osmotic pressure gradients. Patients receiving subcutaneous injections of anticoagulant agents or insulin may show uptake of Tc-99m MDP at the injection sites. These artifacts may obscure the pelvis and lumbar spine on anterior planar imaging, and additional lateral

planar or SPECT imaging may be necessary to differentiate them from real bone lesions (Vallabhajosula et al. 2010).

5.2.1.5 Drug Therapy and Interaction

Drug and radiopharmaceutical interaction can occur due to the pharmacological action of the drug or physicochemical interaction between the drug and radiopharmaceutical. For Tc-99m MDP, these are the most common drug interactions: aluminum-containing drugs, increased hepatic and renal uptake; iron salts, high blood pool and renal activity; amphotericin and other nephrotoxic drugs, increased renal retention; and diphosphonates, reduced bone uptake (Sampson and Cox 1994). Even contamination with antiseptics during preparation or administration of the radiopharmaceuticals can lead to altered biodistribution.

5.2.2 Instrumentation Related

The gamma camera has evolved from a simple analog device of the past into a complex electronic device with an extensive digital supporting system at the present time. Artifacts resulting from an error are easily identified at the level of acquisition of raw data but become extremely difficult to recognize after post-processing, due to data manipulation. Hence, adequate quality control and standardized imaging protocols are mandatory to ensure reliable and reproducible clinical results. Artifacts originating from errors of gamma camera can be grouped under the following categories: (1) uniformity, (2) resolution and linearity, (3) multiple-window spatial registration, (4) collimators, (5) field of view, and (6) computer related (O'Connor 1996).

5.2.2.1 Uniformity

The most sensitive indicator of the performance of a gamma camera system is the measurement of uniformity. This can be affected by faults in the sodium iodide crystal, photomultiplier tube (PMT), and electromechanical circuit (Graham 1984). The most serious cause of nonuniformity is a crack in the sodium iodide crystal, which can

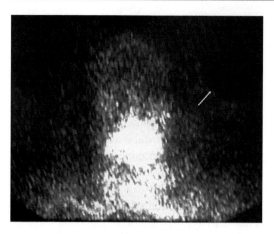

Fig. 5.1 The disk-like area of photopenic artifact (*arrow*) at the *upper right* hand corner was due to drift in the uniformity map

be caused by a sharp blow or a rapid temperature change. The crack in the crystal produces a corresponding cold defect with excess counts at the edge of the defect which is called "edge packing effect" (Fig. 5.1). Apart from the damage by mechanical or thermal stress due to its fragility, sodium crystals may also be damaged by hydration because of its hygroscopic nature. As a gamma camera ages, the hermetic seal of aluminum cover plate may fail and allow moisture to enter the sodium iodine crystal. This results in discoloration of the crystal and produces artifacts of multiple small discrete hot or cold areas affecting commonly the outer rim of field of view with relative sparing of the central portion (Pryma 2014).

The most common cause of the nonuniformity artifact is the malfunction of one or more PMTs in the detector head. Failure of single tube not only affects its field of view because of loss of signal but also causes miscalculation of the energy of an event occurring in the adjacent normal PMT. The artifact produced by PMT malfunction is usually seen as a well-defined round or hexagonal-shaped photopenic area in the field (Fig. 5.2). It is worthy to note that the defects produced by PMT malfunction differ at various energy levels (photo-peak setting) and can be missed if the defective PMT is located peripherally. Another less frequent cause of nonunifor-

mity is produced by a noisy PMT, which produces a confusing pattern of nonuniformity as a result of shift in the positioning of some events toward noisy PMT. It is more difficult to recognize a noisy PMT than a defective PMT, because the artifact of nonuniformity is usually located diametrically opposite to the noisy PMT (Oswald and O'Connor 1987). In addition to the crystal and PMT defects, a large number of electromechanical circuit problems can affect uniformity. These are usually identified easily because the defects produced by them are usually very large (O'Connor 1996).

5.2.2.2 Resolution and Linearity

The principal error affecting the image resolution is spatial distortion. However, many modern gamma cameras have the capability of linearity correction to ensure accurate positioning of the image data. To prevent these types of artifacts, there should be regular updating of linearity correction maps of the system. Occasionally, there is loss or degradation of spatial resolution in one direction only due to analog-to-digital converter problems. These are not usually recognized during the daily quality control and are evident only if resolution tests are performed (O'Connor 1996).

5.2.2.3 Multiple-Window Spatial Recognition

Improperly set pulse height analyzer peak results in degradation of the image and loss of resolution (Fig. 5.3). Artifacts due to multiple-window spatial recognition (MWSR) are not a problem in Tc-99m MDP bone scan but can occur in gallium (Ga)-67 and indium (In)-111 imaging for musculoskeletal infections. Ga-67 and In-117 produce gamma rays of different energy levels; the magnitude of the positioning signals generated by the pulse arithmetic circuitry increases with gamma ray energy. These signals are normalized to reference energy by using MWSR which is usually in the order of 1–3 mm. Larger values of MWSR result in poor co-registration of the images acquired at different energies and degradation of image resolution, especially in the central field of view. Generally, the modern

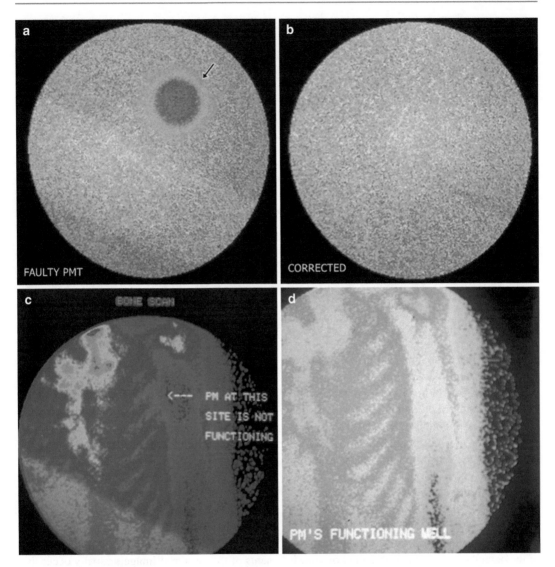

Fig. 5.2 Photomultiplier tube dysfunction created a photopenic artifact at its location on the (**a**) uniformity map and (**c**) bone scintiscan image. When the photomultiplier tube was repaired, the artifact was no longer seen on the (**b**) uniformity map and (**d**) bone scintiscan image

gamma cameras use energy and linear correction maps to improve the MWSR. But there can be errors in the correction map or inappropriate use of a correction map for a given energy level, leading to subtle errors in clinical studies, and these can be avoided by interval checking of MWSR (Kelly and O'Connor 1990).

5.2.2.4 Collimators

Defects of collimators can be mechanical or due to manufacturing. Mechanical defects can be small dents or extensive damage. The visible defects of the collimator correspond to photopenic areas in the extrinsic flood images, and these defects can be distinguished from crystal cracks by the absence of edge packing effect along the margins of cold defects in the flood image. Collimators are manufactured by cast collimation method (mold) or foil method (corrugated strips of lead). Mechanical stress or inadequate bonding may lead to separation of the lead foils; this results in a line of increased

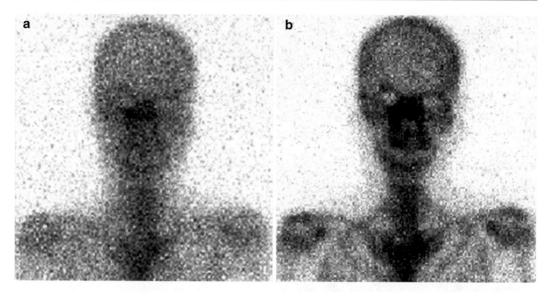

Fig. 5.3 Bone scintiscan image with pulse height analyzer wrongly set at (**a**) cobalt-57 window showed loss of resolution compared to the bone scintiscan image with pulse height analyzer correctly set at (**b**) Tc-99m window

activity on the flood images corresponding to the crack of collimator. Poor matting of collimator to the detector head and gaps between the collimator frame and collimator show hot spots at the edge of the field of view. All these artifacts related to collimator defects can be detected in the extrinsic uniformity image in the presence of a normal intrinsic uniformity image (O'Connor 1996).

5.2.2.5 Field of View

In modern gamma cameras, electronic masking of the outer 1–2 cm of the usable field of view is performed to avoid undesirable edge packing effect along the edges of the crystal. Two most common errors that can occur in electronic masking are over-correction of the edges, resulting in reduced active field of view, and misalignment of mask with actual field, resulting in visualization of a portion of the edge. This should be verified with a point source and a ruler and should be performed after any major servicing (O'Connor 1996). If two or more passes are used to do whole-body sweep scan, incorrect alignment between them results in "zipper" artifacts which are horizontal lines of increased or decreased

activity in the image. Similar banding artifacts can occur in continuous-mode acquisition with electronic timing errors or erratic motion of the gantry. This can be simply and rapidly checked by placing a sheet source on the gantry and acquiring a whole-body sweep image (Standards Publication No.NU 1-1994 1994).

5.2.2.6 Computer Related

With integration of computers into all aspects of nuclear medicine imaging, unexpected artifacts can occur resulting from failure of digital components of the system. Problems usually occur due to corruption of the energy, linearity and uniformity correction maps, or improper application, leading to poor display of digital image. These new-generation digital artifacts can be easily identified with their discrete pixelated appearance (O'Connor 1996).

5.2.3 Patient Related

In general, most of the patient-related artifacts are obvious, but some may be subtle and result in false-positive or false-negative interpretation.

Hence, it is essential for the nuclear medicine physician who is interpreting the scan to be aware of the patient's medical history, and where appropriate, perform a proper physical examination to clarify the abnormality seen on nuclear medicine imaging. Patient-related artifacts can be produced by (1) attenuation, (2) multiple radionuclides and study timing, (3) contamination, (4) patient motion, and (5) extraosseous uptake (Howarth et al. 1996).

5.2.3.1 Attenuation Artifacts

Non-anatomical structures produce artifacts by attenuating gamma photons that can be external or internal to the patient. Usually, before any nuclear medicine scan, patients will be routinely asked to change their clothing and remove any jewelry and coins. Even then, we come across unusual photon-deficient regions suspicious for external artifacts in our scans, and these should prompt us to examine the patients to exclude external items. However, not all external artifacts can be removed from patients before procedures, e.g., limb plaster casts and life-supporting instruments. The most common internal-attenuating structures which we come across in day-to-day nuclear medicine imaging include permanent cardiac pacemakers, ingested radiographic contrast material, prosthesis, orthopedic internal fixation, breast implants, and shunt reservoirs (O'Connor et al. 1991; Storey and Murray 2004).

Sometimes, the patient's anatomical structures can produce attenuation artifacts due to the location; for example, large breasts or malignant pleural effusion tracer uptake can mask subtle rib lesions, and tracer-filled urinary bladder can obscure the lesions of pubic bones in a Tc-99m MDP bone scan. These can be usually avoided by obtaining additional spot images in oblique projections and repeating the scans after catheterization. Occasionally, a 24-h delayed bone scintiscan would be helpful, as soft tissue tracer uptake washes out faster than bone uptake (O'Connor and Kelly 1990; Storey and Murray 2004).

5.2.3.2 Multiple Radionuclides and Study Timing

When multiple studies are to be performed on the same patient, we should be mindful of the physical and biological half-life of radionuclides (Fig. 5.4). For example, if we perform a Tc-99m MDP bone scan after I-131 whole-body scan, the downscatter and septal penetration of I-131 high-energy emissions into the 140 keV energy window of Tc-99m will corrupt the bone scan. Radiocontrast material, medications, and food may compete with radionuclides to bind with target organs, if an adequate time interval is not provided (Howarth et al. 1996).

5.2.3.3 Contamination

Contamination is one of the most commonly encountered causes for artifacts in nuclear medicine imaging. Tracer-mixed urine contamination in the pelvic and thigh region often produces difficulties in evaluating the pelvic bones and proximal femurs. Repeat imaging after removal of clothing and washing of skin, as well as obtaining different views such as lateral projections, is useful to show the superficial nature of the contamination activity (Gnanasegaran et al. 2009). Inadvertent intra-arterial injection of radionuclide will produce unexpected blood flow, blood pool, and delayed imaging findings on bone scintigraphy, resulting in "glove phenomenon" or "glove-like pattern" of radiotracer distribution (Shih et al. 2000).

5.2.3.4 Patient Motion and Positioning Artifacts

Both voluntary and involuntary movements degrade image quality and produce artifacts. Because of movement, overlapping of the moved part over the stationary part can produce false-positive results, or blurring due to constant movements may lead to false-negative results (Fig. 5.5). Patient movements can be identified by cine displays, ultrasound imaging, and summed planar images. We can use software algorithms for correcting patient motion, but the best way is to be aware of its possible occurrence,

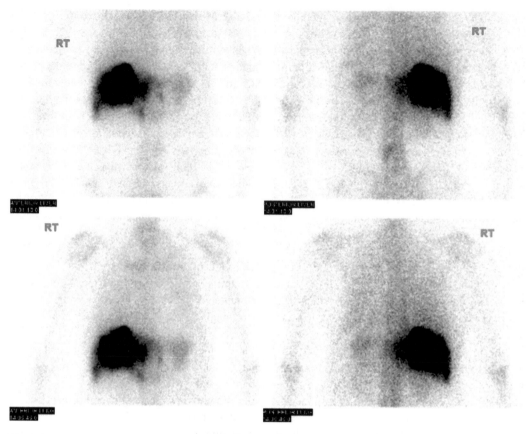

Fig. 5.4 Faint visualization of the bones was noted in the Tc-99m MAA study as part of Y-90 SIRT workup for hepatocellular carcinoma. Bone scintiscan was inadvertently performed a day prior to the MAA scan

minimize patient motion, and repeat the study, when and where necessary (Popilock et al. 2008; Gnanasegaran et al. 2009).

5.2.3.5 Extraosseous Uptake

In nuclear medicine imaging of the musculoskeletal system, we often see unexpected or expected tracer uptake in the non-skeletal tissues (Fig. 5.6). The mechanisms of uptake in soft tissues include (a) tissue necrosis or damage leading to increased calcium deposition, (b) hyperemia, (c) altered capillary permeability, (d) iron deposits, and (f) binding to denatured proteins (Peller et al. 1993). Increased tracer uptake in soft tissues during bone scintigraphy in a few common conditions is mentioned in Table 5.1 (Chew et al. 1981; Gordon et al. 1981; Koizumi et al. 1981; Sherkow et al. 1984; Silberstein et al. 1984; Padhy et al. 1990; Piccolo et al. 1995; Buchpiguel et al. 1996; Maloof et al. 1996; Gnanasegaran et al. 2009; Kannivelu et al. 2013).

5.3 SPECT/CT-Specific Artifacts

Tomographic systems are becoming more complex, with advancements in multi-detector systems, scatter and attenuation correction, and supportive computer system. SPECT/CT artifacts can occur due to errors in the SPECT component or CT component or both. We will discuss them individually, but in day-to-day practice, they are often cumulative and complicated (Gnanasegaran et al. 2009).

5.3.1 SPECT Causes

Artifacts that have minimal impact on the quality of planar studies can seriously compromise the quality of SPECT/CT (tomographic) studies, because the errors are magnified disproportionately in tomography. In addition to the gamma camera artifacts, there are additional artifacts specific to

Fig. 5.5 Motion
artifacts during
whole-body bone
scintiscan acquisition.
The soft tissue uptake
seen over the *left*
anterior chest wall is due
to known breast
carcinoma

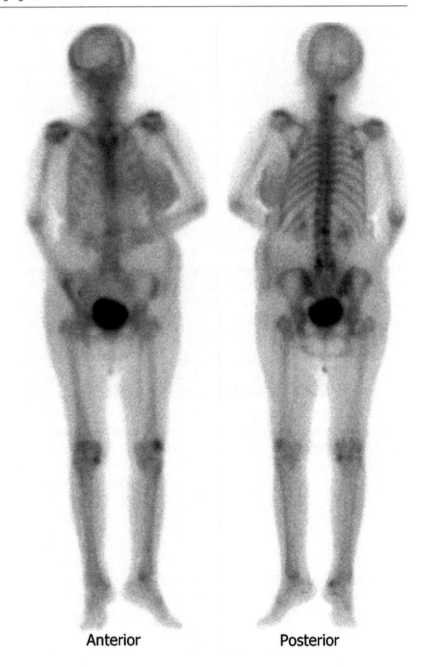

Anterior   Posterior

SPECT due to rotation and alignment, which will be discussed within the following subheadings: (1) Rotational: Uniformity and Center of Rotation and (2) Alignment: Collimator, Gantry, and Gamma Camera (O'Connor 1996).

5.3.1.1 Rotational: Uniformity and Center of Rotation

Photomultiplier tubes are very sensitive to heat and the earth's magnetic field. If there is a varia-

tion in heat distribution generated by the electronics within the head in different angles, the performance of the detector will be affected. Other possibilities of variation in relation to angle of rotation are inadequate magnetic shielding and poor optical coupling of PMT to the light guide or crystal. If the change in uniformity in rotation exceeds 2%, a redesign of the detector head is needed. Similarly, accurate center-of-rotation (COR) correction is very

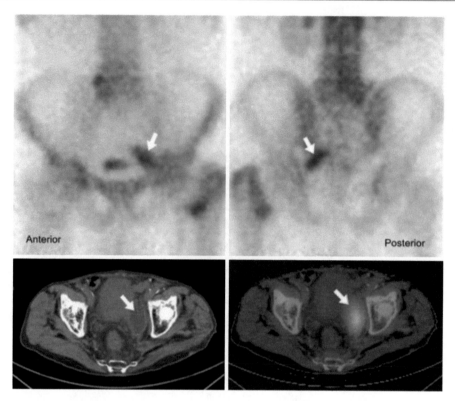

Fig. 5.6 Oval focus of increased tracer uptake projected in the *left* sacroiliac joint region (*arrow*, *top-row* images) is an artifact produced by tracer collection in the urinary bladder diverticulum (*arrow*, *bottom-row* images), which was confirmed on SPECT/CT (*bottom* images)

important for tomography, as even minor changes as little as 0.5% pixel in a 128 × 128 matrix can lead to degradation of image quality (Rogers et al. 1982; Cerqueira et al. 1988; O'Connor 1996).

5.3.1.2 Alignment: Collimator, Gantry, and Gamma Camera

Generally, parallel-hole collimators are used in SPECT, and the holes should be oriented perpendicular to the surface of the crystal. The variations in collimator hole angle can occur locally or globally, which in turn affects the COR. These errors of COR cannot be corrected by standard correction methods, and the only solution for this type of problem is replacement of the collimator. For a tomographic system, the gantry is usually set to 0°, and detector head is leveled before an acquisition. Misalignment of gantry can occur due to incorrect shimming of gantry,

irregularities in the surface of the floor, and sagging of detector arms. The artifacts produced by this misalignment produce variations of COR in the y-axis. Present-day modern systems often use multiple gamma cameras in an integrated scanner. Errors can occur in the alignment of a given detector to itself at different radial positions and the alignment between the different detectors, and resultant artifacts produce variations of COR in both x-axis and y-axis (Busemann-Sokole 1987; Malmin et al. 1990; O'Connor 1996).

5.3.2 CT Causes

The CT applied in SPECT/CT scans uses lower CT current (mAs) and thicker slices than conventional CT, so the chances of usual CT-related noise, beam-hardening artifacts, movement-

Table 5.1 Some common conditions of extra-osseous tracer uptake in bone scintigraphy

Breast	Gynecomastia, benign and malignant tumors
Brain	Cerebral infarct, meningioma
Heart	Myocardial infarct, ventricular aneurysm
Muscle	Trauma, electric burns, polymyositis, dermatomyositis, myositis ossificans
Kidneys	Acute tubular necrosis, glomerulonephritis, obstruction
Lungs	Radiation pneumonitis, bronchogenic carcinoma
Spleen	Sickle cell disease, lymphoma, leukemia
Liver	Metastases, hepatic necrosis
Pleura/peritoneum	Effusion/ascites
Arteries	Atherosclerotic or dystrophic calcifications
Tumors	Neuroblastoma, sarcoma

related artifacts, and partial-voluming artifacts are greater. The CT component of SPECT/CT is mainly used for anatomical localization and attenuation correction; hence, artifacts caused by the CT component in SPECT/CT scans can also be grouped into two broad categories: (1) misregistration artifacts and (2) attenuation errors (Gnanasegaran et al. 2009).

5.3.2.1 Misregistration Artifacts

Dedicated SPECT/CT systems should be able to accurately fuse the SPECT and CT images. But co-registration can be suboptimal, due to instrumental defects or patient movements. The common errors leading to misregistration are (1) change in the SPECT or CT CORs, (2) poor calibration of relative position of the SPECT and CT modalities isocenters, and (3) change in isocenter due to couch movement or sagging. The patient movements causing misregistration can be voluntary or involuntary. Voluntary movements can be accidental or deliberate; they can be minimized by good patient preparation, keeping the patient comfortable and well supported, and keeping the scan time as short as possible. Involuntary movements include respiration, cardiac activity, bowel

movement, and change in size and position of the urinary bladder. Among these, respiration is the most problematic, as the CT component is performed in a single breath-hold in less than a minute and the SPECT component is performed for approximately 20 min with regular breathing. This results in a lot of overlapping of supra- and infradiaphragmatic structures, resulting in unavoidable misregistration (Popilock et al. 2008; Gnanasegaran et al. 2009).

5.3.2.2 Attenuation Errors

High-attenuating materials cause reconstruction problems in CT, with low photon count areas of projections resulting in higher noise, major streaking, and inaccurate calculation of attenuation coefficient. Despite corrections applied for the CT artifacts, SPECT image data can still be corrupted because of error in attenuation coefficient values. Therefore, overall error in attenuation-corrected SPECT/CT is a combination of errors in the CT and SPECT data. Similarly, if the patients keep their arms in the scanned field of view, streaking artifacts of the arms may be seen in the reconstructed field of view, causing truncation artifacts (Howarth et al. 1996; Gnanasegaran et al. 2009).

5.4 PET/CT-Specific Artifacts

The integration of PET and CT allows excellent fusion of the acquired data of both modalities and increases the diagnostic accuracy up to 98% (Hany et al. 2002). CT-based attenuation correction is more rapid than the traditional transmission attenuation correction and reduces overall whole-body PET scanning time by 30–40%. The most common causes of artifacts seen on PET/CT images are metal implants, contrast material, respiratory motion, and truncation (Sureshbabu and Mawlawi 2005). Metallic implants such as dental fillings and skeletal prosthetics and intravenous and oral contrast material produce high CT Hounsfield numbers and streaking artifacts resulting in correspondingly high PET attenuation coefficients and leading to overestimation of PET activity in that region (Fig. 5.7). Evaluation

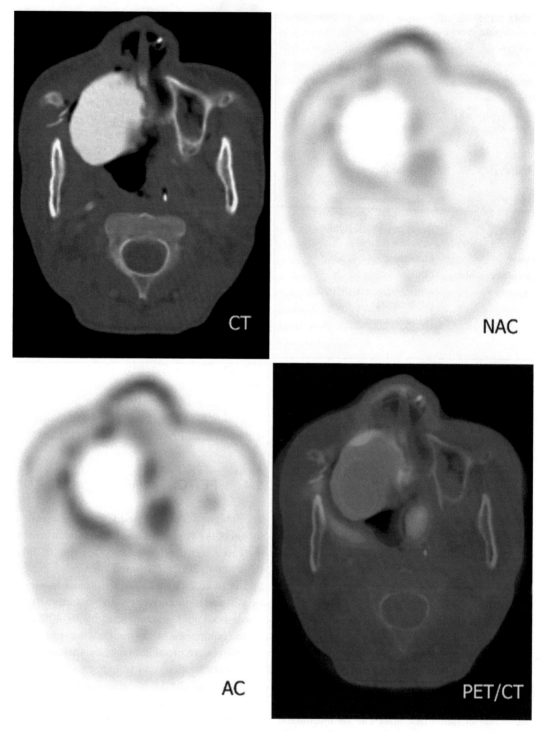

Fig. 5.7 Apparent increased PET tracer activity around the margin of palate metallic prosthesis was produced by attenuation correction artifact

of non-attenuated PET images will help in the interpretation of these high CT density material artifacts, in order to avoid false-positive PET diagnosis (Kamel et al. 2003). Not all metallic implants produce false-positive PET results. Heavy metal implants such as hip prosthetics can attenuate the PET 511 keV photons, resulting in photopenic emission region on PET images (Goerres et al. 2003). Therefore, it is a good practice for technologists to remove all metallic objects possible and document the location of nonremovable metallic objects, in order to identify such artifacts during interpretation.

Similar to SPECT/CT, respiratory motion causes the most prevalent artifact in PET/CT imaging, because the CT scan is acquired in a specific stage of breathing cycle and the PET scan is acquired during free breathing (Figs. 5.8 and 5.9). The most common type of breathing artifact is seen as curvilinear cold areas in the region of the diaphragm. Downward displacement of the diaphragm on CT acquired during inspiration causes underestimation of CT attenuation coefficient of the diaphragm in the normal location, resulting in underestimation of activity on PET image. This also results in misregistration artifacts causing confusion between lung and liver lesions and erroneous calculation of standardized uptake values of lung lesions due to inaccurate attenuation correction; therefore, it is essential to instruct patients about proper breath-hold techniques to minimize such artifacts (Osman et al. 2003). Truncation artifacts in PET/CT are due to the differences in the field-of-view sizes in the CT and PET tomographs. These artifacts frequently occur in large patients and scans performed with the arms-down position. When a part of the patient (arms) extends beyond the CT field of view, the extended part is truncated and not represented in the reconstructed CT image, which results in no attenuation correction values

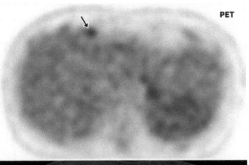

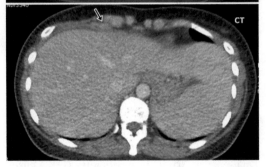

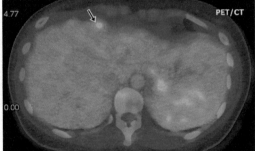

Fig. 5.8 Focus of increased PET tracer activity in liver segment 4a (pseudo-lesion is *arrowed* in *top-row* PET image) was due to misregistration of tracer localization in the nearby enlarged internal mammary lymph node (*arrow* in *bottom-row* CT image)

for the corresponding region and underestimation of standard uptake values. Truncation also produces streaking artifacts at the edges, causing overestimation of attenuation coefficient and creating a rim of high activity along the truncation edge, resulting in misinterpretation of the PET scan (Dizendorf et al. 2003).

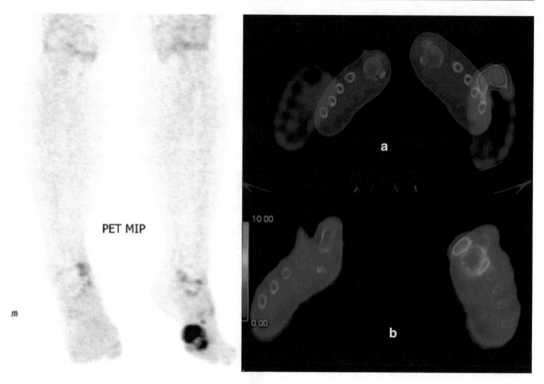

Fig. 5.9 Patient's movements between PET and CT scans produced (**a**) erroneous localization of increased tracer activity laterally. (**b**) Repeated scan after immobilization localized the tracer activity around the first metatarsophalangeal joint and aided the diagnosis of gouty arthritis

5.5 DXA-Specific Artifacts

Dual-energy X-ray absorptiometry (DXA) uses differential attenuation of photons of disparate energies to determine an areal (mass per unit) bone mineral density (BMD) (Blake and Fogelman 1997). Artifactual increase in BMD is possible due to focal increase or diffuse increase of bone sclerosis, leading to underestimation of osteoporosis. The most common sources of artifact are degenerative or osteoarthritic changes. Localized disease is relatively easy to detect. When multiple levels of the lumbar spine exhibit degenerative changes in a fairly homogeneous pattern, it may be difficult to appreciate (Masud et al. 1993). Other causes of focal increase in bone sclerosis are diffuse idiopathic skeletal hyperostosis, ankylosing spondylitis, sclerotic metastases, benign bone neoplasms such as osteoblastoma and exostosis, avascular necrosis, and Paget disease (Martineau et al. 2015).

Vertebral fractures also increase the BMD erroneously. This is not because of increase in calcium content present in the vertebrae but due to relative increase in concentration of bone mass resulting from loss of vertebral height (Ryan et al. 1992). The most common causes of diffuse increase in bone sclerosis are renal dystrophy and fluorosis. Occasionally, non-osseous causes such as heterotopic calcification of the hip, aortic calcifications, soft tissue calcification, and metallic objects within and outside of the patient can show falsely raised BMD values (Schneider 1998). In contrast, dense metallic implants overlying the lumbar spine can result in neighboring "black hole artifact" due to absorption of photons beyond unpredictable levels, which eventually decrease the measured BMD values of the affected vertebrae (Morgan et al. 2008).

Likewise, artifactual decrease of measured BMD levels can occur due to osteolytic bone lesions (especially multiple myeloma), spinal hemangiomas, aneurysmal bone cysts, and fibrous dysplasia. Postsurgical defects, such as laminectomy, and congenital abnormalities, such as spina bifida, lead to decrease in BMD values falsely due to loss of bone mass (Martineau et al. 2015). Another potential cause of pseudo-decrease in BMD is performing BMD scan immediately after other nuclear medicine imaging, because radionuclide photons that downscatter into the DXA windows decrease apparent attenuation, thereby resulting in falsely lowered BMD (Rosenthall 1992). Technical variations in positioning of the patient and assignment of the region of interest can also lead to erroneous BMD values (Jacobson et al. 2000). Interestingly, it has been noted that a rapid change in patient weight (more than 10%) possibly leads to artifactual variation of BMD (Siminoski et al. 2013).

Conclusion

Bone scintigraphy, SPECT/CT, and PET/CT are the most common investigations performed in nuclear medicine departments all over the world for identifying bone metastases and other musculoskeletal problems. Knowledge about the artifacts, pitfalls, and normal variants is necessary to increase the specificity of nuclear medicine imaging interpretation. With rapid evolution of imaging techniques and development of new radiotracers, it is imperative that nuclear medicine physicians should be aware of the artifacts, their sources, and methods to minimize them, in order to make a correct diagnosis.

References

Agrawal K, Marafi F, Gnanasegaran G et al (2015) Pitfalls and limitations of radionuclide planar and hybrid bone imaging. Semin Nucl Med 45:347–372

Blake GM, Fogelman I (1997) Technical principles of dual energy X-ray absorptiometry. Semin Nucl Med 27:210–228

Buchpiguel CA, Roizemblatt S, Pastor EH et al (1996) Cardiac and skeletal muscle scintigraphy in dermato- and polymyositis: clinical implications. Eur J Nucl Med 23:199–203

Busemann-Sokole E (1987) Measurement of collimator hole angulation and camera head tilt for slant and parallel hole collimators used in SPECT. J Nucl Med 28:1592–1598

Cerqueira MD, Matsuoka D, Ritchie JL, Harp GD (1988) The influence of collimators on SPECT center of rotation measurements: artifact generation and acceptance testing. J Nucl Med 29:1393–1397

Chew FS, Hudson TM, Enneking WF (1981) Radionuclide imaging of soft tissue neoplasms. Semin Nucl Med 11:266–276

Davis MA (1975) Particulate radiopharmaceuticals for pulmonary studies. In: Subramanian G, Rodes BA, Cooper JF (eds) Radiopharmaceuticals. Society of Nuclear Medicine, New York

Dizendorf E, Hany TF, Buck A et al (2003) Cause and magnitude of the error induced by oral CT contrast agent in CT-based attenuation correction of PET emission studies. J Nucl Med 44:732–738

Gnanasegaran G, Cook G, Adamson K, Fogelman I (2009) Patterns, variants, artifacts, and pitfalls in conventional radionuclide bone imaging and SPECT/CT. Semin Nucl Med 39:380–395

Goerres GW, Ziegler SI, Burger C et al (2003) Artifacts at PET and PET/CT caused by metallic hip prosthetic material. Radiology 226:577–584

Goldberg E, Lieberman C (1977) "Hot spots" in lung scans. J Nucl Med 18:499–500

Gordon L, Schabel SI, Holland RD, Cooper JF (1981) 99m Tc-methylene diphosphonate accumulation in ascitic fluid due to neoplasm. Radiology 139:699–702

Graham LS (1984) Quality assurance of anger cameras. In: Rao DV, Chandra R, Graham MC (eds) Physics of nuclear medicine – recent advances. American Institute of Physics, New York

Hany TF, Steinert HC, Goerres GW et al (2002) PET diagnostic accuracy: improvement with in-line PET-CT system: initial results. Radiology 225:575–581

Holese C, Kristensen K, Sampson CB (1994) Factors which affect the integrity of radiopharmaceuticals. In: Sampson CB (ed) Textbook of radiopharmacy, theory and practice, 2nd edn. Gordon and Breach Science Publishers, Amsterdam

Howarth DM, Forstrom LA, O'Connor K et al (1996) Patient-related pitfalls and artifacts in nuclear medicine imaging. Semin Nucl Med 26:295–307

Hung JC, Ponto JA, Hammes RJ (1996) Radiopharmaceutical-related pitfalls and artifacts. Semin Nucl Med 26:208–255

Jacobson JA, Jamadar DA, Hayes CW (2000) Dual X-ray absorptiometry: recognizing image artifacts and pathology. AJR Am J Roentgenol 174:1699–1705

Kamel EM, Burger C, Buck A et al (2003) Impact of metallic dental implants on CT-based attenuation correction in a combined PET/CT scanner. Eur Radiol 13:724–728

Kannivelu A, Padhy AK, Srinivasan S, Ali SZ (2013) Extraosseous uptake of technetium-99m methylene diphosphonate by an acute territorial cerebral infarct in a classical biodistribution pattern. Indian J Nucl Med 28:240–242

Kelly BJ, O'Connor MK (1990) Multiple window spatial registration: failure of the NEMA standard to adequately quantitate image misregistration with gallium-67. J Nucl Med Technol 19:92–95

Koizumi K, Tonami N, Hisada K (1981) Diffusely increased Tc-99m-MDP uptake in both kidneys. Clin Nucl Med 6:362–365

Lentle BC, Scott JR, Noujaim AA, Jackson FI (1979) Iatrogenic alterations in radionuclide biodistributions. Semin Nucl Med 9:131–143

Loutfi I, Collier BD, Mohammed AM (2003) Nonosseous abnormalities on bone scans. J Nucl Med Technol 31:149–153

Malmin RE, Stanley PC, Guth WR (1990) Collimator angulation error and its effect on SPECT. J Nucl Med 31:655–659

Maloof J, Hurst J, Gupta N (1996) Diffuse pulmonary uptake of Tc-99m MDP in sarcoidosis. Clin Nucl Med 21:77–79

Martineau P, Bazarjani S, Zuckier LS (2015) Artifacts and incidental findings encountered on dual-energy X-ray absorptiometry: atlas and analysis. Semin Nucl Med 45:458–469

Masud T, Langley S, Wiltshire P et al (1993) Effect of spinal osteophytosis on bone mineral density measurements in vertebral osteoporosis. BMJ 307:172–173

Morgan SL, Lopez-Ben R, Nunnally N et al (2008) Black hole artifacts-a new potential pitfall for DXA accuracy? J Clin Densitom 11:266–275

Morrison RT, Steuart RD (1995) Delayed massive soft tissue uptake of Tc-99m MDP after radiation therapy for cancer of the breast. Clin Nucl Med 20:770–771

Ng DCE, Lam WWC, Goh ASW (2015) Nuclear medicine imaging. In: Peh WCG (ed) Pitfalls in diagnostic radiology. Springer, Berlin/Heidelberg

O'Connor MK, Kelly BJ (1990) Evaluation of techniques for the elimination of "hot" bladder artifacts in SPECT of the pelvis. J Nucl Med 31:1872–1875

O'Connor MK, Brown ML, Hung JC, Hayostek RJ (1991) The art of bone scintigraphy--technical aspects. J Nucl Med 32:2332–2341

O'Connor MK (1996) Instrument- and computer-related problems and artifacts in nuclear medicine. Semin Nucl Med 26:256–277

Ongseng F, Goldfarb CR, Finestone H (1995) Axillary lymph node uptake of technetium-99m-MDP. J Nucl Med 36:1797–1799

Osman MM, Cohade C, Nakamoto Y, Wahl RL (2003) Respiratory motion artifacts on PET emission images obtained using CT attenuation correction on PET-CT. Eur J Nucl Med Mol Imaging 30:603–606

Oswald WM, O'Connor MK (1987) A noisy photomultiplier tube: its unusual effect on gamma camera image uniformity. J Nucl Med 15:157

Padhy AK, Gopinath PG, Amini AC (1990) Myocardial, pulmonary, diaphragmatic, gastric, splenic, and renal uptake of Tc-99m MDP in a patient with persistent, severe hypercalcemia. Clin Nucl Med 15:648–649

Peller PJ, Ho VB, Kransdorf MJ (1993) Extraosseous Tc-99m MDP uptake: a pathophysiologic approach. Radiographics 13:715–734

Piccolo S, Lastoria S, Mainolfi C et al (1995) Technetium-99m-methylene diphosphonate scintimammography to image primary breast cancer. J Nucl Med 36:718–724

Popilock R, Sandrasagaren K, Harris L, Kaser KA (2008) CT artifact recognition for the nuclear technologist. J Nucl Med Technol 36:79–81

Pryma DA (2014) Nuclear medicine: practical physics, artifacts, and pitfalls. Oxford University Press, New York

Rogers WL, Clinthorne NH, Harkness BA et al (1982) Field-flood requirements for emission computed tomography with an Anger camera. J Nucl Med 23:162–168

Rosenthall L (1992) Estimation of the effect of a preinjection of Tc-99m MDP on lumbar spine bone mineral density determinations. Clin Nucl Med 17:195–197

Ryan PJ, Evans P, Blake GM, Fogeman I (1992) The effect of vertebral collapse on spinal bone mineral density measurements in osteoporosis. Bone Miner 18:267–272

Sampson CB, Cox PH (1994) Effect of patient medication and other factors on the biodistribution of radiopharmaceuticals. In: Sampson CB (ed) Textbook of radiopharmacy, theory and practice, 2nd edn. Gordon and Breach Science Publishers, Amsterdam

Schneider DL (1998) Pitfalls in interpretation: calcium that's not bone. J Clin Densitom 1:405–406

Sherkow L, Ryo UY, Fabich D et al (1984) Visualization of the liver, gallbladder, and intestine on bone scintigraphy. Clin Nucl Med 9:440–443

Shih WJ, Wienrzbinski B, Ryo UY (2000) Abnormally increased uptake in the palm and the thumb as the result of a bone imaging agent injection into the radial artery. Clin Nucl Med 25:539–540

Silberstein EB, DeLong S, Cline J (1984) Tc-99m diphosphonate and sulfur colloid uptake by the spleen in sickle disease: interrelationship and clinical correlates: concise communication. J Nucl Med 25:1300–1303

Siminoski K, O'Keeffe M, Brown JP et al (2013) Canadian Association of Radiologists technical standards for bone mineral densitometry reporting. Can Assoc Radiol J 64:281–294

Standards Publication No.NU 1-1994 (1994) NEMA: performance measurements of scintillation cameras. National Electrical Manufactures Association, Washington, DC

Storey G, Murray IPC (2004) Bone scintigraphy: the procedure and interpretation. In: Ell PJ, Gambhir SS (eds) Nuclear medicine in clinical diagnosis and treatment, 3rd edn. Churchill-Livingstone, Philadelphia

Sureshbabu W, Mawlawi O (2005) PET/CT imaging artifacts. J Nucl Med Technol 33:156–161

Tu D-G, Yao W-J, Chang T-W et al (2009) Flare phenomenon in positron emission tomography in a case of breast cancer--a pitfall of positron emission tomography imaging interpretation. Clin Imaging 33:468–470

Vallabhajosula S, Killeen RP, Osborne JR (2010) Altered biodistribution of radiopharmaceuticals: role of radiochemical/pharmaceutical purity, physiological, and pharmacologic factors. Semin Nucl Med 40:220–241

Arthrographic Technique Pitfalls

6

Teck Yew Chin and Robert S.D. Campbell

Contents

6.1   **Introduction** 99

6.2   **General Considerations and Pitfalls** 99
6.2.1   Communication and Consent 100
6.2.2   Anticoagulation 100
6.2.3   Infection 100
6.2.4   Adverse Reactions and/or Allergies 101
6.2.5   Pre-procedural Scan 101

6.3   **General Concepts of Periprocedural
        Arthrographic Technique Pitfalls** 101
6.3.1   Patient Positioning 101
6.3.2   Joint Line Versus Articular Surface 101
6.3.3   Needle Selection and Bevel Positioning 101
6.3.4   Contrast Agent and Mixture 102
6.3.5   Inadvertent Air Instillation 104
6.3.6   Joint Fluid 105
6.3.7   Joint Distension and Manipulation 105
6.3.8   Logistical Issues 106
6.3.9   Ultrasound Imaging Guidance 106

6.4   **Joint-Specific Considerations and
        Pitfalls** 106
6.4.1   Shoulder 106
6.4.2   Elbow 110
6.4.3   Wrist 110
6.4.4   Hip 114
6.4.5   Knee 116
6.4.6   Ankle 118

T.Y. Chin, MBChB, MSc, FRCR (✉)
Department of Diagnostic Radiology, Khoo Teck
Puat Hospital, 90 Yishun Central, Singapore
768828, Republic of Singapore
e-mail: teck.chin82@gmail.com

R.S.D. Campbell, MBChB, DMRD, FRCR
Department of Radiology, Royal Liverpool Hospital,
Prescot Street, Liverpool L7 8XP, UK
e-mail: rsd.campbell@gmail.com

Conclusion 119
References 119

Abbreviations

CT   Computed tomography
Gd   Gadolinium
MRI   Magnetic resonance imaging

6.1   Introduction

Arthrography is the process of introducing contrast material into a joint to optimize visualization of the internal anatomy on cross-sectional imaging with magnetic resonance imaging (MRI) or computed tomography (CT). It is a common procedure performed in many hospitals with a musculoskeletal radiology section within the radiology department. In this chapter, we will discuss the technical and nontechnical pitfalls during the direct arthrographic procedure, with emphasis on the fluoroscopic approach.

6.2   General Considerations and Pitfalls

This section discusses the general pitfalls that pertain to all arthrographic procedures, regardless of joint location.

© Springer International Publishing AG 2017
W.C.G. Peh (ed.), *Pitfalls in Musculoskeletal Radiology*, DOI 10.1007/978-3-319-53496-1_6

6.2.1 Communication and Consent

It is vital that the patient understands the nature of the procedure, the indications for performing the procedure, and the potential risks and complications. Radiology departments should provide explanatory documentation, but it is always good practice to reiterate the key points during patient consultation. Consent may be verbal or written and is dependent on local hospital policy. Communication is key to maintaining good patient-doctor relationships.

6.2.2 Anticoagulation

Review of anticoagulant therapy, in particular warfarin, reduces complication rates of bleeding. A generally accepted standard threshold for joint arthrography in most institutions is an international normalized ratio (INR) of less than 2, although this could be potentially extended safely to an INR <3 for even large joints such as the knee (Conway et al. 2013). A good arthrographic technique is unlikely to result in significant hemarthrosis.

6.2.3 Infection

The risk of joint infection is small with an incidence of 0.003% for septic arthritis and cellulitis in a large retrospective cohort of 126,000 arthrographic procedures (Newberg et al. 1985). However, there have been case series demonstrating much higher incidence clusters of more than 0.6% (Vollman et al. 2013), possibly related to cross contamination from the fluoroscopic image intensifier or contaminated arthrographic trays. All arthrographic procedures should be performed with careful sterile technique to minimize the risk of infection. A sterile arthrographic tray should be prepared (Fig. 6.1). Confusion can be avoided between transparent solutions in syringes, either by labeling or following a standardized preference, e.g., 10 ml syringe for local anesthetic and 5 ml syringe for iodinated contrast agent.

It is also good practice to ensure a thorough wipe down of the fluoroscopic image intensifier and bed in-between patients, particularly in cases of potential splash contamination or in patients with a known infectious pathology. Direct arthrography should never be performed if the patient has

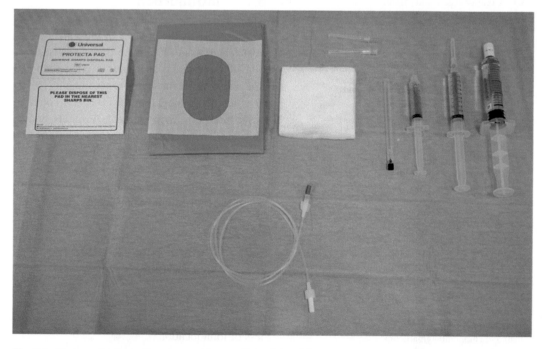

Fig. 6.1 Photograph of a sterile arthrographic tray. Maintaining tidiness and organization will minimize the pitfalls of joint infection and inadvertently injecting a wrong solution

soft tissue infection overlying the site of needle puncture or is known to have an active septic arthritis. Joint injection in patients with reflex sympathetic dystrophy can reactivate or aggravate symptoms (Hodler 2008).

6.2.4 Adverse Reactions and/or Allergies

Minor adverse reactions to the procedure are much more common than true contrast agent allergies, and this includes vasovagal episodes, nausea, and localized pain from a sterile chemical synovitis. True allergies which include laryngeal or angioedema, severe urticaria, and bronchospasm are rare and only applicable to iodinated intra-articular contrast agents. There is currently no documented evidence in the literature of a true allergic reaction to intra-articular gadolinium (Gd)-based contrast agents. There are also no cases of nephrogenic systemic fibrosis attributed to intra-articular Gd administration.

Obtaining a history of such reactions is useful in risk assessment and pre-procedural planning to minimize potential pitfalls and complications. In patients with a known allergic reaction to iodinated contrast agents, the procedure can be performed under fluoroscopic guidance relying on needle guidance alone. Alternatively, ultrasound (US) imaging is an alternative and safe approach to confirm intra-articular placement of the needle. Prophylactic pre-procedural oral steroid cover can also be implemented, depending on local policy. Patients with needle phobia are more likely to experience an exaggerated vasovagal response. They are also more likely to occur in young burly men (Newberg et al. 1985). Positioning the patient in a lying position is recommended, in case of loss of consciousness. Obscuring the arthrographic tray and the needle puncture site from the patient can help reduce anxiety and subsequent incidence of vasovagal reactions (Cerezal et al. 2005).

6.2.5 Pre-procedural Scan

Non-contrast imaging may be required in some CT arthrographic studies. Iodinated contrast material can obscure small calcified intra-articular bodies, and a pre-contrast scan can be helpful when this is a clinical concern. This is not an issue with MR arthrographic studies, although CT may be preferred because it is usually more sensitive for detection of small intra-articular bodies.

6.3 General Concepts of Periprocedural Arthrographic Technique Pitfalls

6.3.1 Patient Positioning

Proper patient positioning optimizes the success rate of the arthrographic procedure, irrespective of joint location. A position which maximizes the articular surfaces for access makes the procedure easier and more comfortable for the patient. Individual positioning for each joint is discussed later on in this chapter.

6.3.2 Joint Line Versus Articular Surface

Although the joint line may provide a landmark for direct needle access in some arthrographic procedures, anatomic restraints may require modification of technique. For example, in arthrography of the radiocarpal joint, the overhanging dorsal lip of the radius will prevent direct access into the joint, unless an oblique approach is utilized (Hodler 2008). In large joints with capacious joint recesses, such as the hip and shoulder, the articular surface can be targeted rather than the joint line. When the tip of the needle is in direct contact with articular cartilage, it must by definition be intra-articular.

6.3.3 Needle Selection and Bevel Positioning

Needle selection depends on the target joint and patient body habitus. Typically, small or superficial joints, such as the wrist, can be performed utilizing a short 23–25 gauge needle. Larger and

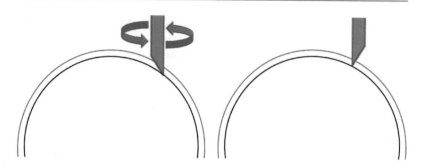

Fig. 6.2 Needle bevel within the articular cartilage. Diagram illustrates that rotating the bevel directs it out of the cartilage, allowing unhindered intra-articular contrast flow

deeper joints, such as the hip, can be assessed by a 20–22 gauge spinal needle, typically 7–12 cm in length. Longer needles are required in patients of large body habitus, and manipulating and directing the needle becomes technically more difficult. Gentle abutment of the needle against the articular surface is commonly employed to confirm intra-articular location. In such instances, resistance to contrast injection may be encountered as the needle tip lies within the hyaline cartilage. Rotating the needle can move the bevel out of the cartilage, whereby a "give" in the syringe pressure will be felt, and there will be unhindered flow into the joint (Fig. 6.2). Similarly, the needle can be withdrawn slightly to displace the bevel out of the cartilage. Needle withdrawal of more than 1–2 mm risks extra-articular positioning and contrast extravasation (Jacobson et al. 2003).

6.3.4   Contrast Agent and Mixture

In CT arthrography, iodinated contrast material should be diluted to 150–300mgI/ml (Winalski and Alparslan 2008). Lower concentrations may improve identification of small intra-articular bodies but will reduce delineation of articular cartilage. Double contrast with air and iodinated contrast material instillation has been historically advocated (Haynor and Schuman 1984) as a method to better delineate the capsulolabral complex. However, this has largely been abandoned as modern CT technology provides high-resolution multi-planar reconstructed images. Single contrast studies using air alone may occasionally be useful in patients with allergic or adverse reactions to contrast agents.

Proprietary Gd solutions are available for intra-articular usage. Although Gd-based contrast agents have not been licensed for intra-artic-

ular usage by the Food and Drug Administration (Peh and Cassar-Pullicino 1999; Steinbach et al. 2002), its excellent safety profile has led to a general and wide acceptance by radiologists for this off-label purpose. If proprietary intra-articular Gd preparations are not available, then it is possible to prepare a dilution of intravenous Gd contrast. The injectate should be diluted to ~2 mmol/L (Kalke et al. 2012; Rhee et al. 2012) using normal saline to achieve satisfactory contrast on T1-weighted sequences. If too concentrated, there is marked T1 and T2 shortening, resulting in low signal intensity of fluid and accompanying susceptibility artifact which will result in a nondiagnostic study (Grainger et al. 2000) (Fig. 6.3).

Iodine can be substituted for saline in the dilution for Gd, as this is useful for confirmation of intra-articular placement, as well as detecting pathology from the pattern of contrast flow during the fluoroscopic procedure. It is also useful for patients who require both CT and MRI, as both arthrographic studies may be acquired at the same attendance. However, iodine produces a greater decrease in signal across T1- and T2-weighted sequences, when compared with saline dilution (Montgomery et al. 2002) and therefore should only be implemented when necessary. A small amount of iodinated contrast agent in a separate syringe can be used to confirm intra-articular location of the needle prior to injection of the Gd preparation, or a small amount can be drawn up within the extension tube attached to the syringe. If there is anticipated delay from injection time to scanning time, epinephrine can be added to the solution to delay resorption of gadolinium, but this is rarely required.

Substitution of Gd-based agents with saline solution alone may be used for MR arthrography,

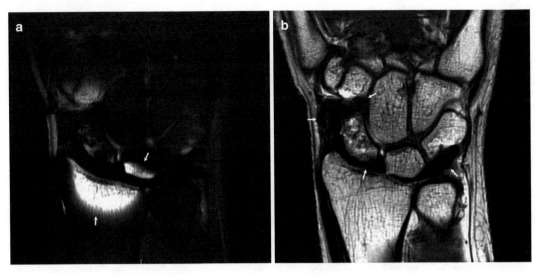

Fig. 6.3 Susceptibility artifact in the wrist from undiluted gadolinium injectate. Coronal (**a**) fat-suppressed T2-W and (**b**) T1-W MR arthrographic images show marked susceptibility artifact from excessive T1 and T2 shortening (*white arrows*) from the undiluted gadolinium preparation. As a result, soft tissue structures are obscured with fluid appearing hypointense, resulting in a nondiagnostic study

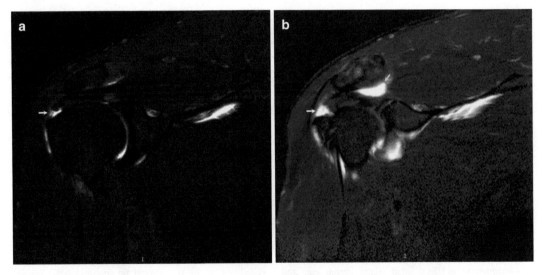

Fig. 6.4 Full-thickness tear of the supraspinatus tendon. (**a**, **b**) Coronal fat-suppressed T1-W MR arthrographic images clearly show the full-thickness defect of the tendon at the footprint (*white arrows*) with contrast agent communicating with the subacromial-subdeltoid bursa (*yellow arrow*)

particularly in patients with a history of previous allergic-like reaction to Gd. The technique of saline arthrography requires the use of T2-weighted sequences only. It can be difficult to distinguish periarticular fluid and native effusions from injected saline, which is not an issue with Gd contrast agents (Grainger et al. 2000). Abnormal communications into the extra-articular bursae are also more conspicuous with gadolinium-based agents which often isolate the underlying pathology (Fig. 6.4). Smaller abnormal communications may be missed on saline arthrograms. Both T1-weighted and fat-suppressed T2-weighted sequences should be obtained in at least one plane in all studies, to help distinguish pathologic fluid collections in or around the joint such as paralabral cysts (Fig. 6.5) or subacromial-subdeltoid bursitis (Fig. 6.6).

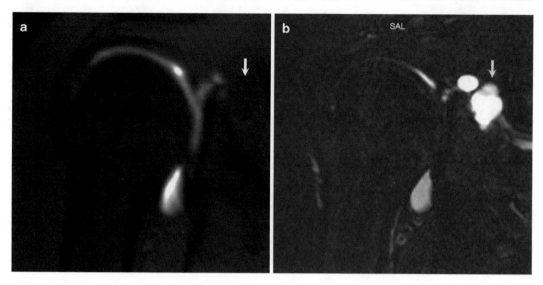

Fig. 6.5 Paralabral cysts. This is easy to miss on the (**a**) coronal fat-suppressed T1-W MR arthrographic image (*white arrow*) but are evident on the (**b**) coronal fat-suppressed T2-W MR arthrographic image (*yellow arrow*) (Courtesy of Dr. A. Grainger)

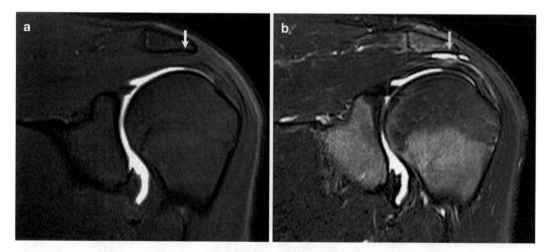

Fig. 6.6 Fluid in the subacromial-subdeltoid bursa accompanied with bursal-sided signal partial tear and fraying of the supraspinatus tendon. These findings are not appreciated on the (**a**) coronal fat-suppressed T1-W MR arthrographic image (*white arrow*) but are easily visualized on the (**b**) coronal fat-suppressed T2-W MR arthrographic image (*yellow arrow*) (Courtesy of Dr. A. Grainger)

6.3.5 Inadvertent Air Instillation

Gas bubble artifacts occur due to the unintentional introduction of air into the joint during the arthrographic procedure. This can mimic intra-articular bodies on both CT and MRI (Fig. 6.7) or create susceptibility artifacts on MRI that can obscure adjacent structures (Hodler 2008). Air bubbles tend to lie in the nondependent upper-most regions of the joint and can also create more pronounced blooming artifacts on certain MRI images, such as gradient-echo sequences. This pitfall can be minimized by employing a technique of filling the needle hub with contrast agent prior to connection to the extension tube. It is also helpful to ensure that all connecting tubes and syringes have been flushed out of any residual bubbles.

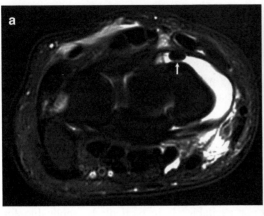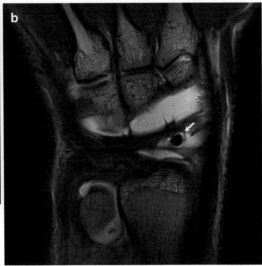

Fig. 6.7 Gas bubble artifact in the wrist. (**a**) Axial fat-suppressed T1-W and (**b**) coronal T1-W MR arthrographic images show a gas bubble in the dorsal dependent position of the radiocarpal joint capsule (*white arrows*)

6.3.6   Joint Fluid

Joint effusions should be aspirated before the administration of intra-articular contrast agent. This helps to preserve optimum joint opacification by preventing over-dilution of the contrast material and also avoids layering between contrast material and native joint fluid.

6.3.7   Joint Distension and Manipulation

Adequate joint distension is required to optimize visualization of intra-articular structures. The contrast agent improves diagnostic quality by filling all the normal joint recesses and outlining normal and abnormal structures. It can also help to identify abnormal communication between anatomical spaces (Morrison 2005). Joint recesses may not be distended if there is inadequate joint distension and may result in false-negative examinations. This is especially true for CT arthrography where the inherent soft tissue contrast is poor. For example, a lack of separation of opposing articular surfaces will obscure chondral defects. Conversely, overdistension can result in unintended capsular rupture with extravasation of contrast material, either obscuring or mimicking pathology.

Table 6.1 Volume capacities for arthrography of various joints

Joint	Volume
Shoulder	12–15 ml
Elbow	8–12 ml
Wrist	3–4 ml radiocarpal and midcarpal, 1–1.5 ml DRUJ
Hip	10–20 ml
Knee	30–50 ml
Ankle	6–10 ml

The optimal volume of injectate required is specific to each joint and varies enormously. The knee is able to accommodate up to 50 ml of injectate (Chung et al. 2005), while the distal radioulnar joint (DRUJ) typically requires only 1.5 ml (Table 6.1). These are general estimates, and other factors may determine the required volume of injectate. For example, adhesive capsulitis will significantly limit the volume of contrast agent that can be injected in a shoulder joint (Fig. 6.8), whereas a full-thickness rotator cuff tear will communicate with the subacromial bursa, and a much greater volume of contrast agent may need to be injected. Other examples include normal anatomical communications, such as that often exists between the ankle joint and subtalar joint which effectively increases the overall joint capacity. Some joints, particularly the wrist and

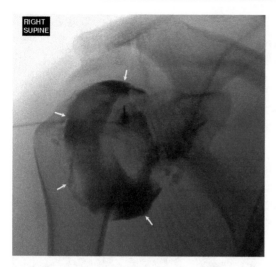

RIGHT
SUPINE

Fig. 6.8 Restrictive pattern of contrast agent flow in the shoulder joint. Fluoroscopic image taken after intra-articular contrast administration through the anterior rotator cuff interval approach shows an abnormal pattern of contrast agent flow with evidence of axillary synovitis and a tight capsule (*white arrows*). The patient was found to have a frozen shoulder

knee, may require post-procedural manipulation in order to distribute the contrast material throughout the joint capsule and to encourage the contrast material to pass through small areas of abnormal communication.

6.3.8   Logistical Issues

Imaging of the joint should take place soon after completion of the arthrogram procedure. Delays in imaging can result in suboptimal studies due to contrast resorption and imbibition, leading to decrease in signal-to-noise and joint distention. Different joints have different tolerances for imaging delay, with successful acquisitions of the knee obtained up to 3.5 h (Wagner et al. 2001), 1.5 h for the shoulder and hip, and 45 min for the wrist postinjection (Andreisek et al. 2007). As a general rule, imaging should ideally be performed relatively soon after the arthrogram. Communication with the CT/MRI sections of the radiology department will help anticipate any potential delays and which can be managed

accordingly. There are also financial implications. Direct arthrography is more expensive than indirect arthrography, requiring additional time, trained personnel, and procedural rooms. Clinical history will help to determine the most appropriate imaging technique.

6.3.9   Ultrasound Imaging Guidance

Ultrasound (US) is a useful alternative modality to guide needle placement when fluoroscopy is not available. It is particularly applicable for joints where the articular surface can be visualized, such as in the shoulder or hip. The tip of the needle can hence be guided onto the chondral surface. It is important to identify a technique where the needle can be kept as horizontal as possible to the probe face, to optimize visualization of the needle tip. Angulation beyond 45° to the probe face will result in very poor visualization of the needle and will increase the incidence of contrast agent extravasation. Joint-specific techniques for US guidance are beyond the scope of this text.

The contrast agent should not pool at the tip of the needle, and if this is identified, the needle should be repositioned. However, it may be difficult to visualize the contrast agent entering the joint, and extravasation may not be appreciated until after cross-sectional imaging has occurred. Furthermore, it may be difficult to estimate the required volume of injectate in patients with extra-compartmental communication into other joints, which can potentially result in a lack of joint distension.

6.4   Joint-Specific Considerations and Pitfalls

6.4.1   Shoulder

The common indications for shoulder arthrography include assessment of the glenolabral complex, rotator cuff and long head of biceps tendon (LHBT), and evaluation of the postoperative

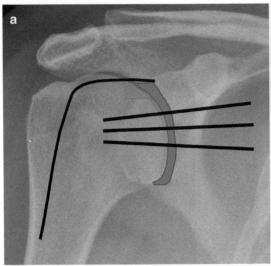
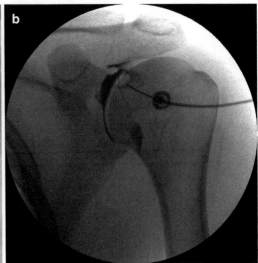

Fig. 6.9 (a) Schematic diagram shows the rotator cuff interval (*red triangle*) with the labral cartilage (*blue outline*) in relation to the long head of biceps and subscapu- laris tendons (*black lines*). (**b**) Postinjection radiograph shows the needle position at the rotator interval and contrast agent flowing away from the joint

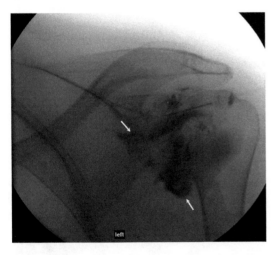

Fig. 6.10 Fluoroscopic image shows extravasation of contrast agent into the subscapularis tendon (*white arrows*) during anterior approach shoulder arthrography with needle placement being too medial

shoulder. Shoulder arthrography is performed either via an anterior or posterior approach. The anterior approach became popular with the Schneider technique (Schneider et al. 1975). Over the years, discussion focused on potential iatrogenic injury and disruption of the anterior stabilizing tendons and anteroinferior labrum, when this method is used. This initiated the development of the modified anterior approach, targeting the rotator cuff interval (Depelteau et al. 2004) and the posterior approach, as typically practiced by orthopedic surgeons during arthroscopy (Farmer and Hughes 2002). More recently, a posterior overhead approach has been used as an alternative to a conventional posterior approach, if access is limited.

6.4.1.1 Anterior Approach

Needle placement with the Schneider technique is at the medial border of the junction of the middle and lower third of the glenohumeral joint. The modified anterior approach targets the triangular space of the rotator cuff interval between the subscapularis tendon and the intra-articular portion of the LHBT and supraspinatus tendons, where there is relative paucity of important anatomical structures (Fig. 6.9). While the patient is in the supine position, the arm remains in external rotation (palm facing upwards) during the procedure as this relocates the tendon laterally, minimizing unintended biceps needle perforation. Both anterior techniques have a common pitfall involving needle malpositioning with contrast agent extravasation, most commonly into the subscapularis tendon (Fig. 6.10) or adjacent bursa and soft tissues. This can obscure underlying anterior capsular abnormalities. Other pitfalls include a long coracoid process which can obscure entry into the rotator cuff interval. If the needle is placed too medially, the capsuloglenolabral complex may be subject to iatrogenic perforation and injury. In patients with proven or suspected rotator cuff injuries, there is a higher risk of needle perforation into a medially displaced LHBT.

6.4.1.2 Posterior Approach

This method avoids potential instrumentation trauma and contrast agent extravasation around the anterior stabilizing structures which are most typically the area of primary interest (Chung et al. 2001; Farmer and Hughes 2002). The patient lies in a prone position with the arm in neutral or external rotation position, with the palm facing medially or toward the bed. The shoulder may be elevated to a slight anterior oblique position to achieve a tangent orientation of the joint space and the X-ray beam. This approach is subject to variations in position and anatomy, which can complicate the procedure. A morphologically normal acromion or posterior glenoid can often overhang the humeral head, obscuring a direct pathway to the joint capsule (Fig. 6.11). In this case, an oblique needle approach under the acromion may be required. Otherwise, a more direct approach can be employed directly onto the articular surface of the posterior humeral head (Fig. 6.12). Repositioning and applying downward traction on the arm can sometimes increase the target area, but this is limited by the mobility of the patient. Alternatively, a posterior overhead approach with the arm above the head may be used (Fig. 6.13). However, this may not be tolerated by the patient if there is significant restriction of shoulder movement or pain. Contrast agent extravasation may occur around the infraspinatus tendon and can potentially mimic tendon pathology. Recognizing this pitfall minimizes interpretative error (Fig. 6.14).

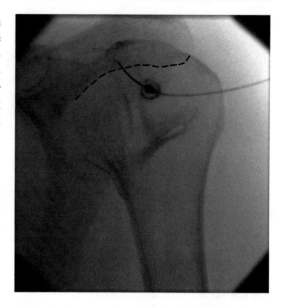

Fig. 6.11 Fluoroscopic image of the shoulder shows the posterior margin of the acromion (*dotted black lines*) overhanging the humeral head. The needle has been angled obliquely in a caudal-cranial direction to negate this

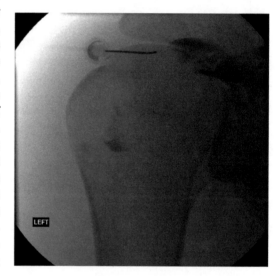

Fig. 6.12 Fluoroscopic image of the shoulder shows the direct posterior approach. In this case, needle access to the posterior humeral head articular surface is straightforward

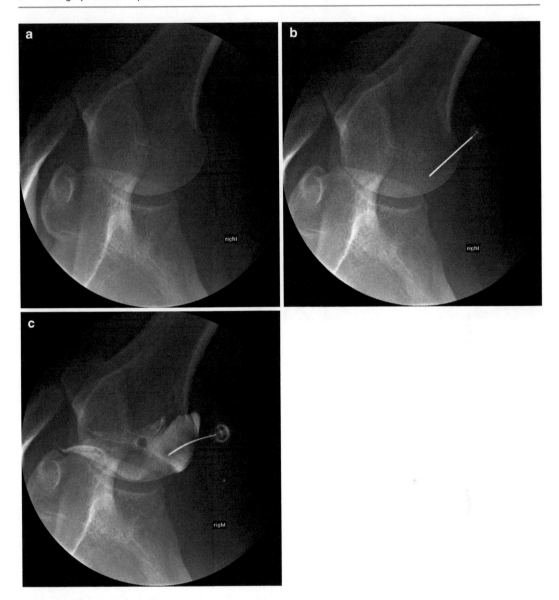

Fig. 6.13 (a–c) Spot fluoroscopic images show the posterior overhead approach with the needle targeting the inferior medial margin of the humeral head

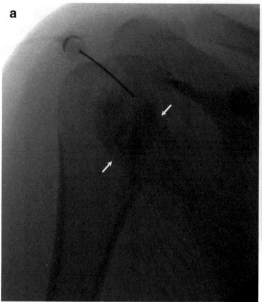

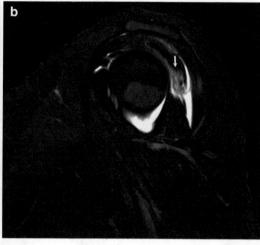

Fig. 6.14 Extravasation of contrast agent into the infraspinatus muscle tendon. (**a**) Fluoroscopic and corresponding (**b**) sagittal fat-suppressed T1-W MR arthrographic images show a large amount of contrast agent extravasation into and around the infraspinatus tendon and muscle belly (*white arrows*). This can mimic or obscure true pathology

6.4.2 Elbow

Elbow arthrography is most useful for identifying intra-articular bodies, ligamentous injury, and subtle chondral abnormalities (Delport and Zoga 2012). The lateral radiocapitellar approach is the most common approach. The patient is seated next to the fluoroscopic table with the upper arm elevated and the elbow flexed at 90° in a true lateral position. If there is a risk of a vasovagal episode, then the procedure can be performed with the patient lying prone. This lateral approach is considered safe as it avoids neurovascular bundles. However, contrast agent extravasation around the lateral stabilizing structures can mimic pathology (Fig. 6.15) and should not be mistaken for tendinosis or pathological ligamentous injuries. A posterior medial approach is an alternative technique, with the needle introduced into the olecranon fossa (Masala et al. 2010). The risk of ulnar nerve injury is increased with this method but can be mitigated by ensuring at least a 1 cm clearance lateral to the medial epicondyle (Fig. 6.16).

6.4.3 Wrist

Wrist arthrography is most usually performed for instability or triangular fibrocartilage complex (TFCC) tears. It can incorporate one or more of the three joint compartments – the radiocarpal joint, the DRUJ, and the midcarpal joint (Fig. 6.17). Practice varies considerably between institutions and is also dependent on the clinical situation. Screening during the procedure can help identify abnormal communication between joint compartments, which may negate the need to perform a second compartment injection. Postinjection wrist manipulation encourages contrast material to pass through small ligament or TFCC defects. A combined radiocarpal and DRUJ injection for evaluation of the TFCC may be preferred, if no abnormal communication is seen on the initial radiocarpal injection. Opacification of the DRUJ can help to demonstrate small partial proximal surface and foveal attachment tears of the TFCC (Fig. 6.18). Radiocarpal and midcarpal injections may be used for assessment of the intrinsic scapholunate and lunotriquetral ligaments (Cerezal et al. 2005).

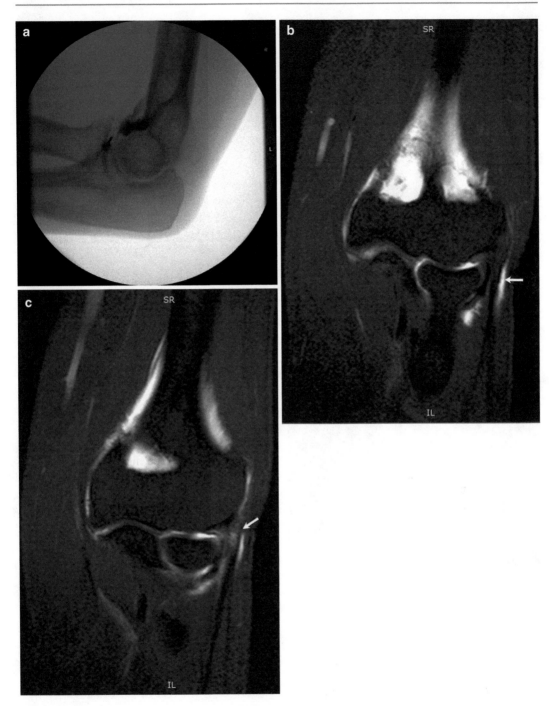

Fig. 6.15 (**a**) Fluoroscopic image shows the direct lateral approach for elbow arthrography. (**b–c**) Corresponding coronal fat-suppressed T1-W MR arthrographic images show signal hyperintensity in and around the radial collateral ligament and the common extensor tendons (*white arrows*). This can be misinterpreted as ligamentous or tendon injuries

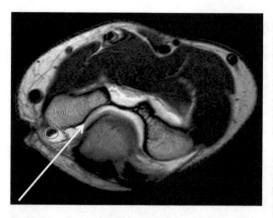

Fig. 6.16 Axial T1-W image with schematic graphic overlay shows the posterior medial approach of the needle (*white arrow*) with a 1 cm clearance required to avoid injury to the ulnar nerve (*red circle*)

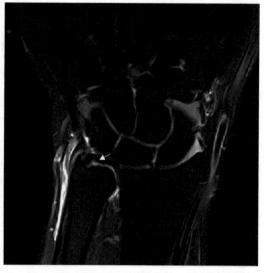

Fig. 6.18 Coronal fat-suppressed T1-W MR arthrographic image of the wrist. Injection into the DRUJ reveals proximal surface irregularity near the foveal attachment of the TFCC indicating a partial tear (Courtesy of Dr. H. Aniq)

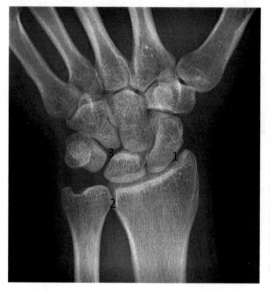

Fig. 6.17 Frontal radiograph of the wrist shows the three main locations for arthrographic puncture: (*1*) radiocarpal, (*2*) distal radioulnar, and (*3*) midcarpal joints

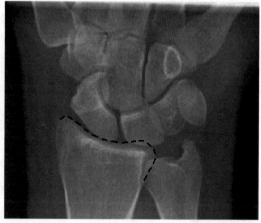

Fig. 6.19 Frontal radiograph of the wrist with schematic overlay (*dotted lines*) shows the dorsal lip of the radius which often prevents direct vertical needle approach into the radiocarpal joint space

However, a single radiocarpal injection in most situations will provide adequate detail to exclude the most significant TFCC and intrinsic ligament injuries.

Wrist arthrography can be performed with the patient sitting with the arm resting palm down on the fluoroscopic table. Alternatively, the patient can lie prone with the arm overhead, elbow partially flexed, and hand in pronated position – the "superman position" – or supine with the arm by the side. The dorsal lip of the radius overlies the radiocarpal joint, limiting joint access on a straight posteroanterior projection (Fig. 6.19). This pitfall can be minimized by using minor wrist flexion with a small wedge placed beneath the wrist. Applying slight ulnar deviation will also maximize access to the radiocarpal joint space. Alternatively, a similar result can be achieved by applying cranial tilt on the imaging intensifier (Cerezal et al. 2012). The path of the needle should subsequently run approximately 5–10 degrees off-tangent to the distal radial artic-

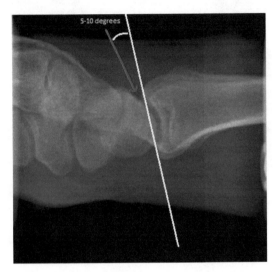

Fig. 6.20 Lateral radiograph of the wrist shows the oblique tilt of the needle (*blue arrow*) required to negate the dorsal lip of the radius

ular surface (Fig. 6.20). A similar pitfall can be encountered with injection of the DRUJ, because the ulnar head lies within the concave articular fossa of the distal radius. The DRUJ is best injected at its proximal margin. The midcarpal joint is accessible via a direct puncture, usually at the junction between the capitate, hamate, lunate, and triquetrum.

The wrist joints require only a small amount of contrast agent, and extravasation can occur very early during injection. It often occurs along the extensor tendon sheaths and should not be misinterpreted as pathology, e.g., tenosynovitis (Fig. 6.21). It is important in MR arthrography not to fill the joint with iodinated contrast agent to confirm intra-articular location of the needle, as this will largely obscure or dilute the Gd contrast material. This pitfall can be avoided with use of a single syringe that contains both iodinated contrast agent and Gd of the appropriate concentration and will also permit dynamic evaluation under fluoroscopy. Observing contrast material flow during the dynamic wrist arthrography procedure can immediately demonstrate abnormal communication between joint com-

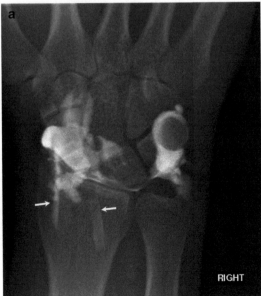

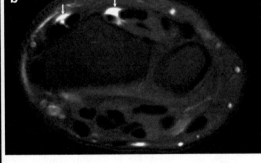

Fig. 6.21 (**a**) Post-arthrographic spot fluoroscopic image of the wrist shows contrast material tracking along the extensor carpi radialis brevis/longus and extensor pollicis longus tendon sheaths (*white arrows*). (**b**) Corresponding

axial fat-suppressed T1-W MR arthroscopic image shows hyperintense contrast material in the tendon sheaths (*white arrows*)

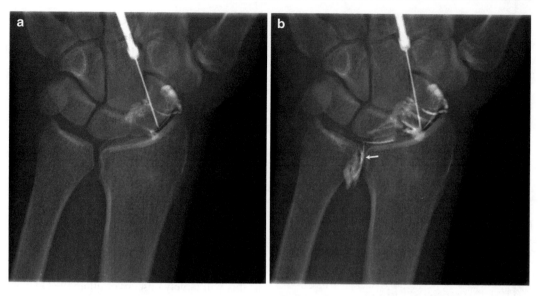

Fig. 6.22 (**a**) Initial spot fluoroscopic image of the wrist taken during radiocarpal arthrographic injection shows contrast agent initially contained within the proximal carpal row. (**b**) Later spot fluoroscopic image shows contrast agent extravasation through the distal radioulnar joint (*white arrow*) indicating an underlying TFC tear or perforation

partments (Figs. 6.22 and 6.23). This may negate the need to perform a second joint injection. Small ligamentous and TFCC tears may not initially demonstrate transcompartmental flow of contrast material. However, this can be achieved by manipulation of the wrist postinjection and therefore helps to avoid a second unnecessary joint injection (Fig. 6.24). Digital subtraction techniques can be applied to make the radiological findings more conspicuous.

6.4.4 Hip

The main indications for hip arthrography are identification of acetabular labral tears and articular cartilage abnormalities. The patient is placed in a supine position. The hip is ideally placed in minor internal rotation and flexion. This position minimizes tension on the anterior joint capsule and may reduce the incidence of contrast agent extravasation. Needle placement should avoid the neurovascular bundle, and clinical palpation of

the femoral artery can be performed. However, unless there is skeletal deformity or hip dysplasia requiring a medial approach, this pitfall is rarely encountered.

There are two main target areas for needle positioning, namely: (1) the femoral neck and (2) superior to the femoral head-neck junction along the lateral edge. A greater rate of contrast agent extravasation occurs with the neck approach, due to the thick underlying annular ligament or zona orbicularis, which encircles the femoral neck (Duc et al. 2006). The lateral aspect of the femoral head is preferred (Fig. 6.25). An oblique needle approach rather than a straight-down perpendicular puncture may also reduce contrast agent extravasation (Llopis et al. 2012), allowing the tip of the needle to slide under the joint capsule. Contrast agent extravasation may occur just around the femoral neck but may also be seen in the iliopsoas tendon sheath. Normal communication between the hip joint and bursa occurs in up to 15% of the population (Llopis et al. 2012) (Fig. 6.26).

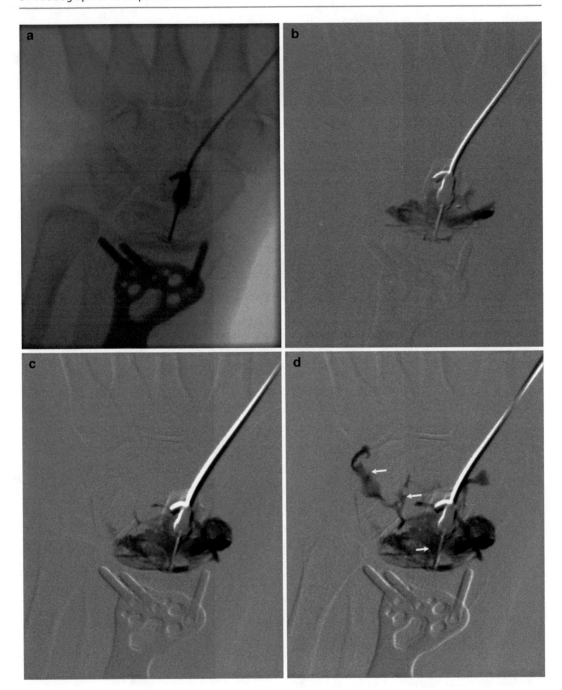

Fig. 6.23 (**a**–**d**) Series of fluoroscopic images acquired during radiocarpal puncture in wrist arthrography with digital subtraction technique. Contrast material can be seen in the last image (**d**, *white arrows*) extravasating into the distal carpal row secondary to a scapholunate ligament injury

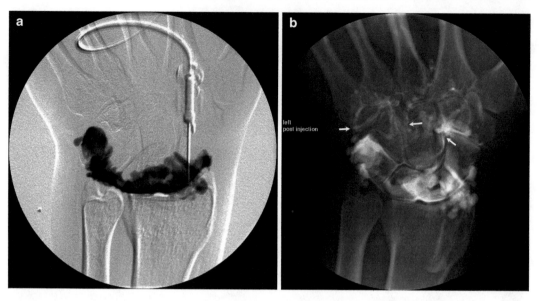

Fig. 6.24 (**a**) Digital subtraction acquisition of a radio-carpal arthrographic puncture. Contrast material is contained on the initial fluoroscopic image. (**b**) Spot fluoroscopic image taken following wrist manipulation after the injection shows extensive contrast material flow into the distal carpal row (*white arrows*) indicating proximal row ligamentous injury and/or perforation

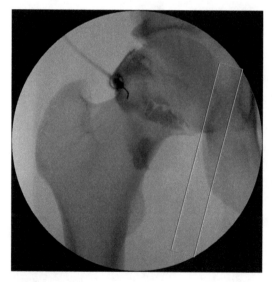

Fig. 6.25 Fluoroscopic image taken during hip arthrography with the needle targeting the lateral edge of the femoral head-neck junction. The femoral vessels (*red rectangle*) are shown in relation to the site of puncture

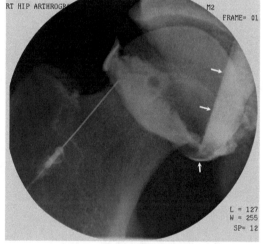

Fig. 6.26 Spot fluoroscopic image taken during hip arthrography shows contrast material from the hip joint communicating with the iliopsoas bursa (*white arrows*)

6.4.5   Knee

Knee arthrography is occasionally utilized for evaluating osteochondral injuries and postoperative menisci (Kalke et al. 2012). This is espe-cially true where MRI is contraindicated and CT arthrography is the only option. The patient is placed in a supine position, with the knee in extension to minimize tension in the extensor mechanism. The joint is usually accessed via a retropatellar approach, either laterally or medi-ally, into the patellofemoral articulation (Shortt

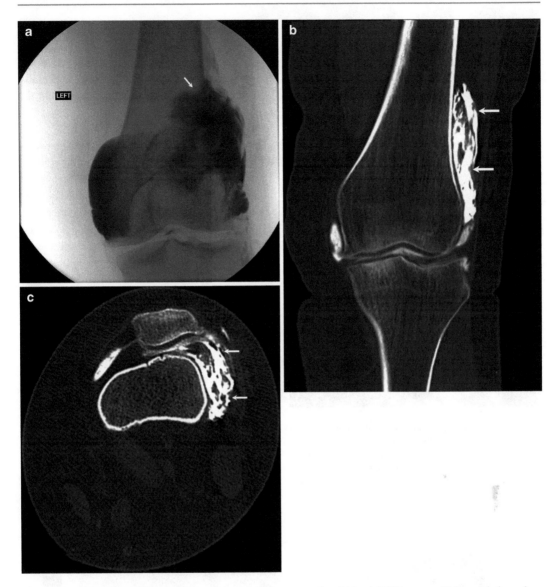

Fig. 6.27 (a) Fluoroscopic image shows abnormal pooling and concentration of contrast material along the lateral edge of the distal femur (*white arrow*). Corresponding (b) coronal and (c) axial CT images with bone windows show contrast extravasation (*white arrows*) into the lateral aspect of the prefemoral fat pad

et al. 2009). The presence of underlying osteoarthritic change will dictate the approach taken, as large osteophytes may obscure joint access.

The main pitfall is an approach that is too cranial in location which can result in injection into the prefemoral fat pad rather than the joint space (Kalke et al. 2012) (Fig. 6.27). Alternative techniques include a direct anterior approach down to the medial femoral condyle (Shortt et al. 2009) or the anterolateral approach down to the lateral

femoral condyle (Moser et al. 2008). This may be of benefit in obese patients where the patella is not easily palpated. Contrast material may pool within the suprapatellar recess, reducing overall joint distension. This effect can be minimized by the application of a tourniquet around the thigh above the patella following joint injection (Grainger et al. 2000). Otherwise, gentle pressure can be applied over the suprapatellar region with the free hand during contrast agent injection.

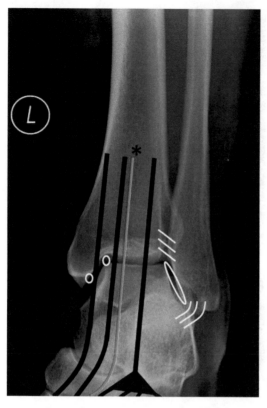

Fig. 6.28 Schematic diagrammatic overlays overlying an AP radiograph of the ankle. Common sites of needle puncture include the medial and lateral clear spaces or anterior puncture into the tibiotalar joint (*white circles* and *white oval*). The extensor tendons (*black lines*) and the dorsalis pedis artery (*red line*) should be avoided during needle puncture. The talofibular/lateral stabilizing ligaments are also shown (*white lines*)

6.4.6 Ankle

Ankle arthrography is occasionally used to assess osteochondral and cartilage lesions, especially with CT where orthopedic metalware limits the use of MRI. Arthrography is much less commonly used for ankle ligament deficiency. The joint is accessed primarily through the anteromedial or anterolateral approach (Chandnani et al. 1994; Fox et al. 2013) (Fig. 6.28), with the patient in a supine position with mild plantar flexion. Clinical palpation (or US imaging guidance) can help avoid puncture of the dorsalis pedis artery. An oblique approach is required to avoid the lip of the anterior tibial plafond and bring the needle tip onto the articular surface of the dome of the talus. Cranial tilt of the X-ray tube (2–5°) may also be helpful.

Large anterior osteophytes can result in a failed procedure, regardless of technique. These may be difficult to appreciate on frontal fluoroscopic images. Lateral fluoroscopy can be utilized when difficulties are encountered. Contrast agent extravasation into the flexor hallucis and digitorum tendon sheaths, and the posterior subtalar joint, is often encountered as a normal variation in up to 25% of cases (Cerezal et al. 2005) (Fig. 6.29). Contrast agent extension into the distal tibiofibular syndesmotic recess should not be misinterpreted as being a syndesmotic injury.

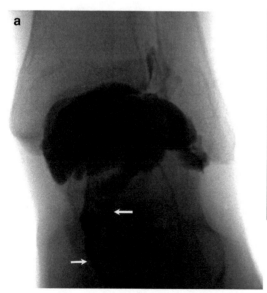

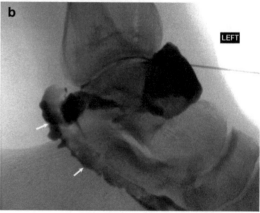

Fig. 6.29 (a) AP and (b) lateral fluoroscopic images taken during ankle arthrography shows contrast agent extravasation into the flexor hallucis tendon sheath (*white arrows*)

Conclusion

In summary, arthrography is widely practiced in most radiology departments with musculoskeletal sections and serves to optimize diagnostic images by better visualization of the internal structures of the joint. As with any procedure, there are technical pitfalls that can result in inadequate outcomes. Understanding these technical pitfalls will help optimize the procedure, maximizing image quality as well as patient comfort.

References

Andreisek G, Duc SR, Froehlich JM (2007) MR arthrography of the shoulder, hip, and wrist: evaluation of contrast dynamics and image quality with increasing injection-to-imaging time. AJR Am J Roentgenol 188:1081–1088

Cerezal L, Abascal F, Garcia-Valtuille R, Canga A (2005a) Ankle MR arthrography: how, why, when. Radiol Clin N Am 43:693–707

Cerezal L, Abascal F, Garcia-Valtuille R, Del Pinal F (2005b) Wrist MR arthrography: how, why, when. Radiol Clin N Am 43:709–731

Cerezal L, Berna-Mestre JD, Canga A et al (2012) MR and CT arthrography of the wrist. Semin Musculoskelet Radiol 16:27–41

Chandnani VP, Harper MT, Ficke JR et al (1994) Chronic ankle instability: evaluation with MR arthrography, MR imaging, and stress radiography. Radiology 192:189–194

Chung CB, Dwek JR, Feng S, Resnick D (2001) MR arthrography of the glenohumeral joint: a tailored approach. AJR Am J Roentgenol 177:217–219

Chung CB, Isaza IL, Angulo M et al (2005) MR arthrography of the knee: know, why, when. Radiol Clin N Am 43:733–746

Conway R, O'Shea FD, Cunnane G, Doran MF (2013) Safety of joint and soft tissue injections in patients on warfarin anticoagulation. Clin Rheumatol 32:1811–1814

Delport AG, Zoga AC (2012) MR and CT arthrography of the elbow. Semin Musculoskelet Radiol 16:15–26

Depelteau H, Bureau NJ, Cardinal E et al (2004) Arthrography of the shoulder: a simple fluoroscopically guided approach for targeting the rotator cuff interval. AJR Am J Roentgenol 182:329–332

Duc SR, Hodler J, Schmid M et al (2006) Prospective evaluation of two different injection techniques for MR arthrography of the hip. Eur Radiol 16:473–478

Farmer KD, Hughes PM (2002) MR arthrography of the shoulder: fluoroscopically guided technique using a posterior approach. AJR Am J Roentgenol 178:433–434

Fox MG, Wright PR, Alford B et al (2013) Lateral mortise approach for therapeutic ankle injection: an alternative to the anteromedial approach. AJR Am J Roentgenol 200:1096–1100

Grainger AJ, Elliott JM, Campbell RSD et al (2000) Direct MR arthrography: a review of current use. Clin Radiol 55:163–176

Haynor DR, Schuman WP (1984) Double contrast CT arthrography of the glenoid labrum and shoulder girdle. Radiographics 4:411–421

Hodler J (2008) Technical errors in MR arthrography. Skeletal Radiol 37:9–18

Jacobson JA, Lin J, Jamadar DA, Hayes CW (2003) Aids to successful shoulder arthrography performed with a fluoroscopically guided anterior approach. Radiographics 23:373–379

Kalke RJ, Di Primio GA, Schweitzer ME (2012) MR and CT arthrography of the knee. Semin Musculoskelet Radiol 16:57–68

Llopis E, Fernandez E, Cerezal L (2012) MR and CT arthrography of the hip. Semin Musculoskelet Radiol 16:42–56

Masala S, Fiori R, Bartolucci DA et al (2010) Diagnostic and therapeutic joint injections. Semin Interv Radiol 27:160–171

Montgomery DD, Morrison WB, Schweitzer ME et al (2002) Effects of iodinated contrast and field strength on gadolinium enhancement: implications for direct MR arthrography. J Magn Reson Imaging 15:334–343

Morrison WB (2005) Indirect MR arthrography: concepts and controversies. Semin Musculoskelet Radiol 9:124–134

Moser T, Moussaoui A, Dupuis M et al (2008) Anterior approach for knee arthrography: tolerance evaluation and comparison of two routes. Radiology 246:193–197

Newberg AH, Munn CS, Robbins AH (1985) Complications of arthrography. Radiology 155:605–606

Peh WCG, Cassar-Pullicino VN (1999) Magnetic resonance arthrography: current status. Clin Radiol 54:575–587

Rhee RB, Chan KK, Lieu JG et al (2012) MR and CT arthrography of the shoulder. Semin Musculoskelet Radiol 16:3–14

Schneider R, Ghelman B, Kaye JJ (1975) A simplified injection technique for shoulder arthrography. Radiology 114:738–739

Shortt CP, Morrison WB, Roberts CC et al (2009) Shoulder, hip, and knee arthrography needle placement using fluoroscopic guidance: practice patterns of musculoskeletal radiologists in North America. Skeletal Radiol 38:377–385

Steinbach LS, Palmer WE, Schweitzer ME (2002) Special focus session. MR arthrography. Radiographics 22:1223–1246

Vollman AT, Craig JG, Hulen R et al (2013) Review of three magnetic resonance arthrography related infections. World J Radiol 5:41–44

Wagner SC, Schweitzer ME, Weishaupt D (2001) Temporal behaviour of intra-articular gadolinium. J Comput Assist Tomogr 25:661–670

Winalski CS, Alparslan L (2008) Imaging of articular cartilage injuries of the lower extremity. Semin Musculoskelet Radiol 12:283–301

Ultrasound-Guided Musculoskeletal Interventional Techniques Pitfalls

7

Gajan Rajeswaran and Jeremiah C. Healy

Contents

7.1 **Introduction** 121

7.2 **Screening for Contraindications/ Consent** 122
7.2.1 Review of Request Form 122
7.2.2 Contraindications to Injection 122
7.2.3 Diagnostic Ultrasound Scan 122
7.2.4 Consent 123
7.2.5 Pre-procedural Check 123

7.3 **Equipment Selection** 123
7.3.1 Probe Selection 123
7.3.2 Syringe Selection 124
7.3.3 Needle Selection 124

7.4 **Needle/Probe Technique** 124
7.4.1 Triangulation 124
7.4.2 In and Out of Plane Needle Approaches 125
7.4.3 Needle Bevel Orientation 126
7.4.4 Needle-Beam Angle 126
7.4.5 Increasing Conspicuity of Needle Using US Machine Settings 128
7.4.6 Expulsion of Gas Within Needle 129
7.4.7 Injection of Local Anesthetic/Normal Saline 129

7.5 **Specific Therapeutic Interventional Techniques** 129
7.5.1 Local Anesthetic Injection 129
7.5.2 Corticosteroid Injection 130
7.5.3 Viscosupplementation 131
7.5.4 Dry Needling 132
7.5.5 Platelet-Rich Plasma (PRP) Injection 132

7.5.6 Management of Achilles/Patellar Tendinopathy 133

7.6 **Post-procedure** 134

Conclusion 134

References 134

G. Rajeswaran, MBBS, FRCR (✉) • J.C. Healy, MA, MBBChir, FRCP, FRCR, FFSEM
Department of Radiology, Chelsea & Westminster Hospital, Imperial College,
369 Fulham Road, London SW10 9NH, UK
e-mail: grajeswaran@hotmail.com; j.healy@ic.ac.uk

Abbreviations

PRP   Platelet-rich plasma
US   Ultrasound

7.1 Introduction

Ultrasound (US) lends itself readily as an ideal modality to guide most musculoskeletal interventions, due to its ease of access, availability at the bedside, dynamic nature, and lack of radiation dose. The ability of US to enable the operator to see the tip of the needle at the intended injection site, as well as its relationship to the adjacent anatomy (such as nearby nerves and blood vessels), allows accurate and safe placement of the needle and minimizes the risk of complications compared with non-guided injections.

In order for US-guided musculoskeletal interventions to be a success, it is important for the operator to consider and address multiple potential pitfalls that could result in complication or error, from the moment the patient arrives to

© Springer International Publishing AG 2017
W.C.G. Peh (ed.), *Pitfalls in Musculoskeletal Radiology*, DOI 10.1007/978-3-319-53496-1_7

the time that they leave the department. The purpose of this chapter is to highlight these potential pitfalls in the chronological order in which the operator would need to address them, including obtaining informed consent, selecting the appropriate equipment, using good needle and probe technique, being aware of specific therapeutic techniques, and providing post-procedural advice. This allows the operator to formulate a systematic approach to evaluate and encourage the highest standard of care for their patients.

7.2 Screening for Contraindications/Consent

7.2.1 Review of Request Form

It is essential for the radiologist to check the patient's details and ensure that the correct patient is being treated. A review of the clinical details provided on the request form with the patient is necessary to prevent wrong side/region intervention.

7.2.2 Contraindications to Injection

A clinical, drug, and allergy history should be obtained. An allergy to an injectate would be an absolute contraindication to using that injectate. Latex and Elastoplast allergies are the most commonly elicited allergies in musculoskeletal intervention, and in this context, latex-free gloves and hypoallergenic plasters should be used, respectively.

A coagulopathy or anticoagulation medication (particularly warfarin) can potentially result in significant peri- or post-procedural bleeding, especially in the context of deep soft tissue or joint injections where the ability to appropriately tamponade bleeding is impaired (Malloy et al. 2009; Taninishi and Morita 2011; Tirado et al. 2013). Ideally, the anticoagulant medication should be stopped for a short period before and after the procedure, and in the con-

text of warfarin, the international normalized ratio (INR) should be 2.0 or less to minimize the risk of significant bleeding (Thumboo and O'Duffy 1998). However, this is not always possible or advisable, depending on the indication for anticoagulation. Discussion with the referring clinician and the patient should take place prior to the procedure so that an appropriate decision can occur regarding whether or not the benefits of the procedure outweigh the risks. In particular, it is important to be aware of national and regional guidelines prior to proceeding. To minimize the risk of post-procedure bleeding, the patient should be appropriately advised regarding actions to take if there are signs of bleeding, including applying pressure to the injection site and attending their general practitioner or accident and emergency department.

Performing an injection in the presence of local cellulitis or ulceration can result in spreading of a superficial infection into deeper structures. Unless a skin entry point can be chosen which avoids the region of skin abnormality, the injection would usually be contraindicated. In particular, the merits of diagnostic aspiration of a joint effusion to exclude septic arthritis in a patient with overlying cellulitis or skin ulceration should be discussed prior to injection. In this situation, an aseptic reactive joint effusion could be converted to a septic arthritis by performing aspiration. For contraindications to specific drugs, please see Sect. 7.5 on Specific Therapeutic Interventional Techniques.

7.2.3 Diagnostic Ultrasound Scan

Prior to the procedure, a preliminary diagnostic ultrasound (US) is usually helpful to check that there has been no change in the diagnosis and also to help plan the procedure. In particular, it is useful to help decide what type of needle to use, what trajectory the needle will need to take, and the skin entry point. It can also be used to document the adjacent neurovascular anatomy and plan a route avoiding these structures (Smith and Finnoff 2009a, b).

7.2.4 Consent

Informed consent should be obtained from the patient, adhering to local standards of practice and federal law. Ideally, the patient should be given an information leaflet on the procedure before attending, to give them a chance to process the information and provide them with a chance to consider questions they may need to be answered at the time of the procedure. Consent should include the reasons for the procedure, its potential risks and complications, and alternative treatment options. If the patient's first language is different to that of the radiologist, an interpreter should be offered.

If the patient's mental capacity is reduced such that they are unable to understand the indications and risks, the procedure should be canceled or deferred until they regain their normal capacity or until formal discussions have occurred with the referring clinician and the patient's family/next of kin and all are agreed that to proceed would be in the patient's best interests. In the latter situation, this should be documented in the patient's notes, and formal written consent should be obtained from the patient's next of kin.

A formal written consent form should also be completed in procedures with significant risks. However, to maintain efficient throughput of patients through the department, written consent is not always feasible, particularly for the procedures with minimal risk (the majority of US-guided intervention). The most important factors are to have the discussion with the patient, to ensure they are fully informed, and to document this in the radiological report. The legal advice in the United Kingdom is that all material risks should be discussed and documented in the patient's report. A material risk is one that might be rare (such as an infection risk of 1 in 3000–4000) but which the patient would consider significant if it occurred.

7.2.5 Pre-procedural Check

Prior to beginning the procedure, a World Health Organization (WHO) surgical safety checklist should be performed if the patient is having a general anesthetic (Haynes et al. 2009). However, this is extremely uncommon in US-guided musculoskeletal intervention and for procedures in which the patient is awake. All that is required is to perform some form of check to minimize the chance of a wrong-sided procedure. This could be as simple as the radiologist confirming with the patient and the healthcare assistant the location and reason for the injection.

7.3 Equipment Selection

7.3.1 Probe Selection

The probe should be selected to provide the best image of the region to be injected. As a result, for diagnosis, a linear high-frequency probe is used in almost all musculoskeletal scenarios. In the main, this is the same for musculoskeletal-guided intervention, as the needle is best seen with the highest frequency probe. In certain areas of the body, the curved contours of soft tissue and bone related to the joints and digits mean that part of the probe may not contact the skin, resulting in no image in this region. In the hands and feet, this is best overcome by using a smaller footplate "hockey stick" high-frequency linear probe. Elsewhere in the body, where the larger imaging window provided by standard footplate high-frequency linear probes is preferred, using a large standoff mound of gel in the gap between the probe and the skin can overcome this.

Curvilinear low-frequency probes can be extremely useful in musculoskeletal intervention as well. Although the resolution of imaging provided is not as good as with the high-frequency probes, there are certain instances where the increased depth of penetration and wider field of view can be more helpful. This includes injection of deep joints (such as the shoulder and hip) and aspiration of deep fluid collections. In these situations, the needle is often inserted at a deeper angle meaning that it is hard to see with linear high-frequency probes but much easier to see with curvilinear low-frequency probes.

7.3.2 Syringe Selection

The decision to use a "Luer lock" or "Luer slip/ slip tip" syringe depends on the preference of the operator. The Luer lock syringe is most advantageous when injecting small compartments such as tendon sheaths and small joints. As these compartments are small, if injection is attempted just outside the compartment, the high resistance often results in the injectate leaking out around the syringe-needle hub interface and spurting onto the patient and/or operator. The Luer lock syringe prevents this by providing a locked seal at the syringe-needle hub interface. This means that the operator can more confidently use the lack of resistance to injection as an additional marker of correct intracompartmental needle position.

Many injectates appear similar to the naked eye once drawn up into the syringe – for example, depomedrone acetate cannot be differentiated from triamcinolone acetonide, and normal saline cannot be differentiated from lidocaine or bupivacaine. In best practice, the syringes should be labeled with the name of the injectate soon after drawing it up. However, this can be time consuming and prevent efficient throughput of patients through the department. An alternative is to get into the habit of using specific syringes for specific injectates, for example, drawing up lidocaine into a 5 ml syringe as opposed to normal saline in a 10 ml syringe. As long as the injectates are drawn up just prior to injection and the operator is consistent with which injectate is drawn into which syringe, the chance of injecting the wrong injectate can be significantly reduced.

7.3.3 Needle Selection

The pre-procedural diagnostic US imaging will help in estimating the depth of tissue to be traversed and the trajectory the needle will take. This then determines the length of needle required. In determining the caliber of needle to use, the larger the caliber of needle, the easier it will be to visualize with US imaging (Bondestam

and Kreula 1989; Schafhalter-Zoppoth et al. 2004). However, larger-caliber needles are more likely to result in a painful procedure and have a higher chance of causing tissue trauma. As such, we tend to use the smallest-caliber needle possible to perform the injection, as the prevention of pain and tissue damage is felt to be most important and even the smallest needles can usually be visualized well. A caveat to this is in the context of aspiration or injection of thick substances such as viscosupplements. In these situations, the fluid passing through the needle is often too thick to pass through the smallest needles, and 21G or 19G needles are preferred.

Ideally, a single needle should be used in one pass to administer the local anesthetic and then the therapeutic injectate. A single-pass technique minimizes the risk of infection compared with two passes. However, when using a 19G needle for the therapeutic injection (such as in aspiration), the benefit of minimizing the infection risk by using a single-pass technique should be weighed against the benefit of minimizing the patient discomfort by using a two-pass technique, with local anesthetic injected in the first pass with a 25G needle followed by the therapeutic injection. Most operators would use a two-pass technique when the therapeutic injection requires a 19G needle, but when it requires a 21G needle, if the operator thinks that the patient will tolerate a single-pass technique, then this should be used.

7.4 Needle/Probe Technique

7.4.1 Triangulation

To accurately land the needle tip at the target site, the US probe should be placed over the target at a site where it is well seen, and the adjacent nerves and blood vessels can be avoided. At this site, the needle skin entry point and trajectory within the tissue can be triangulated by mentally drawing a right-angled triangle over the image (Fig. 7.1). The two fixed points of the triangle are the center of the probe (often marked on the probe by a small line) and the target. The hypotenuse of the

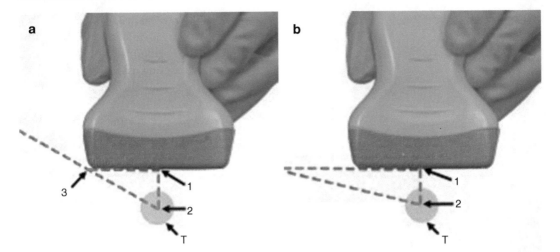

Fig. 7.1 (**a**) Diagram shows the method of "triangulation" to help determine the skin entry point and trajectory of the needle for injection. The US probe is placed over the target (T) at a site where it can be seen well and the adjacent neurovascular structures can be safely avoided. An imaginary right-angled triangle can then be mentally drawn over the image (*red dashed lines*). The fixed points of the triangle are the midpoint of the probe (*1*) and the target (*2*). The skin entry point (*3*) can be varied to produce different potential trajectories (hypotenuse of the triangle) of the needle. Normally, the skin entry point would be relatively close to the probe to allow the whole needle to be seen on the image. As long as the probe remains fixed over the target and the needle is passed along the hypotenuse of the triangle for the given skin entry point, the needle will be seen in its entirety as it is passed toward the target. (**b**) Similar diagram to (**a**) with an altered skin entry point (*3*) which is further from the probe, allowing a shallower trajectory of the needle (hypotenuse of the triangle). As long as the needle is passed from the skin entry point along the trajectory of the hypotenuse of the imaginary triangle, it will be seen in its entirety as it is passed toward the target (*T*)

created right-angled triangle represents the needle, and the third point of the triangle is the skin entry point. By changing the skin entry point, the trajectory of the needle can be altered to reach the target at the preferred needle angle. If the probe position stays the same, by following the imaginary hypotenuse of the triangle from the skin entry point, the needle tip will reach the target and will be visualized on US imaging.

7.4.2 In and Out of Plane Needle Approaches

In order for the needle to be seen, it must pass through the plane of the US beam. With the probe positioned over the target, the needle can be inserted using two approaches. The most commonly used method is the "in plane" approach. Here, the needle is inserted so that its long axis is parallel to the long axis of the probe/beam so that both are collinear (Fig. 7.2). In this approach, the needle is visualized throughout its length as a hyperechoic line, and both the needle tip and shaft can be seen as the needle is advanced. However, if the needle is angled even very slightly out of plane, only part of the shaft of the needle will be visualized, and the tip will usually be out of plane, i.e., not visualized as the needle is advanced (Fig. 7.3a). In this situation, if the probe is moved to the plane of the needle, the needle will be visualized but the target will not. Therefore, the probe should be kept over the target, and the needle should be withdrawn and its angle adjusted so that it lies in plane before readvancing (Fig. 7.3b).

In the "out of plane" approach, the needle is inserted so that its long axis is perpendicular to the long axis of the probe/beam (Fig. 7.4). In this approach, the needle is visualized as a round echogenic dot as only the part of the needle crossing the beam can be seen. The needle shaft and the tip look the same as they pass through the beam, making them difficult to

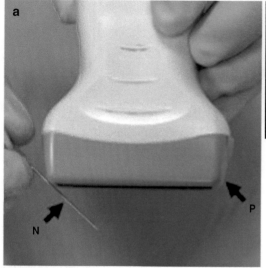
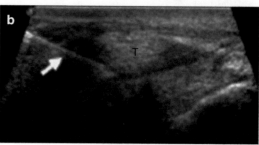

Fig. 7.2 (**a**) Photograph shows the "in plane" approach for needle insertion. The needle (*N*) is passed with its long axis parallel to the probe (*P*) and its beam, both being collinear. (**b**) Resulting US image using the "in plane" approach for needle insertion as in (**a**). The needle (*white arrow*) is passed with its long axis parallel to the probe and its beam, both being collinear. With this approach, the needle can be seen in its entirety on the US image as a hyperechoic line, as long as it remains in the plane of the long axis of the probe. In this example, the needle has been passed into the tendon sheath of the tibialis posterior tendon (*T*) for therapeutic injection

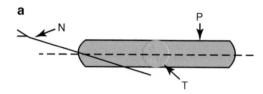
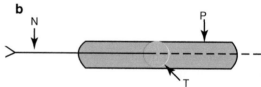

Fig. 7.3 (**a**) Diagram shows that when using the "in plane" approach, if the needle (*N*) is slightly out of plane with the US beam (*dashed line*) of the probe (*P*), it will not be seen as a hyperechoic line on the US image. (**b**) Diagram shows that if the needle is slightly out of plane with the US beam as in (**a**), in order to visualize the needle (*N*) again, it should be withdrawn and reinserted at a different angle in the plane of the beam (*dashed line*) of the probe (*P*). Now the needle will be visualized completely on the US image as a hyperechoic line

differentiate. As such, an echogenic dot at the target site could represent the needle tip or part of the shaft with the actual needle tip beyond the probe. In this situation, moving or angling the probe away from the target site will help to confirm the position of the needle tip, and the probe can then be brought back over the target and the needle adjusted accordingly. The main advantage of the "out of plane" approach versus the "in plane" approach is in visualization of the needle in injections where the trajectory needs to be relatively vertical, such as in small joint injections.

7.4.3 Needle Bevel Orientation

Visualization of the needle tip is enhanced by turning the bevel to face directly toward or directly away from the probe (Bondestam and Kreula 1989; Hopkins and Bradley 2001).

7.4.4 Needle-Beam Angle

The ability to visualize the needle is affected by the needle-beam angle (Chin et al. 2008). This is the angle between the long axis of the needle

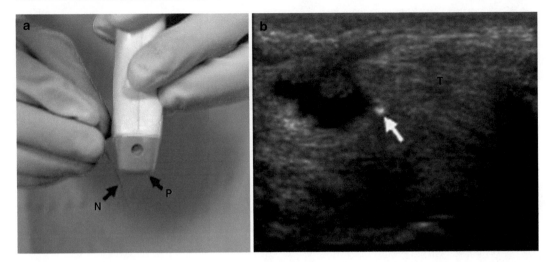

Fig. 7.4 (**a**) Photograph shows the "out of plane" approach for needle insertion. The needle (*N*) is passed with its long axis perpendicular to the probe (*P*) and its beam. (**b**) Resulting US image using the "out of plane" approach for needle insertion as in (**a**). The needle (*white arrow*) is passed with its long axis perpendicular to the probe (*P*) and its beam. With this approach, only the small part of the needle that crosses the US beam can be seen as a round echogenic dot (*white arrow*). In this example, the needle has been passed into the tendon sheath of the peroneus longus tendon (*T*) for therapeutic injection

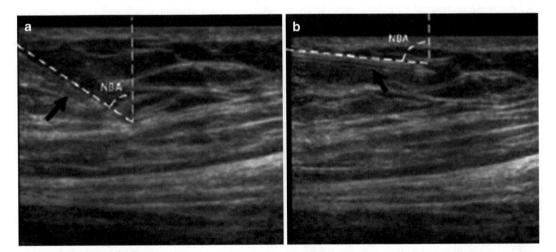

Fig. 7.5 (**a**) US image shows the needle-beam angle (NBA). This is the angle created between the long axis of the needle and the long axis of a line drawn parallel with the US beam/probe. In this case, the needle (*black arrow*) is not well seen as the NBA is less than 55°. Making the NBA greater than 55° makes the needle much easier to see. This can be done by altering the trajectory of the needle or heel-toeing the probe. (**b**) To make the needle easier to see than in (**a**), the NBA is increased to greater than 55° (and to almost 90° in this case) by altering the trajectory of the needle. The needle (*black arrow*) is now much more clearly identified

and a line drawn parallel with the long axis of the US beam/probe (Fig. 7.5a). The needle is better seen when this angle is greater than 55° and best seen when close to 90°, when the needle is essentially parallel to the probe (Bondestam and Kreula 1989; Culp et al. 2000;

Bradley 2001; Schafhalter-Zoppoth et al. 2004; Deam et al. 2007).

Situations in which the injection is deep (such as large joint injections or in large patients) often result in a needle-beam angle of less than 55°, and this makes the needle much more difficult to

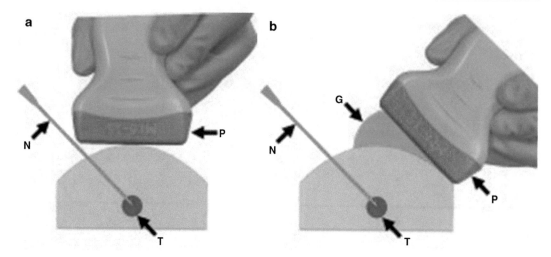

Fig. 7.6 (**a**) Diagram shows the "heel-toe" maneuver to overcome a needle-beam angle of less than 55° by changing the position of the probe. The needle (*N*) has been inserted to the target (*T*), but with the probe (*P*) in this position, the needle is not well seen as the needle-beam angle is too low. Sometimes, the needle can only be inserted at a particular angle due to the location of the injection or the neurovascular structures preventing safe injection at a different angle. In these instances, the probe can be adjusted using the "heel-toe" maneuver as shown in this figure. Here the probe (*P*) is moved so that its long axis is parallel with the needle, making the needle (*N*) much easier to see on the US image. A standoff mound of gel (*G*) may need to be placed on the skin so that when the probe is heel-toed and the probe loses contact with the skin, a good image can still be obtained. (**b**) Diagram shows the "heel-toe" maneuver to overcome a needle-beam angle of less than 55° by changing the position of the probe. In (**a**), the needle (*N*) has been inserted to the target (*T*), but with the probe (*P*) in this position, the needle is not well seen as the needle-beam angle is too low. Sometimes, the needle can only be inserted at a particular angle due to the location of the injection or the neurovascular structures preventing safe injection at a different angle. In these instances, the probe can be adjusted using the "heel-toe" maneuver as in (**b**). Here the probe (*P*) is moved so that its long axis is parallel with the needle, making the needle (*N*) much easier to see on the US image. A standoff mound of gel (*G*) may need to be placed on the skin so that when the probe is heel-toed and the probe loses contact with the skin, a good image can still be obtained

see (Fig. 7.5b). In these situations, the following tips should be considered to increase visibility of the needle:

- *Heel-toe maneuver:* This technique aims to overcome a needle-beam angle of less than 55° by changing the angle of the probe to make it more parallel with the needle (Fig. 7.6). If there is adequate overlying soft tissue coverage, the edge of the probe closest to the needle tip is pushed into the soft tissue. If the underlying anatomy prevents this, the edge of the probe furthest from the needle tip can be raised up. If this results in loss of contact with the skin, the gap between the probe and the skin can be filled with a standoff mound of gel.
- *Electronic beam steering:* This is a machine setting that effectively allows an electronic heel-toe maneuver. The US beam can be electronically angled relative to the probe altering the needle-beam angle without heel-toeing the probe itself (Baker et al. 1999).
- *Use of a curvilinear probe:* The wider field of view and greater depth penetration of lower frequency curvilinear probes mean that they can visualize needles in deeper injections (such as in the shoulder or hip) where linear probes cannot.

7.4.5 Increasing Conspicuity of Needle Using US Machine Settings

Spatial compound imaging combines multiple images of the same target at different angles into a single image in the same plane. It has been shown to increase needle conspicuity compared to conventional B-mode imaging (Cohnen et al. 2003; Saleh et al. 2001). However, frequency compound imaging and tissue harmonic imaging do not enhance visualization of the needle (Karstrup et al. 2002; Mesurolle et al. 2006).

7.4.6 Expulsion of Gas Within Needle

Injected gas results in diffraction of sound and results in poor visualization of the target area. As such, any gas in the syringe or needle should be expelled by flushing the injectate to the needle tip.

7.4.7 Injection of Local Anesthetic/ Normal Saline

When the echogenic needle tip is in a location adjacent to other echogenic structures (such as bone), it may be difficult to see due to a lack of contrast between it and the adjacent structures. In this situation, injecting a small amount of local anesthetic or normal saline can be useful as the hypoechoic fluid collects near the needle tip, contrasting against it and outlining its margin and making it easier to see.

Injecting a small amount of local anesthetic or normal saline can also be useful when injecting into a small cavity such as a tendon sheath. In this situation, the tendon sheath lies directly against the tendon with no separation between the two, unless there is tendon sheath fluid. To prevent the needle tip penetrating the tendon, once the needle tip is near the tendon sheath, a small amount of local anesthetic can be injected. If it is seen to infiltrate along the tendon sheath, correct position is confirmed, and the therapeutic injectate can then be administered.

A similar technique can be used for injecting small joints such as the acromioclavicular joint and the interphalangeal joints of the digits. However, care should be taken to inject only a small amount of local anesthetic or normal saline to confirm the correct position. If too much is injected, given that these joints have small cavities, there may then be no room for the therapeutic injectate to be administered.

7.5 Specific Therapeutic Interventional Techniques

It is outside of the scope of this chapter to discuss all the drugs and types of procedure used in musculoskeletal intervention. Instead, those that are most commonly used or topical will be discussed.

7.5.1 Local Anesthetic Injection

Local anesthetics are used in musculoskeletal intervention to induce cutaneous/subcutaneous analgesia prior to injecting another drug, to provide analgesia at sites of musculoskeletal pain for diagnostic purposes, or to mitigate the symptoms related to a flare from another co-injected drug. In injections of small compartments with high potential resistance, such as small joints and tendon sheaths, there is a risk that the needle tip may appear to be intracompartmental but actually lie just outside. There is therefore a high risk of inadvertent extracompartmental injection with its associated adverse effects. In these situations, a small amount of local anesthetic can be injected first to confirm correct position, prior to injecting the main drug.

The most commonly used local anesthetics in musculoskeletal practice are the amides such as lidocaine, bupivacaine, and ropivacaine, with ropivacaine being the most expensive. Unlike the esters (such as cocaine), they are associated with very little risk of an allergic reaction, although immediate and delayed hypersensitivity reactions (up to 72 h after injection) can occur (Holmdahl 1998; Cox et al. 2003; Duque and Fernandez 2004; Ban and Hattori 2005). Central nervous system toxicity (with symptoms including tremors, respiratory arrest, and generalized convulsions) and cardiac toxicity (with symptoms including arrhythmias and cardiovascular collapse) can occur following inadvertent intravascular or intrathecal injection of local anesthetic.

While bupivacaine is more potentially neurotoxic and cardiotoxic than ropivacaine, ropivacaine is a potent vasoconstrictor and should therefore be used with caution in injections near sites at risk of irreversible ischemia, such as in nerve root and epidural injections (MacMahon et al. 2009).

In the context of joint injections, intra-articular local anesthetic can be chondrotoxic, particularly when used in large volumes such as with orthopedic procedures (Chu et al. 2006, 2008, 2010; Karpie and Chu 2007; Dragoo et al. 2008; Kamath et al. 2008; Piper and Kim 2008). In the context of single intra-articular injections of local anesthetic as used in musculoskeletal radiology (most commonly for diagnostic reasons or with another injectate to mitigate a flare reaction), 0.125% bupivacaine does not appear to have a significant toxic effect on articular cartilage (Chu et al. 2008). We would therefore recommend using 0.25% bupivacaine (rather than 0.5%); as when injected with steroid or another injectate, its effective dose will be 0.125%.

7.5.2   Corticosteroid Injection

Steroids are commonly used in musculoskeletal intervention for their potent anti-inflammatory effect. Synthetic steroids for injection include triamcinolone acetonide, methylprednisolone acetate (depomedrone acetate), betamethasone acetate, dexamethasone sodium phosphate, and hydrocortisone acetate. Triamcinolone acetonide and methylprednisolone acetate are much less water soluble than the other injectable steroids meaning that they are about five times as potent but confer a higher risk of complications/side effects. There is little systematic evidence or national/international guidance on which steroid to select for a particular use, and most decisions relate to the experience and preference of the radiologist and/or referrer (Articular and periarticular corticosteroid injections 1995; Haslock et al. 1995; Stephens et al. 2008).

Contraindications for steroid injection include local or intra-articular sepsis and bacteremia as steroids can potentiate or exacerbate sepsis in this context (Thumboo and O'Duffy 1998). Steroid injections should be avoided in joints that are unstable or potentially unstable, as they can weaken the joint capsule and ligaments and cause avascular necrosis (Padeh and Passwell 1998). The presence of an intra-articular fracture is a relative contraindication to injection as steroids can inhibit bone healing (Aspenberg 2005; Pountos et al. 2008).

Steroids are cytochrome P450 (CYP) substrates metabolized by the CYP3A4 enzyme. Therefore, drugs that inhibit CYP3A4 activity can significantly decrease hepatic clearance of injected steroids and potentially result in adrenocortical suppression and Addisonian crisis. CYP3A4 inhibitors include antifungals (e.g., ketoconazole and itraconazole), antiemetics (e.g., aprepitant and fosaprepitant), immunosuppressants (such as ciclosporin), macrolide antibacterials (e.g., clarithromycin and erythromycin), calcium channel blockers (e.g., diltiazem), oral contraceptives (e.g., ethinylestradiol and norethisterone), and antiretroviral medication (e.g., ritonavir). Patients taking CYP3A4 inhibitors should have the merits and risks of the steroid injection considered by the clinician and the radiologist prior to the procedure and proceed based on local and national guidances. The patient should at least temporarily stop taking the medication for a period before and after the injection. In the literature, the most significant cases of adrenocortical suppression following steroid injection appear to relate to patients with human immunodeficiency virus (HIV) taking ritonavir (Dort et al. 2009; Wood et al. 2015).

Patients with diabetes mellitus should also be counseled before having a steroid injection as it can cause hyperglycemia 2–5 days after the injection (Wang and Hutchinson 2006; Baumgarten et al. 2007; Habib et al. 2008; MacMahon et al. 2009). Steroid injections should be limited to injections no less than 6 weeks apart, with up to three injections per year (Ostergaard and Halberg 1998). If the patient's symptoms are recurrent despite this, alternative management therapy should be considered.

Adverse effects for which patients should be consented include infection (for which the risk of septic arthritis is 0.01–0.03%), postinjection flare/pain (2–25%), skin necrosis and depigmentation, fat atrophy, tendon rupture, cartilage damage (0.7–3% in the context of multiple injections), and facial flushing (15%) up to 2–5 h after injection (Brown et al. 1953; Hollander et al. 1961; Schetman et al. 1963; Iuel and Kryger 1965; Kligman and Willis 1975; Balch et al. 1977; Friedman and Moore 1980; Gray et al. 1981; Jacobs 1986; Rogojan and Hetland 2004).

Skin necrosis and depigmentation, as well as fat atrophy, occur more commonly in superficial injections such as in the hands and feet due to the increased risk of inadvertent steroid infiltration of the skin and subcutaneous fat. The risk can be minimized by using water-soluble steroids in the hands and feet and by flushing the needle with normal saline or local anesthetic after the steroid has been injected, before withdrawing the needle. The appearances usually diminish after 12 months but can last longer (Cassidy and Bole 1966; Jacobs 1986; Rogojan and Hetland 2004). In this instance, normal saline therapy has been shown to be effective as a treatment (Shumaker et al. 2005). In our practice, we tend to use depomedrone in the hands and feet. While not completely water soluble, it is more so than triamcinolone, and there is a lower risk of skin changes, offset by the lower potency of the steroid.

When performing transforaminal nerve root or epidural steroid injections, there is a risk of paraplegia, brain infarction, spinal cord infarction, and rarely death (with cervical injections seemingly most high risk) (Cicala et al. 1989; Brouwers et al. 2001; Houten and Errico 2002; Baker et al. 2003; Rozin et al. 2003; Rathmell et al. 2004; Rosenkranz et al. 2004; Ludwig and Burns 2005; Muro et al. 2007; Suresh et al. 2007; Ruppen et al. 2008). This is postulated to be due to arterial vasospasm or injury, neurotoxicity due to a preservative in the steroid preparation, or embolic infarction by the particulate steroid (MacMahon et al. 2009). The latter seems to be the most common cause (Baker et al. 2003; McMillan and Crumpton 2003; Rathmell et al. 2004). While it would seem prudent to avoid the use of particulate steroids in transforaminal nerve root injections, there is not much evidence relating to the clinical efficacy of non-particulate steroids in this context, and as such, they are used relatively infrequently (MacMahon et al. 2009).

7.5.3 Viscosupplementation

Viscosupplementation refers to intra-articular injection of a hyaluronic acid (a glycosaminoglycan) derivative in patients with osteoarthritis. Hyaluronic acid is viscoelastic at high molecular weights, facilitating lubrication, shock absorption, and fluid retention during movement in weight-bearing joints. It is also thought to inhibit cytokine activity and nociception, reducing inflammation and pain (Lo et al. 2003). There are different licensed hyaluronic acid products, the most common being Durolane, Orthovisc, Synvisc, and Ostenil. Ostenil is of lower molecular weight than the others (Gossec and Dougados 2006).

The main documented adverse effect of hyaluronic acid injection is transient pain and swelling for up to a few days following the injection. This can occur in up to 5–10% of injections and is thought to relate to a foreign body-type reaction which is more common and severe with the higher molecular weight products (Conrozier et al. 2003; Morton and Shannon 2003; Goldberg and Coutts 2004; Pourbagher et al. 2005; Migliore et al. 2006; Qvistgaard et al. 2006; Juni et al. 2007; Rivera 2015; Witteveen et al. 2015). Patients should be consented for this and advised to take analgesia to mitigate the symptoms during the transient postinjection flare. Inadvertent extra-articular injection of hyaluronic acid can result in a similar flare reaction but without the beneficial effects. As such, image guidance with US is recommended, and a small amount of local anesthetic should be injected first to ensure correct intra-articular location of the needle tip prior to injection of hyaluronic acid. Alternatively, if there is a joint effusion, aspiration of joint fluid confirms correct needle tip position. Depending on the clinical presentation, it may be useful to send the aspirate for microscopy, culture and sensitivity, as well as crystal analysis.

7.5.4 Dry Needling

Dry needling (also known as barbotage, fenestration, and tenotomy) is a treatment for tendinopathy which involves passing a needle through an abnormal tendon multiple times to encourage bleeding to change a chronic degenerative process into an acute condition that is more likely to heal (Chiavaras and Jacobson 2013). It is commonly used in the treatment of calcific rotator cuff tendinopathy in the shoulder, common extensor tendinopathy in the elbow, infrapatellar tendinopathy in the knee, and, less commonly, Achilles tendinopathy. The technique involves 20–30 needle passes through the abnormal tendon, along the long axis of the tendon fibers, ensuring that the needle passes through all abnormal areas of the tendon at least once (James et al. 2007; Chiavaras and Jacobson 2013). The presence of a tear in the tendon can be a contraindication to treatment, depending on which tendon is affected and how large the tear is (Chiavaras and Jacobson 2013; Vignesh et al. 2015). In particular, a tear in a rotator cuff or Achilles tendon would usually preclude dry needling. As a general rule, the patient should be advised to avoid sport or overuse activity for 2 weeks following dry needling.

In the context of calcific tendinopathy (most commonly encountered in the rotator cuff tendons of the shoulder), dry needling can be performed in combination with lavage and aspiration. Calcific tendinopathy is a self-limiting condition in most patients, but in some, progression from the symptomatic calcific stage to the asymptomatic post-calcific stage does not occur spontaneously (Vignesh et al. 2015). In these patients, lavage and aspiration can be performed using a single- or two-needle technique to treat the calcification (Farin et al. 1995, 1996; Farin 1996; del Cura et al. 2007; James et al. 2007; Serafini et al. 2009; Yoo et al. 2010; Sconfienza et al. 2011; Saboeiro 2012; Chiavaras and Jacobson 2013; Vignesh et al. 2015). Under US guidance, the needle is used to puncture the calcific deposit, once in the single-needle technique and twice in the two-needle technique.

In the single-needle technique, a small amount of fluid (lidocaine or normal saline) is injected into the calcium, and the plunger is released to allow flow of calcium back into the syringe. In the two-needle technique, the injected fluid is aspirated by the second needle (Greis et al. 2015). The fluid in the syringe should become cloudy due to the presence of the aspirated calcium. Once the aspirated fluid becomes clear or if no cloudy fluid can be aspirated, the calcific deposit is then dry needled repeatedly to break it up. The more chronic the calcification, the less likely aspiration will be possible. The needle is then withdrawn, and a separate needle is used to inject the subacromial-subdeltoid bursa with steroid to either treat concomitant bursitis or for prophylaxis, in case some aspirated calcium is inadvertently deposited into the bursa during the procedure or during withdrawal of the needle.

7.5.5 Platelet-Rich Plasma (PRP) Injection

Platelet-rich plasma (PRP) is defined as having a platelet concentration higher than the physiological concentration of platelets found in healthy whole blood (normally by more than five times) (Marx et al. 1998; Foster et al. 2009). PRP injection has become extremely popular in the management of tendinopathy, muscle tears, and ligament injuries. It is postulated that the intrinsic properties and interplay between the concentrated factors in PRP (such as platelet-derived endothelial growth factor and insulin-derived growth factor) result in a healing response within the tendon, when injected into a region of tendinopathy (Lee et al. 2011).

The procedure for PRP starts with phlebotomy of the patient's vein (usually in the antecubital fossa) to obtain a volume of autologous whole blood in a syringe. The PRP injectate produced will normally comprise 10% of the volume of whole blood obtained, so enough autologous blood should be taken to obtain the desired volume of PRP. The autologous whole blood sample is then placed in a centrifuge for a designated period, separating the blood into three layers: red blood cells (the heaviest and darkest layer), PRP (the middle layer), and platelet-poor plasma which is the buffy coat containing predominantly white blood cells (the lightest layer). The buffy coat should be discarded, allowing the PRP to be extracted. The platelets within the PRP become activated by thrombin and collagen, so dry needling the tendon (producing thrombin as part of the induced bleeding) and injecting the PRP into the dry needling tracts in the tendon (exposing the PRP to intratendinous collagen) facilitate its activation. The PRP injection into small intratendinous spaces has potentially high resistance, so it is recommended that a Luer lock syringe be used to prevent blood spurting onto the operator or patient.

The quality of the PRP is affected by the type of centrifuge, by the duration of spin, and by the composition of the whole blood, which can vary between individuals and even in the same person at different times. As such, the patient should be advised that the effects of the PRP can be variable. The potential adverse effects of PRP injections include infection, bleeding, and post-procedural pain (due to the healing response induced by the injection being inflammatory, at least in part). Nonsteroidal anti-inflammatory drugs (NSAIDs) should be avoided 2 weeks before and after the injection, to prevent inhibition of the effects of the growth factors and healing response (Lee et al. 2011). Patients should be advised to use other forms of analgesia, such as paracetamol, to mitigate postinjection symptoms.

7.5.6 Management of Achilles/ Patellar Tendinopathy

Achilles and patellar tendinopathy are common conditions, with significant functional implications in both athletes and nonathletes. A large variety of injection therapies have been developed to help with the management of patients that are resistant to conventional rehabilitation physiotherapy. These include injections of corticosteroid, high-volume saline, prolotherapy, autologous blood, PRP, aprotinin, botulinum

toxin, sodium hyaluronate, dextrose, and polidocanol, many of which are injected using US guidance (Coombes et al. 2010).

A recent Cochrane review concluded that there is insufficient evidence from randomized controlled trials to support the routine use of injection therapy to treat Achilles tendinopathy and insufficient evidence to support the use of a particular injection therapy over another (Kearney et al. 2015). However, in selected cases, injection therapy might be useful, particularly when the only other management option is surgical. The use of corticosteroid injections is particularly controversial in the management of Achilles tendinopathy, with most studies showing little short-term benefit or no benefit and demonstrating an association with tendon rupture (Shrier et al. 1996; Wong et al. 2004, 2009; Wei et al. 2006; Kearney et al. 2015). Even in the context of treating severe retrocalcaneal bursitis related to insertional Achilles tendinopathy, there is a risk of tendon rupture, as the bursal and Achilles tendon fibers often interdigitate, allowing the injected steroid to reach the tendon from the bursa (Turmo-Garuz et al. 2014).

High-volume image-guided injections (HVIGI) have become relatively popular in the management of Achilles tendinopathy and, more recently, in patellar tendinopathy (Maffulli et al. 2013; Morton et al. 2014). In chronic Achilles and patellar tendinopathy, the ingrowth of new vessels and nerves into and around the tendon can be a source of pain (Longo et al. 2009). The rationale in HVIGI is that the high-volume injection between the Achilles tendon and the paratenon and Kager fat pad (or the patellar tendon and the adjacent Hoffa fat pad) mechanically stretches, breaks, or occludes the neovessels and their accompanying nerve supply, resulting in a reduction in the sensation of pain. The main proponents of HVIGI propose an injection of a 50 ml mixture of normal saline and 0.25% bupivacaine with 25 mg hydrocortisone acetate, the latter to mitigate the effects of the mechanical inflammatory reaction that often follows the high-volume injection (Maffulli et al. 2013). A similar but smaller volume (30 ml) injection is advocated in patellar tendinopathy (Morton et al.

2014). In our practice, we use a more conservative approach, injecting a smaller total volume of the mixture of normal saline and 0.25% bupivacaine (30 ml in Achilles tendinopathy and 15 ml in patellar tendinopathy), and we do not inject corticosteroid due to our concern for the possibility of tendon rupture.

Overall, we would advise that injection therapy should be performed with caution in Achilles and patellar tendinopathy and only following discussion as part of a multidisciplinary team setting involving the sports physician, surgeon, and physiotherapist.

7.6 Post-procedure

After withdrawing the injection needle from the skin, the injection site should be compressed to stop bleeding. It is not uncommon for patients to complain of postinjection bruising, and this can be minimized by pressing over the wound for 10–20 s after the injection. The patient should be advised to press the wound if they notice any swelling or bruising afterward and contact a medical professional if the swelling or bruising continues to increase. The wound should be covered with a plaster. The purpose of the plaster is to keep the wound dry and minimize the risk of post-procedural infection while the skin wound is healing. In most people, a small scab will form very quickly, but in some, it can take several hours and sometimes up to 24 h to form a protective scab. As such, we recommend that patients leave the plaster on for 24 h, although there is no data to support this practice.

Before the patient leaves the room, it is important to reiterate what they should expect to happen afterward, what the likely adverse effects might be, and what to do in the event that they occur. This helps to reduce the risk of complaints related to the procedure. Post-procedural advice should include a discussion regarding exercise following the injection. Most injections would permit normal activity but warrant the cessation of exercise for at least 48 h during the potential

period of flare and synovitis and allow the injected region to settle down. In the context of tendon sheath steroid injections, it is advisable to avoid exercise of the injected area for 2 weeks due to the risk of tendon rupture, as steroids can impair tenocyte proliferation for up to 2 weeks (MacMahon et al. 2009).

Particularly in the context of tendinopathy and impingement, injections should ideally be performed with a plan for rehabilitation. Using both together in the patient's management is usually more successful in treating the condition than either alone. While in general the patient is usually safe to drive home after the injection, they should be advised to check with their insurer whether or not their policy will cover them to do so. The injections in which patients should be advised not to drive on the same day after the injection include spinal injections, large joint arthrographic procedures, and shoulder hydrodilatation. After the patient has left, medicolegal documentation of the procedure should appear in the radiological report. This should include a summary of the risks/complications discussed, the procedural technique, the drugs injected, whether or not there were any immediate complications, and what post-procedural advice was given.

Conclusion

There are multiple potential pitfalls that can occur while performing US-guided musculoskeletal intervention. It is important for the operator to formulate a systematic approach to evaluation from the moment the patient arrives to the moment they leave, to reduce the risk of complications and maximize the chance of a successful injection.

References

(1995) Articular and periarticular corticosteroid injections. Drug Ther Bull 33:67–70

Aspenberg P (2005) Drugs and fracture repair. Acta Orthop 76:741–748

Baker JA, Soo MS, Mengoni P (1999) Sonographically guided percutaneous interventions of the breast using a steerable ultrasound beam. AJR Am J Roentgenol 172:157–159

Baker R, Dreyfuss P, Mercer S, Bogduk N (2003) Cervical transforaminal injection of corticosteroids into a radicular artery: a possible mechanism for spinal cord injury. Pain 103:211–215

Balch HW, Gibson JM, El-Ghobarey AF, Bain LS, Lynch MP (1977) Repeated corticosteroid injections into knee joints. Rheumatol Rehabil 16:137–140

Ban M, Hattori M (2005) Delayed hypersensitivity due to epidural block with ropivacaine. BMJ 330:229

Baumgarten KM, Gerlach D, Boyer MI (2007) Corticosteroid injection in diabetic patients with trigger finger. A prospective, randomized, controlled double-blinded study. J Bone Joint Surg Am 89:2604–2611

Bondestam S, Kreula J (1989) Needle tip echogenicity. A study with real time ultrasound. Invest Radiol 24:555–560

Bradley MJ (2001) An in-vitro study to understand successful free-hand ultrasound guided intervention. Clin Radiol 56:495–498

Brouwers PJ, Kottink EJ, Simon MA, Prevo RL (2001) A cervical anterior spinal artery syndrome after diagnostic blockade of the right C6-nerve root. Pain 91:397–399

Brown EM Jr, Frain JB, Udell L, Hollander JL (1953) Locally administered hydrocortisone in the rheumatic diseases; a summary of its use in 547 patients. Am J Med 15:656–665

Cassidy JT, Bole GG (1966) Cutaneous atrophy secondary to intra-articular corticosteroid administration. Ann Intern Med 65:1008–1018

Chiavaras MM, Jacobson JA (2013) Ultrasound-guided tendon fenestration. Semin Musculoskelet Radiol 17:85–90

Chin KJ, Perlas A, Chan VW, Brull R (2008) Needle visualization in ultrasound-guided regional anesthesia: challenges and solutions. Reg Anesth Pain Med 33:532–544

Chu CR, Izzo NJ, Papas NE, Fu FH (2006) In vitro exposure to 0.5% bupivacaine is cytotoxic to bovine articular chondrocytes. Arthroscopy 22:693–699

Chu CR, Izzo NJ, Coyle CH, Papas NE, Logar A (2008) The in vitro effects of bupivacaine on articular chondrocytes. J Bone Joint Surg Br 90:814–820

Chu CR, Coyle CH, Chu CT, Szczodry M, Seshadri V, Karpie JC, Cieslak KM, Pringle EK (2010) In vivo effects of single intra-articular injection of 0.5% bupivacaine on articular cartilage. J Bone Joint Surg Am 92:599–608

Cicala RS, Westbrook L, Angel JJ (1989) Side effects and complications of cervical epidural steroid injections. J Pain Symptom Manag 4:64–66

Cohnen M, Saleh A, Luthen R, Bode J, Modder U (2003) Improvement of sonographic needle visibility in cirrhotic livers during transjugular intrahepatic portosystemic stent-shunt procedures with use of real-time compound imaging. J Vasc Interv Radiol 14:103–106

Conrozier T, Bertin P, Mathieu P et al (2003) Intra-articular injections of hylan G-F 20 in patients with symptomatic hip osteoarthritis: an open-label, multicentre, pilot study. Clin Exp Rheumatol 21:605–610

Coombes BK, Bisset L, Vicenzino B (2010) Efficacy and safety of corticosteroid injections and other injections for management of tendinopathy: a systematic review of randomised controlled trials. Lancet 376:1751–1767

Cox B, Durieux ME, Marcus MA (2003) Toxicity of local anaesthetics. Best Pract Res Clin Anaesthesiol 17:111–136

Culp WC, McCowan TC, Goertzen TC, Habbe TG, Hummel MM, LeVeen RF, Anderson JC (2000) Relative ultrasonographic echogenicity of standard, dimpled, and polymeric-coated needles. J Vasc Interv Radiol 11:351–358

Deam RK, Kluger R, Barrington MJ, McCutcheon CA (2007) Investigation of a new echogenic needle for use with ultrasound peripheral nerve blocks. Anaesth Intensive Care 35:582–586

del Cura JL, Torre I, Zabala R, Legorburu A (2007) Sonographically guided percutaneous needle lavage in calcific tendinitis of the shoulder: short- and long-term results. AJR Am J Roentgenol 189:W128–W134

Dort K, Padia S, Wispelwey B, Moore CC (2009) Adrenal suppression due to an interaction between ritonavir and injected triamcinolone: a case report. AIDS Res Ther 6:10

Dragoo JL, Korotkova T, Kanwar R, Wood B (2008) The effect of local anesthetics administered via pain pump on chondrocyte viability. Am J Sports Med 36:1484–1488

Duque S, Fernandez L (2004) Delayed-type hypersensitivity to amide local anesthetics. Allergol Immunopathol (Madr) 32:233–234

Farin PU, Jaroma H, Soimakallio S (1995) Rotator cuff calcifications: treatment with US-guided technique. Radiology 195:841–843

Farin PU (1996) Consistency of rotator-cuff calcifications. Observations on plain radiography, sonography, computed tomography, and at needle treatment. Invest Radiol 31:300–304

Farin PU, Rasanen H, Jaroma H, Harju A (1996) Rotator cuff calcifications: treatment with ultrasound-guided percutaneous needle aspiration and lavage. Skeletal Radiol 25:551–554

Foster TE, Puskas BL, Mandelbaum BR, Gerhardt MB, Rodeo SA (2009) Platelet-rich plasma: from basic science to clinical applications. Am J Sports Med 37:2259–2272

Friedman DM, Moore ME (1980) The efficacy of intraarticular steroids in osteoarthritis: a double-blind study. J Rheumatol 7:850–856

Goldberg VM, Coutts RD (2004) Pseudoseptic reactions to hylan viscosupplementation: diagnosis and treatment. Clin Orthop Relat Res 419:130–137

Gossec L, Dougados M (2006) Do intra-articular therapies work and who will benefit most? Best Pract Res Clin Rheumatol 20:131–144

Gray RG, Tenenbaum J, Gottlieb NL (1981) Local corticosteroid injection treatment in rheumatic disorders. Semin Arthritis Rheum 10:231–254

Greis AC, Derrington SM, McAuliffe M (2015) Evaluation and nonsurgical management of rotator cuff calcific tendinopathy. Orthop Clin N Am 46:293–302

Habib GS, Bashir M, Jabbour A (2008) Increased blood glucose levels following intra-articular injection of methylprednisolone acetate in patients with controlled diabetes and symptomatic osteoarthritis of the knee. Ann Rheum Dis 67:1790–1791

Haslock I, MacFarlane D, Speed C (1995) Intra-articular and soft tissue injections: a survey of current practice. Br J Rheumatol 34:449–452

Haynes AB, Weiser TG, Berry WR et al (2009) A surgical safety checklist to reduce morbidity and mortality in a global population. N Engl J Med 360:491–499

Hollander JL, Jessar RA, Brown EM Jr (1961) Intrasynovial corticosteroid therapy: a decade of use. Bull Rheum Dis 11:239–240

Holmdahl MH (1998) Xylocain (lidocaine, lignocaine), its discovery and Gordh's contribution to its clinical use. Acta Anaesthesiol Scand Suppl 113:8–12

Hopkins RE, Bradley M (2001) In-vitro visualization of biopsy needles with ultrasound: a comparative study of standard and echogenic needles using an ultrasound phantom. Clin Radiol 56:499–502

Houten JK, Errico TJ (2002) Paraplegia after lumbosacral nerve root block: report of three cases. Spine J 2:70–75

Iuel J, Kryger J (1965) Local cutaneous atrophy following corticosteroid injection. Acta Rheumatol Scand 11:137–144

Jacobs MB (1986) Local subcutaneous atrophy after corticosteroid injection. Postgrad Med 80:159–160

James SL, Ali K, Pocock C, Robertson C, Walter J, Bell J, Connell D (2007) Ultrasound guided dry needling and autologous blood injection for patellar tendinosis. Br J Sports Med 41:518–521; discussion 522

Juni P, Reichenbach S, Trelle S et al (2007) Efficacy and safety of intraarticular hylan or hyaluronic acids for osteoarthritis of the knee: a randomized controlled trial. Arthritis Rheum 56:3610–3619

Kamath R, Strichartz G, Rosenthal D (2008) Cartilage toxicity from local anesthetics. Skeletal Radiol 37:871–873

Karpie JC, Chu CR (2007) Lidocaine exhibits dose- and time-dependent cytotoxic effects on bovine articular chondrocytes in vitro. Am J Sports Med 35:1621–1627

Karstrup S, Brons J, Morsel L, Juul N, von der Recke P (2002) Optimal set-up for ultrasound guided punctures using new scanner applications: an in-vitro study. Eur J Ultrasound 15:77–84

Kearney RS, Parsons N, Metcalfe D, Costa ML (2015) Injection therapies for Achilles tendinopathy. Cochrane Database Syst Rev (5):CD010960

Kligman AM, Willis I (1975) A new formula for depigmenting human skin. Arch Dermatol 111:40–48

Lee KS, Wilson JJ, Rabago DP et al (2011) Musculoskeletal applications of platelet-rich plasma: fad or future? AJR Am J Roentgenol 196:628–636

Lo GH, LaValley M, McAlindon T, Felson DT (2003) Intra-articular hyaluronic acid in treatment of knee osteoarthritis: a meta-analysis. JAMA 290: 3115–3121

Longo UG, Ronga M, Maffulli N (2009) Achilles tendinopathy. Sports Med Arthrosc Rev 17:112–126

Ludwig MA, Burns SP (2005) Spinal cord infarction following cervical transforaminal epidural injection: a case report. Spine 30:E266–E268

MacMahon PJ, Eustace SJ, Kavanagh EC (2009) Injectable corticosteroid and local anesthetic preparations: a review for radiologists. Radiology 252:647–661

Maffulli N, Spiezia F, Longo UG, Denaro V, Maffulli GD (2013) High volume image guided injections for the management of chronic tendinopathy of the main body of the Achilles tendon. Phys Ther Sport 14:163–167

Malloy PC, Grassi CJ, Kundu S et al (2009) Consensus guidelines for periprocedural management of coagulation status and hemostasis risk in percutaneous image-guided interventions. J Vasc Interv Radiol 20(7 Suppl):S240–S249

Marx RE, Carlson ER, Eichstaedt RM et al (1998) Platelet-rich plasma: growth factor enhancement for bone grafts. Oral Surg Oral Med Oral Pathol Oral Radiol Endod 85:638–646

McMillan MR, Crumpton C (2003) Cortical blindness and neurologic injury complicating cervical transforaminal injection for cervical radiculopathy. Anesthesiology 99:509–511

Mesurolle B, Bining HJ, El Khoury M, Barhdadi A, Kao E (2006) Contribution of tissue harmonic imaging and frequency compound imaging in interventional breast sonography. J Ultrasound Med 25:845–855

Migliore A, Tormenta S, Martin Martin LS et al (2006) The symptomatic effects of intra-articular administration of hylan G-F 20 on osteoarthritis of the hip: clinical data of 6 months follow-up. Clin Rheumatol 25:389–393

Morton AH, Shannon P (2003) Increased frequency of acute local reaction to intra-articular Hylan G-F 20 (Synvisc) in patients receiving more than one course of treatment. J Bone Joint Surg Am 85:2050. author reply 2050–2051

Morton S, Chan O, King J et al (2014) High volume image-guided injections for patellar tendinopathy: a combined retrospective and prospective case series. Muscles Ligaments Tendons J 4:214–219

Muro K, O'Shaughnessy B, Ganju A (2007) Infarction of the cervical spinal cord following multilevel transforaminal epidural steroid injection: case report and review of the literature. J Spinal Cord Med 30:385–388

Ostergaard M, Halberg P (1998) Intra-articular corticosteroids in arthritic disease: a guide to treatment. BioDrugs 9:95–103

Padeh S, Passwell JH (1998) Intraarticular corticosteroid injection in the management of children with chronic arthritis. Arthritis Rheum 41:1210–1214

Piper SL, Kim HT (2008) Comparison of ropivacaine and bupivacaine toxicity in human articular chondrocytes. J Bone Joint Surg Am 90:986–991

Pountos I, Georgouli T, Blokhuis TJ, Pape HC, Giannoudis PV (2008) Pharmacological agents and impairment of fracture healing: what is the evidence? Injury 39:384–394

Pourbagher MA, Ozalay M, Pourbagher A (2005) Accuracy and outcome of sonographically guided intra-articular sodium hyaluronate injections in patients with osteoarthritis of the hip. J Ultrasound Med 24:1391–1395

Qvistgaard E, Christensen R, Torp-Pedersen S, Bliddal H (2006) Intra-articular treatment of hip osteoarthritis: a randomized trial of hyaluronic acid, corticosteroid, and isotonic saline. Osteoarthritis Cartilage 14:163–170

Rathmell JP, Aprill C, Bogduk N (2004) Cervical transforaminal injection of steroids. Anesthesiology 100:1595–1600

Rivera F (2015) Single intra-articular injection of high molecular weight hyaluronic acid for hip osteoarthritis. J Orthop Traumatol. doi:10.1007/s10195-015-0381-8

Rogojan C, Hetland ML (2004) Depigmentation – a rare side effect to intra-articular glucocorticoid treatment. Clin Rheumatol 23:373–375

Rosenkranz M, Grzyska U, Niesen W et al (2004) Anterior spinal artery syndrome following periradicular cervical nerve root therapy. J Neurol 251:229–231

Rozin L, Rozin R, Koehler SA et al (2003) Death during transforaminal epidural steroid nerve root block (C7) due to perforation of the left vertebral artery. Am J Forensic Med Pathol 24:351–355

Ruppen W, Hugli R, Reuss S, Aeschbach A, Urwyler A (2008) Neurological symptoms after cervical transforaminal injection with steroids in a patient with hypoplasia of the vertebral artery. Acta Anaesthesiol Scand 52:165–166

Saboeiro GR (2012) Sonography in the treatment of calcific tendinitis of the rotator cuff. J Ultrasound Med 31:1513–1518

Saleh A, Ernst S, Grust A, Furst G, Dall P, Modder U (2001) Real-time compound imaging: improved visibility of puncture needles and localization wires as compared to single-line ultrasonography. Röfo 173:368–372

Schafhalter-Zoppoth I, McCulloch CE, Gray AT (2004) Ultrasound visibility of needles used for regional nerve block: an in vitro study. Reg Anesth Pain Med 29:480–488

Schetman D, Hambrick GW Jr, Wilson CE (1963) Cutaneous changes following local injection of triamcinolone. Arch Dermatol 88:820–828

Sconfienza LM, Serafini G, Sardanelli F (2011) Treatment of calcific tendinitis of the rotator cuff by ultrasound-guided single-needle lavage technique. AJR Am J Roentgenol 197:W366; author reply 367

Serafini G, Sconfienza LM, Lacelli F et al (2009) Rotator cuff calcific tendonitis: short-term and 10-year outcomes after two-needle us-guided percutaneous treatment – nonrandomized controlled trial. Radiology 252:157–164

Shrier I, Matheson GO, Kohl HW 3rd (1996) Achilles tendonitis: are corticosteroid injections useful or harmful? Clin J Sport Med 6:245–250

Shumaker PR, Rao J, Goldman MP (2005) Treatment of local, persistent cutaneous atrophy following corticosteroid injection with normal saline infiltration. Dermatol Surg 31:1340–1343

Smith J, Finnoff JT (2009a) Diagnostic and interventional musculoskeletal ultrasound: part 1. Fundamentals. PM R 1:64–75

Smith J, Finnoff JT (2009b) Diagnostic and interventional musculoskeletal ultrasound: part 2. Clinical applications. PM R 1:162–177

Stephens MB, Beutler AI, O'Connor FG (2008) Musculoskeletal injections: a review of the evidence. Am Fam Physician 78:971–976

Suresh S, Berman J, Connell DA (2007) Cerebellar and brainstem infarction as a complication of CT-guided transforaminal cervical nerve root block. Skeletal Radiol 36:449–452

Taninishi H, Morita K (2011) Ultrasound-guided peripheral nerve blocks for a patient receiving four kinds of anticoagulant and antiplatelet drugs: a case report. J Anesth 25:318–320

Thumboo J, O'Duffy JD (1998) A prospective study of the safety of joint and soft tissue aspirations and injections in patients taking warfarin sodium. Arthritis Rheum 41:736–739

Tirado A, Nagdev A, Henningsen C, Breckon P, Chiles K (2013) Ultrasound-guided procedures in the emergency department-needle guidance and localization. Emerg Med Clin N Am 3:87–115

Turmo-Garuz A, Rodas G, Balius R et al (2014) Can local corticosteroid injection in the retrocalcaneal bursa lead to rupture of the Achilles tendon and the medial head of the gastrocnemius muscle? Musculoskelet Surg 98:121–126

Vignesh KN, McDowall A, Simunovic N, Bhandari M, Choudur HN (2015) Efficacy of ultrasound-guided percutaneous needle treatment of calcific tendinitis. AJR Am J Roentgenol 204:148–152

Wang AA, Hutchinson DT (2006) The effect of corticosteroid injection for trigger finger on blood glucose level in diabetic patients. J Hand Surg 31:979–981

Wei AS, Callaci JJ, Juknelis D et al (2006) The effect of corticosteroid on collagen expression in injured rotator cuff tendon. J Bone Joint Surg Am 88:1331–1338

Witteveen AG, Hofstad CJ, Kerkhoffs GM (2015) Hyaluronic acid and other conservative treatment options for osteoarthritis of the ankle. Cochrane Database Syst Rev (10):CD010643.

Wong MW, Tang YN, Fu SC, Lee KM, Chan KM (2004) Triamcinolone suppresses human tenocyte cellular activity and collagen synthesis. Clin Orthop Relat Res 421:277–281

Wong MW, Lui WT, Fu SC, Lee KM (2009) The effect of glucocorticoids on tendon cell viability in human tendon explants. Acta Orthop 80:363–367

Wood BR, Lacy JM, Johnston C, Weigle DS, Dhanireddy S (2015) Adrenal insufficiency as a result of Ritonavir and exogenous steroid exposure: report of 6 cases and recommendation for management. J Int Assoc Provid AIDS Care 14:300–305

Yoo JC, Koh KH, Park WH et al (2010) The outcome of ultrasound-guided needle decompression and steroid injection in calcific tendinitis. J Shoulder Elbow Surg 19:596–600

Musculoskeletal Interventional Techniques Pitfalls

8

Paul I. Mallinson and Peter L. Munk

Contents

8.1	**Introduction**	139
8.2	**Vertebroplasty and Bone Augmentation**	140
8.2.1	Variant Anatomy	140
8.2.2	Altered Anatomy	140
8.2.3	Suboptimal Views	141
8.2.4	Needle Malpositioning	142
8.2.5	Cement Placement	142
8.2.6	Equipment Choice	144
8.3	**Fluoroscopically-Guided Injections**	145
8.3.1	Recognizing Different Sides of a Joint/Foramen	145
8.3.2	Sensitive Periosteum	146
8.3.3	Segmentation Anomaly During Spinal Injections	146
8.4	**CT-Guided Bone Tumor Ablation**	147
8.4.1	Slice Thickness	147
8.4.2	Limited Scan Range	147
8.4.3	Needle Retraction During Cryoablation	147
8.4.4	Thermal Ablation Zone Boundaries	147
Conclusion		148
References		148

P.I. Mallinson, MBChB • P.L. Munk, MD, CM, FRCPC, FSIR (✉)
Department of Radiology, University of British Columbia, Vancouver General Hospital, 899 West 12th Avenue, Vancouver, BC V5Z 1M9, Canada
e-mail: dr_pmallinson@hotmail.com; Peter.Munk@vch.ca

Abbreviations

AP   Anteroposterior
CT   Computed tomography

8.1 Introduction

While many of the pitfalls lying in wait for the interventional radiologist are procedure specific, they broadly fall into one of the following categories, namely, planning, perceptual, interpretive, and technical errors.

Planning errors Insufficient knowledge of the case and associated anatomy obtained pre-procedure, prior to entry into the interventional suite. This can be particularly problematic in cases of anatomical variation or anatomy distorted by disease. The presence and location of vital structures must be identified. These errors can often be avoided by ensuring that up-to-date imaging has been performed and all available prior imaging has been thoroughly reviewed.

Perceptual errors These occur when the operator does not recognize visually apparent abnormalities demonstrated during a procedure. These can often occur in the context of suboptimal views; thus, good patient positioning with optimization of image angles and field size prior to commencing intervention is crucial.

© Springer International Publishing AG 2017
W.C.G. Peh (ed.), *Pitfalls in Musculoskeletal Radiology*, DOI 10.1007/978-3-319-53496-1_8

Interpretative errors The significance of an apparent abnormality is not recognized, leading to failure to perform an appropriate action or a continued inappropriate action.

Technical errors Continued development of new products from the industry has led to a great increase in the scope of interventional radiology. However, new and unfamiliar equipment can be challenging for the operator.

This chapter will discuss common and serious pitfalls, which can occur during musculoskeletal intervention. The pitfalls pertaining to arthrography, ultrasound-guided intervention, and biopsy will be discussed elsewhere within the relevant chapters of this book (see Chaps. 6, 7, and 9, respectively). Therefore, the focus of this chapter will be on vertebroplasty and bone augmentation, computed tomography (CT)-guided ablation of musculoskeletal tumors, and spinal injections.

8.2 Vertebroplasty and Bone Augmentation

Vertebroplasty and bone augmentation have become increasingly popular in recent years as methods of treating osteoporotic wedge compression fractures and malignant bone disease, particularly within the axial skeleton. This has been driven by the reported analgesic benefits in the literature, the unwanted side effects of strong opioid analgesia, and limitations of surgery in the palliative care setting (Burton et al. 2005; Taylor et al. 2006; Layton et al. 2007; Chu et al. 2015). Potential complications can be serious however; these include hemorrhage, infection, paralysis from cord injury, worsening pain from neural compression and fatalities relating to embolic phenomenon, and great vessel injury (Nussbaum et al. 2004; Burton et al. 2005). The interventionist should be wary of the following pitfalls, as listed below.

8.2.1 Variant Anatomy

When planning vertebroplasty, familiarization with the pre-intervention imaging and anatomy is essential to choosing a safe access route and avoiding treating the wrong vertebral body level. The lumbar spine is renowned for its variant anatomy with varying numbers of vertebrae, varying levels of the lowest ribs, and ambiguous L5/S1 segments. Additionally, butterfly or hemi-vertebrae may be present. This can result in variation in the described level of an abnormality between different reports and treatment of the incorrect vertebrae. Careful preoperative correlation of reports with images, clinical history, and examination findings when meeting the patient is advised. Discussion with the referring physician may be required for clarification.

8.2.2 Altered Anatomy

Previous spinal procedures and their associated hardware and cement can alter the expected anatomy of the spine and obscure views. In addition, partial destruction may make the pedicle wall hard to identify, leading to misinterpretation of the medial wall location and accidental instrumentation of the spinal canal. In these cases, the pedicle above and below the selected level can be used for reference. It is important to be aware of the dynamic nature of the compression fracture process. Additional fractures may have occurred in the interval since the last imaging was performed. This can lead to confusion, resulting in the wrong level being treated, or the missed opportunity to treat newly affected levels in the same setting, where informed consent was not obtained pre-procedure.

One or more impacted vertebrae may appear to be a single entity. The presence of bone cement from prior vertebroplasty can lead to a confusing appearance whereby part of a treated level may be mistaken for a separate adjacent collapsed vertebral body (Fig. 8.1). Careful review of prior procedural imaging and a low threshold for repeating the patient's cross-sectional imaging are advised, especially if new or significantly worsening symptoms are reported since the current imaging was performed.

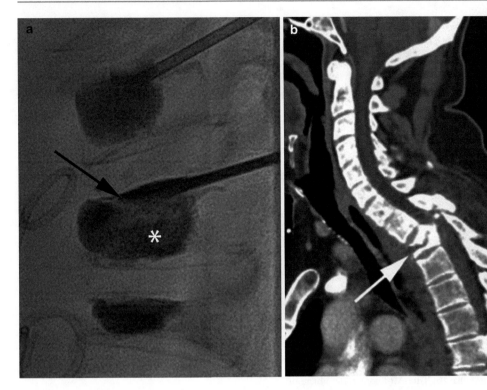

Fig. 8.1 (**a**) Lateral fluoroscopic image shows additional cement placement into the superior vertebral body (*arrow*), which was mistaken for an adjacent vertebra plana. The relatively inferior distribution of the cement after the original procedure contributed to the illusion – this is appreciable as a higher density area (***). This emphasizes the need for careful review of pre-procedure imaging. (**b**) Sagittal reformatted CT image of the thoracic spine shows an apparent wedge fracture of the vertebral body (*arrow*) which was actually two vertebrae partially destroyed and impacted due to infective diskitis

8.2.3 Suboptimal Views

Bone augmentation procedures are most commonly performed under fluoroscopy due to the wide availability and real-time nature of this modality, which is crucial for the safe deployment of bone cement. However, fluoroscopic views must be established and optimized at the start of the procedure, prior to any instrumentation. Major adjustments later risk confusion to the operator as to the location of bony landmarks, instruments, and cement. Marked angulation of the vertebral bodies may vary significantly between levels, especially in the lower lumbar spine or in cases of kyphosis/scoliosis. When multiple vertebrae are treated, this may require correction on a level-by-level basis. Under these circumstances, the technologist can be asked to "remember" set positions using machine presets

or written records of fluoroscopic arm angles and positions. This will allow the operator to return to a previously obtained view quickly with minimal delay to the procedure, which is of particular importance once bone cement has been mixed and is beginning to set.

Initially, a wide field of view is recommended encompassing the lowest ribs and the sacral ala in order to clearly identify the relevant level. This should be followed by magnification and rotational correction of the selected vertebrae. The ribs and lamina should neatly overlap on lateral views, the neural foramen should appear well opened, and the posterior vertebral body wall should appear as a single line. Anteroposterior (AP) views should show well-defined end plates, and the intervertebral joint spaces above and below are usually well visualized. Pedicles should project over the

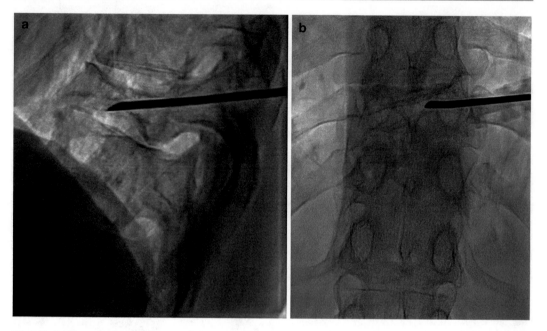

Fig. 8.2 (**a**) Lateral fluoroscopic image shows an optimal view of the thoracic vertebra with overlapping ribs, well-visualized intervertebral disk spaces, and clear view into the neural foramina. (**b**) True AP fluoroscopic image of the thoracic spine shows centralized spinous processes and clear views of the pedicle walls. The intervertebral disk spaces are not well visualized due to the kyphosis

vertebral body. Following this, oblique angulation to find the optimal view of the pedicle can then be performed (Fig. 8.2). Failure to adhere to these principles can result in placement of the needle outside the vertebral body, in locations such as the spinal canal or posterior mediastinum.

8.2.4   Needle Malpositioning

The morphology of the vertebral body must be considered carefully during a vertebroplasty, since the two-dimensional fluoroscopic images can be misleading. The curvature of the anterior vertebral body wall is such that if the needle is placed too laterally, then the lateral view may give the false impression of the needle tip being within the anterior vertebral body, when in fact it has perforated the anterior cortex. This could result in injury to the aorta or vena cava, or deployment of cement outside the vertebral body (Fig. 8.3). A true AP view will reveal the excessively lateral position.

The pedicles are not perfect cylinders and usually taper at the waist. The bone needle may breach the spinal canal while still appearing to be just medial to the medial pedicular wall, especially in the slender thoracic pedicles. A parapedicular approach should be considered for such cases. The vertebroplasty needle may also be placed under cone beam CT guidance, where the equipment is available (Fig. 8.4). This is useful in cases where the pedicle is partially destroyed and difficult to visualize.

8.2.5   Cement Placement

During cement injection, great care must be taken to avoid extravasation into the basilar venous complex and other adjacent vasculature. This is usually achieved by placing the bone needle below the "equator" in the lower half of the vertebral body. On occasion, however, the bone needle may obscure the view of cement entering the basilar venous complex (Fig. 8.5).

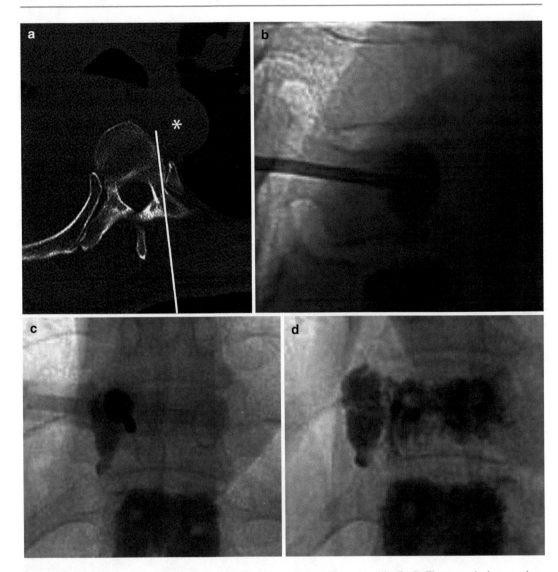

Fig. 8.3 (**a**) Axial CT image shows the hazard of taking a direct AP approach into the vertebral body. The natural curvature of the vertebrae allows the needle to breach the anterior cortex while still appearing to be within the confines of the bone. The needle path in this case (*white line*) ends in the aorta (*). (**b–d**) Fluoroscopic images show cement seemingly within the vertebral bodies (**b, c**) to in fact have been injected adjacent to the vertebral body (**d**) (Reproduced with permission from Klass and Munk 2015)

Extravasation into the disk space may be missed when a vertebral body is asymmetrically wedged. The cement will still appear to be within the confines of the vertebral body seen on the lateral view. Checking the AP as well as lateral views, and prior familiarity with the vertebral body morphology from the planning CT, can help prevent this problem as well as visualizing lateral extravasation.

Calcification from the adjacent aorta and bowel gas shadows can be mistaken for cement extravasation, causing the operator to prematurely terminate the procedure. Careful study of the final needle placement images prior to cement preparation is advised to ensure familiarity with these phenomena (Fig. 8.6). Some fluoroscopy systems allow pre-injection images to be displayed on the screen alongside the current real-time injection images. These provide highly valuable cross-references when a suspected escape of cement is seen on real-time imaging. Cement will follow the paths of least resistance. This can result in sudden and rapid rates of cement flow through narrow cracks. Cement

should be injected with particular care where such cracks are known to communicate with the spinal canal or neural foramina (Fig. 8.7).

8.2.6 Equipment Choice

It is vital to preselect equipment accounting for patient size and the nature of the procedure. Measuring distance from skin to the intended needle tip placement site will allow the correct needle to be selected. For example, a 4-in. needle used in the lower lumbar spine of a patient of large habitus will likely to be of insufficient length to reach a satisfactory location within the vertebral body. Replacing this with a second longer needle then causes unnecessary trauma to the patient. When performing biopsy during vertebroplasty, ensure that the biopsy needle fits through the intended vertebroplasty needle before inserting vertebroplasty needle into the patient. Failure to do so may result in the need for repuncture of the vertebral body via a second site with a larger needle and loss of the original optimal biopsy route, or replacement of the smaller

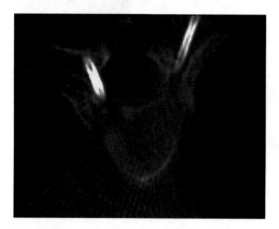

Fig. 8.4 Axial cone beam CT image shows that the medial wall of the spinal canal was perforated by the vertebroplasty needle on the left side of the image. The needle tip did not appear to cross the medial wall during placement under fluoroscopy but passed close to it

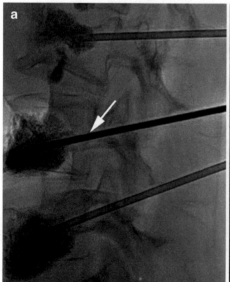
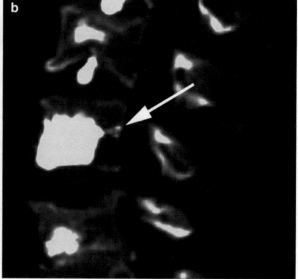

Fig. 8.5 (**a**) Lateral fluoroscopic images do not show extravasation into the venous canal at the posterior vertebral body due to the overlying vertebroplasty needle (*arrow*). (**b**) Subsequent cone beam CT image shows the extravasation (*arrow*), which in this case was minor and of no clinical consequence

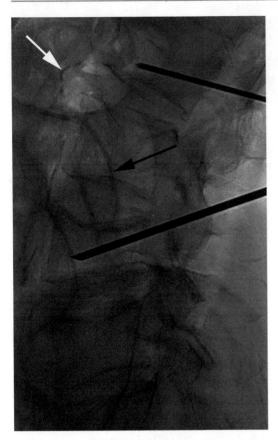

Fig. 8.6 Lateral spine radiograph shows that overlying aortic calcifications (*white arrow*) and bowel gas (*black arrow*) can be mistaken for cement extravasation

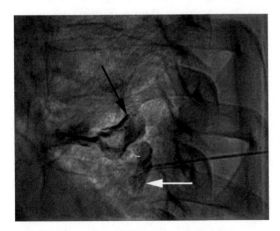

Fig. 8.7 Lateral fluoroscopic image of the thoracic spine shows a narrow crack in continuity with the posterior wall of the vertebral body (*black arrow*) which is rapidly filled with cement during injection. This then extravasated into the spinal canal (*white arrow*)

gauge bone needle with a larger one, risking an iatrogenic fracture.

Finally, the choice of cement kit should be carefully considered. These vary in volume and setting times between manufacturers, and a vendor may provide several volume choices. While waste should be avoided where possible, selecting a kit which is too small can lead to timing problems. The first batch of cement may have set before the second is prepared. It is then no longer possible to inject further cement down the needle. The stylet is likely to become glued in place if replaced into a used needle bore, rendering the needle useless. Operators therefore should avoid beginning to inject cement into any vertebroplasty needle until they are sure that an adequate volume of cement is available. Larger kits are generally desirable when single large quantities of cement are needed, for example, an 11 ml kit in pelvic/acetabular augmentation. However, the use of such a kit in a complex multilevel vertebroplasty may result in the cement being too viscous for effective use by the time the later levels are injected.

8.3   Fluoroscopically-Guided Injections

8.3.1   Recognizing Different Sides of a Joint/Foramen

During facet joint injection, the operator attempts to gain an "end-on" view of the facet joint into which to place the needle. It is important to bear in mind that many of the facet joints have a mild curvature of the articular surface. Therefore, the anteromedial and posterolateral sides of the joints will be visualized at different points of angulation of the image intensifier. This can result in difficulty accessing the joint when the deeper medial side of the joint is mistaken for the superficial lateral side and cortical bone lies between the needle and visualized joint (Fig. 8.8). A similar problem can occur when attempting to access the angulated nerve root foramina in the sacrum. The operator must remember that the deep aspect

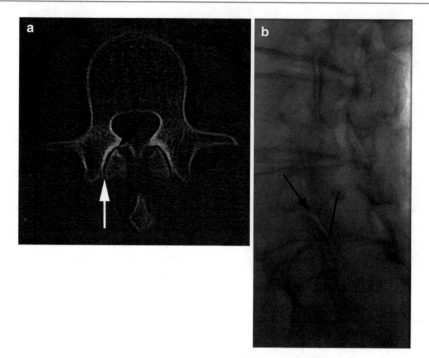

Fig. 8.8 (a) Axial CT image shows the variable angle of the medial (*black arrow*) and lateral aspects (*white arrow*) of the facet joint. (b) Oblique fluoroscopic image shows angulation of the needle to correct for this and enter the facet joint (*black arrow*)

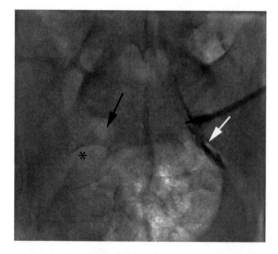

Fig. 8.9 AP fluoroscopic image shows the posteriorly accessible medial aspect of the nerve root foramen (*black arrow*) and the deep lateral aspect covered by the posterior cortex (*). The myelogram (*white arrow*) on the other side shows the course of the nerve root and sacral foramen

lies lateral and superficial and the accessible aspect lies medial. Attempts to access the laterally visualized foramen will encounter the posterior cortex of the sacrum (Fig. 8.9).

8.3.2 Sensitive Periosteum

Care must be taken to avoid contacting the iliac crest during L5 selective nerve root block injection. The sensitivity of the periosteum means that grazing this structure with the needle during attempted access is likely to cause significant discomfort to the patient. Careful identification of this anatomy during intensifier positioning avoids this pitfall.

8.3.3 Segmentation Anomaly During Spinal Injections

Segmentation anomaly will often cause confusion when deciding where to perform a selective nerve root block in the lumbar spine. Where this is being performed to investigate a dermatome-specific pain, the potential for confusion should be explained to the patient and stated in the procedural report. More than one injection performed on different occasions may be required to identify the symptomatic level. Where such an injection is being performed for therapeutic purposes following a previous success, careful review of the prior report and images is required to ensure repetition of the desired result, since different radiologists may describe the anatomy using different nomenclature. Where whole spine images are available, they should be reviewed, since identification and countdown from C2 vertebral level can provide a more definitive numbering system for the levels.

8.4   CT-Guided Bone Tumor Ablation

CT is the modality of choice when performing bone tumor ablation, since it provides sufficient anatomical detail for bone and most soft tissues and allows intra-procedural visualization of the ice ball during cryoablation. However, lack of real-time imaging, limited visualization of smaller soft tissue structures such as nerves, and the need to minimize ionizing radiation exposure can lead to complications.

8.4.1   Slice Thickness

Thicker slices reduce noise and dose but may "miss" the needle tip, making it appear to have retracted or appear to be in a more proximal location than it actually is. In cases where needle movement seems apparent but doubtful, repeating the imaging with thinner slices, e.g., 1 mm versus 3 mm, may reveal the true location.

8.4.2   Limited Scan Range

Only a limited area is typically scanned for each needle movement during placement in order to limit dose. As the tip may fall beyond the limits of the scanned range, the operator should be wary of the needle position when the "tip" appears on the last slice of the series. Range limits can also cause confusion over cranial versus caudal direction due to the limited amount of anatomy on display. Check the CT slice numbers carefully, correlate with the scout guide if available, and

communicate with the CT technologist to avoid directional mishaps, particularly when adjacent to delicate structures.

8.4.3   Needle Retraction During Cryoablation

If a vertebroplasty needle is used as a conduit for a cryoprobe, it must be retracted before performing thermoablation. Failure to do so may lead to thermal conduction along the needle, with unexpected ice ball enlargement and resulting thermal injury to the skin (Fig. 8.10).

8.4.4   Thermal Ablation Zone Boundaries

Manufacturers provide guides as to the size and shape of the expected ablation zones for their equipment. Radiofrequency (RF) ablation zones can be unpredictable and prone to flux with different extents in different tissue types, causing unexpected results. For this reason, the authors favor cryoablation, since the resulting ice balls have more predictable sizes. Virtually all tissue will be ablated at −40 °C

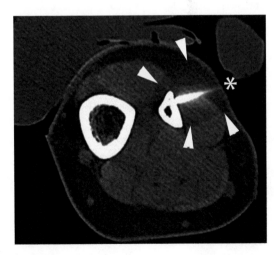

Fig. 8.10 Axial CT image shows a cryoablation probe and overlying vertebroplasty needle *in situ* during the treatment of an osteoid osteoma in the fibula. Failure to retract the vertebroplasty needle resulted in unexpected extension of the ice ball (*arrowheads*) which led to thermal injury to the skin (*asterisk*)

and most at −20 °C. Beyond this, damage level varies. Tissues above 0 °C are generally thought of as being outside the ablation zone; however, caution is advised. Nerves can be damaged at 9 °C and below, so they can theoretically be damaged when "outside" the ablation zone. Hydro-distension with saline is useful to push away these vulnerable structures but should not be used in RF as the electrolytes within provide an electrical conduit.

Conclusion

The benefits of the various musculoskeletal interventions reviewed in this chapter include diagnosis, analgesia, functional improvement, and, in some cases, curative outcomes, making them attractive options for patient care. Awareness of the potential intraoperative pitfalls reduces the risk of patient harm while increasing the likelihood of an effective procedure. Technological advances continue to improve both intraoperative image quality and offer new methods of guidance, such as pre-procedure route planning based on cone beam CT data acquired in the interventional suite. When combined with enhanced operator knowledge of potential errors, this will ensure continued improvement in standards of care in musculoskeletal intervention.

References

Burton AW, Rhines LD, Mendel E (2005) Vertebroplasty and kyphoplasty: a comprehensive review. Neurosurg Focus 18:e1

Chu L, Hawley P, Munk P, Mallinson P, Clarkson P (2015) Minimally invasive palliative procedures in oncology: a review of a multidisciplinary collaboration. Support Care Cancer 23:1589–1596

Klass D, Munk PL (2015) Interventional radiology techniques. In: Peh WCG (ed) Pitfalls in diagnostic radiology. Springer, Berlin/Heidelberg

Layton KF, Thielen KR, Koch CA et al (2007) Vertebroplasty, first 1000 levels of a single center: evaluation of the outcomes and complications. Am J Neuroradiol 28:683–689

Nussbaum DA, Gailloud P, Murphy K (2004) A review of complications associated with vertebroplasty and kyphoplasty as reported to the Food and Drug Administration medical device related web site. J Vasc Interv Radiol 15:1185–1192

Taylor RS, Taylor RJ, Fritzell P (2006) Balloon kyphoplasty and vertebroplasty for vertebral compression fractures: a comparative systematic review of efficacy and safety. Spine 31:2747–2755

Musculoskeletal Biopsy Pitfalls

Mark J. Kransdorf and James S. Jelinek

Contents

9.1   **Introduction** 149

9.2   **History of Musculoskeletal Biopsy** 150
9.2.1   Early Studies Documenting Biopsy
       Complications 150
9.2.2   Recent Studies Documenting Biopsy
       Complications 151

9.3   **Fundamental Biopsy Concepts** 151
9.3.1   Before the Biopsy 151
9.3.2   During the Biopsy 157
9.3.3   After the Biopsy 160

9.4   **Helpful Hints** 162

Conclusion 162

References 162

Abbreviations

CT   Computed tomography
FNA   Fine-needle aspiration
MRI   Magnetic resonance imaging
US   Ultrasound

M.J. Kransdorf, MD, FACR (✉)
Department of Radiology, Mayo Clinic,
5777 East Mayo Boulevard, Phoenix, AZ 85054,
USA
e-mail: kransdorf.mark@mayo.edu

J.S. Jelinek, MD, FACR
Department of Radiology, MedStar Washington
Hospital Center, 110 Irving Street NW,
Washington, DC 20010, USA
e-mail: james.s.jelinek@medstar.net

9.1   Introduction

Image-guided percutaneous biopsy has become the accepted technique for the sampling of a known or suspected musculoskeletal lesion. Although a complete discussion of biopsy techniques is beyond the scope of this text, it is important to emphasize the fundamental concepts which are applicable to the biopsy of musculoskeletal lesions and to highlight the most common pitfalls that may contribute to a less than optimal outcome. This chapter will review the fundamentals of musculoskeletal biopsy that are site independent, emphasizing pre-biopsy planning, biopsy execution, and, finally, post-biopsy follow-up. While there are no absolutes, adherence to simple basic principles will optimize procedure results. In addition, this review will briefly summarize the historical issues associated with the biopsy of musculoskeletal lesions as well as the recent current developments.

It is essential to remember that while image-guided percutaneous biopsy is an extremely safe and accurate procedure, not all lesions or all patients are suitable candidates for this procedure (Fig. 9.1). As emphasized in the American College of Radiology Practice Parameters for the Performance of Image-Guided Percutaneous Needle Biopsy (American College of Radiology 2014), the "...propriety of any specific procedure or course of action must be made by the

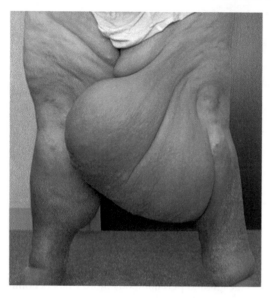

Fig. 9.1 Photograph of a patient who was unable to undergo percutaneous biopsy. Morbidly obese patient estimated to weigh approximately 600 pounds who presented with a slowly-growing soft tissue mass. At the time of his presentation, the patient's weight greatly exceeded the weight limit of all known CT and MRI units. US imaging of the mass was not diagnostic and image-guided biopsy was not possible. Subsequently, the diagnosis of massive localized lymphedema was confirmed surgically

practitioner in light of all the circumstances presented." Although there are no universally applicable techniques, there are general principles which, when followed, will optimize results.

9.2 History of Musculoskeletal Biopsy

The potential hazards associated with the biopsy of musculoskeletal lesions were recognized early on, but the true scope of the problem was not established until the landmark study by Mankin et al. in 1982. Advances in imaging guidance, needle technology, and surgical techniques have markedly improved this situation. Although complications still persist, their character has changed somewhat over the years. A closer look at the history of musculoskeletal biopsy will highlight these changes.

9.2.1 Early Studies Documenting Biopsy Complications

The first study to accurately document the scope of the hazards associated with biopsy of musculoskeletal lesions was based on a survey of members of the Musculoskeletal Tumor Society conducted by Mankin et al. and published in 1982. The authors surveyed 20 Musculoskeletal Tumor Society members at 16 institutions by questionnaire, asking three questions in relation to the efficacy of musculoskeletal tumor biopsy: (1) how accurate was the diagnosis made after biopsy when compared with the so-called definitive diagnosis, (2) what were the complications of the biopsy procedure, and (3) what effect did errors in diagnosis and procedural complications have on the outcome? Mankin et al. (1982) evaluated a total of 329 patients with startling results. Analysis showed major errors in diagnosis in 18.2%, biopsy-related complications in skin, soft tissue or bone in 17.3%, alteration of the optimal treatment plan in 18.2%, unnecessary amputation in 4.5%, and results that adversely affected prognosis and outcome in 8.5%. While the results are quite remarkable, it is important to remember that all patients included in the study had malignant primary bone or soft tissue tumors, required treatment prior to 1979, and were almost all treated by open biopsy. Only 14 (4.3%) of the reported cases were needle biopsies and the guidance for biopsy was not addressed (Mankin et al. 1982).

The authors made several recommendations following their analysis of the results. Many are remarkably still quite appropriate for application to current-day medicine and are summarized (and updated for image-guided procedures) below:

1. Plan the biopsy procedure carefully; as carefully as the definitive surgical procedure.
2. Pay close attention to asepsis, skin preparation, and hemostasis.
3. Place the skin incision or needle in such a manner so as not to compromise a subsequent definitive surgical procedure.
4. Be certain that an adequate amount of representative tissue is obtained.

5. If the surgeon or institution is not equipped to perform accurate diagnostic studies or definitive surgery/treatment, the patient should be referred to a treating center prior to performance of the biopsy.

In 1996, Mankin et al. reported the results of a similar follow-up study with the same objectives as the 1982 study, to determine whether the rates of complications, errors, and deleterious effects related to biopsy had changed. In this new study, there were 597 patients, almost twice as many patients as the initial study, collected from 25 surgeons in 21 institutions. Unfortunately, the results were remarkably similar to those of the original study. Of interest, the accuracy of needle biopsy was compared with that of open incisional or excisional biopsy in this second study. While only 14.2% of patients had needle biopsies, analysis of this subset of patients showed that 40% of needle biopsies were considered nonrepresentative or technically poor, in comparison to 24% of open biopsies (a statistically significant difference). Of greater importance for radiologists was the fact that the rates of altered treatment and altered outcome as a result of needle biopsy were considerably less and statistically significantly lower than those for open biopsy. Although overall analysis showed similar results, the authors did note in their recommendations that while needle biopsy was less accurate than open biopsy, it was associated with fewer complications (Mankin et al. 1996).

9.2.2 Recent Studies Documenting Biopsy Complications

Even prior to the publication of the 1996 follow-up study by Mankin et al., the value of image-guided biopsy was being recognized and evaluated (Fraser-Hill and Renfrew 1992; Fraser-Hill et al. 1992). By the end of the 1990s, percutaneous needle biopsy had established itself as a highly effective technique for the biopsy of musculoskeletal tumors (Ball et al. 1990; Layfield et al. 1993; Dupuy et al. 1998; Yao et al. 1999). A three-year study comparing

the results of computed tomography (CT)-guided biopsy of musculoskeletal neoplasms with the final diagnosis at the time of definitive surgery published in 1998 showed a remarkable accuracy of 93% for needle biopsy and 80% for fine-needle aspiration, with a complication rate for both techniques of less than 1% (Dupuy et al. 1998). A comprehensive 2-year prospective study of the incidence of delayed complications following percutaneous CT-guided biopsy of musculoskeletal bone and soft tissue lesions in 386 patients found no major complications, with only post-procedure fever, pain, bruising, and swelling in 10%, 16%, 16%, and 10%, respectively (Huang et al. 2013). It is of interest that the authors of this 2013 study from a major medical center noted that their results were among the best reported to date and emphasized that "... biopsy of musculoskeletal malignancies is a safe and effective procedure if performed by a team of clinicians, pathologists, and radiologists who possess subspecialty expertise."

9.3 Fundamental Biopsy Concepts

In order to fully avoid pitfalls, it is essential to recognize the basic principles directing the performance of percutaneous biopsy. These were succinctly stated by Mankin et al. in 1982 and are listed in Sect. 9.2.1 above and will not be repeated here. It is convenient to divide potential pitfalls into three separate groups: those associated with preparation for the biopsy, those related to the procedure itself, and those related to follow-up (or more accurately, the absence of follow-up).

9.3.1 Before the Biopsy

Biopsy preparation begins with coordination of the involved physicians. This includes the referring surgeon or clinician and pathologist. While the degree of coordination will vary from case to case, appropriate preparation will minimize unanticipated events.

9.3.1.1 Surgeon or Clinician

Coordination is probably the most important part of any musculoskeletal procedure. As a general rule, it is *absolutely essential* to coordinate with the surgeon who will do the definitive procedure to review the biopsy approach. The traditional teaching for percutaneous or open biopsy has been a strict adherence to a compartmental approach in which the needle path does not transverse any uninvolved anatomic compartments. Anatomic compartments are defined by natural barriers that prevent the spread of tumor (Anderson et al. 1999). These barriers include major fascial septa, periosteum, cortical bone, joint articular cartilage, and joint capsules (Anderson et al. 1999). While this requirement to respect compartmental anatomy has been challenged recently, the compartmental approach is a long accepted dogma in orthopedic oncology, and one is ill-advised to violate it without prior consultation.

In 2012, UyBico et al. reviewed their experience with 363 percutaneous CT-guided needle biopsies of the lower extremities over a 6-year period. All biopsies were done with no direct collaboration with the operating surgeon, and in general, the most direct path was used for the biopsy. For soft tissue lesions, this path was generally the shortest skin-to-lesion distance, whereas for osseous lesions, either the shortest distance or the path to greatest cortical bone loss or soft tissue extension was chosen. Anatomic compartmental boundaries were breached in 13 (3.6%) cases and vital structures (e.g., joints, bursae, neurovascular structures) were violated in 42 cases (11.6%). There was recurrence in 22 of 188 malignant lesions, but no evidence of needle tract seeding or contamination of vital structures. While currently, this is the only study that addresses the use of a non-compartmental approach for the biopsy of musculoskeletal lesions, it provides food for thought that the concern for needle tract seeding is less significant than previously suggested (UyBico et al. 2012).

Despite these study results, caution is still required. As the authors of the above study note, the number of recurrent tumors was small, limiting the ability to definitively evaluate seeding.

Although rare, tumor seeding is a well-recognized phenomenon. It is best documented outside the musculoskeletal system. In a meta-analysis of observational studies, Silva et al. (2008) found that the incidence of needle tract tumor seeding following biopsy of hepatocellular carcinoma was 2.7%. The incidence of seeding in musculoskeletal tumors has not been established. It is likely quite rare, although its existence has been well documented (Davies et al. 1993; Iemsawatdikul et al. 2005; Ofluoglu and Donthineni 2007). It is prudent to take a traditional approach in planning a biopsy. In rare cases, when such an approach is impossible, the study by UyBico et al. (2012) provides support that the adverse consequences previously reported are unlikely.

While the biopsy approach is fundamental to the procedure, determination of the best approach can be problematic for patients referred by medical oncologists, internists, or other nonsurgical specialists. In such cases the results of the biopsy will often determine the patient's treatment; therefore, appropriate planning is critical to ensure optimal care. In the scenario where a patient has a history of a primary malignancy and now is referred for biopsy of one of multiple lesions with similar imaging appearances which are all suspicious for metastatic disease, one can biopsy the most accessible lesion. Patients with a similar history, but only a solitary musculoskeletal lesion, should be approached as if that lesion is a primary tumor. The responsibility to select an appropriate biopsy approach falls to the individual performing the procedure. In such cases, consultation with an orthopedic oncologist for planning the appropriate approach will ensure an optimal result (Fig. 9.2).

9.3.1.2 Pathologist

Coordination with the pathologist is equally as important as consultation with the referring surgeon or clinician. Certain specific diagnoses may require special media. For example, if lymphoma is a diagnostic consideration, biopsy samples may need to be placed in RPMI (Roswell Park Memorial Institute) medium as well as in formalin. RPMI medium is especially suited for cell

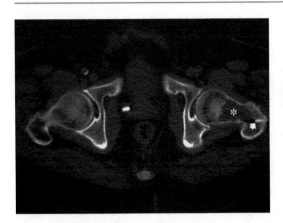

Fig. 9.2 Second malignancy in patient with a history of lung cancer. Axial CT image shows a new osteolytic lesion in the left femoral neck (*asterisk*). Following consultation with an orthopedic oncologist, the biopsy was done with the possibility that the lesion was a primary tumor from a lateral approach (*arrow*). Biopsy revealed clear cell chondrosarcoma

and tissue culture and is used for growth of human lymphoid cells. While practices will vary, many centers find that fine-needle aspiration (FNA) is a useful adjunct to core needle biopsy. Pathologists should be consulted to determine if FNA is appropriate, and if so, will alcohol-fixed slides be sufficient or if air-dried slides are also needed. These can be especially useful in cases in which myeloma or metastatic disease is the prime consideration. All such coordination needs to be completed prior to the procedure.

9.3.1.3 Patient
Pre-procedure laboratory work-up should be ordered and checked and must adhere to the institutional requirements. As a general rule, complete blood count, platelets, prothrombin time (PT), and INR are obtained on all patients. While it is desirable that these are all within normal limits, each case must be evaluated individually. Assessment of patients with abnormal laboratory results should be done in consultation with the referring physician so that the risk of the procedure can be evaluated in the context of its medical necessity.

One must never forget that the patient remains the focus of the procedure. Care must be taken to position the patient in a manner that

allows the planned approach, while ensuring that the patient is comfortable and will be able to maintain that position for the appropriate time anticipated for the procedure. When possible, it is useful to position the patient as they would be positioned during surgery. This facilitates removal of the biopsy track, which is considered contaminated tissue (Aboulafia and Schkrohowsky 2006). When conscious sedation is used, it is prudent to secure the patients' extremities so there will be no movement if they fall asleep.

Many primary bone and soft tissue tumors require multiple cores. Accordingly, we generally recommend moderate (conscious) sedation, although this will vary with the location of the lesion and desires of the patients. Certain specific tumors, such as nerve sheath tumors, can be quite painful, and moderate sedation will optimize both patient comfort and the ability to obtain multiple core samples from different areas of the tumor without undue patient pain.

9.3.1.4 Imaging Review
Review of the pre-procedure imaging is an essential part of biopsy planning. Ideally, this should be done at the time of the initial consultation with the referring surgeon in planning the biopsy approach. It is the responsibility of the radiologist to direct the biopsy to the most aggressive, non-necrotic portion of the tumor. Typically, this is an area that will show the most avid contrast enhancement on magnetic resonance imaging (MRI) (Fig. 9.3), marked hypermetabolic activity on positron-emission tomography (PET) or prominent vascularity on Doppler ultrasound (US) imaging. For osseous lesions, evaluation of radiographic and CT examinations is a useful additional method of identifying the area of greatest biological activity. If adequate pre-procedure images are not available, they should be obtained prior to biopsy.

When reviewing the images to plan the needle approach, one must always plan for "what if..." What if the needle advances further than anticipated? This is critically important in areas such as the skull (Fig. 9.4) or sternum. What

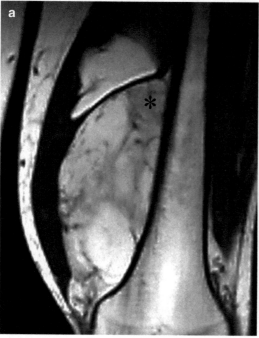

Fig. 9.3 Biopsy site selection. Corresponding coronal (a) T1-W and (b) contrast-enhanced fat-suppressed T1-W images show a predominantly fatty mass with multiple somewhat ill-defined non-adipose areas. Following con-trast agent administration, enhancement is greatest in the proximal aspect of the tumor (*asterisk*). Biopsy of this area revealed atypical lipomatous tumor

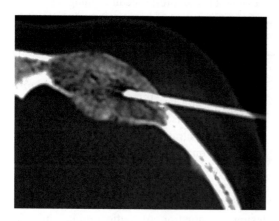

Fig. 9.4 Needle path. CT-guided biopsy of an osteolytic skull lesion which had increased tracer accumulation on bone scintigraphy obtained for staging following diagno-sis of prostate cancer. Note needle path directed to avoid possible injury to brain tissue. Biopsy confirmed inciden-tal hemangioma

vital structures (e.g., nerves, vessels) are adja-cent to the needle path that must be avoided? Addressing these issues in advance will facili-tate the procedure and minimize potential complications.

9.3.1.5 Biopsy Needle Selection

There are a vast number of needles available for both bone and soft tissue biopsies. One size or type is certainly not applicable for all situations. One can only suggest that each individual must find the biopsy systems they are most comfort-able using. In our practice, we stock two coaxial bone biopsy needle systems, one drill system for densely sclerotic osseous lesions, and three coax-ial soft issue biopsy needles. These are available in multiple gauges and lengths.

The diagnosis of metastatic disease and myeloma does not require large cores; in con-trast, primary bone and soft tissue tumors do. Generically speaking, the more hemorrhagic the lesion, the more useful the FNA with a small 22- or 23-gauge needle becomes an adjunct to pro-vide diagnostic tissue samples. For extremely firm and acellular tumors such as fibromatosis or nodular sclerosing Hodgkin lymphoma, large core soft tissue samples can be obtained with a 14- or 16-gauge biopsy systems. In the vast majority of cases, a core sample has greater diag-nostic value than a FNA, increasing yield from

63 to 74% (Hau et al. 2002). However, we routinely do both a fine-needle biopsy and a core biopsy, as both together increase diagnostic yield. In one study, this increased the diagnostic yield of either alone, when compared with both, from 67 to 81% (Ogilvie et al. 2006).

Assessment of lesional vascularity should be part of biopsy planning. Osteolytic lesions, in particular metastatic lesions from primary tumors such as renal cell and thyroid, can be very hypervascular, and for this reason, initial biopsy should be performed with the smallest needle. For hypervascular lesions, this will provide better diagnostic material as well as minimize potential bleeding complications. In contrast, very dense sclerotic lesions may require larger core needles up to 8-gauge size. Such densely sclerotic lesions are often best biopsied using a battery-operated drill (Fig. 9.5). Attempting a biopsy of a densely sclerotic bone lesion with a small-gauge needle is extremely tedious and labor intensive and may result in needle bending or needle fracture. Contrary to previous reports, sclerotic lesions can be readily diagnosed by needle biopsy, provided the proper

needle is used and adequate sample obtained (Leffler and Chew 1999; Jelinek et al. 2002).

9.3.1.6 Special Considerations

While the principles discussed above are valid for both bone and soft tissue lesions, there are certain special considerations for specific types of osseous lesions. This includes lesions that are densely sclerotic or predominantly cystic as well as those involving the "thin" bones such as the rib, fibula, sternum, or skull.

Densely Sclerotic Lesions

With the advent of larger and sharper handheld bone drill tip needles, as well as handheld battery-operated drills, one can now more easily biopsy dense sclerotic lesions (Leffler and Chew 1999). In general, dense sclerotic bone is predominantly less cellular, so that the central portion of sclerotic lesions is not the optimal location for the biopsy; rather, the more peripheral margin of the lesion or an osteolytic component of the lesion should be targeted (Fig. 9.6). Dense sclerotic bone is hard and compact, and whether a large-gauge

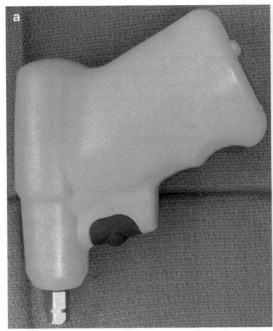
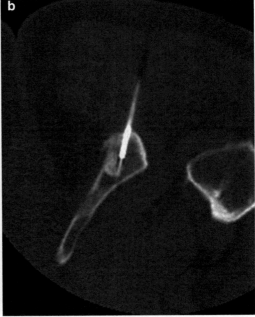

Fig. 9.5 Battery-powered handheld (OnControl, Vidacare Corp) drill. (**a**) Photograph shows a reusable battery-powered drill that can be placed in a sterile bag and utilized with an 11-gauge coaxial biopsy system. (**b**) CT-guided biopsy of new sclerotic lesion in the ischium of patient with a history of prostate cancer. Outer 11-gauge needle is placed at the margin of the sclerotic lesion. The periphery of such lesions are typically (but not invariably) more cellular

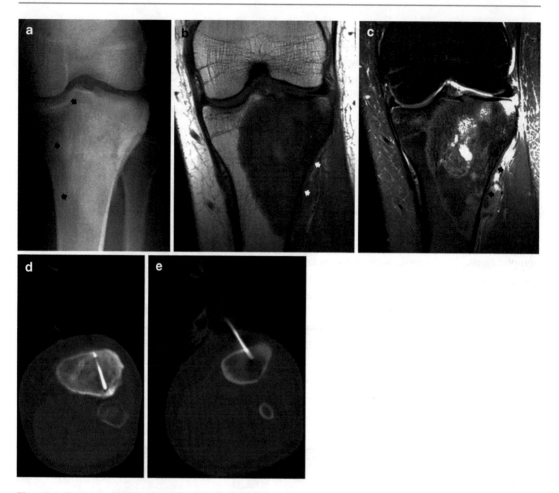

Fig. 9.6 Biopsy of densely sclerotic lesion. (**a**) Radiograph of the proximal tibia shows a predominantly sclerotic lesion in the left proximal tibial metaphysis (*arrows*). Corresponding coronal (**b**) T1-W and (**c**) T2-W MR images show typical features of osteosarcoma. Note predominantly decreased signal due to the dense sclerotic bone as well as subtle lateral periosteal reaction (*arrows*), which was subtly present on the radiograph. (**d**) Axial CT image shows the initial biopsy tract through the superior sclerotic portion of the lesion which had dense osteoid matrix with few low-grade spindle cells. (**e**) Second repeat CT-guided biopsy through the most osteolytic inferior aspect of the tumor closest to the aggressive periosteal reaction and soft tissue extension showed high-grade osteoblastic osteosarcoma

hand needle or power drill is used, the likelihood of the dense sclerotic specimen becoming impacted inside the needle increases with the length of the sample. To avoid this complication, smaller specimen fragments of 3 to 4 mm are preferred rather than those larger than 5 mm.

Cystic Bone Lesions

Cystic bone lesions can be difficult to sample. A large-gauge needle is often required to penetrate the outer cortex in order to enter the lesion. However, it may not be optimal to obtain a satisfactory core of fluid-like or complex cystic contents. In some cases, a soft tissue biopsy needle can be introduced coaxially through the larger bore outer needle to obtain multiple core samples (Fig. 9.7). An additional useful trick for biopsying a cystic or complex bone lesion is to use a much smaller needle in the coaxial approach, for example, using an 18-gauge or smaller needle through a large-gauge introducer. Another advantage to using the smaller coaxial needle is the ability to use it to scrape the osseous margin of a lesion to obtain lining, peripheral cellular material, or possibly osseous fragments from irregular foci of the osseous lesional wall, a process likened to performance of a mini curettage (Jelinek et al. 2002). A small bend can be made in the

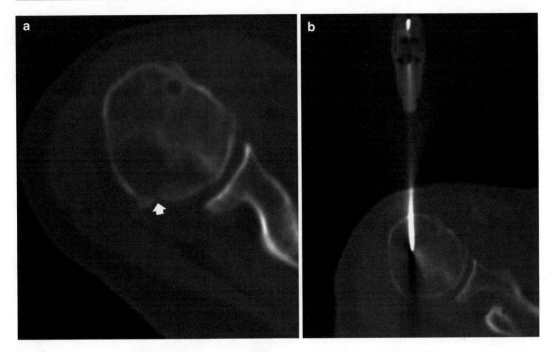

Fig. 9.7 Biopsy of predominantly cystic lesion. (**a**) Axial CT image of the proximal humerus in a patient presenting with shoulder pain shows an osteolytic lesion with posterior pathological fracture (*arrow*) and no associated soft tissue mass. (**b**) CT-guided biopsy was performed through the anterior one-third of the deltoid muscle, as directed by the orthopedic oncologist. An 11-gauge needle was used to penetrate the intact humeral cortex, and initial samples with large-gauge coaxial needle were bloody with no diagnostic material. Additional samples with a coaxial 18-gauge spring-loaded soft tissue needle provided excellent samples, confirming diagnosis of lymphoma

distal aspect of the small-gauge needle to assist in obtaining the optimal positioning.

"Thin" Bone Lesions

Thin bones such as ribs can be safely biopsied (Jakanani and Saifuddin 2013). When biopsying a thin osseous structure such as a rib or sternum, it is often safer to orient the biopsy plane along the long axis of the bone (Fig. 9.4). This will minimize the possibility of inadvertent deep placement of the needle with possible penetration of adjacent more "unforgiving" tissues such as the lung or adjacent neurovascular structure. The same principle applies to a biopsy oriented perpendicular to the sternum or skull, in which deeper penetration can have disastrous consequences.

9.3.2   During the Biopsy

Once committed to perform a biopsy, the overriding goal is to get a representative sample of the tissue in order to allow an accurate diagnosis.

Appropriate planning will usually facilitate sampling at the optimal site, but as with all procedures, sometimes "…best-laid plans of mice and men often go awry…."

9.3.2.1 Sample Site

The target area for the biopsy should be selected during the pre-biopsy planning based on the pre-biopsy imaging. Careful planning increases the diagnostic yield of directed biopsy, and the value of directed biopsies as compared to those without image guidance has been well established (Narvani et al. 2009). Always direct the needle to the area of the most aggressive biological activity as suggested by imaging. As MRI is usually the modality of choice for the diagnosis and local staging of a suspected musculoskeletal tumor, biopsy should be directed to the area of most extensive enhancement. For hypervascular tumors, pre-biopsy enhanced MR (or CT) angiography will identify not only the areas of hypervascularity but feeding and draining vessels. It will also provide superior anatomical detail as to the location of adjacent neurovascular structures (Le et al. 2010).

For hemorrhagic or cystic appearing bone or soft tissue tumors, it may be advisable to perform an unenhanced CT, followed by contrast-enhanced study, at the time of the CT-guided biopsy. In this manner, the most enhancing area of the tumor will be clearly identified and can be appropriately targeted for sampling, avoiding the non-solid components. The number of samples obtained will depend on the type of tumor suspected (primary versus metastatic), as well as its size and location. In general, for primary lesions, at least three or four cores are required.

9.3.2.2 Unanticipated Findings

There are times when, in spite of all the planning, things just do not seem to go right. The needle is exactly in the pre-positioned location, but instead of getting tissue, one gets fluid, blood, or mucoid material.

Fluid

Unexpected fluid of any type, whether it be clear, cloudy, or serosanguineous, should never be discarded. All unexpected fluid should be retained for laboratory analysis. The specific testing will depend on the amount of fluid obtained and the realistic differential for the fluid. The old orthopedic oncology adage of "culture all tumors and biopsy all infections" is still meaningful today.

Just Blood!

When just blood seems to be the only material obtained during a biopsy, that does not necessarily mean the biopsy is nondiagnostic. Focal plasmacytomas and very vascular tumors, for example, may seem to yield just blood. Although biopsy samples appear predominantly bloody, they may still be diagnostic. Sampling an additional site, somewhat remote from the original biopsy site, might also be helpful. In such cases, FNA may be a useful adjunct in providing additional information for the pathologist. If a cytopathologist is not available, the pathology department may be able to provide a cytology technologist to prepare slides from the fine-needle aspirate.

For extremely vascular tumors that have spontaneous bleeding with removal of the trochar from

the outer coaxial biopsy needle, it can be useful to embolize the biopsy site with Gelfoam prior to the completion of the procedure. A larger-diameter needle (14 gauge and larger) can provide access for embolization with Gelfoam pledgets made by rolling small pieces into a thin "torpedo" shape and pushing them into the lesion (Fig. 9.8). This is not practical for smaller needles, and in such cases, a thick slurry of Gelfoam can be made by mixing 1 ml of normal saline with Gelfoam pledgets in two connected small syringes, producing a thick mixture which can be injected directly into the needle. Injected volume should be adjusted for the intensity of the bleeding, location of the needle and possible effect of injected volume. In general, only a small volume of slurry is required.

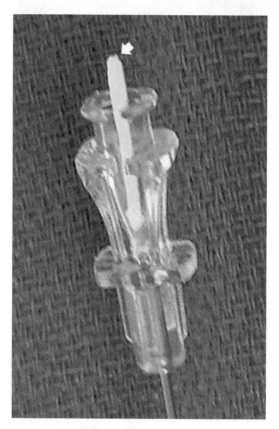

Fig. 9.8 Embolization of biopsy tract for hemorrhagic lesions. Photograph shows Gelfoam pledgets made by rolling thin pieces into a "torpedo" shape (*arrow*). This is not practical for smaller needles. Gelfoam slurry is made by mixing 1 ml of normal saline with Gelfoam pledgets in two connected small syringes. This mixture produces a thick mixture which can be injected directly into the needle. Injected volume should be adjusted for the intensity of the bleeding

These techniques are predominantly for osseous lesions. However, we have occasionally used them in conjunction with soft tissue tumor biopsy. Anecdotally, this likely helps, but in such cases firm direct pressure over the biopsy site is likely the most reliable method for achieving hemostasis.

Mucus

Mucoid material may be difficult to sample, as well as to aspirate. It is common in myxoid tumors which are typically mucus-like in consistency. It is not uncommon in lesions such as myxoid liposarcoma and intramuscular myxoma. Mucoid areas within tumors typically demonstrate hyperintense signal on T2-weighted images and variable enhancement and, as such, may be an unanticipated result at biopsy. When mucoid material is obtained during a biopsy, small quantities should be placed on glass slides and processed as for FNA. Additional material can be placed in forma-lin for pathological evaluation. Depending on the quantity obtained, material can be left in the syringe used for aspiration, capped, and forwarded to pathology. In some cases, sampling of less gelatinous material can be aided by obtaining large core samples. Attention should be focused on trying to obtain the peripheral margins of the tumor without contaminating adjacent compartments.

9.3.2.3 Imaging "Transverse Incision"

Although transverse surgical incisions are ideal for certain types of surgery, they are contraindicated for extremity lesions. Transverse incisions disrupt neurovascular structures and compromise viability of the soft tissue required for coverage following surgery. An equivalent transverse incision can be created during percutaneous biopsy, if a second puncture site is made adjacent to the initial puncture, displaced from it in the transverse plane (Fig. 9.9).

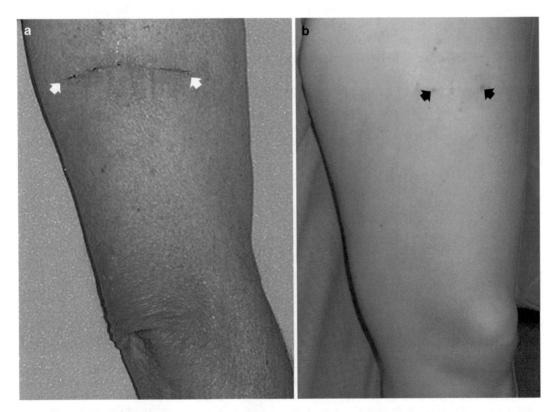

Fig. 9.9 Transverse incision. (**a**) Photograph shows a surgical transverse incision (*arrows*) in the proximal arm. (**b**) Photograph shows a radiological transverse incision (*arrows*) in the thigh. The initial needle biopsy site failed to provide diagnostic tissue, so the puncture site was moved laterally, creating an equivalent "transverse incision"

9.3.2.4 Imaging Documentation

As a general rule, it is accepted practice to document the position of the needle at the time of biopsy. This is easily accomplished during US-guided procedures, as they are done under real-time image guidance. For CT-guided procedures, it is recommended to save images showing the needle tip position. This may be problematic in large patients, when sufficient clearance is not available to allow the patient to move fully into the gantry with the needle in place. In such cases, only the outer coaxial needle position will suffice as appropriate documentation.

9.3.2.5 Ending the Procedure

The procedure is completed when the objectives of the biopsy are met. The true goal of the procedure is not to obtain as large core samples as possible, but to obtain diagnostic tissue. Where possible, it is optimal to have the pathologist review the specimen during the course of the biopsy. This is particularly true when biopsying cystic or hemorrhagic lesions. Large malignant tumors often have a complex morphology with areas of cystic change, necrosis, and hemorrhage. To minimize sampling

errors, it is useful to sample various quadrants of the tumor, rather than obtaining samples from a single location. If a pathologist is not available in the imaging suite for the biopsy, then small core samples can be obtained early in the procedure and sent down to the pathology department to have a pathologist review the specimen to ensure that an adequate sample has been obtained.

Following the procedure, the needle is removed and hemostasis achieved. As a rule, it is not necessary to obtain post-biopsy imaging in all patients. However, it can be useful in specific instances. For example, in cases with prominent bleeding, it may be helpful to identify any hemorrhage at the biopsy site and, if present, to document a baseline size (Fig. 9.10).

9.3.3   After the Biopsy

Review of the biopsy results is an essential component of the procedure. The question one must ask is: "Is the biopsy result consistent with the clinical presentation of the patient and the imaging appearance of the lesion?" If the answer is no,

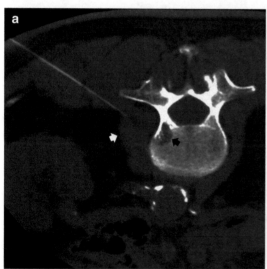
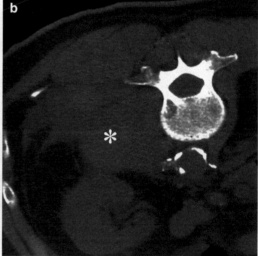
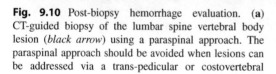

Fig. 9.10 Post-biopsy hemorrhage evaluation. (**a**) CT-guided biopsy of the lumbar spine vertebral body lesion (*black arrow*) using a paraspinal approach. The paraspinal approach should be avoided when lesions can be addressed via a trans-pedicular or costovertebral approach due to the increased vascularity of the paraspinal muscles. A small paraspinal hematoma was identified during the procedure (*white arrow*). (**b**) Repeat CT the following day shows significant enlargement (*asterisk*) of the paraspinal hematoma

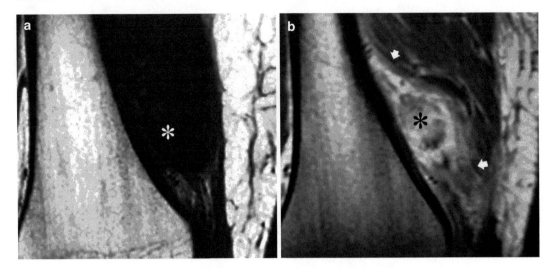

Fig. 9.11 Incomplete communication and misinterpretation of myositis ossificans as osteosarcoma. Corresponding coronal (**a**) T1-W and (**b**) contrast-enhanced fat-suppressed T1-W MR images show a small soft tissue mass (*asterisk*) adjacent to the distal femur. Prominent inflammatory change is noted surrounding the lesion, consistent with early myositis ossificans. There are no changes to suggest in intramedullary, juxtacortical, or soft tissue osteosarcoma. Radiographs (not shown) showed no definitive mineralization

the discrepancy must be resolved. In large institutions, communication among subspecialists may be incomplete; as a result, the pathologist interpreting the case may not be aware of all the case details or the imaging differential. Classic examples are the misinterpretation of myositis ossificans as osteosarcoma (Fig. 9.11), the failure to obtain immunohistochemical evidence of cytokeratin-positive cells in a paucicellular sclerotic metastasis, or interpreting metastatic prostate or breast cancer as reactive bone (Fig. 9.12).

In some specific cases, discussion with the pathologist can change the final diagnosis. The distinction between low-grade chondrosarcoma and enchondroma, or low-grade parosteal osteosarcoma and osteoma of long bone, can be exceedingly difficult; and review of the radiographic features with the pathologist is essential in ensuring an accurate diagnosis. Optimal diagnosis and outcome depends on accurate clinical, pathologic, and radiographic correlation. The radiologist should make sure that the pathologist is aware of the imaging findings and differential diagnosis.

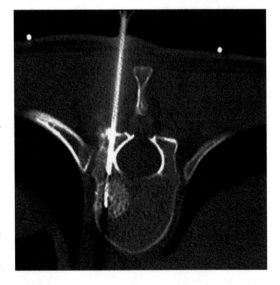

Fig. 9.12 Incomplete communication with history of "suspected bone island" provided to the pathologist rather than the correct history of 26-year-old woman with newly diagnosed breast cancer. CT-guided biopsy of densely sclerotic vertebral spine lesion was performed. Following communication of the suspected diagnosis, immunohistology was performed, revealing cytokeratin-positive cells indicative of metastatic breast cancer

Even under the most optimal circumstances, a false-negative biopsy result is always a possibility. For this reason, a tumor which has been diagnosed on biopsy to have no malignant cells, yet is deemed suspicious by CT or MRI, should not blindly be accepted as benign. Such cases should appropriately be followed, and consultation among all parties (clinician, pathologist, and radiologist) may be helpful in determining the appropriateness of re-biopsy or short-interval follow-up for assessment of tumor stability. Delayed follow-up of the malignant process can have dramatic implications on prognosis. Repeat percutaneous or open biopsies may be required, depending upon the clinical, radiographic, and pathologic correlation of the lesion. Nondiagnostic biopsies are more common with benign lesions, but there is still value in a "nondiagnostic biopsy" as most of these are benign entities (Didolkar et al. 2013).

As radiologists, we are frequently asked to biopsy what appears to be a likely benign lesion. At the time of the initial request, the referring physician should be informed of your differential diagnosis and expectation. When lesional material is required to confirm your expected diagnosis of a benign lesion such as hemangioma, Paget disease, or fibrous dysplasia, it is important to share your suspected diagnosis or differential with the pathologist, so that a firm diagnosis might be obtained rather than "no malignant cells seen." Benign lesion diagnoses are typically difficult to confirm with fine-needle biopsy (Didolkar et al. 2013). With such lesions it is especially important to confirm needle placement so that a follow-up discussion is avoided suggesting the radiologist "missed" the lesion.

9.4 Helpful Hints

We have found the following "hints" to be a useful guide in planning and performing percutaneous biopsy. They are general and applicable to a wide variety of clinical situations:

1. Every biopsy should be planned in detail in consultation with the referring surgeon. This usually occurs while reviewing the images and includes a discussion of the needle path.

2. Always sample the most undifferentiated portion of the tumor. In fatty tumors, for example, place the needle in the dominant non-adipose area. If multiple dominant non-adipose areas are present, PET/CT may be useful to identify the most hypermetabolic focus.

3. It is essential to biopsy viable tissue. This is usually best identified by contrast-enhanced MRI or CT, with biopsy directed to the most extensively enhancing area and avoiding areas of hemorrhage or necrosis.

4. When a request comes from a non-surgeon, determine the objective of the biopsy. If the ultimate goal is diagnosis and referral if "positive," this is a potential for disaster. Biopsy should be done by those who will ultimately do the definitive surgery. Sometimes, the most difficult biopsy is the one you refuse to do.

5. When a patient has a history of previous malignancy and a metastasis is suspected, any solitary lesion should be approached as if it is a primary lesion, until a diagnosis of metastatic disease is confirmed. When such cases are referred from a medical oncologist or primary care physician, a consult with an orthopedic oncologist is important to ensure that the biopsy path will not compromise definitive surgery if the lesion is a primary tumor.

6. For sclerotic lesions, biopsy should be directed to the most osteolytic component of the tumor.

Conclusion

Image-guided percutaneous biopsy is an integral component of the evaluation of suspected musculoskeletal lesion. Adherence to systematic approach to biopsy planning, execution, and follow-up will ensure optimal results.

References

Aboulafia AJ, Schkrohowsky JG (2006) Musculoskeletal tumor biopsy: II. Choosing the appropriate technique. Am J Orthop (Belle Mead NJ) 35:121–124

American College of Radiology (2014) ACR–SIR–SPR practice parameter for the performance of image-guided percutaneous needle biopsy (PNB): https://

www.acr.org/~/media/ACR/Documents/PGTS/guidelines/PNB.pdf

Anderson MW, Temple HT, Dussault RG, Kaplan PA (1999) Compartmental anatomy: relevance to staging and biopsy of musculoskeletal tumors. AJR Am J Roentgenol 173:1663–1671

Ball AB, Fisher C, Pittam M et al (1990) Diagnosis of soft tissue tumours by Tru-cut biopsy. Br J Surg 77:756–758

Davies NM, Livesley PJ, Cannon SR (1993) Recurrence of an osteosarcoma in a needle biopsy track. J Bone Joint Surg Br 75:977–978

Didolkar MM, Anderson ME, Hochman MG et al (2013) Image guided core needle biopsy of musculoskeletal lesions: are nondiagnostic results clinically useful? Clin Orthop Relat Res 471:3601–3609

Dupuy DE, Rosenberg AE, Punyaratabandhu T et al (1998) Accuracy of CT-guided needle biopsy of musculoskeletal neoplasms. AJR Am J Roentgenol 171:759–762

Fraser-Hill MA, Renfrew DL (1992) Percutaneous needle biopsy of musculoskeletal lesions. 1. Effective accuracy and diagnostic utility. AJR Am J Roentgenol 158:809–812

Fraser-Hill MA, Renfrew DL, Hilsenrath PE (1992) Percutaneous needle biopsy of musculoskeletal lesions. 2. Cost-effectiveness. AJR Am J Roentgenol 158:813–818

Hau A, Kim I, Kattapuram S et al (2002) Accuracy of CT-guided biopsies in 359 patients with musculoskeletal lesions. Skeletal Radiol 31:349–353

Huang AJ, Halpern EF, Rosenthal DI (2013) Incidence of delayed complications following percutaneous CT-guided biopsy of bone and soft tissue lesions of the spine and extremities: a 2-year prospective study and analysis of risk factors. Skeletal Radiol 42:61–68

Iemsawatdikul K, Gooding CA, Twomey EL et al (2005) Seeding of osteosarcoma in the biopsy tract of a patient with multifocal osteosarcoma. Pediatr Radiol 35:717–721

Jakanani GC, Saifuddin A (2013) Percutaneous image-guided needle biopsy of rib lesions: a retrospective study of diagnostic outcome in 51 cases. Skeletal Radiol 42:85–90

Jelinek JS, Murphey MD, Welker JA et al (2002) Diagnosis of primary bone tumors with image-guided percutaneous biopsy: experience with 110 tumors. Radiology 223:731–737

Layfield LJ, Armstrong K, Zaleski S, Eckardt J (1993) Diagnostic accuracy and clinical utility of fine-needle aspiration cytology in the diagnosis of clinically primary bone lesions. Diagn Cytopathol 9:168–173

Le HB, Lee ST, Munk PL (2010) Image-guided musculoskeletal biopsies. Semin Interv Radiol 27:191–198

Leffler SG, Chew FS (1999) CT-guided percutaneous biopsy of sclerotic bone lesions: diagnostic yield and accuracy. AJR Am J Roentgenol 172:1389–1392

Mankin HJ, Lange TA, Spanier SS (1982) The hazards of biopsy in patients with malignant primary bone and soft-tissue tumors. J Bone Joint Surg Am 64:1121–1127

Mankin HJ, Mankin CJ, Simon MA (1996) The hazards of the biopsy, revisited. Members of the musculoskeletal tumor society. J Bone Joint Surg Am 78:656–663

Narvani AA, Tsiridis E, Saifuddin A et al (2009) Does image guidance improve accuracy of core needle biopsy in diagnosis of soft tissue tumours? Acta Orthop Belg 75:239–244

Ofluoglu O, Donthineni R (2007) Iatrogenic seeding of a giant cell tumor of the patella to the proximal tibia. Clin Orthop Relat Res 465:260–264

Ogilvie CM, Torbert JT, Finstein JL et al (2006) Clinical utility of percutaneous biopsies of musculoskeletal tumors. Clin Orthop Relat Res 450:95–100

Silva MA, Hegab B, Hyde C et al (2008) Needle track seeding following biopsy of liver lesions in the diagnosis of hepatocellular cancer: a systematic review and meta-analysis. Gut 57:1592–1596

UyBico SJ, Motamedi K, Omura MC et al (2012) Relevance of compartmental anatomic guidelines for biopsy of musculoskeletal tumors: retrospective review of 363 biopsies over a 6-year period. J Vasc Interv Radiol 23:511–518

Yao L, Nelson SD, Seeger LL, Eckardt JJ, Eilber FR (1999) Primary musculoskeletal neoplasms: effectiveness of core-needle biopsy. Radiology 212:682–686

Errors in Radiology

10

Andoni P. Toms

Contents

10.1	**Introduction**	165
10.2	**Prevalence**	167
10.3	**Mechanisms of Visual Perception**	167
10.4	**Errors in Perception**	169
10.5	**External Influences**	172
10.5.1	Fatigue	172
10.5.2	Priming	173
10.5.3	Strain	173
10.5.4	Willpower	174
Conclusion		175
References		175

10.1 Introduction

Error means different things to different people. One of the earliest attempts to define error in medicine was that by Samuel Gorovitz and Alasdair MacIntyre in their 1976 paper "Toward a theory of medical fallibility" (Gorovitz and MacIntyre 1976):

> …where there is scientific activity, there is partial ignorance—the ignorance that exists as a precondition of scientific progress.
>
> (Gorovitz and MacIntyre)

A.P. Toms, BSc, MBBS, PhD, FRCS, FRCR
Radiology Academy, Norfolk and Norwich University Hospital, Cotman Centre, Colney Lane, Norwich, NR4 7UB Norfolk, UK
e-mail: andoni.toms@nnuh.nhs.uk

Gorovitz and MacIntyre (1976) argue that our understanding of medical science and individual patients is always incomplete, and therefore, we are always in a state of partial ignorance when we practice medicine. As individuals, and as a profession, we have some understanding of the extent of our knowledge and expertise. It is not possible to understand the full extent of what we do not know and cannot do:

> There are known knowns. These are things we know that we know. There are known unknowns. That is to say, there are things that we know we don't know. But there are also unknown unknowns. There are things we don't know we don't know.
>
> (Donald Rumsfeld)

This is an essential source of error they term ignorance. It is not a reflection of the medical practitioner but an objective acceptance of the limits of our knowledge. Outside of the limits of medical understanding are other factors that influence the chance of medical error, and these are the good and the bad of human nature, our desire to do good and our desire to be seen to be doing good, our personality, and our physical and mental health:

> … error will arise either from the limitations of the present state of natural science—that is, from ignorance—or from the willfulness or negligence of the natural scientist—that is, from ineptitude.
>
> (Gorovitz and MacIntyre)

These broad categories—ignorance and ineptitude—cover all sources of error. Which of these errors that then become culpable, compensable, or sanctionable depend on the expectations of

© Springer International Publishing AG 2017
W.C.G. Peh (ed.), *Pitfalls in Musculoskeletal Radiology*, DOI 10.1007/978-3-319-53496-1_10

regulatory and legal systems rather than any inherent quality of the error itself (Gorovitz and MacIntyre 1976). In a logical world, we would use those errors that are caused by ignorance to advance the body medical knowledge and those that are caused by ineptitude to advance the performance of the individual medical practitioner.

Having said that, considerable effort has been made, over the past 20 years, to separate ineptitude—the failing of the individual—from failures in the system in which that individual works. This has been popularized as the "person" and the "system" approaches to medical error (Reason 2000). The "person" approach considers error to be caused by "aberrant mental processes such as forgetfulness, inattention, poor motivation, carelessness, negligence, and recklessness." This is a useful approach for medical negligence lawyers seeking compensation for a client; it is easier to bring a case against an individual than it is to sue an institution. It can also be useful for institutions where it may be more convenient to see an individual blamed and punished than it would be to perform detailed analyses of working environments and procedures and then change practice. It is therefore not surprising that this is not conducive to open, frank, and honest analysis of medical error that might then lead to a reduction in the number of patients harmed (Reason 2000).

The argument for attending to the "system" approach is taken from the aviation and other high-risk industries where they recognize that the majority of errors are blameless. In other words, there is no single person at fault for a given error. In these cases, a series of small consecutive failings add up to a significant error, even though each small failing on its own is of little consequence. This now widely recognized as James Reason's Swiss cheese model where each slice of cheese is a safety mechanism blocking the passage of an error. It is only when the holes in each slice line up that the error is made. It is only when every check in a chain of events fails that the system fails.

These system failures can be reduced to a minimum by incorporating open blame-free reporting of all failures into routine working practices. This works in the aviation industry and in the nuclear power industry, where error has catastrophic results but the risk of these errors is very low. The checklist approach to getting it right in these complex high-risk industries can be achieved in medicine and has been popularized in surgery by Atul Gawande where his implementation of aviation style checklists has been adopted by the WHO (Gawande 2011).

Radiologists have acknowledged the truth of these arguments. It is now commonly accepted mandatory practice in the United Kingdom (UK) that discovered errors are reported back to the original reporting radiologist. It is expected that self-directed reflection on these errors is also a mandatory part of the annual appraisal process (The Royal College of Radiologists 2007b). Formal processes for regular anonymized departmental review of discrepancies have been prescribed, and attendance is mandatory (The Royal College of Radiologists 2007a). These are widely considered to be crucial to the good clinical governance of a department of radiology and the best way to learn from our mistakes (Prowse et al. 2014). Despite these good intentions, there is little evidence that the introduction of discrepancy meetings has had an impact on error rates (Bruno et al. 2015). There are a number of reasons why discrepancy meetings might not work to reduce error. The evidence to support the case for discrepancy meetings may not have been gathered robustly, or the changing profile of case mix and technology may not allow us to compare new discrepancy rates with historical data. Or it may be that discrepancy meetings, and the mandatory reporting of discrepancies, do not reduce radiological error rates. As we shall see, there is reason to believe that this last argument may be the case.

As comforting as it might be to a radiologist to attribute an error to a system failure, the truth is that most of our errors belong firmly with the "person," with us as individuals. A very small percentage of errors can be attributed to poor radiographic technique, scheduling errors, uninterpretable clinical details, or other elements of the radiology "system." Most of our errors are errors of perception. They are errors made by every radiologist, however, well trained and maintained. They are the same errors made by all human beings processing visual data. They are errors that result from the strength and weaknesses of the image processing systems that our brains have inherited (Quekel et al. 1999; Donald and Barnard 2012; Berlin 2014).

10.2 Prevalence

Radiological errors are common. The prevalence is derived from estimates that vary for all the usual reasons, such as variation between population samples, imaging techniques, and referral patterns, but error rates of 30% for cases with abnormalities and 4% for mixed caseloads of normal and abnormal studies are generally accepted (Garland 1949; Berlin 2007). As a proportion of an estimated one billion radiological examinations performed worldwide, this translates to a minimum of 40 million errors each year (Bruno et al. 2015). The evidence suggests that these figures have not changed over many years (Stevenson 1969; Berlin 1977; Berlin and Hendrix 1998; Renfrew et al. 1992; Potchen 2006).

As well as making mistakes, we disagree with our colleagues, and with ourselves, about the presence of disease. Interobserver variability for abdominal and pelvic computed tomography (CT) is reported to be higher than 30% in experienced senior radiologists, and intra-observer disagreements can be as high as 25%. These figures suggest that much of the variability is with the individual rather than between observers (Abujudeh et al. 2010). Errors are commonly divided into perceptual—those abnormalities that we miss—and interpretative, the abnormalities we see but misinterpret. Perceptual errors are the most common, accounting for about 60–80% of all errors in radiology (Quekel et al. 1999; Donald and Barnard 2012; Berlin 2014).

Of those perceptual errors, most—two-thirds—are straight misses, with the remaining one-third attributable to satisfaction of search (Kim and Mansfield 2014) (Table 10.1). The satisfaction of search effect can be measured by recording the frequency with which abnormal

Table 10.1 Type and proportion of perceptual errors (Kim and Mansfield 2014)

Error	%
Underreading (missed)	42
Satisfaction of search	22
Faulty reasoning	9
Location	7
Satisfaction of report	6
Prior examination	5

findings are identified in cases with multiple abnormalities. In one study, a single abnormality was identified in 78% of cases, but only 40% of the second and third abnormalities were correctly identified. The logical conclusion is that finding the first abnormality reduces the chances of finding the second (Ashman et al. 2000).

For the rest of this chapter, we will concentrate on the major cause of radiological error, the straight perceptual miss. This is a phenomenon, familiar to all practicing radiologists, that is often accompanied by a feeling of disbelief when presented with an obvious missed scaphoid fracture or Pancoast tumor. And an uncomfortable suspicion that you might not even have looked at the film at all. The following discussion will explain how this happens.

10.3 Mechanisms of Visual Perception

As well as the unexplainable miss, there is another phenomenon, also familiar to the experienced radiologist. This happens the moment you set eyes on an image and you immediately know that something is wrong with it; but you cannot see what that something is. This is an immediate, intuitive, and visceral response to a radiological image. Usually, after a few seconds, an abnormality is found and the problem appears to be solved (Drew et al. 2013b). Is this a real phenomenon? There is evidence that we have selective memory for our successful hunches. In other words, we are better at remembering those gut responses where we have been correct, compared to those where we have been wrong. This selective memory can then reinforce our confidence in our radiological intuition, and this may not be justified (Tversky and Kahneman 1973).

While selective memory may have this effect, there is a substantial and growing body of evidence that humans can extract critical information from scenes in everyday life in the blink of an eye. We can correctly answer certain questions about images of the familiar objects in the world around us after looking at them for as little as 0.025 seconds. We instantly recognize faces we know without having to analyze their features in any systematic way. We immediately recognize when a family member is unhappy by processing subtle facial and behavioral cues, and we do this subconsciously (Fei-Fei et al. 2007; Greene and Oliva 2009). Radiologists can perform similar feats with medical images when they become experts in their field. Human anatomy, as depicted in radiological images with all its normal variations and diseases, becomes as familiar to an expert as other objects and scenes from everyday life. For experienced radiologists, 70% of lesions on chest radiographs are correctly detected within the first 200 milliseconds (Kundel and Nodine 1975).

The speed with which a radiologist can identify an abnormality can be measured using infrared eye-tracking devices. Fitted to the bottom of a monitor, these measure the point of convergence on the screen of the reader's pupils, and they record location and time of the gaze on selected radiological images. The progress from complete novice to expert radiologist can be charted with these techniques. Nonmedical observers demonstrate irrelevant gaze patterns; radiology trainees demonstrate more organized but slow patterns that indicate some knowledge of anatomy and pathology and conscious effort, whereas experts often demonstrate automated and immediate fixation of lesions with more efficient gaze patterns (Kundel and La Follette 1972; Cooper et al. 2009) (Fig. 10.1).

This immediate fixation on an abnormality is too quick to be the result of conscious effort. It is a subconscious and automatic response that can also be described as our instinct or gut feeling for a case. This process, of very rapid detection of anomalies, has now been studied extensively in medical imaging and other settings. The observations about how we perform these automated tasks have been explained as a two-part process. The first part is a nonselective path that informs a second selective pathway (Wolfe et al. 2011). This two-part process has also been described as the global-focal model where an initial global assessment informs, but also restricts, the activity of the subsequent focal pathway (Kundel et al. 1987). The process is too quick to rely entirely on

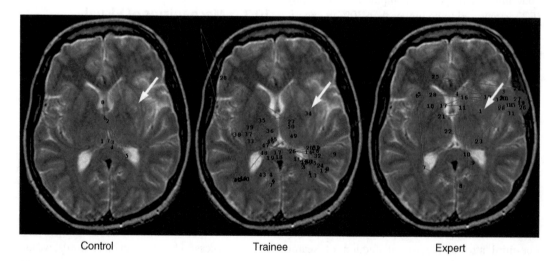

Control   Trainee   Expert

Fig. 10.1 Eye-tracking from nonmedical controls, trainee, and expert radiologists shows evolving ability to detect a small high-intensity lesion in the basal ganglia (*arrow*) on MR images (Reproduced with permission from Cooper et al. 2009)

detailed vision from the fovea and therefore relies on a subtle interaction between the inputs from the fovea and the periphery of the retina (Krupinski 2010). These inputs appear then to be mapped to specific areas of the brain. The parahippocampal cortex is involved in nonselective global scene recognition, and certain parts of the occipitotemporal cortex are used in the recognition of individual objects (Epstein and Kanwisher 1998; Epstein et al. 2003).

The first part of the immediate perception of an image, the nonselective, global, or holistic pathway, is described as that that captures the gestalt or gist of an image. The information obtained is that that leads to assigning the image to a broad category. For example, in an everyday nonmedical situation, this would allow a human to define a scene as urban or rural or a face as male or female. Humans are very good at classifying images into these sorts of broad categories in a fraction of a second but not so good at extracting detailed information in such a short time. While we can reliably tell that a face is female, we may not be able to identify the color of her hair (Greene and Oliva 2009; Joubert et al. 2007).

An example from breast radiology demonstrates this effect. When experienced readers were asked to categorize mammograms as normal or abnormal, after viewing for 500 milliseconds, they were able to do so with reasonable accuracy. They could, more often than not, decide correctly if a mammogram demonstrated a cancer. But when they were asked to localize the lesion into one of four quadrants, they performed poorly. In half a second, their subconscious had enough time to develop the gestalt of an image as either normal or abnormal, but not enough to extract the more specific information about the location of the disease (Drew et al. 2013a).

The importance of this immediate gestalt is that it determines what happens next in that first fraction of a second. The broad category in which we place the image determines how we examine the picture in more detail. In the setting of a psychology laboratory, this is known as contextual cueing. It is a process that is performed subconsciously and probably in part learned subconsciously. It works by influencing which search strategy the brain uses to analyze an image, and it chooses the strategy that is most likely to find the type of lesion most commonly associated with that image (Chun and Jiang 1998).

In a nonmedical setting, this effect can be demonstrated by exposing a research volunteer to a brief glimpse—just 50 milliseconds—of a picture showing a living room. This exposure is too brief for them to be able to describe any detail from the scene. The volunteer is then asked to look for a specific item such as a painting within that scene the next time they are exposed to it (Võ and Henderson 2010). The volunteer will then—too quickly to be the result of conscious action—look to areas of the scene where a painting might be, such as the wall above a fireplace, even if there were no paintings in the original picture. The gestalt of the first exposure has determined the search strategy of the selective or focal phase (Castelhano and Henderson 2007).

The expert radiologist in Fig. 10.1 illustrates this effect. Even without a clinical context, the tissue contrast of the magnetic resonance imaging (MRI) sequence, and the anatomy demonstrated on that single slice, immediately determines a search strategy of the most frequently found lesions in the most frequently involved anatomical locations. In this case, it is a small hyperintense lesion in the basal ganglia (Kundel and La Follette 1972; Kundel et al. 2007; Cooper et al. 2010). While contextual cueing is an effective way of automating subconscious visual search strategies, it has a weakness. The weakness is that while it focuses the visual search, it also restricts it to a limited path and set of expectations. The precise path and expectations are determined by the experience of the reader. This weakness explains one of the more recent, and more infamous, high-profile reports about radiologists' performance.

10.4 Errors in Perception

Trafton Drew's paper entitled "The invisible gorilla strikes again: sustained inattentional blindness in expert observers" was published in

Fig. 10.2 The mainstream media consider why radiologists miss the seemingly obvious dancing gorilla (*arrow*) (Stewart 2013)

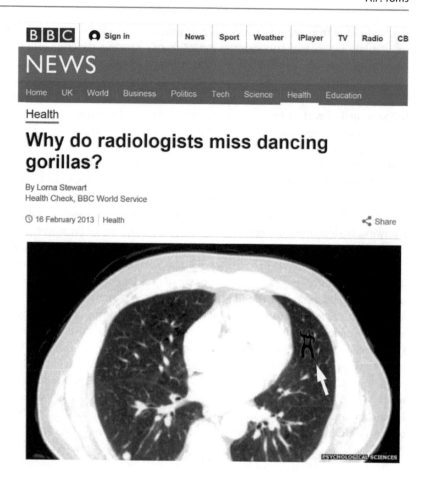

2013 and widely reported in the mainstream media (Fig. 10.2). The strapline was that 80% of radiologists were unable to see a picture of a dancing gorilla pasted onto a CT of the chest and this despite half of the radiologists looking at the gorilla for at least half a second when monitored with eye-tracking equipment (Drew et al. 2013b). Of course the aim of this study was not to denigrate the ability of radiologists, but rather, radiologists were chosen as subjects for study because the nature of their work requires episodes of intense concentration on visual perception tasks. Therefore, radiologists are perfectly suited to studies examining the interplay between different perceptual skills. Professor Daniel Simons, who coauthored the original invisible gorilla study (Chabris and Simons 2010), commented that "Part of the reason that radiologists are so good at what they do is that they are very good at narrowly focusing their attention on these lung nodules. And the cost of that is that they're subject to missing other things, even really obvious large things like a gorilla" (Stewart 2013).

What happens is that the moment that a radiologist sees an axial image through the thorax, set on lung windows, the global assessment of the image triggers the focal search strategy that looks for lung nodules. The search strategy is so narrow that anything that does not fit into the parameters of that strategy is ignored. The result is inattentional blindness, the inability to see an unexpected finding even when it is in plain sight. But is it really blindness? After all, half of the radiologist did look at the gorilla and for about half a second. As we have already discussed, this is much longer than you need to automatically detect abnormalities. Half of the radiologists did see the gorilla, but they denied it, a finding that has also been described in more conventional radiology settings.

In one eye-tracking study, radiologists were asked to look for pulmonary nodules in a set of validated chest radiographs. Seventy percent of all the nodules that were missed by the radiologists—the false negatives—were fixed with a gaze of about 1 s, 40% for 2 s, and 20% for 3 s (Fig. 10.3). And yet when the radiologists were questioned after the study about why they decided not to call the lesion as positive, they denied having seen it (Manning et al. 2004) (Fig. 10.3). Not only do we miss lesions when we have clearly fixed them with our gaze, but we also look at them repeatedly and still miss them (Mallett et al. 2014).

An explanation for this finding—our ability to see an abnormality and then deny we ever did—can be found in the pages of Daniel Kahneman's book *Thinking, Fast and Slow*. This book describes a life's research into the psychology of human judgment and decision-making. In this he divides the brain's functions into two systems: System 1 and System 2 (Table 10.2). System 1 describes the subconscious, effortless, and automatic performance in the first few seconds of a radiologist examining a new case. System 2 is the conscious effort we make to take our observations, the clinical context, the previous radiology, and the expertise of the referrer and create a narrative that responds to the clinical question and ties up all the elements of the case. Kahneman argues that System 1 is always on and easy to use,

whereas System 2 is difficult to rouse and hard work (Kahneman 2011).

Leaving System 1 to process visual data in the form of a series of medical images is fine if, as we have seen, you are an expert in your field, but System 1 has its limitations. It works when the outcomes are obvious, such as "normal wrist radiograph" or "there is a Colles fracture." But when a finding is equivocal, such as "this might be a fracture," then System 1 cannot complete the task on its own. When System 2 is alert and receptive, it will kick in and start a conscious analysis of the radiological findings and make a decision to call the case normal, or a fracture, or sit on the fence and recommend more tests. This analysis and decision-making process requires effort that the brain does not like to expend. Therefore, there is a continuous interplay between System 1 and System 2. System 1 operates for most of the time but calls for help when it cannot

Table 10.2 The features that characterize System 1 and System 2 thinking (Kahneman 2011)

System 1	System 2
Unconscious	Conscious
Intuition	Reasoning
Effortless	Logical
Fast	Effortful
Automatic	Slow
Emotive	Blinkered
Fast	Indecisive

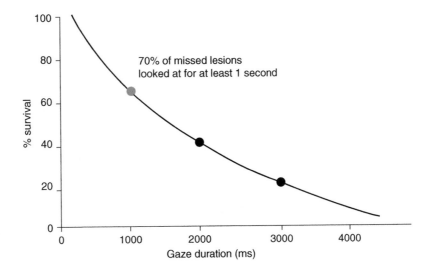

70% of missed lesions looked at for at least 1 second

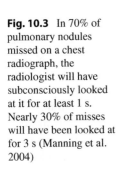

Fig. 10.3 In 70% of pulmonary nodules missed on a chest radiograph, the radiologist will have subconsciously looked at it for at least 1 s. Nearly 30% of misses will have been looked at for 3 s (Manning et al. 2004)

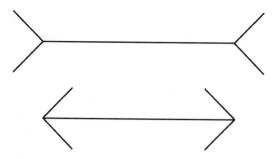

Fig. 10.4 Daniel Kahneman argues that the Müller-Lyer figure illustrates the interplay between System 1 and System 2. Because this optical illusion is so familiar, System 2 tells you that the horizontal lines are the same length. Even so System 1 overwhelms System 2, so that the lines do look as if they are different lengths (Kahneman 2011)

immediately solve the problem. But System 2 does not always respond, and then System 1 solves the problem on its own (Fig. 10.4). It does this by choosing the nearest default position to the problem in question. In a chest radiograph, the default position is that the lungs are normal. If System 1 sees a nodule that does not immediately fall into either the normal or abnormal categories, it calls for help. When it is denied help from System 2, it returns to the default position, i.e., the film is normal. All of this happens in System 1 and therefore, we deny that we have seen anything at all. We have seen the lesion and made a decision about it, all in our subconscious.

The perceptual skill on which this radiological expertise is based is one that is common to all humans and one that is probably widely used to efficiently process the mass of visual data from the world around us. It is apparent that outside the field of radiology, radiologists demonstrate no enhanced powers of image analysis, compared to other people (Nodine and Krupinski 1998). Radiologists have learned to adapt this skill to the analysis of medical images. The question then arises that if we now have some insight into the pathways by which we perceive radiological images, and the process by which we categorize normal from abnormal, and then selectively analyze target areas, can we use this information to enhance the training of radiologists? Indeed there is some early data suggesting that perceptual training with medical images is possible but that

perceptual learning only occurs if feedback is included as part of the learning algorithm (Pauli and Sowden 1997). The power of this perceptual process varies between all humans, and it appears that the perception between radiologists, and between separate reads for the same radiologists, is a fixed entity (Revesz and Kundel 1977; Siegle et al. 1998). However, it is also apparent that there are external influences, some of which we can control, that may allow us to modify our perceptual error rates.

10.5 External Influences

10.5.1 Fatigue

Making difficult decisions is tiring, and making repeated difficult decisions leads to decision fatigue. This effect is nicely illustrated by a study of parole judges in Israel. The judges sat each year to review prisoners' requests for parole, and at the beginning of the day, the chances of being granted early release were about 65%. As the morning progressed, the chances of parole dropped to 0% and then rose back to 60% after a short break. The pattern was repeated until the next break in the working day (Fig. 10.5). The chance of parole was independent of all variables, such as the original length of sentence or race, all except one. The only factor that correlated with a prisoner's chance of release was the time of day that their case was reviewed (Danziger et al. 2011).

The explanation for the judges' behavior is that the process of assessing the suitability of prisoners for parole is an effortful conscious System 2 activity. As the effort is repeated and System 2 tires, then more and more of the decision-making is devolved to System 1. Because these decisions are too complex for System 1, it resorts to the default position. For the judges, the default position is to leave the prisoner's sentence as it is. For radiologists, it is to call the case "normal."

There are two lessons to learn from this. The first is that there is a limit to how many difficult cases we can report back-to-back without increasing the risk of mistakes. A number of radiology

Fig. 10.5 The chances of parole for prisoners, after consideration by a panel of Israeli parole judges, plotted against the time of day (Danziger et al. 2011)

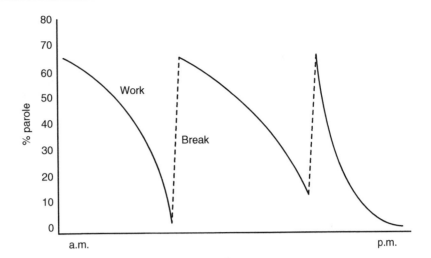

information system (RIS) and picture archiving and communication system (PACS) are starting to address this by incorporating time limits for reporting sessions that force the radiologist to take a break before being allowed to start again. The second lesson is that this break does not have to be a major intervention to return to peak performance. A little food helps but the most important remedy is simply a pause from making repeated judgments. This can take the form of time-out or a change of activity, such as moving from reporting MRI to running an ultrasound list.

10.5.2 Priming

This effect of priming is both subtle and powerful and has long been used by advertisers to sell us things we do not want. For the radiologist, the priming can come in the form of both written and visual stimuli. Psychologists can change the behavior of volunteers by exposing them to simple lists of words masquerading as material in an unrelated psychology experiment. They can elicit aggression and hostility by embedding words associated with rudeness or race. They can make volunteers physically slow down by exposing them to words associated with aging and decrepitude (Bargh et al. 1996).

The clinical history presented with every request for a radiological examination will prime the reader to a given clinical scenario, contributing to the global assessment of the case that determines the search strategy that excludes all other diagnoses. Visual priming is already being used in the airline industry where security workers review hundreds of millions of X-ray images of baggage every year. The chances of finding a serious security threat, such as a gun or a bomb, are so small that each worker knows that most of what they see will not be a threat and therefore System 1 is not alert to the real threat. One company has addressed this by digitally superimposing security threats onto the images that the workers see (Fig. 10.6). The rationale is that seeing these fake threats regularly primes the security teams to recognize the real, but rare, threat when it arrives (Toms 2010).

The same approach could be used in radiology, particularly for uncommon conditions that we often miss, such as Pancoast tumors. A radiologist would know that within a given worklist, there would be a handful of fake cases containing the diagnoses that we most frequently miss. By regularly spotting and missing these, they would be primed to recognize the real cases when they occur.

10.5.3 Strain

Constant interruptions and illegible referrals for imaging examinations are common complaints among radiologists who see these as examples of

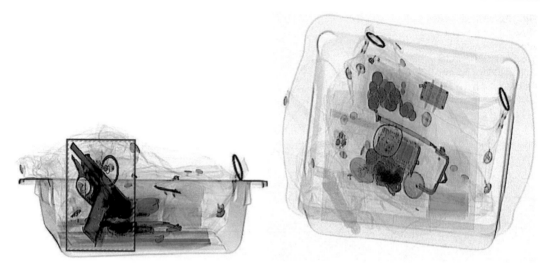

Fig. 10.6 X-ray security image with superimposed handgun used to prime airport security workers (Reproduced with permission from: Toms 2010)

their clinical colleagues conspiring to make the working life of a radiologist more difficult. Evidence from psychologists suggests that, to some degree, the opposite may be true. Shane Frederick's Cognitive Reflection Test is a test that measures the effect of cognitive strain on our ability to use System 2. In other words, what happens to our ability to solve a simple math problem—a cognitive act—when we change the format of the problem by making it more difficult to do. In other words applying strain. Frederick did this by setting questions that could only be answered by using System 2 and then adding cognitive strain by making the typeface of the printed question more difficult to read. 90% of volunteers who saw the normal text made at least one mistake in the attempt to solve the problem, but only 35% of those who could barely read the typeface made a mistake. It appears cognitive strain mobilizes System 2 into action. A bit of low-level irritation makes you work better, but too much and it becomes a distraction (Frederick 2005).

You can also add physical strain to your cognitive action. The standing desks made famous by the likes of Winston Churchill and Donald Rumsfeld have evolved into treadmill desks. These undoubtedly correct the cardiovascular and diabetic risks associated with sitting for long periods of time. However, even though complex

cross-sectional reporting can be performed while walking at a steady 1.5–2 miles per hour, there is no evidence that this physical strain either improves or impedes diagnostic performance (Fidler et al. 2008).

10.5.4 Willpower

In everyday spoken English, the word willpower is not one you hear often. Its meaning is slightly vague and to different people might be the equivalent of self-control, discipline, strength of character, or even "backbone." But to psychologists like Roy Baumeister and John Tierney, it has a specific meaning, and it can be measured and improved (Baumeister and Tierney 2011). The best way to explain their concept of willpower is to describe how they measure it. A volunteer is placed in front of monitor on which flashes the words "Red" or "Blue" in random order. The letters for each word are randomly either red or blue. The subject then has to record the color of the letters as each word appears on the screen. This is a System 2 task. Left to its own devices, System 1 would just read the word on the screen as the answer, but System 2 must overcome this urge, force itself to ignore the meaning of the word, and identify the color of the letters. With repetition, this gets harder and harder. Then, to make the task even more challenging, the researchers play a video of a stand-up comedy performance on a monitor right next to the test screen, for extra distraction.

The measure of the subject's willpower is their ability to correctly identify the color of the letters. In other words, it is the ability of System 2 to perform correctly under cognitive strain. It is your ability to concentrate and ignore distractions. This is a description of the day-to-day activity of a clinical radiologist. Predictably, your willpower fades as you use it but it can be improved with rest and with glucose. Psychologists often use bowls of sweets to achieve rapid rises in blood glucose. Disappointingly, they recommend more complex carbohydrates for sustained fueling of willpower in the real world. They do however suggest that willpower can be trained, like a muscle, to work better and for longer. To study this, volunteers were asked to choose one aspect of their lives over which they were to take more control. These areas included their diet, exercise regimes, their posture, and management of their finances. By following regimes where they exhibited self-control in these areas, the researchers found that the volunteers' measures of willpower also improved. In fact, they found that the self-control in all areas of their lives improved, not just the ones that they had been working on (Oaten and Cheng 2006). This suggests that there is something to be said for the much-derided Victorian ethic of discipline, denial, and self-control.

Conclusion

Most of our radiological mistakes are errors of perception. Many of these errors are the result of unconscious System 1 processes. We do not know that they are happening. These errors happen, and are inevitable, because we are using processing tools that we have inherited from evolution. The way we process visual stimuli has allowed us to flourish in the natural world, but it was not designed to detect disease in radiological images. Therefore we are, as radiologists, necessarily fallible. This limit

of radiology is the ignorance of radiological science that Gorovitz and MacIntyre describe. Differentiating this ignorance from the ineptitude of reporting the wrong radiological image is almost impossible but, unfortunately, that is not a defense in law. Understanding how System 1 and System 2 work gives us insight into what it means to be an expert. While the processes are fixed, we can influence how well they work by using priming effects, paying attention to cognitive strain, mitigating decision fatigue, and exploiting willpower. These elements can inform how we plan our working days, our working environments, and our lives to reduce error in radiology.

References

Abujudeh HH, Boland GW, Kaewlai R et al (2010) Abdominal and pelvic computed tomography (CT) interpretation: discrepancy rates among experienced radiologists. Eur Radiol 20:1952–1957

Ashman CJ, Yu JS, Wolfman D (2000) Satisfaction of search in osteoradiology. AJR Am J Roentgenol 175:541–544

Bargh JA, Chen M, Burrows L (1996) Automaticity of social behavior: direct effects of trait construct and stereotype activation on action. J Pers Soc Psychol 71:230–244

Baumeister RF, Tierney J (2011) Willpower: rediscovering the greatest human strength. Penguin, New York

Berlin L (1977) Does the 'missed' radiographic diagnosis constitute malpractice? Radiology 123:523–527

Berlin L, Hendrix RW (1998) Perceptual errors and negligence. AJR Am J Roentgenol 170:863–867

Berlin L (2007) Radiologic errors and malpractice: a blurry distinction. AJR Am J Roentgenol 189:517–522

Berlin L (2014) Radiologic errors, past, present and future. Diagnosis 1:79–84

Bruno MA, Walker EA, Abujudeh HH (2015) Understanding and confronting our mistakes: the epidemiology of error in radiology and strategies for error reduction. Radiographics 35:1668–1676

Castelhano MS, Henderson JM (2007) Initial scene representations facilitate eye movement guidance in visual search. J Exp Psychol Hum Percept Perform 33:753–763

Chabris C, Simons D (2010) The invisible gorilla: and other ways our intuitions deceive us. Crown, New York

Chun MM, Jiang Y (1998) Contextual cueing: implicit learning and memory of visual context guides spatial attention. Cogn Psychol 36:28–71

Cooper L, Gale A, Darker I et al (2009) Radiology image perception and observer performance: how does expertise and clinical information alter interpretation? Stroke detection explored through eye-tracking. In: Sahiner B, Manning DJ (eds) Medical imaging 2009: image perception, observer performance, and technology assessment. Proc SPIE 7263:2630K

Cooper L, Gale A, Saada J et al (2010) The assessment of stroke multidimensional CT and MR imaging using eye movement analysis: does modality preference enhance observer performance?. In: Manning DJ, Abbey CK (eds) Medical imaging 2010: Image perception, observer performance, and technology assessment. Proc SPIE 7627:76270B

Danziger S, Levav J, Avnaim-Pesso L (2011) Extraneous factors in judicial decisions. Proc Natl Acad Sci 108:6889–6892

Donald JJ, Barnard SA (2012) Common patterns in 558 diagnostic radiology errors. J Med Imaging Radiat Oncol 56:173–178

Drew T, Evans K, Võ MLH et al (2013a) Informatics in radiology: what can you see in a single glance and how might this guide visual search in medical images? Radiographics 33(1):263–274

Drew T, Vo MLH, Wolfe JM (2013b) The invisible gorilla strikes again: sustained inattentional blindness in expert observers. Psychol Sci 24:1848–1853

Epstein R, Kanwisher N (1998) A cortical representation of the local visual environment. Nature 392: 598–601

Epstein R, Graham KS, Downing PE (2003) Viewpoint-specific scene representations in human parahippocampal cortex. Neuron 37:865–876

Fei-Fei L, Iver A, Koch C, Perona P (2007) What do we perceive in a glance of a real-world scene? J Vis 7:10

Fidler JL, MacCarthy RL, Swensen SJ et al (2008) Feasibility of using a walking workstation during CT image interpretation. J Am Coll Radiol 5: 1130–1136

Frederick S (2005) Cognitive reflection and decision making. J Econ Perspect 19:25–42

Garland LH (1949) On the scientific evaluation of diagnostic procedures: presidential address thirty-fourth annual meeting of the Radiological Society of North America. Radiology 52:309–328

Gawande A (2011) The checklist manifesto: how to get things right. Profile, London

Gorovitz S, MacIntyre A (1976) Toward a theory of medical fallibility. J Med Philos 1:51–71

Greene MR, Oliva A (2009) Recognition of natural scenes from global properties: seeing the forest without representing the trees. Cogn Psychol 58:137–176

Joubert OR, Rousselet GA, Fize D, Fabre-Thorpe M (2007) Processing scene context: fast categorization and object interference. Vis Res 47:3286–3297

Kahneman D (2011) Thinking, fast and slow. Farrar, Straus & Giroux/New York

Kim YW, Mansfield LT (2014) Fool me twice: delayed diagnoses in radiology with emphasis on perpetuated errors. AJR Am J Roentgenol 202:465–470

Krupinski EA (2010) Current perspectives in medical image perception. Atten Percept Psychophys 72:1205–1217

Kundel HL, La Follette PS Jr (1972) Visual search patterns and experience with radiological images. Radiology 103:523–528

Kundel HL, Nodine CF (1975) Interpreting chest radiographs without visual search. Radiology 116:527–532

Kundel HL, Nodine CF, Thickman D, Toto L (1987) Searching for lung nodules. A comparison of human performance with random and systematic scanning models. Invest Radiol 22:417–422

Kundel HL, Nodine CF, Conant FF, Weinstein SP (2007) Holistic component of image perception in mammogram interpretation: gaze-tracking study 1. Radiology 242:396–402

Mallett S, Phillips P, Fanshawe TR et al (2014) Tracking eye gaze during interpretation of endoluminal three-dimensional CT colonography: visual perception of experienced and inexperienced readers. Radiology 273:783–792

Manning DJ, Ethell SC, Donovan T (2004) Detection or decision errors? Missed lung cancer from the postero-anterior chest radiograph. Br J Radiol 77:231–235

Nodine CF, Krupinski EA (1998) Perceptual skill, radiology expertise, and visual test performance with NINA and WALDO. Acad Radiol 5:603–612

Oaten M, Cheng K (2006) Improved self-control: the benefits of a regular program of academic study. Basic Appl Soc Psychol 28:1–16

Pauli R, Sowden PT (1997) Role of feedback in learning of screening mammography. Proc Int Soc Opt Engin 3036:205–211

Potchen EJ (2006) Measuring observer performance in chest radiology: some experiences. J Am Coll Radiol 3:423–432

Prowse SJ, Pinkey B, Etherington R (2014) Discrepancies in discrepancy meetings: results of the UK national discrepancy meeting survey. Clin Radiol 69:18–22

Quekel LG, Kessels AG, Goei R, van Engelshoven JM (1999) Miss rate of lung cancer on the chest radiograph in clinical practice. Chest 115:720–724

Reason J (2000) Human error: models and management. Br Med J 320(7237):768–770

Renfrew DL, Franken EA Jr, Berbaum KS et al (1992) Error in radiology: classification and lessons in 182 cases presented at a problem case conference. Radiology 183:145–150

Revesz G, Kundel HL (1977) Psychophysical studies of detection errors in chest radiology. Radiology 123:559–562

Siegle RL, Baram EM, Reuter SR et al (1998) Rates of disagreement in imaging interpretation in a group of community hospitals. Acad Radiol 5:148–154

Stevenson CA (1969) Accuracy of the x-ray report. JAMA 207:1140–1141

Stewart L (2013) Why do radiologists miss dancing gorillas? BBC World Service. Available at: http://www.bbc.co.uk/news/health-21466529. Accessed 27 July 2016

The Royal College of Radiologists (2007a) Standards for radiology discrepancy meetings. The Royal College of Radiologists, London

The Royal College of Radiologists (2007b) Standards for self-assessment of performance. The Royal College of Radiologists, London

Toms AP (2010) The war on terror and radiological error? Clin Radiol 65:666–668

Tversky A, Kahneman D (1973) Availability: a heuristic for judging frequency and probability. Cogn Psychol 5:207–232

Võ ML, Henderson JM (2010) The time course of initial scene processing for eye movement guidance in natural scene search. J Vis 10:14.1–1413

Wolfe JM, Võ ML, Evans KK, Greene MR (2011) Visual search in scenes involves selective and nonselective pathways. Trends Cogn Sci 15:77–84

Part II

Regional and Disease-Based Imaging Pitfalls

Radiographic Normal Variants

11

Mark W. Anderson

Contents

11.1	**Introduction**	181
11.1.1	Identifying a Normal Variant	181
11.2	**Types of Normal Variants**	182
11.2.1	Pseudo-Variants	183
11.2.2	Anatomical Variants	186
11.2.3	Developmental Variants	191
11.2.4	Acquired Variants	196
11.3	**Painful Variants**	198
11.3.1	Spinal	198
11.3.2	Non-spinal	200
11.4	**Variant or Pathology?**	203
Conclusion		204
References		204

11.1 Introduction

Soon after the discovery of X-rays, it became apparent that not everything that looked abnormal on a radiograph was, in fact, pathologic. The term "normal variant" came to be defined as an incidental, usually asymptomatic, imaging finding that simulated true pathology. As the use of diagnostic radiology proliferated in the last century, attempts were made to catalog these variants, and one of the earliest of these, *Borderlands of Normal Variation*, was first published in German in 1910 (Freyschmidt et al. 2003). An updated version is currently available in English, and in 1973, the first edition of the classic text, *Atlas of Normal Roentgen Variants That May Simulate Disease*, was published. This compendium is currently in its ninth edition and has proved to be an invaluable resource for those interpreting radiographs (Keats and Anderson 2013). Because a normal variant often simulates true pathology, it may lead to unnecessary follow-up imaging or intervention. As a result, a basic understanding of these entities is needed to avoid these potential pitfalls. This chapter will attempt to provide just that for the reader, but given the staggering number of variants, this should be considered to be a brief introduction to the topic. Since the vast majority of variants observed on conventional radiographs involve the osseous skeleton, this chapter will concentrate on those entities.

11.1.1 Identifying a Normal Variant

Confirming that an imaging finding is a normal skeletal variant can be challenging. Pathologic proof is rarely acquired, and since these are typically asymptomatic findings, follow-up imaging studies are not often obtained. Certain features can help to differentiate a variant from true pathology.

M.W. Anderson, MD
Department of Radiology, University of Virginia
Health Sciences Center, 1218 Lee Street,
Charlottesville, VA 22908-0170, USA
e-mail: mwa3a@virginia.edu

© Springer International Publishing AG 2017
W.C.G. Peh (ed.), *Pitfalls in Musculoskeletal Radiology*, DOI 10.1007/978-3-319-53496-1_11

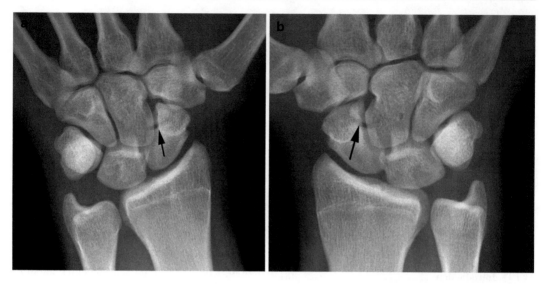

Fig. 11.1 Bilateral ossicles. (**a**) PA radiograph of the left wrist shows a smooth accessory ossicle adjacent to the distal pole the scaphoid (*arrow*). (**b**) PA radiograph of the right wrist shows a symmetrical finding (*arrow*)

A finding that is bilateral and symmetrical is most likely a normal variant (Fig. 11.1). When trying to differentiate a variant from a true fracture, the former will usually demonstrate well-corticated margins (Fig. 11.2), as opposed to an acute fracture in which case the fracture margins are less well defined (although differentiation from an old corticated fracture fragment may be impossible). Other variants can be recognized by their classic location and/or appearance, several of which will be illustrated below. An additional challenge arises in the case of a potential variant found in an area that is clinically painful, and to make things even more confusing, some "normal variants" may become symptomatic. These will be discussed at the end of the chapter along with a few cases illustrating how to determine whether a finding represents a normal variant or true pathology.

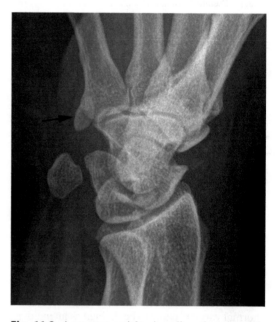

Fig. 11.2 Accessory ossicle. A well-corticated ossicle along the palmar aspect of the hamate (os hamuli proprium) is evident on this oblique radiograph of the wrist (*arrow*)

11.2   Types of Normal Variants

Normal variants can arise from a number of sources. These will be divided into the following categories:

Pseudo-variants – resulting from overlapping anatomical structures or imaging artifacts.
Anatomical variants – related to normal anatomical structures.

Developmental variants – resulting from variability in skeletal development.
Acquired variants – skeletal changes that develop over time.

In each category, spinal and non-spinal examples will be presented.

11.2.1 Pseudo-Variants

Perhaps the most common mimickers of pathology involve "pseudo-variants" that result from either overlapping anatomical structures or technical artifacts. These can occur at any site, so before concluding that a finding is of a pathologic

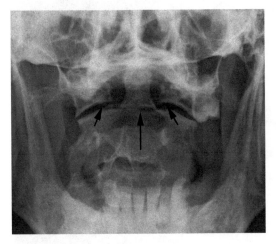

Fig. 11.3 Overlap artifact: pseudo-fracture. A linear lucency at the base of the dens on this open mouth view radiograph (*long arrow*) is the result of an overlap artifact from the posterior arch of the C1 vertebra (*short arrows*)

nature, it is important to consider whether it could be related to this type of pitfall.

11.2.1.1 Spinal

Many overlap artifacts involve the spine. A classic example occurs on an open mouth view radiograph of the cervical spine in which the posterior arch of C1 produces a lucent pseudo-fracture of the base of the dens (Fig. 11.3). Poor patient positioning also may produce artifacts that mimic pathology. A common example of this phenomenon is again seen on the open mouth view radiograph of the cervical spine. Asymmetry in the positions of the lateral masses of C1 vertebra relative to the dens is often related to tilting or rotation of the head rather than true pathology (Lee et al. 1986; Sutherland et al. 1995; Ajmal and O'Rourke 2005; Billmann et al. 2013). A repeat open mouth view radiograph obtained with better head positioning may confirm this, but cross-sectional imaging may be required to completely clear this area (Fig. 11.4).

A pseudo-compression fracture or other artifactual appearance may be produced by the parallax effect of the X-ray beam at the time of image acquisition (Jaremko et al. 2015). This is frequently encountered on a lateral radiograph of the

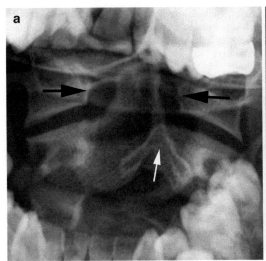
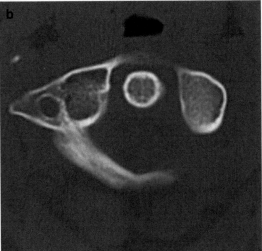

Fig. 11.4 Rotational artifact. (**a**) Open mouth view radiograph of the cervical spine shows asymmetry in the distances between the lateral masses of C1 vertebra (*arrows*) and the dens. Note that the head is rotated as indicated by the lateral position of the C2 spinous process (*small arrow*) and also that the lateral margins of the C1 and C2 lateral masses are well aligned. (**b**) Axial CT image at the level of the dens with the head in neutral position shows normal alignment

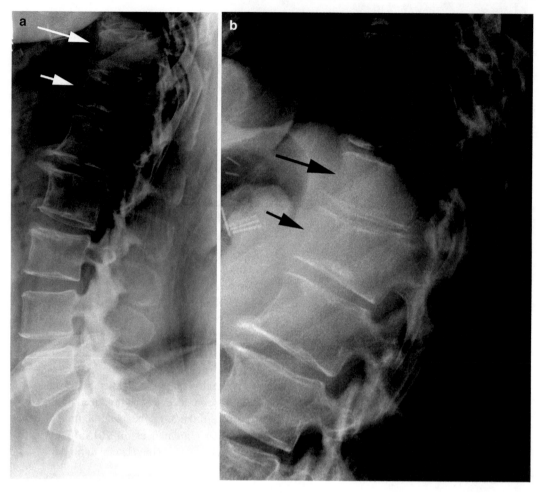

Fig. 11.5 Parallax effect. (**a**) The T11 (*large arrow*) and T12 (*small arrow*) vertebrae appear to be anteriorly wedged on this lateral radiograph of the lumbar spine. (**b**) Lateral radiograph centered at the thoracolumbar junction confirms anterior wedging of T12 (*small arrow*), but there is less prominent deformity of T11 vertebra than initially suspected (*large arrow*). The T12 vertebra was shown to be fractured on a subsequent CT

lumbar spine in which the vertebrae at the thoracolumbar junction, at the upper margin of the image, appear anteriorly wedged. This vertebral distortion occurs because the beam is centered in the mid-lumbar region but diverges with increased distance from this point (parallax) (Fig. 11.5). In these cases, follow-up radiographs centered at the area of interest will usually clarify.

11.2.1.2 Non-spinal

Overlap artifacts may affect any bone (Fig. 11.6). A lucent fat stripe coursing across a bone may mimic a fracture (Fig. 11.7), and overlying bowel gas may be confused with an osteolytic lesion. A normal anatomical structure projected over a bone may produce a similar effect (Fig. 11.8). As in the spine, positioning of the X-ray beam may also produce artifactual distortion of a bone, thereby mimicking pathology (Fig. 11.9). Another imaging artifact that may be problematic is that of the "foreign body" resulting from a contaminated film plate. Imaging plates must be periodically cleaned, or a contaminant may easily mimic a metallic foreign body. In these cases, the abnormality will disappear on subsequent views unless the same plate is used. Even if the same plate is used, the artifact will not overly the same anatomical tissues as on the initial radiograph (Fig. 11.10).

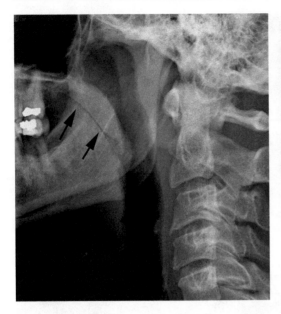

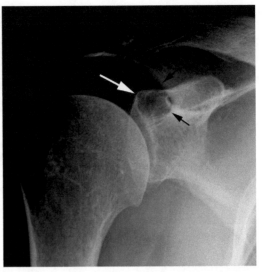

Fig. 11.6 Overlap artifact: pseudo-fracture. An apparent fracture of the mandible on this lateral radiograph of the cervical spine (*arrows*) is the result of air tracking between the soft palate and base of the tongue

Fig. 11.8 Overlap artifact. AP radiograph of the shoulder shows an apparent osteolytic lesion in the superior glenoid (*white arrow*) resulting from overlap of the posterior scapular margin and spinoglenoid notch (*black arrows*). No lesion was found at this site on a subsequent MRI of the shoulder

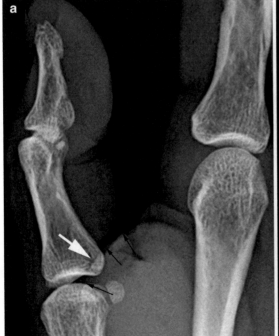

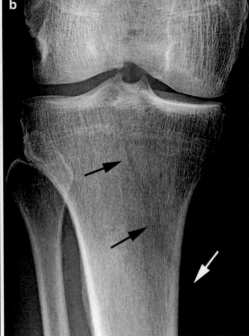

Fig. 11.7 Overlap artifacts: pseudo-fractures. (**a**) A curvilinear lucency simulating a fracture at the base of the first proximal phalanx (*white arrow*) is due to an overlying soft tissue line (*small black arrows*). (**b**) AP radiograph of the proximal tibia shows an oblique linear lucency concerning for a possible fracture (*black arrows*) that is related to a fat stripe in the overlying soft tissues. Note that the lucency continues beyond the medial margin of the bone (*white arrow*)

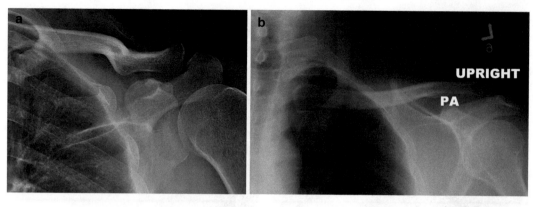

Fig. 11.9 Projectional artifact. (**a**) Radiograph shows apparent deformity of the left clavicle that is related to angulation of the beam at the time of image acquisition. (**b**) Coned-down radiograph from a subsequent chest radiograph shows normal morphology of the clavicle

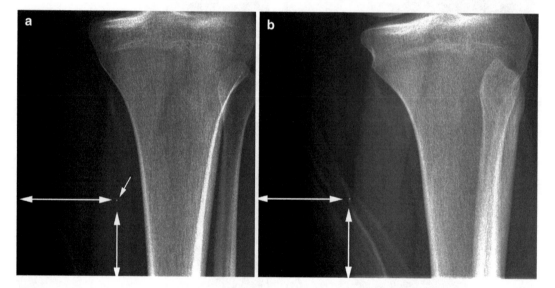

Fig. 11.10 Cassette artifact. (**a**) A punctate metallic density (*small arrow*) suspicious for a foreign body is actually due to a contaminant on the film cassette as evidenced by the fact that it remains in the same location on the cassette on a subsequent (**b**) oblique radiograph

11.2.2 Anatomical Variants

Normal anatomical structures may mimic skeletal pathology.

11.2.2.1 Spinal

It is known that a certain amount of anterior vertebral wedging is commonly seen in asymptomatic patients, especially in the lower thoracic spine (Masharawi et al. 2008; Gaca et al. 2010; Matsumoto et al. 2011). This may be indistinguishable from a compression fracture on radiographs, but an absence of a history of trauma or tenderness in the region suggests a normal variant (Fig. 11.11) (see Sect. 11.4 on "Variant or Pathology?"). Posterior angulation of the dens is another anatomical variant that may mimic a fracture (Fig. 11.12).

11.2.2.2 Non-spinal

In the long bones, penetrating vessels course through nutrient channels that may mimic fractures. These occur at consistent sites and are recognized by their locations as well as the faint sclerosis along their margins. A familiarity with their common locations allows for accurate identification (Fig. 11.13). When seen en face, the radial tuberosity may produce a "lytic" lesion in

Fig. 11.11 Vertebral wedging in a 24-year-old man after rodeo injury. (**a**) Lateral radiograph of the thoracic spine shows mild anterior wedging of T11 vertebra (*arrow*). (**b**) Sagittal STIR MR image shows normal marrow signal intensity and no evidence of vertebral fracture

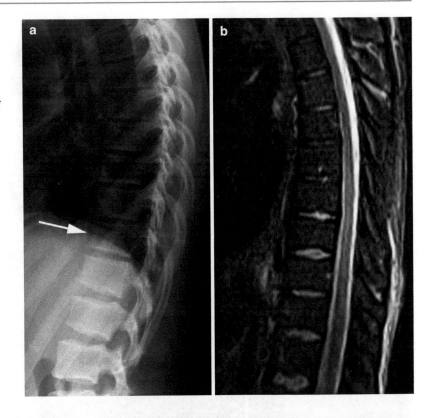

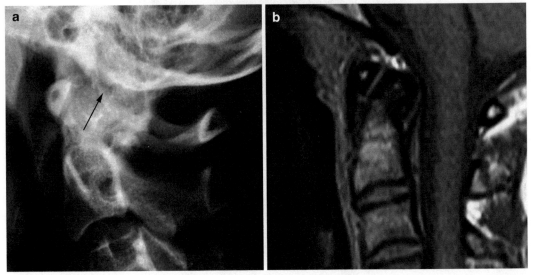

Fig. 11.12 Congenital variant: C2 morphology. (**a**) Lateral radiograph of the upper cervical spine shows posterior inclination of the dens (*arrow*). (**b**) Sagittal MR image shows a similar appearance and no fracture

the proximal radius which can be recognized by its location and absence on a tangential view (Fig. 11.14). A similar finding is commonly observed in the humeral head where a normal paucity of trabecular bone results in a pseudotumor at that site (Helms 1978) (Fig. 11.15).

A sesamoid bone is one that lies within a tendon, the largest of which is the patella. Numerous other sesamoids are located around the body and are most common in the hands and feet (Freyschmidt et al. 2003; Mellado et al. 2003). Given their typical smooth well-corticated margins, these are rarely

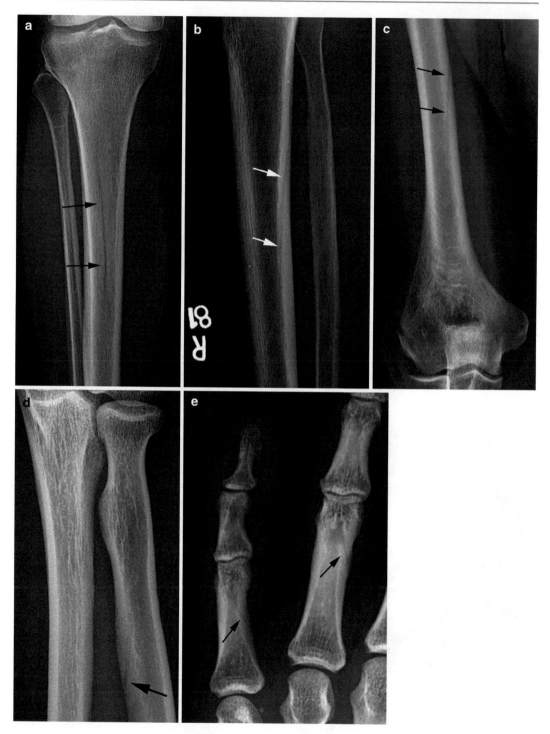

Fig. 11.13 Nutrient channels. (**a**) Vertically oriented lucency in the proximal tibial shaft (*arrows*) concerning for a fracture is shown to be the major nutrient channel traversing the posterior tibial cortex on the lateral radiograph (*arrows* in **b**). There are additional nutrient channels in the (**c**) mid-humerus, (**d**) proximal radius, and (**e**) phalanges

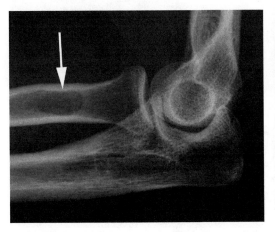

Fig. 11.14 Pseudotumor. Lateral radiograph of the elbow shows an ovoid lucency mimicking an osteolytic lesion (*arrow*) that results from the radial tuberosity seen *en face*

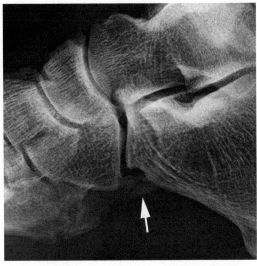

Fig. 11.16 Multipartite ossicle. Lateral radiograph of the foot shows a multipartite os peroneum (*arrow*)

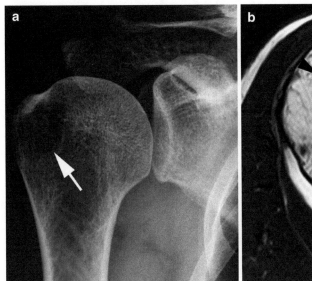
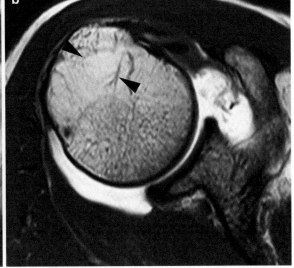

Fig. 11.15 Pseudotumor. (**a**) AP radiograph of the shoulder shows a rounded lucency in the greater tuberosity of the humerus (*arrow*). (**b**) Axial T1-W MR arthrographic image shows a relative lack of trabeculae in that region, accounting for the radiographic appearance (*arrowheads*)

mistaken for an acute fracture. It is, however, common for certain sesamoids to occur in a bipartite or even more multipartite form (Perdikakis et al. 2011) (Fig. 11.16). In these cases, it may be very difficult to differentiate this type of normal variant from an acute or stress-related fracture.

Similarly, numerous accessory ossicles are found throughout the skeleton, and again, these are most common in the hands and feet (Fig. 11.17). An accessory ossicle may simulate a fracture fragment but, like a sesamoid, will usually demonstrate a well-corticated

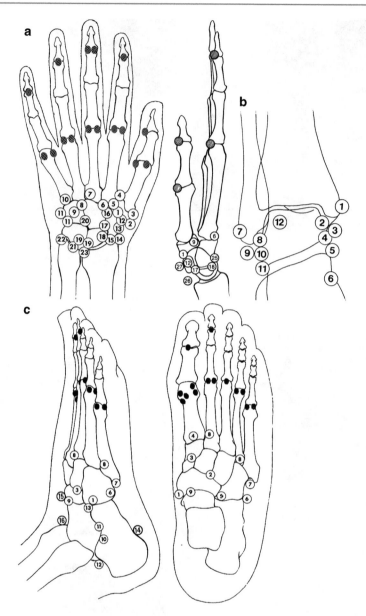

Fig. 11.17 Accessory ossicles. Diagrams of the accessory ossicles of the (**a**) hand, (**b**) ankle, and (**c**) feet. (**a**) *1.* Epitrapezium. *2.* Calcification (bursa, flexor carpi radialis). *3.* Paratrapezium (petrapezium). *4.* Trapezium secundarium. *5.* Trapezoids secundarium. *6.* Os styloideum. *7.* Ossiculum gruberi. *8.* Capitatum secundarium. *9.* Os hamuli proprium. *10.* Os vesalianum. *11.* Os ulnare externum (calcified bursa or tendon). *12.* Os radiale externum. *13.* Fissure of traumatic origin. *14.* Persisting ossification center of the radial styloid process. *15.* Intercalary bone between the navicular and the radius (paranavicular). *16.* Os carpi centrale. *17.* Hypolunatum. *18.* Epilunatum. *19.* Accessory bone between the lunate and the triangular bone. *20.* Epipyramis. *21.* So-called os triangulare. *22.* Persisting center of the ulnar styloid. *23.* Small ossicle at the level of the radioulnar joint. *24.* Avulsion from the triangular bone, no accessory ossicle. *25.* Tendon or bursal calcification. *26.* Calcification of the pisiform. (**b**) *1.* Accompanying shadow on the internal malleolus. *2.* Intercalary bone (or sesamoid) between the internal malleolus and talus. *3.* Os subtibiale. *4.* Talus accessories. *5.* Os sustentaculi. *6.* Os tibiale externum. *7.* Os retinacula. *8.* Intercalary bone (or sesamoid) between the external malleolus and the talus. *9.* Os secundarius. *10.* Talus secundarius. *11.* Os trochleare calcanei. *12.* Os trigonum. (**c**) *1.* Os tibiale externum. *2.* Processus uncinatus. *3.* Os intercuneiforme. *4.* Pars peronea metatarsalia. *5.* Cuboides secundarium. *6.* Os peroneum. *7.* Os vesalianum. *8.* Os intermetatarseum. *9.* Os supratalare. *10.* Talus accessories. *11.* Os sustentaculum. *12.* Os trigonum. *13.* Calcaneus secundarius. *14.* Os subcalcis. *15.* Os supranaviculare. *16.* Os talotibiale (Reproduced with permission from: Keats and Anderson 2013)

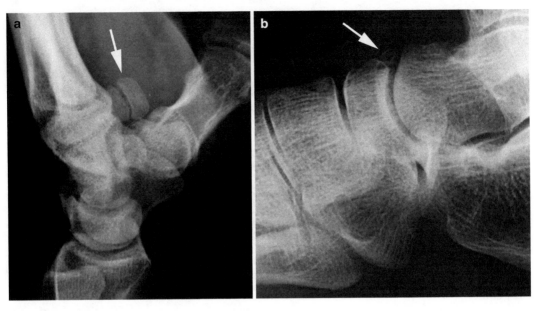

Fig. 11.18 Accessory ossicles. (**a**) Accessory bone (os hamuli proprium, *arrow*) at the tip of the hamate. (**b**) Accessory bone at the dorsal margin of the navicular (os supranaviculare)

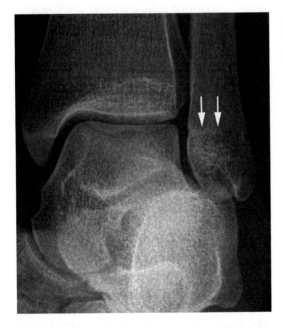

Fig. 11.19 Physeal scar. Mortise view of the ankle shows a sclerotic band (*arrows*) at the site of the fused distal fibular physis, mimicking a stress fracture

mal physis, a sclerotic "scar" is often created which may simulate a stress fracture or cortical injury (Fig. 11.19).

11.2.3 Developmental Variants

Various anomalies of skeletal development may result in radiographic findings that simulate pathology. These often result from a lack of fusion at various apophyses or between ossification centers, but may be due to other processes as well.

11.2.3.1 Spinal

Numerous developmental variants occur in the upper cervical spine, from the skull base through C2 vertebra. A common anomaly involves a lack of fusion in the arch of C1 vertebra (Smoker 1994; Gantopadhyay and Aslam 2003; Doukas and Petridis 2010; Carr et al. 2012). This most commonly occurs in the midline posteriorly, but may involve other parts of the C1 ring and, as such, may mimic a Jefferson burst fracture (Fig. 11.20). Other anomalies in this region include the complete incorporation of C1 verte-

appearance, as opposed to an acute fracture in which case the fracture margins are less well defined (Fig. 11.18). With closure of the nor-

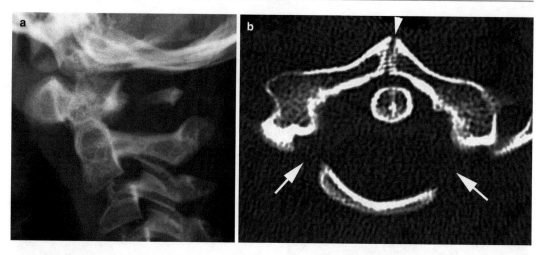

Fig. 11.20 Congenital defects in C1 vertebra. (**a**) Lateral radiograph of the cervical spine shows large defects in the posterior ring of C1 in this 6-year-old girl. (**b**) Axial CT image taken at the same level shows smoothly marginated defects (*arrows*), as well as a midline defect with corticated margins anteriorly (*arrowhead*)

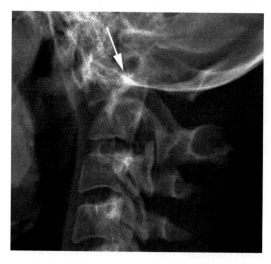

Fig. 11.21 Complete incorporation of C1 vertebra. Lateral radiograph of the craniocervical junction shows complete incorporation of the C1 vertebra into the skull base, with resulting basilar invagination of the dens (*arrow*)

bra into the skull base with associated basilar invagination (Fig. 11.21) or an arcuate foramen ("ponticulus posticus"). This small foramen is formed by a bony bridge along the posterior arch of C1 vertebra through which the vertebral artery passes. It may be complete or incomplete, in which case it may mimic a small fracture fragment in that region (Stubbs 1992) (Fig. 11.22). It may also have rare clinical implications, especially if screw fixation is contemplated in this region (Cushing et al. 2001; Huang and Glaser 2003).

An os odontoideum has been considered to be a normal variant of the C2 vertebra, likely the result of a lack of fusion of the ossification center of the dens at an early age. Others have postulated that it results from a non-united dens fracture (Sankar et al. 2006). Despite the asymptomatic nature of the majority of these ossicles, they can be associated with spinal instability at this level and result in significant neurologic injuries, after even minor trauma (Dai et al. 2000; Arvan et al. 2010; Zhang et al. 2010). As such, active flexion/extension radiographs are often obtained when this "variant" is discovered and if there are neurologic symptoms, magnetic resonance imaging (MRI) is used to evaluate for cord pathology (Fig. 11.23).

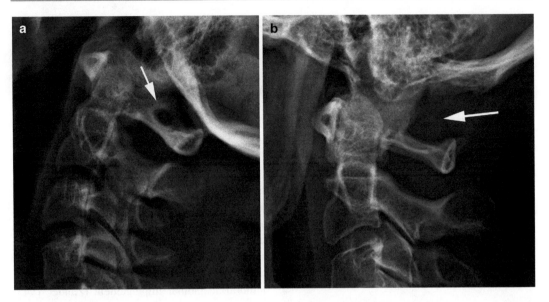

Fig. 11.22 Arcuate foramen. (**a**) Lateral radiograph of the upper cervical spine shows a complete arcuate foramen (*arrow*) of C1 vertebra. (**b**) Lateral radiograph in a different patient shows a partial arcuate foramen mimicking a fracture fragment (*arrow*)

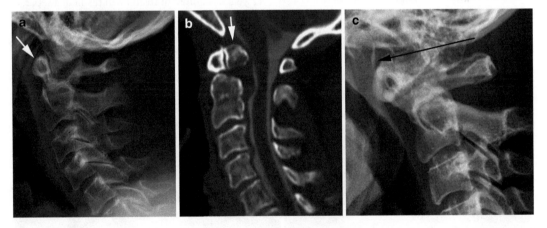

Fig. 11.23 Os odontoideum. (**a**) Lateral radiograph of the cervical spine shows apparent deformity of the dens and hypertrophy of the anterior arch of C1 vertebra (*arrow*). (**b**) Sagittal reconstructed CT myelogram image shows the large os odontoideum (*arrow*) and the associated spinal canal compromise at that level. (**c**) Lateral radiograph obtained in flexion shows anterior displacement of C1 relative to C2 vertebra (*arrow*), indicating associated instability

A lack of fusion between vertebral ossification centers may occur at any level in the spine. Spina bifida occulta refers to a lack of midline fusion in the posterior arch of a vertebra and is very commonly found at the S1 level where it is typically asymptomatic (Fidas et al. 1987) (Fig. 11.24). This may be observed at other vertebral levels (Fig. 11.25), and more unusual forms may involve a lamina or even a pedicle. Non-united transverse processes are often observed at the thoracolumbar junction and are differentiated from a fracture by their corticated margins (Fig. 11.26).

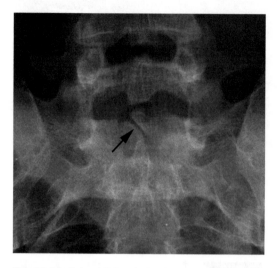

Fig. 11.24 Spina bifida occulta. Spina bifida occulta at S1 segment (*arrow*). Note the smooth corticated margins of the defect

11.2.3.2 Non-spinal

The os acromiale is the apophysis that develops along the anterior margin of the acromion, best seen on an axillary view radiograph. This is a normal finding up until about the age of 25 years when it typically closes. Failure of closure will lead to a persistent apophysis at this site which may mimic a fracture (Sammarco 2000) (Fig. 11.27). The acetabulum develops from numerous ossification centers which typically fuse at 18–24 years of age. An ossific fragment adjacent to the superolateral acetabulum, known as an "os acetabulum," may result from an unfused ossicle or, in some cases, an un-united fracture of the acetabular rim. While these are often quite small, larger ones may contribute to femoral acetabular impingement (Zander 1943; Nguyen et al. 2013) (Fig. 11.28).

The patella also develops from several ossification centers which usually fuse by the age of 12 years. A failure of fusion will result in a separate ossification center that may mimic a fracture fragment (Oohashi et al. 2010). This most commonly involves the upper outer quadrant of the patella

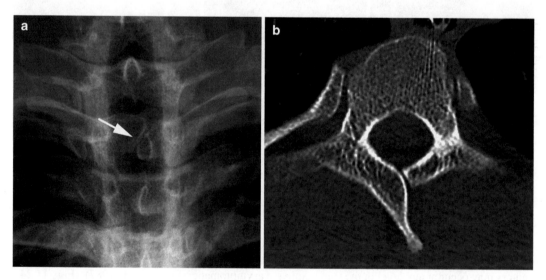

Fig. 11.25 Spina bifida occulta. (**a**) AP radiograph of the upper thoracic spine shows a spina bifida occulta at T2 vertebra (*arrow*), which is also seen on the (**b**) corresponding axial CT image

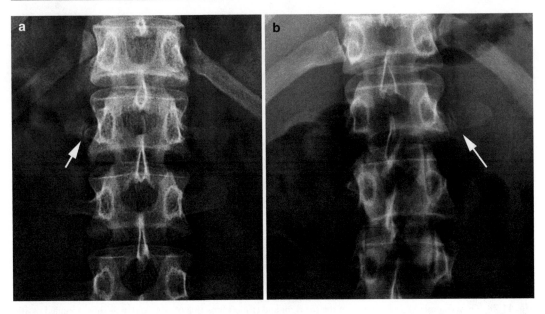

Fig. 11.26 Non-united transverse process. (**a**) Non-united right transverse process at L1 vertebra (*arrow*). Note the sclerotic margins. (**b**) Another example of a non-united left transverse process in a different patient

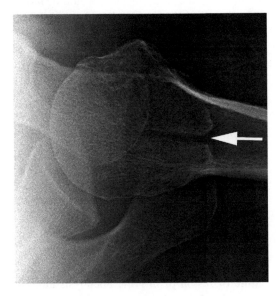

Fig. 11.27 Os acromiale. Axillary view radiograph of the shoulder shows an os acromiale in a 54-year-old man (*arrow*)

(Fig. 11.29). It is present in both knees in up to 50% of cases and is easily recognized by its typical location and well-corticated margins (Kavanagh et al. 2007). A dorsal defect of the patella, another variant that affects the upper outer portion of the patella, may also result from abnormal fusion of the patellar ossification centers (Van Holsbeeck et al. 1987). It appears radiographically as a rounded smoothly marginated lucency in that region (Fig. 11.30a). When viewed on MRI, the smooth defect is typically covered with normal articular cartilage (Ho et al. 1991) (Fig. 11.30b).

An extremely common variant is the bipartite hallux sesamoid (Fig.11.31). This affects the medial hallux sesamoid much more commonly than the lateral, and certain imaging findings have been found to help differentiate this variant from a fracture. As with other variants, the margins of a bipartite sesamoid are

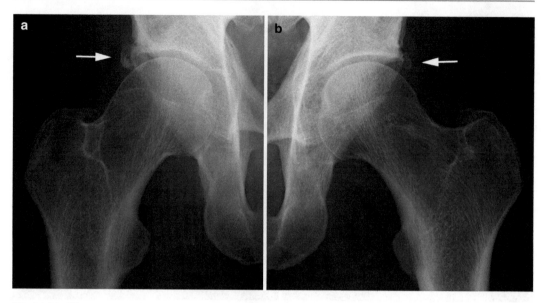

Fig. 11.28 Os acetabuli. AP radiographs of the (**a**) right and (**b**) left hips in a 68-year-old man show rounded ossific densities (os acetabuli) along the superolateral acetabular margins (*arrows*)

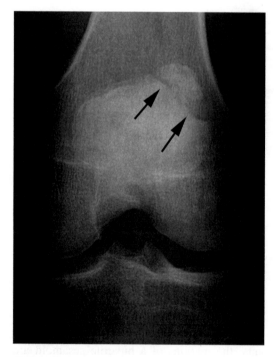

Fig. 11.29 Bipartite patella. AP radiograph of the knee shows a bipartite patella (*arrows*)

usually well corticated, and the margins of a fractured sesamoid will appear to "fit together" whereas those of a bipartite would not. Also,

when both parts of a bipartite sesamoid are "combined," the resulting bone would be larger than the lateral sesamoid (Mellado et al. 2003; Anwar et al. 2005).

11.2.4 Acquired Variants

11.2.4.1 Spinal

A Schmorl node is a common variant found in up to 72% of asymptomatic individuals (Pfirrmann and Resnick 2001; Dar et al. 2010). These "nodes" result from herniation of intervertebral disk material into an adjacent vertebral endplate and are seen as subcortical lucencies on radiographs, usually with sclerotic borders, and are better demonstrated on cross-sectional imaging (Fig. 11.32). A limbus vertebra results from a failure of fusion of the ring apophysis along a vertebral endplate due to intervening disk material that herniates beneath the ring during adolescence. This produces a triangular-shaped ossific density that may mimic a fracture, typically along the anterior superior vertebral endplate, although these can occur posteriorly as well (Henales et al. 1993; Swishchuk et al. 1998) (Fig. 11.33).

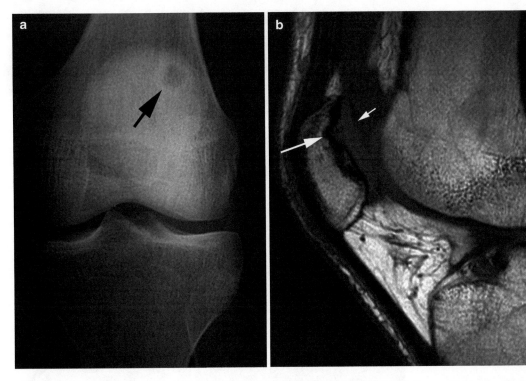

Fig. 11.30 Dorsal defect of the patella. (**a**) AP radiograph of the knee shows a rounded lucency in the superolateral aspect of the patella (*arrow*) compatible with a dorsal defect. (**b**) Corresponding sagittal proton density MR image shows the defect (*large arrow*) and intact overlying cartilage (*small arrow*)

11.2.4.2 Non-spinal

Certain "normal variants" result from acquired conditions. One of the most common is that of a "tug" lesion which produces bone proliferation related to avulsive forces at a tendon attachment. This can occur at any site but is commonly observed at the insertion of the deltoid tendon along the midshaft of the humerus (Fig. 11.34). This may simulate periosteal reaction or even an expansile lesion on radiographs. Other common sites where this occurs include the attachment of the pectoralis major tendon along the proximal humerus, the insertion of the gluteus maximus along the posterior margin of the proximal femur, the linea aspera (the ridge-like structure along the posterior femoral shaft where numerous muscles originate), and the

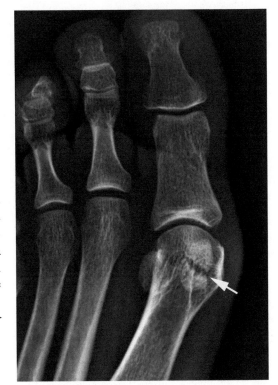

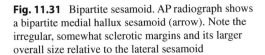

Fig. 11.31 Bipartite sesamoid. AP radiograph shows a bipartite medial hallux sesamoid (arrow). Note the irregular, somewhat sclerotic margins and its larger overall size relative to the lateral sesamoid

Fig. 11.32 Schmorl nodes. (**a**) Lateral radiograph of the lumbar spine shows numerous Schmorl nodes (*arrows*) shown to better advantage on a corresponding (**b**) sagittal T1-W MR image

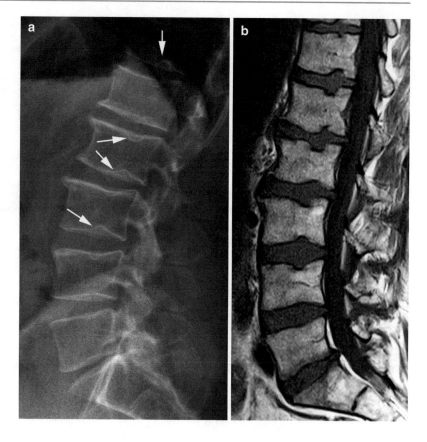

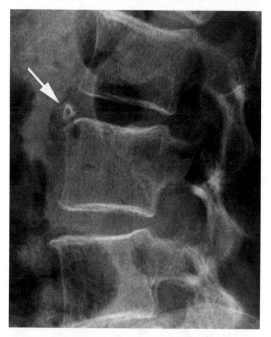

Fig. 11.33 Limbus vertebra. Lateral radiograph of the lumbar spine shows a small, well-corticated limbus vertebra (*arrow*)

origin of the soleus muscle along the posterior proximal tibia (Hoeffel et al. 1993; Gheorghiu and Leinekkugel 2010) (Fig. 11.35).

11.3 Painful Variants

Although most skeletal variants are asymptomatic, some may produce pain and account for a patient's symptoms (Lawson 1994). It is important to be familiar with the most common of these, so as to include this possibility in the imaging report when one of these is identified.

11.3.1 Spinal

While the vast majority of Schmorl nodes are asymptomatic, these endplate herniations may occur acutely and result in back pain in that region. An "acute" Schmorl node cannot be diagnosed radiographically but is suggested when

Fig. 11.34 Deltoid insertion. (**a**) AP radiograph of the humerus shows prominent corticoperiosteal thickening along its lateral midshaft at the insertion site of the deltoid. (**b**) Coronal T1-W MR image shows the humeral finding (*arrow*) as well as the deltoid muscle (*D*)

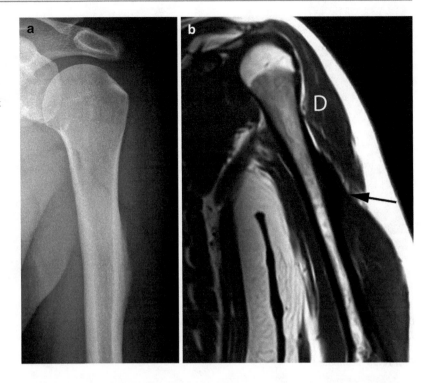

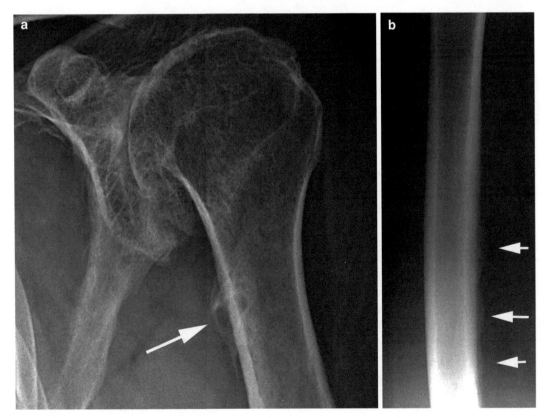

Fig. 11.35 Bone proliferation at tendon attachments. Radiographs show (**a**) proliferative ossification at the pectoralis major insertion along the proximal humeral shaft (*arrow*), (**b**) along the posterior femoral shaft (linea aspera – *arrows*), and at the site of the tibial attachment of the soleus muscle on both (**c**) lateral and (**d**) AP radiographs (*arrows*)

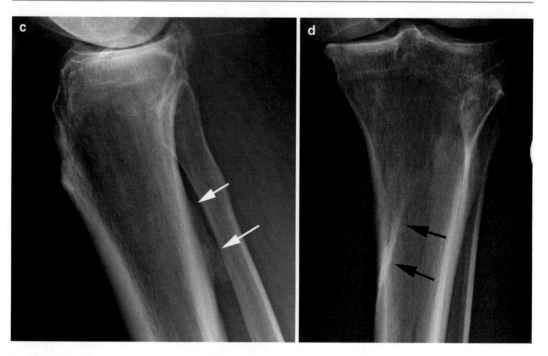

Fig. 11.35 (continued)

extensive edema-like signal intensity and enhancement is observed in the adjacent marrow on MRI (Walters et al. 1991; Stabler et al. 1997; Wagner et al. 2000) (Fig. 11.36).

11.3.2 Non-spinal

As discussed above, a bipartite patella results from a lack of fusion between patellar ossification centers, producing a separate fragment, typically along its superolateral aspect. While this is typically asymptomatic, it may be a source of pain, possibly owing to instability and/or motion along the synchondrosis in some cases from direct trauma. Marrow edema along its margins is often seen in those patients in which this is the source of their pain (Kavanagh et al. 2007) (Fig. 11.37).

While a variety of variants may produce pain, some of the accessory ossicles are among the most common to do so. The accessory navicular is a common accessory bone found along the medial aspect of the tarsal navicular. Three types have been described: type 1, the ossicle lies within the distal posterior tibial tendon; type 2, the ossicle is separate from, but in close proximity to, the navicular where it forms a synchondrosis; and type 3, an enlarged tubercle at the site of the tendon insertion along the medial navicular, also known as a "cornu-ate" navicular (Bernaerts et al. 2004) (Fig. 11.38). Types 2 and 3 have been reported as the most common to be associated with pain ("accessory navicular syndrome"). MRI can be useful for diagnosis by demonstrating the associated marrow edema commonly encountered in these patients (Miller et al. 1995; Mosel et al. 2004). Another ossicle that may be a source of pain is the os trigonum along the posterior ankle, where it produces the "os trigonum syndrome" (Karasick and Schweitzer 1996; Nault et al. 2014) (Fig. 11.39).

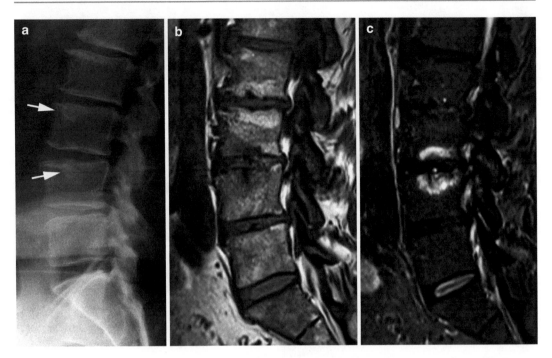

Fig. 11.36 Acute Schmorl nodes. (**a**) Lateral radiograph of the lumbar spine shows typical Schmorl nodes in a 64-year-old man (*arrows*). These are also seen on the (**b**) corresponding sagittal T1-W MR image. These were not present on the MRI from 2 years earlier. (**c**) Sagittal STIR MR image shows prominent focal marrow edema surrounding the nodes at the L3–4 vertebral level, suggesting these are of an acute nature

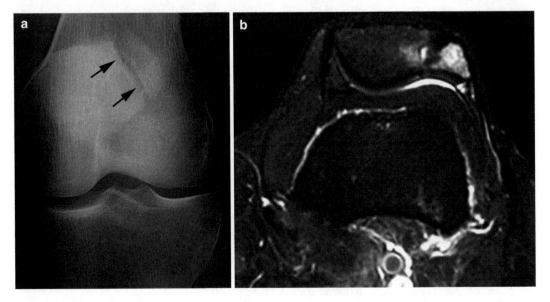

Fig. 11.37 Painful bipartite patella. (**a**) AP radiograph of the knee shows a bipartite patella (*arrows*), while (**b**) corresponding axial fat-suppressed T2-W MR image shows prominent edema within the ossicle and adjacent patella

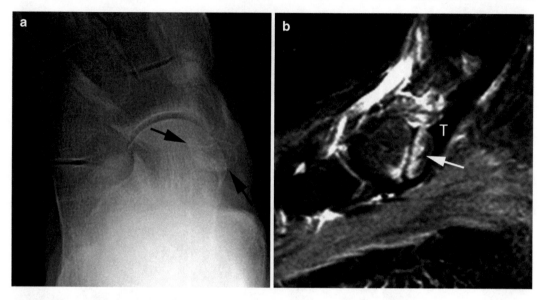

Fig. 11.38 Accessory navicular syndrome. (**a**) Oblique radiograph of the foot shows a large accessory navicular bone (*arrows*). (**b**) Sagittal STIR MR image shows a type 2 accessory navicular within the distal posterior tibial tendon (*T*), as well as edema within it and the adjacent navicular (*arrow*)

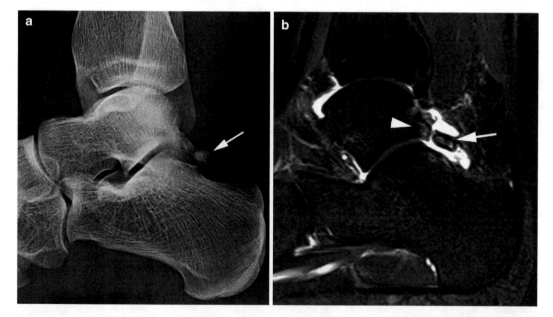

Fig. 11.39 Os trigonum syndrome. (**a**) Lateral radiograph of the hindfoot shows an os trigonum (*arrow*) in this dancer with posterior ankle pain. (**b**) Corresponding sagittal fat-suppressed T2-W MR image shows marrow edema within the ossicle (*arrow*) and adjacent talus (*arrowhead*)

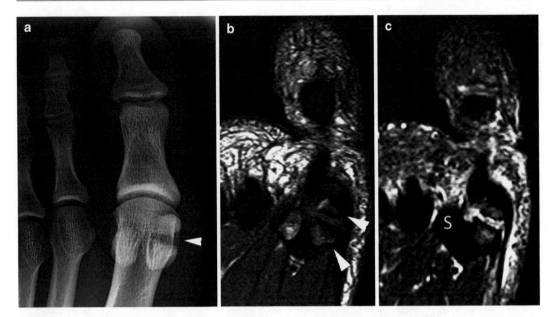

Fig. 11.40 Symptomatic hallux sesamoid. (**a**) AP radiograph of the great toe in a 19-year-old runner who presented with forefoot pain shows a bipartite medial hallux sesamoid with apparently increased distance between its two segments (*arrowhead*). (**b**) Long-axis T1-W MR image shows mildly decreased signal intensity within the marrow of these segments (*arrowheads*) and (**c**) corresponding long-axis STIR MR image confirms hyperintense edema in these regions compatible with injury. Note the normal signal hypointensity within the lateral sesamoid (*S*)

The hallux sesamoids may become painful due to stress injury or osteonecrosis, despite appearing normal on radiographs. As with other types of painful variants, MRI demonstrates abnormal marrow signal intensity in these cases (Karasick and Schweitzer 1998; Anwar et al. 2005) (Fig. 11.40). Similarly, the os peroneum, another sesamoid which lies within the peroneus longus tendon, may result in lateral forefoot pain, producing what is known as the painful os peroneum syndrome ("POPS") (Sobel et al. 1994; Wang et al. 2005).

11.4 Variant or Pathology?

The determination of whether a finding is simply an asymptomatic variant or a source of the patient's symptoms is usually impossible based on radiographic findings alone, but there are principles that will help make this differentiation. Correlation with clinical findings is essential, and if there are symptoms in that region, further imaging is usually warranted. In most cases, MRI will provide the most useful information in this scenario, but other modalities may be more appropriate. As an example, anterior vertebral wedging is a common asymptomatic variant that is often observed in the lower thoracic spine. However, a traumatic or insufficiency fracture may present with an identical appearance. As such, if the clinical examination reveals pain in this region, further evaluation with MRI can differentiate a variant from true pathology by demonstrating the marrow edema associated with an acute injury (Fig. 11.41).

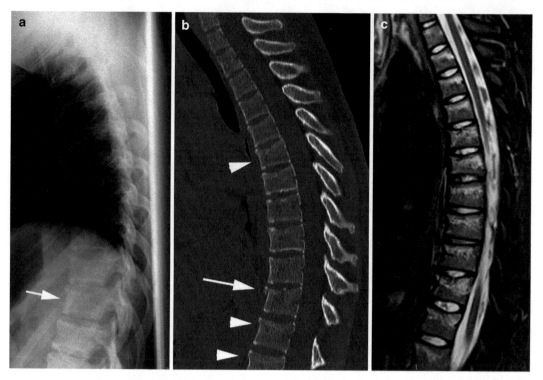

Fig. 11.41 (a) Lateral radiograph of the thoracic spine in an 18-year-old woman obtained after trauma shows anterior wedging of the T12 vertebra (*arrow*). Other vertebrae appear mildly wedged as well but were difficult to evaluate due to technique. (**b**) Sagittal reconstructed CT image confirms an acute fracture at T12 (*arrow*) and probably at T7, L1, and L2 vertebrae as well (*arrowheads*). (**c**) However, corresponding sagittal STIR MR image shows fracture-related edema at virtually all thoracic levels

Conclusion

Given the ubiquitous nature of skeletal variation, a solid understanding of commonly encountered normal radiographic variants is essential to avoid mistaking one for true pathology. Similarly, familiarity with those "normal" variants that are known to occasionally become symptomatic is essential to help direct further work-up when the clinical findings are suggestive. Since an exhaustive treatment of this topic beyond the scope of this chapter, familiarity with some of the more comprehensive texts on this subject is indispensable!

References

Ajmal M, O'Rourke SK (2005) Odontoid lateral mass interval (OLMI) asymmetry and rotary subluxation: a retrospective study in cervical spine injury. J Surg Orthop Adv 14:23–26

Anwar R, Anjum SN, Nicholl JE (2005) Sesamoids of the foot. Curr Orthop 19:40–48

Arvan B, Fournier-Gosselin MP, Fehlings MG (2010) Os odontoideum: etiology and surgical management. Neurosurgery 66:A22–A31

Bernaerts A, Vanhoenacker FM, Van de Perre S et al (2004) Accessory navicular bone: not such a normal variant. JBR-BTR 87:250–252

Billmann F, Bokor-Billmann T, Burnett C et al (2013) Occurrence and significance of odontoid lateral mass interspace asymmetry in trauma patients. World J Surg 37:1988–1995

Carr RB, Tozer Fink KR, Gross JA (2012) Imaging of trauma: part 1, pseudotrama of the spine – osseous variants that may simulate injury. AJR Am J Roentgenol 199:1200–1206

Cushing KE, Ramesh V, Gardner-Medwin D et al (2001) Tethering of the vertebral artery in the congenital arcuate foramen of the atlas vertebra: a possible cause of vertebral artery dissection in children. Dev Med Child Neurol 43:491–496

Dai L, Yuan W, Ni B et al (2000) Os odontoideum: etiology diagnosis and management. Surg Neurol 53:106–109

Dar G, Masharawi Y, Peleg S et al (2010) Schmorl's nodes distribution in the human spine and its possible etiology. Eur Spine J 19:670–675

Doukas A, Petridis AK (2010) A case of aplasia of the posterior arch of the atlas mimicking fracture: review of the literature. Clin Anat 23:881–882

Fidas A, McDonald HL, Elton RA et al (1987) Prevalence and patterns of spina bifida occulta in 2707 normal adults. Clin Radiol 38:537–542

Freyschmidt J, Brossmann J, Wiens J, Sternberg A (eds) (2003) Borderlands of normal and early pathological findings in skeletal radiography. Thieme, New York

Gaca AM, Barnhart HX, Bisset GS (2010) Evaluation of wedging of lower thoracic and upper lumbar vertebral bodies in the pediatric population. AJR Am J Roentgenol 194:516–520

Gantopadhyay S, Aslam M (2003) Posterior arch defects of the atlas: significance in trauma and literature review. Eur J Emerg Med 10:238–240

Gheorghiu D, Leinekkugel A (2010) The linea aspera-pilaster complex as a possible cause of confusion with the 'flame sign': a case report. Acta Orthop Traumatol Turc 44:254–256

Helms CA (1978) Pseudocysts of the humerus. AJR Am J Roentgenol 131:287–288

Henales V, Hervas JA, Lopez P et al (1993) Intervertebral disc herniations (limbus vertebrae) in pediatric patients: report of 15 cases. Pediatr Radiol 23:608–610

Ho VB, Kransdorf MJ, Jelinek JS et al (1991) Dorsal defect of the patella: MR feature. J Comput Assist Tomogr 15:474–476

Hoeffel C, Munier G, Hoeffel JC (1993) The femoral linea aspera: radiological pattern. Eur Radiol 3:357–358

Huang MJ, Glaser JA (2003) Complete arcuate foramen precluding C1 lateral mass screw fixation in a patient with rheumatoid arthritis: case report. Iowa Orthop J 23:96–99

Jaremko JL, Siminoski K, Firth GB et al (2015) Common normal variants of pediatric vertebral development that mimic fractures: a pictorial review from a national longitudinal bone health study. Pediatr Radiol 454:593–605

Karasick D, Schweitzer ME (1996) The os trigonum syndrome: imaging features. AJR Am J Roentgenol 166:125–129

Karasick D, Schweitzer ME (1998) Disorders of the hallux sesamoid complex: MR features. Skeletal Radiol 24:411–418

Kavanagh EC, Zoga A, Omar I et al (2007) MRI findings in bipartite patella. Skeletal Radiol 36:209–214

Keats TE, Anderson MW (eds) (2013) Atlas of normal roentgen variants that may simulate disease, 9th edn. Philadelphia, Elsevier

Lawson JP (1994) Clinically significant radiologic anatomic variants of the skeleton. AJR Am J Roentgenol 163:249–255

Lee S, Joyce S, Seeger J (1986) Asymmetry of the odontoid-lateral mass interspaces: a radiographic finding of questionable clinical significance. Ann Emerg Med 15:1173–1176

Masharawi Y, Salame K, Mirovsky Y et al (2008) Vertebral body shape variation in the thoracic spine: characterization of its asymmetry and wedging. Clin Anat 21:46–54

Matsumoto M, Okada E, Kaneko Y et al (2011) Wedging of vertebral bodies at the thoracolumbar junction in asymptomatic healthy subjects on magnetic resonance imaging. Surg Radiol Anat 33:223–228

Mellado JM, Ramos A, Salvado E et al (2003) Accessory ossicles and sesamoid bones of the ankle and foot: imaging findings, clinical significance and differential diagnosis. Eur Radiol 13:L164–L177

Miller TT, Staron RB, Feldman F et al (1995) The symptomatic accessory tarsal navicular bone: assessment with MR imaging. Radiology 195:849–853

Mosel LD, Kat E, Voyvodic F (2004) Imaging of the symptomatic type II accessory navicular bone. Australas Radiol 48:267–271

Nault M-L, Kocher MS, MIcheli LJ (2014) Os trigonum syndrome. J Am Acad Orthop Surg 22:545–553

Nguyen MS, Kheyfits V, Giordano BD et al (2013) Hip anatomic variants that may mimic pathologic entities on MRI: nonlabral variants. AJR Am J Roentgenol 201:W401–W408

Oohashi Y, Koshino T, Oohashi Y (2010) Clinical features and classification of bipartite or tripartite patella. Knee Surg Sports Traumatol Arthrosc 18:1465–1469

Perdikakis E, Grigoraki E, Karantanas A (2011) Os naviculare: the multi-ossicle configuration of a normal variant. Skeletal Radiol 40:85–88

Pfirrmann CW, Resnick D (2001) Schmorl nodes of the thoracic and lumbar spine: radiographic-pathologic study of prevalence, characterization, and correlation with degenerative changes of 1,650 spinal levels in 100 cadavers. Radiology 219:368–374

Sammarco VJ (2000) Os acromiale: frequency, anatomy, and clinical implications. J Bone Joint Surg Am 82:394–400

Sankar WN, Wills BPD, Dormans JP et al (2006) Os odontoideum revisited: the case for a multifactorial etiology. Spine 31:979–984

Smoker WRK (1994) Craniovertebral junction: normal anatomy, craniometry, and congenital anomalies. Radiographics 14:255–277

Sobel M, Pavlov H, Geppert MJ et al (1994) Painful os peroneum syndrome: a spectrum of conditions responsible for plantar lateral foot pain. Foot Ankle Int 15:112–124

Stabler A, Belian M, Weiss M et al (1997) MR imaging of enhancing intraosseous disk herniation (Schmorl's nodes). AJR Am J Roentgenol 168:933–938

Stubbs DM (1992) The arcuate foramen. Variability in distribution related to race and sex. Spine 17:1502–1504

Sutherland JP, Yaszemski MJ, White AA (1995) Radiographic appearance of the odontoid lateral mass interspace in the occiptoatlantoaxial complex. Spine 20:2221–2225

Swishchuk LE, John SD, Allbery S (1998) Disk degenerative disease in childhood: Scheuermann's disease, Schmorl's nodes, and the limbus vertebra: MRI findings in 12 patients. Pediatr Radiol 28:334–338

Van Holsbeeck M, Vandamme B, Marchal G et al (1987) Dorsal defect of the patella: concept of its origin and relationship with bipartite and multipartite patella. Skeletal Radiol 16:304–311

Wagner AL, Murtagh FR, Arrington JA et al (2000) Relationship of Schmorl's nodes to vertebral body endplate fractures and acute endplate disk extrusions. AJNR Am J Neuroradiol 21:276–281

Walters G, Coumas JM, Akins CM et al (1991) Magnetic resonance imaging of acute symptomatic Schmorl's node formation. Pediatr Emerg Care 7:294–296

Wang XT, Rosenberg ZS, Mechlin MB et al (2005) Normal variants and diseases of the peroneal tendons and superior peroneal retinaculum: MR imaging features. Radiographics 25:587–602

Zander G (1943) Os acetabuli and other bone nuclei; periarticular calcifications at the hip joint. Acta Radiol 24:317–327

Zhang Z, Zhou Y, Wang J et al (2010) Acute traumatic cervical cord injury in patients with os odontoideum. J Clin Neurosci 17:1289–1293

Long Bone Trauma: Radiographic Pitfalls

12

Robert B. Uzor, Johnny U.V. Monu, and Thomas L. Pope

Contents

12.1 **Introduction** 208

12.2 **General Considerations** 208
12.2.1 Errors in Perception and Interpretation 209
12.2.2 Satisfaction of Search 209
12.2.3 Availability of Clinical Information 210

12.3 **Practical Approaches for Combating Errors** 210

12.4 **Radiographic Signs** 211
12.4.1 Atypical Radiographic Signs 211
12.4.2 Avulsion Fractures 211
12.4.3 Stress Fractures 211
12.4.4 Abnormal Underlying Bone 211

12.5 **Shoulder Trauma** 212
12.5.1 Radiographic Examination 212
12.5.2 Commonly Missed Injuries 212

12.6 **Elbow Trauma** 221
12.6.1 Non-displaced Radial Head Fractures 221
12.6.2 Coronoid Process Fractures 221

12.7 **Wrist and Hand Trauma** 222

12.7.1 Distal Radial Fractures 222
12.7.2 Scaphoid Fractures 224
12.7.3 Avulsion Fractures 224
12.7.4 Triquetral Fractures 224
12.7.5 Disorders of Alignment in the Wrist and Carpus 225
12.7.6 Carpal Instability 225
12.7.7 Lunate and Perilunate Injuries 226

12.8 **Finger Trauma** 229

12.9 **Pelvic Trauma** 231

12.10 **Hip and Femoral Neck Trauma** 232

12.11 **Knee Trauma** 234
12.11.1 Avulsions Related to the Distal Femur 234
12.11.2 Segond Fracture 234
12.11.3 Arcuate Complex Avulsion Fracture 235
12.11.4 Patellar Avulsion Fractures 236
12.11.5 Osteochondral Impaction Fracture 236
12.11.6 Stress Fractures 236
12.11.7 Soft Tissues 237
12.11.8 Tibial Plateau Fractures 238

12.12 **Ankle Trauma** 238
12.12.1 Soft Tissue Signs 240
12.12.2 Talar and Peritalar Fractures 242
12.12.3 Anterior Process of Calcaneum Fractures 242
12.12.4 Lateral Process of Talus Fractures 242
12.12.5 Posterior Talar Process Fractures 242
12.12.6 Talar Neck Fractures 244
12.12.7 Osteochondral Injuries 244
12.12.8 Dislocations 245

12.13 **Foot Trauma** 245
12.13.1 Base of Fifth Metatarsal Fractures 246
12.13.2 Lisfranc/Chopart Injury 246
12.13.3 Stress Fractures 249
12.13.4 Calcaneal Fractures 251
12.13.5 Hallux Sesamoid Bones 252

Conclusion 252

References 253

R.B. Uzor, MD, MRCS (✉)
J.U.V. Monu, MBBS, MSc
Department of Imaging Sciences,
University of Rochester,
601 Elmwood Avenue, Rochester, NY 14642, USA
e-mail: Saturn7t@gmail.com;
Johnny_monu@urmc.rochester.edu

T.L. Pope, MD, FACR
Radisphere National Radiology Group,
Candescent Health,
221 Crescent Street, Suite 301,
Waltham, MA 02453, USA
e-mail: tommy.pope@gmail.com

© Springer International Publishing AG 2017
W.C.G. Peh (ed.), *Pitfalls in Musculoskeletal Radiology*, DOI 10.1007/978-3-319-53496-1_12

Abbreviations

CT   Computed tomography

12.1   Introduction

> You only see what you look for; you recognize
> only what you know. Professor Thomas MacRae.

According to Dictionary.com, the definition of "pitfall" is "any trap or danger for the unwary." In the interpretation of all radiographic images, the "trap" or "danger" is likely determined by the level of training, confidence, and experience of the radiologist/imager. Presumably, the more experience and the more images in that subspecialty area that the individual has interpreted, the less "unaware" he/she is and, thus, the less errors are generated in reports. Of course, one has to be willing to study and be willing to learn. The concept of lifelong learning is an excellent one as it encourages (in some cases mandates) an individual to continue to study and learn as he/she progresses through their career. Long bone trauma is commonly encountered in emergent and non-emergent clinical scenarios, and so one should be quite familiar with the lesions with which one is most likely to be confronted. In the long bones, the feet and the hands have many different bones, and attention to all of them can be tough, especially in a busy clinical practice.

In the digital age, however, it is very easy to magnify the images and look closely at all of the visualized bones and soft tissues. This one simple and quick standard practice can minimize the errors in this setting. Unfortunately, most studies show that we as radiologists miss about 25–30% of pathology encountered in our daily practice. However, in the ideal situation, each of us would eventually become as educated and "perfect" as the average commercial pilot who really cannot afford to make one serious error as it has wide-ranging consequences. Fortunately, our daily misses in our practice (at least for most of us) do not have such devastating effects. This chapter will present some of the most common long bone pitfalls encountered in clinical practice and outline some of the clinical and technical clues to help minimize mistakes. The most important role, however, for each of us is to commit to personal professional individual study for our futures to try to achieve that goal of diagnostic perfection.

12.2   General Considerations

Radiography is the first-line imaging modality for evaluating the trauma patient. It is quick, is relatively inexpensive, and detects the majority of traumatic lesions in the appendicular skeleton. The radiologist interpreting trauma radiographs is often faced with the pressures of making rapid and accurate diagnoses in the emergency setting. The impact for the patient of missed injuries may be significant, including the complications of delayed treatment and the risk of exacerbating the underlying injury.

Missed fractures are the second most common reason for litigation in radiology, after missed diagnosis of cancer. In a study of the causes of medical malpractice suits against radiologists in the United States, Wang et al. (2013) identified errors in diagnosis as the most common general cause of malpractice suits, with missed non-spinal fractures coming second only to breast cancer in frequency. Missed orthopedic injuries are also the leading cause of malpractice claims in emergency medicine (Moore 1988). Data shows that extremity fractures occur most frequently in the wrist, elbow, foot, and ankle (Emergency Department Visits 1998–2006). Litigation resulting from missed fractures occurs most commonly in the foot, knee, elbow, hand, and wrist, in order of decreasing frequency (Wei et al. 2006; Baker et al. 2014), while the individual bones most commonly involved in malpractice suits are the tarsal navicular, scaphoid, and calcaneal bones (Baker et al. 2014).

In a systematic analysis of missed extremity fractures in emergency radiology, Wei et al. (2006) detected a 3.7% missed fracture rate overall; however, only a third of these missed fractures were truly imperceptible radiographically.

About two-thirds (64–66%) of the missed fractures in the study were correctly identified on a subsequent radiologist review – with the single most common category of missed fractures being the "subtle but still visible" group. This study suggests that perceptual and interpretative errors are a more significant contributing fracture to missed diagnosis of fractures in radiography than any shortcomings of the modality itself. Other less common cited factors contributing to missed diagnosis of fractures in this study include obscuration by splinting devices, multiplicity of fractures, problems with radiographic technique, lack of relevant clinical information, and severe osteoporosis.

Addressing each of these factors would be a worthwhile strategy to help reduce diagnostic errors in trauma radiography. However, most benefit would probably derive from increasing our ability to look for traumatic lesions in the "subtle but visible" category. To this end, the incorporation into our own radiographic analysis of a "second look," targeted toward the identification of potentially subtle lesions, as well as having awareness of the potential sources of diagnostic error, would be helpful.

12.2.1 Errors in Perception and Interpretation

In general, errors in diagnosis include errors in *perception* and errors in *interpretation*, with the former occurring four times more frequently than the latter. In particular, in the appendicular skeleton, errors in perception accounted for the majority (54%) of errors found in a study (Donald and Barnard 2012; Roddie 2015). A study evaluating reader performance (analysis of eye position and movement to evaluate search patterns in identifying trauma indicators) in acute skeletal trauma showed 29% search errors (eyes failed to fixate on lesion), 29% recognition errors (lesion seen but not recognized), and 51% decision errors (erroneous interpretation) (Lund et al. 1997). A similar study by Hu et al. (1994) identified 9%, 56%, and 35% search, recognition, and decision errors, respectively. From these studies, we may deduce that errors in both perception and interpretation are a significant occurrence, and combating both these types of error is a logical approach in our quest to improve accuracy.

Errors in perception may occur due to multiple factors, including radiologist workload and speed of reporting, level of alertness/fatigue, viewing conditions, distraction factors, and – last but not least – the conspicuity of the abnormality (Donald and Barnard 2012). Unduly increasing the speed of interpretation under the pressures of high-volume reading can have adverse effects – critically reducing the time spent viewing and interpreting each image – and can lead to an increase in the miss rate; such a phenomenon was proven to occur in a study by Oestmann et al. (1988) with respect to lung lesion detection in chest radiology, which showed that the detectability of lesions decreased considerably as image viewing time dropped below 4 s. The true relationship between rate of error and the actual total number of studies reported is however unclear (Berlin 2013). Radiologist fatigue and level of alertness also affect diagnostic accuracy – studies show that the ability to focus and detect fractures diminishes at the end of the working day (Krupinski et al. 2010).

Errors in judgment have to do with the interpretation ascribed to perceived findings, which in turn depends on the radiologist's level of training and education, knowledge base, previous experience, and, once again, levels of alertness or fatigue. It is an important factor, estimated to account for 10% of all errors in radiology (Smith 1967). It may be attributed to "faulty reasoning," where the radiologist relies on the first interpretation which jumps to mind when confronted with a perceived abnormality, without devoting time to systematically work through all the diagnostic possibilities available (Berlin 1996).

12.2.2 Satisfaction of Search

The satisfaction of search effect occurs when the identification of one radiographic abnormality tends to hinder the subsequent identification of other abnormalities on the same study. Its occurrence in chest radiography is well demonstrated (Berbaum et al. 1990, 1991). However, Ashman et al. (2000) also demonstrated a strong satisfaction of search effect in the interpretation of skeletal radiographs, implicating it as a cause of inaccuracies especially in cases with multiple findings. Having a comprehensive and consistent search pattern will help us achieve satisfaction of search, as well as adopting the mindset that there may be multiple findings on the image. In addition to these, however, the radiologist must also examine the images in their entirety, taking care to review the edges of the film where subtle abnormalities may be missed (Fig. 12.1a–b).

12.2.3 Availability of Clinical Information

The availability of accurate clinical information is essential for an accurate interpretative process and helps us render reports which are relevant for the management of the patient. It provides the context under which we interpret a radiographic study and influences our search patterns and thought processes. In particular, it has been shown by Berbaum et al. (1993) that availability of clinical history helps alleviate the satisfaction of search effect for the pertinent abnormality. Even if radiographs are initially evaluated without looking at the clinical history in an attempt to eliminate "framing bias," a reevaluation of the images in the light of the clinical history is still necessary both as an aid to the detection of abnormalities and for structuring relevant radiology reports.

12.3 Practical Approaches for Combating Errors

Some practical ways in which we may help reduce diagnostic errors include obtaining as much clinical information as possible, review of prior studies and reports if available, examining the entire radiograph utilizing our predetermined search algorithms – including the edges of the image – allotting adequate time for interpretation of the findings and for due consideration of all the diagnostic possibilities, and, when necessary, targeted research of relevant radiology textbooks and consultation with colleagues and/or the referring physician to increase our interpretative accuracy (Berlin 1996). Knowing where to look is especially important in skeletal radiography – some institutions make use of ink stamps on which the

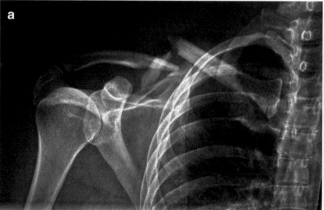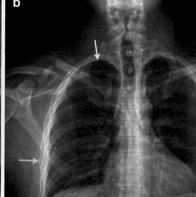

Fig. 12.1 Frontal radiograph of the right shoulder of a motor vehicle accident victim. (**a**) Note the obvious comminuted right clavicular fracture. Did you also notice the small right apical pneumothorax (*white arrow* in **b**)?

Further evaluation of **b** shows right-sided rib fractures (*yellow arrow*). We must not stop searching till everything on the radiograph is evaluated!

technologist may indicate the site at which the patient feels pain (Riddervold and Pope 1981), and the site of tenderness may be requested of the referring physician if not initially indicated. Obtaining high-quality radiographs with appropriate radiographic technique/exposure values optimized for displaying bones, and including all relevant anatomy on the image(s) is essential. Radiographs of joints should ideally include a tangential view through the articular surface and be centered on the joint. Radiographs of long bones should include the relevant proximal and distal joints. Orthogonal projections should be used, as well as the intelligent use of special additional views where required – including oblique views and axial and stress views – and the use of follow-up radiographs or other modalities where appropriate for the clinical indication (Gertzben and Barrington 1975).

12.4 Radiographic Signs

12.4.1 Atypical Radiographic Signs

When searching for fractures, we need to look not only for the typical linear lucency traversing bone and the cortical disruption which highlight a displaced fracture, but we must also look for certain atypical or subtle signs of fracture. These include areas of abnormal increased density due to fracture impaction or overlapping fragments, subtle cortical buckling or angulation, step deformity in an articular surface, and subchondral bone abnormalities (crescents of sclerosis or lucency). Careful analysis of the soft tissues can, in many cases, highlight an underlying subtle osseous or articular injury. Certain dislocations or malalignment may be subtle. To identify them, we should routinely assess the defined anatomic relationships between bones at an articulation with the help of various defined "lines" and "arcs," to help us detect otherwise subtle forms of malalignment. This is especially important in areas of complex anatomy, such as in the carpus, foot, and pelvis. The following fracture categories or clinical situations may constitute pitfalls to radiographic diagnosis.

12.4.2 Avulsion Fractures

Avulsion fractures are often subtle due to their small size. They result from traction injuries at ligamentous, capsular, and tendinous attachments. Therefore, to identify them, we need to carefully scrutinize the periarticular or periapophyseal locations for small fragments of bone. They may be mimicked by accessory ossicles or sesamoid bones, posing a further pitfall to their diagnosis as fractures. Acute avulsion fragments may be distinguished by fragment irregularity and lack of cortication (if large enough to see these features); also helpful for their diagnosis is the identification of an obvious donor site or overlying soft tissue abnormalities, and positive correlation with a location of point tenderness.

12.4.3 Stress Fractures

Stress fractures may present as bands of sclerosis in cancellous bone (thickening of trabeculae from microcallus) or fusiform cortical thickening (endosteal/periosteal callus apposition). They may be subtle in their early stages, presenting as subtle blurring of cortex (gray cortex sign). Stress fractures in cancellous bone may be hard to identify, as up to 50% change in bone density is required for them to be rendered visible radiographically (Greenspan 2011).

12.4.4 Abnormal Underlying Bone

The state of the underlying bone must be specifically assessed. The fracture margins and surrounding bone should be evaluated for any permeative or osteolytic changes which may potentially indicate an underlying pathologic fracture. Careful review in this fashion would help avoid potentially disastrous consequences (Fig. 12.2 a–c). This assessment may be difficult if the fracture is subacute and when bone resorption has usually occurred at the fracture margins, rendering them ill-defined (Russe 1960).

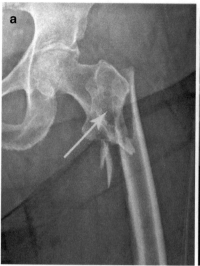
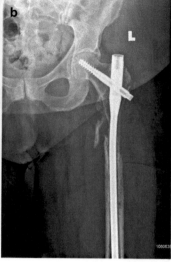
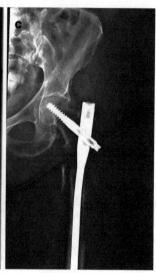

Fig. 12.2 (**a**) Frontal radiograph of the left hip shows a comminuted intertrochanteric fracture of the left femur. Careful review of the fracture site shows a subtle lytic lesion in the central intertrochanteric region (*arrow*), which was not initially identified. Follow-up radiographs after internal fixation at (**b**) 2 months and (**c**) 6 months show dissemination of disease into the femoral shaft with osteolytic destruction following intramedullary nail fixation. Pathology revealed a rare primary bone sarcoma

In osteoporotic patients, detection of non-displaced fractures is rendered difficult, and careful evaluation of cortical margins is essential, as well as having a high index of suspicion for fractures at such sites as the distal radius and femoral neck. A third of all fractures are truly occult radiographically, due to the limitations of this modality (Wei et al. 2006). Therefore, if high clinical suspicion persists despite negative radiographs, we have recourse to other imaging modalities such as computed tomography (CT), magnetic resonance imaging (MRI), or nuclear scintigraphy. In certain cases, radiographs may be repeated in 7–10 days from the injury, the rationale being that bone resorption occurs at the fracture margins in the hyperemic phase of fracture evolution, rendering fracture lines more visible by 1–2 weeks (Russe 1960).

12.5 Shoulder Trauma

12.5.1 Radiographic Examination

A typical radiographic trauma series for the shoulder may include anteroposterior (AP), Grashey (true AP), and axillary and/or scapular "Y" views (Goud et al. 2008). The Grashey (true AP) view is useful in patients with instability and subtle malalignment, particularly patients with persistent subluxation due to post-traumatic glenoid defects; glenohumeral congruity is optimally assessed – any overlap on this view suggests a subluxation or dislocation. Special views which may also find use in patients with shoulder dislocation include the West Point axillary view (which displays glenoid rim fractures), the Garth view (anterior glenohumeral dislocation, profile of anteroinferior glenoid, and posterosuperior tuberosity), and the Stryker Notch view (posterosuperior humeral head/Hill-Sachs deformity) (Greenspan 2011) (Fig. 12.3a–d).

12.5.2 Commonly Missed Injuries

12.5.2.1 Posterior Dislocation

Posterior dislocations of the shoulder account for less than 5% of shoulder dislocations, being much less common than anterior dislocations. However, they are much more frequently missed – in a series of 41 locked posterior dislocations of the shoulder, the injury was missed on initial assessment in the majority of cases. The average time to diagno-

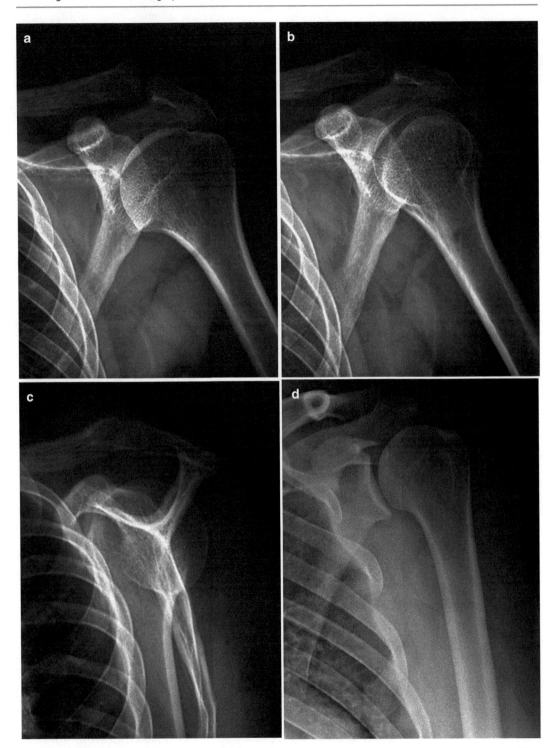

Fig. 12.3 Commonly used projections in shoulder radiography. (**a**) AP view with external rotation. (**b**) AP view with internal rotation. (**c**) Scapular Y view. (**d**) Grashey or "true AP" view

sis in the missed cases was 1 year, and the diagnosis was confirmed on the axillary projection in all cases (Hawkins et al. 1987). Another study reported that posterior dislocations are missed on initial examination in up to 50% of cases (Arndt and Sears 1965). This high miss rate may in part be due to clinical attention being diverted to the causative conditions (such as seizures or electrocution) and in part due to the subtlety of the findings on standard AP projections. Gaining familiarity with the subtle signs of posterior shoulder dislocation will help spot this easily missed diagnosis (Fig. 12.4a–d).

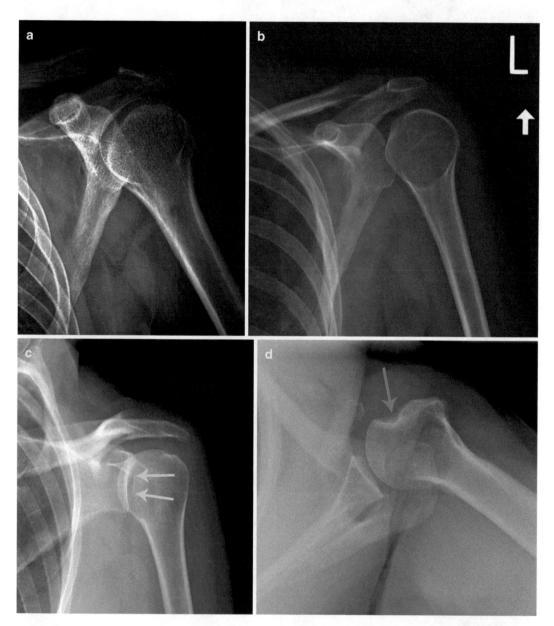

Fig. 12.4 (a) Standard AP view in internal rotation of a normal shoulder shows the lesser tuberosity in profile. Note degree of overlap of humeral head with glenoid, with "half-moon" shape of overlap. (b) Externally rotated view of the shoulder shows persistent internal rotation (appears like an internally rotated view) and characteristic shape of proximal humerus – "light bulb" sign. Compared with a, there is loss of normal overlap of the humeral head with glenoid (overlap sign) – a subtle but important sign – in b. (c) Grashey view of the shoulder shows a posteriorly dislocated shoulder. Note the linear vertical indentation/density on the humeral head (arrows) – "trough line" sign. Note glenohumeral overlap – an abnormal finding on a Grashey view. (d) Axillary view of the shoulder, postreduction, shows the trough sign (arrow) – a "reverse" Hill-Sachs deformity

12.5.2.2 Anterior Dislocation

In anterior dislocations, the humeral head is often directed to a subcoracoid position due to the constraint of the coracoid process, rendering the diagnosis of dislocation more obvious on AP radiographs. However, associated fractures may not be so obvious – including greater tuberosity fractures, glenoid rim fractures, and Hill-Sachs lesions. These fractures may be missed on the initial radiographs in more than one-third of cases and may appear only on the postreduction radiographs, suggesting the need to obtain and to carefully scrutinize postreduction radiographs (Kahn and Mehta 2007) (Fig. 12.5a–b).

Careful evaluation of the glenoid may reveal loss of the anterior sclerotic line of the inferior

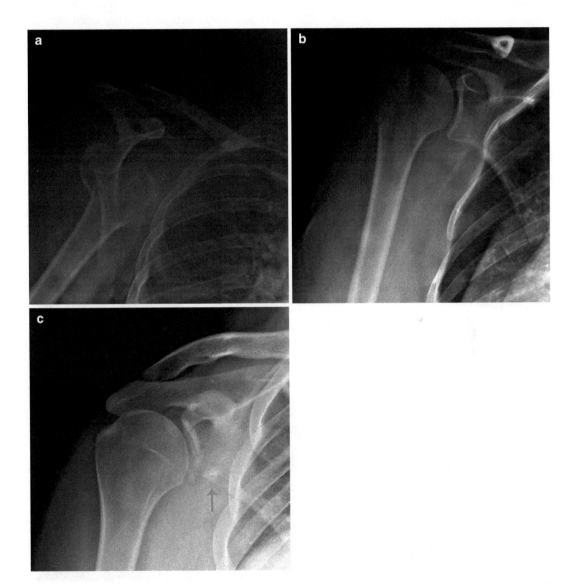

Fig. 12.5 (a) AP view of the shoulder shows anterior dislocation. But look carefully, do you see the displaced greater tuberosity fracture projecting over the glenoid? (b) Postreduction Grashey view of the shoulder shows clearly the greater tuberosity fracture which is spontaneously reduced. (c) Grashey view of the shoulder, following reduction of an anterior dislocation (not shown). Note the poor definition of the inferior half of the anterior glenoid rim, with loss of the sclerotic line – a subtle sign of an osseous Bankart fracture. Compare this with the sclerotic complete glenoid rim in **b** above. The nearby Bankart fragment can also be seen in this case (*arrow*), but is not always seen

half of the glenoid on the AP radiograph, which is a subtle sign specific for anterior glenoid rim fracture (Jankauskas et al. 2010) (Fig. 12.5c). Searching for this sign could help determine the need for special projections to better evaluate the anteroinferior glenoid rim such as the West Point axillary view (variant of axillary view for cases where pain is a limitation) or the Garth view (AP apical oblique view).

12.5.2.3 Proximal Humeral/Greater Tuberosity Fractures

These are the most common fracture type involving the shoulder girdle in adults (Nordqvist and Petersson 1995). Radiographs are valuable in the initial diagnosis of proximal humeral fractures. Lesser tuberosity fractures may be identified on axillary views (Fig. 12.6). Greater tuberosity fractures may occur as avulsion fractures in the setting of glenohumeral dislocation or as direct impaction injuries during hyperabduction of the shoulder. A high miss rate has been reported for greater tuberosity fractures, with up to 75% of missed fractures reported in one study (Gumina et al. 2009). This has been partly attributed to the fact that due to limited external rotation in these patients on account of pain, the greater tuberosity is not shown in profile on the externally rotated AP view and therefore the fractures are not seen (Mason et al. 1999). In elderly or osteoporotic patients, trabecular resorption limits

evaluation particularly for non-displaced fractures of the greater tuberosity – and special attention needs to be paid to the cortical margins on the externally rotated view in such patients. Close attention to the contours of the greater tuberosity facets, especially on the scapular Y view, is also helpful for detecting non-displaced fractures. Since non-displaced fractures of the greater tuberosity are treated conservatively, the AP view in external rotation may be repeated after 7 days, when the pain may have lessened (Ogawa et al. 2003) (Fig. 12.7a–b). The presence of calcific tendinopathy around the greater tuberosity may provide a pitfall to diagnosis of fractures; the often globular shape of the calcific deposit may be a clue to the correct diagnosis in this regard (Fig. 12.8).

12.5.2.4 Acromioclavicular Joint

Acromioclavicular injuries account for 12% of injuries to the shoulder girdle (Cave et al. 1974). They may be classified according to the direction and degree of displacement of the distal end of the clavicle relative to the acromion (Rockwood classification) (Rockwood 1984). To obtain good-quality radiographs, the standard shoulder radiographic technique needs to be adjusted – otherwise, the AC joint may be over-penetrated. Assessment of acromioclavicular congruity may be done on routine AP views. However, the difficulty with this view is that the AC joint projects

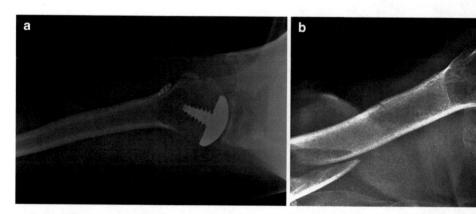

Fig. 12.6 (a) Axillary view of the shoulder following glenohumeral resurfacing arthroplasty. This view is necessary to show the lesser tuberosity osteotomy which would not be well seen on standard AP views. Any abnormal displacement of the osteotomy fragment should be sought for in this view on follow-up radiographs of shoulder arthroplasties. (b) Lesser tuberosity fractures will be also well demonstrated on this view. Note also the humeral shaft fracture at the edge of the radiograph

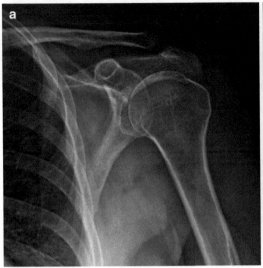
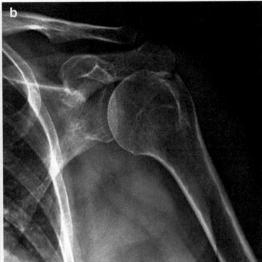

Fig. 12.7 (**a**) Initial AP radiograph following trauma to shoulder. Non-displaced greater tuberosity fracture is barely visible. Voluntary external rotation is limited, and there is relative osteopenia at the greater tuberosity, both of which render fracture detection difficult. (**b**) Repeat radiograph taken 2 weeks later shows the occult greater tuberosity fracture to better advantage. There are better external rotation and osseous resorption at the fracture line, both of which expose the underlying fracture

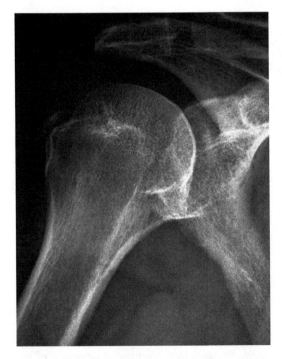

Fig. 12.8 AP radiograph of the shoulder. Calcific tendinopathy may mimic a greater tuberosity avulsion fracture, especially if it does not present with a typical globular appearance

over the spine of the scapula, which may obscure small periarticular avulsion fragments. A modified "Zanca view" with 10–15° of cephalic tilt provides an unobscured view of the joint, standardizes the coracoclavicular distance better than the AP view, and is particularly useful to exclude potential occult avulsion fractures related to the AC joint or coracoid process. Comparison with the contralateral side is very useful in examination of the AC joint, since the standard metrics of coracoclavicular and acromioclavicular distance may vary from person to person.

12.5.2.5 Scapular Fractures

Scapular fractures are relatively uncommon, accounting for less than 1% of all fractures and 3–5% of all fractures of the shoulder girdle (Bartonicek 2015), and include fractures of the glenoid, scapular neck and body, and the acromion and coracoid process. The acromion and coracoid process and acromioclavicular regions should be surveyed to identify potentially occult avulsion fractures. Unfused ossification centers may constitute a potential diagnostic pitfall to

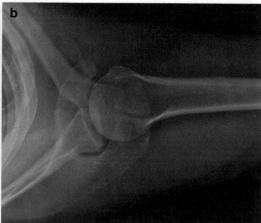

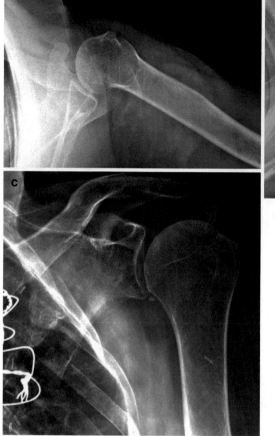

Fig. 12.9 (**a**) Axillary view of the shoulder shows a displaced acute acromial avulsion fracture, with irregular sharp margins and lack of cortication. (**b**) Similar projection shows an os acromiale – with smooth corticated margins. (**c**) Grashey view of the shoulder shows an acute displaced acromial avulsion fracture at the deltoid attachment, which may be easy to miss. Note the sharp irregular non-corticated fracture edges

diagnosis of these injuries, e.g., os acromiale (Fig. 12.9a–c).

12.5.2.6   Coracoid Process Fractures

Coracoid process fractures may be associated with glenohumeral or acromioclavicular joint dislocations and may be missed without appropriate satisfaction of search. An important clue to their presence in the setting of grade 3 acromioclavicular dislocation is the presence of a normal coracoclavicular distance equal to the contralateral side (Edgar et al. 2015) (Fig. 12.10a–c). Coracoid and acromial fractures may occur in the setting of shoulder dislocation and may be missed if not specifically searched for (Goss 1996).

The scapular body is obscured by the rib cage on frontal view, which may hinder easy identification of scapular body fractures on radiography. Scapular fractures often occur in the setting of high-impact trauma and are often associated with other significant injuries which may serve as distractors. Rib fractures may be associated in as many as 65% of cases of scapular fracture (Bartonicek 2015). A systematic assessment of the entire scapular body, glenoid, spine/acromion, and coracoid process would help reveal potentially occult fractures in this setting. Assessment of the glenopolar angle is a useful aid; this is described as the angle between a line connecting the most cranial and caudal poles of the glenoid and a line connecting the cranial pole of the glenoid and the most

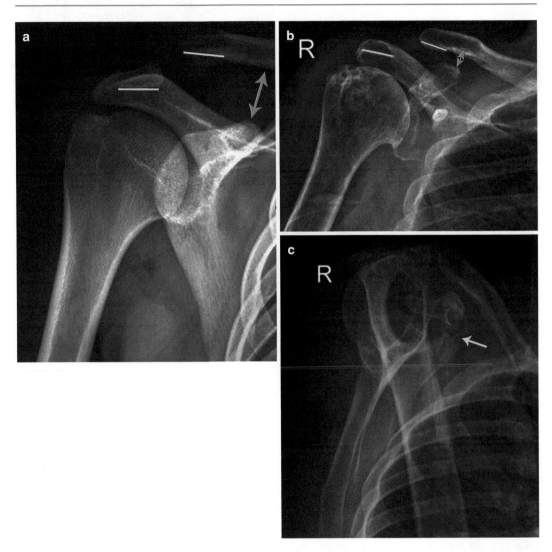

Fig. 12.10 (a) Frontal radiograph of the shoulder shows typical grade 3 acromioclavicular separation. There is complete dissociation of the acromion from the distal clavicle (*yellow lines*), with associated widened coracoclavicular distance (*double arrow*). (b) Frontal view of the shoulder shows grade 3 acromioclavicular separation, but with a normal coracoclavicular distance (*double arrow*). An occult coracoid avulsion fracture should be suspected and sought on the axillary or scapular Y view in such cases. (c) Axillary view of shoulder (poorly oblique) (same case as b) shows a non-united fracture at base of coracoid process (*arrow*)

caudal point of the scapular body. It usually ranges between 30 and 45°; if it is <20 °, it indicates operative management (Tuček et al. 2014). Even if overt scapular fracture lines are not seen on radiography, scrutinizing this angle may help reveal an underlying scapular fracture (Fig. 12.11a–c).

12.5.2.7   Sternoclavicular Joint

The sternoclavicular joint is the only true joint connecting the shoulder girdle with the axial skeleton. The larger bulbous head of the clavicle articulates with the small clavicular notch of the sternum. Much of the stability of the joint is afforded by powerful ligaments. Sternoclavicular dislocations are rare, accounting for only 3% of shoulder girdle injuries in one series (Cave et al. 1974), and are usually the result of significant trauma. Dislocation may occur anteriorly or posteriorly, with anterior dislocations being 20 times more

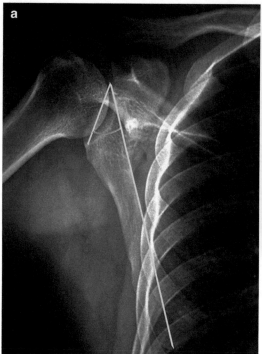

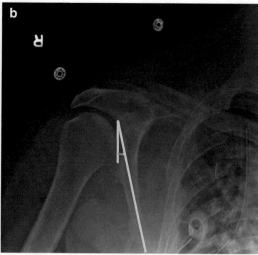

Fig. 12.11 (**a**) AP view of the scapula shows a normal glenopolar angle. (**b**) Comminuted scapular fracture with abnormally small glenopolar angle (less than 5°). Though the scapular fracture lines are not well seen in this image, the presence of a significant fracture can be inferred from the abnormal glenopolar angle in this case. Note associated rib fractures and clavicular fracture

common, but with posterior dislocations carrying potential for significant neurovascular or visceral injury (Ernberg and Potter 2003).

Radiographic imaging of the sternoclavicular joint presents difficulties. The joint is not well visualized on the lateral projection; therefore, true radiographic assessment of anterior-posterior translation is not possible. This is done indirectly through AP views and special oblique projections. Side-to-side comparison is important, as the sign may be subtle and easily missed – both joints need to be included on the study. On the AP view, a difference between the relative craniocaudal positions of the medial ends of the clavicles of greater than 50% of the clavicular heads is suggestive of dislocation (McCulloch et al. 2001). The Rockwood/serendipity view may be helpful, with the affected clavicle being displaced cephalad or caudad in anterior or posterior dislocations, respectively. Whichever view is used, radiography is at best only suggestive of the type of injury, and CT provides the mainstay of

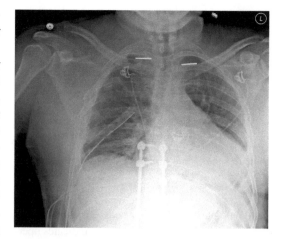

Fig. 12.12 Right sternoclavicular dislocation. Note the relative elevation of the right clavicular head on this AP radiograph of the chest. Also note multiple rib fractures, ipsilateral grade 3 acromioclavicular separation, and right pneumothorax, all compatible with high-energy impact trauma

diagnosis, determining the direction/degree of dislocation and potential complications more accurately (Fig. 12.12).

12.6   Elbow Trauma

In a study of the most frequently overlooked fractures, Freed and Shields (1984) reported that fractures about the elbow ranked second in frequency,
particularly the fractures of the proximal radius.
Radial head fractures are also the most common
fractures of the elbow, commonly arising from a fall
on an outstretched hand (Duckworth et al. 2012).
Standard radiographic examination of the elbow
includes an AP view with the elbow fully extended
and forearm in supination and a lateral view with 90°
of elbow flexion with the forearm in neutral position.
The radiocapitellar view is a useful additional view
which improves visualization of the radial head,
capitellum, coronoid process, and proximal radioulnar articulation (Greenspan and Norman 1982).

12.6.1   Non-displaced Radial Head
Fractures

Non-displaced radial head fractures may be difficult to diagnose. The presence of an elbow joint
effusion, indicated by the sail sign and posterior fat

pad sign, raises suspicion for non-displaced radial
head fracture in adults. In patients with radial head
fractures who also present with wrist pain, bilateral
wrist radiographs should be obtained to exclude
associated distal radioulnar joint instability which
would suggest an associated Essex-Lopresti injury.
The radial head-neck junction should be surveyed
carefully for angulation or step deformity; the presence of radial head osteophytes may create diagnostic confusion in this regard (Fig. 12.13).

12.6.2   Coronoid Process Fractures

Coronoid process fractures are important to identify, as they do not commonly occur in isolation and
may occur in up to 15% of elbow dislocations
(Wells and Ablove 2008). In cases with spontaneous reduction of an elbow dislocation, they may be
the only sign that a significant injury has occurred.
The association of a coronoid tip fracture with a
radial head fracture is radiographic evidence of the
terrible triad injury of the elbow, associated with lateral collateral ligament injury; if missed, significant
instability of the elbow may result (Beingessner

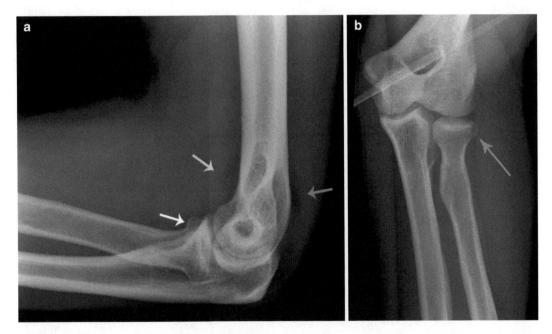

Fig. 12.13 (a) Lateral radiograph of the elbow shows the
sail sign (*yellow arrow*) and posterior fat pad sign (*red
arrow*), indicating joint effusion/hemarthrosis. There is
the need to check for intra-articular fractures such as a

partly visualized non-displaced radial head fracture (*white
arrow*). (b) AP view of the elbow better shows the radial
head fracture, with subtle step deformity (*arrow*)

et al. 2015). Radiocapitellar and humeroulnar congruity should also be assessed in order to detect subtle signs of instability. The identification of a

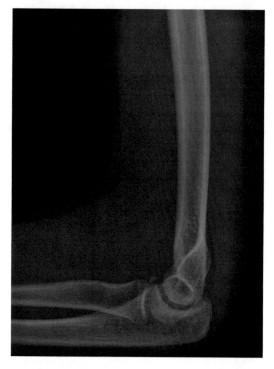

Fig. 12.14 Lateral radiograph of the elbow shows acute avulsion fracture of coronoid process. Note the associated joint effusion, with sail sign and posterior fat pad sign. The elbow joint is congruent

coronoid tip fracture is best done on the lateral view, but visualization may be hindered due to the overlapping radial head or trochlea. In such cases, adding a radiocapitellar view would be helpful (Fig. 12.14).

Coronoid tip avulsion fractures may occur in isolation; avulsion of the sublime tubercle have been described in throwing athletes, due to traction injury at the attachment of the anterior bundle of the ulnar collateral ligament (Glajchen et al. 1998). 25% of these injuries may be missed on radiographs; they are best identified on the AP projection (Salvo et al. 2002). A persistent ossification center may be found at the tip of the coronoid process and may mimic an avulsion fracture (Fig. 12.15).

12.7   Wrist and Hand Trauma

12.7.1 Distal Radial Fractures

Distal radial fractures are the fractures most frequently encountered by orthopedic trauma surgeons, accounting for 16% of all adult fractures (McQueen 2015). They most commonly occur following a fall from standing height onto the outstretched hand. A study investigating the reasons for litigation claims related to

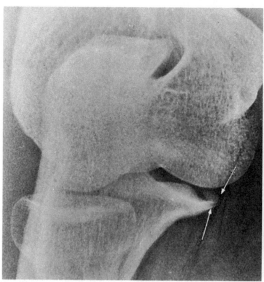
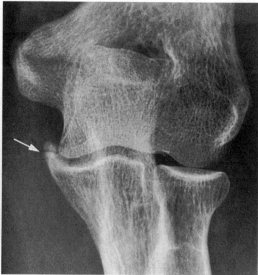

Fig. 12.15 Two examples of persistent ossification center of the coronoid process which could be mistaken for an avulsion fracture – contrast its smooth corticated appear-ance with the sharp-edged non-corticated avulsion fragment in Fig. 12.14 (Reproduced with permission from Keats and Anderson 2013)

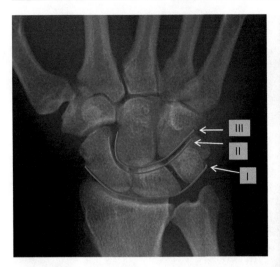

Fig. 12.16 AP radiograph of a normal wrist tracing the arcs of Gilula. Arc I traces the proximal convexities of the proximal carpal row bones. Arc II traces the distal concavities of the proximal carpal row bones. Arc III traces the proximal convexities of the capitate and hamate. These arcs should be assessed on every wrist radiograph to detect potential carpal malalignment

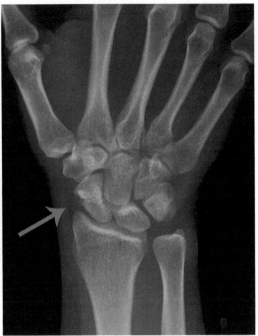

Fig. 12.17 AP radiograph of the wrist shows a non-displaced scaphoid waist fracture, with associated blurring of the scaphoid fat stripe (*arrow*)

the wrist and hand cited fractures of the wrist and scaphoid in 36.3% of cases, with almost half of these resulting from incorrect, missed, or delayed diagnosis (Ring et al. 2015). The wrist and carpus constitute an area of complex anatomy, and the assessment for subtle fractures or malalignment needs to be systematic (Fig. 12.16).

Furthermore, distal radial fractures are highly associated with osteoporosis, which may also hinder detection of subtle fractures. Wei et al. (2006) identified the wrist as the site at which fractures were most frequently missed, in terms of absolute number of fractures missed, perhaps because they are such common fractures. A study of the sensitivity of radiography for identifying wrist fractures and the pattern of missed fractures showed that 30% of wrist fractures were not prospectively identified on radiography, necessitating further imaging; this study also demonstrated a high rate of occult fractures involving the triquetrum, hamate, capitate, and lunate (Welling et al. 2008).

The standard radiographic series for evaluating the traumatized wrist includes the PA, lateral, semiprone oblique (45°) views. Special views such as the scaphoid view, semisupine oblique

view, and the carpal tunnel view may be added if clinically warranted (American College of Radiology 2001). Searching for associated injuries is a key concept when evaluating radiographs of the wrist and hand, as many injury patterns/associations occur here particularly in the radius and ulna, carpus, and metacarpal/carpometacarpal articulations.

The assessment of soft tissue fat planes for bulging, blurring, or obliteration provides valuable clues to underlying osseous injury of the wrist, even when no fracture is immediately evident. The navicular fat stripe and the pronator fat pad in particular may be abnormal in cases of occult scaphoid and distal radial fractures, respectively (Figs. 12.17 and 12.18). These signs are not entirely specific, e.g., the navicular fat strip may be obliterated in cases of radial styloid fractures, other carpal fractures, scapholunate ligament tears, or regional inflammation. The pronator fat pad sign is 65% sensitive and 69% specific for occult wrist fracture detection, being also seen in cases of wrist sprain (Zimmers 1984; Fallahi et al. 2013).

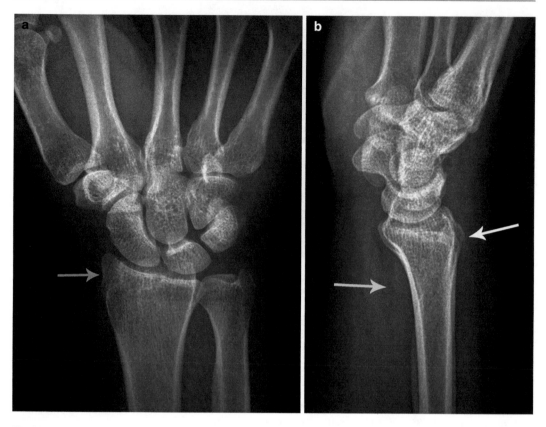

Fig. 12.18 (**a**) AP radiograph of the wrist shows a subtle non-displaced radial styloid fracture (*blue arrow*) with blurred scaphoid fat stripe. (**b**) Lateral radiograph shows an obliterated pronator fat pad (*yellow arrow*). Note also the non-displaced dorsal radial tubercle fracture (*white arrow*)

12.7.2 Scaphoid Fractures

The scaphoid is the most commonly fractured carpal bone, constituting 60–70% of all osseous injuries to the carpus (Geissler 2001). They may be difficult to identify radiographically, regardless of the view, and may be occult in 20% of cases. Because of the limitations of radiography in diagnosis of scaphoid fractures, even with the best technique, the standard practice in patients with clinical suspicion for scaphoid fracture and negative radiographs is to immobilize in a cast and to repeat clinical and radiographic evaluation in 7–10 days (American College of Radiology 2001). A specific type of avulsion fracture, the dorsal avulsion fracture of the scaphoid, may be occult since it will not be seen on standard radiographic projections. A semisupine oblique or ball catcher view would be needed to identify it. It, however, tends to have a good prognosis (Compson et al. 1993; Welling et al. 2008) (Fig. 12.19).

12.7.3 Avulsion Fractures

The periarticular regions should be scrutinized for avulsion fractures around the wrist and carpus, including the radial styloid (Fig. 12.18a), ulnar styloid, dorsal triquetral avulsion fractures, and dorsal scaphoid avulsion fractures.

12.7.4 Triquetral Fractures

The triquetrum is the second most commonly fractured carpal bone. Fractures mostly occur in form of dorsal avulsion. Three ligaments converge to attach to the dorsal surface of the triquetrum – the dorsal intercarpal/scapho-triquetral ligament, the dorsal radiocarpal ligament, and the triquetro-hamate ligament – predisposing the triquetrum to an avulsion fracture of the dorsal cortical surface. This fracture is usually seen tangentially in standard radiographic projections – particularly on the

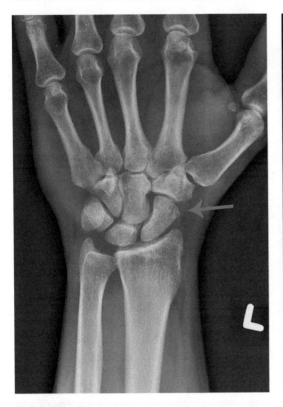

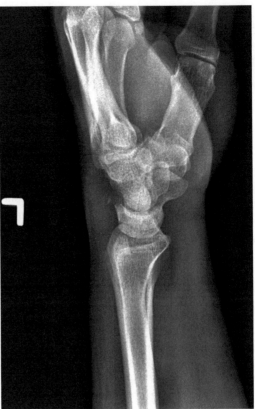

Fig. 12.19 AP radiograph of the wrist shows a dorsal avulsion fracture of the distal pole of the scaphoid, which is non-displaced (*arrow*). Note associated blurring of the scaphoid fat stripe

Fig. 12.20 Lateral radiograph of the wrist shows a triquetral avulsion fracture, seen tangentially dorsal to the carpus. Overlying dorsal soft tissue swelling of the wrist is present

lateral view. The oblique projection is useful as the flake avulsion may be difficult to accurately localize on the lateral projection (De Beer and Hudson 1987) (Fig. 12.20). If there are clinical signs such as tenderness in or around the hypothenar eminence with no obvious fractures on standard radiographs, then special views may be obtained such as the semisupinated oblique view to look for a pisiform fracture and a carpal tunnel view to look for the otherwise occult hook of hamate fracture.

Joint widening is found associated with a displaced radial fracture and no obvious ulnar styloid avulsion, suggesting underlying triangular fibrocartilage complex (TFCC) injury. If there is distal radioulnar joint widening without an obvious distal radial fracture on radiography, attention should be drawn to the elbow to exclude a radial head fracture (Essex-Lopresti injury) and to the radial shaft (Galeazzi injury).

12.7.5 Disorders of Alignment in the Wrist and Carpus

Distal radial fractures have a very high association with distal radioulnar joint injury, as evidenced by concomitant distal radioulnar joint widening, usually with an ulnar styloid avulsion fracture. Distal radioulnar joint widening is an important sign to identify, as its presence can direct the search for important associated injuries.

12.7.6 Carpal Instability

Just over 50% of patients with acute distal radial fracture have concomitant signs of scapholunate instability, demonstrating abnormal scapholunate widening and an increased scaphocapitate angle. These signs should be sought for in cases of acute distal radial fracture (Lee et al. 1995). If scapholunate instability is suspected clinically but initial radiographs are negative, closed-fist views or radial deviated views of the wrist may reveal occult scapholunate dislocation. Lunotriquetral instability may be occult on standard AP views; however, the presence of VISI on the lateral view may be a clue to its presence.

12.7.7 Lunate and Perilunate Injuries

Carpal dislocations occur in a spectrum of injury including perilunate dislocation, midcarpal dislocation, and lunate dislocation. Fractures are a common association – a study showed that perilunate fracture dislocations are twice as common as perilunate dislocations alone (Herzberg et al. 1993), with the trans-scaphoid perilunate fracture dislocation being the most common pattern. Fractures also occur through the radial styloid, capitate, hamate, lunate, and triquetrum. Up to 25% of perilunate dislocations may be missed on initial assessment (Herzberg et al. 1993), particularly lesser arc injuries which usually occur without

obvious fractures. If undetected, these injuries can lead to a high incidence of long-term functional disability and chronic pain (Perron et al. 2001).

Carpal alignment should be carefully studied in every case: on the AP projection, the use of Gilula lines helps navigate the complex anatomy of the carpus and detects subtle carpal malalignment (Gilula and Weeks 1978; Gilula and Totty 1992). The intercarpal joint spaces should be of uniform dimension (2 mm or less). Change in the shape and orientation of the lunate to a more triangular configuration is a suggestive but subtle sign. On the lateral projection, assessing the collinearity between the radius, lunate, and capitate enables characterization of the subtype of carpal dislocation. Palmar rotation of the lunate – the "spilled teacup sign" (O'brien 1984) – indicates lunate-capitate disruption. Preservation of collinearity between the lunate and the radius indicates a perilunate dislocation, while preservation of collinearity between the capitate and the radius indicates a lunate dislocation (Alexander and Lichtman 1997) (Figs. 12.21 and 12.22).

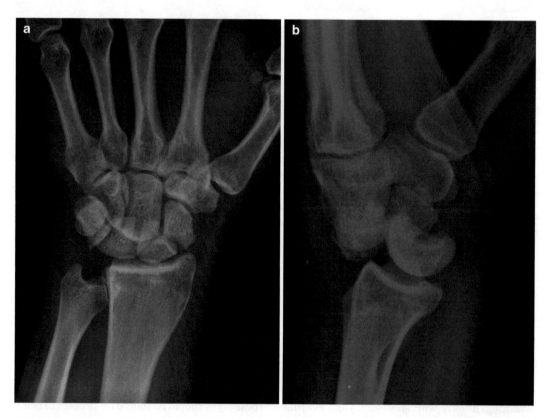

Fig. 12.21 Perilunate dislocation (trans-scaphoid). (**a**) AP radiograph of the wrist shows disruption of Gilula arcs I and II, which should raise suspicion for carpal malalignment (compare with Fig. 12.16). Note the displaced fracture through the waist of the scaphoid. (**b**) Lateral radiograph of the wrist shows that the colinearity between the lunate and radius is maintained, and the capitate is dislocated dorsally, indicating a perilunate dislocation

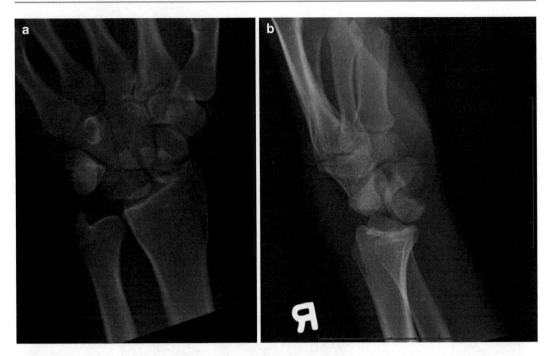

Fig. 12.22 Lunate dislocation. (**a**) AP radiograph of the wrist shows disruption of Gilula arcs and triangular shape of the lunate (which should normally be quadrangular), signifying carpal malalignment. Also note the displaced scaphoid waist fracture. (**b**) Lateral radiograph of the wrist shows maintained colinearity between the radius and the capitate, with volar dislocation of the lunate with its distal concave surface facing anteriorly – diagnosis is lunate dislocation. Contrast Fig. 12.21b with Fig. 12.22b

The standard radiographic examination includes posteroanterior (PA), semipronated oblique, and lateral projections, which suffice for identification of most injuries of the hand. However, evaluation of metacarpals is often limited on the lateral projection due to bony overlap. The semisupinated oblique/ ball catcher view is a useful complement to the standard oblique view when metacarpal or carpometacarpal injury is suspected clinically, and its use in this regard is advocated by various authors (Stapczynski 1991; Lane et al. 1992). It is particularly useful for demonstrating and for quantifying angulation in metacarpal neck fractures.

The fifth metacarpal is the most frequently fractured metacarpal bone (boxer fracture), followed by the fourth metacarpal. With appropriate radiographic technique, these fractures are easy enough to identify. However, a pitfall lies here if the search for other injuries is terminated. There is an association of fractures of the fourth and fifth metacarpals with carpometacarpal joint dislocations – with or without fractures of the metacarpal bases or hamate (Liaw et al. 1995). Therefore, carpometacarpal relationships should be specifically evaluated in all cases of obvious metacarpal fracture, particularly the articulation between the fourth/fifth metacarpals and the hamate, to avoid missing associated fracture dislocations. The oblique views are especially useful in this regard (Stapczynski 1991).

Carpometacarpal dislocations are easy to miss if not specifically sought for (Henderson and Arafa 1987). The key to detecting this injury is careful assessment of the carpometacarpal joints on the PA projection, examining for uniformity of the joint spaces and for parallel alignment of the articular surfaces (parallelism) (Gilula and Totty 1992). Overlap between the metacarpal bases and the carpus, as well as the presence of fractures at the metacarpal bases, should arouse suspicion for carpometacarpal joint injury. Evaluating the metacarpal convergence on the PA view is another helpful sign for subtle carpometacarpal injury, done by tracing the "metacarpal cascade lines" to a point proximal to the distal articular surface of the radius (Hodgson and Shewring 2007) (Fig. 12.23).

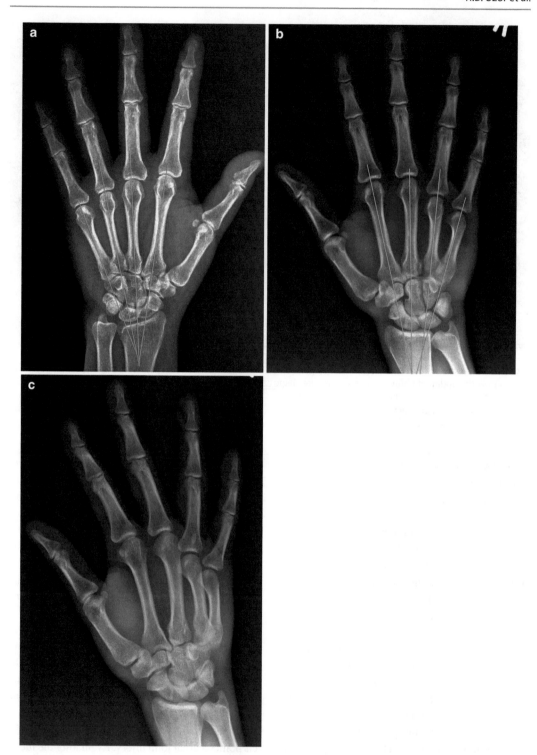

Fig. 12.23 (a) AP radiograph of the hand shows normal metacarpal convergence. The axes of the metacarpal shafts roughly converge proximally at a point in the distal radial metaphysis. (b) AP radiograph of the hand shows non-convergence of the axes of the fourth and fifth metacarpal shafts, relative to the second and third. (c) Semi-pronated oblique radiograph shows fourth and fifth carpometacarpal fracture dislocations

12.8   Finger Trauma

In the fingers and thumb, careful attention to detail is required to a greater extent since there is a multiplicity of smaller bones and joints involved. Standard radiographic examination includes a true AP and true lateral view of the fingers, with an externally rotated oblique view (Tuncer et al. 2011). A second oblique projection perpendicular to the first may also be obtained to improve fracture detection where warranted (Street 1993). Meticulous radiographic technique is essential to display the bones and joints in their minute detail, as well as the liberal use of coned radiographs of the individual digits and use of picture archiving and communication system (PACS) magnification tools when injury of the digit is suspected clinically (Fig. 12.24).

The lateral view of the fingers may produce difficulties with interpretation if technique is sub-optimal, due to the potential for overlapping of structures on these views. A study showed that inadequate technique in these particular radiographs resulted in 71% of missed or misdiagnosed fractures; therefore, inadequate views of the digits should not be accepted for interpretation or use as basis for management (Tuncer et al. 2011). Coned radiographs of the individual injured digit would be preferable to improve radiographic detail.

Detection of avulsion fractures is another diagnostic pitfall in the digits, particularly due to their small size. The sites at which avulsion

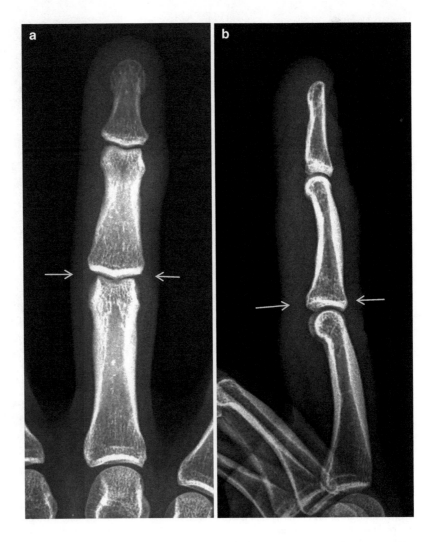

Fig. 12.24 Normal (**a**) AP and (**b**) lateral radiographs of a digit. Good technique would afford a tangential view through the joints on all the views, without digit overlap, coned to the digit of interest. The periarticular areas (*arrows*) should be searched for the presence of subtle avulsion fragments in the interphalangeal and metacarpophalangeal joints of the digits

fractures typically occur include the insertions of the digital flexor and extensor tendons at the bases of phalanges (volar plate avulsion fracture and dorsal avulsion fracture/mallet finger, respectively) and the attachments of the collateral ligaments to the radial and ulnar sides of the phalangeal bases/metacarpal heads. These four categories of avulsion fracture are periarticular in location and may be seen related to the metacarpophalangeal or interphalangeal joints. Freed and Shields (1984) evaluated all the sites at which fractures are missed in the body and cited periar-

ticular fractures of the phalanges as the third most common site of missed fractures (in terms of absolute number). The periarticular areas should therefore be carefully scrutinized for potential tiny avulsions (Fig. 12.25).

The common occurrence of sesamoid bones and accessory ossicles in the periarticular regions of the digits may serve as a diagnostic pitfall. Here, as in the rest of the body, they may be distinguished from acute cortical avulsions by their smooth, rounded, and corticated configuration and the absence of abnormal clinical signs at such locations. Hence, communication with the referring physician and targeted clinical exam are helpful (Fig. 12.26).

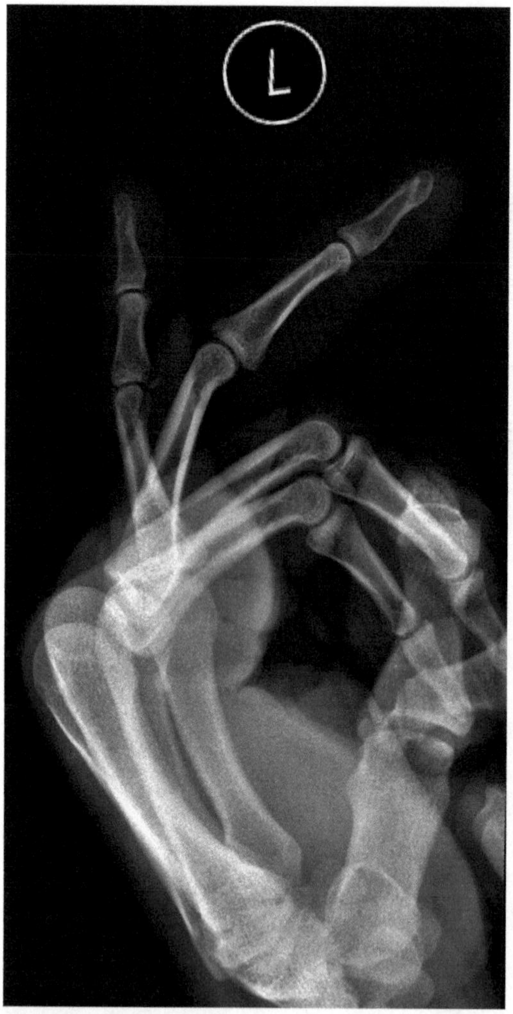

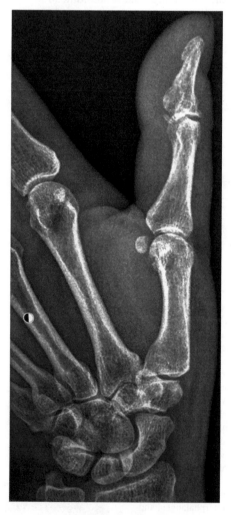

Fig. 12.25 Lateral radiograph shows the ring and little fingers. Note the volar plate avulsion fracture of the base of the little finger middle phalanx. Scrutinize the periarticular regions – did you notice the subtle non-displaced mallet avulsion fracture of the dorsal base of the ring finger middle phalanx? Note the sentinel sign of dorsal soft tissue swelling at the fourth proximal interphalangeal joint

Fig. 12.26 Lateral radiograph of the thumb shows a sesamoid bone at volar base of distal phalanx of the thumb, which may be confused for volar plate avulsion fracture by the unwary

12.9 Pelvic Trauma

The pelvis is a ring structure composed of paired lateral innominate bones which articulate anteriorly at the pubic symphysis. Each innominate bone articulates posteriorly through a sacroiliac joint with the centrally located sacrum, thus completing the pelvic ring. The radiographic anatomy is complex, and only with a thorough evaluation will we avoid missing potentially serious injuries. The first step in evaluating the pelvis is a standard AP radiograph, which is obtained as part of the primary trauma survey. The limitations of evaluating with a single radiographic projection include the risk of missing minimally displaced fractures and certain dislocations. But the value of this projection lies not only in its ability to detect major displaced pelvic fractures, which could be life-threatening due to the associated blood loss, but also in the simplicity with which it is obtained in the supine position without disturbing the patient. The evaluation of the pelvis is completed with inlet and outlet views to aid detection of more subtle pelvic ring fractures and/or oblique (Judet) views for detection of acetabular fractures where suspected.

Systematic evaluation of the pelvic ring includes tracing the outline of the pelvic brim on each side and its continuity with the outline of the superior borders of the second sciatic notches bilaterally and examining for any pubic symphyseal or sacroiliac incongruity or widening (Jackson et al. 1982). Evaluate the L5 transverse processes for avulsion fractures, which are a sign of posterior ring disruption, and evaluate other sciatic notches for sacral alar fractures. If a pubic ramus fracture is seen, special attention must be paid to the posterior ring. A study showed that 97% of patients with pubic rami fractures have a concomitant posterior ring injury, with transforaminal fractures predominating (Scheyerer et al. 2012) (Fig. 12.27).

Evaluation of the acetabulum includes tracing key "lines" on the radiograph which help to identify otherwise potentially subtle injuries to the acetabular walls and columns (Armbuster et al.

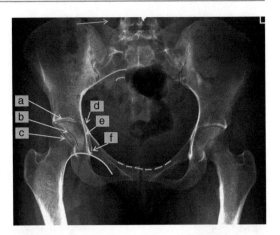

Fig. 12.27 AP radiograph of the normal pelvis – checklist for assessment. Assessment of pelvic ring: alignment of pelvic brim with S2 sciatic notch (*long green curve*). Alignment of pelvic brim at pubic symphysis (*broken green curve*). Intact sacral alae: (*short green curves*). Intact L5 transverse process (*green arrow*) Six blue items: assessment of intact acetabulum – acetabular roof (*a*), anterior and posterior acetabular walls (*b* and *c*), and iliopectineal and ilioischial lines (*d* and *e*); assessment for intra-articular fragments in hip joint, teardrop distance (*f*). Shenton line, assessment of hip joint congruity (*yellow curve*)

1978). These include the ilioischial line (posterior column of acetabulum), iliopectineal line (anterior iliopubic column of acetabulum), anterior and posterior outlines of acetabulum (anterior and posterior acetabular walls), roof of acetabulum, and teardrop (anterior acetabular fossa laterally and quadrilateral surface medially, connected inferiorly by the inferior margin of the acetabular notch). To help identify subtle cases of hip dislocation, Gregory (1973) described specific radiographic signs. These include (a) identifying a discontinuity of Shenton line and (b) disparity in the size of the femoral heads – a dislocated femoral head will project differently as it is located either closer to or further away from the cassette, thus appearing smaller or larger than the contralateral one (Fig. 12.28). Widening of the "teardrop distance" is helpful in suggesting the presence of an intra-articular osseous fragment in the setting of a reduced hip dislocation and would help identify what would otherwise be a subtle injury (Fig. 12.29).

12.10 Hip and Femoral Neck Trauma

Displaced fractures of the femoral neck are usually readily identified on radiography. The standard radiographic projections in this setting are the AP (taken with 15° of internal rotation of the limb – to display the femoral neck in profile) and the lateral (usually with cross-table technique to minimize pain). Careful evaluation

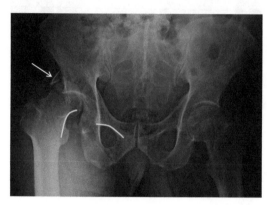

Fig. 12.28 AP radiograph of the pelvis shows posterior dislocation of the right hip. Note the apparently smaller size of the dislocated right femoral head (marked "*x*") compared to the contralateral side. Also note the disruption in Shenton line (*gray curved lines*). There is a shear fracture of the right femoral head (medially), a subtle finding, and a displaced fracture of the posterior acetabular wall (*arrow*)

of the AP projection involves tracing the smooth S-shaped or reverse S-shaped outline of the femoral head and neck, to identify any angulation which may point to a fracture (Lowell's alignment theory) (Wheeless 2015) (Fig. 12.30). A common pitfall to be wary of in such cases is the presence of marginal osteophytes at the femoral head-neck junction (Fig. 12.31). In a pilot study, Chiang et al. (2012) reviewed the initial radiographs of patients with "occult" hip fractures (with radiographs initially labeled as "negative") and found that in 87.5% of these cases, there was at least one radiographic sign which could have indicated the diagnosis on the initial radiograph. They proposed the use of three signs to potentially increase the detection rate on initial radiographs. These were the lateral sign, posterior sign (signs of cortical disruption in the lateral and posterior cortices of the femoral neck on the AP and lateral views, respectively), and the elevation of fat pad sign, indicating joint effusion/hemarthrosis (Chiang et al. 2012) (Fig. 12.32).

Femoral neck fractures are osteoporosis-related fractures, and unfortunately, osteopenia limits radiographic detection of non-displaced and subtle fractures. Therefore, a certain number of these fractures, studies estimate between 2 and 9% of fractures, will be radiographically

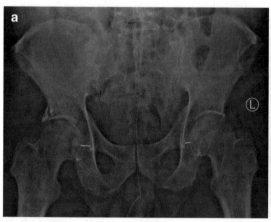

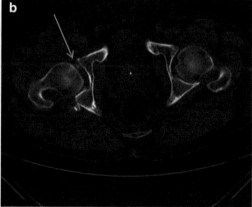

Fig. 12.29 Intra-articular fracture fragment. (**a**) AP radiograph of the pelvis of the same case in Fig. 12.28, postreduction. Note the relatively widened teardrop distance on the right (*yellow line* – between the lateral border of the teardrop and the medial border of the femoral head), which suggests the presence of an intra-articular fracture fragment in the reduced hip joint. (**b**) This is confirmed on CT (*arrow*). Note also the shear fracture of the right femoral head

occult (Perron et al. 2002; Dominguez et al. 2005). When no obvious fracture is seen, but a femoral neck fracture is suspected clinically, the recommendation is to proceed with further

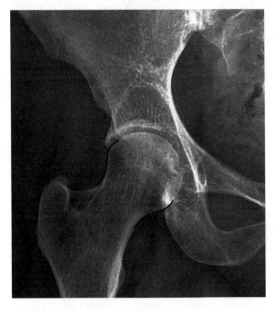

Fig. 12.30 AP radiograph of normal hip shows a smooth curved S-shaped outline of the femoral head and neck (*dark curved lines*)

imaging – usually fast MRI – so as to facilitate early surgical treatment (Rizzo et al. 1993). This is because if it is not diagnosed, an occult hip fracture could become displaced with continued ambulation and lead to disastrous consequences. Blickenstaff and Morris (1966) found that when undiagnosed, many occult hip fractures proceeded to displacement, and on follow-up even after eventual treatment, many of these patients developed the sequelae of prolonged incapacity, nonunion, and avascular necrosis. In osteoporotic patients, other insufficiency fractures of the pelvis may mimic hip fractures clinically, presenting with pain in the pelvic/hip region. Therefore, it is important to routinely search the pelvic radiograph for these other fractures, especially in the osteopenic patient with no radiographic signs of a femoral neck fracture. Sites to be surveyed include the femoral neck, pubic rami, sacrum, intertrochanteric region, and the greater trochanter. Most fatigue fractures in the proximal femur are intracapsular in location, located either on the superior cortex (tension side) or the inferior cortex (compression side) of the femoral neck, and may be subtle (Fig. 12.32).

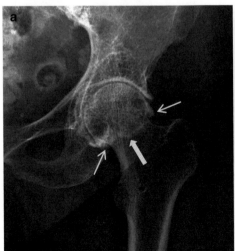
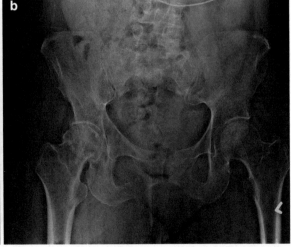

Fig. 12.31 Mach band. (a) AP radiograph of the osteoarthritic hip shows apparent angulation at femoral head-neck junction due to marginal osteophytes (*outer arrows*) and the resulting Mach band across the femoral neck (*middle arrow*), which may mimic a fractured femoral neck. (b) AP radiograph of an impacted right femoral neck fracture. There are disruption in the primary compressive trabeculae of the right femoral neck, compared to normal trabeculae as seen on the left, and the angulation at the femoral head-neck junction

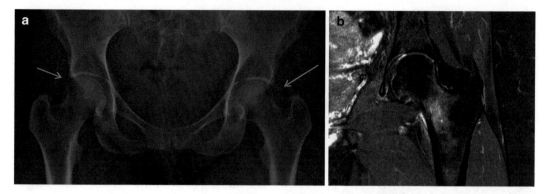

Fig. 12.32 Stress fracture. (**a**) AP radiograph of the pelvis. Subtle cortical thickening is present in the medial aspect of the left femoral neck – is this a real finding? Note the ipsilateral elevation of the left hip fat pad indicative of a joint effusion/hemarthrosis, compared with normal hip fat pad on the right (*arrows*), indicating that a left hip abnormality is likely. (**b**) An underlying stress fracture was confirmed on MRI

12.11 Knee Trauma

Cockshott et al. (1983) recommended that two standard radiographic projections of the knee, AP and lateral, are sufficient for initial assessment and that if a fluid collection is evident on a lateral view with no fracture seen on the standard projections, clinical evaluation would then determine which additional views would be most appropriate to detect the occult fracture, with a choice of oblique, tunnel, and skyline projections. Other authors have demonstrated that four radiographic views – AP, lateral, and both obliques (medial and lateral 45° obliques) – are more sensitive for the detection of fractures (Gray et al. 1997). The oblique views are especially helpful for the detection of certain subtle avulsion fractures around the knee, as these fractures are often only seen when the X-ray beam is tangential to the fracture line. Avulsion injuries are especially important to detect, as they may indicate the presence of often severe underlying soft tissue injuries in the knee (Singer et al. 2014). Missing such injuries may lead to significant morbidity to the patient, such as early post-traumatic knee degeneration. Knowledge of the key ligamentous and tendinous attachments around the knee will help to predict which underlying soft tissue structures are injured with each particular avulsion fracture.

12.11.1 Avulsions Related to the Distal Femur

Popliteal tendon avulsion fracture occurs at the tendon origin on the lateral femoral condyle, presenting with osseous fragment(s) lateral to the popliteal groove. A single fragment in this location may resemble a cymella – a rare sesamoid bone of the popliteus tendon origin.

12.11.2 Segond Fracture

Segond fracture is a well-known fracture present on the AP radiograph as a vertical sliver of bone just below and lateral to the articular margin of the lateral tibial plateau (Fig. 12.33). It had previously been thought to result from avulsion of the middle third of the lateral capsular ligament. However, recently, cadaveric studies have shown it to be related to the so-called anterolateral ligament of the knee (Claes et al. 2013). There is a very high association with underlying anterior cruciate ligament (ACL) tear and a high association with underlying meniscal injury. Failure to identify this injury may result in instability, cartilage damage, and early osteoarthritis.

A *reverse Segond fracture* is a similar appearing sliver of bone located just medial to the

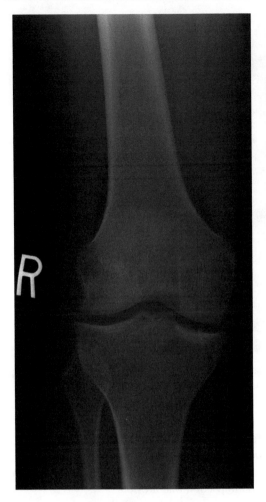

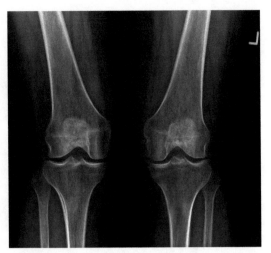

Fig. 12.34 AP radiograph of the knee shows a minimally displaced avulsion fracture superior to the *left* tibial eminence, indicating avulsion at the distal attachment of the ACL

This is an avulsion of the distal attachment of the iliotibial band and also indicates risk for associated ACL injury. On the lateral projection, avulsions of the tibial attachments of the ACL and PCL may be identified superior to the tibial eminence or superior to the posterior aspect of the medial tibial plateau, respectively (Fig. 12.34). The location of the latter avulsion of the PCL should be correlated on the AP radiograph so as not to confuse it with a fabella or the rare "meniscal ossicle."

Fig. 12.33 Segond fracture. AP radiograph of the knee shows a small curvilinear vertically oriented bone fragment lateral to lateral tibial plateau. This is indirect evidence of underlying ACL tear

12.11.3 Arcuate Complex Avulsion Fracture

medial tibial plateau. This fracture results from avulsion of the deep fibers of the medial collateral ligament (MCL) from their tibial attachment. Its presence may signify that a dislocation has taken place (Escobedo et al. 2002), even though the knee may be reduced at the time of imaging; this should raise suspicion for concomitant risk of vascular injury. It is associated with tears of the PCL and medial meniscus. *Gerdy tubercle avulsion* occurs at the anterolateral aspect of the tibial plateau, more anterior and inferior in relation to the Segond fracture, and is best seen on a medial oblique view of the knee.

The arcuate sign, a horizontally oriented elliptical bone fragment arising from the fibular styloid process, results from avulsion of the arcuate ligament complex insertion and signifies injury to the important posterolateral corner stabilizers of the knee (Gottsegen et al. 2008). This injury, along with the more laterally located fibular head avulsion of the conjoint tendon insertion, may be hidden on an AP radiograph by the overlapping tibial plateau; they may be well seen on trauma oblique views (Fig. 12.35).

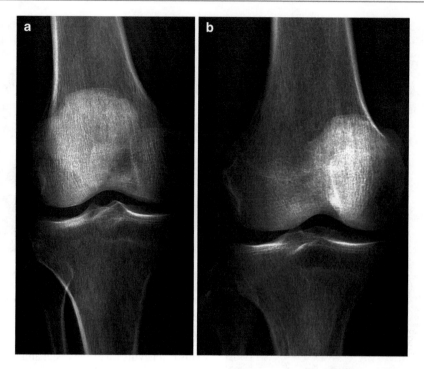

Fig. 12.35 Arcuate sign. There is a small crescentic bone fragment from the tip of the fibular styloid process, indicating avulsion at the insertion of the arcuate ligament complex. It may be obscured on the (**a**) AP view, but is well profiled on the (**b**) oblique projection

12.11.4 Patellar Avulsion Fractures

The main forces acting through the patella are superior and inferior forces of the extensor mechanism (quadriceps and patellar tendons) and medial and lateral stabilizing forces (medial and lateral patellar retinacula). Patellar avulsion fractures may occur at the attachments of each of these structures. Quadriceps and patellar tendon avulsions may be suggested by fragments at the superior and inferior poles of the patella, respectively, on the lateral radiograph (Fig. 12.36). Medial and lateral patellar avulsion fractures may be occult on standard AP and lateral radiographs, but are shown to advantage on trauma oblique views or a patellar view (Fig. 12.37). Aside from a survey of the knee for the above avulsion fractures, the articular surfaces and subchondral bone should be scrutinized for the following radiographic signs: step or notched deformity in the articular surface, focal changes in subchondral bone density to either subchondral lucency or subchondral sclerosis, or a frank focal defect in the articular bone, to help identify potentially subtle minimally displaced tibial plateau fractures and femoral condylar osteochondral impaction fractures.

12.11.5 Osteochondral Impaction Fracture

Osteochondral impaction fracture occurs during the course of a pivot shift injury and is a sign indicating underlying ACL tear. It is identified through abnormal deepening of the normal lateral condyle-patellar sulcus of the lateral femoral condyle to a depth of more than 2 mm (Pao 2001).

12.11.6 Stress Fractures

Proximal tibial cortical stress fractures commonly occur at the popliteal-soleal line of the posteromedial tibial surface and involve cortical bone, manifesting as periosteal reaction,

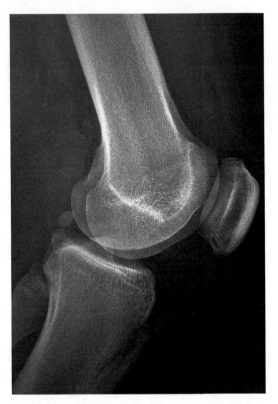

Fig. 12.36 Lateral radiograph of the knee shows an unfused ossification center of the tibial tuberosity. Note also the tiny acute avulsion fracture of the inferior pole of the patella, identifiable through fulfilling satisfaction of search

without or with a fracture line (Engber 1977; Daffner et al. 1982). Conversely, insufficiency fractures of the proximal tibia involve the cancellous bone of the proximal tibia and instead may be seen on knee radiographs as a transverse sclerotic band on the standard views (Manco et al. 1983) (Fig. 12.38). An unusual type of stress fracture is the longitudinal stress fracture. This occurs due to repetitive twisting-type forces on the involved long bone, with the unusually oriented longitudinal fracture. It may be missed because of its relative rarity and subtle appearance (Fig. 12.39).

12.11.7 Soft Tissues

Evaluation of prepatellar soft tissues is especially helpful for identifying occult patellar fractures and indicates the need for further patellar views, where these are not routinely obtained (Fig. 12.37a). Identification of lipohemarthrosis, indicated by the presence of joint effusion with a fat-fluid level on a cross-table lateral radiograph, helps raise suspicion for underlying intra-articular fractures such as the tibial plateau fracture.

Fig. 12.37 (**a**) Cross-table lateral radiograph of the knee shows prepatellar soft tissue swelling and large joint effusion – raising suspicion for underlying injury – but no fracture was evident on this view or on the AP view (not shown).
(**b**) Further patellar view radiograph clearly shows an avulsion fracture of the medial pole of the patella; this fracture may also be well seen on a trauma oblique view

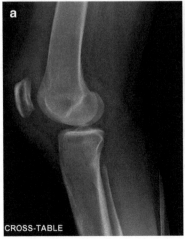

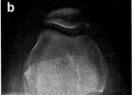

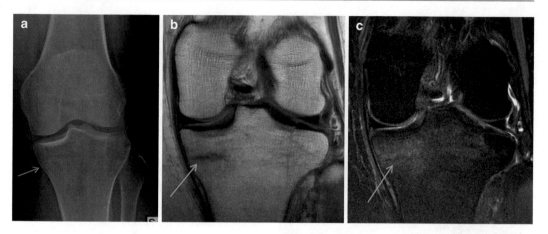

Fig. 12.38 (a) AP radiograph of the knee shows a very subtle transverse sclerotic band in the proximal medial tibial plateau, indicating an underlying stress fracture of cancellous bone (*arrow*). This was confirmed on coronal (**b**) T1-W and (**c**) fat-suppressed T2-W MR images (*arrows*)

12.11.8 Tibial Plateau Fractures

Displaced impacted tibial plateau fractures with obvious comminution, and fractures with a vertical split component, would likely be easily detected in most radiographic examinations. However, minimally depressed tibial plateau fractures – with less than 4 mm of depression – may be subtle on standard AP radiographs (Capps and Hayes 1994). This is due to the obliquity of the articular surface of the tibial articular surface, which has a slight posterior decline. A modified plateau view, taken with 10–15° caudal tube angulation, tangentially outlines the articular surface of the tibial plateau and enables identification and measurement of the degree of articular surface depression (Moore and Harvey 1974). Complete preoperative characterization of comminuted fractures is usually done with the help of CT (Fig. 12.40).

12.12 Ankle Trauma

Ankle injuries are particularly common, with up to 12% of emergency visits involving an ankle injury (Cockshott et al. 1983). Foot fractures are found to be the most commonly missed fractures, with ankle fractures being the seventh most commonly missed fracture (Wei et al. 2006). However, ankle fractures have been found to incur the highest malpractice awards in a study (Baker et al. 2014). Certain severe and disabling foot injuries may present with very subtle radiographic signs which may be easy to miss in the background of complex ankle and foot anatomy. Subtle fractures around the ankle may often be misdiagnosed as ankle or foot "sprains" (Mansour et al. 2011). For these reasons, heightened vigilance is needed when interpreting ankle and foot radiographs, with particular attention to the areas where subtle radiographic signs of injury lend themselves to detection. Brandser et al. (1997) found in a study of consecutive ankle radiographic series for trauma that the most commonly missed fractures were talar fractures, base of fifth metatarsal fractures, calcaneal stress fractures, syndesmotic injury, as well as incorrect classification of old fractures as acute.

The standard radiographic evaluation of the ankle includes a minimum of AP, lateral, and oblique "mortise" radiographic projections. Many ankle fractures will be easily evident on these standard radiographs. However, even when none are found at first pass, paying special

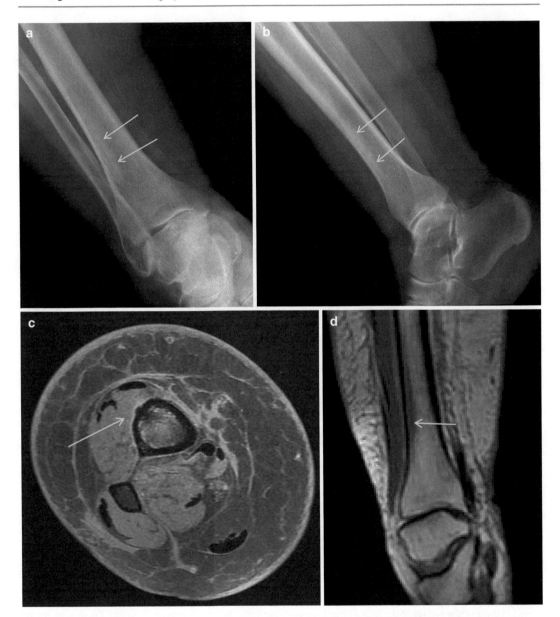

Fig. 12.39 Longitudinal stress fracture in the distal tibia. (**a**) AP and (**b**) lateral radiographs of the distal tibia and fibula show a subtle longitudinally oriented sclerotic band in the distal metadiaphysis of the tibia. (**c**) Axial fat-suppressed T2-W MR image shows corresponding perios- teal and endosteal callus formation (*arrow*), with bone marrow edema and periosteal edema. (**d**) Coronal T1-W MR image shows a longitudinally oriented hypointense sclerotic line (*arrow*)

attention to sites of commonly missed injury would help improve diagnostic accuracy. To detect subtle syndesmotic injury in the ankle, evaluation of certain radiographic measurements is key. These include measuring the tibiofibular overlap, medial clear space, and lateral syndes- motic clear space and checking for any malalign- ment between the lateral border of the talus and

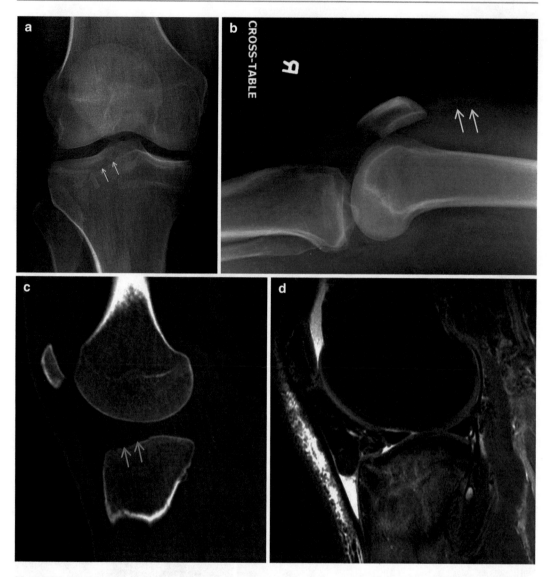

Fig. 12.40 (**a**) AP radiograph of the knee shows focal depression (*yellow arrows*) and step deformity (*blue arrow*) in the articular surface of the lateral tibial plateau, which may only be identified with careful evaluation of the articular surface. For reference, see the normal appearance of the lateral tibial plateau articular surface in

Fig. 12.35a–b. (**b**) Cross-table lateral radiograph of the knee shows a large lipohemarthrosis with fat-blood level (*arrows*), indirect supporting evidence for an intra-articular fracture. Subtle minimally depressed tibial plateau fracture is confirmed on (**c**) CT (*arrows*) and (**d**) MRI

the lateral anterior border of the distal tibia, as seen on the mortise view (Fig. 12.41a). In the event that no fracture is found on initial assessment, a targeted evaluation for signs of the subtle injuries – small avulsion fractures, stress fractures or osteochondral injury, soft tissue signs, and subtle malalignment – may be performed.

12.12.1 Soft Tissue Signs

Clark et al. (1995) demonstrated, in a series of patients with ankle trauma and negative initial radiographic examination, that one-third of patients with an ankle joint effusion as demonstrated on the lateral projection actually had

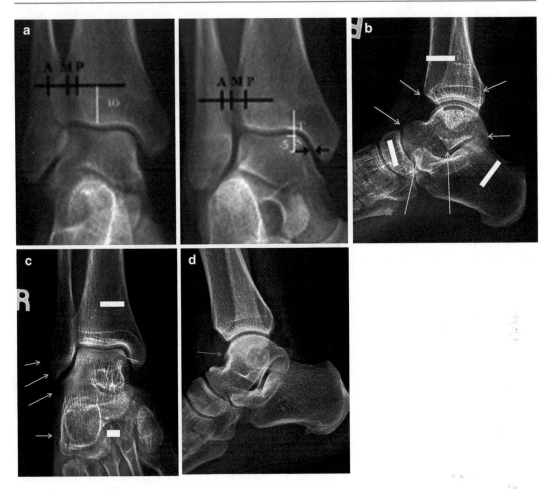

Fig. 12.41 (a) AP radiograph depicting ankle metrics and dimensions (Reproduced with permission from Pope TL, Bloem HL, Beltran J, Morrison WB, Wilson DJ (eds) (2015) *Musculoskeletal imaging*, 2nd edn. Elsevier Saunders, Philadelphia). (b) Lateral and (c) oblique (mortise) views of ankle, with suggested search pattern for potentially subtle injuries. (b) Lateral projection. *Yellow arrows* – "marching" around the talus, searching for avulsion injuries: dorsal avulsion of talar head, anterior process of calcaneus, lateral process of the talus (better seen on AP/oblique), posterior process of the talus, posterior malleolus, and anterior lip of tibial plafond. And don't forget the fifth metatarsal base (*red star*). *White bands* – bones around the talus searching for sclerotic bands indicating stress fractures of calcaneus, distal tibia, and tarsal navicular. *Purple crescent* – check talar dome for subchondral lucent crescent, osteochondral lesion. (c) Mortise projection. *Yellow arrows* – avulsion fractures: laterally, lateral malleolus, lateral process of the talus, anterior process of the calcaneus (extensor digitorum brevis avulsion), and the fifth metatarsal base, from superior to inferior. *White bands* – stress fractures of distal tibia and metatarsals. *Purple crescent* – osteochondral lesion of talar dome. (d) Lateral radiograph of the ankle shows convex anterior bulge of an ankle joint effusion (*arrow*)

occult fractures and that a joint effusion of greater than 13 mm in total capsular distension has an 82% positive predictive value for the presence of an underlying fracture, highlighting the importance of this sign (Clark et al. 1995) (Fig. 12.41d). Identification of edema in Kager fat pad may raise suspicion for underlying acute or stress fractures of the calcaneus and occult ankle and talar posterior process fractures (Ly and Bui-Mansfield 2004). The presence of dorsal soft tissue swelling in the foot may direct attention to the presence of metatarsal stress fractures and Lisfranc injuries.

12.12.2 Talar and Peritalar Fractures

Talar and peritalar fractures may be easy to miss and may masquerade as ankle sprains. The points of tenderness resulting from talar/peritalar injury are not routinely assessed in accordance with the Ottawa ankle rules and are sometimes relatively nonspecific, resulting in a lower index of suspicion for these hindfoot injuries. In a study of missed peritalar injuries, Matuszak et al. (2014) found that talar fractures were the most commonly missed injury.

The talus has an important position and role in the foot and ankle. It is the bone through which axial weight forces are transmitted from the tibia to the calcaneus and forefoot and is the axis through which complex subtalar motion occurs. It is connected to the neighboring tarsal bones and the tibia through a multitude of ligaments, but has no tendinous attachments. As this bone is secondarily mobilized in relation to the surrounding bones, it is no surprise that many fractures occur either through or around it, and this knowledge would help more accurately assess foot and ankle radiographs. A careful search for avulsion fractures by "marching around the talus" and following the cortical margin in a complete circle would help detect subtle fractures of the ankle and hindfoot. Furthermore, when talar fractures are identified, a targeted search for adjacent navicular fractures and calcaneocuboid dislocations must be performed, as these abnormalities have a high association with talar fractures (Matuszak et al. 2014; Robinson and Davies 2015). It is useful to have a dedicated search template for detection of injuries to the ankle, in which several key points need to be assessed for signs of subtle injury (Fig. 12.41b–c); one such template has been proposed by Yu (2015).

12.12.3 Anterior Process of Calcaneus Fractures

Avulsion fractures of the anterior process of the calcaneus result from traction injury at the attachment of the bifurcate ligament during forced ankle inversion (Yu 2015). They may be seen on a lateral radiograph of the ankle or an oblique view of the foot. On the lateral radiograph of the foot, they may be obscured by the overlying talus. It is possible to confuse them with the accessory ossicle – the os calcaneus secundarius (Hodge 1999) (Fig. 12.42). Accessory ossicles occur very frequently as a normal variant in the ankle and foot. They may be difficult to distinguish from avulsion fragments, but accessory ossicles are generally smooth and well corticated, unlike avulsion fractures which are irregular and sharp-edged (Mellado et al. 2003). Symmetry is a feature which supports the diagnosis of an accessory ossicle (Fig. 12.43).

12.12.4 Lateral Process of Talus Fractures

The lateral process of the talus projects from the talar body. Several ligaments, including the lateral talocalcaneal and anterior talofibular ligaments, attach to this important lateral stabilizing structure; as such, it is prone to avulsion injury during ankle eversion/dorsiflexion (snowboarder fracture) (DiGiovanni et al. 2007). Avulsion fractures at this location are best seen on the frontal or mortise views as a fragment arising lateral to the lateral talar process, inferior to the tip of the lateral malleolus. Extensor digitorum brevis avulsion fractures arise from the calcaneus and may be found further inferior to this (Fig. 12.44). An important aid to diagnosis of the above two tarsal avulsion fractures that enables distinction from lateral malleolar avulsion fractures is that the epicenter of soft tissue swelling is inferior to the lateral malleolus, rather than over it (Yu 2015) (Fig. 12.45).

12.12.5 Posterior Talar Process Fractures

The posterior talar process comprises of two tubercles, namely, medial and lateral. The lateral process projects more posteriorly and is the structure

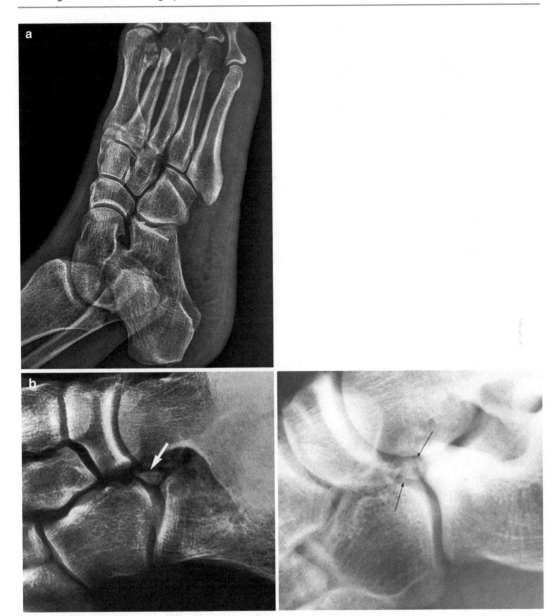

Fig. 12.42 (a) Oblique radiograph of the foot shows an avulsion fragment of the anterior process of the calcaneus, with sharp, irregular, and poorly corticated margins (*arrow*). (b) Oblique radiographs of the foot in two different patients show a well-corticated accessory ossicle of the anterior process of the calcaneus – os calcaneus secundarius (*arrows*). This may mimic an avulsion fracture (Reproduced with permission from Keats and Anderson 2013)

better seen on the lateral view. The posterior talofibular ligament attaches here and may contribute to avulsion injury of this process. Avulsion fractures of the posterior talar process may be con-

fused with the os trigonum; this accessory ossicle occurs in 50% of normal individuals and is characterized by a smooth and corticated appearance, while fractures may demonstrate rough irregular

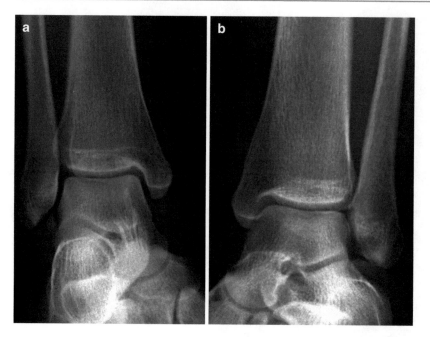

Fig. 12.43 (**a**) Oblique radiograph of the ankle in a patient following a recent ankle injury. Lateral malleolar soft tissue swelling is present. A corticated ossific fragment projects medial to the lateral malleolar tip – is this a chronic avulsion fracture or an os subfibulare? No donor site defect is present in the fibula. (**b**) Contralateral view shows symmetry of the finding – indicating an os subfibulare. This illustrates the value of comparison views

edges. Imaging the contralateral ankle may help corroborate the presence of an os trigonum but not always – as it may be a unilateral finding (McDougall 1955) (Fig. 12.46).

12.12.6 Talar Neck Fractures

Talar neck fractures are somewhat analogous to scaphoid fractures. The detection of non-displaced talar neck fractures may be hindered due to the oblique orientation of the talus relative to the standard radiographic projections, thus necessitating special views. Canale and Kelly (1978) modified the AP radiographic projection of the foot to focus on the talar neck by inverting the foot by 15° and also angling the X-ray tube 15° cephalad. If missed, talar neck fractures may become displaced and may confer a risk of avascular necrosis to the talar body.

12.12.7 Osteochondral Injuries

Osteochondral fractures involving the foot and ankle generally occur through impaction or shearing injury and most commonly involve the talar dome. In the foot, they may involve the head of the second metatarsal bone (Freiberg infraction) and the navicular bone. Tarsal osteochondral shear fractures may accompany Lisfranc injury. Radiographic detection depends on the plane of projection being tangential to the plane of the osteochondral fracture line. Osteochondral lesions of the talus are relatively common and may occur in up to 50% of acute ankle sprains

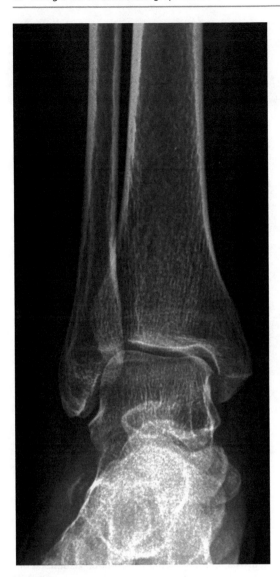

Fig. 12.44 Frontal radiograph of the ankle shows a small avulsion fracture projecting lateral to the hindfoot, at a level inferior to lateral process of the talus. This is an extensor digitorum brevis avulsion fracture from the anterior process of the calcaneum. Note soft tissue swelling is maximal at a level inferior to the lateral malleolus

and fractures (Saxena and Eakin 2007). About 50% of osteochondral lesions of the talus are radiographically occult (O'Loughlin et al. 2010). Searching the joint space and recesses for bone

fragments, articular incongruity, and subchondral lucencies or focal articular surface defects will help in detection of these subtle injuries. Attention should be paid to the mortise ankle view, as the distal fibula partly obscures the lateral talar dome on the AP view (Fig. 12.47).

12.12.8 Dislocations

Subtalar or peritalar dislocations may be missed on standard ankle radiographs. Attention to the talonavicular alignment is key – the talar head should fit within the navicular "cup." If there is concern for such injuries, dedicated radiographs of the foot may be obtained. This injury is often associated with avulsion fractures, as well as subtle osteochondral shear injuries to the talus, navicular, and calcaneus. Associated injuries occur in 45% of patients and are often radiographically occult (DeLee and Curtis 1982).

12.13 Foot Trauma

The foot is an area of anatomic complexity. Almost a quarter of all the bones in the body are located in the feet. In addition, there is a multitude of sesamoid bones and accessory ossicles which occur naturally in the foot, which may mimic avulsion fractures. Standard radiographic examination of the foot includes the AP, oblique, and lateral projections. If injury to the toes is suspected, coned views of the respective digit would increase sensitivity for detecting potentially subtle injuries. It is highly recommended to use the magnification tool on PACS on all foot exams to minimize errors. Doing this causes one to look more closely as in the majority of cases, the exact location of the injury/pain is not given. In the authors' experience in these areas, the most common history is "pain."

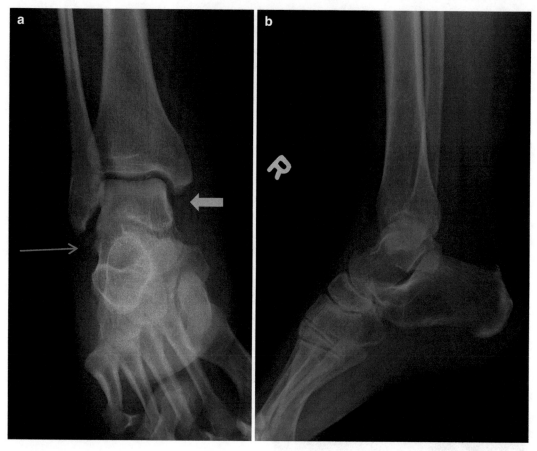

Fig. 12.45 (**a**) Frontal radiograph of the ankle shows a lateral talar process avulsion fracture (*blue arrow*). Note also the medial malleolar avulsion fracture (*white solid arrow*). (**b**) Lateral radiograph of the foot shows a dorsal avulsion fracture of the head of the talus

12.13.1 Base of Fifth Metatarsal Fractures

Fractures of the fifth metatarsal are the most common traumatic injuries encountered in the foot (Pao et al. 2000). Two main categories of fractures of the base of the fifth metatarsal exist. These are the avulsion fractures of the styloid process of the fifth metatarsal and the transversely oriented fracture involving a 1.5 cm segment of the fifth metatarsal base distal to the styloid process, the Jones fracture. The former is much more common, but the latter is prone to long-term complications resulting from nonunion. According to Pao et al. (2000), avulsion fracture of the base of the fifth metatarsal results from traction injury at the attachment of the lateral cord of the plantar apo-

neurosis and may actually be better visualized on radiographs of the ankle than on standard radiographs of the foot. The base of the fifth metatarsal should always be included on standard ankle radiographs and must be carefully reviewed in every case (Fig. 12.48).

12.13.2 Lisfranc/Chopart Injury

The Lisfranc articulation is the tarsometatarsal osteoligamentous complex between the cuneiform bones and cuboid proximally and the metatarsal bases distally. There is a mortise configuration where the base of the second metatarsal is wedged between the medial and

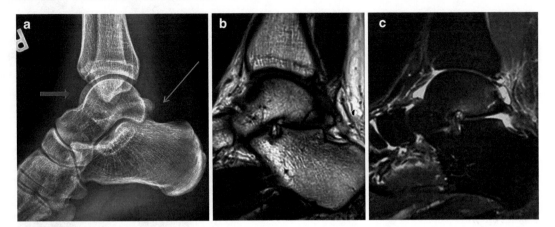

Fig. 12.46 (**a**) No fracture line is seen on the lateral radiograph of the ankle. However, infiltration of the anteroinferior corner of Kager fat pad (*long arrow*) and ankle joint effusion (*solid short arrow*) are seen. The patient experienced difficulty with weight-bearing, which increased suspicion for occult injury and prompted further imaging. Sagittal (**b**) T1-W and (**c**) fat-suppressed T2-W MR images of the ankle show an occult non-displaced fracture of the posterior process of the talus, illustrating the importance of paying attention to the soft tissue signs

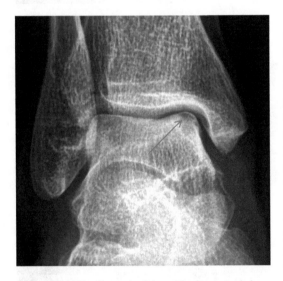

Fig. 12.47 AP radiograph of the ankle shows a subchondral crescent of lucency involving the medial talar dome (*arrow*) – indicating an osteochondral lesion of the talus

lateral cuneiform bones, which, together with the array of tarsometatarsal and intermetatarsal ligaments, contributes to the stability of the joint complex. Lisfranc fracture dislocations usually occur through a variety of mechanisms, including crush or twisting injury or forced plantar flexion of the forefoot, and result in three injury patterns: homolateral, divergent, and isolated.

Though Lisfranc injuries are relatively rare, accounting for only about 0.2% of all fractures, it may be missed on initial examination in as many as 20% of cases (Trevino and Kodros 1995; Gupta et al. 2008; Yu 2015). A key to their accurate diagnosis is paying special attention to the tarsometatarsal relationships when evaluating foot radiographs. Due to the complex configuration of the midfoot, tarsometatarsal congruity needs to be assessed on both the AP and oblique views of the foot (Figs. 12.49, 12.50, and 12.51).

The "fleck sign" – identification of a small flake avulsion fragment in the Lisfranc interval – is a pathognomonic sign indicating underlying Lisfranc fracture dislocation. Other periarticular avulsion fractures may be seen. On a lateral view of the foot, the dorsal border of the second metatarsal base should never be dorsal to the intermediate cuneiform bone. Even where no fracture or malalignment is identified on standard imaging, if there is high clinical suspicion due to such signs as significant midfoot soft tissue swelling or plantar ecchymosis, imaging may proceed with weight-bearing radiographs to demonstrate stress-induced widening of the Lisfranc interval, indicating Lisfranc ligament injury (Englanoff et al. 1995) (Fig. 12.51c).

The Chopart joint or midtarsal joint consists of the talonavicular joint and the calcaneocuboid joint. Injuries to this joint are rare and are often combined with other injuries to the foot

Fig. 12.48 History of "twisted ankle." (**a**) Oblique radiograph of the ankle shows lateral malleolar soft tissue swelling, but no lateral malleolar fracture. Did you look at the edge of the radiograph? Note the tiny avulsion fracture of the fifth metatarsal base. Dedicated (**b**) oblique foot radiograph subsequently obtained showed not only the above avulsion fracture but also a comminuted fracture of the cuboid and a calcaneal avulsion fracture at the calcaneocuboid joint

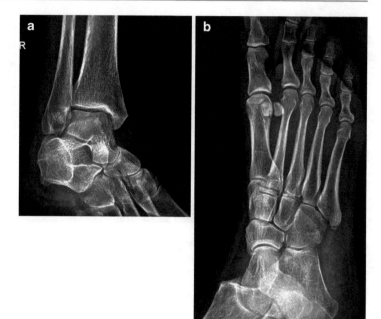

Fig. 12.49 (**a**) Frontal radiograph of a normal foot shows normal first and second tarsometatarsal alignment and a preserved intermetatarsal fat pad (*arrow*). (**b**) Oblique radiograph of a normal foot shows congruity of the third metatarsal – lateral cuneiform and fourth metatarsal – cuboid alignment. No avulsion fragment at the proximal intermetatarsal spaces or at medial/lateral ends of the Lisfranc articulation

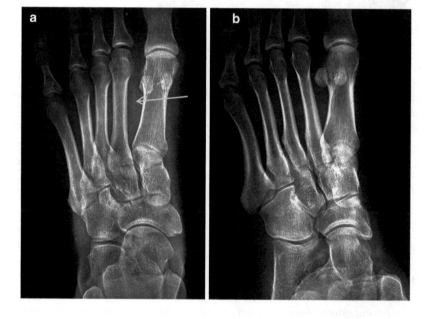

Fig. 12.50 (**a**) Frontal, (**b**) oblique, and (**c**) lateral radiographs of the foot show a Lisfranc fracture dislocation. There is significant malalignment/ incongruity at the tarsometatarsal joints, loss of the first intermetatarsal fat pad, gross soft tissue swelling in the foot, and significant widening of the Lisfranc interval (*yellow line*)

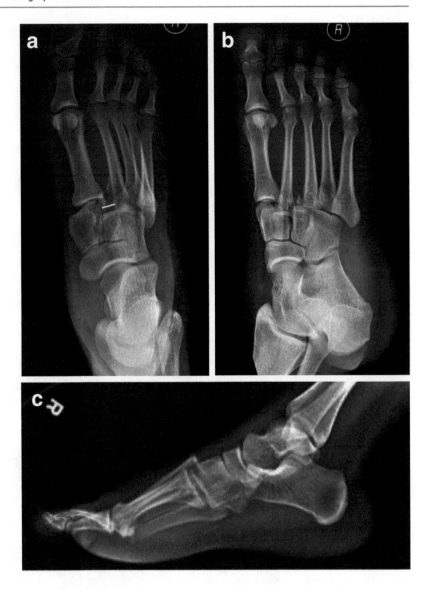

(Benirschke et al. 2012). Evaluation of this joint is often sufficient on standard radiographs and consists of tracing the S-shaped cyma line to detect malalignment, as well as evaluation for small talonavicular and/or calcaneocuboid avulsion fractures (Dewar and Evans 1968) (Fig. 12.52).

12.13.3 Stress Fractures

Stress fractures in the foot commonly involve the calcaneus, tarsal navicular, talus, and metatarsal bones. Stress fractures result from repetitive trauma to normal bone. They are typically radiographically occult in their early stages and often do not become visible until healing begins. The resulting periosteal reaction is generally much easier seen. In the foot, these lesions most commonly involve the shafts of the metatarsals (Forrester and Kerr 1990). They present with periosteal reaction or cortical hyperostosis of the metatarsal shaft, with or without a hairline fracture. Even in the absence of obvious osseous signs, the presence of soft tissue swelling in the dorsum of the foot may be a clue to their presence. A potential pitfall is the normal cortical hyperostosis which occurs in the metatarsal shafts due to muscle attachments (Figs. 12.53

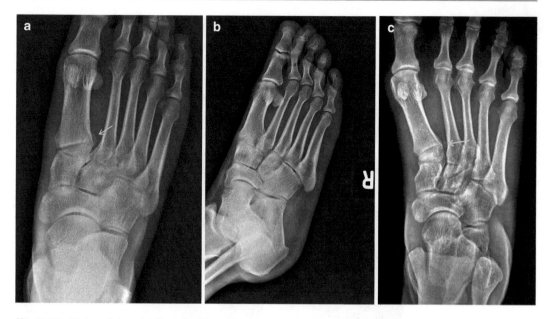

Fig. 12.51 Lisfranc injury. (**a**) Frontal radiograph of the foot shows the "fleck" sign, with an avulsion fragment in the first-second proximal intermetatarsal space (*arrow*). (**b**) Oblique radiograph shows small avulsion fragments medial to the first tarsometatarsal articulation and in the proximal second-third intermetatarsal space. Unlike the case in Fig. 12.50, no significant disturbance of Lisfranc joint congruity is seen in this case; the avulsion fractures are a key but subtle sign that a Lisfranc injury has occurred. (**c**) Frontal radiograph of the foot shows an os intermetatarseum (*arrow*), a normal variant, which may mimic the fleck sign of a Lisfranc fracture dislocation. Note the normal Lisfranc interval in this case

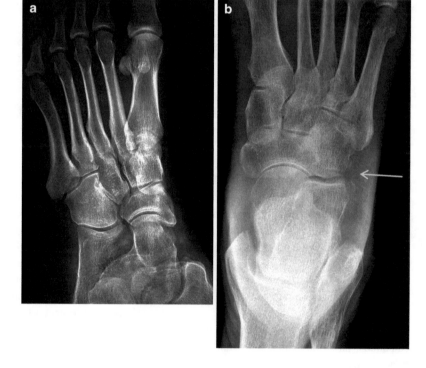

Fig. 12.52 (**a**) Oblique radiograph of the foot shows a normal Chopart joint with the S-shaped cyma line formed by the calcaneocuboid and talonavicular joint spaces. (**b**) Frontal radiograph of the foot shows the cyma line – there is widening of the calcaneocuboid joint space and calcaneocuboid avulsion fractures (*arrow*) secondary to Chopart joint injury

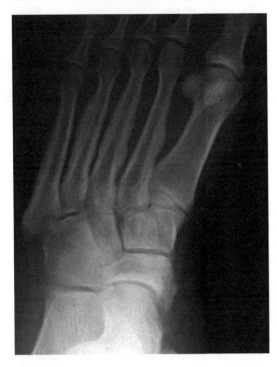

and 12.54). In the base of the metatarsals, they may present as a medullary band of sclerosis, from healing of microtrabecular fractures. In the calcaneus, a stress fracture presents as a band of sclerosis perpendicular to the plane of the trabeculae (Fig. 12.55); and in the navicular bone, it presents as a perpendicular lucency through the mid-navicular seen on the AP radiograph of the foot.

12.13.4 Calcaneal Fractures

Calcaneal fractures are often visible on the lateral radiograph. Carefully evaluating the position of the posterior facet and assessing for loss of calcaneal height (Bohler angle) assist in detection of subtle calcaneal fractures. If there is strong clinical suspicion for calcaneal fracture and the lateral radiograph is negative, an axial (Harris) view may be obtained to evaluate the calcaneal tuberosity, sustentaculum tali, and posterior facet (Germann et al. 2004) (Fig. 12.56).

Fig. 12.53 Oblique radiograph of the foot shows age-related cortical thickening in the metatarsal shafts of no pathologic significance (Reproduced with permission from Keats and Anderson 2013)

Fig. 12.54 (a) Frontal radiograph of the foot shows very subtle periosteal reaction involving the mid-shaft of the third metatarsal. (b) Repeat radiograph 6 weeks later shows callus formation, indicating non-displaced stress fracture

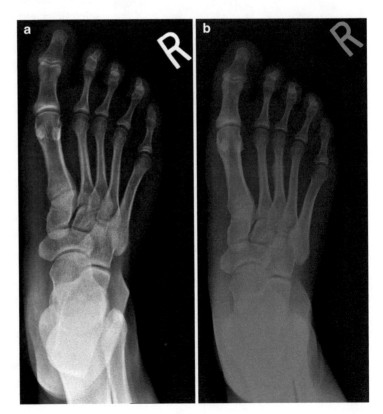

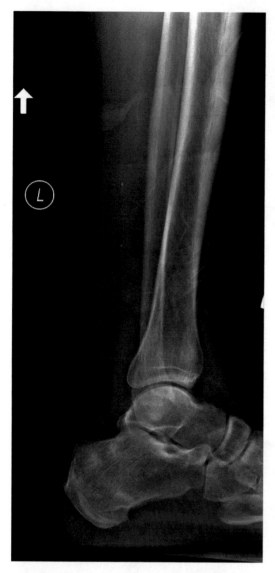

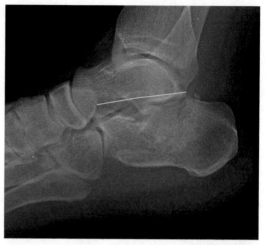

Fig. 12.56 Lateral radiograph of the ankle shows subtle calcaneal fracture, best identified through flattening of Bohler angle (*yellow line*)

be confounded by the presence of a bipartite sesamoid. The medial sesamoid is more commonly bipartite than its lateral counterpart and is more commonly fractured (Uri and Umans 2015). In contrast to the irregular sharp margins of an acute fracture, the bipartite sesamoid has smooth and sclerotic margins, and the sum of the members is often, but not always, larger than the counterpart sesamoid (Burgener and Kormano 2008; Keats and Anderson 2013).

Fig. 12.55 Lateral radiograph of the ankle shows transverse sclerotic bands in the posterior process of the calcaneum, perpendicular to the compressive trabeculae, indicating calcaneal stress fracture

12.13.5 Hallux Sesamoid Bones

The hallux sesamoid bones may be prone to direct trauma on account of their location, and trauma may result in a range of injury from acute fracture to stress fracture and sesamoiditis. Sesamoid injury may be detected on standard projections of the foot and on the special sesamoid view. Diagnosis of sesamoid fracture may

Conclusion

In the setting of trauma, radiography remains the modality of choice for initial imaging evaluation of the appendicular skeleton. Factors which may constitute pitfalls to diagnosis include certain fractures and dislocations which are subtle by nature or which are obscured in areas of complex anatomy, lack of available clinical information, radiologist's fatigue, satisfaction of search effect, and a defective knowledge base. Strategies to help improve radiologist's perceptual and interpretative accuracy include adhering to a consistent search pattern, looking for the subtle and atypical signs of fractures such as avulsion fractures and stress fractures, and close scrutiny of anatomical locations at which fractures and other traumatic lesions are commonly missed. This chapter presented some of the most common long bone pitfalls encountered in clinical practice and outlined some of the clinical and technical clues to help minimize mistakes.

References

Alexander CE, Lichtman DM (1997) Triquetrolunate instability. In: Lichtman DM, Alexander AH (eds) The wrist and its disorders, 2nd edn. Saunders, Philadelphia

American College of Radiology (2001) Expert panel on musculoskeletal imaging, ACR appropriateness criteria. Acute hand and wrist trauma. American College of Radiology, Reston, pp 1–7

Armbuster TG, Guerra J Jr, Resnick D et al (1978) The adult hip: an anatomic study. Radiology 128:1–10

Arndt JH, Sears AD (1965) Posterior dislocation of the shoulder. AJR Am J Roentgenol 94:639–645

Ashman CJ, Yu JS, Wolfman D (2000) Satisfaction of search in osteoradiology. AJR Am J Roentgenol 175:541–544

Baker SR, Patel RH, Lelkes V et al (2014) Non-spinal musculoskeletal malpractice suits against radiologists in the USA--rates, anatomic locations, and payments in a survey of 8,265 radiologists. Emerg Radiol 21:29–34

Bartonicek J (2015) Scapular fractures. In: Court-Brown CM, Heckman JD, McQueen MM et al (eds) Rockwood and Green's fractures in adults, 8th edn. Lippincott, Philadelphia

Beingessner DM, Whitcomb Pollock J, King GJW (2015) Elbow fractures and dislocations. In: Court-Brown CM, Heckman JD, McQueen MM et al (eds) Rockwood and Green's fractures in adults, 8th edn. Lippincott, Philadelphia

Benirschke SK, Meinberg E, Anderson SA (2012) Fractures and dislocations of the midfoot: Lisfranc and Chopart injuries. J Bone Joint Surg Am 94:1325–1337

Berbaum KS, Franken EA Jr, Dorfman DD et al (1990) Satisfaction of search in diagnostic radiology. Invest Radiol 25:133–140

Berbaum KS, Franken EA Jr, Dorfman DD et al (1991) Time course of satisfaction of search. Invest Radiol 26:640–648

Berbaum KS, Franken EA Jr, Anderson KL et al (1993) The influence of clinical history on visual search with single and multiple abnormalities. Invest Radiol 28:191–201

Berlin L (1996) Errors in judgment. AJR Am J Roentgenol 166:1259–1261

Berlin L (2013) Medicolegal-malpractice and ethical issues in radiology: does interpreting too many radiologic studies increase the chance of error? AJR Am J Roentgenol 201:W357

Blickenstaff LD, Morris JM (1966) Fatigue fracture of the femoral neck. J Bone Joint Surg Am 48:1031–1047

Brandser EA, Braksiek RJ, El-Khoury GY et al (1997) Missed fractures on emergency room ankle radiographs: an analysis of 433 patients. Emerg Radiol 4:295–302

Burgener FA, Kormano M (2008) Differential diagnosis in conventional radiology, 3rd edn. Thieme, New York

Canale ST, Kelly FB (1978) Fractures of the neck of the talus. Long-term evaluation of seventy-one cases. J Bone Joint Surg Am 60:143–156

Capps GW, Hayes CW (1994) Easily missed injuries around the knee. Radiographics 14:1191–1210

Cave ER, Burke JF, Boyd RJ (1974) Trauma management. Year Book Medical, Chicago, pp 409–411

Chiang CC, Wu HT, Lin CF et al (2012) Analysis of initial injury radiographs of occult femoral neck fractures in elderly patients: a pilot study. Orthopedics 35:e621–e627

Claes S, Vereecke E, Maes M et al (2013) Anatomy of the anterolateral ligament of the knee. J Anat 223:321–328

Clark TW, Janzen DL, Ho K (1995) Detection of radiographically occult ankle fractures following acute trauma: positive predictive value of an ankle effusion. AJR Am J Roentgenol 164:1185–1189

Cockshott WP, Jenkin JK, Pui M (1983) Limiting the use of routine radiography for acute ankle injuries. Can Med Assoc J 129:129–131

Compson JP, Waterman JK, Spencer JD (1993) Dorsal avulsion fractures of the scaphoid: diagnostic implications and applied anatomy. J Hand Surg Br 18:58–61

Daffner RH, Martinez S, Gehweiler JA et al (1982) Stress fractures of the proximal tibia in runners. Radiology 142:63–65

De Beer JD, Hudson DA (1987) Fractures of the triquetrum. J Hand Surg Br 12:52–53

DeLee JC, Curtis R (1982) Subtalar dislocation of the foot. J Bone Joint Surg Am 64:433–437

Dewar FP, Evans DC (1968) Occult fracture-subluxation through the mid-tarsal joint. J Bone Joint Surg Br 50:386–388

DiGiovanni CW, Langer PR, Nickisch F (2007) Proximity of the lateral talar process to the lateral stabilizing ligaments of the ankle and subtalar joint. Foot Ankle Int 28:175–180

Dominguez S, Liu P, Roberts C et al (2005) Prevalence of traumatic hip and pelvic fractures in patients with suspected hip fracture and negative initial standard radiographs - a study of emergency department patients. Acad Emerg Med 12:366–369

Donald JJ, Barnard SA (2012) Common patterns in 558 diagnostic radiology errors. J Med Imaging Radiat Oncol 56:173–178

Duckworth AD, Clement ND, Jenkins PJ et al (2012) The epidemiology of radial head and neck fractures. J Hand Surg Am 37:112–119

Edgar C, DeGiacomo A, Lemos MJ et al (2015) Acromioclavicular joint injuries. In: Court-Brown CM, Heckman JD, McQueen MM et al (eds)

Rockwood and Green's fractures in adults, 8th edn. Lippincott, Philadelphia

Emergency Department Visits – National Hospital Ambulatory Medical Care Survey 1998–2006. Number (in thousands) of emergency department visits for fracture. http://www.aaos.org/research/stats/ ER_Visits_Fracture.pdf. American Academy of Orthopedic Surgeons

Engber WD (1977) Stress fractures of the medial tibial plateau. J Bone Joint Sung Am 59:767–769

Englanoff G, Anglin D, Hutson HR (1995) Lisfranc fracture-dislocation: a frequently missed diagnosis in the emergency department. Ann Emerg Med 26:229–233

Ernberg LA, Potter HG (2003) Radiographic evaluation of the acromioclavicular and sternoclavicular joints. Clin Sports Med 22:255–275

Escobedo EM, Mills WJ, Hunter JC (2002) The "reverse Segond" fracture: association with a tear of the posterior cruciate ligament and medial meniscus. AJR Am J Roentgenol 178:979–983

Fallahi F, Jafari H, Jefferson G et al (2013) Explorative study of the sensitivity and specificity of the pronator quadratus fat pad sign as a predictor of subtle wrist fractures. Skeletal Radiol 42:249–253

Forrester DM, Kerr R (1990) Trauma to the foot. Radiol Clin N Am 28:423–433

Freed HA, Shields NN (1984) Most frequently overlooked radiographically apparent fractures in a teaching hospital emergency department. Ann Emerg Med 13:900–904

Geissler WB (2001) Carpal fractures in athletes. Clin Sports Med 20:167–188

Germann CA, Perron AD, Miller MD et al (2004) Orthopedic pitfalls in the ED: calcaneal fractures. Am J Emerg Med 22:607–611

Gertzben SD, Barrington TW (1975) Diagnosis of occult fractures and dislocations. Clin Orthop Relat Res 108:105–109

Gilula LA, Weeks PM (1978) Post-traumatic ligamentous instabilities of the wrist. Radiology 129:641–651

Gilula LA, Totty WG (1992) Wrist trauma: roentgenographic analysis. In: Gilula LA (ed) The traumatized hand and wrist: radiographic and anatomic correlation. WB Saunders, Philadelphia

Glajchen N, Schwartz ML, Andrews JR et al (1998) Avulsion fracture of the sublime tubercle of the ulna: a newly recognized injury in the throwing athlete. AJR Am J Roentgenol 170:627

Goss TP (1996) The scapula: coracoid, acromial, and avulsion fractures. Am J Orthop 25:106–115

Gottsegen CJ, Eyer BA, White EA et al (2008) Avulsion fractures of the knee: imaging findings and clinical significance. Radiographics 28:1755–1770

Goud A, Segal D, Weissman BN et al (2008) Radiographic evaluation of the shoulder. Eur J Radiol 68:2–15

Gray SD, Kaplan PA, Dussault RG et al (1997) Acute knee trauma: how many plain film views are necessary for the initial examination? Skeletal Radiol 26:298–302

Greenspan A, Norman A (1982) The radial head, capitellum view: useful technique in elbow trauma. AJR Am J Roentgenol 138:1186–1188

Greenspan A (2011) Radiologic evaluation of trauma. In: orthopedic imaging, a practical approach, 5th edn. Lippincott Williams and Wilkins, Philadelphia

Gregory CF (1973) Fractures and dislocations of the hip and fractures of the acetabulum. Part I. Early complications of dislocation and fracture-dislocations of the hip joint. Instr Course Lect 22:105–115

Gumina S, Carbone S, Postacchini F (2009) Occult fractures of the greater tuberosity of the humerus. Int Orthop 33:171–174

Gupta RT, Wadhwa RP, Learch TJ et al (2008) Lisfranc injury: imaging findings for this important but often-missed diagnosis. Curr Probl Diagn Radiol 37:115–126

Hawkins RJ, Neer CS 2nd, Pianta RM et al (1987) Locked posterior dislocation of the shoulder. J Bone Joint Surg Am 69:9–18

Henderson JJ, Arafa MA (1987) Carpometacarpal dislocation – an easily missed diagnosis. J Bone Joint Surg Br 69:212–214

Herzberg G, Comtet JJ, Linscheid FL et al (1993) Perilunate dislocations and fracture-dislocations: a multicenter study. J Hand Surg Am 18:768–779

Hodge JC (1999) Anterior process fracture or calcaneus secundarius: a case report. J Emerg Med 17: 305–309

Hodgson PD, Shewring DJ (2007) The 'metacarpal cascade lines'; use in the diagnosis of dislocations of the carpometacarpal joints. J Hand Surg Eur 32:277–281

Hu CH, Kundel HL, Nodine CF et al (1994) Searching for bone fractures: a comparison with pulmonary nodule search. Acad Radiol 1:25–32

Jackson H, Kam J, Harris JH Jr et al (1982) The sacral arcuate lines and upper sacral fractures. Radiology 145:35–39

Jankauskas L, Rüdiger HA, Pfirrmann CWA et al (2010) Loss of the sclerotic line of the glenoid on anteroposterior radiographs of the shoulder: a diagnostic sign for an osseous defect of the anterior glenoid rim. J Shoulder Elbow Surg 19:151–156

Kahn JH, Mehta SD (2007) The role of post-reduction radiographs after shoulder dislocation. J Emerg Med 33:169–173

Keats TE, Anderson MW (2013) Atlas of normal roentgen variants that may simulate disease, 9th edn. Elsevier Saunders, Philadelphia

Krupinski EA, Berbaum KS, Caldwell RT (2010) Long radiology workdays reduce detection and accommodation accuracy. J Am Coll Radiol 7:698–704

Lane CS, Kennedy JF, Kuschner SH (1992) The reverse oblique x-ray film: metacarpal fractures revealed. J Hand Surg Am 17:504–506

Lee JS, Gaalla A, Shaw RL et al (1995) Signs of acute carpal instability associated with distal radial fracture. Emerg Radiol 2:77–83

Liaw Y, Kalnins G, Kirsh G et al (1995) Combined fourth and fifth metacarpal fracture and fifth carpometacarpal joint dislocation. J Hand Surg Br 20:249–252

Lund PJ, Krupinski EA, Pereles S et al (1997) Comparison of conventional and computed radiography: assessment of image quality and reader performance in skeletal extremity trauma. Acad Radiol 4:570–576

Ly JQ, Bui-Mansfield LT (2004) Anatomy of and abnormalities associated with Kager's fat pad. AJR Am J Roentgenol 182:147–154

Manco LG, Schneider R, Pavlov H (1983) Insufficiency fractures of the tibial plateau. AJR Am J Roentgenol 140:1211–1215

Mansour R, Jibri Z, Kamath S (2011) Persistent ankle pain following a sprain: a review of imaging. Emerg Radiol 18:211–225

Mason BJ, Kier R, Bindleglass DF (1999) Occult fractures of the greater tuberosity of the humerus: radiographic and MR imaging findings. AJR Am J Roentgenol 172:469–473

Matuszak SA, Baker EA, Stewart CM et al (2014) Missed peritalar injuries: an analysis of factors in cases of known delayed diagnosis and methods for improving identification. Foot Ankle Spec 7:363–371

McCulloch P, Henley BM, Linnau KF (2001) Radiographic clues for high-energy trauma: three cases of sternoclavicular dislocation. AJR Am J Roentgenol 176:1534

McDougall A (1955) The os trigonum. J Bone Joint Surg Br 37:257–265

McQueen MM (2015) Fractures of the distal radius and ulna. In: Court-Brown CM, Heckman JD, McQueen MM et al (eds) Rockwood and Green's fractures in adults, 8th edn. Lippincott, Philadelphia

Mellado JM, Ramos A, Salvado E et al (2003) Accessory ossicles and sesamoid bones of the ankle and foot: imaging findings, clinical significance and differential diagnosis. Eur Radiol 13:L164–L177

Moore TM, . Harvey PJ Jr (1974) Roentgenographic measurement of tibial-plateau depression due to fracture. J Bone Joint Surg Am 56:155–160

Moore MN (1988) Orthopedic pitfalls in emergency medicine. South Med J 81:371–378

Nordqvist A, Petersson CJ (1995) Incidence and causes of shoulder girdle injuries in an urban population. J Shoulder Elbow Surg 4:107–112

O'brien ET (1984) Acute fractures and dislocations of the carpus. Orthop Clin N Am 15:237–258

Oestmann JW, Greene R, Kushner DC et al (1988) Lung lesions: correlation between viewing time and detection. Radiology 166:451–453

Ogawa K, Yoshida A, Ikegami H (2003) Isolated fractures of the greater tuberosity of the humerus: solutions to recognizing a frequently overlooked fracture. J Trauma 54:713–717

O'Loughlin PF, Heyworth BE, Kennedy JG (2010) Current concepts in the diagnosis and treatment of osteochondral lesions of the ankle. Am J Sports Med 38:392–404

Pao DG, Keats TE, Dussault RG (2000) Avulsion fracture of the base of the fifth metatarsal not seen on conventional radiography of the foot: the need for an additional projection. AJR Am J Roentgenol 175:549–552

Pao DG (2001) The lateral femoral notch sign. Radiology 219:800–801

Perron AD, Brady WJ, Keats TE et al (2001) Orthopedic pitfalls in the ED: lunate and perilunate injuries. Am J Emerg Med 19:157–162

Perron AD, Miller MD, Brady WJ (2002) Orthopedic pitfalls in the ED: radiographically occult hip fractures. Am J Emerg Med 20:234–237

Riddervold HO, Pope TL Jr (1981) Detection of easily missed fractures. Curr Probl Diagn Radiol 10: 1–50

Ring J, Talbot C, Price J et al (2015) Wrist and scaphoid fractures: a 17-year review of NHSLA litigation data. Injury 46:682–686

Rizzo PF, Gould ES, Lyden JP et al (1993) Diagnosis of occult fractures about the hip. Magnetic resonance imaging compared with bone-scanning. J Bone Joint Surg Am 75:395–401

Robinson KP, Davies MB (2015) Talus avulsion fractures: are they accurately diagnosed? Injury 46: 2016–2018

Rockwood CA (1984) Injuries to the acromioclavicular joint. In: Rockwood CA, Green DP (eds) Fractures in adults, vol 1, 2nd edn. JB Lippincott, Philadelphia

Roddie ME (2015) Approach to characterizing radiological errors. In: Peh WCG (ed) Pitfalls in diagnostic radiology. Springer, Berlin/Heidelberg

Russe O (1960) Fracture of the carpal navicular: diagnosis, non-operative treatment and operative treatment. J Bone Joint Surg Am 42:759–768

Salvo JP, Rizio L 3rd, Zvijac JE et al (2002) Avulsion fracture of the ulnar sublime tubercle in overhead throwing athletes. Am J Sports Med 30:426–431

Saxena A, Eakin C (2007) Articular talar injuries in athletes: results of microfracture and autogenous bone graft. Am J Sports Med 35:1680–1687

Scheyerer MJ, Osterhoff G, Wehrle S (2012) Detection of posterior pelvic injuries in fractures of the pubic rami. Injury 43:1326–1329

Singer A, Tresley J, Dalal R et al (2014) Tip of the iceberg: subtle findings on traumatic knee radiographs portend significant injury. Am J Orthop 43: E48–E56

Smith MJ (1967) Error and variation in diagnostic radiology. CC Thomas, Springfield

Stapczynski JS (1991) Fracture of the base of the little finger metacarpal: importance of the "ball-catcher" radiographic view. J Emerg Med 9:145–149

Street JM (1993) Radiographs of phalangeal fractures: importance of the internally rotated oblique projection for diagnosis. AJR Am J Roentgenol 160: 575–576

Trevino SG, Kodros S (1995) Controversies in tarsometatarsal injuries. Orthop Clin N Am 26:229–238

Tuček M, Naňka O, Bartoníček J et al (2014) The scapular glenopolar angle: standard values and side differences. Skeletal Radiol 43:1583–1587

Tuncer S, Aksu N, Dilek H et al (2011) Fractures of the fingers missed or misdiagnosed on poorly positioned or poorly taken radiographs: a retrospective study. J Trauma 71:649–655

Uri IF, Umans HR (2015) Imaging of the forefoot. In: Pope TL, Bloem HL, Beltran J et al (eds) Musculoskeletal imaging, 2nd edn. Elsevier Saunders, Philadelphia

Wei CJ, Tsai WC, Tiu CM et al (2006) Systemic analysis of missed extremity fractures in emergency radiology. Acta Radiol 47:710–717

Welling RD, Jacobson JA, Jamadar DA et al (2008) MDCT and radiography of wrist fractures: radiographic sensitivity and fracture patterns. AJR Am J Roentgenol 190:10–16

Wells J, Ablove RH (2008) Coronoid fractures of the elbow. Clin Med Res 6:40–44

Whang JS, Baker SR, Patel R et al (2013) The causes of medical malpractice suits against radiologists in the United States. Radiology 266:548–554

Wheeless CR III (2015) Wheeless' textbook of orthopedics. Orthopedic references and discussions for physicians. Wheelessonline.com

Yu JS (2015) Easily missed fractures in the lower extremity. Radiol Clin N Am 53:737–755

Zimmers TE (1984) Fat plane radiological signs in wrist and elbow trauma. Am J Emerg Med 2:526–532

Spine Trauma: Radiographic and CT Pitfalls

13

Prudencia N.M. Tyrrell and Naomi Winn

Contents

13.1   **Introduction** 257

13.2   **Pitfalls Due to Technical Factors** 258
13.2.1 Radiography 258
13.2.2 CT 259

13.3   **Pitfalls Due to Overlapping Tissues
        and Artifacts** 262
13.3.1 Radiography 263
13.3.2 CT 263

13.4   **Pitfalls Due to Normal Ossification
        and Developmental Appearances** 263
13.4.1 Normal Ossification 264
13.4.2 Ossicles 265
13.4.3 Synchondroses 270
13.4.4 Vertebral Morphology/Shape 270
13.4.5 Pseudo-Subluxation 271

13.5   **Pitfalls Due to Abnormal
        Development/Normal Variants** 271
13.5.1 Segmentation Anomalies 271
13.5.2 Fusion Defects 273
13.5.3 Vertebral Transition 273
13.5.4 Scoliosis 274

13.6   **Pitfalls Due to Acquired Disease** 274

Conclusion 275

References 275

P.N.M. Tyrrell, FRCR (✉) • N. Winn, FRCR
Department of Diagnostic Imaging, Robert Jones and
Agnes Hunt Orthopaedic Hospital, Gobowen,
Oswestry, SY10 7AG Shropshire, UK
e-mail: Prudencia.Tyrrell@rjah.nhs.uk;
Naomi.Winn@rjah.nhs.uk

Abbreviations

AP   Anteroposterior
CT   Computed tomography
MRI   Magnetic resonance imaging

13.1   Introduction

Imaging of spinal injury frequently involves the modalities of conventional radiography, computed tomography (CT), and magnetic resonance imaging (MRI). Sometimes, these are used in isolation but more often in combination. Depending on the clinical scenario, radiographs may be the preliminary and indeed sole investigation, whereas at the other end of the clinical spectrum, imaging may commence immediately with CT, closely followed by MRI. The modalities of CT and MRI are truly complementary, with CT allowing detection of the more subtle fractures which are often poorly appreciated or overlooked on MRI, while MRI facilitates detection of soft tissue and ligamentous injury which can be difficult to appreciate on CT unless there is associated disturbance in alignment (Tins and Cassar-Pullicino 2006). The nature of injury to the cord itself is also well defined on MRI, and cord contusion and disruption can be readily visualized on MRI when CT can seem normal. There are limitations with any imaging modality and appreciation of this will help avoid potential pitfalls.

© Springer International Publishing AG 2017
W.C.G. Peh (ed.), *Pitfalls in Musculoskeletal Radiology*, DOI 10.1007/978-3-319-53496-1_13

Pitfalls in imaging essentially refer to imaging findings which could be misinterpreted as pathology, when in fact they may be a normal appearance or of a less significant etiology than originally thought. Although bone injury with fracture can often be clearly appreciated on radiographs and CT, soft tissue disruption can also be deducted through disturbances in alignment of the vertebral column and processes. Unrecognized physiological movement can be misinterpreted as being due to ligamentous injury. Many potential pitfalls in spinal injury imaging are related to normal developmental anatomy and normal developmental variance. Familiarity with normal ossification of the spine, normal anatomy, and knowledge of normal variants will help to avoid many pitfalls (Juhl et al. 1962; Davies 1963; Kattan and Pais 1982; Schmidt and Freyschmidt 1993; Keats 1996; Lustrin et al. 2003). This chapter addresses the potential pitfalls in the interpretation of radiographs and CT of the spine, obtained during workup for potential spinal injury. Pitfalls related to radiographic normal variants of the spine are also addressed in Chap. 11 and those related to MRI in spinal injury are addressed in Chap. 14.

13.2 Pitfalls Due to Technical Factors

13.2.1 Radiography

Radiographic assessment of the spine requires a minimum of anteroposterior (AP) and lateral projections of the part of the spine under investigation. Some areas need additional views as a routine, such as the open mouth view to assess the odontoid peg and a coned lateral projection of the lumbosacral junction. High-quality radiographs require careful patient positioning relative to the X-ray tube and appropriate exposure factors (kV and mAs). Underexposure can diminish bone detail, and overexposure can obscure soft tissue signs which could facilitate diagnosis and injury detection. Poor patient positioning for radiographs may lead to obscuration of normal anatomical landmarks and result in unfamiliar bone and/or soft tissue overlap, or failure of superimposition of normal structures may distort normal anatomical appearances and interfere with image interpretation (Fig. 13.1).

Abnormal tilt of the spine or undue rotation can lead to loss of normal bony landmarks.

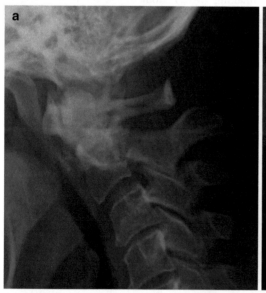 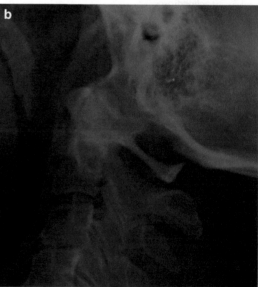

Fig. 13.1 (a) Lateral radiograph shows a simulated fracture through the lamina of C2 vertebra owing to the overlapping soft tissue shadow of the pinna of the ear. There is also a simulated fracture of the posterior arch of C1 vertebra due to rotation. (b) Repeat radiograph of the same patient with a true lateral projection does not show any fracture

A rotated spine can result in loss of superimposition of endplate margins and poor visibility of facet joints. In the cervical region, this can simulate facet joint subluxation if one fails to follow the line of all of the visualized rotated facets. Rotation can lead to asymmetry in the dens-lateral mass interval which could be misinterpreted as a sign of fracture of the atlas ring. In the cervical spine, a view of the odontoid peg is obtained by angling the X-ray tube through an open mouth. In this projection, if the mouth is not open wide enough to visualize the peg, the radiograph may be obtained with the incisor teeth overlying the peg, with potential for misinterpretation of a rare vertical fracture of the peg (Fig. 13.2). If there is too much or too little tilt of the X-ray tube through the open mouth, there is superimposition of the occiput or the anterior arch of the atlas, respectively, on the base of the odontoid peg which can simulate a fracture, unless the arch of C1 is followed across and beyond the peg (Fig. 13.2).

In evaluation of the cervical spine in the trauma setting, it is mandatory to visualize the cervicothoracic junction (Rogers 1992). This can be a difficult area to visualize radiographically in some patients. Failure to do so however will risk missing a fracture, and possibly also dislocation,

at the C7/T1 level (Figs. 13.3 and 13.4). Even in the absence of a fracture, appreciation of disturbances in normal bone alignment can be difficult, and this is an area particularly at risk of potential pitfalls in image interpretation. Alternatively, where radiographic visualization proves difficult, CT (and/or MRI) can be employed, usually with satisfactory results.

13.2.2 CT

Technical factors associated with pitfalls in interpretation of CT are less likely with the advent of third generation and more modern multi-detector CT (MDCT) scanners. These have the ability to rapidly acquire an isotropic volume of fine multi-slice images, with facility to reconstruct high-resolution sagittal and coronal reconstructions within seconds. These can be acquired with a high-definition bone algorithm with high contrast and high spatial resolution. The images can however be downgraded by movement artifact which although not common due to rapid image acquisition, nonetheless can and does occur, especially in the traumatized spinal injury patient who may also have associated brain injury. Movement

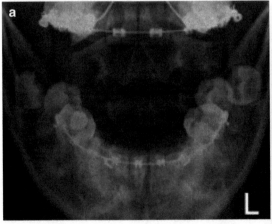
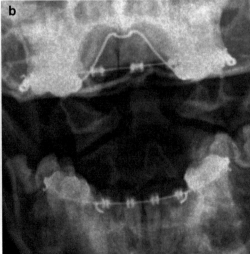
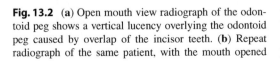

Fig. 13.2 (**a**) Open mouth view radiograph of the odontoid peg shows a vertical lucency overlying the odontoid peg caused by overlap of the incisor teeth. (**b**) Repeat radiograph of the same patient, with the mouth opened wider for the examination such that the incisor teeth no longer overlap the peg. In this projection, however, there is faint linear lucency traversing the base of the odontoid peg, similar to that demonstrated in Fig. 13.6a

Fig. 13.3 (**a**) Lateral radiograph of the cervical spine of a patient following a fall. The cervicothoracic junction is not visualized. (**b**) Sagittal reformatted CT image shows a fracture through the anteroinferior corner of the C7 vertebral body

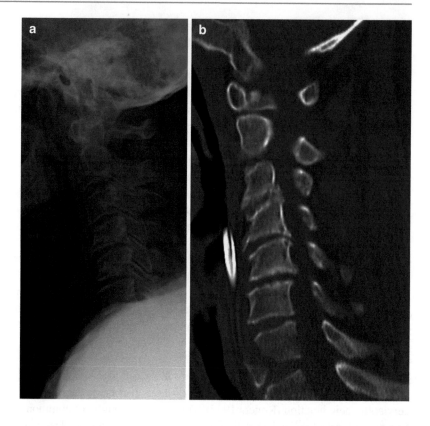

during image acquisition can give rise to streak artifact interfering with image interpretation, and breathing motion can give rise to apparent fractures, particularly of the sternum on reformatted images (sternal fractures often being associated with major thoracic injury). There is potential for fracture to be missed or at the other end of the spectrum, overread, in such a scenario.

On reading a CT examination, there is often a tendency to initially view the sagittal reconstructions (Begemann et al. 2004). CT scanners of different manufacturers and individual setups vary as to whether sagittal studies are read from right to left or vice versa. Clarity on which side of an imaging study is right or left can usually be obtained by viewing the axial images, assuming that these have been obtained in correct topographic format and this should be done in every case, to confirm right and left. Images should ideally be labeled or right-left orientation indicated on a scout or pilot image accompanying the study. This is a basic point but a potential pitfall for those unfamiliar with reading CT images.

The presence of metalwork in the spine, e.g., previous surgery, can result in significant arti-

facts. This is especially the case with instrumentation made from stainless steel. However, titanium results in rather less artifact. Imaging techniques, such as slight angulation of the gantry and altered exposure factors, can help to reduce the degree of artifact and improve interpretation. The use of ultrafine slice thickness, slice overlap, and appropriate windowing will facilitate high-resolution sagittal and coronal reconstructions, which will help to increase fracture detection and minimize the risk of missed fracture. Newer CT scanners with iterative reconstruction software can also help reduce the artifact from metalwork and thus aid in image interpretation.

A significant pitfall with CT imaging is identifying soft tissue injuries. Often, the only clue on CT of a soft tissue injury is malalignment. If the patient is immobilized and correctly positioned on the CT scanner, it may be very difficult to detect a soft tissue injury if one is simply looking for soft tissue swelling or altered attenuation. Ligamentous injury on CT can be easily missed (Fig. 13.4). Interrogation of the images for subtle signs indicating ligamentous disruption such as

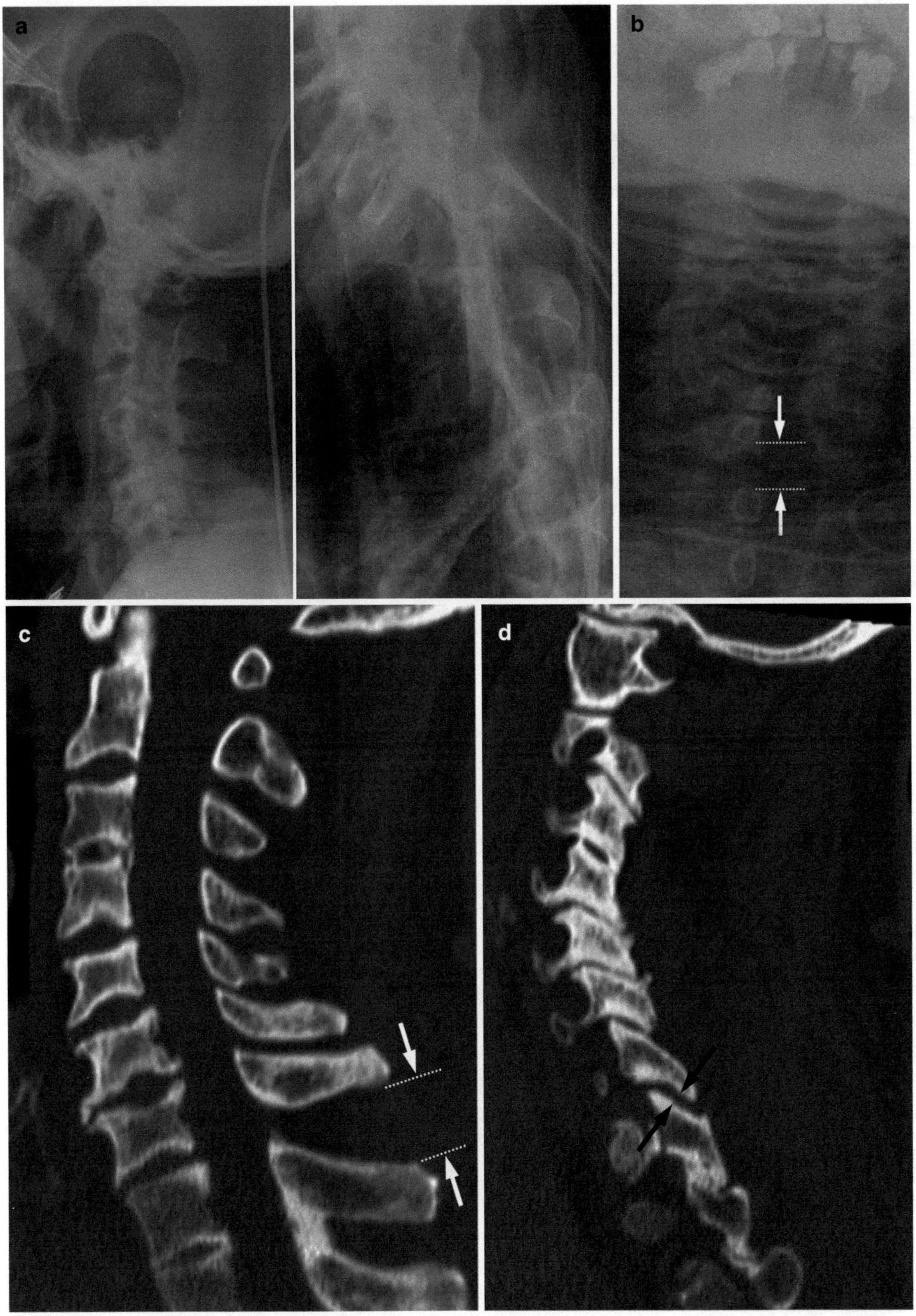

Fig. 13.4 The cervicothoracic junction can be difficult to evaluate on radiographs. (**a**) On the lateral radiographs, the vertebral body alignment appears satisfactory. (**b**) The AP projection shows widening (*arrows*) of the C7-T1 spinous process distance, highly suspicious for ligamentous injury. (**c**) Sagittal reformatted CT image taken in the midline shows widening of the C7/T1 spinous process distance (*arrows*). (**d**) Parasagittal reformatted CT image also shows widening (*arrows*) of the C7/T1 facet joints indicative of ligamentous injury

widening of facet joints or widening of the inter-spinous distance needs to be actively sought. It is a pitfall in itself to fail to recognize the limitations of the different imaging modalities. A clinical review on clearing of the cervical spine in adult obtunded patients found MRI to be inferior to MDCT for detecting bone injury, but superior for detecting soft tissue injury. MRI following "normal" CT may detect up to 7.5% of missed injuries (Plumb and Morris 2012). If a soft tissue injury is suspected and no significant abnormality is detected on CT or radiography, MRI is the next investigation of choice (Plumb and Morris 2012; Badhiwala et al. 2015).

13.3 Pitfalls Due to Overlapping Tissues and Artifacts

An awareness of the effect of overlapping tissues in the interpretation of radiographs can help minimize the risk of pitfalls, especially in the setting of potential spinal injury.

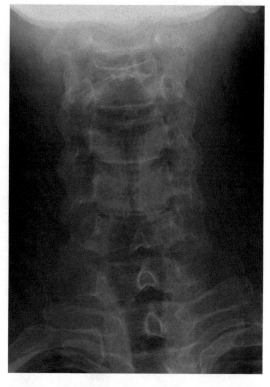

Fig. 13.5 AP radiograph shows a simulated vertical fracture through the body of C5 vertebra, due to air within the larynx. The fine column of air is continuous with the air shadow both proximal and distal to the endplate margins

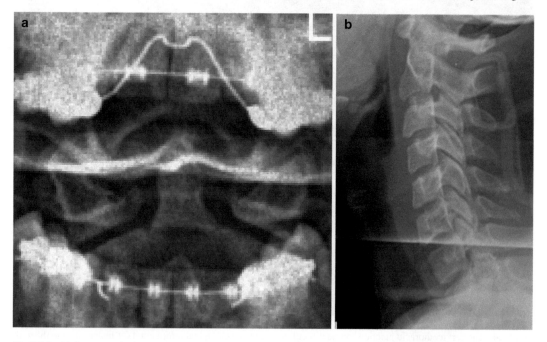

Fig. 13.6 (**a**) Open mouth view radiograph of the odontoid peg shows a simulated fracture through the base of the odontoid peg due to the overlapping shadow of the posterior arch of C1 vertebra. This has also been alluded to as the Mach effect. (**b**) Lateral radiograph of the cervical spine shows that the base of the odontoid peg is intact. There is no prevertebral soft tissue swelling. If there is still concern, the situation can be further clarified with a targeted CT scan

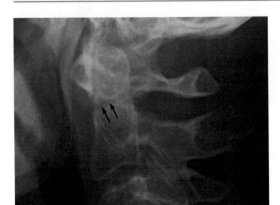

Fig. 13.7 Lateral radiograph of the cervical spine coned to the C1/C2 level shows a fine lucency projected over the base of C2 vertebra (*arrows*). This is projectional and related to the overlapping C1/C lateral mass articulation. The clinical history will be helpful, but if in doubt, CT can confirm normality

13.3.1 Radiography

In the cervical spine, air, either within or between structures, can be projected over the spine and simulate a fracture line. This can occur especially with regard to the larynx overlying the cervical spine (Fig. 13.5). Recognition that this is not a sagittal spinal fracture is achieved by following the lucent line of air either above or below the superimposed endplate margin of the vertebral body. The air gap between the two incisor teeth can be projected as a vertical lucency over the odontoid peg. A vertical fracture would be very unusual but following identification of the vertical lucency, appreciation of the incisor teeth on either side allows one to recognize the potential pitfall. Air related to the pinna of the ear can be recognized by the lucency extending beyond the bony margin and also by appreciating the soft tissue shadow of the pinna in this location once recognized (Fig. 13.1).

Normal anatomical structures may mimic pathology on radiographs due to superimposition of structures. Dark and light lines, named Mach bands, that appear on radiographs at the borders of structures of different densities may give the impression of a fracture. A result of this Mach effect can often be seen at the base of the odontoid peg, where superimposition of the posterior arch of the atlas can give the impression of a fracture (Kattan and Pais

1982) (Figs. 13.2b and 13.6). On the lateral radiograph of the cervical spine, the transverse processes projected over the vertebral body, especially at C2 level, should not be mistaken for a fracture (Fig. 13.7). A horizontal lucency between contiguous osteophytes at the uncinate process/vertebral articulations that simulates a fracture on a lateral radiograph is well described (Goldberg et al. 1982). The radiolucency created by bowel gas on a lumbar spine radiograph may give the spurious impression of a fracture. Another example includes a pseudo-fracture of the proximal thoracic spine from superimposition of the glenoid, especially apparent on a swimmer's projection.

13.3.2 CT

Pitfalls due to overlapping tissues are rarely an issue on CT, due to the facility of multiplanar interrogation of abnormalities seen on preliminary axial, sagittal, or coronal images. Normal anatomical structures can usually be clearly identified. Abnormal structures, including the soft tissue signs of trauma allied to the spine, are usually identified by disruption or loss of anatomical fat planes, altered attenuation characteristics of tissues, possible associated fracture of bone, and disturbances in alignment.

13.4 Pitfalls Due to Normal Ossification and Developmental Appearances

In the developing skeleton, an understanding and recognition of normal appearances at different stages of growth together with knowledge of normal variants is vital in order to avoid pitfalls of interpretation in spinal injury (Tyrrell and Cassar-Pullicino 2006). Familiarity with the normal progression of ossification in the developing skeleton will help minimize misinterpretation (Bailey 1952; Cattel and Filtzer 1965; Lustrin et al. 2003). In the immature skeleton, areas of lucency may be representative of cartilaginous development. The expected sites of secondary ossification centers and their expected time of

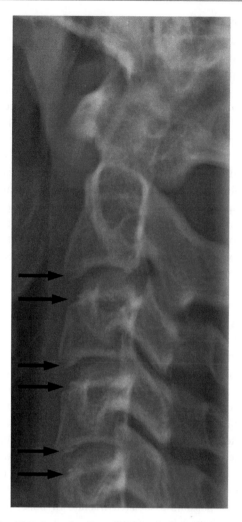

Fig. 13.8 Lateral radiograph of the upper cervical spine shows normal cervical ring apophyses (*arrows*) in this 14-year-old boy – not to be confused with avulsion injury

appearance will help to avoid their misinterpretation as fractures. Synchondroses tend to be symmetrical in location, occur at typical sites, and have smooth well-corticated margins.

13.4.1 Normal Ossification

Primary ossification centers begin to appear by the ninth fetal week. Each typical vertebra ossifies from three primary ossification centers – one in each half of the vertebral neural arch and one in the body, termed the centrum. Ossification starts at different times in the vertebral arches and vertebral bodies in different areas of the spine; but by the 7th month, centers have been established in all areas. Generally, the vertebral arches unite between 1 and 3 years of age, while the centrum unites with the arches at the neurocentral synchondroses between 3 and 6 years of age. In the upper cervical spine, the centrum unites with the posterior neural arch at approximately the 3rd year; but in the lumbar spine, this may be not completed until the 6th year. Ossification tends to progress cranio-caudally (Lustrin et al. 2003).

The ring apophysis appears around the age of 12 years and is identified on the radiograph as a small triangular-shaped bone focus adjacent to the vertebral body margin, often being best appreciated at the anterosuperior corner of the vertebral body (Fig. 13.8). It fuses with the body itself around 15–18 years. Recognition of this ring apophysis is important to ensure that its normal appearance is recognized, and also that any variance from its normal and expected location at the vertebral body corner margin is also recognized, as this could imply epiphyseal injury. At puberty, three further secondary centers of ossification appear – one for each of the transverse processes and one for the spinous process.

Exceptions to the above ossification process occur in the first and second cervical vertebrae. The C1 vertebra ossifies from three centers. Initially, there is an ossification center for each lateral mass which gradually extends into the posterior arch, where the two usually fuse later than in other vertebrae at about the age of 3 or 4 years. At birth, the anterior arch consists of fibrocartilage between the two lateral masses. Toward the end of the 1st year, a third center of ossification appears within the anterior arch and unites with the lateral masses between the ages of 6 and 8 years. Failure of fusion or congenital absence of any of these ossification centers can simulate a fracture, but awareness of the normal developmental process, the typical location, and the smooth margins at the defect site will help to avoid misinterpretation of this entity.

The central pillar of the axis (C2) develops from three segments, namely, the tip of the dens, the base of the dens, and the centrum

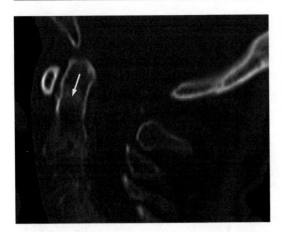

Fig. 13.9 Sagittal reformatted CT image taken through C2 vertebra shows a fine sclerotic line (*arrow*). This likely represents an old syndesmotic scar but an old healed fracture could also be within the differential diagnosis

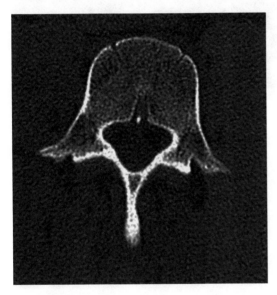

Fig. 13.10 Axial CT image shows a lucency at the posterior aspect of the vertebral body correlating with the site of the basivertebral venous plexus and the peripherally extending venous channels, not to be mistaken as a fracture line

(the body). Ossification occurs in the order of the centrum, the base of the dens, and the tip of the dens. The basilar odontoid synchondrosis usually fuses between 3 and 6 years but may be delayed. This should not be mistaken for a fracture. The vestigial form may persist, being represented by a fine sclerotic line, and

not to be misinterpreted as a fracture line, which would appear clearly lucent with an irregular margin (Fig. 13.9).

With maturation, there is a normal variation in contour of the vertebral bodies which could be mistaken for a fracture. In the lower thoracic spine, the anterior vertebral height is normally less than the posterior vertebral body height, which may be mistaken for a vertebral compression fracture (Black et al. 1991). Other potential pitfalls in the normally developed spine include prominent lucency of the posterior border of the vertebral body, at the site of the basivertebral venous plexus, and also venous channels within the vertebral body as seen on axial CT images which may simulate a fracture. The typical Y configuration extending to the basivertebral venous plexus almost confirms the venous nature and excludes a fracture (Helms et al. 1987; Schmidt and Freyschmidt 1993) (Fig. 13.10).

13.4.2 Ossicles

Secondary centers of ossification occur at typical locations, as do accessory ossicles, and should not be confused with fracture fragments. Typically, ossicles are corticated and usually have a smooth margin although occasionally, they may have a very subtle marginal irregularity. Secondary centers of ossification (apophyses) form along the tips of the spinous processes. The Bergman ossicle at the proximal tip of the odontoid peg is a developmental ossicle (the primordial proatlas) and forms the tip of the dental axis (Fig. 13.11). It is frequently located in a V-shaped vertical cleft at the apex of the dens. It usually fuses between the ages of 2 and 12 years, but may remain as a separate ossicle and not to be confused with an avulsion injury (Schmidt and Freyschmidt 1993).

The os odontoideum is not a true accessory ossicle but rather the result of multiple minor avulsion injuries in childhood with a resultant appearance (Fig. 13.12a, b). While this is usually readily identified as being a long-standing ossicle, in the adolescent patient, perhaps being seen for the first time

Fig. 13.11 (**a**) Axial, (**b**, **c**) coronal reformatted, and (**d**) sagittal reformatted CT images show normal developmental appearances of C2 vertebra, including a fragmented apical ossicle, and the fusing syndesmosis between the C2 vertebral body and the odontoid peg. Note also the rather flattened normal developmental appearance of the vertebral bodies in this 6-year-old girl who complained of neck pain following trampolining

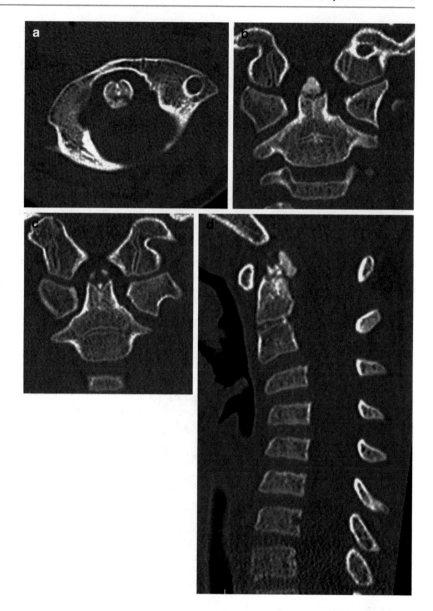

following a cervical spine injury, their presence on the radiograph may cause alarm until full interrogation of the radiograph possibly supplemented by CT identifies the smooth corticated margin of the long-standing ossicle, as opposed to the irregular margin of a fresh fracture with cortical break/disruption. The os odontoideum can be stable (Fig. 13.12c, d) or unstable. The unstable os odontoideum is associated with abnormal movement which can be readily detected on flexion and extension radiographs (Fig. 13.13a, b), but on MRI, secondary effects on the cord can be seen in the form of focal atrophy of

the cord and intrinsic cord signal change, and fluid signal between the ossicle and the parent bone can also be seen (Fig. 13.13c, d). Again, these features are usually as a result of chronic instability rather than due to any acute event. While recognition of the unstable os odontoideum is important for the patient, it is equally important to recognize that it is not related to an acute injury.

Other ossicles seen in the spine are usually as a result of failure of fusion of a secondary ossification center – often without known cause – and are not infrequently seen adjacent to the tip of the spi-

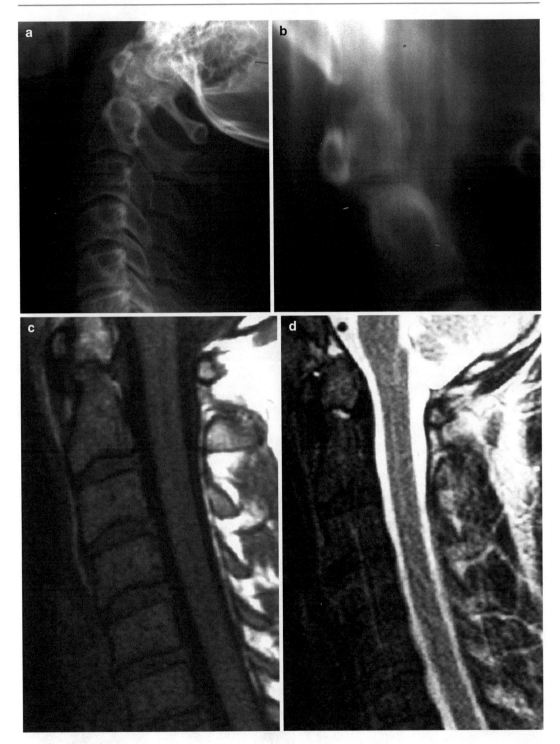

Fig. 13.12 The os odontoideum should not be mistaken for an acute fracture. (**a**) Lateral radiograph shows the well-corticated margins of the ossicle but if in doubt can be more readily appreciated on a (**b**) cervical spine tomo-gram, or if more readily available, CT. Note the smooth well-corticated margins of the ossicle. Sagittal (**c**) T1-W and (**d**) GRE T2*-W MR images show a stable os odontoideum

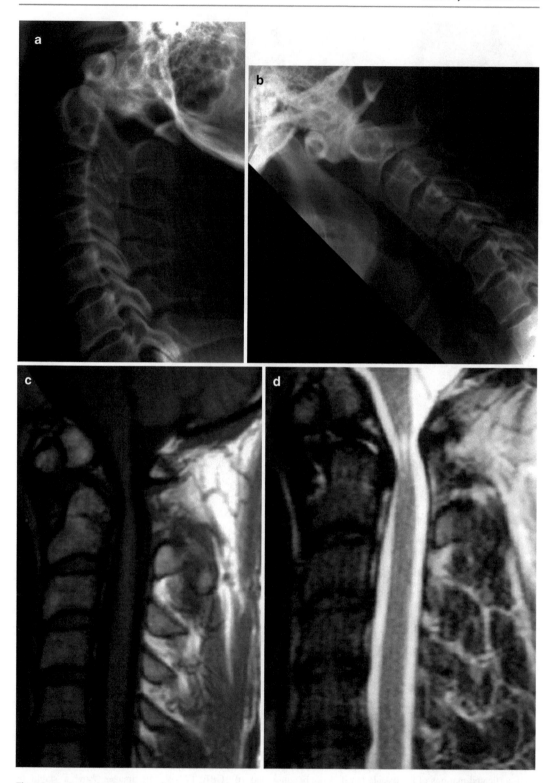

Fig. 13.13 Lateral radiographs of the cervical spine taken in (**a**) extension and (**b**) flexion show abnormal movement of the os odontoideum indicating an unstable ossicle. Sagittal (**c**) T1-W and (**d**) GRE T2*-W MR images show the secondary effects on the cervical cord of an unstable os odontoideum. The cord is thinned and demonstrates abnormal increased myelomalacic type signal as a result of repetitive impingement during flexion and extension movements of the cervical spine (**a**, **c** are reproduced with permission from: Tyrrell and Cassar-Pullicino 2006)

nous process, or adjacent to the tip of a transverse process, where they can mimic an avulsion fracture. In the child, sacral ossification centers should not be confused with fracture. The limbus vertebra is the term applied to small triangular-shaped bone fragment at the anterosuperior margin of the vertebral body. This represents a portion of the ring apophysis, through which there has been herniation of disk material, likely as a result of a single or more commonly multiple minor traumatic events during childhood, and which failed to fuse with the rest of the vertebra (Goldman et al. 1990). The limbus vertebra is most commonly seen in the lumbar spine (Fig. 13.14) but is also seen on occasion in the cervical spine. It can mimic a vertebral body fracture. The development of multiple limbus vertebrae in a 15-year-old male patient with chronic back pain is shown in Fig. 13.15.

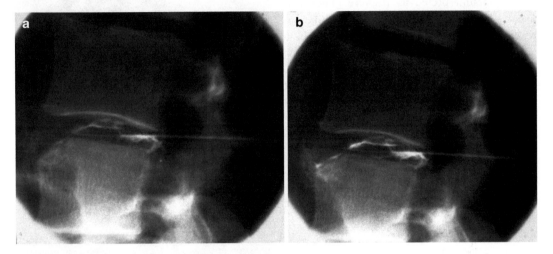

Fig. 13.14 (**a**) Coned lateral radiograph shows a limbus vertebra in a patient undergoing diskography. (**b**) The injected contrast agent is seen tracking into the herniated disk material between the parent bone and the unossified secondary center (bone fragment)

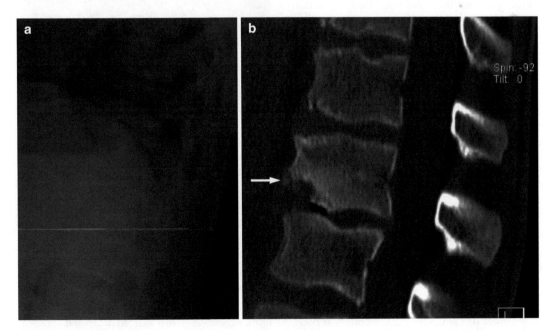

Fig. 13.15 (**a**) Lateral radiograph and (**b**) sagittal reformatted CT image shows irregularity and fragmentation of the apophyses at multiple vertebral levels. There is a developing limbus vertebra (*arrow*) in this 15-year-old male patient with chronic back pain. Gas is also seen within the disk, indicative of degeneration

13.4.3 Synchondroses

Developmental anomalies related to incomplete fusion or failure of fusion at the synchondroses can result in osteolytic defects. The smooth margins should highlight the anomalous nature of the persistent synchondrosis or developmental cleft. On CT, the normal synchondrosis in the developing skeleton should not be misinterpreted as fracture. They can usually be readily identified by their bilateral and symmetrical appearance, occurring in a typical location, with smooth tapered margins. Congenital absence of structures, for example, congenital absence of a pedicle, results not only in a lucent area but may be associated with abnormal motion at a segment. With the clinical history of potential spinal injury, the abnormal movement and lucent area could be confused with a fracture-dislocation. Congenital spondylolysis should not be confused with persistent synchondrosis (Schwartz 2001).

13.4.4 Vertebral Morphology/Shape

With growth, the vertebral body gradually changes shape. In early infancy, the vertebral body appears oval. With growth, it gradually assumes a slightly flattened rectangular shape with rounded corners and sometimes, with a variable degree of wedging. With further growth, it develops a more rectangular or square shape with sharper corners. It starts to assume the adult shape around the age of 8 years (Schmidt and Freyschmidt 1993). A wedging deformity involving the anterosuperior corner of the vertebral body is a well-recognized normal developmental appearance in the young child, described by Swischuk et al. (1993). It occurs most commonly at the level of C3 vertebra (Fig. 13.16) but can occasionally involve the C4 vertebra. This anterior wedging is due to chronic exaggerated hypermobility, causing chronic repetitive impaction of the anterosuperior corner of the C3 by the C2 vertebral body.

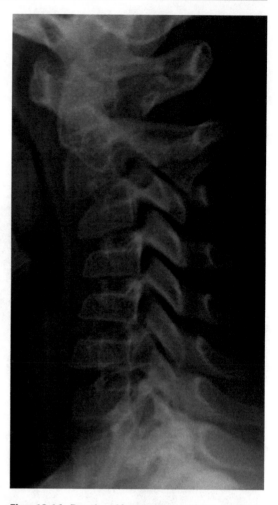

Fig. 13.16 Pseudo-subluxation at C2/C3 vertebra. Lateral radiograph of the cervical spine shows mild anterior subluxation of C2 on C3 vertebra. Note also the wedging of C3 vertebra. Same patient as in Fig. 13.11 where these features are also demonstrated on the sagittal reformatted CT images

Recognition of this appearance helps to avoid the pitfall of diagnosing a compression fracture. However, if there is a history of cervical spine trauma, CT can help to confirm the normal variant, with no fracture being seen. As the child grows older, the wedging disappears as the bone remodels in the absence of hypermobility (Swischuk et al. 1993). The same phenomenon has also been documented in infants at the T12 to L1 vertebral levels due to normal hyperflexion at the T12/L1 level, which results in a wedged or tapered vertebral body. As the child grows and hyperflexion in this part of the body diminishes, so the vertebral body wedging also disappears (Swischuk 1970).

13.4.5 Pseudo-Subluxation

Hypermobility of the upper cervical spine is most pronounced at the C2/C3 level (Sullivan et al. 1958). This hypermobility is due to the fact that the fulcrum for motion of the upper cervical spine in the young child is at the C2/C3 level and laxity of the ligaments of the cervical spine in childhood. The hypermobility can be so marked as to take the form of actual subluxation at C2/C3 level (Swischuk 1977). A potential pitfall is in the recognition or differentiation of physiological from pathological subluxation of C2 on C3 vertebra (Fig. 13.16). Swischuk (Swischuk et al. 1993) described the posterior cervical line as being valuable in this regard. Physiological subluxation can occur in the adult. This is differentiated from a true subluxation by observing the normal smooth curve of the spine by following its anterior and posterior vertebral body lines without interruption. In a true subluxation, a slight step deformity will be observed. With physiological slipping, there is correction with the opposite movement (Scher 1979). Many of the features described above will be appreciable on both radiographs and CT. Because of its axial cross-sectional capability, CT will be able to demonstrate many developmental clefts to better advantage. The differentiation from a fracture is highlighted by the typical location and often symmetrical appearance, together with the smooth margins which are usually corticated.

13.5 Pitfalls Due to Abnormal Development/Normal Variants

13.5.1 Segmentation Anomalies

Segmentation anomalies resulting in congenital block vertebrae can distort the normal anatomy and hinder interpretation (Fig. 13.17). While

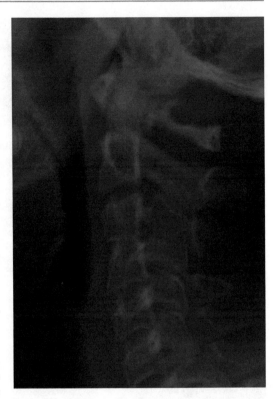

Fig. 13.17 Lateral radiograph of the cervical spine shows a segmentation anomaly at the C3/C4 level – congenital block vertebrae – not to be confused with a diskovertebral injury

such anomalies can usually be recognized as such, when there is a history of trauma, there may be doubt, and depending on the clinical scenario, further imaging for clarification may be required. It is noteworthy that segmentation anomalies are often associated with other features in the spinal dysraphism spectrum. With segmentation anomalies, disturbances in vertebral body shape or complete failure of formation may lead to initial difficulties with interpretation of the radiograph. CT is particularly helpful in such a situation, providing clarification of osseous anatomy and architecture (Fig. 13.18).

Developmental anomalies giving rise to a butterfly vertebra can be well appreciated on radiographs. This is a situation, however, where viewing the AP and lateral radiographs together, rather than the lateral projection in

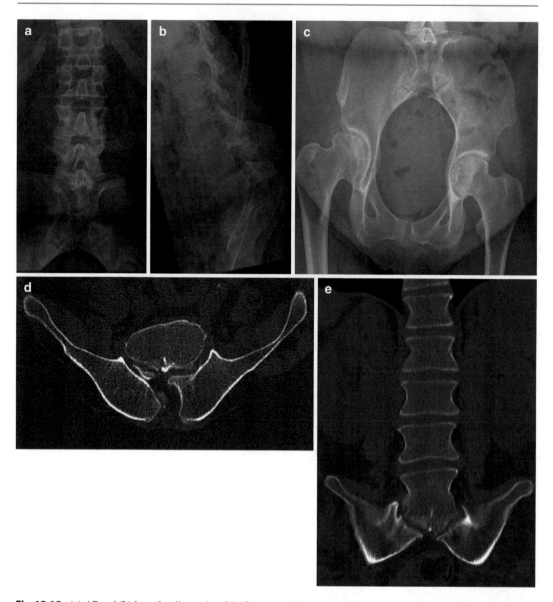

Fig. 13.18 (**a**) AP and (**b**) lateral radiographs of the lumbosacral junction show abnormality at the lumbosacral junction which might be interpreted as being related to trauma in the trauma setting. (**c**) AP radiograph of the pelvis shows sacral agenesis which accounts for the unusual shape and orientation of the pelvis. (**d**) Axial and (**e**) coronal reformatted CT images confirm the osseous features of sacral agenesis, a developmental anomaly

isolation, allows one to appreciate the diagnosis. Viewing the lateral projection in isolation could be a pitfall. In the assessment of spinal trauma, if the immediate imaging is undertaken with CT, care to view all the imaging planes will help to avoid the pitfall of diagnosing a compression fracture in the case of a butterfly vertebra (Fig. 13.19). MRI will also be beneficial in such a case by demonstrating normal marrow signal.

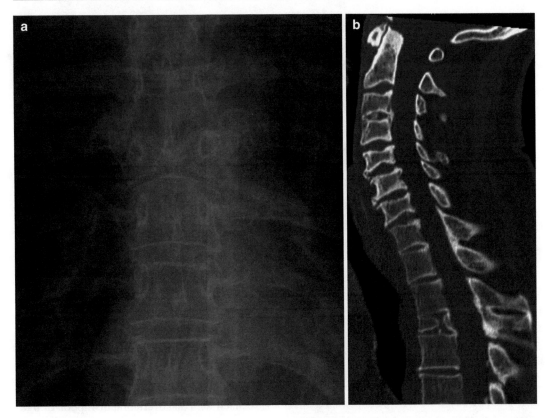

Fig. 13.19 (**a**) Coned AP radiograph of the thoracic spine shows a butterfly vertebra (developmental anomaly). This should not be confused on sagittal CT or MR images with a collapsed vertebra. (**b**) Sagittal reformatted CT image shows a butterfly vertebra at T4 vertebral level which may simulate fracture in the acute setting. This example also shows incomplete segmentation of the T3-T5 spinous processes

13.5.2 Fusion Defects

In spina bifida, the underdevelopment or absence of the posterior elements may be mistaken for a fracture. The smooth corticated margin of the defect, however, should allow recognition of this developmental anomaly (Fig. 13.20). A chronic spondylolysis may be mistaken for an acute fracture. A helpful feature for distinguishing between the two entities is the remodeling that occurs in a chronic spondylolysis, with enlargement of the inferoposterior border of the vertebral body, mainly at L5 level (Wiltse and Winter 1983).

13.5.3 Vertebral Transition

Within the spine, there are many normal variants which may simulate pathology. Anatomy at the lumbosacral junction is often transitional, with the lower lumbar vertebra sharing characteristics with sacral vertebra, and vice versa. Sometimes, an L5 transverse process can be elongated and articulate with the sacrum, which may simulate a fracture in the acute trauma setting (Fig. 13.21). The corticated margins and typical appearance of the lumbosacral transition should be readily recognized.

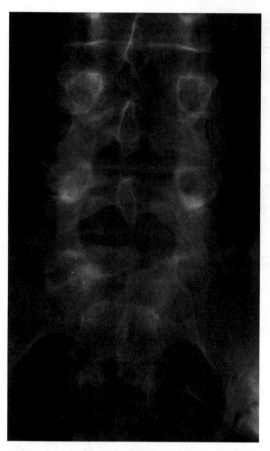

Fig. 13.20 Coned AP radiograph of the lumbosacral region shows a posterior fusion defect of the S1 segment (spina bifida occulta)

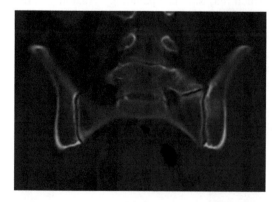

Fig. 13.21 Coronal reformatted CT image shows the elongated left transverse process of L5 vertebra which forms a pseudo-articulation with the sacrum, not to be confused with a fracture, in this case of lumbosacral transition

13.5.4 Scoliosis

Congenital anomalies may be difficult to distinguish from acute trauma, particularly if there are no prior radiographs or CT for comparison. On an AP image, an idiopathic scoliosis may give the impression of a fracture or pedicle erosion, owing to the rotation and oblique profile on the frontal image.

13.6   Pitfalls Due to Acquired Disease

Degenerative disease, either at intervertebral disks or at uncovertebral joint, can result in pseudo-fractures, often due to the presence of osteophytes with air trapped between, which simulates a fracture line (Goldberg et al. 1982). Certain acquired disease processes can hinder interpretation of both the radiographs and CT in the diagnosis of spinal injury. Widespread osteoarthritic changes can result in loss of disk height, such that the subtle abnormal disk widening associated with diskovertebral disruption or ligamentous injury with associated disk space or interspinous widening may not be fully appreciated. This is where MRI can be very valuable as a supplementary imaging modality to avoid the missed injury.

In ankylosing spondylitis, many pitfalls exist. The osteoporotic spine and limited mobility often pose difficulty to obtain adequate radiographs, and thus there is an increased risk of missing an injury. A high index of suspicion of fracture in this patient group will help to minimize the risk of pitfall. Fracture of the rigid spine invariably affects all three columns. While displacement may be obvious, and on occasion extreme, there may also be minimal displacement. The pattern of injury in ankylosing spondylitis is often different, compared with patients whose spine is not fused. Fracture through the disk or mid-vertebral body may occur, as these areas can be the weakest points in an otherwise ankylosed spine. These fractures may be mistaken for degenerative disk disease with vacuum phenomenon, if the radiographs are not fully assessed (Fig. 13.22). In patients with anky-

Fig. 13.22 (**a**) AP and (**b**) lateral radiographs of an adult patient with ankylosing spondylitis. There is a fused spine and sacroiliac joints. Trauma in this patient resulted in a fracture through T11 mid-vertebral body and posterior elements, giving an unusual appearance on the lateral projection. At first glance, this transverse lucent line through the vertebral body could be dismissed as vacuum phenomenon in a degenerative disk. However, full assessment of the radiograph shows this to be an unstable vertebral fracture with important negative consequences for the patient, if missed

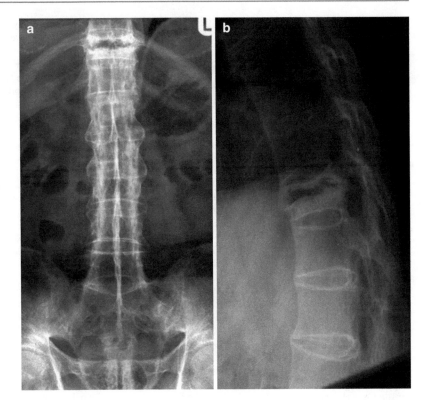

losed spines where a serious injury is suspected from the mechanism of injury, CT is mandatory (Harrop et al. 2005).

Close attention to imaging technique, whether with radiography or CT, is important. Depending on the clinical scenario, follow-up imaging with MRI including a STIR sequence will help to minimize the potential pitfall of missed injury in this group of patients in whom standard radiography can be particularly challenging, as regards to obtaining diagnostic images of high quality.

interpretation, and knowledge of normal ossification and normal variants will minimize the risk of over- or, indeed more seriously, under-reporting radiological findings. There are several substantive textbooks available, covering the very wide and extensive normal variants which may act as a potential pitfall for the unwary and even the more experienced, in the scenario of spinal injury, and which will act as a bench-book for many (Schmidt and Freyschmidt 1993; Keats 1996).

Conclusion

Imaging evaluation of the spine can be challenging. Awareness of the limitations of the different imaging modalities allows one to take a considered approach to their interpretation. Often the modalities of radiographs, CT, and MRI are complementary to each other in the information they provide. There are many pitfalls to be avoided. Familiarity with normal radiological anatomy, an awareness of technical factors which can lead to confusion in

References

Badhiwala JH, Lai CK, Alhazzani W et al (2015) Cervical spine clearance in obtunded patients after blunt traumatic injury: a systematic review. Ann Intern Med 162:429–437

Bailey DK (1952) The normal cervical spine in infants and children. Radiology 59:712–719

Begemann PGC, Kemper J, Gatzka C et al (2004) Value of multiplanar reformations (MPR) in multidetector CT (MDCT) of acute vertebral fractures. J Comput Assist Tomogr 28:572–580

Black DM, Cummings SR, Stone K et al (1991) A new approach to defining normal vertebral dimensions. J Bone Miner Res 6:883–892

Cattel HS, Filtzer DL (1965) Pseudosubluxation and other normal variants in the cervical spine in children. J Bone Joint Surg Am 47:1295–1309

Davies DV (ed) (1963) Grays anatomy, 34th edn. Longmans, Green and Co, London

Goldberg RP, Vine HS, Sacks BA, Ellison HP (1982) The cervical split: a pseudofracture. Skeletal Radiol 7:267–272

Goldman AB, Ghelman B, Doherty J (1990) Posterior limbus vertebrae: a cause of radiating back pain in adolescents and young adults. Skeletal Radiol 19:501–507

Harrop JS, Sharan A, Anderson G et al (2005) Failure of standard imaging to detect a cervical fracture in a patient with ankylosing spondylitis. Spine (Phila Pa 1976) 30:E417–E419

Helms CA, Vogler JB III, Hardy DC (1987) CT of the lumbar spine: normal variants and pitfalls. Radiographics 7:447–463

Juhl JH, Miller SM, Roberts GW (1962) Roentgenographic variations in the normal cervical spine. Radiology 78:591–597

Kattan KR, Pais MJ (1982) Some borderlands of the cervical spine. Skeletal Radiol 8:1–6

Keats TE (1996) Atlas of normal roentgen variants that may simulate disease, 6th edn. Mosby-Year Book, St Louis

Lustrin ES, Karakas SP, Ortiz AO et al (2003) Paediatric cervical spine: normal anatomy, variants and trauma. Radiographics 23:539–560

Plumb JO, Morris CG (2012) Clinical review: spinal imaging for the adult obtunded blunt trauma patient: update from 2004. Intensive Care Med 38:752–771

Rogers LF (1992) Radiology of skeletal trauma, 2nd edn. Churchill Livingstone, New York

Scher AT (1979) Anterior cervical subluxation: an unstable position. AJR Am J Roentgenol 133:275–280

Schmidt H, Freyschmidt J (eds) (1993) Koehler/Zimmer's borderlands of normal and early pathological findings in skeletal radiography, 4th edn. Thieme, Stuttgart

Schwartz JM (2001) Case 36: bilateral cervical spondylolysis of C6. Radiology 220:191–194

Sullivan CR, Bruwer AJ, Harris LE (1958) Hypermobility of the cervical spine in children: a pitfall in the diagnosis of cervical dislocation. Am J Surg 95: 636–640

Swischuk LE (1970) The beaked, notched or hooked vertebra: its significance in infants and young children. Radiology 95:661–664

Swischuk LE (1977) Anterior displacement of C2 in children: physiologic or pathologic? A helpful differentiating line. Radiology 122:759–763

Swischuk LE, Swischuk PN, John SD (1993) Wedging of C3 in infants and children: usually a normal finding and not a fracture. Radiology 188:523–526

Tins B, Cassar-Pullicino VN (2006) Optimising the imaging options. In: Cassar-Pullicino VN, Imhof H (eds) Spinal trauma - an imaging approach. Georg Thieme Verlag, Stuttgart

Tyrrell PNM, Cassar-Pullicino VN (2006) Trauma to the paediatric spine. In: Cassar-Pullicino VN, Imhof H (eds) Spinal trauma - an imaging approach. Georg Thieme Verlag, Stuttgart

Wiltse LL, Winter RB (1983) Terminology and measurement of spondylolisthesis. J Bone Joint Surg Am 65:768–772

Spine Trauma: MRI Pitfalls

14

Sri Andreani Utomo, Paulus Rahardjo,
Swee Tian Quek, and Wilfred C.G. Peh

Contents

14.1 **Introduction** 277

14.2 **Fracture Mimics** 278
14.2.1 Normal Anterior Wedging 278
14.2.2 Limbus Vertebra 279
14.2.3 Congenital Anomalies 279
14.2.4 Segmentation Anomalies 284

14.3 **Acute Compression Fracture: Benign
    Versus Malignant** 286

Conclusion 290

References 291

S.A. Utomo, MD • P. Rahardjo, MD
Department of Radiology, Airlangga University,
Surabaya, Indonesia
e-mail: sriandreaniutomo@gmail.com;
paulus.r.rahardjo@gmail.com

S.T. Quek, MBBS, FRCR
Department of Diagnostic Radiology, National
University of Singapore, National University Health
System, Singapore, Republic of Singapore
e-mail: swee_tian_quek@nuhs.edu.sg

W.C.G. Peh, MD, FRCPE, FRCPG, FRCR (✉)
Department of Diagnostic Radiology, Khoo Teck
Puat Hospital, 90 Yishun Central, Singapore 768828,
Republic of Singapore
e-mail: Wilfred.peh@alexandrahealth.com.sg

Abbreviations

CT   Computed tomography
MRI   Magnetic resonance imaging

14.1 Introduction

Spinal trauma is a potentially devastating injury (Parizel et al. 2010) that may be accompanied by significant neurological damage such as paraplegia, quadriplegia, or even death. Imaging studies are often essential to determine the nature and extent of the injury. While computed tomography (CT) plays a critical role in the rapid assessment of patients with trauma (Linsenmaier et al. 2002) and is often the primary imaging modality employed in spinal trauma, magnetic resonance imaging (MRI) frequently plays an important role as well (Bagley 2006). This is especially so given the increased availability of MRI worldwide and in cases where the clinical concern requires the assessment of subtle bone marrow, soft tissue, and/or spinal cord injuries that are usually not so apparent on the other imaging modalities. Accurate MRI assessment requires not only a good understanding of the mechanism of injury but also knowledge of some of the normal variants that may mimic pathology as well as pitfalls in interpretation. Pitfalls related to radiographic normal variants of the spine are also addressed in Chap. 11,

© Springer International Publishing AG 2017
W.C.G. Peh (ed.), *Pitfalls in Musculoskeletal Radiology*, DOI 10.1007/978-3-319-53496-1_14

and those related to the use of radiographs and CT in spinal trauma are addressed in Chap. 13.

14.2 Fracture Mimics

A number of normal variants and congenital and developmental anomalies that occur in the spine may mimic fractures. Many of these potential mimics may only be discovered when a patient undergoes MRI during adulthood, often for assessment following trauma, leading to greater likelihood for misinterpretation and misdiagnosis of fracture when none exists.

14.2.1 Normal Anterior Wedging

As loss of anterior vertebral body height is the most common radiographic finding for compression fracture, this normal variant is frequently mistaken for a fracture, often by those who are unaware of this variant. The normal vertebral bodies from T11 to L2 levels have a slight anterior wedge shape. Compared to the posterior vertebral body height, the anterior body height is typically

1–3 mm (approximately 10–15%) less. A study of dissected thoracic and lumbar (T1–L5) vertebrae in 240 individuals measured using a three-dimensional (3D) digitizer showed that the vertebral body size was anteriorly wedged from T1 through L2 (peak at T7) levels (Masharawi et al. 2008).

Even in asymptomatic children, it is not rare to see mild anterior wedging of vertebral bodies at the thoracolumbar junction. This normal variant of mild anterior wedging, misdiagnosed as the sequelae of trauma, may result in unnecessary imaging of these patients, with unnecessary radiation exposure (Gaca et al. 2010). Osteoporosis in elderly patients would result in more severe anterior wedging and, eventually, senile kyphosis.

On MRI, normal anterior vertebral wedging shows normal marrow signal, and the adjacent intervertebral disks should be normal in shape and signal (Fig. 14.1). An acute compression fracture will show a T1-hypointense fracture line and adjacent T2-hyperintense bone marrow edema (Fig. 14.2). In older healed compression fractures, although the marrow signal may be normal, the anterior wedge deformity is typically greater than 15%, and there may be remnant disk damage (Fig. 14.3).

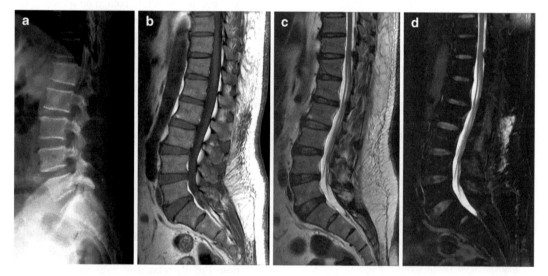

Fig. 14.1 (a) Lateral radiograph shows normal anterior wedging of T12 and L1 vertebral bodies. Sagittal (b) T1-W, (c) T2-W, and (d) fat-suppressed T2-W MR images also show normal anterior wedging. No fracture line or bone marrow edema is detected

Fig. 14.2 Acute compression fracture of T12 vertebral body. Sagittal (**a**) T1-W and (**b**) fat-suppressed T2-W MR images show a fracture line and adjacent bone marrow edema that is T1-hypointense and T2-hyperintense

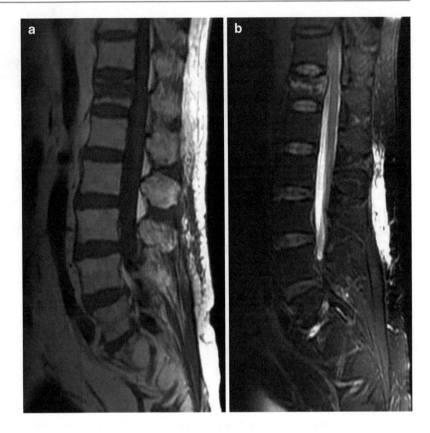

14.2.2 Limbus Vertebra

Limbus vertebra can be mistaken for a fracture involving the vertebral body. Limbus vertebra was first described by Schmorl and is believed to arise as a result of mechanical stress to the spine (Shikhare et al. 2014). The limbus vertebra is a fairly commonly encountered radiological finding. It occurs most frequently in the mid-lumbar spine and appears as a well-corticated osseous fragment, usually at the anterosuperior vertebral body corner. These are the sites of epiphyseal centers of the vertebra, where the vertebral ring apophysis (which ossifies between the ages of 6 and 13 years) fuses with the vertebral body by the time of skeletal maturation at approximately 18 years of age (Edelson and Nathan 1988).

However, a weak point exists between the ring apophysis and the adjacent vertebral body before physis fusion (Akhaddar et al. 2011). If disk her-

niation were to occur at this weak point, there is isolation and non-fusion of the ring apophysis, giving rise to the limbus vertebra, which may be easily confused with an avulsion fracture of the vertebral body. A limbus vertebra is usually recognized by its characteristic appearance and location at the anterosuperior vertebral body. The absence of adjacent marrow edema, as demonstrated by MRI (Fig. 14.4), can help confirm that the abnormality is developmental in nature rather than related to trauma (Ghelman and Freiberger 1976), particularly in the clinical setting of acute injury.

14.2.3 Congenital Anomalies

Although congenital anomalies can occur anywhere in the spine, those that cause confusion with pathology are most frequently found in the

Fig. 14.3 Chronic healed mild compression fracture of T12 vertebral body with fatty marrow changes. Sagittal (**a**) T1-W and (**b**) fat-suppressed T2-W MR images show T1-hyperintense and T2-hypointense signal changes due to fatty marrow with the T12 chronic compression fracture. L2 superior endplate Schmorl node is also seen

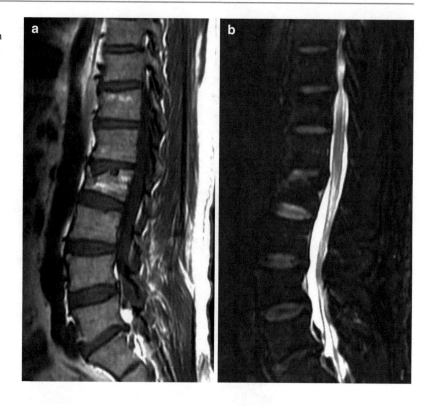

cervical region. Many of these relate to synchondroses which are mistaken for fractures in patients with acute trauma. Knowledge of the normal embryologic development and anatomy of the spine is useful to avoid this pitfall. Familiarity with anatomical variants is also important for correct image interpretation. These variants include pseudo-subluxation (Shaw et al. 1999), absence of cervical lordosis, wedging of the C3 vertebra, widening of the atlanto-axial space, or prevertebral soft tissue widening, and these are most frequently seen in children. Many of these diagnostic pitfalls are not peculiar to MRI alone but are also seen on radiographs or CT. However, the practice in many communities is to proceed directly to MRI without performing other imaging modalities, particularly so in the pediatric patient, in order to minimize radiation exposure. Some of the more interesting or important congenital anomalies are outlined below.

14.2.3.1 Congenital Basilar Impression

Cranio-cervical junction malformation (CCJM) often refers to the Chiari malformation and/or basilar invagination. CCJM is derived from mesodermal malformations that result in underdevelopment of the occipital bone, with subsequent herniation of the cerebellar tonsils and/or invagination of the upper cervical spine toward the base of the skull (Botelho and Ferreira 2013). This entity should not be mistaken for traumatic injuries.

Basilar invagination may be divided into two types:

(a) Type I: with dens invagination into the foramen magnum
(b) Type II: with invagination of the dens toward the base of the skull rather than inside the foramen magnum (Fig. 14.5)

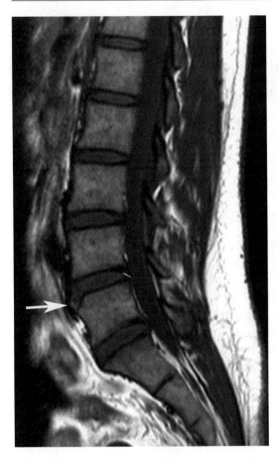

The C2 vertebra (axis) has the most complex development of all the vertebrae. It has four ossification centers: one for each of the two neural arches, one for the body, and the last for the odontoid process. Prior to fusion of these ossification centers, they may be easily mistaken for fractures in the setting of acute trauma. MRI may be helpful in these instances, by demonstrating the absence of marrow edema that helps in making a more confident distinction from acute fractures. An os odontoideum can be confused with a type 2 odontoid fracture and is seen as an oval bony structure cranial to the body of atlas, associated with the hypoplastic odontoid process of the axis (Shikhare et al. 2014).

Os odontoideum is an ossicle of variable size, with smooth circumferential cortical margins, separated from the foreshortened odontoid peg (Arvin et al. 2010). It stands apart from the hypoplastic dens and can be divided into two types:

(a) Orthotopic: when the ossicle is located in the position of the normal odontoid
(b) Dystopic: if the ossicle is situated near the occiput in the region of the foramen magnum

Fig. 14.4 A 20-year-old woman who fell from height. Sagittal T1-W MR image shows a well-corticated osseous lesion (*arrow*) at the anterosuperior corner of the L4 vertebral body due to a limbus vertebra. This can be easily confused with an avulsion fracture, but note that the fragment shows normal marrow signal with no marrow edema that would be expected if it were an acute fracture

14.2.3.2 C2 and Os Odontoideum

Several congenital abnormalities of the axis (C2) are well recognized. These include the Bergman ossicle (persistent ossiculum terminale) and os odontoideum. A Bergman ossicle is due to nonfusion of the terminal ossicle of the odontoid and appears as a small pyramidal or triangular well-corticated fragment, just cranial to the odontoid process. It can be confused with a type 1 odontoid fracture.

The presentation of an os odontoideum can vary from an incidental radiographic finding, which is the usual case, to more severe symptoms with varying degree of myelopathy, vertebral artery compression, and intracranial manifestations (Warner 2007). While its true incidence is unknown, recognition of this entity is important to distinguish it from an acute odontoid fracture. There is some debate as to its etiology. It was originally thought to be a congenital/developmental lesion secondary to failure of the center of ossification of the dens to fuse with the body of C2, but some believe that it may actually represent an old fracture through the C2 dens growth plate before the age of 5 or 6 years. Whatever its true etiology, it should not be confused with an acute traumatic injury. CT with reconstructed

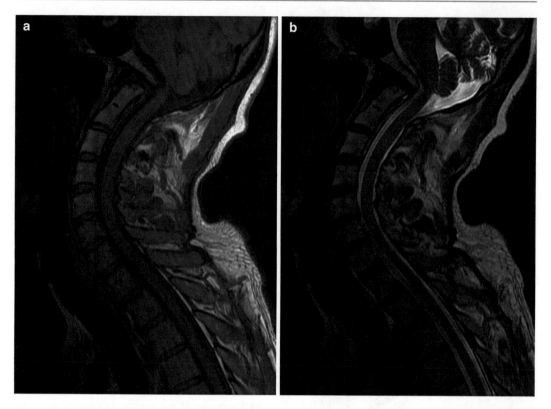

Fig. 14.5 Sagittal (**a**) T1-W and (**b**) T2 W MR images show type II basilar impression. The tip of the dens abuts the clivus, preventing cranial migration. The acute angula-tion and orientation of the cranio-cervical junction is developmental rather than traumatic

images and MRI are helpful in making the diagnosis (Fig. 14.6), but initial routine cervical spine radiographs with a well-taken open mouth odontoid view may also be useful.

14.2.3.3 Congenital Ligamentous Laxity

Ligaments are major stabilizers of the upper cervical spine. Hence, ligamentous laxity, whether physiological as may be seen in the pediatric age group or associated with conditions like Down syndrome and mucopolysaccharidosis, may result in widened intervertebral distance that may be misinterpreted as soft tissue or ligamentous inju-ries in acute trauma. This tends to be more common at the C1/2 level as this region is subject to higher torque and shear forces in the hypermobile immature spine. Besides ligamentous laxity, other factors include shallow and angled facet joints, underdeveloped spinous processes, and physiological anterior wedging of the lower cervical vertebral bodies (Lustrin et al. 2003). Such physiological widening of intervertebral distance is a normal finding and should not be misinterpreted as ligamentous injury. In more severe cases, they may even predispose to nontraumatic subluxation or dislocation that can be difficult to distinguish from traumatic injuries (Fig. 14.7).

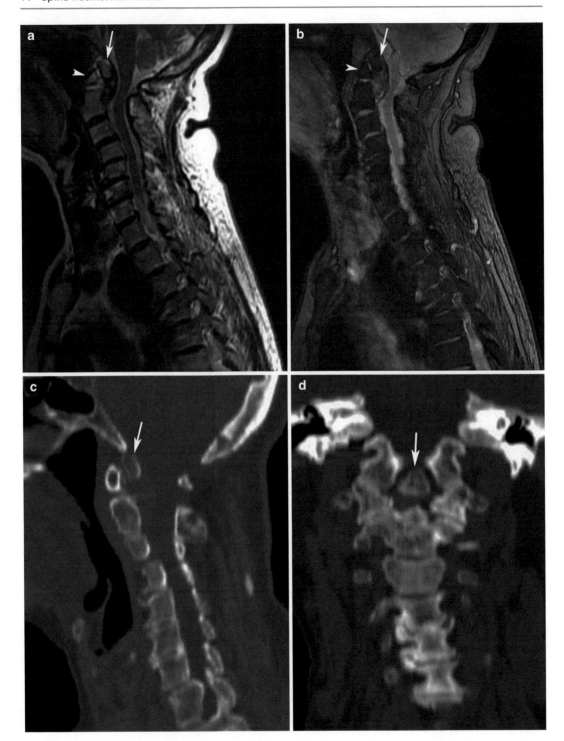

Fig. 14.6 Incidental finding in a 60-year-old man who presented with a minor head injury. Sagittal (**a**) T2-W and (**b**) GRE MR images show abnormal posterior translation of C1 arch (*arrowhead*) and an os odontoideum (*arrow*) in relation to the remainder of the C2 vertebral body. (**c**) Sagittal and (**d**) coronal reformatted CT images confirm the presence of an os odontoideum with well-corticated margins (*arrow*)

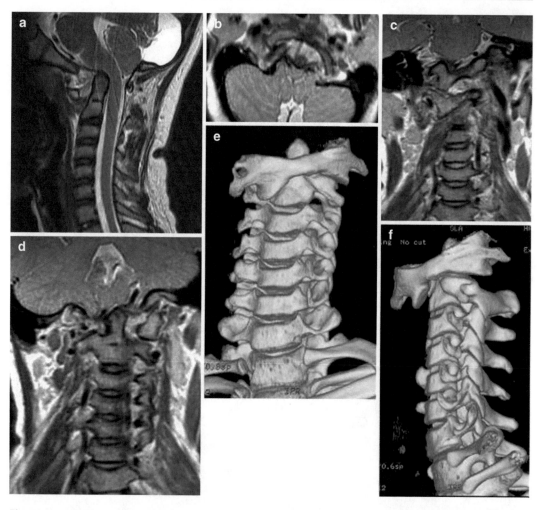

Fig. 14.7 A 12-year-old boy with atlanto-axial disloca- tion, basilar impression, and C1–C2 facet dislocation due to nontraumatic transverse ligament laxity. (**a**) Sagittal T2-W MR image shows widening of the atlanto-axial space and posterior dislocation of C2 odontoid peg. (**b**) Axial T2-W MR image shows transverse ligament lax- ity with widened atlanto-axial space. (**c, d**) Coronal T2-W MR images and (**e, f**) volume-rendered 3D reformatted CT images show bilateral C1–C2 facet dislocations

14.2.4 Segmentation Anomalies

Of the segmentation anomalies (Fig. 14.8), those that are most frequently confused with traumatic injuries include hemivertebra and but- terfly vertebra. A hemivertebra is a congenital defect of the vertebral column in which one side of the vertebra fails to develop completely due to failure of the chondrification center to form on that side, while a butterfly vertebra is thought to occur between the third and sixth week of embryonic development due to failure of fusion of the two lateral sclerotomes that derive from the somites.

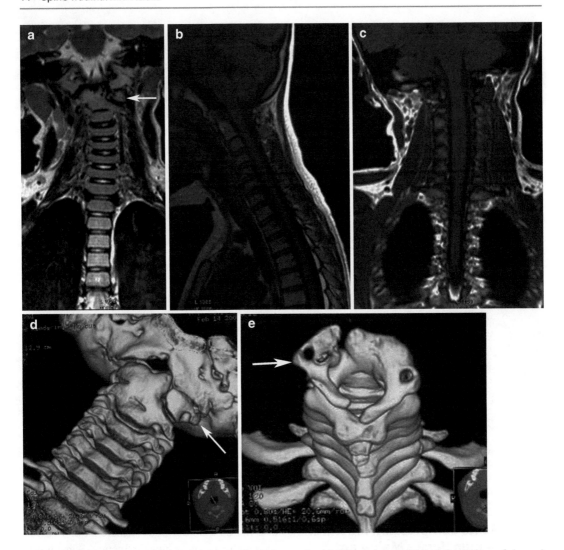

Fig. 14.8 Segmentation anomaly mimicking a fracture. (**a**) Coronal T2-W, (**b**) sagittal T1-W, and (**c**) coronal T1-W MR images and (**d**, **e**) volume-rendered 3D reformatted CT images show hemifusion of the C1 anterior arch with C2 vertebra, while the left anterior arch (*arrow*) has been separated from C2 vertebra, mimicking a fracture

Both these anomalies may present with wedge-shaped deformities (Fig. 14.9) or, in the case of a butterfly vertebra, vertebral fragmentation that may be mistaken for a compression or even a burst fracture (Karargyris et al. 2015). While most hemivertebrae or butterfly vertebrae are usually asymptomatic, incidental and isolated findings, the latter may be rarely associated with other congenital anomalies such as Müllerian hypoplasia/aplasia and Alagille syndrome. Evaluation with MRI may be useful to look for the uncommon associated anomalies such as supernumerary lumbar vertebrae, spina bifida, diastematomyelia, and kyphoscoliosis.

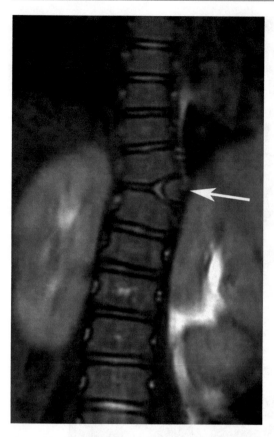

Fig. 14.9 A 7-year-old boy with a T11 hemivertebra. Coronal T2-W MR image shows failure of development of the right side of T11 vertebra. The remnant left hemivertebra (*arrow*) may mimic a compression fracture

14.3   Acute Compression Fracture: Benign Versus Malignant

Compression fracture due to osteoporosis most often occurs in the spine and should be differentiated from a traumatic compression or burst fracture from a fall. For a start, the clinical history (such as patient's age, severity of the trauma, site and severity of symptoms, predisposing factors for osteoporosis) is often helpful. In cases of chronic compression fracture, the distinction from an acute traumatic injury is easily made by looking at the marrow signal, particularly on the T1-weighted and STIR images. In chronic compression fractures, the normal fatty marrow signal should be preserved on all sequences (Fig. 14.3).

In an acute vertebral compression fracture, the distinction of an osteoporotic from a traumatic fracture on MRI alone may be difficult, as there will almost certainly be marrow edema in both instances (Fig. 14.10). As it is likely that both the trauma and the osteoporosis have contributory roles leading to the fracture in the elderly, the clinical management is likely to be the same in stable fractures. Without the benefit of other correlative imaging modalities, such as radiographs and in particular CT, injuries to the smaller but vital stabilizing structures of the posterior column, such as facet dislocations, pars articular process, and neural arch fractures, may be missed (Fig. 14.11).

Pathological fractures may be due to a number of causes, the most common of which are malignancy and infection. Differentiating pathological fractures from traumatic fractures is clinically important due to the vastly different management implications. As in the case of osteoporotic fractures, the underlying pathology is already present, but the fracture itself may be either precipitated by, or brought to, clinical attention, due to the trauma. When assessing patients with traumatic injuries, it is therefore important to exclude an underlying cause for the fracture rather than cursorily attributing it to trauma without a more detailed review of all the images. This is particularly important when the trauma sustained is mild or minimal.

Where the underlying cause is infection, there may be clinical signs to suggest the true etiology, but, often, these clues may be subtle. The soft tissue component associated with the infection may also mimic the soft tissue hematoma and edema seen with an acute traumatic fracture. Some imaging clues that may help make the distinction include the signal differences between a fluid collection within an abscess and acute or subacute hematoma (with characteristic signals of blood products) and, in case of infection, infection of the adjacent disk or adjacent endplates, subligamentous spread, and involvement of contiguous vertebral segments. To this end, adding sequences after intravenous contrast agent injection is useful where there is suspicion of possible infective etiology (Fig. 14.12).

Where the pathological fracture is due to malignancy, distinction from a traumatic fracture is relatively straightforward if there are "classic" signs of a pathological fracture (Yuh et al. 1989) and/or involvement of other parts of the skeleton (Fig. 14.13). Morphological

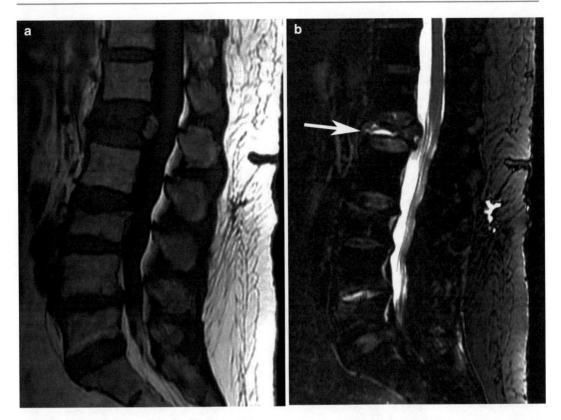

Fig. 14.10 A 63-year-old woman with a compression fracture due to osteoporosis. This may mimic a traumatic burst fracture. Sagittal (**a**) T1-W and (**b**) fat-suppressed T2-W MR images show diffuse fatty marrow changes reflecting the patient's age in all the vertebral bodies except for L1 level where there is a severe L1 vertebral compression fracture, a T2-hyperintense fluid cleft (*arrow*), adjacent marrow edema, and posterior bulging with canal encroachment. Mild L3 compression fracture is also noted

changes of malignant vertebral compression fractures consist of complete replacement of the vertebral body marrow by tumor, involvement of the posterior elements, and associated epidural or paraspinal mass. Occasionally, however, these morphological changes may be seen in benign fractures, so these changes are not specific (Ishiyama et al. 2010). On the contrary, absence of these changes does not exclude underlying malignancy. Involvement of other parts of the skeleton or multiplicity of lesion is however not exclusive for malignancy – it can also occur with trauma (Fig. 14.14), and a detailed review for underlying marrow replacement is required.

Although malignant fractures typically show strong enhancement after intravenous contrast injection, benign fractures may also enhance (Shih et al. 1999; Jung et al. 2003). If there is solitary involvement of a vertebra, the distinction can be even more problematic. Finally, it should be remembered that both benign traumatic fractures and pathological fractures may coexist, with benign vertebral compression fractures being present in approximately one-third of cancer patients (Fornasier and Czitrom 1978). Given these scenarios, what are reliable signs on MRI that we can depend on to distinguish malignant from benign acute compression fractures?

A reliable sign of benignity is the presence of a fracture line, seen as an area of linear hypointensity in the middle of a compressed vertebral body or adjacent to a compressed endplate on both T1-weighted and T2-weighted MR images (Jung et al. 2003) (Figs. 14.2 and 14.10). Other MRI features of benignity described are presence of intravertebral fluid (Figs. 14.2 and 14.10),

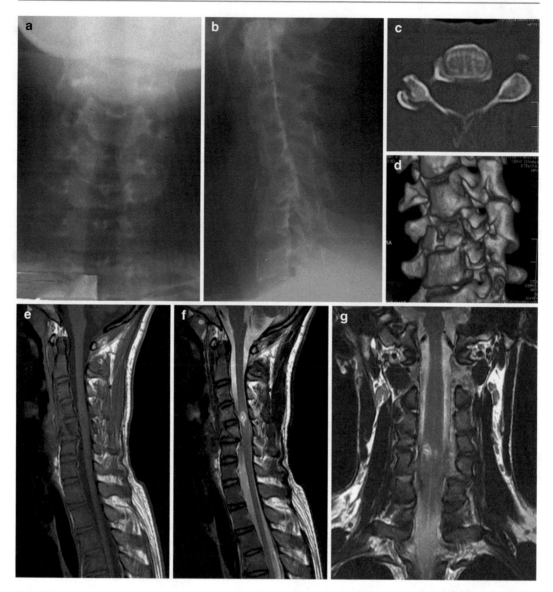

Fig. 14.11 (a) Anteroposterior and (b) lateral radiographs show fracture-dislocation of C5 vertebral body with unilateral facet dislocation and increased interspinous distance at C5–C6 and C6–C7 levels. (c) Axial and (d) volume-rendered 3D reformatted CT images are better than (e–g) MR images for showing the fracture and unilateral dislocation. However, sagittal (e) T1-W, (f) T2-W, and (g) coronal T2-W MR images are better for showing the ligament tear, subligamentous hemorrhage, cord contusion, and hematomyelia

intravertebral vacuum cleft, and lack of pedicle involvement (Baur et al. 2002). In acute benign fractures, there is usually some spared areas of normal bone marrow signal within the compressed vertebral body (Figs. 14.2 and 14.14) and retropulsion of a posterior bone fragment (Jung et al. 2003).

Reliable MRI features of malignant vertebral compression fractures consist of convex posterior contour of the involved vertebral body, epidural mass, encasing epidural mass, focal paraspinal mass, and presence of other spinal metastases (Jung et al. 2003) (Fig. 14.13). With application of the abovenamed morphological

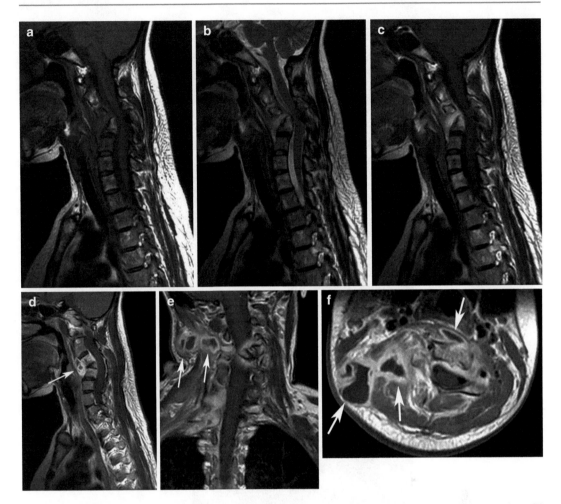

Fig. 14.12 A 29-year-old woman with tuberculous spondylodiskitis at C3–C4 level resulting in destruction of the C3–C4 disk with pathological compression of the C3 and C4 vertebrae. The sharp angulation or gibbus formation should be differentiated from fracture-dislocation caused by trauma. Sagittal (**a**) T1-W, (**b**) T2-W, (**c, d**) contrast-enhanced T1-W, (**e**) coronal contrast-enhanced T1-W, and (**f**) axial contrast-enhanced T1-W MR images show C3 and C4 vertebral body destruction, C3–C4 disk destruction with gibbus formation, and a paravertebral as well as subligamentous rim-enhancing abscess formation (*arrows*) and anterior cervical cord compression. Enhancing infective tissue and abscesses were key features in differentiation from traumatic vertebral fracture-dislocations

criteria, MRI has been found to have an accuracy of 79–94% in distinguishing between malignant and acute benign compression fractures (Yuh et al. 1989; An et al. 1995; Cuenod et al. 1996), although with addition of adequate scan quality and clinical history, the diagnostic confidence probably exceeds 90% (Finelli 2001).

To better assess indeterminate vertebral compression fractures, several advanced MRI techniques such as diffusion-weighted imaging (DWI) (Baur et al. 1998), quantitative DWI assessment (Chan et al. 2002; Herneth et al. 2002; Zhou et al. 2002), and chemical shift imaging (Zajick et al. 2005; Erly et al. 2006) have been developed, and currently, the search for this "holy grail" is still ongoing (Geith et al. 2012, 2014). If these advanced MRI techniques are unavailable or not helpful, a commonsense approach would be to repeat the MRI after a reasonable interval (e.g., 4–8 weeks). In a patient

Fig. 14.13 A 58-year-old man with multiple myeloma. Sagittal (**a**) T1-W and (**b**) fat-suppressed T2-W MR images show multiple vertebral body compression fractures with endplate depression. (**c**) Axial contrast-enhanced T1-W MR images show destruction of right iliac wing with bulging soft tissue mass and extensive bone marrow replacement by tumor

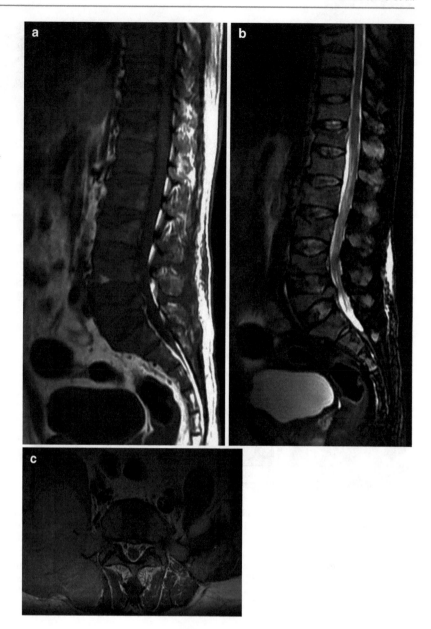

who is not actively mobilizing, the vertebral signal changes should improve in acute osteoporotic fractures, whereas it should remain unchanged or progress in malignancy. For more pressing cases, imaging-guided biopsy can be considered and should provide a definitive answer.

Conclusion

MRI is increasingly used for imaging patients with acute spinal trauma. While the diagnosis is usually straightforward in most cases, there are a few normal variants as well as some pathological conditions that can create diag-

Fig. 14.14 Multiplicity of lesions is not exclusive for malignancy. In this case, it is secondary to trauma sustained from a fall from height. Sagittal (**a**) T1-W and (**b**) STIR MR images show the classical appearance of fluid within the fracture lines at typical locations near the vertebral endplates (*arrow*), making the diagnosis simple

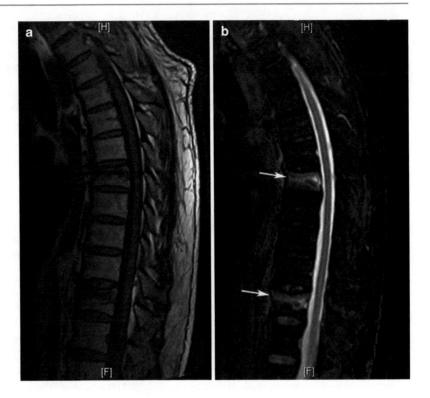

nostic confusion in interpretation. Knowledge of these potential diagnostic pitfalls will aid accurate assessment and appropriate management of the patient with spinal trauma undergoing MRI evaluation.

References

Akhaddar A, Belfquih H, Oukabli M et al (2011) Posterior ring apophysis separation combined with lumbar disc herniation in adults: a 10-year experience in the surgical management of 87 cases. J Neurosurg Spine 14:475–483

An HS, Andreshak TG, Nguyen C et al (1995) Can we distinguish between benign versus malignant compression fractures of the spine by magnetic resonance imaging? Spine 20:1776–1782

Arvin B, Fournier-Gosselin MP, Fehlings M (2010) Os odontoideum: etiology and surgical management. Neurosurgery 66:A22–A31

Bagley LJ (2006) Imaging of spinal trauma. Radiol Clin N Am 44:1–12

Baur A, Stabler A, Bruning R et al (1998) Diffusion-weighted MR imaging of bone marrow: differentiation of benign versus pathologic vertebral compression fractures. Radiology 207:349–356

Baur A, Stabler A, Arbogast S et al (2002) Acute osteoporotic and neoplastic vertebral compression fractures: fluid sign at MR imaging. Radiology 225:730–735

Botelho RV, Ferreira EDZ (2013) Angular craniometry in craniocervical junction malformation. Neurosurg Rev 36:603–610

Chan JHM, Peh WCG, Tsui EYK et al (2002) Acute vertebral body compression fractures: discrimination between benign and malignant causes using apparent diffusion coefficients. Br J Radiol 75:207–214

Cuenod CA, Laredo JD, Chevret S et al (1996) Acute vertebral collapse due to osteoporosis or malignancy: appearance on unenhanced and gadolinium-enhanced MR images. Radiology 199:541–549

Edelson JG, Nathan H (1988) Stages in the natural history of the vertebral end-plates. Spine 13:21–26

Erly WK, Oh ES, Outwater EK (2006) The utility of in-phase/opposed-phase imaging in differentiating malignancy from acute benign compression fractures of the spine. Am J Neuroradiol 27:1183–1188

Finelli DA (2001) Diffusion-weighted imaging of acute vertebral compressions: specific diagnosis of benign versus malignant pathologic fractures. AJNR Am J Neuroradiol 22:241–242

Fornasier VL, Czitrom AA (1978) Collapsed vertebrae: a review of 659 autopsies. Clin Orthop Relat Res 131:261–265

Gaca AM, Barnhart HX, Bisset GS (2010) Evaluation of wedging of lumbar vertebral bodies in children. AJR Am J Roentgenol 194:516–520

Geith T, Schmidt M, Biffar A et al (2012) Comparison of qualitative and quantitative evaluation of diffusion-weighted MRI and chemical-shift imaging in the differentiation of benign and malignant vertebral body fractures. AJR Am J Roentgenol 199:1083–1092

Geith T, Schmidt G, Biffar A et al (2014) Quantitative evaluation of benign and malignant vertebral fractures with diffusion-weighted MRI: what is the optimum combination of b values for ADC-based lesion differentiation with the single-shot turbo spin-echo sequence? AJR Am J Roentgenol 203:582–588

Ghelman B, Freiberger RH (1976) The limbus vertebra: an anterior disc herniation demonstrated by discography. AJR Am J Roentgenol 127:854–855

Herneth AM, Philipp MO, Naude J et al (2002) Vertebral metastases: assessment with apparent diffusion coefficient. Radiology 225:990–894

Ishiyama M, Fuwa S, Numaguchi Y et al (2010) Pedicle involvement on MR imaging is common in osteoporotic compression fractures. Am J Neuroradiol 31:668–673

Jung HS, Jee WH, McCauley TR et al (2003) Determination of metastatic from acute compression spinal fractures with MR imaging. Radiographics 23:179–187

Linsenmaier U, Krotz M, Hauser H et al (2002) Whole-body computed tomography in polytrauma: techniques and management. Eur Radiol 12:1728–1740

Lustrin ES, Karakas SP, Ortiz AO et al (2003) Pediatric cervical spine: normal anatomy, variants, and trauma. Radiographics 23:539–560

Karargyris O, Lampropoulou-Adamidou K, Morassi LG et al (2015) Differentiating between traumatic pathology and congenital variant: a case report of butterfly vertebra. Clin Orthop Surg 7:406–409

Masharawi Y, Salame K, Mirovsky Y et al (2008) Vertebral body shape variation in the thoracic and lumbar spine: characterization of its asymmetry and wedging. Clin Anat 21:46–54

Parizel PM, Van Der Zijden T, Gaudino S et al (2010) Trauma of the spine and spinal cord: imaging strategies. Eur Spine J 19(Suppl 1):8–17

Shaw M, Burnett H, Wilson A et al (1999) Pseudosubluxation of C2 on C3 in polytraumatized children: prevalence and significance. Clin Radiol 54:377–380

Shih TT, Huang KM, Li YK (1999) Solitary vertebral collapse: distinction between benign and malignant causes using MR patterns. J Magn Reson Imaging 9:635–642

Shikhare SN, Singh DR, Peh WCG (2014) Variants and pitfalls in MR imaging of the spine. Semin Musculoskelet Radiol 18:23–35

Tehranzadeh J, Andrews C, Wong E (2000) Lumbar spine imaging. Normal variants, imaging pitfalls, and artifacts. Radiol Clin N Am 38:1207–1253

Warner W (2007) Pediatric cervical spine. In: Canale ST, Beaty JH (eds) Campbell's operative orthopaedics, 11th edn. Mosby, Philadelphia

Yuh WT, Zachar CK, Barloon TJ et al (1989) Vertebral compression fractures: distinction between benign and malignant causes with MR imaging. Radiology 172:215–218

Zajick DC, Morrision WB, Schweitzer ME et al (2005) Benign and malignant processes: normal values and differentiation with chemical shift MR imaging in vertebral marrow. Radiology 237:590–596

Zhou XJ, Leeds NE, Mckinnon GC et al (2002) Characterization of benign and metastatic vertebral compression fractures with quantitative diffusion MR imaging. Am J Neuroradiol 23:165–170

Shoulder Injury: MRI Pitfalls

15

Josephina A. Vossen and William E. Palmer

Contents

15.1	**Introduction**	293
15.2	**Normal Anatomic Structures That May Mimic Pathology**	293
15.2.1	Labrum	293
15.2.2	Cartilage	295
15.2.3	Ligaments	296
15.2.4	Osseous Structures	297
15.2.5	Rotator Cuff, Rotator Cable, and Rotator Interval	298
15.3	**Postoperative Findings**	300
15.4	**Pitfalls Due to Imaging Techniques**	302
Conclusion		303
References		304

Abbreviations

ABER Abduction and external rotation
IGHL Inferior glenohumeral ligament
MGHL Middle glenohumeral ligament
MRI Magnetic resonance imaging
SGHL Superior glenohumeral ligament

J.A. Vossen, MD, PhD • W.E. Palmer, MD (✉)
Department of Musculoskeletal Imaging and
Intervention, Massachusetts General Hospital and
Harvard Medical School, 55 Fruit St., YAW 6030,
Boston, MA 02114, USA
e-mail: josephina.vossen@gmail.com;
wpalmer@mgh.harvard.edu

15.1 Introduction

Magnetic resonance imaging (MRI) of the shoulder is a reliable and accurate method for the assessment of the shoulder in the setting of pain and instability. There has been a steady increase in the number of shoulder MRI studies performed over the last decades, attributable to improvements in MRI technique, spatial resolution, as well as advancement in clinical treatment. It is important for the radiologist involved in the interpretation of these studies to be aware of the imaging pitfalls that can be encountered during routine clinical practice. This awareness will lead to the improvement of diagnostic accuracy in MRI interpretation and avoidance of diagnostic errors. In this chapter, we present an overview of pitfalls that can confound the assessment of conventional and arthrographic shoulder MRI. Pitfalls include normal anatomic structures that may mimic pathology and technical challenges relating to artifacts. Additionally, strategies for addressing these challenges will be suggested.

15.2 Normal Anatomic Structures That May Mimic Pathology

15.2.1 Labrum

The glenoid labrum is a fibrocartilaginous rim that marginates the glenoid cavity. The labrum contributes to shoulder stability by providing attachments for the glenohumeral ligaments and adding to the glenoid surface and depth. The normal labrum is low in MR signal intensity on all pulse sequences and has firm attachments to the glenoid bone and articular cartilage posteriorly and inferiorly. At the chondrolabral junction, an intermediate signal transition zone can be present (Zanetti et al. 2001). This type of junction is seen between the 11 o'clock and the 1 o'clock position. In order to decrease the likelihood of false-positive diagnosis of labral tears, the use of T2-weighted imaging is recommended, providing increased contrast between the cartilage surface and joint effusion, when compared to gradient-echo (GRE) and proton density (PD) pulse sequences. Additionally, arthrographic MR images may increases diagnostic confidence.

The long head of the biceps attaches to the supraglenoid tubercle and merges with the superior glenoid labrum to form the biceps labral complex. The sublabral sulcus, or recess, can be present between the capsulolabral complex and the superior glenoid cartilage. Typically, the sulcus is confined to the superior labrum between the 11 o'clock and the 1 o'clock position, has smooth margins, measures less than 2 mm in width, follows the surface of the glenoid rim medially, and does not extend posterior to the biceps anchor (Smith et al. 1996) (Fig. 15.1a). The sublabral sulcus should not be mistaken for a superior labral with anterior and posterior extension (SLAP) tear (Chang et al. 2008) (Fig. 15.1b, c).

The sublabral foramen, or hole, can be seen anterior to the biceps tendon attachment at the anterior labrum. This sublabral foramen provides a

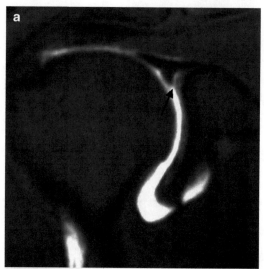

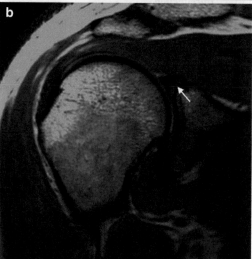

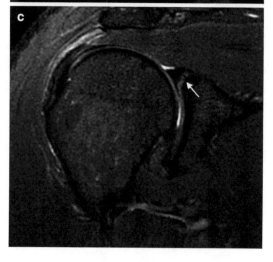

Fig. 15.1 Sublabral recess versus SLAP tear. (**a**) Coronal oblique fat-suppressed T1-W MR arthrographic image shows linear intermediate signal undercutting the contour of the superior glenoid labrum (*black arrow*), following the contour of the glenoid cartilage, without extension posterior to the biceps anchor. This represents a sublabral recess. Coronal oblique (**b**) T1-W and (**c**) T2-W MR images show an irregular defect (*white arrow*) extending into the substance of the superior labrum with extension posterior to the biceps anchor. This represents a SLAP tear

communication between the glenohumeral joint and the subscapularis recess. Conventionally, the foramen is located between the 1 o'clock and the 3 o'clock position, has smooth edges, measures less than 1.5 mm in width, and is oriented medially and posteriorly toward the glenoid (Cooper et al. 1992; Rao et al. 2003) (Fig. 15.2a). In younger patients, the degree of labral displacement is minimal. In older patients, the sublabral foramen can increase in size, giving the appearance of a torn, displaced labral fragment. The sublabral foramen should not be confused with an anterior labral tear (Fig. 15.2b, c). A true tear typically propagates a greater distance superiorly into the bicipital anchor or inferiorly into the inferior glenohumeral ligament attachment site.

15.2.2 Cartilage

Hyaline cartilage lines the articular surfaces of the humeral head and glenoid fossa. The humeral head articular cartilage is thicker centrally and thinner peripherally. The glenoid articular cartilage is relatively thinner centrally and thicker peripherally. Variations in cartilage coverage should not be mischaracterized as osteochondral injuries. The tubercle of Assaki is a focal thickening of the subchondral bone at the central aspect of the glenoid fossa, with an area of overlying cartilage thinning termed the bare spot (De Wilde et al. 2004). Expected locations for true glenoid cartilage defect include the superior cartilage adjacent to a superior labral tear and the anteroinferior cartilage in the setting of a Bankart lesion. These defects often demonstrate chondral delamination and are accompanied by underlying bone marrow edema. Known bare areas of the humeral head include a bare area posteriorly

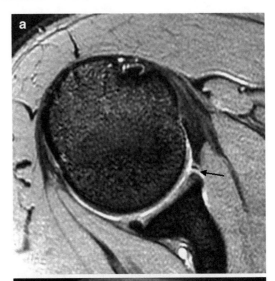
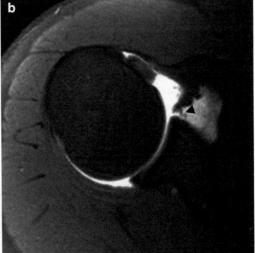
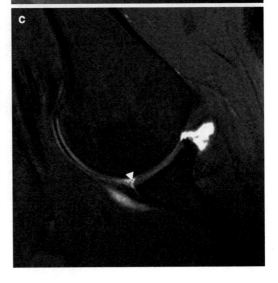

Fig. 15.2 Sublabral hole versus anterior labral tear. (**a**) Axial fat-suppressed GRE MR image shows a sublabral hole (*black arrow*) located in a typical position between the 1 o'clock and 3 o'clock position. (**b**) Axial and (**c**) axial ABER position fat-suppressed T1-W MR arthrographic images show an avulsion of the anterior labrum (*arrowheads*)

between the posterior insertion of the joint capsule and synovial membrane and the adjacent articular cartilage and a bare area superiorly between the supraspinatus insertion on the greater tuberosity and the adjacent articular cartilage. True humeral head cartilage defects are often located in the posterosuperior portion of the humeral head, medial to the location of the bare areas.

15.2.3 Ligaments

The glenohumeral ligaments are discrete capsular thickenings that provide primary passive anterior and inferior joint stabilization (Yeh et al. 1998). Awareness of the normal anatomic variants of these ligaments helps to prevent diagnostic errors. The superior glenohumeral ligament (SGHL) extends from the superior glenoid margin and base of the coracoid and courses inferolaterally to the anterior humerus just superior to the lesser tuberosity at the anatomic neck. Variant origins of the SGHL include a common origin with the middle glenohumeral ligament (MGHL) and/or direct origin from the biceps tendon.

The MGHL extends from the anterior margin of the anterior labrum or scapular neck, and courses oblique inferolaterally along the posterior margin of the subscapularis tendon, and inserts on the neck of the humerus (Beltran et al. 2002). Variant appearances of the MGHL include absence of the MGHL, a conjoint origin with either the SGHL or inferior glenohumeral ligament (IGHL), and a cord-like thickening of the MGHL (Buford complex) (Williams et al. 1994). The Buford complex can be present in combination with an absent anterosuperior labrum (Fig. 15.3).

The IGHL complex consists of an anterior and posterior band with the axillary recess in-between. The anterior band arises from the inferior glenoid rim at the 2 o'clock to 4 o'clock position. The posterior band arises from the inferior glenoid rim at the 7 o'clock to 9 o'clock position. Both the anterior and posterior bands of the IGHL insert at the anatomical neck of the humerus. Variant anatomy of the IGHL includes a high origin above the level of the anterior equator (Ramirez Ruiz et al. 2012). The IGHL should not be mistaken for a displaced labral fragment. Prominent

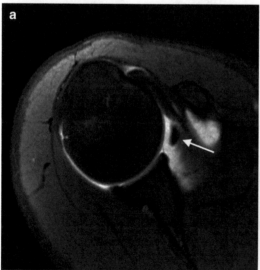
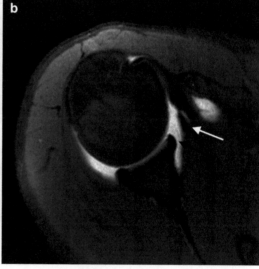

Fig. 15.3 Buford complex. (**a**) Axial fat-suppressed T1-W MR arthrographic image shows a cord-like middle glenohumeral ligament (*white arrow*) associated with an absent anterior superior labrum, mimicking a labral tear.

(**b**) Axial fat-suppressed T1-W MR arthrographic image obtained at a more inferior level shows a normal anterior inferior labrum (*black arrow*) and thickened middle glenohumeral ligament (*white arrow*)

synovial folds of the axillary recess may stimulate loose bodies on MRI. The fact that these folds are in the nondependent position of the recess will help distinguish them from true loose bodies.

15.2.4 Osseous Structures

An os acromiale is an accessory bone that results from failure of osseous fusion of one of the acromial ossification centers with the scapular spine. Although often asymptomatic, an os acromiale may contribute to clinical symptoms of impingement and might be painful due to mechanical instability and pseudarthrosis formation (Sammarco 2000). Both instability and pseudarthrosis formation can be exacerbated by acromioplasty. Therefore, documenting its presence is important. Because an os acromiale can be mistaken for the normal acromioclavicular joint, coronal and axial images should be examined routinely for an unfused acromial ossification center (Fig. 15.4).

Physiological flattening of the humeral head can be seen at the posterolateral position below the level of the coracoid process (Fig. 15.5a, b). This should be distinguished from a Hill-Sachs compression fracture as a sequela of anterior shoulder dislocation, which is seen in the most superior 2 cm of the humeral head, at or above the level of the coracoid process (Richards et al. 1994) (Fig. 15.5c, d).

Rounded cystic structures in the posterior aspect of the greater tuberosity might be seen and likely represent developmental pseudocysts or vessels entering the humeral head (Williams et al. 2006) (Fig. 15.6). They can

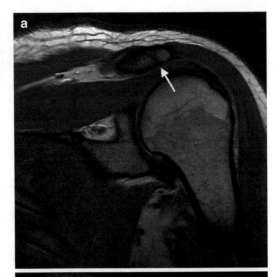

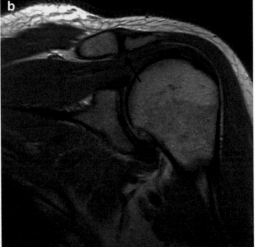

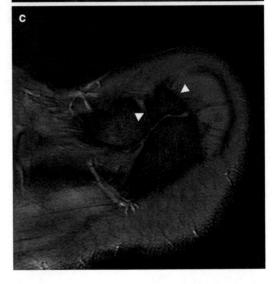

Fig. 15.4 Os acromiale. (**a**) Coronal oblique fat-suppressed T1-W MR image shows the os acromiale (*white arrow*) mimicking the acromioclavicular joint. (**b**) Coronal oblique fat-suppressed T1-W MR image obtained slightly more anteriorly shows the acromioclavicular joint (*black arrow*). (**c**) Axial fat-suppressed gradient echo MR image shows an unfused anterior acromial ossification center (*white arrowheads*)

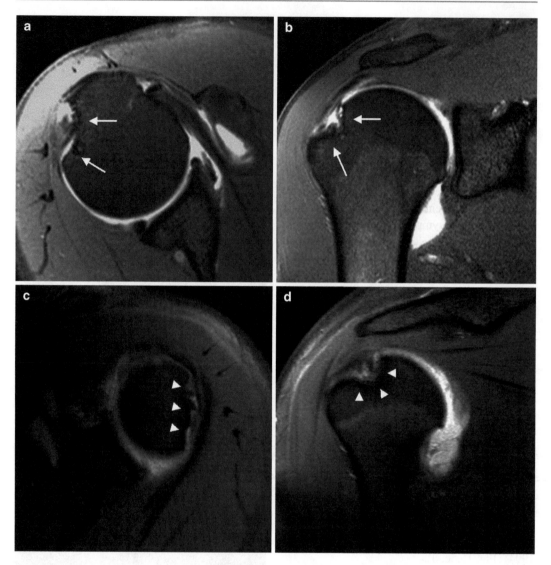

Fig. 15.5 Normal humeral head flattening versus Hill-Sachs lesion. (**a**) Axial and (**b**) coronal oblique fat-suppressed T1-W MR arthrographic images show physiological flattening of the posteroinferior aspect of the humeral head (*white arrows*) below the level of the coracoid process. (**c**) Axial and (**d**) coronal oblique fat-suppressed T1-W MR arthrographic images show a bony defect involving the posterosuperior humeral head (*white arrowheads*) in a patient with prior anterior shoulder dislocation – typical of a Hill-Sachs lesion

become substantially increased in size in over-head athletes, such as baseball and tennis players. These cystic changes are not associated with rotator cuff pathology and should not be confused with reactive subchondral cysts of the lesser tuberosity and anterior aspect of the greater tuberosity related to rotator cuff tendinopathy and tears (Sano et al. 1998; Fritz et al. 2007).

15.2.5 Rotator Cuff, Rotator Cable, and Rotator Interval

The rotator cuff is a group of muscles, and their tendons act to stabilize the shoulder. The four muscles of the rotator cuff are the supraspinatus, infraspinatus, teres minor, and subscapularis muscles. The anterosuperior margin of the infraspinatus tendon partially overlaps the supraspinatus

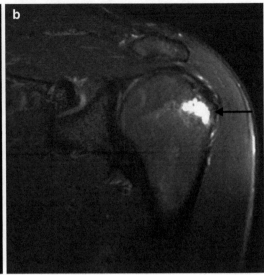

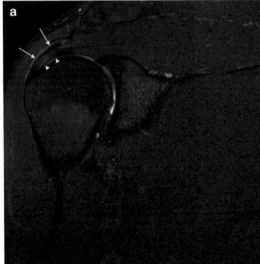
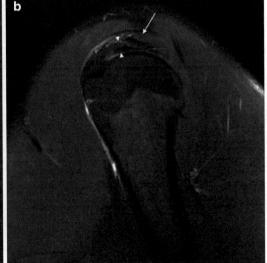

Fig. 15.6 Humeral head cysts. (**a**) Axial fat-suppressed GRE and (**b**) coronal oblique fat-suppressed T2-W MR images show cysts (*black arrows*) at the posterior supero-lateral humeral head margin. These cysts should be distinguished from the more anteriorly located cysts associated with adjacent rotator cuff pathology

Fig. 15.7 Supraspinatus-infraspinatus interdigitation. (**a**) Coronal oblique and (**b**) sagittal oblique fat-suppressed T2-W MR images show the superposition of the infraspinatus (*white arrows*) and supraspinatus (*white arrow-heads*) tendons. The linear hyperintense signal area between two hypointense tendons could be due to the interposition of muscle fibers, creating a three-layer appearance

tendon before inserting laterally at the superior humeral facet (Michelin et al. 2014) (Fig. 15.7). This interdigitation is more prominent with the shoulder internally rotated and should not be confused with tendinopathy.

Partial-thickness tears of the rotator cuff may occur at the articular surface, bursal surface, or within the substance of the tendon. A delaminated tear refers to a longitudinal split of the rotator cuff tendons. The identification and

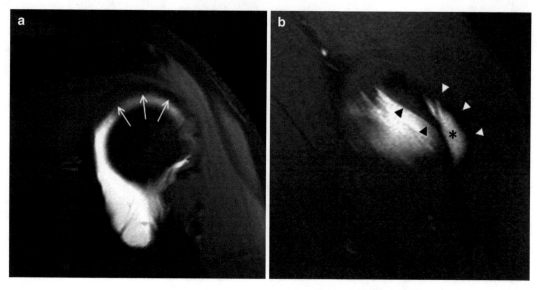

Fig. 15.8 Interstitial partial-thickness infraspinatus tendon tear visualized on the ABER view only. (**a**) Coronal oblique fat-suppressed T1-W MR arthrographic image shows minimal irregularity of the articular surface of the infraspinatus tendon (*white arrows*). (**b**) Fat-suppressed T1-W MR arthrographic image with the patient in the ABER position shows intratendinous contrast (*). The articular surface (*black arrowheads*) and bursal surface (*white arrowheads*) fibers appear intact

accurate description of a delaminating interstitial tear by the radiologist are important, since these tears can be concealed and difficult to visualize during arthroscopy. When identified, they may require a more complicated treatment approach. The use of the abduction and external rotation (ABER) position at MR arthrography can be beneficial in the detection of a horizontal component in partial-thickness tears (Lee and Lee 2002) (Fig. 15.8).

The rotator cable or ligamentum semicirculare humeri is a linear condensation of fibers extending in an oblique direction from the coracohumeral ligament along the articular surface of the supraspinatus and infraspinatus fibers (Clark and Harryman 1992). Recognition of the cable is important in order to distinguish it from a tear. The normal rotator cable is often better identified on ABER images (Sheah et al. 2009) (Fig. 15.9).

The rotator interval is a triangular space defined superiorly by the anterior border of the supraspinatus tendon, inferiorly by the superior border of subscapularis tendon, and by the cor-

acoid process at the base (Cole et al. 2001). Rotator interval abnormalities, including tear, capsulitis and adjacent bursal scarring, are difficult to visualize during arthroscopy. Identification of these findings on MRI is valuable because surgical repair can help glenohumeral stabilization and decrease pain (Krych et al. 2013) (Fig. 15.10).

15.3 Postoperative Findings

The evaluation of the postoperative shoulder on MRI can be complicated. Susceptibility artifact represents a distortion of the MR images caused by inhomogeneity of the local magnetic field. Adaptation of the standard MRI protocols can improve imaging quality. The metal artifact reduction sequence (MARS) is intended to reduce the size and intensity of susceptibility artifacts resulting from magnetic field distortion and signal loss (Fig. 15.11). Technique changes include the use of inversion recovery instead of fat suppression, the

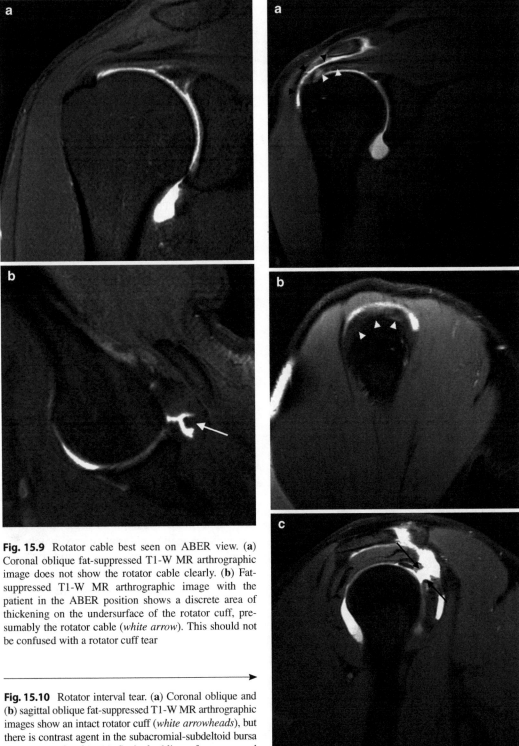

Fig. 15.9 Rotator cable best seen on ABER view. (**a**) Coronal oblique fat-suppressed T1-W MR arthrographic image does not show the rotator cable clearly. (**b**) Fat-suppressed T1-W MR arthrographic image with the patient in the ABER position shows a discrete area of thickening on the undersurface of the rotator cuff, presumably the rotator cable (*white arrow*). This should not be confused with a rotator cuff tear

Fig. 15.10 Rotator interval tear. (**a**) Coronal oblique and (**b**) sagittal oblique fat-suppressed T1-W MR arthrographic images show an intact rotator cuff (*white arrowheads*), but there is contrast agent in the subacromial-subdeltoid bursa (*black arrowheads*). (**c**) Sagittal oblique fat-suppressed T1-W MR arthrographic image shows a tear of the rotator interval with contrast material in the defect (*black arrows*)

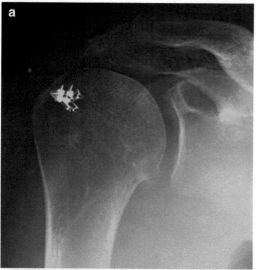

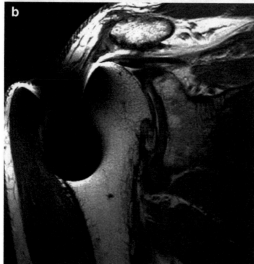

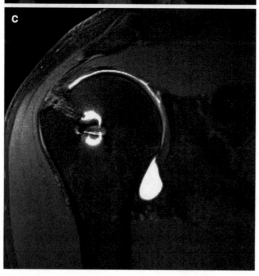

increase of bandwidth and matrix size, and the decrease of slice thickness and time to echo (Lee et al. 2007).

Knowledge of the operative techniques and commonly expected postoperative findings is important to avoid interpretation errors. Small residual defects of the rotator cuff contour can be seen without association with clinical symptoms. The signal intensity of the cuff tendons returns to normal in only 10% of cases. Persistent intra-substance increased T2 signal is often present, representing fibrosis and granulation tissue. This abnormal signal intensity within the repaired tendons may be seen for months or years after repair and should not be mistaken for recurrent/residual tendinopathy (Beltran et al. 2014) (Fig. 15.12). Subacromial bursal edema and fibrosis are routinely seen after rotator cuff repair and are probably irrelevant clinically in the absence of other signs of capsular arthrofibrosis (Zanetti et al. 2000).

15.4 Pitfalls Due to Imaging Techniques

Magic angle phenomenon refers to the artifactual-increased signal on sequences with short echo time (TE) in tissues with well-ordered collagen fibers in one direction (e.g., tendon or articular hyaline cartilage). This artifact occurs when the angle of these fibers with the main magnetic field is at approximately 55° (Erickson et al. 1993; Navon et al. 2001). Magic angle phenomenon can be decreased by lengthening the TE (Peh and Chan 1998) or changing the orientation of the structure relative to the magnetic field of the scanner. Additionally, evaluation for secondary signs of injury and use

Fig. 15.11 Effect of metal artifact reduction sequence (MARS) on metal-related artifacts on MRI. (**a**) Radiograph of the right shoulder shows metallic anchors in the humeral head. (**b**) Coronal oblique T1-W MR image shows a large artifact from metallic anchors. (**c**) Coronal oblique MR image employing MARS parameters shows decrease in artifact

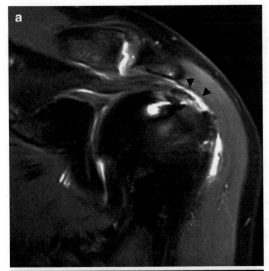

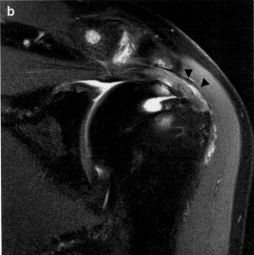

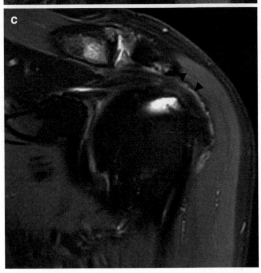

of the ABER position may be helpful in resolving magic angle artifact. Common locations for magic angle phenomenon in the shoulder include the supraspinatus tendon, the posterior superior and anterior inferior labrum, and the intra-articular long head of the biceps tendon (Fig. 15.13).

Intra-articular air bubbles introduced during contrast injection can create artifacts on MR arthrography. Proper technique during the procedure usually prevents noticeable accumulation of intra-articular gas. Air bubbles are located in the nondependent aspect of the joint and should not be misinterpreted as intra-articular bodies, metal, chondrocalcinosis, or possible labral tear. Small air bubbles in the biceps tendon sheath can cause a rope-ladder artifact characterized by variably sized and shaped signal abnormalities (Gückel and Nidecker 1997) (Fig. 15.14). Recognition of this artifact will prevent overdiagnosis of bicipital pathology.

Conclusion

MRI is often the modality of choice for the assessment of shoulder disorders and internal derangements. In this chapter, we reviewed several pitfalls that challenge the interpretation of shoulder MR images, including structural variations of the glenoid and glenoid labrum, articular cartilage, capsular ligaments, and rotator cuff tendons. By standardizing MR image acquisition and the design of pulse sequences, common artifacts can be avoided or recognized.

Fig. 15.12 Postoperative rotator cuff. Coronal oblique fat-suppressed T2-W MR images obtained at (**a**) 4 and (**b**) 6 months after rotator cuff repair show abnormal hyperintense signal in the supraspinatus tendon (*black arrowheads*). (**c**) Coronal oblique fat-suppressed T2-W image obtained at 12 months after rotator cuff repair shows return of normal supraspinatus tendon appearance (*black arrowsheads*). There is no defect within the tendon to indicate a re-tear

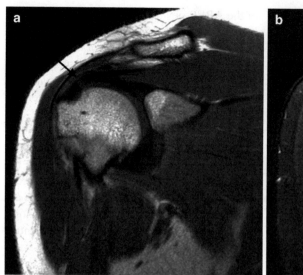

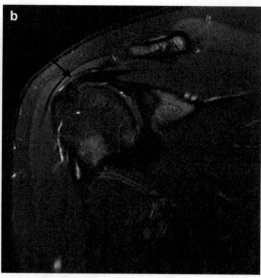

Fig. 15.13 Magic angle phenomenon. (**a**) Coronal oblique T1-W MR image shows a focal hyperintense area in the supraspinatus tendon 1–2 cm from the insertion site (*black arrow*), due to magic angle phenomenon.

(**b**) Coronal oblique fat-suppressed T2-W MR image in the same patient shows normal appearance of the supraspinatus tendon (*black arrow*)

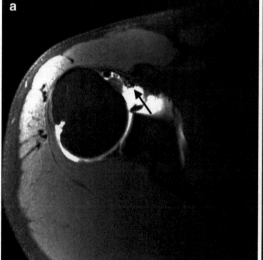

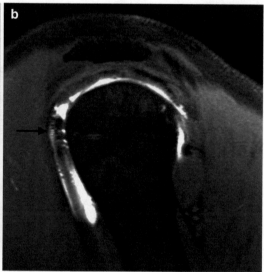

Fig. 15.14 Intra-articular air bubbles. (**a**) Axial fat-suppressed T1-W MR arthrographic image shows several rounded hypointense areas (*black arrow*) in the nondependent aspect of the joint. (**b**) Sagittal oblique fat-suppressed T1-W MR arthrographic image shows air bubbles along the long head of the biceps tendon (*black arrow*)

References

Beltran J, Bencardino J, Padron M et al (2002) The middle glenohumeral ligament: normal anatomy, variants and pathology. Skeletal Radiol 31:253–262

Beltran LS, Bencardino JT, Steinbach LS (2014) Postoperative MRI of the shoulder. J Magn Reson Imaging 40:1280–1297

Chang D, Mohana-Borges A, Borso M, Chung CB (2008) SLAP lesions: anatomy, clinical presentation, MR imaging diagnosis and characterization. Eur J Radiol 68:72–87

Clark JM, Harryman DT (1992) Tendons, ligaments, and capsule of the rotator cuff. Gross and microscopic anatomy. J Bone Joint Surg Am 74:713–725

Cole BJ, Rodeo SA, O'Brien SJ et al (2001) The anatomy and histology of the rotator interval capsule of the shoulder. Clin Orthop Relat Res 390:129–137

Cooper DE, Arnoczky SP, O'Brien SJ et al (1992) Anatomy, histology, and vascularity of the glenoid labrum. An anatomical study. J Bone Joint Surg Am 74:46–52

De Wilde LF, Berghs BM, Audenaert E et al (2004) About the variability of the shape of the glenoid cavity. Surg Radiol Anat 26:54–59

Erickson SJ, Prost RW, Timins ME (1993) The 'magic angle' effect: background physics and clinical relevance. Radiology 188:23–25

Fritz LB, Ouellette HA, O'Hanley TA, Kassarjian A, Palmer WE (2007) Cystic changes at supraspinatus and infraspinatus tendon insertion sites: association with age and rotator cuff disorders in 238 patients. Radiology 244:239–248

Gückel C, Nidecker A (1997) The rope ladder: an uncommon artifact and potential pitfall in MR arthrography of the shoulder. AJR Am J Roentgenol 168:947–950

Lee SY, Lee JK (2002) Horizontal component of partial-thickness tears of rotator cuff: imaging characteristics and comparison of ABER view with oblique coronal view at MR arthrography initial results. Radiology 224:470–476

Lee MJ, Kim S, Lee SA et al (2007) Overcoming artifacts from metallic orthopedic implants at high-field-strength MR imaging and multi-detector CT. Radiographics 27:791–803

Krych AJ, Shindle MK, Baran S, Warren RF (2013) Isolated arthroscopic rotator interval closure for shoulder instability. Arthrosc Tech 3:e35–e38

Michelin P, Trintignac A, Dacher JN et al (2014) Magnetic resonance anatomy of the superior part of the rotator cuff in normal shoulders, assessment and practical implication. Surg Radiol Anat 36:993–1000

Navon G, Shinar H, Eliav U, Seo Y (2001) Multiquantum filters and order in tissues. NMR Biomed 14:112–132

Peh WCG, Chan JHM (1998) The magic angle phenomenon in tendons: effect of varying the MR echo time. Br J Radiol 71:31–36

Ramirez Ruiz FA, Baranski Kaniak BC, Haghighi P et al (2012) High origin of the anterior band of the inferior glenohumeral ligament: MR arthrography with ana-tomic and histologic correlation in cadavers. Skeletal Radiol 41:525–530

Richards RD, Sartoris DJ, Pathria MN, Resnick D (1994) Hill-Sachs lesion and normal humeral groove: MR imaging features allowing their differentiation. Radiology 190:665–668

Rao AG, Kim TG, Chronopoulos E, McFarland EG (2003) Anatomical variants in the anterosuperior aspect of the glenoid labrum: a statistical analysis of seventy-three cases. J Bone Joint Surg Am 85:653–659

Sammarco VJ (2000) Os acromiale: frequency, anatomy, and clinical implications. J Bone Joint Surg Am 82:394–400

Sano A, Itoi E, Konno N et al (1998) Cystic changes of the humeral head on MR imaging. Relation to age and cuff-tears. Acta Orthop Scand 69:397–400

Sheah K, Bredella MA, Warner JJP, Halpern EF, Palmer WE (2009) Transverse thickening along the articular surface of the rotator cuff consistent with the rotator cable: identification with MR arthrography and relevance in rotator cuff evaluation. AJR Am J Roentgenol 193:679–686

Smith DK, Chopp TM, Aufdemorte TB et al (1996) Sublabral recess of the superior glenoid labrum: study of cadavers with conventional nonenhanced MR imaging, MR arthrography, anatomic dissection, and limited histologic examination. Radiology 201:251–256

Williams MM, Snyder SJ, Buford D (1994) The Buford complex – the 'cord-like' middle glenohumeral ligament and absent anterosuperior labrum complex: a normal anatomic capsulolabral variant. Arthrosc J Arthrosc Relat Surg 10:241–247

Williams M, Lambert RGW, Jhangri GS et al (2006) Humeral head cysts and rotator cuff tears: an MR arthrographic study. Skeletal Radiol 35:909–914

Yeh L, Kwak S, Kim YS et al (1998) Anterior labroligamentous structures of the glenohumeral joint: correlation of MR arthrography and anatomic dissection in cadavers. AJR Am J Roentgenol 171:1229–1236

Zanetti M, Jost B, Hodler J, Gerber C (2000) MR imaging after rotator cuff repair: full-thickness defects and bursitis-like subacromial abnormalities in asymptomatic subjects. Skeletal Radiol 29:314–319

Zanetti M, Carstensen T, Weishaupt D, Jost B, Hodler J (2001) MR arthrographic variability of the arthroscopically normal glenoid labrum: qualitative and quantitative assessment. Eur Radiol 11:559–566

Shoulder Injury: US Pitfalls

16

Richard W. Fawcett, Emma L. Rowbotham,
and Andrew J. Grainger

Contents

16.1	**Introduction**	307
16.2	**Normal Anatomy and Physiology**	308
16.2.1	Normal Tendon	308
16.2.2	Musculotendinous Junction and Tendinous Attachment	308
16.2.3	Rotator Interval	309
16.2.4	Deltoid Muscle	309
16.3	**Technical Factors**	310
16.3.1	Transducers	310
16.3.2	Focus	310
16.3.3	Anisotropy	310
16.4	**Scanning Technique**	311
16.4.1	Scrupulous Technique	311
16.4.2	Complete Rotator Cuff Evaluation	311
16.4.3	Dynamic Examination	312
16.4.4	Transducer Handling and Doppler Imaging	312
16.5	**Patient Factors**	313
16.5.1	Limitation of Movement	313
16.5.2	Obesity and Muscularity	313
16.6	**Full-Thickness Tendon Tears**	314
16.6.1	Small Full-Thickness Tears	314
16.6.2	Nonvisualization of the Rotator Cuff	314
16.7	**Partial-Thickness Tendon Tears**	315
16.7.1	Partial-Thickness Tears	315
16.7.2	Tendon Thinning	315
16.7.3	Tendinosis	315
16.8	**Calcific Tendinosis**	315
16.9	**Trauma**	316
16.9.1	Fractures	316
16.9.2	Hemorrhage and Edema	316
16.10	**Other Related Lesions**	317
16.10.1	Bursal Effusion	317
16.10.2	Osteoarthritis	318
16.10.3	Synovitis	318
16.10.4	Postoperative Shoulder	318
Conclusion		319
References		319

Abbreviation

US   Ultrasound

R.W. Fawcett, MBChB, FRCR • E.L. Rowbotham,
FRCS, FRCR • A.J. Grainger, FRCP, FRCR (✉)
Department of Musculoskeletal Radiology, Chapel
Allerton Hospital, Leeds Teaching Hospitals,
Leeds LS7, UK
e-mail: richardfawcett@doctors.org.uk;
emma.rowbotham@nhs.net; andrewgrainger@nhs.net

16.1   Introduction

An understanding of the normal anatomy of the shoulder joint together with the normal ultrasound (US) imaging appearances and associated artifacts is paramount to avoid potential diagnostic pitfalls. Appreciating basic US physics and utilizing it to improve image quality will aid diagnostic accuracy. The pathological appearances of the rotator cuff tendons present particular difficulty, with pitfalls predominantly relating to the more subtle findings.

© Springer International Publishing AG 2017
W.C.G. Peh (ed.), *Pitfalls in Musculoskeletal Radiology*, DOI 10.1007/978-3-319-53496-1_16

The US imaging appearances of a range of different pathological entities can overlap with imaging artifacts. Close scrutiny of every abnormality needs to be made in two planes, utilizing dynamic assessment, where necessary, in order to avoid pitfalls.

16.2 Normal Anatomy and Physiology

16.2.1 Normal Tendon

The accurate assessment of superficial tendons with US requires an appreciation of their histological composition. They are composed of ordered bundles of collagen fibers known as fascicles, and on US imaging, these are demonstrated as an internal network of fine parallel and linear fibrillar echoes which relate to reflections at the interface between collagen bundles and internal septa (Martinoli et al. 1993). Optimal visualization of tendons requires modern US systems with high frequency transducers allowing resolution of these fibrillary echoes, which are optimally visualized if the US beam is transmitted and received in a plane perpendicular to the fibers. The rotator cuff tendons do not display the homogeneous echotexture of simpler tendons. The supraspinatus tendon, in particular, shows a complex microanatomical pattern, appearing heterogeneous due to fanning and interdigitation of fibers in a complex histological structure involving layers of fibers with collagen bundles in differing planes (Clark and Harryman 1992). This complex microstructure is especially evident at the interface between the supraspinatus and infraspinatus tendons. An appreciation of these appearances will help to avoid the overdiagnosis of tendinosis and tears (Fig. 16.1). If scanning is undertaken too far laterally in the short axis plane, the tendon complex appears thin at this site, due to the presence of the normal bony protuberance between the anterior and middle facets of the greater tuberosity. This should not be interpreted as focal tendon thinning.

16.2.2 Musculotendinous Junction and Tendinous Attachment

It is important to understand the normal appearance of the musculotendinous junction of the rotator cuff tendons. The musculotendinous junction appears as an interdigitation of muscle and tendon fibers, giving a slightly heterogeneous appearance that can be mistaken for tendinosis (Fig. 16.2). Further medially, toward the muscle, the appearance will become more hypoechoic with linear clefts of hypoechogenicity interspersing with tendon fibers. Care is needed not to misinterpret this as a longitudinal split tear of the tendon (Fig. 16.3). Fibrocartilage is normally found at the point where tendons attach to the bone, termed the enthesis. In the case of tendons attaching close to the margin of articular cartilage, such as the rotator cuff tendons, the fibrocartilage insertion is in continuity with the articular cartilage (Benjamin 1986) and appears as a hypoechoic line at the enthesis. This may mimic a rim of fluid, and knowledge of its presence will prevent overdiagnosis of tears and tendinosis at this site (Rutten et al. 2006) (Fig. 16.4).

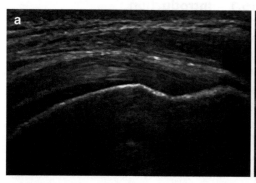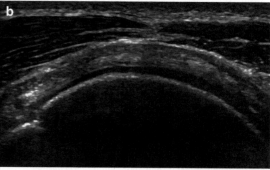

Fig. 16.1 The normal appearance of the supraspinatus tendon in both (**a**) long and (**b**) short axes US imaging. Both images show a layered appearance to the tendon due to the normal tendon microstructure. Fibrillar bundles give the short axis image a particularly heterogeneous appearance

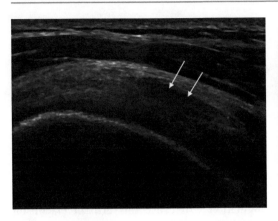

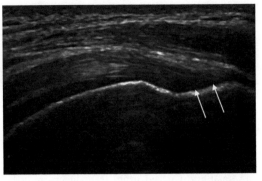

Fig. 16.2 The normal musculotendinous junction. Long-axis US image of the supraspinatus tendon shows focal regions of hypoechogenicity at the musculotendinous junction (*arrows*) that can mimic tendinopathic change

Fig. 16.4 Normal fibrocartilaginous tendon insertion of the supraspinatus tendon on US imaging. A thin hypoechoic line at the insertion of the tendon onto the greater tuberosity (*arrows*) should not be misinterpreted as a tear

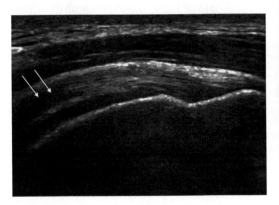

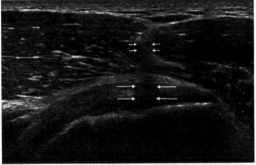

Fig. 16.3 Interdigitation of tendon and muscle fibers should not be misinterpreted as a longitudinal split tear of the tendon (*arrows*) on US imaging

Fig. 16.5 US image shows the normal subscapularis tendon in its long axis. Focal acoustic shadowing in the subscapularis tendon (*arrows*) from septa (*short arrows*) within the overlying musculature may not only obscure the tendon fibers beneath it but also mimic tendinopathic change

16.2.3 Rotator Interval

The rotator interval is increasingly recognized as an important component of the rotator cuff, and far from representing an "empty space" in the cuff, between the supraspinatus and subscapularis, it is integral to shoulder stability (Harryman et al. 1992; Jost et al. 2000; Petchprapa et al. 2010). It contains the biceps tendon, coracohumeral ligament, and the superior glenohumeral ligament. The interval, on US imaging, appears as a hypoechoic triangle forming a small gap on either side of the biceps tendon which can be misinterpreted as a tear. However, the interval also represents an important landmark for the anterior free edge of the supraspinatus tendon and the superior

border of subscapularis which must be visualized if cuff tears are not to be missed.

16.2.4 Deltoid Muscle

The deltoid muscle consists of anterior, central, and posterior parts, with a complex arrangement of tendinous intersections within the muscle substance. If these intersections are especially thick or are scanned in a tangential plane, they may cast an acoustic shadow on the underlying supraspinatus tendon (Rutten et al. 2006). This can result in focal regions of hypoechogenicity in the underlying rotator cuff tendons that can mimic a tear or focal tendinosis (Fig. 16.5).

16.3   Technical Factors

16.3.1 Transducers

The choice of transducer is instrumental in determining the image quality of a shoulder US examination. There is a requirement for high-resolution imaging and also a moderately large field of view in order to completely assess larger structures in their entirety and their relationship to surrounding anatomy. Curved array transducers may be prone to increased anisotropic artifact, and skin contact can be problematic; therefore, a high frequency, large field-of-view, linear array transducer is advised.

16.3.2 Focus

Modern transducers will optimize parameters, such as focusing, by digital management of the signal (Rizzatto 1999). However, manual adjustment is also advised as examination of the shoulder requires evaluation of structures at varying depths, for example, assessment of the more superficially located tendons and the more deeply located rotator cuff muscles.

16.3.3 Anisotropy

Anisotropy is a form of artifact that results in a tendon appearing abnormally hypoechoic due to suboptimal scanning technique. The structural organization of tendons renders them highly susceptible to this, and in order to reliably image tendons, the incident US beam must be perpendicular to the tendinous fibrils in both the longitudinal and transverse planes (Fornage 1987). As little as 2 to 3 degrees of angulation will cause this artifact (Jacobson 2011). The curvilinear nature of the rotator cuff tendons and their oblique position relative to the skin surface necessitates skilled control of the probe. If a careful technique is not used, the resultant pitfall is the overdiagnosis of tendon pathology, especially tendinosis and partial-thickness tears (Fig. 16.6). In particular, intrasubstance tears may be misdiagnosed. Their appearance is of a focal intra-tendinous cleft of fluid that is visible in both planes and persists with angulation of the probe. They will lack the helpful diagnostic features of focal tendon thinning seen in bursal surface tears, or continuity with joint fluid seen in articular surface tears.

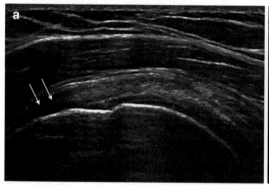 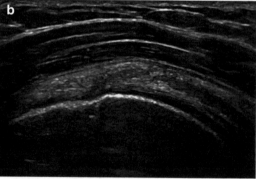

Fig. 16.6 US images show the effect of anisotropy in the normal supraspinatus tendon. (**a**) The hypoechoic region within the tendon at the insertion is artifactual due to the direction of the fibers in the tendon (*arrows*). (**b**) Angling the probe to ensure the tendon fibers are more perpendicular to the beam minimizes this artifact

16.4   Scanning Technique

16.4.1 Scrupulous Technique

A full assessment of all structures of a shoulder US examination is required in what is often a short amount of time. A protocol-driven systematic approach helps ensure that omissions are not made. This should include a focused patient history and clinical examination if required (Jamadar et al. 2010). Each practitioner will have their own preferred technique; however, the focus for the practitioner should be on completeness and reproducibility.

16.4.2 Complete Rotator Cuff Evaluation

When diagnosing rotator cuff tendon abnormalities, the tendon should always be examined in its entirety in both the longitudinal and transverse planes, avoiding anisotropy by angling the probe (Jacobson et al. 2011; Gupta and Robinson 2015). If an apparent abnormality is visualized in one plane and close inspection of the same region in the perpendicular plane reveals no abnormality, the finding should be attributed to artifact. A common reason will be anisotropy mimicking tendon tears or tendinosis.

Each tendon should be visualized in its entirety using a sweeping motion, from the musculotendinous junction to the osseous insertion, as far as possible. This can be particularly difficult with the supraspinatus tendon, but is of the utmost importance. Care should be taken when scanning the supraspinatus tendon in the transverse plane at its insertion onto the greater tuberosity, as no tendon will be visualized if the transducer is positioned too laterally, and thus a full-thickness tendon tear may be erroneously diagnosed. To allow complete visualization of the tendon, the shoulder should be internally rotated and extended to displace the tendon from under

the acromion. The degree of internal rotation and extension can be varied allowing demonstration of the whole of the supraspinatus and also the infraspinatus.

Although both the modified Crass position, hand on the ipsilateral buttock (the "back pocket") (Ferri et al. 2005), and the Crass position, dorsum of the hand over the mid-back, with the fingers pointing toward the contralateral scapula (Crass et al. 1987), have been described, in practice, the authors will usually move the arm between the two positions during examination to ensure complete assessment of the cuff has been undertaken. Positioning the shoulder, as described, also applies stress to the supraspinatus tendon which may help identify subtle pathological findings (Bianchi and Martinoli 2007).

Assessment of subscapularis requires external rotation with arm adduction for optimal assessment. A potential pitfall is misinterpreting the normal multipennate appearance of the subscapularis in its short axis as tearing (Fig. 16.7). When assessing the rotator cuff, particular attention should be paid to the cuff immediately adjacent to the rotator interval, the anterior border of supraspinatus, and the superior border of sub-

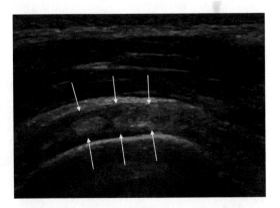

Fig. 16.7 US image shows the normal subscapularis tendon in short axis. The tendon has a multipennate appearance (*arrows*) which should not be confused with tendinosis

scapularis. These are sites where tears are commonly seen and represent parts of the rotator cuff which can be easily missed on US imaging assessment (Jacobson et al. 2011; Gupta and Robinson 2015).

16.4.3 Dynamic Examination

While static assessment reveals much of the relevant pathology during shoulder US imaging, a few dynamic maneuvers ensure that certain findings are not missed. The long head of the biceps tendon can appear correctly sited in the bicipital groove at rest; however, on dynamic assessment with external rotation of the forearm, it may sublux or dislocate (Jacobson et al. 2011). Secondary signs of impingement exist on static US examination, but assessment of subacromial impingement can be enhanced if the movement of the tendon and bursa relative to the coracoacromial arch is visualized dynamically as the patient abducts the arm. The subacromial bursa will bunch as the patient reports pain during this maneuver, suggesting the diagnosis. Difficulty in evaluating the insertion points of the infraspinatus and the teres minor tendons can arise, as these tendons may appear lateral rather than posterior. Assessment during both internal and external rotation can allow a more complete visualization of the tendons at their insertions.

16.4.4 Transducer Handling and Doppler Imaging

Sweeping the probe along the length and width of tendons ensures their full evaluation. While good skin contact is necessary, light pressure is encouraged as it ensures minimal distortion of the underlying tissues. The most important example is the subacromial/subdeltoid bursa, where a heavy hand may lead to underdiagnosing fluid in the bursa (Fig. 16.8). While a bursal effusion has a multitude of causes, it has been shown that the presence of both a bursal effusion and a glenohumeral joint effusion has a specificity of 99% for the diagnosis of a rotator cuff tear in patients with a painful shoulder (Hollister et al. 1995). Application of more pressure (sonopalpation) does have its uses, for example, in clarifying the presence of a nonretracted full-thickness rotator cuff tear by using superficial pressure to push overlying intact fibers into the defect or by moving overlying bursal fluid into the defect (Fig. 16.9).

While power Doppler imaging is not commonly used in everyday practice during examination of the shoulder, it can act as a useful adjunct to confirm or refute-specific findings and avoid pitfalls. Hyperemia may be seen in relation to tendon tears or be associated with tendinitis (Newman et al. 1994). Demonstration of hyperemia at the rotator interval has also been described as a feature of adhesive capsu-

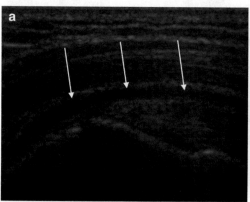 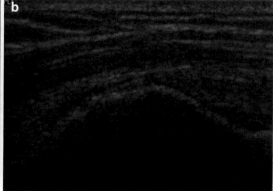

Fig. 16.8 The effect of too much downward pressure with the probe can underestimate or even obscure the presence of subacromial/subdeltoid bursitis. (**a**) US image shows a bursal effusion when minimal probe pressure is applied (*arrows*). (**b**) Repeat US image shows that the effusion is obscured with firm sonopalpation

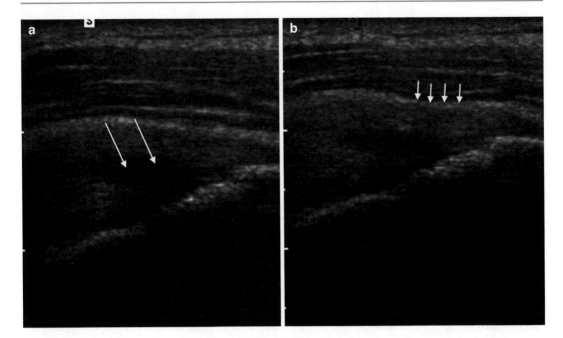

Fig. 16.9 The usefulness of sonopalpation in a partial-thickness tear. (**a**) US image shows a focal hypoechoic region in the supraspinatus tendon that is suspicious for a partial tear (*long arrows*). (**b**) The use of sonopalpation during US imaging confirms the presence of a tear by forcing fibers into the defect and thus creating a focal depression (*short arrows*) in the bursal surface of the tendon

litis (Lee et al. 2005). Comparison with the contralateral side is advised.

16.5 Patient Factors

16.5.1 Limitation of Movement

The cause of a decreased range of movement may be directly due to the underlying pathology, for example, in adhesive capsulitis, or may be indirectly due to pain, for which there are many causes. There should be a degree of acceptance that some patients will find a shoulder US examination painful, in which case it is helpful to be quick and efficient. While discomfort is often accepted by the patient and the clinician, there may occasionally be a compromise in the quality of the examination. Conditions limiting shoulder movement, such as adhesive capsulitis, can be more difficult to deal with. A "frozen" shoulder manifests as limitation in external rotation, flexion, and internal rotation (Manske and Prohaska 2008). It is specifically the external rotation that

may limit accurate assessment, particularly affecting full assessment of the subscapularis tendon. External rotation causes the most medial part of the tendon to move laterally, exposing the proximal tendon and musculotendinous junction. Limitation of this movement may lead to tears missed at these sites, although this loss of external rotation can be an important sign to the examining radiologist that the problem may be an adhesive capsulitis.

16.5.2 Obesity and Muscularity

The presence of a thickened subcutaneous fat layer, a large deltoid muscle, or fatty infiltration of the deltoid causes attenuation of the US beam. While gross abnormalities such as full-thickness rotator cuff tears will normally still be visible, diagnostic confidence may be reduced, and more subtle findings such as partial-thickness tears and tendinosis may be missed. Measures can be taken to increase diagnostic accuracy, such as decreasing the frequency or changing the transducer, but the key is recognition of these features and the reduction in diagnostic accuracy. If necessary, this should be stated in the examination report. An important observation is that an abnormal cuff will rarely look normal, but it is very easy to make a normal cuff look abnormal.

16.6　Full-Thickness Tendon Tears

16.6.1　Small Full-Thickness Tears

The common site for small full-thickness rotator cuff tears is the insertion point of the anterior supraspinatus tendon onto the greater tuberosity of the humerus. Small tears at this site should be carefully evaluated in two planes. The tear will appear as a hypoechoic cleft extending from the bursal surface to the articular cartilage but may only measure a few millimeters in the short or long axis, and therefore the majority of the tendon will appear normal. Visualizing a focal hypoechoic or anechoic region in isolation is not reliable for diagnosing tears that will be visible at arthroscopy. Searching for the additional presence of irregular margins can be helpful to confirm the diagnosis (Jacobson 2004), as well as fluid present focally over the region of suspicion or focal thickening of the overlying bursa. Care must be taken to accurately measure the tear size, which can be reliably done in the right hands. Ferri et al. (2005) demonstrated that the modified Crass position, which involves forced external rotation, may increase the longitudinal tension on the tendon and overestimate the size of the tear in the longitudinal plane. Positioning the arm in internal rotation behind the back (the Crass position) gives a more accurate measurement, when correlated surgically.

16.6.2　Nonvisualization of the Rotator Cuff

A massive rotator cuff tear results in diastasis of the tendon margins. Often, the medial part of the ten-

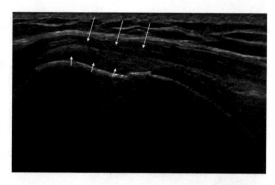

Fig. 16.10 US image shows a full-thickness supraspinatus tear with no tendon fibers over the humeral head. The deltoid muscle fibers (*long arrows*) and a thickened subacromial bursa (*short arrows*) lie against the humeral head (*arrows*) and should not be mistaken for intact tendon fibers

don will retract medially beneath the acromion and may not be visualized. The US imaging appearance in this setting is that of an uncovered or "naked" humeral head, and there will often be an absence of joint or bursal fluid, if the tear is chronic (Teefey et al. 2000). With no rotator cuff directly overlying the articular cartilage and no joint or bursal fluid to suggest the presence of a recent tear, the deltoid muscle descends to make direct contact with the humeral head cartilage. Two pitfalls to avoid here are interpreting the cartilage as a thinned cuff and interpreting the intact deltoid muscle fibers as intact tendon fibers (Fig. 16.10). Awareness of the capability of the deltoid muscle to mimic intact tendon is important. The normal fibrillar pattern of tendon fibers should be actively looked for, and if there is diagnostic doubt, the deltoid muscle should be tracked proximally or distally to visualize its insertion or origin.

An interesting pitfall involves the overdiagnosis of a massive cuff tear and emphasizes the necessity of scrupulously scanning in two planes. Transverse plane scanning of the supraspinatus at a site lateral to the tendon will demonstrate a bare humeral head and an appearance that will mimic a "naked" head and potential overcalling of a large cuff tear (Fig. 16.11). Correlation with longitudinal images and ensuring the articular cartilage is visualized should help avoid this pitfall.

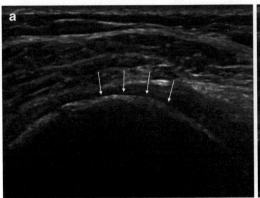
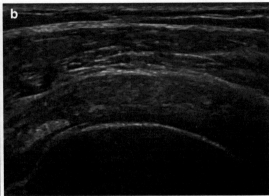

Fig. 16.11 US imaging of a rotator cuff that is scanned too far laterally in this patient. (**a**) The probe is positioned too far lateral where there is no rotator cuff overlying the greater tuberosity. This appearance mimics the "naked" humeral head sign (*arrows*) seen with a full-thickness cuff tear; but note the absence of articular cartilage. (**b**) Moving the probe medially shows the normal supraspinatus tendon in short axis

16.7 Partial-Thickness Tendon Tears

16.7.1 Partial-Thickness Tears

US imaging has become increasingly accurate and reliable at diagnosing partial-thickness rotator cuff tears (van Holsbeeck et al. 1995). The appearance is of a focal fluid-filled cleft, often extending from the articular or bursal surface. The tears can also be intrasubstance, which is a more difficult diagnosis to make. Again, confirmation of the abnormality in two planes is advised to avoid pitfalls.

16.7.2 Tendon Thinning

A normal-looking tendon that is thinned should not be overanalyzed. While the average thickness of an intact rotator cuff in patients with a painful shoulder is 4.7 mm (Yamaguchi et al. 2006), there are multiple other causes of rotator cuff tendon thinning such as rheumatoid arthritis, disuse, nerve impingement, or surgery (Rutten et al. 2006). It is focal tendon thinning that may be significant and represent a tear; however, the presence of an underlying fluid-filled cleft is required to confirm the diagnosis. If there is diagnostic doubt, it may be helpful to compare with the contralateral side.

16.7.3 Tendinosis

The presence of superadded tendinosis can make diagnosing partial-thickness tears more difficult. A tendinopathic tendon is more likely to tear, and the pitfall is differentiating a partial-thickness tear from tendinosis, which can be very difficult. The US imaging appearance of tendinosis is that of a heterogeneous and thickened tendon. However, an isolated measurement of tendon thickness should be interpreted with care, and correlation with other findings is essential. These may include, in the setting of tendinosis, increased bursal fluid and bursal wall thickening and US imaging evidence of impingement. There is an overlap in the diagnostic features, as increased bursal fluid can also be seen with a partial-thickness cuff tear. The concomitant findings may help if there is diagnostic doubt, and consideration of clinical symptoms and signs is also invaluable. In reality, the differentiation may not influence the management of the patient, but diagnostic doubt should be communicated in the report.

16.8 Calcific Tendinosis

It has been suggested that calcific tendinosis has an incidence of 2.7% in adults. Three distinct phases have been proposed, namely, the pre-calcific, calcific, and post-calcific stages, with a predisposition for degenerative tendons and those subjected to impingement (Kachewar 2013). The resultant appearance on US imaging varies from amorphous mildly hyperechoic foci to a dense echogenic focus with posterior acoustic shadowing and obscuration of the structures deep to this. The most common site of occurrence is within the supraspinatus tendon. It is important not to misinterpret a large calcific focus as cortical irregularity or a fracture. However, in the authors' experience, it is more common to mistake an unsuspected and undisplaced greater tuberosity avulsion fracture for calcific tendinopathy.

In cases of suspected calcific tendinopathy, the concomitant finding of a degenerative-appearing tendon should be looked for. Occasionally, fine linear calcifications representing enthesophytes are seen within the rotator cuff at the enthesis, paralleling the tendon fibers. These should not be over-interpreted as calcium deposition (Fig. 16.12). Reviewing conventional radiographs will often help, and if none are available, they should be obtained. If the disease process is in the earlier stages, then the appearance will be less convincing for calcific tendinosis. Patchy echogenic foci with a faint or absent shadow may mimic tendinosis or fibrosis, but the application of power Doppler imaging may demonstrate hyperemia to add weight to the diag-

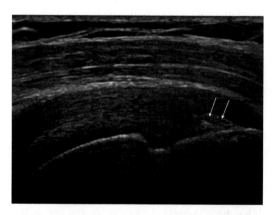

Fig. 16.12 Long-axis US image of the supraspinatus tendon shows enthesophytes at its insertion (*arrows*). It is important not to over-interpret this as calcific tendinosis or a fracture

nosis, especially if the patient reports pain (Chiou et al. 2002).

16.9 Trauma

16.9.1 Fractures

Radiographically occult fractures of the greater tuberosity can represent another pitfall. If a fracture of the proximal humerus is suspected clinically but is not visualized on the radiograph, then it should be looked for on US imaging. The US imaging signs include cortical irregularity or discontinuity of the greater tuberosity, elevation of the periosteum, and the double-line sign (Rutten et al. 2007) (Fig. 16.13). In particular, the double-line sign has been shown to be a reliable indicator of fracture and may aid in differentiating the cortical irregularity of a fracture from foci of calcification in the adjacent rotator cuff tendon at its insertion, an appearance seen with calcific tendinosis.

The Hill-Sachs lesion is an important hallmark of previous anterior shoulder dislocation, and it is important to identify this abnormality and obtain an accurate measurement for prognostic value. Cortical irregularity associated with tendinosis may cause confusion; however, looking for medialization of the defect and possible contact between the defect and the glenoid during external rotation is usually seen with a Hill-Sachs lesion (Fig. 16.14). A history of trauma should always lead to close scrutiny of the cortical surfaces of the proximal humerus to identify any associated fracture.

16.9.2 Hemorrhage and Edema

While hemorrhage and edema in the soft issues around the shoulder joint are likely to be present in the setting of a recent fracture, these entities may be present in isolation. The appearance of a hypoechoic or mixed echogenicity soft tissue fluid collection in the setting of trauma may obscure underlying structures. A hematoma will appear as a focal collection of mixed echogenicity

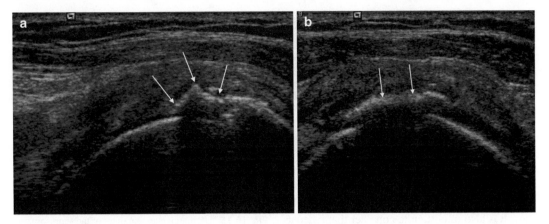

Fig. 16.13 Fracture of the greater tuberosity. (**a**) US image shows cortical irregularity (*arrows*) associated with a fracture of the greater tuberosity. The fracture was not visible on radiographs. (**b**) The fracture is shown in the short-axis US image. The cortical irregularity can mimic dense calcification in the overlying tendon (*arrows*). This abnormality should always be examined in two planes and correlated with available previous imaging

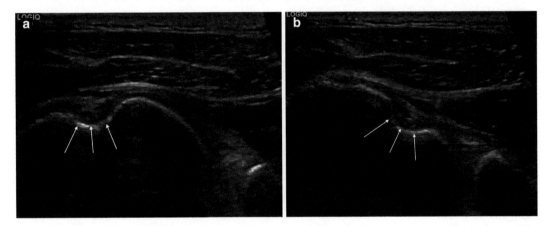

Fig. 16.14 A Hill-Sachs lesion is shown on US images taken in (**a**) internal and (**b**) external rotation. Note how the defect (*arrows*) moves toward the posterior joint space in external rotation

and, if the injury is long-standing, may demonstrate peripheral calcification.

16.10 Other Related Lesions

16.10.1 Bursal Effusion

The presence of subacromial/subdeltoid bursal effusion is well described as part of the shoulder impingement syndrome. Increased fluid in the bursa in addition to bursal wall thickening, changes in the supraspinatus tendon, and associated bursal bunching on abduction suggest the diagnosis of bursitis. If clinically suspected and if these findings are present, the diagnosis of impingement is often straightforward. However, interpreting too much fluid in the bursa as an apparent isolated finding can be more difficult, as this can occur with a number of other abnormalities. Inflammatory arthropathies such as rheumatoid arthritis may cause a bursal effusion in isolation, and in the right clinical setting, infection should be considered. Moreover, bursal fluid can be seen in the shoulders of asymptomatic patients (Awerbuch 2008), but a supraspinatus tear must be excluded (Hollister et al. 1995). Compression of the fluid-filled bursa into the bursal surface of the tear may suggest the diagnosis.

16.10.2 Osteoarthritis

Conventional radiographs remain the modality of choice for diagnosing glenohumeral osteoarthritis, and if this diagnosis is a concern, these should be obtained. The diagnosis on US imaging can be more challenging, and changes associated with osteoarthritis may be mistaken for other pathologies. It is also important to consider that osteoarthritis can be present alongside cuff pathology, and its presence may influence management. In cases of osteoarthritis, joint effusion and the irregular cortex of the articular surface can be incorrectly interpreted as relating to cuff damage or a tear. The biceps tendon sheath is a common site for joint fluid to collect, and loose bodies may also be seen here. Care must be taken to accurately evaluate the biceps tendon itself to allow correct differentiation of a joint-based pathology from biceps tendinosis.

16.10.3 Synovitis

Bursal effusion has been found to be the most common finding in arthritic shoulder joints (Alasaarela 1998). Recognition of the additional expected findings will help to avoid diagnoses such as impingement or bursitis. These include glenohumeral joint effusion, fluid in the sheath of the long head of the biceps tendon, and visualization of the synovitis itself, for which the use of power Doppler imaging may be helpful.

16.10.4 Postoperative Shoulder

The assessment of the postoperative shoulder requires an understanding of findings that should be considered within normal limits and knowledge of the type of surgery performed. Appearances that may be considered pathologi-

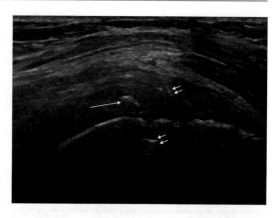

Fig. 16.15 US imaging appearances of the supraspinatus tendon 8 months following surgical repair. The heterogeneous appearance of the tendon is considered to be within normal limits in the postoperative rotator cuff. Note the small calcific focus (*long arrow*) and suture material in the tendon and suture anchor in the bone (*short arrows*)

cal in a normal shoulder may in fact be normal in the postoperative one. For example, the repair of a tendon after a tear will render the tendon more heterogeneous and, hence, should not be diagnosed as tendinosis (Fig. 16.15). In the initial stages after repair, the tendon may be hypoechoic and appear thinner between the suture anchors at the greater tuberosity (Jacobson et al. 2011), an appearance that should not be interpreted as a re-tear. Over time, the tendon will develop a fibrillar pattern again, but during healing, persistent echogenicity may also mimic small tears and disruption of soft tissue planes may mask more subtle findings (Crass et al. 1986).

Fortunately, US imaging does not suffer from the same artifacts from orthopedic hardware that are seen with magnetic resonance imaging (MRI). Sutures and suture anchors should be easily recognized, especially with the relevant clinical information at hand, and should not be misinterpreted as loose bodies or calcific foci. Focus should remain on the reliable US imaging findings used in a nonoperated shoulder, i.e., complete cuff retraction and a focal cleft in the tendon to indicate full-thickness and partial-thickness tears, respectively. Overall, US imaging has been shown to be highly effective in assessing the postoperative rotator cuff (Prickett et al. 2003).

Conclusion

While a multitude of diagnostic pitfalls exist when performing a shoulder US imaging examination, they can be avoided with a good understanding of the anatomy, correct technique, and an awareness of the pathologies that are most prone to misdiagnosis. Comparison with previous imaging, particularly conventional radiographs, is often helpful, as well as comparison with the contralateral side. A brief relevant clinical history and physical examination can add weight to the suspected diagnosis. While a scrupulous approach combined with an experienced understanding of a range of normal appearances of structures about the shoulder joint will maximize diagnostic accuracy, a good report will always mention limitations to diagnostic accuracy that have been encountered.

References

Alasaarela E (1998) Ultrasound and operative evaluation of arthritic shoulder joints. Ann Rheum Dis 57:357–360

Awerbuch M (2008) The clinical utility of ultrasonography for rotator cuff disease, shoulder impingement syndrome and subacromial bursitis. Med J Aust 188:50–53

Benjamin M (1986) The histology of tendon attachments to bone in man. J Anat 149:89–100

Bianchi S, Martinoli C (2007) Shoulder. In: Ultrasound of the musculoskeletal system. Springer-Verlag, Berlin/Heidelberg

Chiou HJ, Chou YH, Wu JJ et al (2002) Evaluation of calcific tendonitis of the rotator cuff: role of color Doppler ultrasonography. J Ultrasound Med 21:289–295

Clark JM, Harryman DT (1992) Tendons, ligaments, and capsule of the rotator cuff Gross and microscopic anatomy. J Bone Joint Surg Am 74:713–725

Crass JR, Craig EV, Feinberg SB (1986) Sonography of the postoperative rotator cuff. AJR Am J Roentgenol 146:561–564

Crass JR, Craig EV, Feinberg SB (1987) The hyperextended internal rotation view in rotator cuff ultrasonography. J Clin Ultrasound 15:416–420

Ferri M, Finlay K, Popowich T et al (2005) Sonography of full-thickness supraspinatus tears: comparison of patient positioning technique with surgical correlation. AJR Am J Roentgenol 184:180–184

Fornage BD (1987) The hypoechoic normal tendon: a pitfall. J Ultrasound Med 6:19–22

Gupta H, Robinson P (2015) Normal shoulder ultrasound: anatomy and technique. Semin Musculoskelet Radiol 19:203–211

Harryman DT, Sidles JA, Harris SL et al (1992) The role of the rotator interval capsule in passive motion and stability of the shoulder. J Bone Joint Surg Am 74:53–66

Hollister MS, Mack LA, Patten RM et al (1995) Association of sonographically detected subacromial/subdeltoid bursal effusion and intraarticular fluid with rotator cuff tear. AJR Am J Roentgenol 165:605–608

Jacobson JA, Lancaster S, Prasad A et al (2004) Full-thickness and partial-thickness supraspinatus tendon tears: value of US signs in diagnosis. Radiology 230:234–242

Jacobson JA (2011) Shoulder US: anatomy, technique, and scanning pitfalls. Radiology 260:6–16

Jacobson JA, Miller B, Bedi A et al (2011) Imaging of the postoperative shoulder. Semin Musculoskelet Radiol 15:320–339

Jamadar DA, Robertson BL, Jacobson JA et al (2010) Musculoskeletal sonography: important imaging pitfalls. AJR Am J Roentgenol 194:216–225

Jost B, Koch PP, Gerber C (2000) Anatomy and functional aspects of the rotator interval. J Shoulder Elbow Surg 9:336–341

Kachewar S (2013) Calcific tendinitis of the rotator cuff: a review. J Clin Diagn Res 7:1482–1485

Lee JC, Sykes C, Saifuddin A et al (2005) Adhesive capsulitis: sonographic changes in the rotator cuff interval with arthroscopic correlation. Skeletal Radiol 34:522–527

Manske R, Prohaska D (2008) Diagnosis and management of adhesive capsulitis. Curr Rev Musculoskelet Med 1:180–189

Martinoli C, Derchi LE, Pastorino C (1993) Analysis of echotexture of tendons with US. Radiology 186:839–843

Newman JS, Adler RS, Bude RO et al (1994) Detection of soft-tissue hyperemia: value of power Doppler sonography. AJR Am J Roentgenol 163:385–389

Petchprapa CN, Beltran LS, Jazrawi LM et al (2010) The rotator interval: a review of anatomy, function, and normal and abnormal MRI appearance. AJR Am J Roentgenol 195:567–576

Prickett WD, Teefey SA, Galatz LM et al (2003) Accuracy of ultrasound imaging of the rotator cuff in shoulders that are painful postoperatively. J Bone Joint Surg Am 85:1084–1089

Rizzatto G (1999) Evolution of US transducers: 1.5 and 2D arrays. Eur Radiol 9:304–306

Rutten MJ, Maresch BJ, Jager GJ et al (2006) From the RSNA refresher courses: US of the rotator cuff: pitfalls, limitations, and artifacts. Radiographics 26:589–604

Rutten MJ, Jager GJ, de Waal Malefijt MC et al (2007) Double line sign: a helpful sonographic sign to detect occult fractures of the proximal humerus. Eur Radiol 17:762–767

Teefey SA, Middleton WD, Bauer GS (2000) Sonographic differences in the appearance of acute and chronic full-thickness rotator cuff tears. J Ultrasound Med 19:377–378

van Holsbeeck MT, Kolowich PA, Eyler WR et al (1995) US depiction of partial-thickness tear of the rotator cuff. Radiology 197:443–446

Yamaguchi K, Ditsios K, Middleton WD (2006) The demographic and morphological features of rotator cuff disease A comparison of asymptomatic and symptomatic shoulders. J Bone Joint Surg Am 88: 1699–1704

Elbow Injury: MRI Pitfalls

17

Mark Harmon, Elaine NiMhurchu,
Gordon Andrews, and Bruce B. Forster

Contents

17.1   **Introduction** 321

17.2   **Pitfalls from MRI Technique and
       Patient Positioning** 322
17.2.1   Sequences and Positioning 322
17.2.2   Magic Angle Phenomenon 323
17.2.3   Arthrography 324

17.3   **Pitfalls in Normal Anatomy** 325
17.3.1   Capitellar Pseudo-Defect 325
17.3.2   Pseudo-Lesions of the Trochlear Notch 327
17.3.3   Synovial Folds 328
17.3.4   Elbow Fat Pads 329
17.3.5   Triceps Insertion 329
17.3.6   Ulnar Collateral Ligament 330
17.3.7   Lateral Collateral Ligaments 330

17.4   **Pitfalls in Normal Variant Anatomy** 332
17.4.1   Distal Biceps Insertion 332
17.4.2   Bicipitoradial Bursa 334
17.4.3   Anconeus Epitrochlearis 334
17.4.4   Cubital Tunnel and the Ulnar Nerve 334
17.4.5   Red Marrow 335
17.4.6   Supracondylar Process 336

Conclusion 336

References 336

M. Harmon, MBBCh, MRCPI, FFRRCSI, FRCR
E. NiMhurchu, MBBCh, MRCPI, FFRRCSI
G. Andrews, MD, FRCPC • B.B. Forster, MSc, MD,
FRCPC (✉)
Department of Radiology, University of British
Columbia, Vancouver General Hospital,
899 West 12th Avenue, Vancouver, BC V5Z 1M9,
Canada
e-mail: dr.markharmon@gmail.com;
elainenimhurchu@hotmail.com;
gordon.andrews@vch.ca; bruce.forster@vch.ca

Abbreviations

MRA   Magnetic resonance arthrography
MRI   Magnetic resonance imaging

17.1   Introduction

The elbow is a complex hinge synovial joint. It is comprised of three bones and three articulations, allowing for flexion, extension, supination, and pronation of the forearm. The elbow is less commonly imaged than many of the other large joints in the musculoskeletal system, usually limited to competitive and recreational athletes, as well as those sustaining chronic repetitive occupational injuries. The combination of complex bony and soft tissue anatomy, as well as inexperience related to the lower frequency of imaging, can render interpretation of elbow magnetic resonance imaging (MRI) particularly vulnerable to mistakes in interpretation.

In this chapter, we review many of the common pitfalls representing normal or variant anatomy and many pitfalls related to the technical aspects of MRI of the elbow, all of which can lead to misdiagnosis. We also highlight several pitfalls in the interpretation of true pathologic findings that may occasionally be misinterpreted or overlooked, particularly at sites where variant anatomy is common. We hope that the information provided will improve the interpretive abilities of the general radiologist who may be

© Springer International Publishing AG 2017   321
W.C.G. Peh (ed.), *Pitfalls in Musculoskeletal Radiology*, DOI 10.1007/978-3-319-53496-1_17

struggling with the evaluation of this less frequently imaged and technically difficult joint.

17.2 Pitfalls from MRI Technique and Patient Positioning

17.2.1 Sequences and Positioning

The field of view should routinely cover the distal humeral metaphysis to the bicipital tuberosity of the radius, in order to adequately assess the biceps tendon insertion. Imaging should be performed in all three planes. The choice of sequences varies by institution but should include both nonfat-suppressed T1-weighted and proton density (PD)-weighted sequences and fat-suppressed T2-/PD-weighted or short tau inversion recovery (STIR) sequences, which are essential for the evaluation of marrow edema. Gradient-echo sequences are not routinely used but can be added

if there is a specific clinical suspicion for loose bodies or synovial abnormality, such as seen with pigmented villonodular synovitis or hemophilia. In these cases, three- dimensional (3D) sequencing is suggested to optimize spatial resolution (Kijowski et al. 2004; Sampath et al. 2013).

Proper patient positioning is essential for MRI assessment of the elbow. The first consideration in any position should be to maximize patient comfort; this will in turn minimize motion artifact. Conventional positioning is performed supine with the arm relaxed at the side. This is well tolerated by patients but has the disadvantage of the elbow not positioned isocenter within the magnet. This negatively affects signal-to-noise ratio and field homogeneity, which will have an effect on image quality. In particular, inhomogeneous fat suppression can occur (Figs. 17.1 and 17.2).

Therefore, prone positioning with the arm over the head in the so-called "superman" position can be performed. This places the elbow joint close to

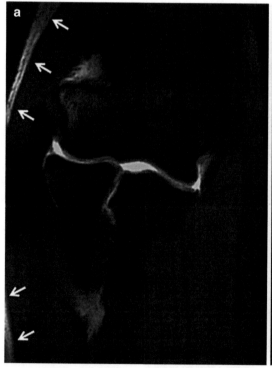
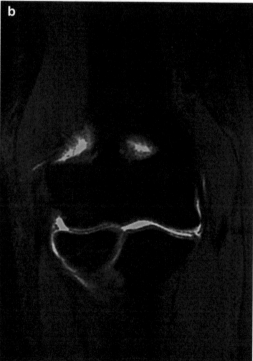

Fig. 17.1 Coronal fat-suppressed T1-W MRA images obtained in the same patient in the (**a**) supine and (**b**) "superman" positions show the effect of inhomogeneous fat suppression. In (**a**), the arm is positioned by the patients' side, and there is incomplete fat suppression at lateral aspect of the arm (*arrows*) as it is furthest from isocenter. In the "superman" position (**b**), the elbow is at isocenter, and the fat suppression is homogeneous

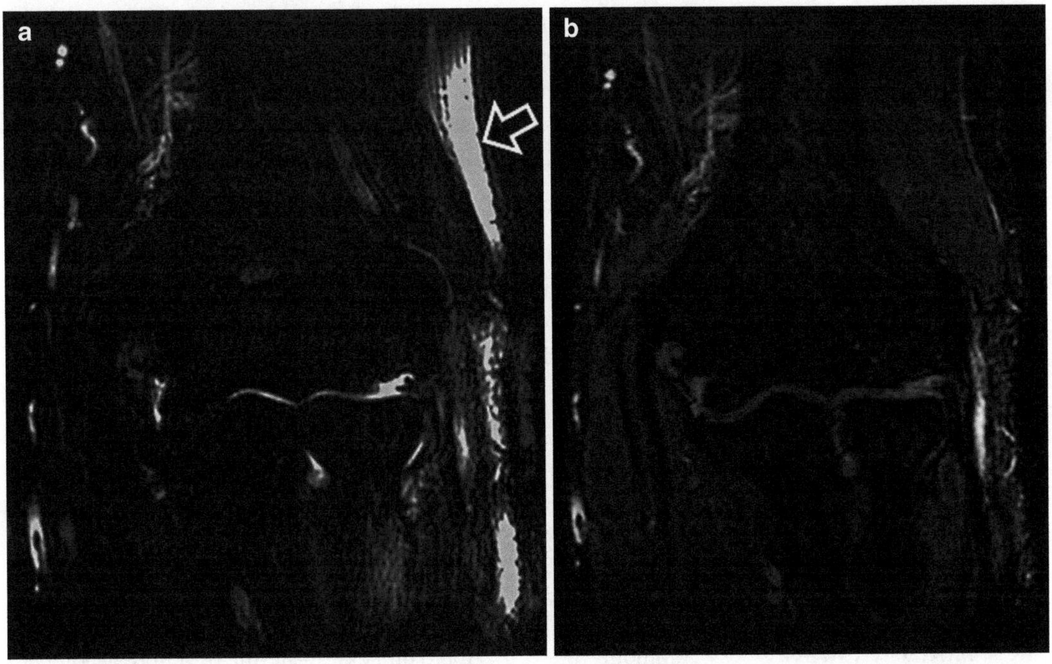

Fig. 17.2 Coronal (**a**) fat-suppressed T2-W and (**b**) STIR MR images obtained in the same patient in the supine position. The STIR image is not affected by field inhomogeneity and results in more homogeneous fat suppression than the T2-W image (*open arrow*). Both images also demonstrate the poor signal-to-noise ratio that may be an issue when the elbow is imaged in this position

the isocenter of the scanner and thereby improves image quality. However, the prone position is relatively uncomfortable for the patient, which increases the likelihood of patient motion during the examination. This position also results in forearm pronation and radioulnar joint rotation, making it somewhat more difficult to evaluate the collateral ligaments as well as the common flexor and extensor tendons in the coronal plane. If the elbow is to be positioned by the patients' side, STIR is superior to fat-suppressed T2-weighted imaging when trying to reduce uneven fat suppression, as the STIR sequence is not affected by field inhomogeneity (Delfaut et al. 1999) (Fig. 17.2).

Special consideration may be given to alternative positioning when partial tears of the biceps brachii tendon are suspected clinically or on routine elbow MRI. Although MRI is extremely sensitive for diagnosing complete tears, it is less sensitive in diagnosing partial tears (Festa et al. 2010). Guiffre and Moss (2004) described a novel technique to obtain a long axis view of the entire tendon on one or two slices, which involves the patient

being positioned with the shoulder abducted, elbow flexed, and forearm supinated (FABS). This has advantages over conventional direct sagittal images with the elbow extended, where the distal biceps tendon may suffer from partial volume average effects due to its oblique course to its insertion (Giuffrè and Moss 2004). However, this increases imaging time and is not performed routinely.

Take-Home Points The choice of supine or "superman" positioning may affect the homogeneity of fat suppression and can result in artifacts. This may be further compounded by the choice of spectral versus inversion recovery fat suppression techniques.

17.2.2 Magic Angle Phenomenon

The magic angle phenomenon affects structures that contain ordered collagen. These include nerves, tendons, ligaments, and cartilage. These tissues normally should have low signal at all echo time (TE) values. However, when fibers of these structures are oriented at 55° to the main magnetic field, there is increased T2 relaxation time, and this produces artifactual increased signal in images with short TE values (i.e., T1, GRE, PD) (Erickson et al. 1991). Sequences with a longer TE (T2 including fat-suppressed sequences) can be used to avoid this artifact. This artifact is less common in the elbow. It is more often seen elsewhere, for example, in the supraspinatus tendon in the shoulder. However, in theory, it could be seen in the elbow when imaged in the previously described FABS position.

17.2.3 Arthrography

17.2.3.1 Indications for Arthrography

Compared with the other larger joints of the body, MR arthrography (MRA) is less commonly utilized in elbow imaging. The main indications for MRA in the elbow are for the assessment of partial ligamentous injury and the evaluation of osteochondral defects and loose bodies. A common use of MRA is for the diagnosis of a partial versus complete tear of the ulnar collateral ligament (UCL) in throwing athletes, when surgical reconstruction is considered (Grainger et al. 2000).

Initially 3 T (3 Tesla) scanning was touted as possibly replacing the need for arthrography; however, this has been shown not to be the case. MRA remains superior at diagnosing full- and partial-thickness ligamentous and tendinous tears with a higher sensitivity and specificity, when compared with non-arthrographic studies (Magee 2015).

17.2.3.2 Arthrogram Technique and Protocol

The patient lies prone on the X-ray table with the elbow flexed 90 degrees, in the FABS position. The lateral aspect of the elbow is facing upward, and the radiocapitellar joint is accessed with a 22G needle under fluoroscopy guidance (Steinbach and Schwartz 1998). An alternative access site is posterior, between the bony prominences of the medial and lateral epicondyles, and proximal to the olecranon (Lohman et al. 2009).

Approximately 8–12 ml of 1:200 gadolinium contrast agent is injected and should be visualized around the radial neck and within the anterior recess of the elbow (Steinbach and Schwartz 1998) (Fig. 17.3). Sequences should include fat-suppressed sequences in all three planes, as well as T1-weighted and STIR sequences without fat suppression. One study has recommended the use of coronal oblique images obtained in a 20° posterior oblique plane

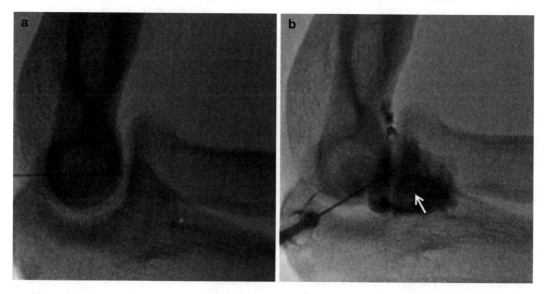

Fig. 17.3 Lateral radiograph shows the normal arthrographic technique. (**a**) Normal needle position within the radiocapitellar joint. (**b**) Expected contrast agent filling around the radial neck (*arrow*) and anterior joint

(or parallel to the humeral shaft with slight elbow flexion) for best demonstrating the collateral ligaments; however again, this increases imaging time and is not routinely used (Cotten et al. 1997).

17.2.3.3 Pitfalls Associated with Arthrography

It is important to take all precautions to ensure that no air bubbles are injected at time of arthrography, since they may mimic loose bodies. However, air bubbles have a characteristic margin of signal hyperintensity surrounding the signal void, due to the magnetic susceptibility artifact (Fig. 17.4a). They may also be distinguished from intra-articular loose bodies by their location, as air bubbles will usually rise to a non-dependent position in the joint (Steinbach et al. 1997). Extravasation of contrast material outside the joint, possibly as a result of overdistension, can be confused with capsular disruption or injury (Fig. 17.4a, b). The inadvertent use of incorrectly diluted gadolinium can cause T1 and T2 shortening, with fluid appearing very low in signal on these sequences (Grainger et al. 2000).

17.3 Pitfalls in Normal Anatomy

17.3.1 Capitellar Pseudo-Defect

The pseudo-defect of the capitellum can be seen on coronal and sagittal MRI of the elbow and is due to partial volume averaging through the complex bony anatomy of the capitellum (Rosenberg et al. 1994). The capitellum is a smooth bony protuberance arising anteriorly from the distal humerus. At the posterior junction of the humeral lateral epicondyle and the capitellum, there is a small posterior bony groove with irregular margins. The anterior articular surface of the capitellum overhangs this groove. Therefore, partial volume averaging between this rough bony groove that is devoid of articular cartilage and the smooth articular surface of the overhanging capitellum results in a pseudo-defect. The pseudo-defect is seen in 85% of normal individuals (Husarik et al. 2010), usually on coronal and sagittal MR images of the elbow, depending on patient anatomy, slice selection, and slice thickness (Fig. 17.5a–c).

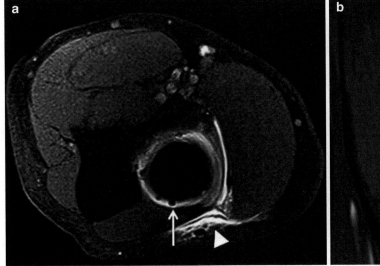
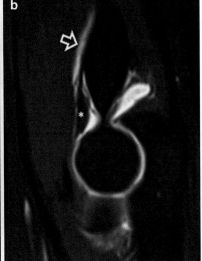

Fig. 17.4 Potential artifacts in MRA of the elbow. (**a**) Axial fat-suppressed T1-W MRA image shows air bubbles within the joint (*arrow*), which could be misinterpreted as loose bodies. However note how the regions of signal void are not lying dependently as would be expected with loose bodies. There is also a margin of signal hyperintensity due to magnetic susceptibility artifact. This image also demonstrates extra-articular contrast material (*arrowhead*) due to injection technique. This may mimic a capsular injury. (**b**) Sagittal fat-suppressed T1-W MRA image shows extra-articular contrast material (*open arrow*). There is contrast material on both sides of the anterior fat pad (*asterisk*)

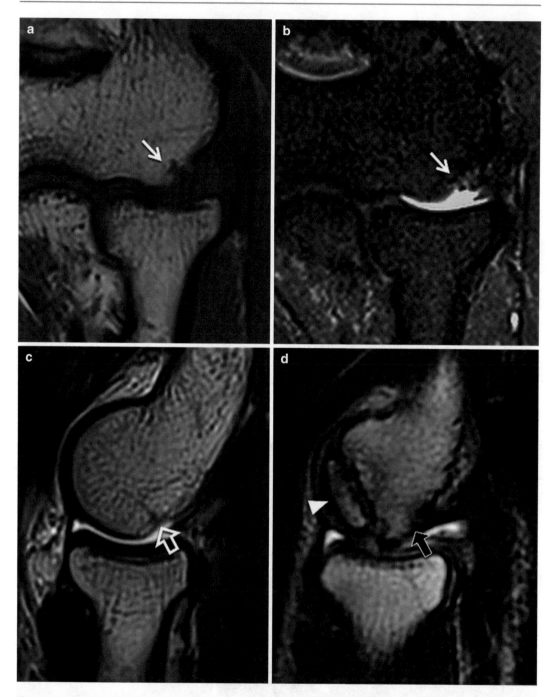

Fig. 17.5 Capitellar pseudo-defect. (**a**) Coronal T1-W, (**b**) coronal STIR, and (**c**) sagittal T2-W images show the capitellar pseudo-defect (*arrows*). Cross-reference with sagittal images will confirm the posterior position (*open arrow*) of this normal finding. This is in contrast to a find-

ing in a different patient (**d**) who has an osteochondral lesion (*arrowhead*). Note this is located anteriorly. The posteriorly located pseudo-defect is also seen on the same image (*black arrow*)

The significance of the capitellar pseudo-defect is that it can lead to the misdiagnosis of an osteochondral lesion. Importantly, review of other sequences will demonstrate that this pseudo-lesion is situated posteriorly. This is in contrast to almost all osteochondral lesions (osteochondritis dissecans, Panner disease, and subchondral cysts/geodes from arthritis) of the capitellum, which are located anteriorly (Kijowski and De Smet 2005) (Fig. 17.5d). The one exception to the anterior location of osteochondral lesions is the rare posterior impaction injury to the capitellum that can occur following transient subluxations and posterolateral rotatory instability, in which demonstration of marrow edema on fluid-sensitive sequences or ligamentous injury is helpful in distinguishing points (Rosenberg et al. 2008).

Take-Home Points Pseudo-defects of the capitellum occur posteriorly. With the exception of rare posterior impaction injuries from transient subluxation, all capitellar osteochondral pathology is found anteriorly.

17.3.2 Pseudo-Lesions of the Trochlear Notch

The trochlear notch is the proximal aspect of the ulna that articulates with the distal humerus. It is formed by the confluence of the olecranon and coronoid processes of the ulna. A small bony ridge lies along a narrow waist between these two articular surfaces, known as the trochlear ridge. The trochlear ridge lacks articular cartilage and is approximately 2–3 mm wide and 4–5 mm in height (Rosenberg et al. 2013). When viewed on sagittal MRI, this structure may mimic a central osteophyte or a stress fracture. However, it is a common normal finding, seen in more than 80% of elbow MRIs in normal volunteers (Rosenberg et al. 1997) (Fig. 17.6).

As this bony ridge approaches the edges of the waist between the articular surfaces, it begins to taper. On sagittal MRI, there will be images on either side of the trochlear ridge where the nar-

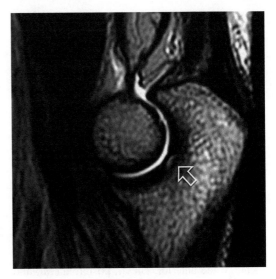

Fig. 17.6 Sagittal T2-W MR image shows a trochlear ridge (*open arrow*)

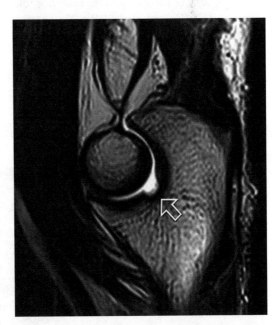

Fig. 17.7 Sagittal T2-W MR image shows a trochlear groove (*open arrow*)

row waist containing the ridge is no longer in the image, but the olecranon and coronoid articular processes still are; this can mimic an osteochondral defect. This is known as the trochlear groove and can be distinguished from pathology based on this characteristic location (Fowler and Chung 2004) (Fig. 17.7).

Take-Home Point The two pseudo-lesions of the trochlear notch are seen on sagittal MR images.

17.3.3 Synovial Folds

Embryologically, the elbow joint forms by mesenchymal cavitation, initially in the radiohumeral site, followed by the ulnohumeral and radioulnar sites. These three cavities merge, and synovial folds, or plicae, are the septal remnants of this process (Mérida-Velasco et al. 2000). The radiohumeral synovial fold is a consistent anatomical structure found in 100% of cadaveric studies and has four portions that can be differentiated by location: the anterior, lateral, posterolateral, and lateral olecranon folds (Isogai et al. 2001). The most common location is posterolateral, being present in 98% of MRIs, while the posterior fold is seen in 33% (Husarik et al. 2010). The anterior fold lies in the radiocapitellar joint and is present in approximately two-thirds of individuals. These three folds occur along the cranial margin of the annular ligament, blending with the capsule. The lateral olecranon fold is seen in about one-third of people, and although it runs posteriorly along the lateral margin of the olecranon recess, it originates from the posterolateral fold. There is no consensus regarding the shape and size of these folds.

Cadaveric work on 50 specimens revealed that the folds were comprised of either a rigid fibrous structure or a thin layer of fatty tissue, both of which are surrounded by synovial layers. Except in extremely rare circumstances, they do not contain fibrocartilage and should not ordinarily be thought of as meniscal equivalents (Duparc et al. 2002; Huang et al. 2005). On MRI, the folds/plicae can be seen as a tongue of tissue, surrounded by synovial fluid, extending from the capsule between the radial head and the capitellum, or within the olecranon recess. The folds are typically thin, measuring 1–2 mm in thickness. They should be smooth and they should be hypointense in signal on MRI. More than one fold may be present and folds can merge. Depending on the location and plane, they may mimic loose bodies within the joint (Fig. 17.8). Review of other imaging planes and knowledge of the typical locations for folds should be sufficient to exclude loose bodies.

Of note, cadaveric studies have shown that there are nerve fibers within the folds and this is felt to reflect an association with pain in some

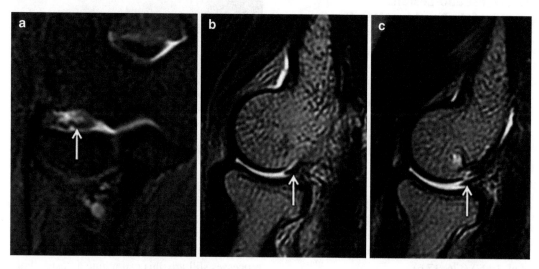

Fig. 17.8 (**a**) Coronal STIR MR image shows an apparent abnormality within the radiocapitellar joint (*arrow*). Cross-reference with contiguous (**b**, **c**) sagittal T2-W MR images in the same patient shows normal posterolateral synovial fold/plica (*arrows*)

patients. Resected folds in symptomatic patients with lateral elbow pain have shown a thickened synovial lining and an increased number of nearby nerve fibers (Duparc et al. 2002). Therefore, although the folds are normal variants in most people, the presence of thickened folds (>3 mm) that are abnormal in signal or irregular in patients with lateral elbow pain, snapping, locking, or catching may reflect synovial fold/plica syndrome/impingement. Synovitis and joint effusions are not always present, especially in the early stage of disease. This entity is frequently under- or misdiagnosed, as the findings are often subtle. Additionally, there may be considerable overlap in the imaging findings between symptomatic and asymptomatic individuals (Awaya et al. 2001; Cerezal et al. 2013).

Take-Home Points Synovial folds/plica are normal embryological remnants found in all subjects, most commonly the posterolateral to the radiohumeral joint. Although they are a normal finding in most people, they can be associated with lateral elbow pain or snapping in some individuals. This can lead to two potential contrasting pitfalls: misinterpreting normal folds/plica for intra-articular loose bodies and underdiagnosing thickened or abnormal folds/plica in elbow synovial fold syndrome.

17.3.4 Elbow Fat Pads

There are three major fat pads in the elbow. Two anterior fat pads correspond to the capitellar and trochlear fossae; a single posterior fat pad is present within the olecranon fossa. The fat pads are located between the synovial and deep fibrous layers; thus, they are intra-articular, but extrasynovial (Fowler and Chung 2004). It is well known from radiography that in the presence of a joint effusion confined to the synovial capsule, the extra-synovial fat pads are elevated.

While the presence of a displaced fat pad on conventional elbow MRI is not normal and should not be overlooked, on MRA, the fat pads will be displaced due to joint distension from the intra-articular contrast agent. They can occasionally be misinterpreted as loose bodies as the fat pads will appear dark on the fat-suppressed T1-weighted images used in MRA. This is particularly true if there is extracapsular contrast material due to injection technique; contrast material on both sides of the fat-suppressed (hypointense) fat pad can make it appear intrasynovial and mimic a loose body (Fig. 17.4b). Review of the nonfat-suppressed images will usually confirm this as artifact.

Take-Home Point Elbow fat pads are extrasynovial and will be elevated and displaced during MR arthrography. This can potentially be misinterpreted as an intra-articular loose body on fat-suppressed T1-weighted MR images.

17.3.5 Triceps Insertion

The triceps arises from three heads, namely, the long head from the infraglenoid tubercle of the scapula, the lateral head from the posterolateral humerus, and the medial head from the distal posterior humerus. The triceps insertion on the olecranon can have a variable appearance on imaging. The long and lateral heads appear to form a common tendon that inserts more superficially on the olecranon than the medial head, which is seen to insert deeper and appears mainly muscular. A small area of fat signal is often seen between the medial head and common tendon, which can mimic a tendon tear or tendon degeneration (Fig. 17.9).

The anatomy of the triceps insertions has been studied in cadavers, and it was found that on gross dissection, the medial head and common tendon appear to have separate insertions. On histological analysis, there is no separation between the deep and superficial tendons at the insertion on the olecranon. Although the muscle of the medial head appears to insert directly onto the bone, no muscle was found attached to the bone at the insertion (Madsen et al. 2006; Belentani

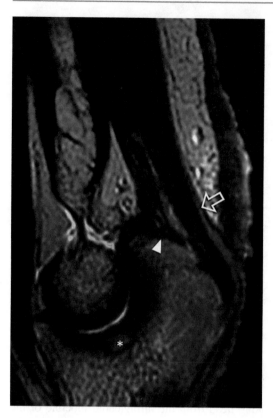

Fig. 17.9 Sagittal T2-W MR image shows a normal distal triceps insertion. The common long head and lateral head tendon is seen to insert on the olecranon (*open arrow*). The medial head muscle appears to insert more anteriorly, directly onto the bone (*arrowhead*). Anatomical analysis has shown that this is not the case and the medial head blends with the common tendon and all three heads insert a single unit. The fat signal between both muscles is normal and should not be interpreted as a tear. Note the incidental trochlear ridge on this image (*asterisk*)

et al. 2009) (Fig. 17.9). The triceps tendon insertion also has a striated/fasciculated appearance on axial imaging, similar to the quadriceps tendon, and should not be mistaken for tendinopathy.

Take-Home Points On sagittal MRI, hyperintense signal and fat signal between the deeper medial head of triceps and the more superficial common tendon of the long and lateral heads can mimic a tear or degeneration of the distal triceps insertion. This is a normal finding, and, histologically, all three heads insert as a single functional unit without discernable separation.

17.3.6 Ulnar Collateral Ligament

The ulnar (medial) collateral ligament is composed of the anterior, posterior, and transverse bands. The anterior band is the strongest, most important, and most frequently injured of the three and is the primary stabilizer of the elbow to valgus stresses. The anterior band is best appreciated on coronal imaging as a discrete focal thickening of the medial joint capsule that extends from the inferior margin of the medial epicondyle and inserts at the sublime tubercle of the ulna, or 3–4 mm distal to it (Munshi et al. 2004). It is important to be aware of this variation, as a small amount of fluid can be seen between the sublime tubercle and the distal ligament in this setting, and this may mimic a tear or partial tear. This can also be seen on arthrography of the elbow, leading to the "false-positive T-sign." In this setting, the ligament will appear normal and hypointense and will have a smooth insertion on the medial aspect of the ulna (Fig. 17.10).

Interdigitation of fat is frequently seen at the wider proximal insertion of the anterior bundle. This can lead to signal alteration at the proximal ligament attachment on both fat-suppressed and nonfat-suppressed sequences, and caution should be used calling partial-thickness tears (Munshi et al. 2004). The ulnar collateral ligament may also appear heterogeneous at its origin and insertion, on T1-weighted and gradient-echo imaging in adolescents. This is a normal finding and is due to a combination of an immature ligament and incomplete ossification. The signal abnormality resolves as the growth plate closes (Rosenberg et al. 1997).

Take-Home Points The anterior bundle of the ulnar collateral ligament may insert 3–4 mm distal to the sublime tubercle, and this may be mistaken for a tear on conventional MR and MRA.

17.3.7 Lateral Collateral Ligaments

The lateral collateral ligamentous complex is composed of the radial collateral ligament (RCL), the lateral ulnar collateral ligament (LUCL), and

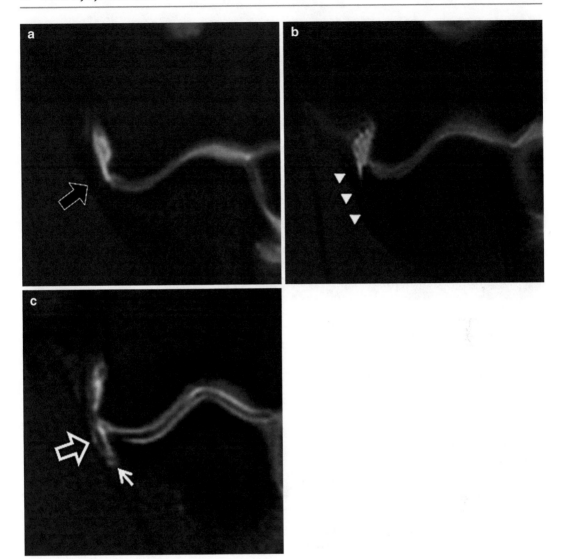

Fig. 17.10 Coronal fat-suppressed T1-W MRA images show (**a**) normal insertion of the ulnar collateral ligament, (**b**) "false-positive T-sign," and a (**c**) "true-positive T-sign." (**a**) shows the normal insertion of the ulnar collateral ligament on the sublime tubercle of the ulna (*black arrow*). (**b**) shows normal variant anatomy where the anterior band of the ulnar collateral ligament (*arrowheads*) may insert 3–4 mm distal to sublime tubercle of the ulna. A small cleft of fluid (or in this case contrast material) may be seen between the ligament and the tubercle. Note that the ligament (*arrowheads*) is smooth and homogeneously hypointense. It has a smooth insertion onto the ulna, close to the sublime tubercle. This is in contrast to the "true-positive T-sign" in a partial ulnar collateral ligament tear (**c**), where the ligament appears thin and irregular (*open arrow*) and there is wide gap filled with contrast material (*arrow*) where the ligament should have attached

the annular ligament. The normal ligaments are hypointense on all sequences, and the RCL, LUCL, and common extensor origin are usually inseparable as discrete structures at the lateral epicondyle. In some instances, a bilaminar appearance may be seen which delineates the ligamentous from the overlying tendinous structures and should not be confused with a tear or tendinopathy in the common extensor origin (Fig. 17.11).

The LUCL may not be visualized on a single plane due to the obliquity of its course, cradling

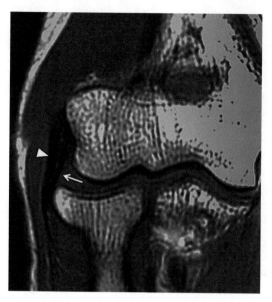

Fig. 17.11 Coronal T1-W MR image shows the bilaminar appearance delineating the common extensor origin (*arrowhead*) and the radial collateral ligament (*arrow*). These structures are usually inseparable, but can occasionally have this appearance. It should not be confused with a tear or tendinopathy

the posterior radial head. Assessment of the ligament requires careful cross-referencing with sagittal and axial images. For example, volume averaging from the posterior capsule and anconeus muscle can be mistaken for pathology at the LUCL origin, particularly on gradient-echo imaging. This is important to recognize, as the most common injury to the LUCL is an avulsion of the proximal ligament from the distal humerus (McKee et al. 2003). As the LUCL passes posterolateral to the radius, it will usually partially blend with the annular ligament and is indistinguishable. The LUCL insertion posteriorly on the supinator crest of the ulna is often indistinguishable from the more anteriorly inserting annular ligament. If LUCL injury is suspected, coronal oblique imaging is most useful to demonstrate a greater length of the ligament on a single image.

Take-Home Points The lateral ulnar collateral ligament is often difficult to evaluate due to its oblique course and blending with the annular ligament. When injured, it is most commonly an avulsion from the lateral epicondyle.

17.4 Pitfalls in Normal Variant Anatomy

17.4.1 Distal Biceps Insertion

The biceps tendons originate from the supraglenoid tubercle (long head) and the coracoid process of the scapula (short head). The common distal tendon inserts on the radial tuberosity. The bicipital aponeurosis (lacertus fibrosus) is a consistent finding that arises from the superficial tendinous fibers of both muscle bellies and inserts over the medial aspect of the proximal forearm and elbow (Dirim et al. 2008). The distal biceps tendon has a variable appearance. Although it usually appears to insert as a common tendon, it is often macroscopically separable into distinct long and short head components.

It can also have a completely bifid appearance on imaging and insert as two separate tendons, the short head inserting more distally on the radial tuberosity (Dirim et al. 2008; Koulouris et al. 2009) (Fig. 17.12a). It is important to be aware of the appearances of this common variant, particularly in the setting of trauma. Isolated rupture of the short head can occur and should not be interpreted as a partial-thickness tear of a common tendon insertion or tendinosis (Fig. 17.12b, c). This has important management implications, as the former may be managed surgically and the latter two conservatively (Koulouris et al. 2009). Imaging in the FABS position, as described previously in the chapter, may be used as an adjunct if isolated tendon rupture is suspected, but not clear on conventional positioning.

It is also worth noting that the bicipital aponeurosis or lacertus fibrosus can act to restrict proximal retraction of a completely torn tendon. Therefore, the degree of retraction is an imperfect indicator of complete versus partial tear, and a complete biceps tendon tear may retract only slightly if the lacertus remains intact. Conversely, significant retraction of a complete biceps tendon tear may imply injury to the lacertus fibrosus (Fitzgerald et al. 1994).

Take-Home Points The distal biceps can insert as two distinct long and short head tendons on the

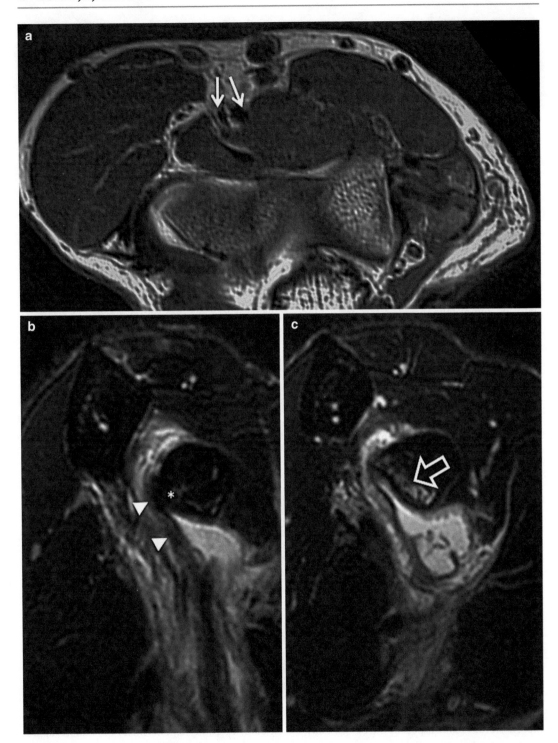

Fig. 17.12 (**a**) Axial T1-W MR image shows the normal bifid appearance of the distal biceps tendon which may occasionally be seen. (**b, c**) Fat-suppressed T2-W MR images obtained in the FABS position show the long head tendon (*arrowheads* in **b**) attached to radial tuberosity (*asterisk*). There is complete avulsion of the short head with marrow edema in the distal radial tuberosity (*open arrow* in **c**)

radial tuberosity. It is particularly important to be aware of and assess for this variant in the setting of distal biceps tendon trauma. Complete tendon tears may only retract slightly, if the lacertus fibrosus remains intact.

17.4.2 Bicipitoradial Bursa

The bicipitoradial bursa is located between the radial tuberosity and the biceps tendon. As the forearm moves from supination to pronation, the radial tuberosity rotates from a medial to a posterior position. The function of the bursa is to reduce local friction effects (Skaf et al. 1999). Although the distal tendon of the biceps does not have its own tendon sheath, the bursa can partially or completely surround the distal tendon close to its insertion and can give the appearance of a synovial sheath. Enlargement of the bicipitoradial bursa should therefore be recognized as bursitis and not due to tenosynovitis, or indeed a neoplasm. Knowledge of its anatomical position allows distinction from a ganglion or synovial cyst (Skaf et al. 1999). It is not usually visualized unless inflamed; therefore, it is usually considered by most to be pathological. Bicipitoradial bursitis can be a useful sign of partial tearing of the distal biceps tendon (Fitzgerald et al. 1994).

Take-Home Points The distal biceps tendon does not have a synovial sheath, and bicipitoradial bursitis should not be misinterpreted as tenosynovitis. The bursa is not seen unless inflamed, and when it is seen, a partial distal biceps tendon tear should be suspected.

17.4.3 Anconeus Epitrochlearis

Anconeus epitrochlearis, not to be confused with the anconeus muscle, is an atavistic accessory muscle on the medial aspect of the elbow. It arises from the medial epicondyle and passes over the ulnar nerve to insert on the olecranon, following the same course as the cubital tunnel retinaculum. The retinaculum is postulated to be the remnant of the anconeus epitrochlearis muscle. It has a

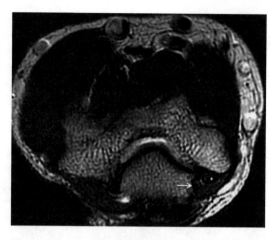

Fig. 17.13 Axial T2-W MR image shows the anconeus epitrochlearis muscle (*arrow*). This is an atavistic muscle seen in approximately 23% of people. Its remnant is believed to be the cubital tunnel retinaculum. It is a normal finding, although it may predispose to compressive neuritis of the ulnar nerve (*asterisk*)

reported incidence of 23% on MRI of the elbow in asymptomatic individuals (Husarik et al. 2009) and 4–34% in cadaveric studies (Dahners and Wood 1984; O'Hara and Stone 1996; Jeon et al. 2005). It may be unilateral or bilateral. Although it may be a source of ulnar nerve compression and ulnar neuritis in some individuals, particularly if edematous or thickened, it is a normal anatomical variant in most cases (Fig. 17.13).

Take-Home Point The anconeus epitrochlearis muscle is a normal variant that may replace the cubital tunnel retinaculum in approximately 20% of normal individuals.

17.4.4 Cubital Tunnel and the Ulnar Nerve

The cubital tunnel is the fibro-osseous conduit for the ulnar nerve as it passes across the elbow joint. It lies along the posterior aspect of the medial epicondyle. The posterior bundle of the ulnar collateral ligament forms the floor, and the roof is formed by the arcuate ligament/cubital tunnel retinaculum. A number of variations of the retinaculum have been described. The retinaculum may be absent (Type 0), a normal thin structure (Type 1a), thickened (Type 1b), or replaced by the anconeus epitrochlearis (O'Driscoll et al. 1991). However, the significance of these subtypes in now less clear as work by Kawahara et al. (2016) has shown that the ulnar nerve subluxes or dislocates from the cubital tunnel in 49% of asymptomatic elbows, all of which had a cubital tunnel retinaculum. Signal hyperintensity is only seen in the ulnar nerve of patients that had an anconeus epitrochlearis muscle during elbow flexion, when the nerve was compressed (Kawahara et al. 2016). This study supports previous data that the anconeus epitrochlearis muscle, although a normal structure, may predispose to ulnar neuritis in some patients.

Regarding the ulnar nerve itself, there are a number of potential pitfalls that lead to the overdiagnosis of ulnar neuritis and ulnar nerve compression. Husarik et al. (2009) showed that in 60% of normal asymptomatic individuals, the ulnar nerve demonstrated increased signal intensity on fluid-sensitive MR sequences; this was not seen in the radial and median nerves and may lead to overdiagnosis of ulnar neuritis (Husarik et al. 2009). Earlier work by Rosenberg et al. (2013) described the presence of deep posterior recurrent ulnar veins that also run in the cubital tunnel with the ulnar nerve. These may become engorged and be mistaken for a thickened hyperintense ulnar nerve (Fig. 17.14). This confusion can be avoided by recognizing that an engorged vein should be homogeneous and isointense to the cubital veins, whereas a diseased nerve should be of heterogeneous signal hyperintensity and individual fascicles can sometimes be seen (Rosenberg et al. 2013).

Lastly, the ulnar nerve is usually round or oval in its appearance when the elbow is imaged in extension. In elbow flexion, the pressures in the cubital tunnel are increased and the nerve becomes flat. If the patient is imaged in elbow flexion, this is an important pitfall to avoid, as it does not always indicate the presence of cubital tunnel syndrome (Sampaio and Schweitzer 2010). In extension, the maximum diameter of the normal ulnar nerve should be 7 mm or less (Husarik et al. 2009).

Take-Home Points The cubital tunnel retinaculum can be congenitally absent, thickened, or

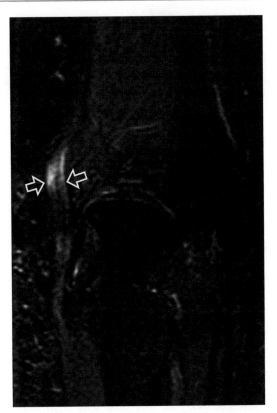

Fig. 17.14 Coronal STIR MR image shows the deep posterior recurrent ulnar veins (*arrows*) running in the cubital tunnel. This may mimic ulnar neuritis. Note that there are two vessels running together

replaced by the anconeus epitrochlearis muscle. It is normal to see ulnar nerve subluxation or dislocation in almost half of normal individuals during flexion of the elbow. However, the presence of an anconeus epitrochlearis muscle may predispose some people to ulnar neuritis. Hyperintense signal in the cubital tunnel does not always mean ulnar neuritis. Inherent signal hyperintensity can be seen in the ulnar nerve in 60% of normal asymptomatic individuals, and engorged deep posterior recurrent ulnar veins in the cubital tunnel may also mimic ulnar pathology.

17.4.5 Red Marrow

Bone marrow occupies approximately 85% of the medullary bone cavities, with the rest being composed of a network of trabecular bone. Normal bone marrow is divided into red marrow and yellow marrow, both of which are composed of the same constituents, but are differentiated based on their fat content. Approximately 95% of yellow marrow is fat cells, compared to 40% in red marrow (Snyder et al. 1975). This can lead to a heterogeneous appearance of marrow on T1- and fat-suppressed sequences where both yellow and red marrows coexist. In infancy, red marrow occupies the entire ossified skeleton, except for the epiphyses and apophyses. Red marrow gradually retreats from the central skeleton and, in adulthood, is commonly found in axial skeleton, notably in the femoral necks and proximal humeri. Islands of red marrow however can be found anywhere in the skeleton (Vande Berg et al. 1998a; Vande Berg et al. 1998b). Yellow marrow may be reconverted to red marrow in times of hematopoietic need, such as in chronic anemia.

In the elbow, red marrow may be commonly seen in the distal humeral metaphysis or at the radial neck. These red marrow islands will appear hyperintense on fat-suppressed fluid-sensitive sequences (Sampaio and Schweitzer 2010). Red marrow should always be hyperintense to muscle on T1-weighted MR images (due to its fat content); this will help differentiate it from other pathologies. Red marrow at the radial neck may mimic a fracture or reactive changes from a biceps tendinosis. In the diaphysis and metaphysis of professional tennis players, marrow edema from stress injury to the humerus can occur, and hyperintensity in the marrow should not always be discounted as red marrow in this select group (Hoy et al. 2006).

Take-Home Point Red marrow is common on fat-suppressed fluid-sensitive sequences, particularly in the distal humeral metaphysis and sometimes at the radial neck.

17.4.6 Supracondylar Process

The supracondylar process is a congenital bony projection on the anteromedial distal humerus, approximately 5–6 cm proximal to the epicondyle. It is seen in approximately 2% of the population and is usually asymptomatic (Opanova

and Atkinson 2014). Occasionally, a ligamentous attachment between the spur and the medial epicondyle exists, called the ligament of Struthers. This fibrous connection between the process and medial epicondyle forms an osteofibrous tunnel over the median nerve and may lead to symptomatic compression of the traversing median nerve or brachial artery. The humeral cortex remains intact beneath the supracondylar process. The supracondylar process should not be confused with an osteochondroma. The latter often points away from its adjacent joint and will show contiguity with the underlying humeral medullary bone (Al-Qattan and Husband 1991).

Take-Home Points Supracondylar processes arise from the distal anterior humeral cortex and point toward the joint. Osteochondromas have a variable location around the metaphysis, are contiguous with the medullary cavity, and are oriented away from the joint.

Conclusion

The complex and variable bony and soft tissue anatomy of the elbow joint can predispose to the misinterpretation of MRI. In this chapter, we have dealt with many of the common pitfalls representing normal or variant anatomy and many pitfalls related to the technical aspects of imaging the elbow, all of which can lead to misdiagnosis. We have also highlighted several pitfalls in the interpretation of true pathologic findings that may occasionally be misinterpreted or overlooked, particularly at sites where variant anatomy is common. We hope that the information provided in this chapter will improve the interpretive abilities of the general radiologist who may be struggling with the evaluation of this less frequently imaged and technically difficult joint.

References

Al-Qattan MM, Husband JB (1991) Median nerve compression by the supracondylar process: a case report. J Hand Surg Br 16:101–103

Awaya H, Schweitzer ME, Feng SA et al (2001) Elbow synovial fold syndrome. MR imaging findings. Am J Roentgenol 177:1377–1381

Belentani C, Pastore D, Wangwinyuvirat M et al (2009) Triceps brachii tendon: anatomic-MR imaging study in cadavers with histologic correlation. Skeletal Radiol 38:171–175

Cerezal L, Rodriguez-Sammartino M, Canga A et al (2013) Elbow synovial fold syndrome. AJR Am J Roentgenol 201:W88–W96

Cotten A, Jacobson J, Brossmann J et al (1997) Collateral ligaments of the elbow: conventional MR imaging and MR arthrography with coronal oblique plane and elbow flexion. Radiology 204:806–812

Dahners LE, Wood FM (1984) Anconeus epitrochlearis, a rare cause of cubital tunnel syndrome: a case report. J Hand Surg Am 9:579–580

Delfaut EM, Beltran J, Johnson G et al (1999) Fat suppression in MR imaging: techniques and pitfalls. Radiographics 19:373–382

Dirim B, Brouha SS, Pretterklieber ML et al (2008) Terminal bifurcation of the biceps brachii muscle and tendon: anatomic considerations and clinical implications. AJR Am J Roentgenol 191:W248–W255

Duparc F, Putz R, Michot C et al (2002) The synovial fold of the humeroradial joint: anatomical and histological features, and clinical relevance in lateral epicondylalgia of the elbow. Surg Radiol Anat 24:302–307

Erickson SJ, Cox IH, Hyde JS et al (1991) Effect of tendon orientation on MR imaging signal intensity: a manifestation of the "magic angle" phenomenon. Radiology 181:389–392

Festa A, Mulieri PJ, Newman JS et al (2010) Effectiveness of magnetic resonance imaging in detecting partial and complete distal biceps tendon rupture. J Hand Surg Am 35:77–83

Fitzgerald SW, Curry DR, Erickson SJ et al (1994) Distal biceps tendon injury: MR imaging diagnosis. Radiology 191:203–206

Fowler KAB, Chung CB (2004) Normal MR imaging anatomy of the elbow. Magn Reson Imaging Clin N Am 12:191–206

Giuffrè BM, Moss MJ (2004) Optimal positioning for MRI of the distal biceps brachii tendon: flexed abducted supinated view. AJR Am J Roentgenol 182:944–946

Grainger AJ, Elliott JM, Campbell RSD et al (2000) Direct MR arthrography: a review of current use. Clin Radiol 55:163–176

Hoy G, Wood T, Phillips N, Connell D (2006) When physiology becomes pathology: the role of magnetic resonance imaging in evaluating bone marrow oedema in the humerus in elite tennis players with an upper limb pain syndrome. Br J Sports Med 40:710–713

Huang G-S, Lee C-H, Lee H-S, Chen C-Y (2005) A meniscus causing painful snapping of the elbow joint: MR imaging with arthroscopic and histologic correlation. Eur Radiol 15:2411–2414

Husarik DB, Saupe N, Pfirrmann CW et al (2009) Elbow nerves: MR findings in 60 asymptomatic subjects - normal anatomy, variants, and pitfalls. Radiology 252:148–156

Husarik DB, Saupe N, Pfirrmann CWA et al (2010) Ligaments and plicae of the elbow: normal MR imaging variability in 60 asymptomatic subjects. Radiology 257:185–194

Isogai S, Murakami G, Wada T, Ishii S (2001) Which morphologies of synovial folds result from degeneration and/or aging of the radiohumeral joint: an anatomic study with cadavers and embryos. J Shoulder Elbow Surg 10:169–181

Jeon I-H, Fairbairn KJ, Neumann L et al (2005) MR imaging of edematous anconeus epitrochlearis: another cause of medial elbow pain? Skeletal Radiol 34:103–107

Kawahara Y, Yamaguchi T, Honda Y et al (2016) The ulnar nerve at elbow extension and flexion: assessment of position and signal intensity on MR images. Radiology 280:483–492

Kijowski R, Tuite M, Sanford M (2004) Magnetic resonance imaging of the elbow. Part I: Normal anatomy, imaging technique, and osseous abnormalities. Skeletal Radiol 33:685–697

Kijowski R, De Smet AA (2005) MRI findings of osteochondritis dissecans of the capitellum with surgical correlation. AJR Am J Roentgenol 185:1453–1459

Koulouris G, Malone W, Omar IM et al (2009) Bifid insertion of the distal biceps brachii tendon with isolated rupture: magnetic resonance findings. J Shoulder Elbow Surg 18:e22–e25

Lohman M, Borrero C, Casagranda B et al (2009) The posterior transtriceps approach for elbow arthrography: a forgotten technique? Skeletal Radiol 38:513–516

Madsen M, Marx RG, Millett PJ et al (2006) Surgical anatomy of the triceps brachii tendon: anatomical study and clinical correlation. Am J Sports Med 34:1839–1843

Magee T (2015) Accuracy of 3-T MR arthrography versus conventional 3-T MRI of elbow tendons and ligaments compared with surgery. AJR Am J Roentgenol 204:W70–W75

McKee MD, Schemitsch EH, Sala MJ, O'Driscoll SW (2003) The pathoanatomy of lateral ligamentous disruption in complex elbow instability. J Shoulder Elbow Surg 12:391–396

Mérida-Velasco JA, Sánchez-Montesinos I, Espín-Ferra J et al (2000) Development of the human elbow joint. Anat Rec 258:166–175

Munshi M, Pretterklieber ML, Chung CB et al (2004) Anterior bundle of ulnar collateral ligament: evaluation of anatomic relationships by using MR imaging, MR arthrography, and gross anatomic and histologic analysis. Radiology 231:797–803

O'Driscoll SW, Horii E, Carmichael SW, Morrey BF (1991) The cubital tunnel and ulnar neuropathy. J Bone Joint Surg Br 73:613–617

O'Hara JJ, Stone JH (1996) Ulnar nerve compression at the elbow caused by a prominent medial head of the triceps and an anconeus epitrochlearis muscle. J Hand Surg Br 21:133–135

Opanova MI, Atkinson RE (2014) Supracondylar process syndrome: case report and literature review. J Hand Surg Am 39:1130–1135

Rosenberg ZS, Beltran J, Cheung YY (1994) Pseudodefect of the capitellum: potential MR imaging pitfall. Radiology 191:821–823

Rosenberg ZS, Bencardino J, Beltran J (1997) MR imaging of normal variants and interpretation pitfalls of the elbow. Magn Reson Imaging Clin N Am 5:481–499

Rosenberg ZS, Blutreich SI, Schweitzer ME (2008) MRI features of posterior capitellar impaction injuries. AJR Am J Roentgenol 190:435–441

Rosenberg ZS, Beltran J, Cheung Y et al (2013) MR imaging of the elbow: normal variant and potential diagnostic pitfalls of the trochlear groove and cubital tunnel. AJR Am J Roentgenol 164:415–418

Sampaio ML, Schweitzer ME (2010) Elbow magnetic resonance imaging variants and pitfalls. Magn Reson Imaging Clin N Am 18:633–642

Sampath SC, Sampath SC, Bredella MA (2013) Magnetic resonance imaging of the elbow: a structured approach. Sports Health 5:34–49

Skaf AY, Boutin RD, Dantas RWM et al (1999) Bicipitoradial bursitis: MR imaging findings in eight patients and anatomic data from contrast material opacification of bursae followed by routine radiography and MR imaging in cadavers. Radiology 212:111–116

Snyder WS, Cook MJ, Nasset ES et al (1975) Report of the task group on reference man. Pergamon Press, Oxford

Steinbach LS, Fritz RC, Tirman PFJ et al (1997) Magnetic resonance imaging of the elbow. Eur J Radiol 25:223–241

Steinbach LS, Schwartz M (1998) Elbow arthrography. Radiol Clin N Am 36:635–649

Vande Berg BC, Malghem J, Lecouvet FE, Maldague B (1998a) Magnetic resonance imaging of normal bone marrow. Eur Radiol 8:1327–1334

Vande Berg BC, Malghem J, Lecouvet FE, Maldague B (1998b) Magnetic resonance imaging of the normal bone marrow. Skeletal Radiol 27:471–483

Elbow Injury: US Pitfalls

18

Graham Buirski and Javier Arnaiz

Contents

18.1   **Introduction** 339

18.2   **Technique-Specific Pitfalls** 340
18.2.1   Equipment/Transducer Selection 340
18.2.2   Operator Training 340
18.2.3   Anisotropy 341
18.2.4   Transducer Pressure 342
18.2.5   Dynamic Imaging 342

18.3   **Diagnostic-Specific Pitfalls:**
         Normal Variants 343

18.4   **Diagnostic-Specific Pitfalls:**
         Pathological Misinterpretations 345
18.4.1   Triceps Tendon Injury 345
18.4.2   Cubital Tunnel Syndrome 345
18.4.3   Elbow Snapping Syndrome 346
18.4.4   Acute Elbow Trauma 347
18.4.5   Elbow Plica Syndrome 348
18.4.6   Elbow Soft Tissue Masses 348
18.4.7   Medial or Lateral Epicondylar Pain 349
18.4.8   Medial Collateral Ligament Injury 350
18.4.9   Anterior Elbow Pain 351

Conclusion 352

References 352

G. Buirski, MD (✉)
Department of Radiology, Sidra Medical and
Research Center, Al Dafna, Doha, Qatar
e-mail: gbuirski@me.com

J. Arnaiz, MD
Department of Radiology, Aspetar Orthopaedic
and Sports Medicine Hospital,
Sports City Street, Doha, Qatar
e-mail: javierarnaiz@outlook.com

Abbreviations

POC   Point-of-care
US   Ultrasound

18.1   Introduction

Injuries to the elbow are common. Elbow fractures account for up to 15% of all fractures in children (Rabiner et al. 2013). Some injuries may be due to chronic repetitive strain, leading to partial or complete tears of tendons or tendon degeneration (tendinopathy). Concerns of radiation exposure and the increased availability of portable and inexpensive ultrasound (US) imaging equipment are providing the clinical care physician an alternative imaging modality to assess their patients. This has led to an increase in the use of "point-of-care" US (POCUS) assessment in traumatic injuries to the upper limb (Patel et al. 2009; Shen et al. 2012; Rabiner et al. 2013).

Apart from the lack of radiation, US imaging also allows comparison with the contralateral normal side and dynamic and stress imaging. Correlation with US findings and clinical symptoms can be obtained at the time of the imaging examination. Despite the increasing use of POCUS, the diagnostic radiologist still has a significant role in assessing injuries to the upper limb and where necessary, helping POC physicians in confirming their findings. This chapter

© Springer International Publishing AG 2017
W.C.G. Peh (ed.), *Pitfalls in Musculoskeletal Radiology*, DOI 10.1007/978-3-319-53496-1_18

attempts to provide information for both the POC physician and the diagnostic radiologist. Pitfalls in the production of US images (including the role of dynamic imaging) of the elbow will be discussed. Operator knowledge of local anatomy is paramount in correct interpretation. Certain relevant anatomical variations as well as common misinterpretations of US imaging pathology will be highlighted.

18.2 Technique-Specific Pitfalls

18.2.1 Equipment/Transducer Selection

There is now a wide range of US equipment available, ranging from stand-alone stationary scanners to small handheld fully mobile machines. Each machine will come with certain transducers, all having different resolution capabilities (Kane et al. 2010). However, the smaller machines may not have the same diagnostic capabilities compared to more costly dedicated stationary equipment. Potential pitfalls can be expected if physicians have higher diagnostic

expectations than their scanner can deliver. For instance, small portable machines may not provide the diagnostic resolution for small tendons or ligaments.

Selection of the most optimal transducer will deliver the most detailed diagnostic image. In musculoskeletal US imaging, the most common transducers used are linear arrays of varying frequency and footprint size. The larger lower-frequency transducers provide better field of view (FOV) and depth of resolution; this is useful for providing a general "road map" of pathology. Any abnormality identified can then be further interrogated in higher resolution by using a smaller higher frequency transducer (Fig. 18.1).

18.2.2 Operator Training

Modern US machines are complex pieces of computerized equipment. Although the manufacturer's goal is to make them as simple as possible for operators, there is still a requirement for users to understand basic operational principles. These include the use of:

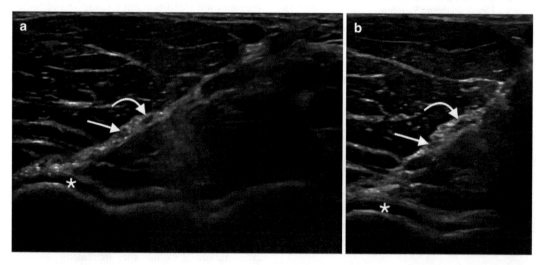

Fig. 18.1 US images show improved resolution and detail with different transducers. (**a**) Longitudinal 9 MHz linear array transverse US image of the antecubital fossa shows the superficial (*curved arrow*) and deep branches (*straight arrow*) of the radial nerve. Note the width of the image reflecting the larger footprint of the transducer. (**b**) Hockey stick 15 MHz US image. Due to the smaller transducer size, the width of the image is reduced, but detail has improved. The radial nerve branches are seen with more clarity, and there is better definition of the articular cartilage/bone interphase (*)

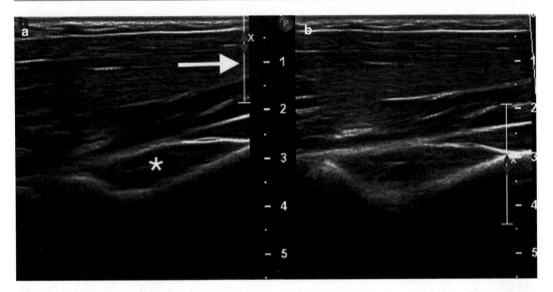

Fig. 18.2 Image resolution and focus. (**a**) The position of the focal zone is superficial (*arrow*) in relation to the supinator muscle (*). (**b**) Anatomical muscle fiber detail of the

supinator has improved now that the focal zone has been positioned to correspond to the area of interest

- Depth. Changes in transducer frequency or focus optimize US imaging of soft tissue at different depths. Anatomy and consequently pathology may be missed when only superficial structures are optimized (Fig. 18.2).
- Gain and frequency adjustment. Required for optimal image contrast.
- Color and power Doppler. Neovascularity is an important sign of underlying pathology and may help in differential diagnosis (see below).
- Recording dimensions and distance.
- Panoramic imaging. This technique allows correct measurement of lengths greater than the footprint of the transducer. Consecutive images of distances using only single frames from the transducer may be inaccurate, e.g., length of tendon ruptures (Fig. 18.3).

Probably one of the most important factors distinguishing the POC physician from the diagnostic radiologist is the examiner's knowledge of anatomy. The POC physician will scan focally to target certain pathologies suggested by the patients' clinical presentation, e.g., tendon rupture or fracture. Pitfalls will occur when unexpected pathologies involving other anatomical structures go unrecognized: a normal POC scan

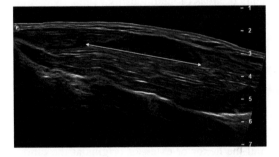

Fig. 18.3 Panoramic view. Large field of view shows the extent of the superficial muscle tear (*double arrow*) on one image. Accurate assessment of size can be obtained using extended fields of view rather than sequential standard images

or one that does not correlate with the patient's symptoms should always be followed by a formal diagnostic scan by a trained diagnostic radiologist. The radiologist usually has a greater understanding of local anatomy and will have a more holistic approach to the diagnostic assessment.

18.2.3 Anisotropy

A full discussion of US artifacts is beyond the scope of this chapter and has been discussed in Chap. 2. However, the anisotropic artifact is

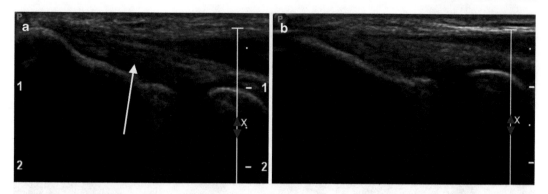

Fig. 18.4 Anisotropy. (**a**) Hypoechoic artifact (*arrow*) of the common extensor origin is due to anisotropy. (**b**) Changing transducer inclination shows normal fiber structure

worth further consideration as it has significant implications in US assessment of musculoskeletal structures. Anisotropy is an artifact where tendons and ligaments become hypoechoic due to the non-perpendicular inclination of the US beam. It can mimic partial or complete tendon tears or areas of tendinopathy (Taljanovic et al. 2014). This can be a significant issue when structures follow an oblique course going from superficial to deep or when they surround normal anatomical structures, e.g., in the elbow (Arend 2013). The artifact can be removed by changing the transducer's angle of inclination. Examples of tendons that are particularly prone to anisotropy include the distal biceps brachii and the flexor or extensor origins at the elbow (Fig. 18.4).

18.2.4 Transducer Pressure

One of the "golden rules" in musculoskeletal US imaging is the use of light or no transducer pressure on the patient's skin when assessing superficial structures. Excess pressure during the examination may displace fluid in areas of traumatic pathology, leading to a missed diagnosis. US can demonstrate small elbow effusions (1–3 ml), but care must be taken not to use too much transducer pressure; otherwise, the effusion can be displaced (De Maeseneer et al. 1998). Fluid in tendon sheaths can be easily compressed and displaced. Tendon or muscle tears can be missed, if

sufficient transducer pressure is used to displace the fluid from the gap between the torn fibers or from within the muscle fascia. Increased Doppler blood flow is a useful sign reflecting neovascularity or inflammation in chronic tendinopathy of the extensor (tennis elbow) or flexor (golfer elbow) tendon origins. Excess transducer pressure may eliminate this finding and diminish diagnostic accuracy (Fig. 18.5).

18.2.5 Dynamic Imaging

The use of dynamic and stress imaging is an integral part of the musculoskeletal US examination (Bouffard and Goitz 2010; Jacobson 2013). Excluding dynamic imaging from the study may limit demonstration and lead to diagnostic pitfalls in:

- abnormal movement of structures
- determining the difference between partial and complete tears

Around the elbow joint, dynamic subluxation of the ulnar nerve (Fig. 18.6) and medial head of the triceps tendon (triceps snapping) during flexion and extension (see Sect. 18.4.3 on snapping elbow syndrome) can predispose to traumatic ulnar nerve damage and neuritis. Dynamic imaging is important to distinguish partial from complete tears of the distal biceps, ulnar collateral ligament (Bouffard and Goitz 2010), and

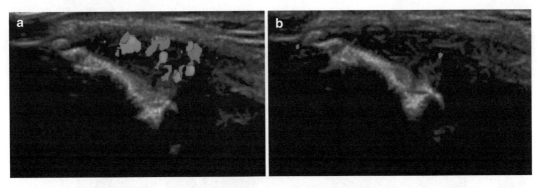

Fig. 18.5 Neovascularity of the common extensor origin. (**a**) Color Doppler US image shows extensive vascular flow within the extensor origin. (**b**) If there is excess transducer pressure, the neovascularity can be compressed and disappears. Note the flattening of the superficial surface of the extensor tendon reflecting the increase transducer pressure by the operator

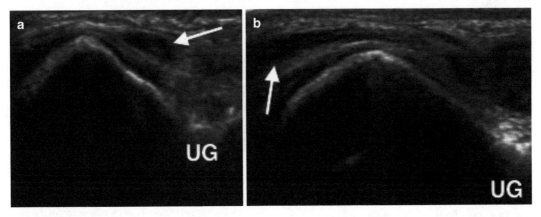

Fig. 18.6 Ulnar nerve medial subluxation. (**a**) Transverse US image in the neutral position shows the ulnar nerve (*arrow*) lying in the ulna groove (*UG*). (**b**) Dynamic US image after flexion shows that the nerve has now dislocated medially

muscle ruptures. Movement on both sides of the muscle tear indicates only a partial disruption, whereas no movement on one or either side indicates a complete tear.

18.3 Diagnostic-Specific Pitfalls: Normal Variants

Many osseous and soft tissue anatomical variants have been described around the elbow (Sookur et al. 2008; Tomsick and Petersen 2010). Although many have no clinical relevance, they need to be recognized so as not to be mistaken for post-traumatic pathology. Furthermore, pitfalls may also occur when normal anatomical variants are identified, but imaging physicians fail to realize that they could be responsible for clinical symptoms.

A supracondylar process is seen in 1–3% of the population, projecting from the anterior surface of the distal humerus (Fig. 18.7). Sometimes, this process communicates with the medial epicondyle by a fibrous band (ligament of Struthers) and may result in median nerve compression. Failure to recognize a supracondylar process could lead to a US diagnostic pitfall of a distal humeral fracture with cortical elevation. Radiographic evaluation will confirm this as a normal finding. An accessory ossification center

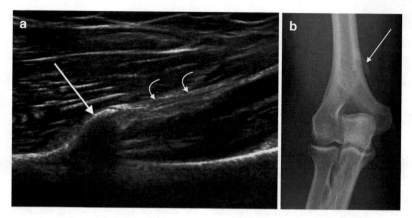

Fig. 18.7 Supracondylar process of distal humerus. (**a**) Longitudinal US image shows deformity of humeral shaft (*straight arrow*) suggestive of a possible cortical fracture. Note the ligament of Struthers extending distally (*curved arrows*). (**b**) Radiograph confirms the supracondylar process (*arrow*) (Courtesy of Dr. S. Wu)

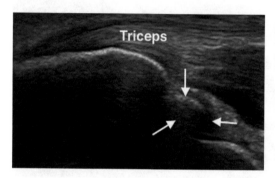

Fig. 18.8 Os supratrochleare dorsale. Posterior sagittal US image of the elbow shows an echogenic soft tissue mass in the olecranon fossa (*arrows*)

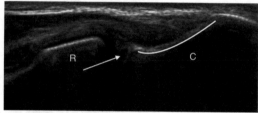

Fig. 18.9 Pseudo-defect of the capitellum. Posterior sagittal US image of the radius (*R*) and capitellum (*C*) shows normal hypoechoic capitellar articular cartilage (*arrow*) beneath the normal concavity or pseudo-defect of the posterior cortical surface (*line*)

in the olecranon fossa (os supratrochleare dorsale) can be mistaken for an intra-articular loose body (Fig. 18.8). Dynamic imaging in extension will show that the ossicle moves out of the fossa, allowing the olecranon process to sit in its correct position.

In comparison, fluid seen surrounding a posterior echogenic fragment suggests that it is likely to represent an intra-articular loose body, possibly arising from an area of osteochondritis dissecans (OCD). Dynamic imaging will show that the intra-articular loose body remains in the fossa and limits full extension. Furushima et al. (2015) showed that US imaging is clinically useful in identifying sites of origin of OCD involving the anterior articular surface of the humerus. The normal "pseudo-defect" and bony irregularity seen on the coronal and sagittal flexed elbow scans of the posterior aspect of the capitellum should not be interpreted as a site of OCD (Fig. 18.9).

Multiple accessory muscles have been described around the elbow (Sookur et al. 2008) and should not be mistaken for soft tissue masses or pathology. The anconeus epitrochlearis is seen in 11–23% of the population. The muscle arises from the medial epicondyle of the elbow and passes inferiorly and medially to insert into the olecranon, forming the roof of the cubital tunnel. Although it may be asymptomatic, if large enough, it can cause compression of the ulnar nerve (Fig. 18.10). Symptoms can be further exacerbated by repetitive low-grade trauma. Other accessory muscles include the accessory head of the flexor pollicis longus and accessory

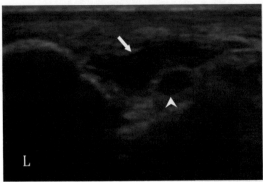
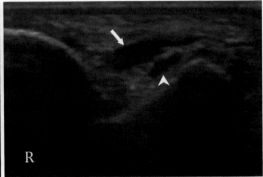

Fig. 18.10 Bilateral anconeus epitrochlearis muscles (*arrows*). On the left, the muscle is hypertrophic, and the ulnar nerve is thickened due to chronic neuritis (*arrow-* *head*). Normal right ulnar nerve is shown for comparison (Courtesy of Dr. Yalcin)

brachialis; however, these are usually identified with magnetic resonance imaging (MRI) rather than US imaging. Anatomical variations in normal tendon structure should not be misinterpreted as traumatic tears. The distal biceps tendon may be bifurcated, simulating a longitudinal tear, but the tendon is of normal size and echogenicity and moves as expected on dynamic imaging.

18.4 Diagnostic-Specific Pitfalls: Pathological Misinterpretations

Misinterpretations of US imaging findings may lead to incorrect pathological diagnoses which may impact on patient management. A number of clinical presentations will be discussed, illustrating potential pitfalls in image analysis.

18.4.1 Triceps Tendon Injury

The triceps tendon is composed of three heads, namely, the superficial long and lateral heads and a deeper medial head which is present in 53% of individuals. The muscle of the medial head extends further distally than the superficial heads (Madsen et al. 2006; Athwal et al. 2009). Other than triceps muscle contusions, distal tendon tears may occur at or close to the olecranon process of the ulna. Tears of the distal tendon require either forced flexion of the elbow against a contracting

triceps, as occurs during a fall on an outstretched arm, or are secondary to a direct blow onto the olecranon process at the tendon insertion.

US imaging is excellent in delineating the degree of tendon retraction, aiding in differentiating partial from complete tears. In a partial tear, focal discontinuity of fibers within the triceps tendon is seen. In cases of a complete tendon tear involving all three heads, full discontinuity and retraction of the triceps is present. The retracted muscle/tendon complex has a wavy appearance, with surrounding fluid and variable proximal migration. However, an isolated rupture of the superficial triceps insertion (long and lateral heads) can mimic a complete tear of the tendon, due to its degree of retraction and wavy appearance. The examiner should ensure that the medial head is identified and remains intact, confirming only a partial tear (Fig. 18.11). A complete tear requires immediate surgery to avoid retraction of the tendon, whereas a partial tear may be treated conservatively.

18.4.2 Cubital Tunnel Syndrome

Patients with cubital tunnel syndrome present with medial elbow pain, weakness, and numbness in the fourth and fifth fingers. This is normally due to compression of the ulnar nerve in cubital tunnel. The ulnar nerve arises from the medial cord of brachial plexus (C8, T1) and lies within the fibro-osseous cubital tunnel formed by

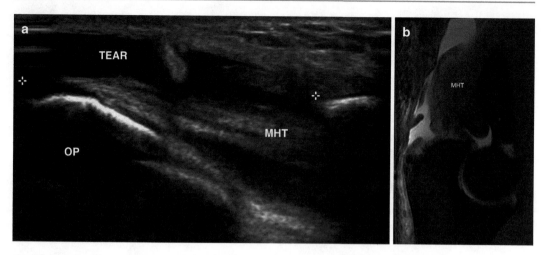

Fig. 18.11 Rupture of superficial lateral and long heads of triceps. (**a**) Longitudinal US image of superficial tear of triceps with an intact medial head (*MHT*). Note the tendon retraction forming an echogenic soft tissue mass. (**b**) Comparative sagittal fat-suppressed T2-W MR image confirms the intact medial head

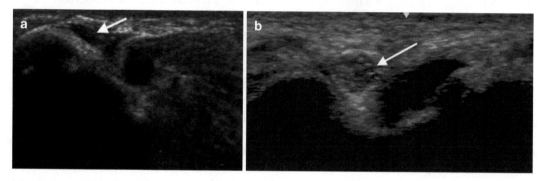

Fig. 18.12 Cubital tunnel syndrome. (**a**) Normal transverse US image of the ulnar nerve (*arrow*). (**b**) The nerve is significantly enlarged in this symptomatic patient

medial epicondyle, olecranon, and cubital retinaculum. Although the diagnosis is essentially based on electrophysiological studies, US imaging can show features suggesting the diagnosis. These include abrupt narrowing and displacement of the nerve within the tunnel, associated with proximal swelling and loss of normal fascicular pattern.

It should be remembered that the normal ulnar nerve is mildly enlarged within the cubital tunnel but not as much as in cubital tunnel syndrome. The circumferential area of the nerve at the level of the epicondyle is significantly larger in patients with cubital tunnel syndrome (Fig. 18.12), compared to healthy subjects or the contralateral normal elbow (Thoirs et al. 2008). However, quantitative measure analysis with US imaging is not reproducible, and threshold values are unreliable (Jacob et al. 2004; Thoirs et al. 2008). Most cases of cubital tunnel syndrome are idiopathic and are associated with repetitive flexion of the elbow and chronic low-grade trauma, resulting in increased tensile load on the ulnar nerve (e.g., baseball pitchers and constant cell-telephone users). However, in some cases, US imaging may demonstrate a definite cause of nerve compression such as ganglion cyst or an accessory anconeus epitrochlearis muscle (Fig. 18.10).

18.4.3 Elbow Snapping Syndrome

Patients with "snapping syndrome" mainly complain of pain on the medial side of the elbow. Sometimes, the patient can willingly reproduce the characteristic "snap" when asked to do so. Clinically, it can be associated with or without ulnar neuropathy symptoms (sensory deficit or paresthesia in the distribution of the ulnar nerve). The symptoms are often more prominent with physical activities such as push-ups, weightlifting, and swimming. US imaging is useful in differentiating causes of "snapping" elbow, such as ulnar nerve instability or abnormal mobility of the medial head of the triceps.

Ulnar nerve instability is secondary to congenital, partial, or complete absence of the cubital tunnel retinaculum. This may predispose to ulnar nerve subluxation over the anterior aspect of the medial epicondyle in 16–20% of asymptomatic elbows during flexion (Miller and Reinus 2010). Dynamic US imaging may show anterior dislocation of the ulnar nerve with a transient "snapping" sensation during elbow flexion (Fig. 18.6). The nerve returns to its normal anatomical position inside the tunnel when the joint is extended. Repeated translocation of ulnar nerve may lead to ulnar neuritis, functional impairment, and symptoms of cubital tunnel syndrome.

The snapping triceps syndrome is a rare and often unknown cause of medial elbow pain. It is a condition in which the distal portion of the triceps (medial head muscle belly) dislocates anteriorly over the medial epicondyle during flexion and extension of the elbow (Jacobson et al. 2001). It may be associated with ulnar nerve dislocation (Fig. 18.13). The muscle structure of the medial head should be distinguished from the fibrillar structure of an accessory triceps tendon which extends distally to form an arch over the ulnar groove.

18.4.4 Acute Elbow Trauma

POCUS imaging is being increasingly utilized by physicians in the assessment of pediatric trauma around the elbow. The ability to use US as part of the clinical examination without radiation risks makes this modality an attractive option. It has been shown to be accurate and reliable in detecting

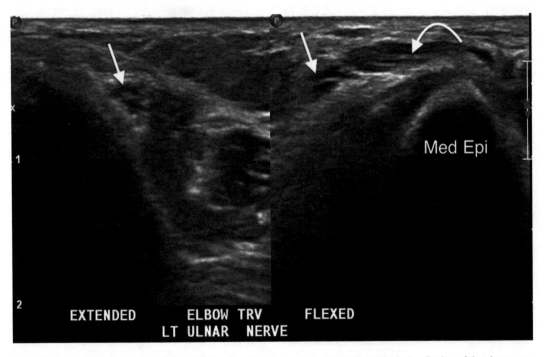

Fig. 18.13 Snapping elbow. Transverse US images show dynamic medial dislocation during flexion of the ulnar nerve (*straight arrow*) and medial head of triceps (*curved arrow*) (Courtesy of Dr. W. Breidahl)

forearm fractures (Patel et al. 2009), where discontinuity and angulation can be easily assessed in the long tubular bones of the forearm. However, due to the curved orientation of the bones around the elbow joint, the identification of fractures around this joint is more difficult.

The presence of a joint effusion in the adult population on lateral radiography (fat pad sign) has >80% likelihood of a fracture. In the pediatric population, US imaging has been shown to be more sensitive than radiography in identifying small effusions (as little as 1–3 ml) with associated elevation of the posterior fat pad (De Maeseneer et al. 1998). But unlike adults, the presence of an elbow effusion in children is nonspecific and may not necessarily be associated with an underlying fracture (Rabiner et al. 2013). Echogenic material within the effusion reflects the presence of fat (lipohemarthrosis). It may be diffuse or form a fat/fluid level within the joint but is highly specific for an intra-articular fracture.

Demonstration of elbow effusion by US needs to be performed posteriorly over the olecranon fossa in the sagittal plane (Fig. 18.14). Scanning over the posterior joint in the transverse plane may show asymmetric elevation of the posterior fat pad which can be normal. The whole fat pad needs to be elevated by the effusion to be confident that this is abnormal (Rabiner et al. 2013). Careful "light touch" scanning is recommended to avoid compression and displacement of small amounts of fluid. In all patients with a joint effusion and no trauma, color Doppler US interrogation to determine the presence of synovitis is recommended. Unfortunately, as there are no pathognomonic US finding of an infected effusion, when there is any clinical concern, then the joint needs to be aspirated to exclude septic arthritis.

18.4.5 Elbow Plica Syndrome

The elbow plica syndrome (also called synovial fold syndrome or posterolateral impingement) arises from an injury, such as a direct blow or repetitive flexion and extension and overloading in athletes (low-grade trauma). It results in inflammatory thickening and focal synovitis of a congenital synovial fold/plica in the lateral compartment of the elbow between the radial head and capitellum. Occasionally, there may be no predisposing factors for this syndrome (Cerezal et al. 2013). Symptoms include lateral elbow pain mimicking epicondylitis, snapping, or locking. Careful US imaging evaluation is required to obtain the correct diagnosis.

On US imaging, the normal synovial fold shows a hyperechoic triangular shape partially surrounded by a thin hypoechoic ring of articular cartilage (Fig. 18.15a). A pathological synovial fold appears thickened on US imaging with irregular echogenicity and margins (Fig. 18.15b). In addition, the abnormal fold is now fully surrounded by a hypoechoic rim due to the addition of synovial thickening superficial to the fold. Color Doppler US imaging readily identifies this associated active focal synovitis and excludes other more common conditions of the elbow, such as lateral epicondylitis.

18.4.6 Elbow Soft Tissue Masses

Clinical history is important for differentiating soft tissue masses around the elbow. An acute traumatic hematoma is usually readily distinguishable on US imaging from other muscle masses such as abscess and tumor. It is initially hyperechoic or isoechoic, becoming more hypoechoic with increasing liquefaction after

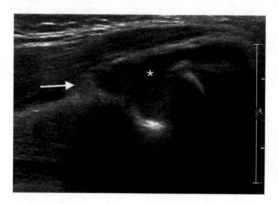

Fig. 18.14 Elbow effusion. Sagittal posterior US image shows the effusion (*) and elevation of the posterior fat pad (*arrow*)

several days to weeks (Fig. 18.16). Other than trauma, a hematoma may be due to anticoagulation or vascular malformation. Soft tissue sarcoma is seen as a large well-defined, hypoechoic mass within the muscle which is moderately to highly vascular but is occasionally hypovascular. Abscess is more frequent in immunosuppressed patients and has many variable appearances but normally shows a thick-walled, irregular hypervascular outline with a hypoechoic/anechoic

avascular necrotic center with edema and hyperemia of adjacent inflamed tissues.

Adjacent to the medial epicondyle and just proximal to the elbow, enlarged regional lymph nodes may simulate a mass (Fig. 18.16). Reactive hyperplasia or septic inflammation may be seen in "cat-scratch" disease. Other disorders of lymph nodes in this area must be considered including benign and malignant diseases. Whatever the cause of epitrochlear lymphadenopathy, US imaging can confirm the nodal anatomy and exclude other local soft tissue masses (e.g., neurogenic tumor or sarcoma). Typical US imaging appearances of a reactive lymph node consist of an oval hypoechoic mass with an echogenic hypervascular hilum on color Doppler imaging, which regresses over weeks to months (Fig. 18.16).

In chronic reactive lymphadenopathy, the lymph node may undergo diffuse massive adipose infiltration, leading to an extensive and hyperechoic medulla with atrophy of the cortex. In these cases, the examiner should be careful not to mistake these atrophic nodes for lipomas. Detection of a thin continuous hypoechoic rim related to the atrophic cortex and a vascularized hilum may help the diagnosis. US-guided biopsy may be required to provide a more definitive diagnosis.

18.4.7 Medial or Lateral Epicondylar Pain

Acute traumatic injury to the common extensor or flexor origins is unusual. The clinical presentation should not cause any diagnostic difficulty,

Fig. 18.15 US imaging of the synovial fold syndrome. (a) Normal appearances of the synovial fold (*) lying between the radial head (*R*) and capitellum (*C*). (b) Abnormal synovial plica. The synovial fold is thickened and hypoechoic with synovial thickening deep to the plica (*curved arrow*) and extending around the adjacent annular ligament (*straight arrows*)

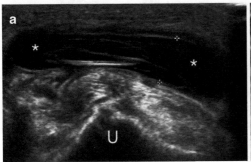

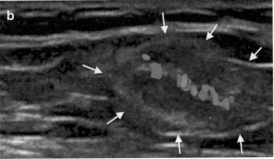

Fig. 18.16 US imaging of soft tissue masses around elbow. (a) Liquifying hematoma is seen as a loculated fluid collection (*) superficial to the ulna (*U*). (b) Solid echogenic lesion (*arrows*) with central color Doppler US flow is typical of an epitrochlear lymph node

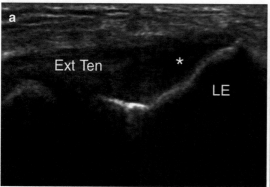

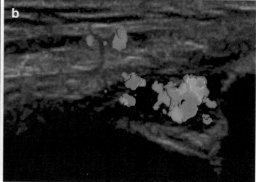

Fig. 18.17 Chronic extensor tendinosis. (**a**) The common extensor tendon (*Ext Ten*) origin from the lateral epicondyle (*LE*) is thickened and hypoechoic with poor fiber definition. A more focal hypoechoic area (*) due to marked tendinosis is seen and shows (**b**) marked neovascularity on Doppler flow US imaging

and US imaging will show either complete or partial tear of the tendon origins. A complete tear is defined as complete discontinuity of the tendon fibers. Any associated epicondylar fracture will be seen on radiography. However, epicondylar pain due to chronic low-grade trauma is more frequent. Medial pain (golfer elbow) and lateral pain (tennis elbow) may radiate down into the forearm and be exacerbated by activity.

The main US imaging features of epicondylitis are insertional swelling of the tendon which contains focal or diffuse areas of decreased reflectivity with loss of the normal fibrillary pattern, i.e., tendinopathy. Fluid adjacent to the common tendons and ill-defined tendon margins may also be seen. In chronic high-grade tendinosis, there is angiofibroblastic infiltration causing a striking hypervascular pattern within the intratendinous hypoechoic areas on color and power Doppler imaging (Fig. 18.17). Identification of this neovascular pattern provides an opportunity for intratendinous injection therapy which is not usually performed in partial tears.

In practice, US imaging discrimination of focal tendinosis and small partial tears can be difficult. The diagnosis of a partial tear is recommended only when discrete anechoic cleavage planes are demonstrated with loss of fiber continuity (Fig. 18.18) and absent Doppler flow. These tears may appear as longitudinal splits originating from the bony enthesis and extend-

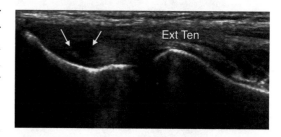

Fig. 18.18 Partial tendon tear. There is abrupt intrasubstance discontinuity (*arrows*) of the fibers of the extensor tendon (*Ext Ten*) due to a partial tear

ing distally. Thickening of peritendinous soft tissues and a thin layer of superficial fluid over the extensor tendon are also more often observed with partial tears. As discussed earlier, care should be taken to avoid any anisotropy artifact, as this may be misinterpreted as a partial or complete tear of the tendon.

18.4.8 Medial Collateral Ligament Injury

Acute or chronic repetitive overstretching during valgus stress can occur in the acceleration phases of throwing, resulting in degeneration and tears of the medial collateral ligament. Acute traumatic tears of the ligament may also be secondary to posterior dislocation of the elbow. These ligament injuries may be associated with or

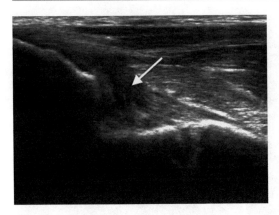

Fig. 18.19 Complete rupture of the medial collateral ligament. US imaging shows that the ligament is thickened and hypoechoic. A complete tear (*arrow*) is seen at the humeral insertion (Courtesy of Dr. W. Breidahl)

without injury to the adjacent origin of the common flexor tendon. When the medial collateral ligament is injured, it becomes diffusely thickened and hypoechoic on US imaging, with a surrounding effusion posteriorly and deep to the medial epicondyle. In cases of complete rupture, US imaging may show either a gap or focal hypoechoic areas in the proximal and distal portions of the ligament (Fig. 18.19).

However, occasionally, distinguishing between partial and complete tears can be difficult. In order to improve the diagnostic accuracy, dynamic US examination can provide assessment of the degree of medial joint laxity in both neutral and valgus stressed positions. Widening of the trochlea-ulna joint with soft tissue falling into the distracted joint space indicates a complete rather than partial tear of the ligament. Examination of the non-injured elbow should be obtained to compare the amount of joint widening that occurs during valgus stressing.

18.4.9 Anterior Elbow Pain

Patients with a complete tear of the distal biceps brachii tendon normally present with pain and swelling in the antecubital fossa, following a popping sensation at the time of acute injury.

Physical examination demonstrates weakness and limited elbow flexion. As expected, US imaging in complete tears shows fiber discontinuity of the tendon in the antecubital fossa. Unfortunately, this diagnosis can be difficult due to a number of factors. The distal biceps tendon is particularly prone to anisotropy due to its anatomical course anterior across the elbow. This is further compounded due to the contour surface of the elbow, making positioning of the transducer difficult in some patients. In addition, the tendon is composed of both long and short heads with different fiber orientation. Changing transducer angle inclination and dynamic imaging showing that the tendon moves normally on pronation/supination throughout its length will exclude anisotropy and confirm that the tendon is intact.

Occasionally, anisotropy may only affect one head, and the operator must be cautious in reporting this as a partial tear. Although in both these situations the tendon is hypoechoic, a partial tear is usually focally larger than the normal adjacent tendon. Distinction between a partial tear and tendinopathy can be subjective. Pathologically, tendinopathy often includes areas of micro-tearing of the tendon; these are best demonstrated on axial rather than longitudinal US imaging of the tendon.

Bicipitoradial bursitis is a focal fluid collection that forms around the distal biceps tendon or between distal biceps tendon and radial neck. It is typically seen as a hypoechoic or anechoic mass with through transmission; the shape of which often changes with pronation/supination. Although this may be seen as a solitary finding, it is often associated with partial or complete tears of the distal biceps tendon (Fig. 18.20). It is therefore important that in the presence of an enlarged bursa, the distal biceps tendon should be evaluated for injury. US imaging evaluation of the distal tendon and bursa using an anterior approach is often difficult because of technical factors. In a posterior approach with the forearm pronated, the radial tuberosity faces posteriorly, bringing the distal biceps tendon insertion into view, enabling a better visualization of this area.

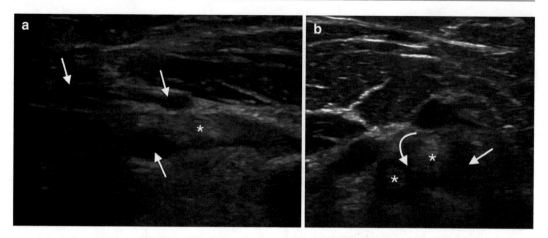

Fig. 18.20 Bicipitoradial bursitis. (**a**) Longitudinal and (**b**) transverse US images of the distal biceps tendon (*). Fluid due to bursitis surrounds the distal tendon (*straight* *arrows*). The tendon is thickened and hypoechoic due to tendinopathy, and there is a longitudinal tear distally (*curved arrow*)

Conclusion

Pitfalls in US imaging of the elbow can be avoided, if attention is given to appropriate equipment setup and examination technique, particularly dynamic imaging. The examiner should perform US imaging and techniques reflecting the patient's symptoms and signs. Knowledge of the appearances of normal anatomical structures and anatomical variants is essential to avoid pitfalls in pathological misinterpretation.

References

Arend CF (2013) Top ten pitfalls to avoid when performing musculoskeletal ultrasound: what you should know before entering the examination. Eur J Radiol 82:1933–1939

Athwal GS, McGill RJ, Rispoli DM (2009) Isolated avulsion of the medial head of the triceps tendon: an anatomic study and arthroscopic repair in 2 cases. Arthroscopy 25:983–988

Bouffard JA, Goitz H (2010) Ultrasound in sports medicine. In: Essential applications of musculoskeletal ultrasound in rheumatology. Elsevier, Philadelphia

Cerezal L, Rodriquez-Sammartino M, Canga A et al (2013) Elbow synovial fold syndrome. AJR Am J Roentgenol 201:W88–W96

De Maeseneer M, Jacobson JA, Jaovisidha S et al (1998) Elbow effusions: distribution of joint fluid with flexion and extension and imaging implications. Invest Radiol 33:117–125

Furushima K, Iwabu S, Itoh Y (2015) Osteochondritis dissecans of the throwing elbow. In: Park JY (ed) Sports injuries to the shoulder and elbow. Springer-Verlag, Berlin

Jacob D, Creteur V, Courthaliac C et al (2004) Sonoanatomy of the ulnar nerve in the cubital tunnel: a multicentre study by the GEL. Eur Radiol 14:1770–1773

Jacobson JA, Jebson PJL, Jeffers AW et al (2001) Ulnar nerve dislocation and snapping triceps syndrome: diagnosis with dynamic sonography – report of three cases. Radiology 220:601–605

Jacobson JA (2013) Elbow ultrasound. In: Fundamentals of musculoskeletal ultrasound, 2nd edn. Elsevier, Philadelphia

Kane D, Kitchen J, Hammer HB (2010) Purchasing ultrasound equipment. In: Essential applications of musculoskeletal ultrasound in rheumatology. Elsevier, Philadelphia

Madsen M, Marx RG, Millett PJ et al (2006) Surgical anatomy of the triceps brachii tendon: anatomical study and clinical correlations. Am J Sports Med 34:1839–1843

Miller TT, Reinus WR (2010) Nerve entrapment syndromes of the elbow, forearm and wrist. AJR Am J Roentgenol 195:585–594

Patel DD, Blumberg SM, Crain EF (2009) The utility of bedside ultrasonography in identifying fractures and guiding fracture reduction in children. Paed Emerg Care 25:221–225

Rabiner JE, Khine H, Avner JR et al (2013) Accuracy of point-of-care ultrasonography for diagnosis of elbow fractures in children. Ann Emerg Med 61:9–17

Shen X, Zhou Z, Yu L et al (2012) Ultrasound assessment of the elbow joint in infants and toddlers and its clinical significance. Acta Radiol 55:745–752

Sookur PA, Naraghi AM, Bleakney RR et al (2008) Accessory muscles: anatomy symptoms and radiologic evaluation. Radiographics 28:481–499

Taljanovic MS, Melville DM, Scalcione LR et al (2014) Artifacts in musculoskeletal ultrasonography. Semin Musculoskelet Radiol 18:3–11

Thoirs K, Williams MA, Phillips M (2008) Ultrasonographic measurements of the ulnar nerve

at the elbow: role of confounders. J Ultrasound Med 27:737–743

Tomsick SD, Petersen BD (2010) Normal anatomy and anatomical variants of the elbow. Semin Musculoskelet Radiol 14:379–393

Wrist and Hand Injuries: MRI Pitfalls

19

Mingqian Huang and Mark E. Schweitzer

Contents

19.1	**Introduction**	355
19.2	**Technical Factors**	356
19.2.1	Magic Angle Phenomenon	356
19.2.2	Chemical Shift Artifacts	356
19.2.3	Susceptibility Artifacts	356
19.2.4	Motion Artifacts	357
19.2.5	Wraparound Artifacts	357
19.2.6	Partial Volume Averaging Artifacts	358
19.2.7	Saturation Artifacts	358
19.2.8	Truncation Artifacts	358
19.2.9	Shading Artifacts	358
19.2.10	Radio-Frequency Interference Artifacts/ Zipper Artifacts	358
19.3	**Osseous Injuries**	358
19.3.1	Carpal Fractures	358
19.3.2	Marrow Edema	358
19.3.3	Scaphoid Fractures	360
19.3.4	Scaphoid Osteonecrosis	361
19.3.5	Other Carpal Bone Fractures	362
19.3.6	Stress Fractures	363
19.3.7	Mimickers of Osseous Trauma	363
19.4	**Wrist Ligamentous Injury**	363
19.4.1	Interosseous Ligaments	364
19.4.2	Wrist Extrinsic Ligaments	368
19.4.3	Triangular Fibrocartilage Complex (TFCC)	369
19.5	**Finger Ligamentous Injury**	372
19.5.1	Ulnar Collateral Ligament of the Thumb	372
19.5.2	Finger Tendon-Related Injury	373
Conclusion		375
References		375

Abbreviation

MRI   Magnetic resonance imaging

19.1 Introduction

The wrist is an interesting joint. It does not have the intrinsic lack of stability of the shoulder, but is yet quite mobile. Nor does it have the frequency of injury of the ankle or the knee, but injuries are nonetheless quite frequent. In the following pages, we will discuss wrist and finger injuries beginning with optimizing techniques and minimizing artifacts. We will not be encyclopedic but intend to provide a clinically relevant overview, with an emphasis on normal anatomy of what we think clinicians will see most frequently. We will also aim to help radiologists to avoid some of the pitfalls that are commonly encountered in daily practice.

M. Huang, MD (✉)
M.E. Schweitzer, MD, FRCPSC
Department of Radiology, Stony Brook University,
Stony Brook University Hospital,
101 Nicolls Road, Stony Brook,
New York, NY 11794-8460, USA
e-mail: Mingqian.Huang@stonybrookmedicine.edu;
Mark.schweitzer@stoneybrookmedicine.edu

© Springer International Publishing AG 2017
W.C.G. Peh (ed.), *Pitfalls in Musculoskeletal Radiology*, DOI 10.1007/978-3-319-53496-1_19

19.2 Technical Factors

Magnetic resonance imaging (MRI) has proven to be a valuable tool at diagnosing a variety of wrist and finger injuries, ranging from osseous contusion and fracture to ligamentous and tendon injuries (Gold et al. 2003; Mosher 2006; Ahn and El-Khoury 2007). However, MRI of the wrist and finger is subject to several artifacts. Some of these artifacts are more prominent with increasing utilization of high-field-strength scanners. Thus, a thorough knowledge of these artifacts is quite important at avoiding pitfalls for diagnosing pathologies in the wrist and finger. In general, MRI artifacts arise from interactions between the magnet, coils, and radio-frequency (RF) transmitter and receiver, either worsened or minimized based on the reconstruction algorithm used (Zhuo and Gullapalli 2006). They can also be patient related, hardware related, and protocol related. For further information on MRI artifacts, also see Chap. 4.

19.2.1 Magic Angle Phenomenon

Tendons and hyaline cartilage may be affected by the magic angle phenomenon on short echo time sequences, such as gradient-echo and T1- and some proton density (PD)-weighted sequences (Peh and Chan 2001). The magic angle phenomenon occurs when collagen fibers are oriented at a 55-degree angle to the static magnetic field. At this angle, the spin-spin interactions from the static local field are nullified, resulting in T2 decay being controlled only by the dynamic local field. As a result, the T2 relaxation time rises while the T2 decay is not as rapid, causing anisotropic structures, such as tendon and hyaline cartilage, to appear speciously bright at short TE (echo time) values (Peh and Chan 2001).

In the wrist, the third extensor compartment of extensor pollicis longus tendon has an oblique course distal to the Lister tubercle. Due to the magic angle phenomenon, there may be high signal within this tendon distal to the Lister tubercle. The flexor pollicis longus tendon has a similar course as the extensor pollicis longus tendon distal to the carpal tunnel, making it also susceptible to pronounced magic angle phenomenon and sometimes hardly visible within the thenar muscles. This artifact can be corrected by closely comparing abnormalities with those on T2-weighted images, repeating the scan with a TE value of 37 milliseconds or more (Peh and Chan 1998), or by repositioning the patient.

19.2.2 Chemical Shift Artifacts

This artifact has sometimes been referred to as the India ink artifact as it causes semicircumferential black borders around images. The resonance frequencies of protons are different between fat and water, about 224 Hz at 1.5 T (Peh and Chan 2001). This difference is directly proportional to the magnetic field strength and is thus higher on 3 T imaging (Smith and Nayak 2010). This artifact is seen in the frequency-encoding direction as high signal areas where fat and water overlap and low signal where they separate (Soila et al. 1984). In- and opposed-phase imaging sequences have been developed based on the principles of chemical shift. Switching the frequency- and phase-encoding gradient directions, using fat-suppression techniques, and increasing the receiver bandwidth are ways to reduce this artifact (Peh and Chan 2001). In the wrist MRI, chemical shift artifact occurs at the cartilage-bone marrow interface, possibly leading to overestimation or underestimation of cartilage thickness (Weissman 2009). When noted, an advantage of this artifact is that the reader knows that the lesion has clear borders and hence is likely benign.

19.2.3 Susceptibility Artifacts

This artifact arises due to the inhomogeneity of the local magnetic field at the interface of structures with different magnetic susceptibilities. It produces spatial misregistration as a result of distortion of the magnetic field (Peh and Chan 2001). This is proportional to the magnetic field strength and thus is twice as large on 3 T when compared to 1.5 T scanners (Dietrich et al. 2008). Magnetic susceptibility artifacts cause a shift in resonance frequency of lipid and water, reducing the efficacy of fat suppression. This is of particular importance in interpreting postoperative studies, as well as MR arthrographic images, as introduction of air into the joint space may cause susceptibility artifacts and be misinterpreted as a lesion (Gückel and Nidecker 1997).

Using fast spin-echo sequences with short echo times; increasing the bandwidth; using small field-of-view (FOV), high-resolution matrix; and decreasing the inter-echo space (with high gradient strength) are ways to reduce susceptibility artifacts (Lee et al. 2007). Additionally, newer MRI techniques have been developed to address the increasing prevalence of prosthetic joints and implants in patients. These include slice encoding for metal artifact correction (SEMAC) and multi-acquisition variable-resonance image combination (MAVRIC) (Koch et al. 2009; Lu et al. 2009).

19.2.4 Motion Artifacts

Motion artifacts are the most common and easily recognized MR artifacts. These artifacts occur because the phase gradient cannot predictably encode the radio waves arising from moving structures (Peh and Chan 2001). The type of motion, moving object speed, and magnetic field strength are the factors controlling motion artifacts (Taber et al. 1998). Ghosting and smearing are the common artifacts arising from voluntary or involuntary patient motions (Morelli et al. 2011). There are varieties of ways to reduce these artifacts, such as using sequences with shorter acquisition time and using soft pads between the inner surface of coil and the patient's skin.

With advances of MRI, there has been significant progress made in reducing imaging time, and this is made possible with the use of higher magnetic field strengths, stronger gradients, multichannel coils, and newer image acquisition techniques (Morelli et al. 2011). Continuous motion, like blood flow, can cause artifacts that are best seen on T2-weighted images. It can also appear as ghosting in pulsatile flow and as increased signal on gradient-echo images due to inflowing blood (Peh and Chan 2001). Currently,

motion artifacts occur only occasionally in spine images, unless the patient is uncooperative.

19.2.5 Wraparound Artifacts

This is also known as aliasing artifacts. It is usually seen in the phase-encoding direction. This is because when imaging a small FOV that is insufficient to encompass the tissues being imaged, there will be superimposition of the phase-encoded signals from outside and within the FOV, creating wraparound of a structure to the opposite side of the image. It is important to eliminate and recognize this artifact to avoid misinterpretation of underlying abnormalities. When imaging the wrist, wraparound artifact usually occurs when the wrist is positioned by the patient's side. The abdominal and pelvic lateral body wall may be mapped into the wrist images (Fig. 19.1). Sometimes, if the phase-encoding direction is oriented parallel to

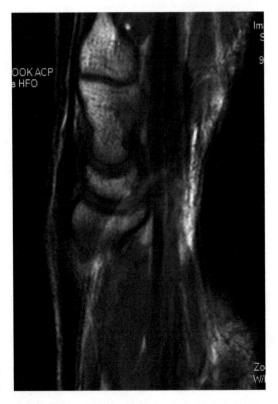

Fig. 19.1 Wraparound artifact. Sagittal PD-W MR image of the wrist shows wraparound artifact from the adjacent thorax

long axis of the wrist, the more proximal and distal aspects of the wrist, hand, and forearm may become mapped into the section of interest. Using a larger FOV and oversampling are techniques that can address this artifact. A rectangular FOV and switching the frequency- and phase-encoding directions also reduce these artifacts (Peh and Chan 2001). With proper protocoling, these artifacts are quite rare currently, but occasionally are seen when one leg is imaged in the body coil.

19.2.6 Partial Volume Averaging Artifacts

This artifact occurs when a single voxel contains signal from tissues of different MR properties. This is particularly troublesome when evaluating small structures, such as cartilage and ligament in the wrist. Using a smaller FOV and thinner slices can reduce the artifacts (Peh and Chan 2001). This type of artifact is often seen when tissues are obliquely oriented in their axis.

19.2.7 Saturation Artifacts

This is usually due to overlapping intersection of the imaging slices (Peh and Chan 2001). This happens when imaging slices intersect due to different obliquities, resulting in repeated RF excitation of the overlapping central tissues (Singh et al. 2014). Thus, it is often seen on axial images.

19.2.8 Truncation Artifacts

Also known as Gibbs phenomenon or ringing, truncation artifacts are usually seen at tissue interfaces with an abrupt change in intensity of the MR signal and occur with under-sampling of several phase-encoding steps of high spatial resolution (Peh and Chan 2001). The artifact is seen as dark or bright lines that appear parallel to the margin of the area showing an abrupt change in signal intensity (Smith and Nayak 2010). Truncation artifacts usually occur at fat-muscle interfaces and can result in an area of false high signal intensity. However, with modern sequences, they have become rare.

19.2.9 Shading Artifacts

Nonuniformity of the RF field causes this artifact, which is also known as intensity gradient artifact. This is especially seen with the use of surface coil (Smith and Nayak 2010). These artifacts result in loss of brightness, variable image contrast, and deterioration of the image quality from decreasing RF signal in the structures located further away from the coil. This artifact can be corrected by using a larger surface coil or a whole-volume coil (Peh and Chan 2001).

19.2.10 Radio-Frequency Interference Artifacts/ Zipper Artifacts

This artifact is commonly seen due to leakage of electromagnetic waves in the scan room (Zhuo and Gullapalli 2006). This will cause image distortion, usually as linear band of increased noise and perpendicular to the frequency-encoding direction.

19.3 Osseous Injuries

19.3.1 Carpal Fractures

Early and accurate diagnosis of carpal fractures is critical for appropriate and timely management to minimize complications such as delayed union, nonunion, osteonecrosis, and secondary osteoarthritis (Tibrewal et al. 2012). Besides providing early diagnosis of osseous contusion and fracture, MRI has the added benefit of no ionizing radiation. Additionally, MRI can also provide alternative diagnoses, such as unsuspected distal radius/ulna or hand fractures, osseous contusion, and soft tissue injuries.

19.3.2 Marrow Edema

Bone marrow edema is the most frequent finding in acute or subacute osseous injury. Without marrow edema, an acute fracture and osseous contusion can be confidently excluded. Fracture can be confidently diagnosed with the presence of linear hypointense signal abnormality in the carpal bones, especially on T1-weighted sequences, together with marrow edema. Without the linear area of hypointense signal, the marrow edema could represent microtrabecular injury or osseous contusion in the traumatic setting. However, sometimes fractures of the wrist may not demonstrate MRI-visible fracture lines. In this case, even without a visible fracture line, if there is overt marrow edema on a T1-weighted image, we should err on the side of calling a fracture rather than a bone bruise.

The distinction between nondisplaced fracture and osseous contusion is important, as it affects clinical management. MRI can also assist in gauging the acuity of the injury. Fractures with more avid marrow edema usually represent acute injury. However, there are a variety of causes of marrow edema, with trauma being one of the main ones. Marrow edema from osseous injury is usually focal and accompanied by adjacent soft tissue swelling (Fig. 19.2). On the other hand, reactive marrow edema from inflammation or infection tends to be more diffuse (Fig. 19.3). Marrow edema from cartilage loss could be focal and often located at the edges of a bone. However, when there is adjacent cartilage abnormality, the edema tends to be subchondral in location, such as in hamate chondromalacia in patients with type 2 lunate (Fig. 19.4).

In childhood, hyperintensity of the marrow on fluid-sensitive sequences can be seen on MRI, even in the absence of bone pathology. Hyperintensity on fat-suppressed fluid-sensitive sequences can be normally seen around the physis (Laor and Jaramillo 2009). The bones in the wrist are considered epiphysis equivalent; hence, hyperintense signal within these bones may also represent vascular channels (Shabshin and Schweitzer 2009). All these pose a challenge in differentiating between pathological and physiological causes of marrow edema. Shabshin and Schweitzer (2009) described a pattern with maturation: frequency and intensity decrease and distal-to-proximal resolution. This pattern is quite similar to normal marrow conversion. Usually by the age of 5 years, the marrow conversion in the hands is complete with residual red marrow in the distal forearm metaphysis. The marrow conver-

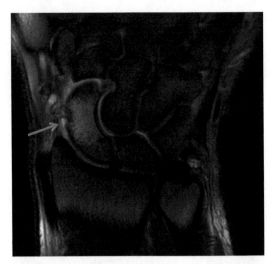

Fig. 19.2 Coronal fat-suppressed PD-W MR image of the left wrist shows marked marrow edema of the scaphoid including distal pole and waist with adjacent soft tissue edema (*arrow*), consistent with scaphoid fracture

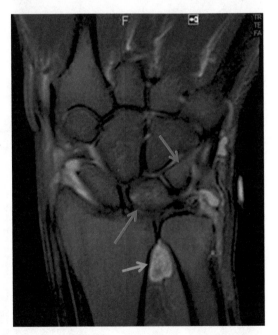

Fig. 19.3 Coronal fat-suppressed T2-W MR image of the wrist in a patient with history of rheumatoid arthritis shows marrow edema in multiple carpal bones including lunate, and triquetrum (*blue arrows*), accompanied by distal radioulnar and radiocarpal joint complex effusions (*orange arrow*) consistent with chronic synovitis. Fluid is noted in the prestyloid recess as well

sion of the metaphysis is completed by the age of 15 years (Taccone et al. 1995). They observed that marrow edema is most commonly seen in the distal radius and ulna and the first carpal row, when compared to the rest of the osseous structures in the wrist (Fig. 19.5). Most carpal bone fractures occur along the zone of vulnerability, which follow the direction of the major volar wrist ligaments starting at the radial styloid, traversing the waist and proximal pole of the scaphoid, and the body of the capitate, before turning ulnarly to include the base of the hamate and the ulnar styloid (Johnson 1980).

19.3.3 Scaphoid Fractures

Scaphoid fractures account for 58–89% of all carpal fractures (Van Onselen et al. 2003; Green et al. 2011) and can be complicated by nonunion in 10–12% of cases (Herbert and Fisher 1984; Steinmann and Adams 2006). The most common mechanism of injury is a fall onto an outstretched hand, resulting in wrist dorsiflexion, exerting palmar tensile and dorsal compressive forces on the scaphoid (Green et al. 2011). The scaphoid can be divided into the distal pole, tubercle on the volar aspect of the distal pole immediately proximal to the trapezium, the waist, and proximal pole (Karantanas

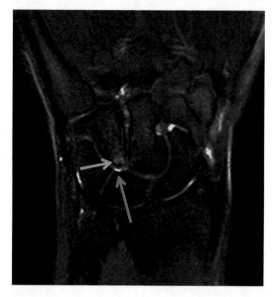

Fig. 19.4 Coronal fat-suppressed T2-W MR image of the wrist shows a type II lunate (*blue arrow*) with chondromalacia (*orange arrow*) at the articulating proximal hamate and associated subchondral marrow edema

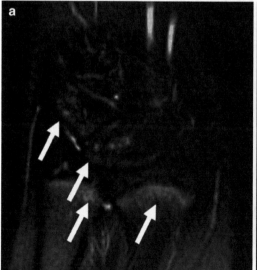
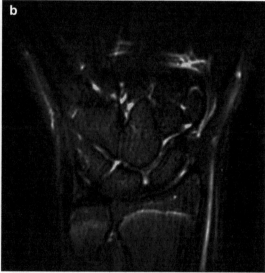

Fig. 19.5 Interval resolution of hyperintense bone marrow seen on fluid-sensitive MR images of the wrist. (**a**) At 12 years of age: regions of hyperintense bone marrow seen on fluid-sensitive sequences of the distal radius and ulna (*arrows*), representing normal appearance of the metaphysis, and in the lunate and triquetrum,the later possibly representing normal penetrating vessels in the carpal bones. (**b**) At 14 years of age: only minimal residual hyperintense changes of the bone marrow are seen in the distal forearm. The hyperintense bone marrow seen on fluid-sensitive sequences of carpal bones has decreased

et al. 2007). Most of scaphoid fractures (65%) involve the waist, 15% involve the proximal pole, 10% the distal body, 8% the volar tubercle, and 2% the distal articular surface (Cooney et al. 1996).

Scaphoid fractures can be classified by location, by plane of the fracture with respect to the long axis of the scaphoid, or by time since injury. The Herbert classification combines the above information and emphasizes acute stable and unstable fractures. With a stable fracture, the overlying cartilage is usually intact and there is no associated ligamentous injury. These are often treated with immobilization alone. Tubercle fractures and nondisplaced waist fractures are considered stable. Findings that might indicate instability include cortical offset of more than 1 mm, fracture angulation, associated ligamentous injury, or fracture fragment motion with ulnar or radial deviation, thus requiring fixation.

The standard four-view wrist radiographs, including a scaphoid view, are the first-line method of evaluation of suspected acute scaphoid fractures. In a large meta-analysis, 84% of initial radiographs correctly diagnosed the presence or absence of a scaphoid fracture (Hunter et al. 1997). Unenhanced MRI for evaluation of suspected, radiographically occult, scaphoid fracture has a sensitivity of 100% and specificity of 95–100% (Gaebler et al. 1996; Breitenseher et al. 1997; Hunter et al. 1997) with high interobserver reliability ($k = 0.8$–0.96) (Breitenseher et al. 1997; Hunter et al. 1997; Bretlau et al. 1999). Dorsay et al. (2001) demonstrated cost-effectiveness of a limited protocol MRI examination compared to casting and repeat radiograph in 10–14 days.

19.3.4 Scaphoid Osteonecrosis

The unique retrograde nature of the blood supply from the dorsal branch of the radial artery to the scaphoid makes it vulnerable to developing osteonecrosis. Hence, depending on the location of the fracture, there are different likelihoods. The incidence of osteonecrosis is 30% for fractures involving the middle third of the

scaphoid, up to 100% when fractures involve the proximal one fifth (Inoue and Sakuma 1996). Determination of the viability of the proximal fragment is of clinical significance, for it determines whether a non-vascularized or vascularized bone graft is used.

MRI is the imaging modality of choice for assessment of proximal fragment viability in scaphoid nonunion (Cerezal et al. 2000; Anderson et al. 2005; Fox et al. 2010; Donati et al. 2011; Schmitt et al. 2011; Ng et al. 2013). However, the most efficacious MRI protocol for this purpose is not universally agreed upon. Imaging of scaphoid fracture follow-up can be performed with or without intravenous gadolinium. After administration of the contrast agent, images can be obtained in a delayed fashion at single time point or dynamically over multiple early time points to generate a perfusion curve. There are conflicting results in the literature at comparing the efficacy of these different imaging protocols. We use mostly the severity of the hypointense signal in the proximal pole to determine viability (Fig. 19.6).

There are some theories that may help us understand the inconsistencies of these imaging research results. Firstly, observation of intraoperative punctate bleeding at the debrided fracture margin is considered the reference standard. This, however, is not entirely reliable and accurate (Urban et al. 1993). Histopathologic findings of osteonecrosis can be interposed with the "normal" bone (Sakai et al. 2000), leading to potential sampling error. Secondly, confluent loss of the normal high T1 signal of fat in the medullary cavity has long been considered diagnostic of osteonecrosis (Anderson et al. 2005; Fox et al. 2010). However, the central necrotic region in femoral head osteonecrosis maintains bright T1 fat signal due to the presence of fatty acids from hydrolyzed triglycerides (Vande Berg et al. 1992; Cerezal et al. 2000; Sakai et al. 2000). This same process could conceivably occur in the scaphoid. Thirdly, contrast enhancement of proximal fragment on delayed contrast-enhanced MRI does not necessarily indicate preserved vascularity. Contrast diffusion across the fracture can cause false-positive results on these delayed

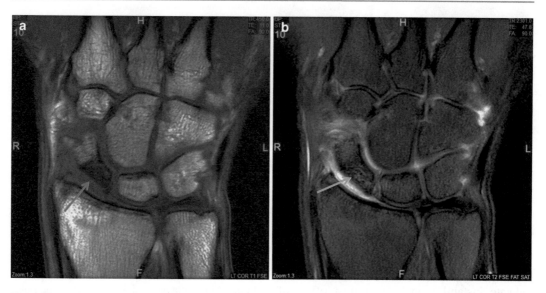

Fig. 19.6 Avascular necrosis of the scaphoid. (**a**) Coronal T1-W MR image of the wrist shows marked loss of normal T1 signal at the proximal pole of the scaphoid including the waist (*blue arrow*), indicating avascular necrosis. (**b**) Coronal fat-suppressed PD-W MR image of the same wrist shows only mild marrow edema (*orange arrow*) in the same region, consistent with chronicity

images (Sebag et al. 1997; Fox et al. 2010). Also, fibrous tissue from healing response may enhance, leading to potential false-positive results. Lastly, caution must be taken in interpreting the enhancement curve, especially with a long time period between injuries and imaging (Ng et al. 2013). Comparison of the curve should be carried out between the proximal pole, the adjacent capitate, and the distal pole.

19.3.5 Other Carpal Bone Fractures

The other carpal bones account for 11–42% of carpal bone fractures, and most of these involve the triquetrum and the hamate (Van Onselen et al. 2003; Raghupathi and Kumar 2014). This group of fractures account for 4–10% of injuries identified in the work-up of suspected radiographically occult scaphoid fractures (Brydie and Raby 2003; Tibrewal et al. 2012). MRI is particularly useful in the pediatric population, with partially ossified or non-ossified bones (Obdeijn et al. 2010).

19.3.5.1 Triquetral Fractures

The most common pattern of triquetral fracture is at the dorsal cortex. Dorsal triquetral fractures only rarely lead to nonunion (Suh et al. 2014). However, they are frequently associated with ligament injuries, which can lead to instability and early arthritis. The commonly involved ligaments are dorsal radiocarpal, ulnotriquetral, and intercarpal ligaments.

19.3.5.2 Hamate Fractures

Hamate fractures can involve the body or the hook, with hook fractures being more common (Milch 1932). This injury is common in racket sports from direct compression and repetitive microtrauma. It can also be seen in golfers. Hence, many of these are actually stress rather than acutely traumatic injuries. Hamate fractures should therefore be suspected in athletes participating in racket sports, golf, or baseball who are seen with ulnar-sided wrist pain. Early diagnosis can reduce the risk of complications, including nonunion, flexor digitorum profundus tendon rupture, ulnar neuritis, and ulnar artery injury (Kato et al. 2000; Suh et al. 2014). Both axial and sagittal images should be obtained before excluding fractures of hook of the hamate. The T1-weighted and proton density images should be carefully evaluated to avoid missing fractures without marrow edema. A pitfall to avoid is bipartite hamate hook (os hamuli proprium), which may mimic a hamate fracture. This ossicle is usually oval or pyramidal in shape and is typically embedded in the pisohamate ligament.

19.3.6 Stress Fractures

Stress fractures occur when repetitive force is applied to a bone. If the bone is softened mechanically, the injuries are termed insufficiency fractures. If the bone is of normal strength, then injuries are termed fatigue fractures. All stress fractures are more common in weight-bearing parts of the skeleton, but they can rarely be seen in the wrist and hand. In the upper extremity, most stress fractures are fatigue fractures.

Stress fractures of the scaphoid are usually from repeated dorsiflexion of the wrist, commonly seen in shot-putting and gymnastics. Other much less common stress fractures include hook of the hamate in racket sports, the pisiform in volleyball, the triquetrum in breakdancing, the second metacarpal in tennis, and the fifth metacarpal in softball pitchers (Waninger and Lombardo 1995; Jowett and Brukner 1997; Guha and Marynissen 2002; Blum et al. 2006). There is a continuum of stress injury from altered mechanics to stress response. On imaging, early stress response is usually demonstrated as marrow edema with periosteal edema. When a hypointense T1 line is identified, progression to a stress fracture has occurred.

A particular variant of stress injury, epiphysiolysis, is seen in adolescent gymnasts at the distal radius. It can be bilateral. It is thought to be due to repeated compressive forces causing stress fracture of the distal growth plate or metaphyseal failure (Shih et al. 1995). Widening of the growth plate,

extending of the physeal cartilage into the metaphysis, and bruising of metaphyseal bone are the common imaging findings. Liebling et al. (1995) described physeal widening as a thin irregular line of hyperintense signal located just proximal to the normal high signal region of the physis. This linear region of increased signal was thought to represent persistent chondrocytes and cartilaginous matrix in the primary spongiosa of the metaphysis, similar to physeal stress injuries of little league shoulder. This stress injury can lead to premature physeal closure and worsened prognosis.

19.3.7 Mimickers of Osseous Trauma

Carpal boss refers to a dorsal fragment located in between the base of the second and third metacarpals and distal to the capitate and trapezoid, which can cause pain or limiting mobility (Fig. 19.7). It could be from degenerative osteophytes or an os styloideum, an ossicle. This should not be mistaken for fracture. Pain related to os styloideum may be caused by overlying ganglion, bursitis, or extensor tendon subluxation (Conway et al. 1985). Soft tissue edema can often be seen adjacent to the os styloideum.

19.4   Wrist Ligamentous Injury

Injury to the wrist ligaments is a common cause of chronic wrist pain and carpal instability. MRI is an established method for the detection, evaluation, and follow-up of disorders of the wrist ligaments (Hobby et al. 2001; Nikken et al. 2005). The ligaments of the wrist guide and constrain the complex motion of the carpus relative to the forearm and metacarpals and facilitate transmission of force between carpal bones (Berger 1996; Berger 1997; Berger 2001). They are divided into intrinsic and extrinsic groups (Taleisnik 1976). Intrinsic ligaments arise and insert entirely within carpal bones, whereas extrinsic ligaments arise in the forearm or extend onto metacarpals or have

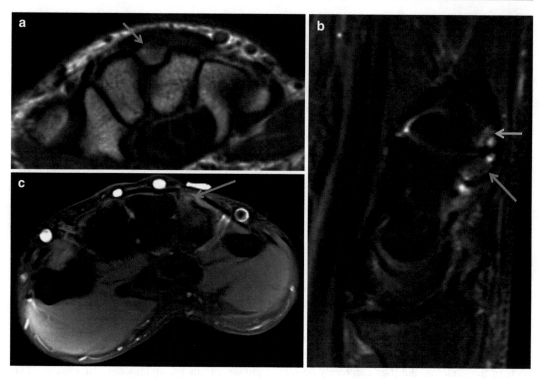

Fig. 19.7 Carpal boss. (**a**) Axial PD-W MR image shows an ossicle in between the capitate and trapezoid (*arrow*). (**b**) Sagittal fat-suppressed T2-W MR image of the wrist shows marrow edema within the ossicle dorsal to the capitate (*blue arrow*) compatible with carpal boss and also marrow edema at base of the 3rd metacarpal (*orange arrow*). (Courtesy Dr. Y.M. Ying) Carpal boss. (**c**) Axial fat-suppressed T2-W MR image of the wrist shows focal marrow edema around the dorsal base of 2nd metacarpal with slight cortical protuberance (*arrow*). Note the adjacent marker. Patient complains of chronic discomfort in the region with no history of trauma. Carpal boss was suggested by the radiologist and confirmed by the hand surgeon at surgery. (Courtesy Dr. K.R. Desai)

additional attachments to retinacular and/or tendon sheaths (Taleisnik 1976; Bateni et al. 2013). The accepted nomenclature is to name the ligaments for the bones from which they originate and onto which they insert, proximal to distal and radial to ulnar (Taleisnik 1988).

19.4.1 Interosseous Ligaments

The two most clinically important intrinsic wrist ligaments are the scapholunate and lunotriquetral ligaments. In contradistinction to other ligaments, these intrinsic wrist ligaments are vulnerable to attritional wear (Viegas and Ballantyne 1987). In general, ligament tears manifest as ligament discontinuity (especially at their osseous insertions), fluid signal violating the ligament, or altered morphology. Knowledge of the precise anatomy, as well as variant patterns of signal and morphology changes, can help increase sensitivity and specificity of the diagnosis.

19.4.1.1 Anatomy

Scapholunate Ligament (SLL)
The SLL has three distinct components, namely, dorsal, volar, and membranous (proximal). Together they form a C-shaped structure, which is 18 mm in length and 2–3 mm in thickness (Daunt 2002), and connect the articulating surface of the ulnar scaphoid and radial lunate. The thicker trapezoidal-shaped (axial plane) dorsal SLL and the much thinner volar SLL are true collagenous ligaments, whereas the membranous portion is fibrocartilaginous.

The dorsal component of the SLL is the strongest and most important for carpal stability

(Bencardino and Rosenberg 2006). It has an intimate relationship with the dorsal joint capsule. The volar segment is obliquely oriented. The proximal or membranous component of the SLL varies in shape from its volar to dorsal aspect on coronal images. The volar aspect of the membranous component has a trapezoidal shape and attaches directly to both scaphoid and lunate cortex. The central portion of the membranous component becomes triangular in shape and attaches to the hyaline cartilage of the scaphoid and lunate. The dorsal aspect of the membranous component is more band-like on coronal images as it approaches the dorsal component and is variable in attachment.

Lunotriquetral Ligament (LTL)

The LTL is slightly longer compared to SLL, measuring 20 mm in length, and is more V shaped. Similar to the scapholunate ligament, it has three histologically and functionally distinct segments (Berger et al. 1999; Daunt 2002). Unlike the SLL, the volar component is thicker and more important (Berger 2001). The dorsal component is made of transverse fibers and covered by the dorsal radiocarpal ligament. It is only 1–1.5 mm in thickness, making it challenging to identify on MRI. It is important functionally to restrain rotation. The volar segment is the thickest with transverse fibers interweaved with the ulnocapitate ligament, measuring up to 2.5 mm in thickness. It transits the extension moment of the triquetrum. The membranous (proximal) portion is very thin, no more than 1–1.5 mm. It is composed of fibrocartilaginous tissue, similar to that of triangular fibrocartilage.

19.4.1.2 Normal MRI Appearances

Scapholunate Ligament (SLL)

The dorsal component of SLL usually shows band-like hypointense signal on axial MR images, likely due to the majority of homogeneous transversely oriented collagen fascicles. However, in the coronal images, the dorsal component usually shows a striated pattern. The volar component can show hypointense to striated heterogeneous hyperintense signal, because of the

close proximity to loose vascular connective tissue. The progression from trapezoidal shape in the volar aspect to central triangular shape and dorsal band-like appearance of the membranous portion explains the variable signal intensities ranging from the hyperintense-intermediate signal in the volar aspect to signal hypointensity to the dorsal aspect (Totterman and Miller 1996).

Lunotriquetral Ligament (LTL)

The dorsal and volar portions of the LTL are the biomechanically more important part of the LTL. Diagnosing LTL injury can be challenging, with reported sensitivities at 0–56% and specificities ranging from 46–100% (Zlatkin et al. 1989; Schweitzer et al. 1992; Johnstone et al. 1997). One factor contributing to this challenge is the variable appearances at the ligament-bone interface (Smith and Snearly 1994). Yoshioka et al. (2006) reported shape and signal intensity of the membranous portion of the LTL with high-resolution MRI and concluded that it is important to gain familiarity with normal MRI appearance of LTL membranous portion using high-resolution techniques to improve diagnosis of LTL injury.

The membranous portion has a triangular or deltoid shape of hypointense signal in >85% of subjects on gradient-echo (GRE) images. The triangular geometry is classified as regular (essentially an equilateral triangle) (41.1%), a broad-based isosceles triangle (20%), a narrow-based isosceles triangle (6.7%), or an asymmetric (scalene) triangle (17.8%) (Yoshioka et al. 2006). An alternative linear or bar-like morphology may mimic a tear, owing to the absence of its distal vertex (Yoshioka et al. 2006). An amorphous shape may be seen in older patients and likely due to degenerative changes with chronic incomplete collagen disruption. Thus, the membranous component of the LTL demonstrates a spectrum of normal variants in shape on coronal images (Smith and Snearly 1994).

There are also variations in signal intensity of the membranous component of the LTL. It can be classified into type 1 variant as uniform signal hypointensity (33.8%), type 2 variant as a thin line of signal hyperintensity inside the triangular body of the ligament that traverses the distal margin of the membranous component (45.5%), and type 3 variant as linear signal hyperintensity extending through the triangle and traversing both the proximal (base) and distal margins of the membranous component (20.8%) (Yoshioka et al. 2006). The curvilinear signal hyperintensity classified as type 2 or 3 may be further subclassified according to its orientation relative to the lunate and triquetrum (Yoshioka et al. 2006).

The LTL is a flexible structure, with change in shape and signal intensity depending on the position of the wrist during imaging. Therefore, it is important to first evaluate the position of the wrist when considering LTL pathology. In wrist ulnar deviation, there is distortion of the triangular shape and decrease in the size, compared to the neutral position. In wrist radial deviation, the triangular body becomes wider and higher in internal signal intensity, compared to the neutral position.

19.4.1.3 Pathology

Wrist injuries are one of the most common injuries of the musculoskeletal system. Among wrist injuries, lesions to the scapholunate joint are the most frequent cause of carpal instability (Manuel and Moran 2007; Kuo and Wolfe 2008). A tear that involves one or two of the three components of either the SLL or LTL is considered a partial tear, whereas a tear of all three components is a complete tear (Manton et al. 2001; Zlatkin and Rosner 2004; Theumann et al. 2006). A partial-thickness tear may show the presence of fluid through a portion of the ligament or partially altered ligament morphology (Manton et al. 2001). A full-thickness tear will show a completely abnormal ligament morphology, even with rare absence of the entire ligament or the presence of fluid violating all three portions of the ligament on T2-weighted images (Schweitzer et al. 1992). Radiologists should be aware that the widely accepted Geissler arthroscopic grading scale which quantifies carpal instability, rather than the extent or size of the SLL or LTL tear (Slutsky 2008). Note the combination of interosseous ligamentous tear, which may be partial, together with deficient secondary stabilizers or extrinsic liga-

ment tears would cause instability (Timins et al. 1995; Linkous et al. 2000; Mitsuyasu et al. 2004; Theumann et al. 2006).

In general, an absent ligament or fluid-filled gap is a reliable sign of tear on MRI. Distortion of morphology such as fraying, thinning or thickening, irregularity, elongation or stretching, abnormal course, or focal increased fluid signal has all been reported as evidence for tear (Zlatkin et al. 1989; Manton et al. 2001; Daunt 2002; Zlatkin and Rosner 2004). However, there is considerable overlap with asymptomatic degeneration. Thus MRI has higher sensitivity than specificity. To increase specificity, it should be noted that, often, these ligament disruptions manifest at their insertion and fit into the spectrum of avulsion injuries. Specific secondary MRI findings that may increase specificity include widening of the intercarpal interval, focal osseous offset or incongruous joint, carpal arc disruption, associated ganglion cyst, or focal chondromalacia/osteoarthritis (Manton et al. 2001; Daunt 2002; Zlatkin and Rosner 2004). However, there is suboptimal interobserver consistency of these secondary signs. To ensure reliability, as the proximal carpal row has curved morphology in the coronal plane, only midline images should be used for assessment. Carpal arc disruption is offset in the cranial-caudal axis. Osseous offset is offset at the articulation between two carpal bones. Secondary signs are of limited use in the diagnosis of partial thickness tear. However, the absence of secondary signs may help the radiologist to exclude a full thickness tear.

SLL Tear

The sensitivities of diagnosing SLL tear on MRI are quoted as 40–88%, with specificities being 60–100% at 1.5 T (Zlatkin et al. 1989; Schweitzer et al. 1992; Potter et al. 1997). Direct MR arthrography appears to be more sensitive (86–92%) but is not necessarily more specific (46–100%) than conventional MRI. In symptomatic patients, the dorsal component is often completely torn (Fig. 19.8) and typically avulsed from the scaphoid attachment. Isolated dorsal or volar tears are unusual, probably because such tears quickly propagate into the proximal segment (Schmid

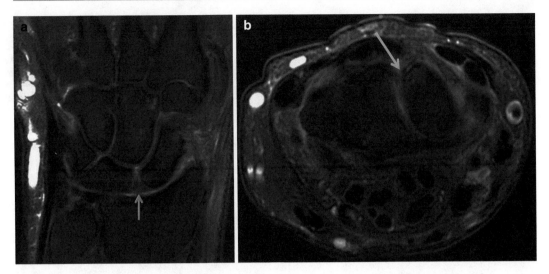

Fig. 19.8 (**a**) Coronal fat-suppressed T2-W MR image of the wrist shows a widened scapholunate interval (*blue arrow*). (**b**) Axial fat-suppressed T2-W MR image of the wrist shows tear of the dorsal and membranous components of the scapholunate ligament (*orange arrow*)

et al. 2005; Lee et al. 2013). While isolated membranous portion tears are common, they do not cause carpal instability. Although rarely present before the age of 20 years, half of all adults have SLL communicating defects by the age of 70 years, and 65% to 70% of those are bilateral (Viegas et al. 1993; Wright et al. 1994). However, membranous defect can be symptomatic and does respond to surgical debridement (Ruch and Poehling 1996; Weiss et al. 1997) in the absence of scapholunate dissociation. There is usually excellent relief of pain and crepitant symptoms after debridement.

LTL Tear

These patients usually present with ulnar-sided wrist pain. Similar to SLL tear, isolated asymptomatic membranous portion defects are common and often bilateral and are increased with age (Cantor et al. 1994; Yin et al. 1996). Volar and dorsal tears nearly always extend to the membranous portion (Schmid et al. 2005). However, even with the LTL completely torn, the lunotriquetral interval is typically not widened, but there is disruption of the normal proximal carpal row arc (Ringler 2013). LTL tear should be carefully assessed in the presence of a visible TFCC disorder.

19.4.1.4 Wrist Dynamic and Instability

The proximal carpal row is considered an "intercalated segment" because it is located between the radius and the distal carpal row with no attaching tendons. The lunate is in the center, with the scaphoid and triquetrum on the sides exerting opposing volar flexion and dorsiflexion tendencies upon it. The natural tendency of the unopposed scaphoid is volar flexion (rotatory subluxation). This is the dorsal intercalated segmental instability (DISI) pattern. The unopposed triquetrum pulls the lunate into dorsiflexion. A tear of the lunotriquetral ligament produces the opposite pattern, volar intercalated segmental instability (VISI), since the lunate is freed from the triquetrum and pulled volarly by the scaphoid.

When assessing DISI on sagittal MR images, caution should be applied to distinguish normal dorsal tilt of the lunate that can occur with normal ulnarly deviated or hyperextended wrist positions (Fig. 19.9). The normal scapholunate angle is between 30° and 60°. A measurement over 80 degrees indicates dorsiflexion instability. On MRI, this angle can be calculated by combining the dorsal tilt angle of the lunate and volar tilt angle of the scaphoid relative to the vertical plane on sagittal images.

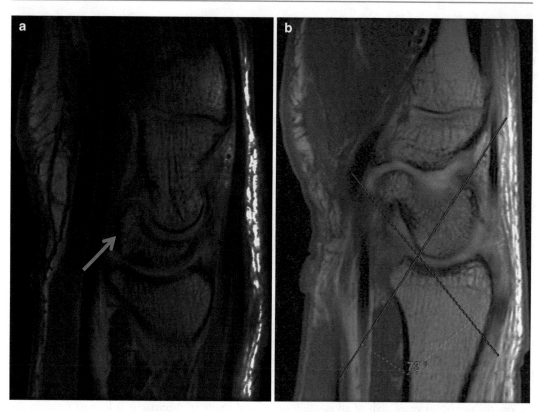

Fig. 19.9 (**a**) Sagittal T1-W MR image of the wrist shows "dorsal tilt" of the lunate (*arrow*) in a patient with ulnar deviated wrist. (**b**) Sagittal T1-W MR image of the same patient shows a scapholunate angle of 73 degrees, less than 80 degrees, thus confirming the positional artifact and the absence of a true DISI deformity

19.4.2 Wrist Extrinsic Ligaments

Extrinsic ligament injuries in the wrists are equally common clinically as are intrinsic ligament tears. Studies have shown that together with intrinsic ligament, they played a vital role in maintaining wrist stability. Taneja et al. (2013) found that 60% of patients who had wrist MRI exam after trauma demonstrated intrinsic ligament injury and 75% had extrinsic ligament injury. The most frequently injured extrinsic ligaments are the radioscaphocapitate ligament (RSL), the long radiolunate ligament (LRL), and the dorsal radiocarpal ligament (DRL) (Taneja et al. 2013). The RSL and LRL are often injured together (Mak et al. 2012). Extrinsic ligaments are intracapsular and extrasynovial. These ligaments connect the radius and ulna to the carpal bones. They are made up of radiocarpal and ulnocarpal ligaments, both at palmar and dorsal aspects of the wrist. Palmar ligaments are thicker and

stronger than dorsal ligaments in general. Capsular ligaments generally appear as predominant linear hypointense structures on MRI with alternating bands of intermediate signal intensity within, producing a striated appearance (Ringler 2013).

The RSL arises from the tip of the radial styloid process, passing the scaphoid fossa, attaches to proximal cortex of the distal scaphoid pole, and distally interdigitates with fibers from ulnocapitate ligament (UCL) and palmar scaphotriquetral ligament, with only about 10% of fibers ultimately inserting on the capitate (Berger 2001) (Fig. 19.10). It acts like a sling at the scaphoid wrist. In general, it is easily seen on arthroscopy, except for the radial styloid attachment where it crosses the scaphoid wrist, making tears in these areas difficult to diagnose (Mak et al. 2012). The LRL arises from palmar rim of the scaphoid fossa, passing anterior to proximal scaphoid pole, and attaches to radial volar lunate cortex. It serves

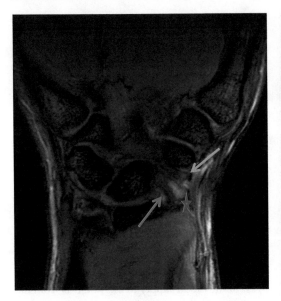

Fig. 19.10 Coronal gradient-echo MR image of the wrist shows the radioscaphocapitate (RSL) (*orange arrow*) and, long radiolunate ligament (LRL) (*blue arrow*) at the volar aspect of the wrist with an inter-ligamentous sulcus (star) filled with fluid

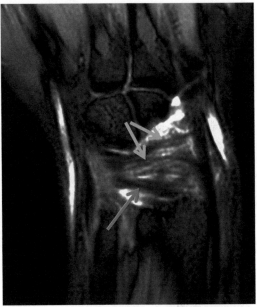

Fig. 19.11 Coronal gradient-echo MR image of the wrist (dorsal aspect) shows the dorsal radiotriquetral ligament (DRL) as a single band that arises from distal radius to triquetrum (*blue arrow*). The dorsal intercarpal ligament (*orange arrows*) is seen as a broad fused band with triquetroscaphoid and triquetrotrapezoid fasciles

as a volar sling for the lunate. The radial and palmar origins of the RSL and LRL on the radial styloid process cannot be distinguished on MRI (Ringler 2013). Proximally, they run parallel to each other. There is an inter-ligamentous sulcus between the ligaments that can be seen on both coronal and sagittal images (Fig. 19.10).

The DRL is also known as dorsal radiotriquetral ligament. Most often, it originates from the dorsal rim of the distal radius, spanning the Lister tubercle to the sigmoid notch (Berger 2001). Then it passes obliquely distally and ulnarly to attach to the dorsal ulnar horn of the lunate, dorsal LTL, and fourth and fifth extensor compartment septa, terminating just proximal to the radial dorsal ridge of the triquetrum. This ligament is usually well seen on thin coronal 3D MR images (Fig. 19.11). The dorsal intercarpal ligament extends from dorsal tubercle of the triquetrum to the dorsal groove of the scaphoid and attaches to both scapholunate and lunotriquetral ligaments. Together, the DRL and dorsal intercarpal ligaments form a zigzag or V shape (Fig. 19.11). They function as a radioscaphoid stabilizer on the dorsal side.

19.4.3 Triangular Fibrocartilage Complex (TFCC)

19.4.3.1 Anatomy

The TFCC is centered between the distal ulna, lunate, and triquetrum. This complex is composed of a fibrocartilage disk and multiple surrounding ligaments (Vezeridis et al. 2010). The TFCC is central to the stability of the distal radioulnar joint, functions in axial loading from the carpus to ulna, and is a predominant stabilizer for ulnar-sided carpal stability (Bencardino and Rosenberg 2006). There is some controversy about the exact components of the TFCC. The general consensus is that TFCC is made up of TFC proper including the triangular fibrocartilage, ulnar collateral ligament, ulnotriquetral ligament (UTL), ulnolunate ligament (ULL), the meniscus homologue, and the sheath of extensor carpi ulnaris tendon and capsule of the distal radioulnar joint.

The TFC proper is composed of dorsal and volar radioulnar ligaments and the fibrocartilage central disk (Brown et al. 1998). It is thinner at its fibrocartilaginous center and may even show fenestrations in middle-aged and elderly patients (Metz et al. 1993a, b). It becomes thicker at the periphery; this is called the limbus. The thickness of the TFC is related to the length of the ulna relative to the distal radius. At its palmar side, the ulnolunate and ulnotriquetral ligaments attach to the TFC proper. The fibrocartilaginous TFC proper is hypointense on fat-suppressed PD and T1-weighted images (Totterman and Miller 1995) but may be more hyperintense on GRE sequences (Friedrich et al. 2009), depending on the specific TE and flip angle selected. In older patients, mucoid degeneration may lead to increased signal on fat-suppressed PD sequences (Mikić 1978). Both UTL and ULL are palmar stabilizers of the TFCC. They both originate from palmar radioulnar ligament. The ULL is an enforcement of the joint capsule, with fibers joining the lunotriquetral ligament. Their size shows considerable anatomical variability. In most cases, they appear as inhomogeneous small structures which cannot be clearly differentiated (Zlatkin and Rosner 2004). The TFCC may be further divided into its volar and dorsal as well as radial and ulnar components.

Radial Attachment

There is broad attachment of the TFCC to the radius. The dorsal and volar distal radioulnar ligaments anchor the fibrocartilage disk to the distal radius around the sigmoid notch. There is a transition from the central fibrocartilage to hyaline cartilage between these two ligaments. Thus, we usually can observe curvilinear intermediate signal at this transition from the hypointense central disk to the hyaline cartilage on coronal MR images.

Ulnar Attachment

The triangular ligament connects the fibrocartilage to the ulna. This is a V-shaped ligament with its apex pointing toward the fibrocartilage and base along the distal ulna. The triangular ligament is made up of two laminae, which attach to the ulnar styloid and ulnar fovea, respectively. The lamina connecting to the ulnar styloid is consid-

ered distal and more horizontal in orientation, and the lamina connecting to the fovea is considered proximal and more vertical. In between these two laminae, there is a region called the ligamentum subcruentum. The triangular ligament usually demonstrates a striated appearance on MRI due to its collagen fiber composition and vascular connective tissue. The ligamentum subcruentum also often shows hyperintense signal (Fig. 19.12). This increased signal should not be mistaken as tear. There is hyaline cartilage at the tip of the ulnar styloid process, with intermediate signal on PD and GRE images, and this should not be mistaken for partial tear of the ligamentous attachment.

Vascularity to the TFCC

Most of the blood supply to the TFCC is from the ulnar artery, directly and indirectly. The central portion of the TFCC and the radial attachments are relatively avascular, while the peripheral aspect of the disk is more vascular (Bednar et al. 1991). At the most ulnar aspect of the TFCC near the styloid process, the ulnar artery proper supplies most of the blood through penetrating end

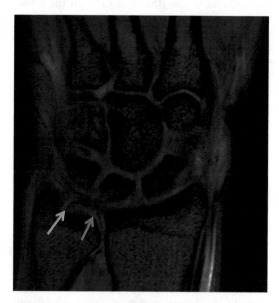

Fig. 19.12 Coronal gradient-echo MR image of the wrist shows the ligamentum subcruentum having increased signal intensity (*orange arrow*). This ligament lies between the two ulnar insertions of the triangular ligament, to the fovea of ulnar styloid process and the tip of the ulnar styloid process. Additionally, note the small incomplete undersurface perforation at the radial aspect of the central disk (*blue arrow*)

vessels (Cody et al. 2015). More radially, the TFCC receives blood through dorsal and volar branches of the anterior interosseous artery, an early branch of the ulnar artery distal to the elbow (Cody et al. 2015).

TFCC Shape During Rotation

The distal radioulnar joint is a pivot joint. The radius moves around the ulna during both pronation and supination. The shape of the disk of the TFCC has been found to show little change between supinated and pronated positions of the wrist on high-resolution MRI with a specially designed surface coil (Nakamura et al. 1999). No significant shape variation mimicking a tear of the disk should be expected as result of wrist positioning during MRI, in contradistinction to the carpal ligaments.

Ulnar Variance

Ulnar variance is measured at the center of the distal articular surfaces of the radius and ulna in a neutral position (Palmer et al. 1984; De Smet 1994; De Smet 1999; Cerezal et al. 2002). If the radius and ulna are of same length, this is termed neutral ulnar variance. In this case, most of the axial loading is transmitted from the ulna to the radius, with ulna only carrying about 20% of the load (Palmer and Werner 1981; Palmer et al. 1984). If the ulna is >2 mm longer than the radius, this is called ulnar-positive variance. The TFC proper is usually thin in this circumstance, and also the axial loading forces transmitted by ulna are higher and hence predisposing to tear. This positive variance also predisposes the patient to the related ulnocarpal impaction syndrome. The ulnocarpal impaction syndrome can be seen in patients with ulnar neutral variance, but only rarely with ulnar-negative variance (Tomaino 1998). The TFCC is thicker with a relatively decreased load on the ulna and lower incidence of TFCC lesions in the cases of ulnar-negative variance. However, there is a somewhat weak association of Kienböck disease with ulnar-negative variance. Ulnar impingement is a condition of a short ulna impinging on the radius with a pseudoarthrosis. This is the opposite of ulnar impaction in many ways.

19.4.3.2 Pathology

Patients with TFCC pathology usually present with ulnar-sided or diffuse wrist pain, with and without clicking or snapping sensations during rotation. The most common mechanism of traumatic injury to the TFCC is axial loading to an extended wrist with forearm pronation, e.g., fall onto an outstretched hand. Racket sports with distraction forces applied to the volar wrist predispose patients to TFCC injury. Although atraumatic tears are much more common, anatomical factors such as ulnar variance also predispose patients to both acute injuries and chronic degenerative changes. Palmar classified TFCC tears into traumatic (class 1) or degenerative (class 2). Further, traumatic lesions are subdivided according to the location of the injury into 1A, central perforation; 1B, ulnar avulsion; 1C, distal avulsion; and 1D, radial avulsion.

Class IA tear is most common traumatic subtypes of TFCC tears (Sachar 2008). The tear is usually at the radial half of the disk, even though it is called central perforation (Fig. 19.12). The tear can have a complex configuration. There are two types of disk injuries, i.e., perforation and linear tear. With perforation, the linear hyperintense signal is perpendicular to the disk, whereas in the case of linear tear, the linear hyperintense signal is parallel to the disk. Degenerative perforation is more common in elderly patients, while linear tears are more common in trauma settings.

Evaluation of peripheral TFCC tear is challenging due to the inherent striated appearance along the ulnar attachment of the TFCC. Haims et al. (2002) reported that the sensitivity for evaluation of peripheral TFCC tear was 17%, with a specificity of 63% and an accuracy of 64%. When signal hyperintensity was used as marker for peripheral tear, they found that the sensitivity improved to 42%, while the specificity and accuracy dropped to 63% and 55%, respectively. Class IC tear involves tears of the volar ligaments, particularly the UTL and ULL. These ligaments are relatively robust; thus, this type of tear is uncommon. This type of injury can lead to ulnar carpal instability with palmar migration of the ulnar carpus.

Class ID tear involves avulsion of the TFCC from the radial attachment to the sigmoid notch. It can be seen with avulsion fracture of the sigmoid notch. With this type of tear, abnormal fluid extends between the TFCC and hyaline cartilage of the distal radius (communicating). This is different from class IA lesion, where the abnormal fluid signal is within the TFCC disk proper (noncommunicating). Zanetti et al. (2000) showed that radial-sided communicating TFC defects are commonly seen bilaterally and are often asymptomatic. Noncommunicating and communicating defects of TFC near the ulnar attachment are more reliable associated with symptomatic wrists than the radial communicating defects.

Many TFCC abnormalities fall outside of this classification system (Daunt 2002). Extensor carpi ulnaris tendon sheath injury and injury to the ulnar collateral ligament complex are not included in this classification system. Overall, knowledge of the detailed normal appearances of TFCC on MRI and grasp of the impact of anatomical variants are the basis for avoiding pitfalls at diagnosing TFCC injury.

19.5 Finger Ligamentous Injury

19.5.1 Ulnar Collateral Ligament of the Thumb

Gamekeeper thumb was first described by Campbell in Scottish gamekeepers, where there was a high incidence of deficient metacarpophalangeal (MCP) ulnar collateral ligament (UCL) of the thumb among them. Currently, acute injuries to the UCL of the thumb at MCP level are more common in ski injuries with some calling "skier thumb." The main vector of injury is sudden valgus stress to the UCL.

19.5.1.1 Anatomy and Mechanism of Injury

The UCL consists of the UCL proper and the accessory UCL, which are taut during flexion and extension, respectively. The proper UCL attaches to the base of the proximal phalanx, and the accessory UCL attaches to the volar plate and ulnar sesamoid. The adductor pollicis longus muscle is composed of transverse and oblique

muscle heads. The tendons form an aponeurosis that attaches at the ulnar aspect of the proximal phalanx, superficial to the UCL.

A wedge-shaped fibrocartilage plate surrounds the joint and strengthens the joint capsule (Rozmaryn and Wei 1999; Drapé and Le Viet 2007) and is prominent on the volar and dorsal side. A full thickness synovial recess between the base of the phalanx and plate at the dorsal side of the metacarpophalangeal joint is seen in nearly all healthy volunteers in a study by Hirschmann et al. (2014). This should be avoided for misinterpretation as a tear or avulsion of the attachment of the dorsal plate (Drapé and Le Viet 2007). A full thickness recess means 100% relative length to the length of the distal part of the plate. At the volar aspect, the recess was only seen in a minority of volunteers and differs in length (Hirschmann et al. 2014).

Injuries usually begin with abduction and rotatory force at the MCP, initially stretching and eventually rupturing the proper UCL and joint capsule (Tsiouri et al. 2009). With additional force, the volar plate and embedded sesamoids rotate radially, and finally there is disruption of the accessory UCL. Thus, there can be secondary radial subluxation of the proximal phalanx, leading to adductor aponeurosis slides distal to and/or beneath portions of the disrupted UCL (Stener lesion).

19.5.1.2 MRI

Proper positioning is critical at diagnosing and characterizing UCL tears. Coronal images are most helpful in evaluating the UCL. Emphasis should be placed at obtaining proper coronal plane images, which parallel the dorsal cortex of the metacarpal head. At this level, the metacarpal head is rectangular or trapezoidal in shape (Fig. 19.13). The next most distal cut typically includes the sesamoids. Axial images are especially useful for the identification of Stener lesions. The proper and accessory components of the UCL are not readily separable on MRI. Their distinction lies in understanding of their normal course. The proper UCL extends obliquely from dorsal ulnar aspect of the metacarpal head to the volar portion of the proximal phalanx. It inserts

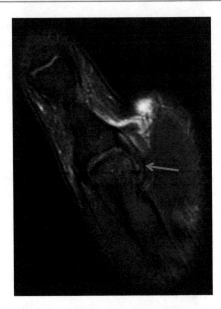

Fig. 19.13 Coronal fat-suppressed T2-W MR image of the thumb shows complete tear of the ulnar collateral ligament from its metacarpal insertion (*arrow*). Note the proper positioning of the thumb with metacarpal head in rectangular shape

proximal to the adductor pollicis attachment at the ulnar tubercle of the proximal phalanx.

Hirschmann et al. (2014) found that the proper UCL and adductor aponeurosis usually have a striated appearance on fat-suppressed fluid-sensitive sequences, while the radial collateral ligament was mainly of hypointense signal, and the accessory UCL showed variable signal intensity (Hirschmann et al. 2014). Thus, we evaluate the UCL abnormality for size, contour, and signal. Tears of the UCL are most common at the proximal phalangeal attachment, but can occur at metacarpal origin or within the ligament substance (Fig. 19.13).

For the Stener lesion, the classic description is "yo-yo on a string" appearance. The adductor aponeurosis is the string, and the balled-up and proximally retracted UCL represents the yo-yo. As the balled-up ligament is blocked from re-approximating at the proximal phalangeal insertion, normal healing and stability cannot be achieved, and thus surgery is required. However, the balled-up appearance is not specific because a proximally retracted UCL in the absence of a Stener lesion can be seen deep to the adductor aponeurosis.

Approximately 60% of collateral ligament injuries involve the thumb, whereas only 39% involve the remaining fingers (Delaere et al. 2003). In a study of small series of ten patients, Delaere et al. (2003) reported the distribution of collateral ligament injury by finger and location. They showed that the fourth and fifth fingers were more likely to have radial collateral ligament (RCL) injuries, and the second digit was more likely to have UCL injury, whereas the third finger has an equal distribution of RCL and UCL lesions (Delaere et al. 2003). MRI is the imaging modality of choice for detection of UCL and RCL injuries of the fingers. Findings include frank discontinuity or detachment, ligament thickening with T2-hyperintense intraligamentous signal, or extravasation of joint fluid into adjacent soft tissues (Clavero et al. 2003).

19.5.2 Finger Tendon-Related Injury

19.5.2.1 Finger Flexor Tendon Injuries

Related Anatomy

Flexor tendon Each finger receives attachment of both flexor digitorum superficialis (FDS) and flexor digitorum profundus (FDP) tendons. However, the thumb only receives the flexor pollicis longus (FPL). The FDS is superficial and volar to the FDP tendons to the level of metacarpal. The FDS tendon then splits at the level of mid-diaphysis of the proximal phalanges to allow the FDP tendons to pass superficially. At the level of the proximal interphalangeal (PIP) joint, the two slips of each FDS tendon reunite deep to the FDP to form the Camper chiasm. The FDS tendon slips then insert on the middle phalanx (P2) in close proximity to A4 pulley. The FDP tendons become superficial and insert distally at the volar base of the distal phalanx. The relationship of FDS and FDP tendons is better evaluated by following the tendon on contiguous axial images on both PD and fat-suppressed fluid-sensitive sequences. The insertion of the flexor tendons can be better seen on sagittal images. The vincula tendinum are thin bands of synovial tissue that attach the tendons to the dorsal fibro-osseous tunnel near its attachment. Delivery of nutrients to the tendons is accomplished by blood supply via vinculae and from the synovial fluid in the tendon sheath.

Pulley system The second to fifth fingers usually contain five annular (A1 to A5) and three cruciate (C1 to C3) pulleys (Doyle 1988; Lin et al. 1989; Hauger et al. 2000). These pulleys are numbered from proximal to distal. The digital pulleys are condensations of transversely oriented fibrous bands. The A2 pulley (at proximal aspect of proximal phalanx) and A4 pulley (at mid-aspect of the middle phalanx) are the key stabilizing digital annular pulleys. They function to stabilize the flexor tendons during flexion and resist ulnar/radial displacement as well as palmar bowing.

Flexor Tendon Injury

In partial tears, the smooth contour of the tendon is disrupted. Axial images enable us to estimate the amount of fiber that is involved in the injury. Sharp margin and linear interposed fluid signal can be seen in lacerations and usually accompanied by soft tissue injuries. MRI can also provide information on tendon retraction in cases of complete rupture, which are critical for management of these injuries. Avulsions (closed injuries) and lacerations are common injuries of the flexor tendons. The FDP tendon is avulsed more commonly than the FDS tendon, especially among football and rugby players when the player grabs the jersey of the opponent (also known as "jersey finger"). This injury occurs with forced hyperextension at the DIP joint during active finger flexion. The ring finger is the most common digit to be affected.

Leddy and Packer (1977) first classified tendon injury into three types. Type 1 injury with tendon retraction into the palm is associated with tear of the vincula blood supply and requires urgent surgical repair. In type 2 injury, the tendon is retracted to level of PIP joint and is usually associated with some degree of intact direct vascular perfusion. Type 3 injuries are avulsion fractures, which do not lead to tendon retraction

proximal to the A4 pulley. Three additional avulsion types have been subsequently described (Leddy and Packer 1977). Type 4 injuries are avulsion fractures of the FDP with the fragment no longer attached to the torn FDP tendon. Type 5 injuries are avulsion fractures of FDP with an extra-articular (type 5a) or intra-articular (type 5b) fracture of the proximal phalanx. Type 6 injuries are open avulsion fractures of the FDP with a lost fragment (Al-Qattan 2001; Al-Qattan 2005). Small cortical avulsions are usually difficult to identify on MRI, and correlation with radiographs and CT images is useful in this situation.

Associated tenosynovial fluid can be seen with flexor tendon tears. When chronic, the sheath can fibrose in reaction to the blood, with subsequent thickening of the tendon sheath and pulleys, potentially presenting clinically as trigger finger (McAuliffe 2010). Lacerations are the most common cause of flexor tendon ruptures and typically affect the midsubstance of the tendon, rather than at the site of insertion. Kleinert and Verdan (1983) classified tendon injuries into five anatomical zones. Zone 2–5 injuries involve both flexor tendons and neurovascular bundle. Zone 2 extends from the A1 pulley to distal insertion of the FDS and was historically considered surgically irreparable due to high complication rate. In current practice, primary surgical repair (within 24 h) is preferred for injury in any of the five zones. Emergency repair is indicated when there are associated neurovascular bundle injuries (Momeni et al. 2010; Wolfe et al. 2011).

Pulley Injuries

Pulley injuries can be commonly seen in rock climbers. However, they can occur in anyone who abruptly injuries a flexed digit. The A2 pulley of the ring finger is the most commonly injured pulley (Crowley 2012). For evaluation of the pulley system, T1-weighted MR images are better than intermediate-weighted fat-suppressed sequences for these thin structures which are surrounded by fat (Hauger et al. 2000; Goncalves-Matoso et al. 2008). Axial and partially flexed sagittal images are recommended. Pulley disruption can be identified on

MRI as focal discontinuity or secondary bow-string of the flexor tendon. The longitudinal extent and degree of the bowstring are related to the number of the pulleys torn and finger position during the imaging. Thus, when we estimate the bowstring, we need to bear in mind that there would be increased bowstringing with finger flexion. It is equally important to realize that partial pulley tears may not result in bowstringing (Hauger et al. 2000). Other secondary signs of pulley injury include soft tissue edema around the pulley and fluid in the tendon sheath (Scalcione et al. 2010).

19.5.2.2 Finger Extensor Mechanism

Related Anatomy

Finger extension involves the coordinated action of both extrinsic and intrinsic extensor muscles. They are coordinated by an array of fibrous structures known as the extensor mechanism. The extensor mechanism in the hand is very complex. At the level of the MCP joint, the extensor digitorum tendon is joined by sagittal bands. The sagittal bands, as main components of the extensor hood, attach volarly to the palmar plate of the MCP joint. The sagittal bands prevent medial to lateral translation of the extensor tendons. Distal to the MCP joint, the extensor digitorum tendon divides into three slips, with a central slip and two lateral bands. The central slip inserts at base of the middle phalanx. Combined with fibers from intrinsic tendons, the lateral band forms the conjoined tendon and inserts at the base of the distal phalanx. The triangular ligament is located between the conjoined tendons.

Injuries

We stress the two main types of traumatic injuries regarding the extensors, namely, the injury to the extensor mechanism and mallet finger. Injury to extensor mechanism of the radial sagittal band is more common, when compared to the ulnar side, because the radial fibers are thinner and longer (Rayan et al. 1997). The middle finger is the most commonly injured finger, due to its long radial sagittal band and big metacarpal head (Lisle et al. 2009). Injury to the extensor hood usually is from direct blow and sudden forced flexion of MCP (Lisle et al. 2009). Mallet finger typically occurs when there is direct trauma to the dorsal aspect of the distal phalanx while the DIP is in extension, thus resulting in forced flexion. There may or may not be associated bony avulsion at the dorsal base of the distal phalanx.

Imaging

Discontinuity, thickening, or attenuation of the extensor hood is seen in injury. Secondary signs include edema of the dorsal soft tissue. Subluxation or dislocation of the extensor tendon can also be seen in patients who suffer from sagittal band injuries. These are best seen on axial MR images. Using a small field-of-view and dedicated wrist coil or wrap coil, MRI with MCP joints in flexion is recommended for detection of extensor hood injuries.

Conclusion

Wrist injuries are common. Finger injuries are perhaps even more common, but much less frequently go onto advanced imaging. We have provided an overview of these injuries that may be detected by MRI.

References

Ahn JM, El-Khoury GY (2007) Role of magnetic resonance imaging in musculoskeletal trauma. Top Magn Reson Imaging 18:155–168

Al-Qattan MM (2001) Type 5 avulsion of the insertion of the flexor digitorum profundus tendon. J Hand Surg Br 26:427–431

Al-Qattan MM (2005) Type 6 avulsion of the insertion of the flexor digitorum profundus tendon. Injury Extra 36:19–21

Anderson SE, Steinbach LS, Tschering-Vogel D et al (2005) MR imaging of avascular scaphoid non-union before and after vascularized bone grafting. Skeletal Radiol 34:314–320

Bateni CP, Bartolotta RJ, Richardson ML et al (2013) Imaging key wrist ligaments: what the surgeon needs the radiologist to know. AJR Am J Roentgenol 200:1089–1095

Bednar MS, Arnoczky SP, Weiland AJ (1991) The micro-vasculature of the triangular fibrocartilage complex: its clinical significance. J Hand Surg Am 16:1101–1105

Bencardino JT, Rosenberg ZS (2006) Sports-related injuries of the wrist: an approach to MRI interpretation. Clin Sports Med 25:409–432

Berger RA (1996) The anatomy and basic biomechanics of the wrist joint. J Hand Ther 9:84–93

Berger RA (1997) The ligaments of the wrist. A current overview of anatomy with considerations of their potential functions. Hand Clin 13:63–82

Berger RA, Imeada T, Berglund L et al (1999) Constraint and material properties of the subregions of the scapholunate interosseous ligament. J Hand Surg Am 24:953–962

Berger RA (2001) The anatomy of the ligaments of the wrist and distal radioulnar joints. Clin Orthop Relat Res 383:32–340

Blum AG, Zabel JP, Kohlmann R et al (2006) Pathologic conditions of the hypothenar eminence: evaluation with multidetector CT and MR imaging. Radiographics 26:1021–1044

Breitenseher MJ, Trattnig S, Gäbler C et al (1997) MRI in radiologically occult scaphoid fractures. Initial experiences with 1.0 tesla (whole body-middle field equipment) versus 0.2 tesla (dedicated low-field equipment). Radiologe 37:812–818

Bretlau T, Christensen OM, Edström P et al (1999) Diagnosis of scaphoid fracture and dedicated extremity MRI. Acta Orthop Scand 70:504–508

Brown RR, Fliszar E, Cotten A et al (1998) Extrinsic and intrinsic ligaments of the wrist: normal and pathologic anatomy at MR arthrography with three compartment enhancement. Radiographics 18:667–674

Brydie A, Raby N (2003) Early MRI in the management of clinical scaphoid fracture. Br J Radiol 76:296–300

Cantor RM, Stern PJ, Wyrick JD et al (1994) The relevance of ligament tears or perforations in the diagnosis of wrist pain: an arthrographic study. J Hand Surg Am 19:945–953

Cerezal L, Abascal F, Canga A et al (2000) Usefulness of gadolinium-enhanced MR imaging in the evaluation of the vascularity of scaphoid non-unions. AJR Am J Roentgenol 174:141–149

Cerezal L, del Piñal F, Abascal F et al (2002) Imaging findings in ulnar-sided wrist impaction syndromes. Radiographics 22:105–121

Clavero JA, Golanó P, Fariñas O et al (2003) Extensor mechanism of the fingers: MR imaging-anatomic correlation. Radiographics 23:593–611

Cody ME, Nakamura DT, Small KM, Yoshioka H (2015) MR imaging of the triangular fibrocartilage complex. Magn Reson Imaging Clin N Am 23:393–403

Conway WF, Destouet JM, Gillula LA et al (1985) The carpal boss: an overview of radiographic evaluation. Radiology 156:29–31

Cooney WP, Linscheid RL, Dobyns JH (1996) Fractures and dislocations of the wrist. In: Rockwood CA Jr, Green DP (eds) Fractures in adults, 4th edn. Lippincott, Philadelphia

Crowley TP (2012) The flexor tendon pulley system and rock climbing. J Hand Microsurg 4:25–29

Daunt N (2002) Magnetic resonance imaging of the wrist: anatomy and pathology of interosseous ligaments and the triangular fibrocartilage complex. Curr Probl Diagn Radiol 31:158–176

De Smet L (1994) Ulnar variance: facts and fiction review article. Acta Orthop Belg 60:1–9

De Smet L (1999) Ulnar variance and its relationship to ligament injuries of the wrist. Acta Orthop Belg 65:416–417

Delaere OP, Suttor PM, Degolla R et al (2003) Early surgical treatment for collateral ligament rupture of metacarpophalangeal joints of the fingers. J Hand Surg Am 28:309–315

Dietrich O, Reiser MF, Schoenberg SO (2008) Artifacts in 3-T MRI: physical background and reduction strategies. Eur J Radiol 65:29–35

Donati OF, Zanetti M, Nagy L et al (2011) Is dynamic gadolinium enhancement needed in MR imaging for the preoperative assessment of scaphoidal viability in patients with scaphoid non-union? Radiology 260: 808–816

Dorsay TA, Major NM, Helms CA (2001) Cost-effectiveness of immediate MR imaging versus traditional follow-up for revealing radiographically occult scaphoid fractures. AJR Am J Roentgenol 177:1257–1263

Doyle JR (1988) Anatomy of the finger flexor tendon sheath and pulley system. J Hand Surg Am 13:473–484

Drapé JL, Le Viet D (2007) Traumatic finger injuries. In: Stoller DW (ed) Magnetic resonance imaging in orthopaedics and sports medicine, 3rd edn. Lippincott Williams & Wilkins, Philadelphia

Fox MG, Gaskin CM, Chhabra AB et al (2010) Assessment of scaphoid viability with MRI: a reassessment of findings on unenhanced MR images. AJR Am J Roentgenol 195:W281–W286

Friedrich KM, Chang G, Vieira RLR et al (2009) In vivo 7.0-tesla magnetic resonance imaging of the wrist and hand: technical aspects and applications. Semin Musculoskelet Radiol 13:74–84

Gaebler C, Kukla C, Breitenseher M et al (1996) Magnetic resonance imaging of occult scaphoid fractures. J Trauma 41:73–76

Gold GE, Hargreaves BA, Beaulieu CF (2003) Protocols in sports magnetic resonance imaging. Top Magn Reson Imaging 14:3–23

Goncalves-Matoso V, Guntern D, Gary A et al (2008) Optimal 3-T MRI for depiction of the finger A2 pulley: comparison between T1-weighted and gadolinium-enhanced fat saturated T1-weighted sequences. Skeletal Radiol 37:307–312

Green DP, Hotchkiss RN, Pederson WC et al (2011) Green's operative hand surgery. Elsevier/Churchill Livingstone, Philadelphia

Gückel C, Nidecker A (1997) The rope ladder: an uncommon artifact and potential pitfall in MR arthrography of the shoulder. AJR Am J Roentgenol 168:947–950

Guha AR, Marynissen H (2002) Stress fracture of the hook of the hamate. Br J Sports Med 36:224–225

Haims AH, Schweitzer ME, Morrison WB et al (2002) Limitations of MR imaging in the diagnosis of peripheral tears of the triangular fibrocartilage of the wrist. AJR Am J Roentgenol 178:419–422

Hauger O, Chung CB, Lektrakul N et al (2000) Pulley system in the fingers: normal anatomy and simulated lesions in cadavers at MR imaging, CT, and US with and without contrast material distention of the tendon sheath. Radiology 217:201–212

Herbert TJ, Fisher WE (1984) Management of the fractured scaphoid using a new bone screw. J Bone Joint Surg Br 66:114–123

Hirschmann A, Sutter R, Schweizer A, Pfirrmann CWA (2014) MRI of the thumb: anatomy and spectrum of findings in asymptomatic volunteers. AJR Am J Roentgenol 202:819–827

Hobby JL, Dixon AK, Bearcroft PW et al (2001) MR imaging of the wrist: effect on clinical diagnosis and patient care. Radiology 220:589–593

Hunter JC, Escobedo EM, Wilson AJ et al (1997) MR imaging of clinically suspected scaphoid fractures. AJR Am J Roentgenol 168:1287–1293

Inoue G, Sakuma M (1996) The natural history of scaphoid non-union. Radiographic and clinical analysis in 102 cases. Arch Orthop Trauma Surg 115:1–4

Johnson RP (1980) The acutely injured wrist and its residuals. Clin Orthop Relat Res 149:33–44

Johnstone DJ, Thorogood S, Smith WH, Scott TD (1997) A comparison of magnetic resonance imaging and arthroscopy in the investigation of chronic wrist pain. J Hand Surg Br 22:714–718

Jowett AD, Brukner PD (1997) Fifth metacarpal stress fracture in a female softball pitcher. Clin J Sport Med 7:220–221

Karantanas A, Dailiana Z, Malizos K (2007) The role of MR imaging in scaphoid disorders. Eur Radiol 17:2860–2871

Kato H, Nakamura R, Horii E et al (2000) Diagnostic imaging for fracture of the hook of the hamate. Hand Surg 5:19–24

Kleinert HE, Verdan C (1983) Report of the committee on tendon injuries (International Federation of Societies of surgery of the hand). J Hand Surg Am 8:794–798

Koch KM, Lorbiecki JE, Hinks RS, King KF (2009) A multispectral three-dimensional acquisition technique for imaging near metal implants. Magn Reson Med 61:381–390

Kuo CE, Wolfe SW (2008) Scapholunate instability: current concepts in diagnosis and management. J Hand Surg Am 33:998–1013

Laor T, Jaramillo D (2009) MR imaging insights into skeletal maturation: what is normal? Radiology 250:28–38

Leddy JP, Packer JW (1977) Avulsion of the profundus tendon insertion in athletes. J Hand Surg Am 2:66–69

Lee MJ, Kim S, Lee SA et al (2007) Overcoming artifacts from metallic orthopedic implant at high-field-strength MR imaging and multidetector CT. Radiographics 27:791–803

Lee RK, Ng AW, Tong CS et al (2013) Intrinsic ligament and triangular fibrocartilage complex tears of the wrist: comparison of MDCT arthrography, conventional 3-T MRI, and MR arthrography. Skeletal Radiol 42:1277–1285

Liebling MS, Berdon WE, Ruzal-Shapiro C et al (1995) Gymnasts' wrist (pseudorickets growth plate abnormality) in adolescent athletes: findings on plain films and MRI imaging. AJR Am J Rosentgenol 164:157–159

Lin GT, Amadio PC, An KN, Cooney WP (1989) Functional anatomy of the human digital flexor pulley system. J Hand Surg Am 14:949–956

Linkous MD, Pierce SD, Gilula LA (2000) Scapholunate ligamentous communicating defects in symptomatic and asymptomatic wrists: characteristics 1. Radiology 216:846–850

Lisle DA, Shepherd GJ, Cowderoy GA, O'Connell PT (2009) MR imaging of traumatic and overuse injuries of the wrist and hand in athletes. Magn Reson Imaging Clin N Am 17:639–654

Lu W, Pauly KB, Gold GE, Pauly JM, Hargreaves BA (2009) SEMAC: slice encoding for metal artifact correction in MRI. Magn Reson Med 62:66–76

Mak WH, Szabo RM, Myo GK (2012) Assessment of volar radiocarpal ligaments: MR arthrographic and arthroscopic correlation. AJR Am J Roentgenol 198:423–427

Manton GL, Schweitzer ME, Weishaupt D et al (2001) Partial interosseous ligament tears of the wrist: difficulty in utilizing either primary or secondary MRI signs. J Comput Assist Tomogr 25:671–676

Manuel J, Moran SL (2007) The diagnosis and treatment of scapholunate instability. Orthop Clin N Am 38:261–277

McAuliffe JA (2010) Tendon disorders of the hand and wrist. J Hand Surg Am 35:846–853

Metz VM, Mann FA, Gilula LA (1993a) Three-compartment wrist arthrography: correlation of pain site with location of uni- and bidirectional communications. AJR Am J Roentgenol 160:819–822

Metz VM, Mann FA, Gilula LA (1993b) Lack of correlation between site of wrist pain and location of noncommunicating defects shown by three-compartment wrist arthrography. AJR Am J Roentgenol 160:1239–1243

Mikić ZD (1978) Age changes in the triangular fibrocartilage of the wrist joint. J Anat 126:367–384

Milch H (1932) Fracture of the hamate bone. J Bone Joint Surg Am 16:459–462

Mitsuyasu H, Patterson RM, Shah MA et al (2004) The role of the dorsal intercarpal ligament in dynamic and static scapholunate instability. J Hand Surg Am 29:279–288

Momeni A, Grauel E, Chang J (2010) Complications after flexor tendon injuries. Hand Clin 26:179–189

Morelli JN, Runge VM, Ai F et al (2011) An image-based approach to understanding the physics of MR artifacts. Radiographics 31:849–866

Mosher TJ (2006) Musculoskeletal imaging at 3T: current techniques and future applications. Magn Reson Imaging Clin N Am 14:63–76

Nakamura T, Yabe Y, Horiuchi Y (1999) Dynamic changes in the shape of the triangular fibrocartilage complex during rotation demonstrated with high resolution magnetic resonance imaging. J Hand Surg Br 24:338–341

Ng AW, Griffith JF, Taljanovic MS et al (2013) Is dynamic contrast-enhanced MRI useful for assessing proximal fragment vascularity in scaphoid fracture delayed and non-union? Skeletal Radiol 42:983–992

Nikken JJ, Oei EH, Ginai AZ et al (2005) Acute wrist trauma: value of a short dedicated extremity MR imaging examination in prediction of need for treatment 1. Radiology 234:116–124

Obdeijn MC, van der Vlies CH, van Rijn RR (2010) Capitate and hamate fracture in a child: the value of MRI imaging. Emerg Radiol 17:157–159

Palmer AK, Werner FW (1981) The triangular fibrocartilage complex of the wrist—anatomy and function. J Hand Surg Am 6:153–162

Palmer AK, Glisson RR, Werner FW (1984) Relationship between ulnar variance and triangular fibrocartilage complex thickness. J Hand Surg Am 9:681–682

Peh WCG, Chan JHM (1998) The magic angle phenomenon in tendons: effect of varying the MR echo time. Br J Radiol 71:31–36

Peh WCG, Chan JHM (2001) Artifacts in musculoskeletal magnetic resonance imaging: identification and correction. Skeletal Radiol 30:179–191

Potter HG, Asnis-Ernberg L, Weiland AJ et al (1997) The utility of high-resolution magnetic resonance imaging in the evaluation of the triangular fibrocartilage complex of the wrist. J Bone Joint Surg Am 79:1675–1684

Raghupathi AK, Kumar P (2014) Nonscaphoid carpal injuries-incidence and associated injuries. J Orthop 11:91–95

Rayan GM, Murray D, Chung KW, Rohrer M (1997) The extensor retinacular system at the metacarpophalangeal joint. Anatomical and histological study. J Hand Surg Br 22:585–590

Ringler MD (2013) MRI of wrist ligaments. J Hand Surg Am 38:2034–2046

Rozmaryn LM, Wei N (1999) Metacarapophalangeal arthroscopy. Arthroscopy 15:333–337

Ruch DS, Poehling GG (1996) Arthroscopic management of partial scapholunate and lunotriquetral injuries of the wrist. J Hand Surg Am 21:412–417

Sachar K (2008) Ulnar-sided wrist pain: evaluation and treatment of triangular fibrocartilage complex tears, ulnocarpal impaction syndrome, and lunotriquetral ligament tears. J Hand Surg Am 33:1669–1679

Sakai T, Sugano N, Nishii T et al (2000) MR findings of necrotic lesions and the extralesional area of osteonecrosis of the femoral head. Skelet Radiol 29:133–141

Scalcione LR, Pathria MN, Chung CB (2010) The athlete's hand: ligament and tendon injuries. Semin Musculoskelet Radiol 16:338–350

Schmid MR, Schertler T, Pfirrmann CW et al (2005) Interosseous ligament tears of the wrist: comparison of multi-detector row CT arthrography and MR imaging 1. Radiology 237:1008–1013

Schmitt R, Christopoulos G, Wagner M et al (2011) Avascular necrosis (AVN) of the proximal fragment in scaphoid non-union: is intravenous contrast agent necessary in MRI? Eur J Radiol 77:222–227

Schweitzer ME, Brahme SK, Hodler J et al (1992) Chronic wrist pain: spin-echo and short tau inversion recovery MR imaging and conventional and MR arthrography. Radiology 182:205–211

Sebag G, Ducou Le Pointe H, Klein I et al (1997) Dynamic gadolinium-enhanced subtraction MR imaging–a simple technique for the early diagnosis of Legg-calve´-Perthes disease: preliminary results. Pediatr Radiol 27:216–220

Shabshin N, Schweitzer ME (2009) Age dependent T2 changes of bone marrow in pediatric wrist MRI. Skeletal Radiol 38:1163–1168

Shih C, Chang CY, Penn IW et al (1995) Chronically stressed wrists in adolescent gymnasts: MR imaging appearance. Radiology 195:855–859

Singh DR, Chin MSM, Peh WCG (2014) Artifacts in musculoskeletal MR imaging. Semin Musculoskelet Radiol 18:12–22

Slutsky DJ (2008) Incidence of dorsal radiocarpal ligament tears in the presence of other intercarpal derangements. Arthroscopy 24:526–533

Smith DK, Snearly WN (1994) Lunotriquetral interosseous ligament of the wrist: MR appearances in asymptomatic volunteers and arthrographically normal wrists. Radiology 191:199–202

Smith TB, Nayak KS (2010) MRI artifacts and correction strategies. Imaging Med 2:445–457

Soila KP, Viamonte M Jr, Starewicz PM (1984) Chemical shift misregistration effect in magnetic resonance imaging. Radiology 153:819–820

Steinmann SP, Adams JE (2006) Scaphoid fractures and non-unions: diagnosis and treatment. J Orthop Sci 11:424–431

Suh N, Ek ET, Wolfe SW (2014) Carpal fractures. J Hand Surg Am 39:785–791

Taber KH, Herrick RC, Weathers SW et al (1998) Pitfalls and artifacts encountered in clinical MR imaging of the spine. Radiographics 18:1499–1521

Taccone A, Oddone M, Dell'Acqua AD et al (1995) MRI "roadmap" of normal age related bone marrow. II. Thorax and extremities. Pediatr Radiol 25:588–595

Taleisnik J (1976) The ligaments of the wrist. J Hand Surg Am 1:110–118

Taleisnik J (1988) Current concepts review. Carpal instability. J Bone Joint Surg Am 70:1262–1268

Taneja AK, Bredella MA, Chang CY et al (2013) Extrinsic wrist ligaments: prevalence of injury by magnetic resonance imaging and association with intrinsic ligament tears. J Comput Assist Tomogr 37:783–789

Theumann NH, Etechami G, Duvoisin B et al (2006) Association between extrinsic and intrinsic carpal ligament injuries at MR arthrography and carpal instability at radiography: initial observations 1. Radiology 238:950–957

Tibrewal S, Jayakumar P, Vaidyas et al (2012) Role of MRI in the diagnosis and management of patients with clinical scaphoid fracture. Int Orthop 36:107–110

Timins ME, Jahnke JP, Krah SF et al (1995) MR imaging of the major carpal stabilizing ligaments: normal anatomy and clinical examples. Radiographics 15:575–587

Tomaino MM (1998) Ulnar impaction syndrome in the ulnar negative and neutral wrist. Diagnosis and patho-anatomy. J Hand Surg Br 23:754–757

Totterman SMS, Miller RJ (1995) Triangular fibrocarti-lage complex: normal appearance on coronal three-dimensional gradient-recalled-echo MR images. Radiology 195:521–527

Totterman SM, Miller RJ (1996) Scapholunate ligament: normal MR appearance on three-dimensional gradient-recalled-echo images. Radiology 200:237–241

Tsiouri C, Hayton MJ, Baratz M (2009) Injury to the ulnar collateral ligament of the thumb. Hand 4:12–18

Urban MA, Green DP, Aufdemorte TB (1993) The patchy configuration of scaphoid avascular necrosis. J Hand Surg Am 18:669–674

Van Onselen EB, Karim RB, Hage JJ et al (2003) Prevalence and distribution of hand fractures. J Hand Surg Br 28:491–510

Vande Berg B, Malghem J, Labaisse MA et al (1992) Avascular necrosis of the hip: comparison of contrast-enhanced and nonenhanced MR imaging with histologic correlation. Work in progress. Radiology 182:445–450

Vezeridis PS, Yoshioka H, Han R et al (2010) Ulnar-sided wrist pain. Part I: anatomy and physical examination. Skeletal Radiol 39:733–745

Viegas SF, Ballantyne G (1987) Attritional lesions of the wrist joint. J Hand Surg Am 12:1025–1029

Viegas SF, Patterson RM, Hokanson JA et al (1993) Wrist anatomy: incidence, distribution, and correlation of anatomic variations, tears, and arthrosis. J Hand Surg Am 18:463–475

Waninger KN, Lombardo JA (1995) Stress fracture of index metacarpal in an adolescent tennis player. Clin J Sport Med 5:63–66

Weiss AP, Sachar K, Glowacki KA (1997) Arthroscopic debridement alone for intercarpal ligament tears. J Hand Surg Am 22:344–349

Weissman BN (2009) Expert consult. In: Imaging of arthritis and metabolic bone disease. Saunders/Elsevier, Philadelphia

Wolfe SW, Hotchkiss RN, Pederson WC, Kozin SH (2011) Flexor tendon injury. In: Green's operative hand surgery, 6th edn. Elsevier/Churchill Livingstone, Philadelphia

Wright TW, Charco MD, Wheeler D (1994) Incidence of ligament lesions and associated degenerative changes in the elderly wrist. J Hand Surg Am 19:313–318

Yin YM, Evanoff B, Gilula LA et al (1996) Evaluation of selective wrist arthrography of contralateral asymp-tomatic wrists for symmetric ligamentous defects. AJR Am J Roentgenol 166:1067–1073

Yoshioka H, Tanaka T, Ueno T et al (2006) High-resolution MR imaging of the proximal zone of the lunotriquetral ligament with a microscopy coil. Skeletal Radiol 35:288–294

Zanetti M, Linkous MD, Gilula LA, Hodler J (2000) Characteristics of triangular fibrocartilage defects in symptomatic and contralateral asymptomatic wrists. Radiology 216:840–845

Zhuo J, Gullapalli RP (2006) AAPM/RSNA physics tuto-rial for residents: MR artifacts, safety, and quality con-trol. Radiographics 26:275–272

Zlatkin MB, Chao PC, Osterman AL et al (1989) Chronic wrist pain: evaluation with high-resolution MR imag-ing. Radiology 173:723–729

Zlatkin MB, Rosner J (2004) MR imaging of ligaments and triangular fibrocartilage complex of the wrist. Magn Reson Imaging Clin N Am 12:301–331

Wrist and Hand Injuries: US Pitfalls

20

Graham Buirski and Javier Arnaiz

Contents

20.1   **Introduction** 381

20.2   **Selected Technique-Specific Pitfalls** 382
20.2.1   Equipment/Transducer Selection 382
20.2.2   Dynamic Imaging 382

20.3   **Diagnostic-Specific Pitfalls: Normal Variants** 382

20.4   **Diagnostic-Specific Pitfalls: Pathological Misinterpretations** 384
20.4.1   Dorsal Wrist Tenosynovitis 384
20.4.2   Extensor Carpi Ulnaris Instability 384
20.4.3   Trigger Finger 386
20.4.4   Flexor Tendon Tear 387
20.4.5   Pulley Tear 387
20.4.6   Boxer Knuckle 387
20.4.7   Gamekeeper Thumb (Skier Thumb) 388

Conclusion 389

References 389

G. Buirski, MD (✉)
Department of Radiology, Sidra Medical
and Research Center, Al Dafna, Doha, Qatar
e-mail: gbuirski@me.com

J. Arnaiz, MD
Department of Radiology, Aspetar Orthopaedic
and Sports Medicine Hospital,
Sports City Street, Doha, Qatar
e-mail: javierarnaiz@outlook.com

Abbreviation

US   Ultrasound
POC   Point-of-care

20.1 Introduction

Injuries to the wrist and hand are common and are responsible for 28% of all musculoskeletal trauma (Karabay 2013). Some injuries may be due to chronic repetitive strain, leading to partial or complete tears of tendons or tendon degeneration (tendinopathy). As in all other areas of the body, concerns of radiation exposure and the increased availability of "point-of-care" ultrasound (US) (POCUS) allow the treating physician immediate imaging assessment in cases of trauma to the wrist and hand (Patel et al. 2009).

Correlation with the clinical symptoms and comparison imaging with the normal contralateral side provide the physician a unique opportunity to enhance their physical examination. Stress and dynamic US imaging is an important part in assessing the complex mobile anatomy of the wrist and hand. Due to this anatomical complexity, the radiologist still has an important diagnostic role in soft tissue injuries and patient management.

Following the same format as Chap. 18 on elbow injuries, selected pitfalls in the production of US images (including the role of dynamic imaging) of the wrist and hand will be discussed. Operator knowledge of local complex anatomy is

© Springer International Publishing AG 2017
W.C.G. Peh (ed.), *Pitfalls in Musculoskeletal Radiology*, DOI 10.1007/978-3-319-53496-1_20

important in correct interpretation of wrist and hand pathology. Certain relevant anatomical variations as well as common misinterpretations of US imaging pathology will be highlighted.

20.2 Selected Technique-Specific Pitfalls

Most of the technique-selected pitfalls related to US imaging have been covered in Chap. 18 on elbow injuries. A few selected pitfalls specific to the wrist and hand are highlighted below.

20.2.1 Equipment/Transducer Selection

There is a wide range of US equipment available, with each machine having certain transducers

with different resolution capabilities (Kane et al. 2010). Physicians need to be continually mindful of the diagnostic capabilities of their US machines. For instance, small portable machines may not provide enough diagnostic resolution for small tendons or ligaments in the hand. The complex superficial anatomy of the wrist and hand is ideally suited to the small "hockey stick" transducer; its high-resolution capabilities and small area of skin contact allows focused dynamic and stress imaging to be performed (Fig. 20.1).

20.2.2 Dynamic Imaging

The use of dynamic and stress imaging is a vital part of musculoskeletal US imaging (Bouffard and Goitz 2010; Jacobson 2013). Dynamic imaging is important in the hand and wrist (Jacobson 2013). Stress imaging of the flexor tendons of the fingers may be the only way to demonstrate pulley rupture (see below Sect. 20.4.5). Flexion and extension of the fingers under US imaging is used to confirm extensor hood rupture and dynamic dislocation of the extensor tendon (boxer knuckle: see below Sect. 20.4.6).

20.3 Diagnostic-Specific Pitfalls: Normal Variants

Many osseous and soft tissue anatomical variants have been described around the wrist and hand (Martinoli et al. 2000; Sookur et al. 2008).

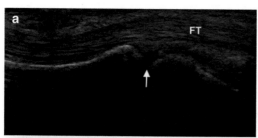
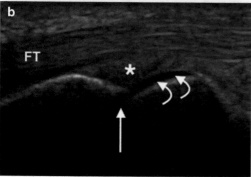

Fig. 20.1 US images show improved resolution and detail with different transducers. (**a**) Longitudinal 12 MHz linear array image of flexor tendon (*FT*) and PIPJ (*straight arrow*) of the finger. Note the long length of the tendon imaged using the large footprint. (**b**) Hockey stick 15 MHz image of the same joint. Although the length of tendon imaged is reduced, detail has improved. The volar plate (*) and articular cartilage of the metacarpal head are now clearly visible (*curved arrows*)

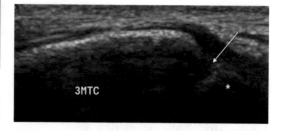

Fig. 20.2 US image of os styloideum. Dorsal prominence of the base of the third metacarpal (*MTC*) is seen. The os styloideum (*) is separated from the metacarpal base (*arrow*), and this should not be mistaken for a fracture

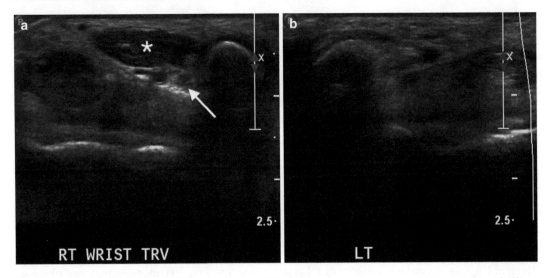

Fig 20.3 Abductor digiti minimi muscle in Guyon canal. (**a**) Transverse US image shows the accessory muscle (*) on the right with posterior displacement of the ulna nerve (*arrow*) (**b**) Normal left side is shown for comparison (Courtesy of Dr. W. Breidahl)

Although many of these variants may not have any clinical significance, they need to be recognized so as not to be mistaken for posttraumatic lesions. Normal variants can sometimes be responsible for clinical symptoms, leading to potential pitfalls in diagnosis and interpretation.

In the hand, the os styloideum on the dorsal aspect of the base of the third metacarpal may cause swelling and soft tissue deformity (Fig. 20.2). US imaging may show prominence of the metacarpal base with a separated bone fragment; this should not be misinterpreted as a fracture. Radiographs or computed tomography (CT) will confirm this as a normal variant.

Accessory muscles have been identified around the wrist and hand (Sookur et al. 2008). Although most are not clinically relevant, when they extend into osteofibrous anatomical tunnels, they may simulate soft tissue masses and cause nerve compression (Martinoli et al. 2000). An accessory flexor carpi ulnaris, abductor digiti minimi (Fig. 20.3), or anomalous hypothenar adductor may all extend into Guyon canal with subsequent compression of the ulnar nerve. Extensor digitorum brevis manus in extensor compartment 4 can simulate a soft tissue mass on the dorsum of the wrist (Fig. 20.4). The median nerve can be compressed in the carpal tunnel by palmaris longus variants. Neurological symp-

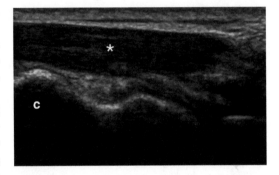

Fig 20.4 US image shows the extensor digitorum brevis manus muscle (*) lying dorsal to the capitate (*C*). The patient presented with pain and a soft tissue mass

toms may be worsened by exercise, chronic low-grade trauma, or repetitive movements causing increased swelling, venous congestion, and edema of theses muscles. Variations of tendon anatomy may occur around the wrist and hand.

The median nerve can divide into two nerve bundles in the distal forearm (high division) and appear as a bifid median nerve in the carpal tunnel. It has an incidence of 3%. A bifid median nerve may be accompanied by an accessory artery (median artery), which lies in between the two nerve bundles (Fig. 20.5). This normal variant should not be mistaken for median nerve thickening secondary to carpal tunnel syndrome. The associated median artery can be easily detected on

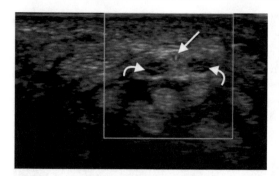

Fig. 20.5 US image shows bifid median nerve (*curved arrows*) with accessory median artery (*straight arrow*) between the nerve bundles

Doppler US imaging, and it is essential that this is mentioned in the radiologist's report to avoid injury to the nerve and artery during surgical release of the transverse carpal ligament.

20.4 Diagnostic-Specific Pitfalls: Pathological Misinterpretations

20.4.1 Dorsal Wrist Tenosynovitis

The tendons of the dorsal wrist are invested by a synovial sheath. Any of the dorsal compartments of the wrist can develop tenosynovial inflammation (tenosynovitis), which is normally due to overuse or chronic low-grade trauma secondary to sport or occupational activities. Diagnosis of tenosynovitis with US imaging is not difficult. The affected tendons are typically swollen and have a larger cross-sectional area than in normal subjects or when compared to the contralateral normal side. The synovial sheath is thickened, with or without an associated effusion, and has increased vascularity on color Doppler US imaging. Transducer compression will help distinguish between fluid and synovial thickening. Care must be taken to avoid anisotropy of the normal extensor retinaculum which might be mistaken for tenosynovitis or fluid. Compression and changes in inclination of the probe will demonstrate the absence of fluid and normal retinacular appearances.

The most frequently affected site of dorsal wrist tenosynovitis is extensor compartment 1, namely, de Quervain disease (Fig. 20.6). The other three most commonly affected extensor tendon complexes are:

- At the level where the extensor carpi radialis brevis (ECRB) and longus (ECRL) are crossed superficially by the abductor pollicis longus and extensor pollicis brevis (proximal intersection syndrome)
- Where the extensor pollicis longus crosses superficial to ECRB and ECRL (distal intersection syndrome)
- In the ulnar groove involving the extensor carpi ulnaris (extensor compartment 6)

The extensor digitorum and extensor indicis tendons occupy extensor compartment 4 and are surrounded by a thick fibrillar retinaculum that prevents bowstringing during extension. This retinaculum can mimic tenosynovitis on US imaging as it appears as a thick hypoechoic rim surrounding the tendon, particularly when lower-frequency transducers are used. Its tapered normal anatomical morphology distally on longitudinal scans (Fig. 20.7) distinguishes it from true tenosynovitis. In rare cases of extensor digitorum tenosynovitis, longitudinal scans show a characteristic "dumbbell" appearance as the fluid and inflamed tenosynovium are compressed by the retinaculum (Fig. 20.8).

20.4.2 Extensor Carpi Ulnaris Instability

A unique anatomical characteristic of the extensor carpi ulnaris (ECU) is its fibro-osseous tunnel, which stabilizes the tendon at the level of the distal ulna. This fibro-osseous tunnel is formed by the distal ulna and connective tissue referred to as the ECU subsheath. This retains the ECU tendon in its correct position during forearm rotation and flexion-extension. An ECU subsheath tear is a result of acute trauma, chronic overuse, and inflammatory changes (e.g., rheumatoid disease) in the ECU tendon sheath. Acute and

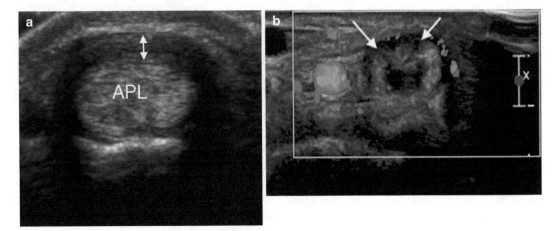

Fig. 20.6 de Quervain tenosynovitis. (**a**) The abductor pollicis longus tendon (*APL*) is thickened and hypoechoic due to tendinopathy. Associated synovial thickening is seen (*double head arrow*). (**b**) In another patient, the synovitis shows increased Doppler flow around an enlarged hypoechoic tendon. Note the normal variant of multiple tendon slips (*arrows*) which should not be mistaken for multiple longitudinal tears

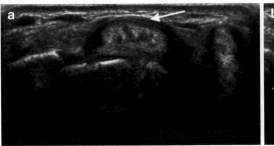

Fig. 20.7 Normal extensor retinaculum. (**a**) Transverse and (**b**) longitudinal US images show the normal hypoechoic fibrillar structure of the retinaculum (*straight arrow*) which tapers distally on the longitudinal images (*curved arrow*). This should not be mistaken for a thickened synovial sheath

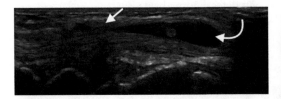

Fig. 20.8 US of extensor tenosynovitis. Rather than tapering, the distal synovial sheath is distended with an effusion (*curved arrow*) but proximally remains constricted by the retinaculum (*straight arrow*)

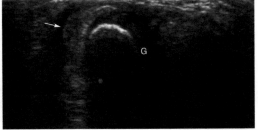

Fig. 20.9 ECU dislocation. US image shows that the ECU tendon (*arrow*) lies anterior and medial to the ulnar groove (*G*). The tendon is thickened and hypoechoic due to associated tendinopathy

chronic tears can be observed in sport injuries, including tennis, when the player performs a powerful pronation from a supinated position. This causes a sudden contraction of the ECU, which stabilizes the ulnar head, and may lead to stripping of the subsheath. Regardless of the cause of the tear, the ECU tendon undergoes anterior (volar) dislocation (Fig. 20.9).

Chronic instability of the ECU may result in either subluxation, when the flattened tendon moves over the medial aspect of the ulna, or intermittent dislocation, when there may be either spontaneous phases of dislocation and reduction or permanent dislocation. Because of its high-resolution and dynamic capabilities, US imaging is the ideal imaging tool to confirm instability of the ECU tendon. Permanent dislocation of the ECU is uncommon and can best be identified on transverse rather than sagittal imaging obtained over the posteromedial aspect of the ulna. Transient dislocation may cause symptoms, and this possibility needs to be considered during the examination. To avoid false-negative results, care should be taken not to limit the US examination to the static assessment of the tendon. Transverse imaging during progressive pronation of the forearm can reveal the progressive displacement of the ECU tendon over the ulnar head. Once again, it is important not to use too much transducer pressure, as this may prevent visualization of abnormal ECU motion.

The main difficulty with assessing tendon instability is the large variation of movement seen in asymptomatic volunteers. ECU tendon displacement of up to 50% of the tendon width from the ulnar groove may be observed in asymptomatic patients and is greatest in supination, flexion, and ulnar deviation (Lee et al. 2009). Features of associated tendinopathy, tendon fiber disruption, and correlation with clinical symptoms would support the diagnosis of symptomatic ECU subluxation.

20.4.3 Trigger Finger

Trigger finger is the term given to reflect a restricted range of motion which can be confirmed on dynamic US imaging. It may or may not be associated with locking or catching during movement. It is predominately due to a focal stenosing tenosynovitis of any finger, with hypertrophy of a flexor pulley or retinaculum (thickness 1–1.5 mm measured at the 10 o'clock and 2 o'clock positions on axial images; normal thickness <0.5 mm). This is usually localized to the A1 pulley but occasionally involves A2 (Fig. 20.10). An associated tendon sheath effusion and adjacent focal tendinopathy may be seen. Thickening of the pulley should be differentiated from a more diffuse tenosynovitis. The latter shows enlargement of the tendon sheath due to fluid or synovial thickening associated with variable focal or diffuse tendon enlargement. There may be associated diffuse soft tissue inflammatory edema around the tendon. Examination of the full length of tendon or group of tendons is required in the axial plane using minimal transducer pressure to avoid effacing tendon sheath effusion or vascularity. Always include evaluation with color Doppler imaging to help distinguish vascular synovial proliferation from synovial fluid. Examine nearby joints for synovitis or effusion to exclude underlying inflammatory joint disease and compare with contralateral normal side.

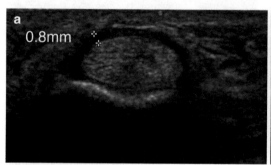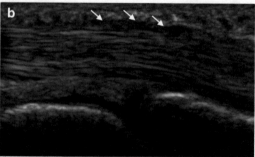

Fig. 20.10 Trigger finger. Abnormally thickened A1 pulley (0.8 mm; normal <0.5 mm) of the flexor tendon seen on the (**a**) transverse and (**b**) longitudinal US images (*arrows*)

20.4.4 Flexor Tendon Tear

Flexor tendon tears can be partial or complete, and they are usually the result of penetrating injuries. More rarely, tendon tears are caused by rheumatoid arthritis or closed trauma. A partial tear presents as a fusiform hypoechoic swelling of the tendon with focal interruption of the internal fibrillar pattern. It may be difficult to differentiate from focal tendinopathy based on US imaging findings alone. Clinical findings and history are essential for this purpose. When doubts arise, dynamic US scanning should be done during passive and active movements of the finger to evaluate the continuity of tendons and to differentiate between partial and complete ruptures.

In complete tears, the ruptured tendon may not be visualized at the site of injury. The retracted tendon forms an irregular hyperechoic mass with loss of fibrillar echoes and, in many cases, posterior acoustic shadowing. Acute tears are frequently associated with a tendon sheath effusion; while in chronic tears, the retracted tendon is surrounded by a hypoechoic area that reflects perilesional adhesions and fibrosis. US imaging plays a dual role in assessing complete tendon tears. It serves not only to confirm the clinical diagnosis but also to demonstrate and quantify the length of retraction of the proximal tendon stump. This is particularly helpful since tendon retraction is difficult, if not impossible, to assess clinically (Bianchi et al. 2007). It is therefore essential that scanning is extended proximally in order to identify the position of the retracted tendon (Fig. 20.11). In the presence of a flexor tendon

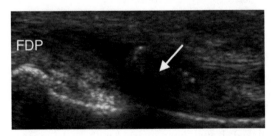

Fig. 20.11 US image shows complete tear and retraction of the superficial flexor tendon. Only the profunda tendon (*FDP*) is intact with the superficial tendon (*straight arrow*) retracted into the palm forming an echogenic mass-like structure (Courtesy of Dr. W. Breidahl)

injury, the volar plate and collateral ligament complexes need to be assessed to exclude associated abnormalities.

20.4.5 Pulley Tear

Acute tears of the annular pulleys are among the most frequent lesions in elite climbers. They most commonly involve the ring and middle fingers. Tears are commonly seen in free climbers who use handgrips in which the entire weight of the body is borne by a single finger (Bianchi et al. 2007). Stress US imaging of the flexor tendons is an integral part of this examination. A partial pulley tear consists of pulley thickening (usually A2) without bowstringing of flexor tendon during isometric flexion stress. Normally the clinical history is essential to differentiate partial pulley tear from trigger finger.

If the tendon separates in a volar direction away from proximal phalanx (bowstringing), then this indicates complete pulley tear. An increased distance of the flexor tendon to the mid-volar cortical surface of the proximal phalanx of more than 1 mm indicates a pulley injury. Klauser et al. (2002) showed that increasing bowstring distances reflect the number of pulley ruptures. When the distance is greater than 3 mm, then this indicates complete A2 pulley rupture (Fig. 20.12). If the distance is greater than 5 mm with forced isometric flexion, the A2 and A3 pulleys are torn. If the distance at the middle phalanx is more than 2.5 mm, then this indicates A4 pulley rupture.

20.4.6 Boxer Knuckle

Boxer knuckle is the term used to describe an extensor hood sagittal band tear at the MCP joint with subluxation/dislocation of the common extensor tendon during finger flexion (Lopez-Ben et al. 2003). This is normally due to a direct blow, while the joint is flexed and finger ulnarly deviated. Static US images normally demonstrate swelling of the soft tissues with normal

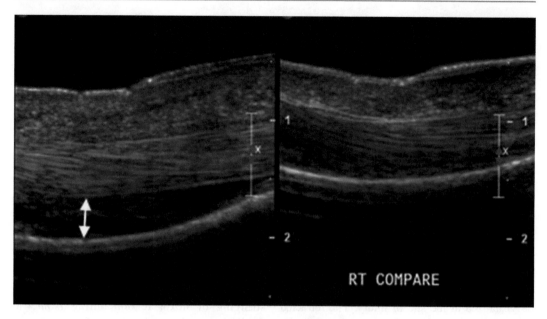

Fig. 20.12 Ruptured A2 flexor pulley. Stress longitudinal US images show displacement (bowstringing) of the flexor tendon away from the phalanx due to pulley rupture (*double arrow*). Normal right side is shown for comparison (Courtesy of Dr. B. Giuffre)

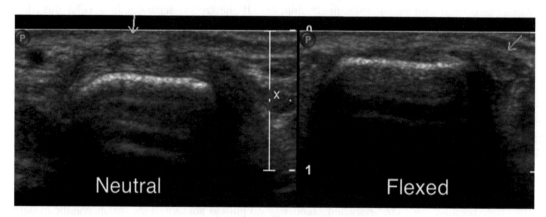

Fig. 20.13 US imaging of extensor hood rupture. In the neutral position, the extensor tendon (*arrow*) lies in its correct position. During flexion, the tendon dislocates in an ulnar direction (Courtesy of Dr. W. Breidahl)

echogenicity in the common extensor tendon that may mimic tenosynovitis. Dynamic imaging of the extensor tendons is essential to confirm this condition. The extensor tendon sheath of the knuckle may be displaced slightly from the dorsum toward the ulna when the fingers are fully extended. With flexion of the MCP joint, ulnar subluxation or dislocation of the common extensor tendon with respect to the dorsal metacarpal bone is visualized, reflecting the tear of the extensor hood (Fig. 20.13).

20.4.7 Gamekeeper Thumb (Skier Thumb)

Rupture of the ulnar collateral ligament (UCL) of the metacarpophalangeal joint of the thumb is caused by hyperabduction, while the thumb is flexed. It may be associated with avulsion fracture at the ligament insertion. Partial or complete tears can be easily differentiated using dynamic stress US scanning. A partial tear is seen as ligament thickening, whereas a complete tear is a

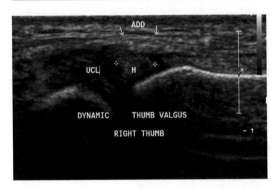

Fig. 20.14 US imaging of complete ulnar collateral ligament tear. The MCPJ is widened with the valgus stress and the tear is filled with hematoma (*H*). Note the normal appearances and position of the adductor (*ADD*) aponeurosis (*arrows*)

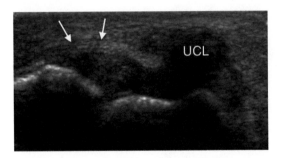

Fig. 20.15 Stener lesion. US image shows that the ulnar collateral ligament (*UCL*) is completely torn and retracted proximally, lying partially superficial to the adductor aponeurosis (*arrows*)

detached, discontinuous ligament with significant widening of the joint during abduction stress maneuvers (Fig. 20.14).

Occasionally, the UCL ligament retracts, allowing interposition of adductor pollicis aponeurosis between UCL and first metacarpal head (Stener lesion) (Fig. 20.15). The retracted ligament fibers appear "mass-like" with acoustic shadowing similar to a bone avulsion fragment. However, its position superficial to the adductor aponeurosis should allow identification of this lesion. The aponeurosis can be identified by passive flexion and extension movement of the distal phalanx, as there is a connection between the adductor pollicis insertion and extensor pollicis tendon. It is important to recognize a Stener lesion, as surgery is required to reattach the ligament. A small "hockey stick" high-frequency (10 MHz) transducer is recom-

mended for high-resolution US imaging and to obtain adequate anatomical access to the ligament.

Conclusion

Complex superficial anatomy of the wrist and hand is ideally suited to high-resolution dynamic US imaging. Imaging should be always be performed and reconciled with the patient's clinical history and examination. Understanding the normal anatomical structures, movement, and anatomical variants in the hand and wrist is essential in avoiding misinterpretation of pathology and injury.

References

Bianchi S, Martinoli C, de Gautard R, Gaignot C (2007) Ultrasound of the digital flexor system: normal and pathological findings. J Ultrasound 10:85–92

Bouffard JA, Goitz H (2010) Ultrasound in sports medicine. In: Essential applications of musculoskeletal ultrasound in rheumatology. Elsevier, Philadelphia

Jacobson JA (2013) Wrist and Hand Ultrasound. In: Fundamentals of Musculoskeletal Ultrasound, 2nd edn. Elsevier, Philadelphia

Kane D, Kitchen J, Hammer HB (2010) Purchasing ultrasound equipment. In: Essential applications of musculoskeletal ultrasound in rheumatology. Elsevier, Philadelphia

Karabay N (2013) US findings in traumatic wrist and hand injuries. Diagn Interv Radiol 19:320–325

Klauser A, Frauscher F, Bodner G et al (2002) Finger pulley injuries in extreme rock climbers: depiction with dynamic US. Radiology 222:755–761

Lee KS, Ablove RH, Singh S et al (2009) Ultrasound imaging of normal displacement of the extensor carpi ulnaris tendon within the ulnar groove in 12 forearm-wrist positions. AJR Am J Roentgenol 193:651–605

Lopez-Ben R, Lee DH, Nicolodi DJ (2003) Boxer knuckle (injury of the extensor hood with extensor tendon subluxation): diagnosis with dynamic ultrasound – report of three cases. Radiology 220:642–646

Martinoli C, Bianchi S, Gandolfo N et al (2000) US of nerve entrapments in osteofibrous tunnels of the upper and lower limbs. Radiographics 20:S199–S217

Patel DD, Blumberg SM, Crain EF (2009) The utility of bedside ultrasonography in identifying fractures and guiding fracture reduction in children. Paed Emerg Care 25:221–225

Sookur PA, Naraghi AM, Bleakney RR et al (2008) Accessory muscles: anatomy symptoms and radiologic evaluation. Radiographics 28:481–499

Taljanovic MS, Melville DM, Scalcione LR et al (2014) Artifacts in musculoskeletal ultrasonography. Semin Musculoskelet Radiol 18:3–11

Hip Injury: MRI Pitfalls

21

Lauren M. Ladd, Donna G. Blankenbaker,
and Michael J. Tuite

Contents

21.1 **Introduction** 391

21.2 **Intra-articular Hip Anatomy, Injuries,
 and Mimics** 392
21.2.1 Acetabular Labrum 392
21.2.2 Hip Cartilage 396
21.2.3 Ligamentum Teres 397

21.3 **Muscle and Soft Tissue Injuries and
 Mimics** 399
21.3.1 Tendon Tears and Avulsions 399
21.3.2 Myotendinous Strain 401
21.3.3 Muscle Contusion 403
21.3.4 Pitfalls and Mimics of Acute Muscle and
 Tendon Injuries 404
21.3.5 Other Soft Tissue Normal Variants and
 Mimics 406

21.4 **Osseous Injuries and Mimics** 406
21.4.1 Fatigue and Insufficiency Fractures 407
21.4.2 Contusions 408
21.4.3 Pitfalls and Mimics of Acute Osseous
 Injury 409

Conclusion 411

References 411

L.M. Ladd, MD (✉)
Department of Radiology, Indiana University School
of Medicine, 1701 North Senate Boulevard,
MH1238A, Indianapolis, IN 46202, USA
e-mail: LMLadd@iupui.edu

D.G. Blankenbaker, MD • M.J. Tuite, MD
Department of Radiology, University of Wisconsin,
School of Medicine and Public Health,
E3/366 Clinical Science Center, 600 Highland
Avenue, Madison, WI 53792-3252, USA
e-mail: DBlankenbaker@uwhealth.org;
MTuite@uwhealth.org

Abbreviation

MRI   Magnetic resonance imaging

21.1 Introduction

The hip joint is a complex articulation of important osseous and soft tissue structures and is the key to movement between the torso and lower extremities. Many everyday functions, such as walking and sitting/standing, as well as athletic activities, depend on proper alignment and function of the structures in and about the hip. Trauma, from acute injury or chronic overuse, may limit these essential functions and result in significant morbidity. Thus, prompt and accurate diagnosis of the source of hip pain is vital to improving quality of life and preventing further joint damage. After initial radiographic evaluation, magnetic resonance imaging (MRI) is generally the imaging method of choice for the hip, due to its superior soft tissue contrast. An in-depth knowledge of the MRI appearance of normal hip structures, as well as injuries and mimics of abnormalities, is crucial to correctly evaluate the hip and diagnose sources of pain. MRI of normal hip structures, common hip injuries, and hip imaging pitfalls will be reviewed in this chapter.

21.2 Intra-articular Hip Anatomy, Injuries, and Mimics

21.2.1 Acetabular Labrum

The acetabular labrum is a horseshoe-shaped fibrocartilaginous structure attached to the rim of the bony acetabulum. The transverse ligament creates a complete ring inferiorly, attaching to the anterior and posterior margins of the inferior labrum (Fig. 21.1). The labrum is composed of type I collagen fibers that predominantly parallel the acetabular rim (Hodler et al. 1995; Nguyen et al. 2013) with little internal vascularity. What vascular nourishment that is present arises from a network of small peripheral capsular vessels (McCarthy et al. 2003; Petersen et al. 2003) and supplies predominantly the peripheral third of the labral tissue, limiting potential primary and postoperative healing (Seldes et al. 2001; McCarthy et al. 2003). Despite a limited vascu-

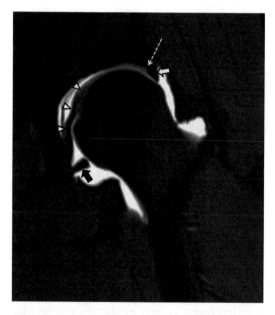

Fig. 21.1 Coronal fat-suppressed T1-W MR arthrographic image of normal hip anatomy. The hypointense fibrocartilaginous labrum (*thick white arrow*) is intact and triangular, and the transverse ligament is seen inferiorly (*thick black arrow*). Normal appearance of the cartilage and hyperintense chondrolabral transition zone (*long dashed arrow*). The ligamentum teres is intact, originating from the fovea of the femoral head and inserting inferomedially on the transverse ligament (*arrowheads*)

lar supply, there is an ample network of nerve endings with nociceptive and proprioceptive functions, explaining why labral tears may be painful (Kim and Azuma 1995). The cross-section shape of the labrum is triangular in the majority of individuals, with the base attached to the bony acetabulum and acetabular cartilage (Lecouvet et al. 1996). A normal transitional zone of 1–3 mm between the labral fibrocartilage and adjacent articular hyaline cartilage (Fig. 21.1) is important to recognize, when evaluating for labral tears or chondrolabral separation, so as not to confuse for a labral tear (Hodler et al. 1995; Seldes et al. 2001).

21.2.1.1 Labral Tears

Injury of the labrum may be acute due to trauma or chronic from ongoing "wear and tear." Labral tears are common, particularly in patients with hip or groin pain, and lead to greater loss of time from sport in athletes than any other lower extremity injuries (Narvani et al. 2003). Overall, there is an increase in incidence of labral tears with age, and degenerative tearing is believed to be a part of normal aging, exemplified by an incidence as high as 96% in cadaveric specimens (Schmerl et al. 2005). Although nerve endings within the labrum may contribute to pain when the labrum is torn, MRI studies of asymptomatic patients have demonstrated a high incidence of labral tears that are not symptomatic, including a study by Register and colleagues that documented labral tears by MR arthrography in 69% of asymptomatic patients (Register et al. 2012).

Given the high prevalence, it is important to be able to identify labral tears and to distinguish them from normal variants and mimickers of tears. Labral tears are most common in the anterior or anterosuperior quadrant (Blankenbaker et al. 2007) (Fig. 21.2). Posterior tears may be seen with posterior dislocations or subluxations, as well as with acetabular retroversion. Because there is poor correlation between MRI and surgical arthroscopic labral tear classification systems, it is recommended to report labral tear morphology, extent, and location, rather than specific labral tear classification (Blankenbaker et al. 2007).

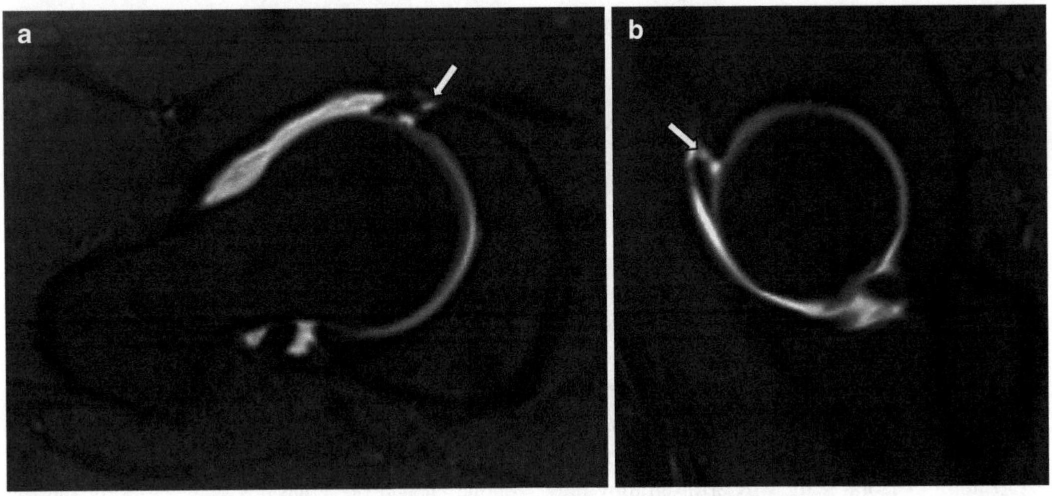

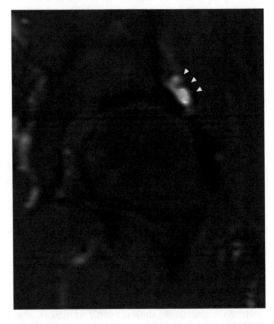

Fig. 21.2 33-year-old woman presenting with left hip and groin pain. (**a**) Oblique axial and (**b**) sagittal fat-suppressed T1-W MR arthrographic images show a complete tear of the anterior labrum with contrast cleft extending across labral base at its expected attachment to the bony acetabulum (*thick white arrow*)

Imaging findings of labral tears include linear hyperintense signal or contrast agent extending into or through the labral substance, a blunted or rounded labral margin, or complete detachment from the acetabulum (Fig. 21.2). Despite differences in technology, such as magnet strength and improving image resolution, MR arthrography has greater accuracy for detection of labral tears (90–95% sensitivity) than conventional MRI (30–87% sensitivity) and is favored for detailed evaluation of the labrum and intra-articular structures (Czerny et al. 1996; Smith et al. 2010; Tian et al. 2014; Naraghi and White 2015). Secondary signs of labral tears include paralabral cysts and adjacent cartilage damage. Paralabral cysts typically extend extra-articularly into the perilabral recess between the labrum and joint capsule or external to the joint capsule (Fig. 21.3). However, intraosseous extension can also be seen. These cysts may or may not fill with intra-articular contrast material (Thomas et al. 2013).

21.2.1.2 Normal Variants and Tear Mimics

Although labral signal and morphologic abnormalities may be due to labral tears, there are several anatomical variants that mimic labral pathology and may be mistaken for tears, if not

Fig. 21.3 45-year-old man with hip pain. Coronal STIR MR image shows a prominent left lateral acetabular paralabral cyst (*arrowheads*), resulting from an underlying labral tear. Note the rounded cyst-like shape, which helps differentiate this from the normal perilabral recess

understood and accurately recognized. Potentially confusing variants include labral signal intensity, labral shape and symmetry, chondrolabral junction, sublabral sulci, labroligamentous sulcus, perilabral recess, and os acetabuli.

Because it is fibrocartilage, the labrum is expected to be hypointense on all MRI sequences. However, intermediate labral signal may be seen in up to 40–60% of "normal" patients without symptoms, labral tear, or histologic degeneration (Hodler et al. 1995; Cotten et al. 1998). This is more frequently noted on T1-weighted and proton density (PD) pulse sequences (short echo time). However, a small percentage of these patients may also have corresponding altered T2 signal as well (Cotten et al. 1998). The abnormal signal may be globular, linear, or curvilinear and is more commonly seen in the anterior and superior labrum, which unfortunately corresponds to the commonest location of labral tears. MR arthrography may be useful to help differentiate from a labral tear.

As previously described, the labrum is most commonly triangular in cross section. This triangular configuration, however, is only seen in approximately 66% of asymptomatic patients, according to Lecouvet et al. (1996). Normal variations in shape include a rounded (~10%) or flattened (~10%) labrum. Labral hypoplasia or absence is described by some as a normal phenomenon, reportedly found in 1–10% of the population (Lecouvet et al. 1996; Cotten et al. 1998). In general though, absence of the labrum is more commonly seen in older individuals and is considered abnormal, likely due to degeneration or a chronic tear. In addition to general shape variability, the labra may vary in shape and size by 25% and 15%, respectively, in the contralateral hips of the same patient (Aydingöz and Oztürk 2001).

Hyperintense signal at the chondrolabral junction is another commonly misinterpreted imaging finding (Fig. 21.1). Mildly hyperintense signal at the articular surface of the labral base may be seen with cartilage undercutting (DuBois and Omar 2010) and the previously described transition zone of the labral attachment to the articular cartilage. Relatively fluid-dense hyaline cartilage has higher signal intensity than the labrum and may extend beneath the labral base, resulting in linear intermediate to hyperintense signal at the chondrolabral junction. This is differentiated from a labral tear because the signal is hypointense to fluid or contrast material, and it smoothly parallels the labral base and acetabular rim.

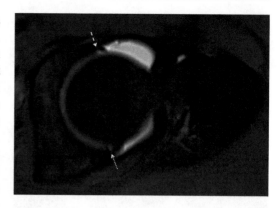

Fig. 21.4 25-year-old woman with history of fall. Oblique axial fat-suppressed T1-W MR arthrographic image shows a small smooth cleft at the articular surface of the chondrolabral junction both anteriorly (*dashed arrow*) and posteriorly (*dotted arrow*), consistent with small anteroinferior and posterior sublabral sulci

Another cause of hyperintense signal at the chondrolabral junction may be due to a sublabral sulcus (Fig. 21.4). This normal variant sulcus is located where the labrum meets the adjacent cartilage but is not directly attached at the articular surface. This sulcus is present in approximately 20–25% of the normal population and should not be confused with a labral tear (Dinauer et al. 2007; Studler et al. 2008). Studler et al. (2008) best described the sublabral sulcus as a smooth shallow defect at the labral base along the articular surface, which involves less than one-third of the labral thickness and often has a larger width than depth. Keys to differentiating the normal variant sulcus from a tear include its smooth contour, limited depth, and lack of secondary abnormalities, such as chondral damage or paralabral cysts. Although described in a variety of locations, sublabral sulci are most commonly found at the posterior and anteroinferior labrum.

Similar to the sublabral sulcus, another smooth shallow cleft at the chondrolabral base may be seen at the junction of the anterior labrum and transverse ligament. This is referred to as the labroligamentous sulcus and is found in up to one-third of normal, asymptomatic individuals (Dinauer et al. 2007). Recognition of this variant is largely based on its location and helps to avoid mistaking it for a labral tear.

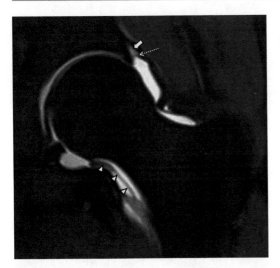

Fig. 21.5 17-year-old girl with a history of persistent left hip pain and popping after falling down stairs. Coronal fat-suppressed T1-W MR arthrographic image shows the normal perilabral recess (*thick white arrow*) with contrast material between the lateral margin of the labrum and the joint capsule, extending a few millimeters cranial to the labrum along the lateral acetabulum. Additional normal variants noted include a labral plica (*dotted white arrow*) and pectinofoveal fold (*arrowheads*), which should not be confused for a labral tear or displaced ligamentum teres tear, respectively

Another normal potential fluid-filled cleft to recognize is the perilabral recess, which is located between the joint capsule and labrum at its superficial, non-articular surface (Fig. 21.5). At the superolateral acetabulum, the joint capsule attaches to the bony acetabulum about 2–3 mm superior to the osseous-labral attachment. The potential space between the capsule and labrum may fill with joint fluid or contrast agent, often in a linear or rounded configuration (DuBois and Omar 2010). Thus, this may be confused for a labral tear or paralabral cyst. Anteriorly and posteriorly, the capsule attaches more directly to the labrum, so the perilabral recess should only be identified superiorly. Further, within this recess, a thin linear hypointense band of tissue may be seen, known as a labral plica, which may further complicate the appearance and mimic a circumscribed paralabral cyst or a torn labrum (Fig. 21.5).

The last and commonly overlooked mimicker of a labral tear is an os acetabuli (Fig. 21.6). This entity is often considered as a normal variant and is found in 2–3% of asymptomatic patients. It may be a developmental labral calcification,

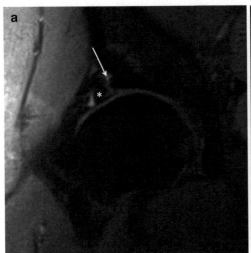

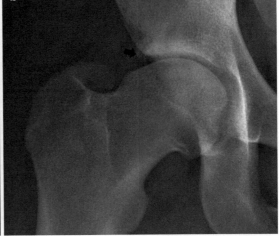

Fig. 21.6 22-year-old male football player with hip pain for several years. (**a**) Coronal fat-suppressed PD-W MR image shows a prominent os acetabuli (*asterisk*), mimicking a labral tear, with a fluid-filled cleft (*thin white arrow*) between the ossicle and the remaining acetabulum. (**b**) Frontal radiograph confirms the os acetabuli (*thick black arrow*) and can be key in helping make this diagnosis

sequela of a secondary ossification center non-union, or result of an incompletely healed acetabular rim fracture (DuBois and Omar 2010). Because the ossification demonstrates hypointense signal on MRI, particularly on fat-suppressed sequences, it may blend with the hypointense labral fibrocartilage and be unrecognized. If the ossification is not identified, the relatively high signal interface with the adjacent acetabular rim and chondrolabral junction may be mistaken for a labral tear.

In summary, labral signal intensity and shape, sulci, and os acetabuli are important variations in hip anatomy to recognize and understand for accurate interpretation of MRI of the hip labrum.

21.2.2 Hip Cartilage

Unlike the fibrocartilage of the labrum, the articular cartilage of the acetabulum and femoral head is hyaline cartilage, which is made up of predominantly water (80%) reinforced by chondrocytes and a type II collagen and proteoglycan matrix (Petchprapa and Recht 2013). This hyaline cartilage covers the majority of the femoral head, sparing only the fovea superomedially where the ligamentum teres attaches. The articular cartilage of the acetabulum covers the bony surface, otherwise known as the lunate surface. Therefore, the cartilage creates a horseshoe-shape configuration with discontinuity medially at the acetabular fossa and inferiorly at the acetabular notch. In general, the cartilage is thickest at the superolateral acetabulum and anterosuperior femoral head, where there is greatest contact and need for load-bearing support.

21.2.2.1 Cartilage Injury

Chondral damage may be caused by shearing, impact, or routine wear on an incongruent joint. Because of its high water content, cartilage is generally hyperintense on T2-weighted MR images and intermediate signal on proton density and fat-suppressed MR arthrographic images (Fig. 21.1). Injury to the cartilage is identified on MRI as generalized thinning, surface irregularity,

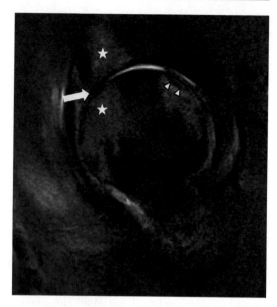

Fig. 21.7 44-year-old man with primary osteoarthritis of the right hip. Sagittal fat-suppressed PD-W MR image shows full-thickness cartilage loss of the anterosuperior acetabulum and femoral head (*thick white arrow*), resulting in bone-on-bone articulation and subchondral bone marrow edema (*white stars*). Posterior cartilage loss with a subchondral insufficiency fracture (*white arrowheads*) and adjacent bone marrow edema of the posterior femoral head are also present

fissures, delamination, chondral flaps, or full-thickness cartilage defects (Bharam 2006) (Fig. 21.7). Most cartilage injuries involve the anterior acetabulum, followed by the superior and posterior acetabulum, and chondral lesions are often accompanied by labral pathology, particularly when higher grade cartilage damage is present (Yen and Kocher 2010).

The cartilage grading systems of the knee, including the modified Outerbridge and modified Noyes criteria, can be applied to the hip. However, there is limited accuracy, largely due to the rounded contours of the hip joint and difficulty obtaining tangential imaging planes. Although limited in accuracy, MR arthrography is superior to conventional MRI for detection of cartilage damage, similar to labral tear identification, with 71–92% sensitivity for MR arthrography and 58–83% for conventional MRI (Schmid et al. 2003; Mintz et al. 2005; Sutter et al. 2014).

21.2.2.2 Normal Variants and Injury Mimics

Although a focal gap or fluid-filled defect is considered a finding of cartilage damage, there are several normal anatomical variants that present as focal gaps or indentations of the articular cartilage, which should not be confused for cartilage pathology. Two normal variations of the articular cartilage include the supraacetabular fossa and the stellate crease.

The supraacetabular fossa is a focal cavity in the superior weight-bearing region of the acetabulum, located at approximately the 12 o'clock position (Fig. 21.8). This focal indentation may be associated with a defect of the underlying bone and may or may not be filled with fibrous tissue, excluding it from filling with fluid or contrast agent (Dietrich et al. 2012). It has been identified in up to 10% of the normal population and is often seen in individuals less than 30 years of age, suggesting a developmental etiology (Byrd 2012). According to Dietrich et al. (2012), the average fossa measures 3 mm in depth and 4.5 mm in width. This normal variant can be

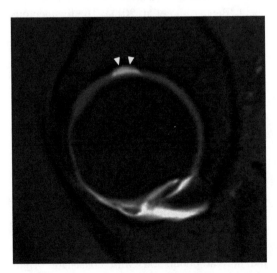

Fig. 21.8 25-year-old woman with left hip pain and popping. Sagittal fat-suppressed T1-W MR arthrographic image shows a small focal, smooth fossa at the superior acetabulum, demonstrating indentation of the subchondral bone and absence of normal cartilage, consistent with a normal variant supraacetabular fossa. This should not be confused for an abnormal cartilage defect or injury

differentiated from cartilage defects and osteochondral lesions because it is a smooth focal indentation in a characteristic location without associated subchondral bone marrow edema or adjacent cartilage irregularity.

In a similar but separate superior central acetabular location, the other normal variant cleft is the stellate crease. Described by arthroscopists in the early 1990s, this is a bare area at the anterosuperior margin of the acetabular fossa (Keene and Villar 1994). It is linear in configuration and located closer to the acetabular fossa than the previously described supraacetabular fossa (DuBois and Omar 2010). The lack of underlying subchondral bone abnormality helps differentiate it from a true cartilage defect.

21.2.3 Ligamentum Teres

The ligamentum teres is composed of two to three bundles of connective tissue, including randomly organized collagen, fibrous tissue, and fat, with interspersed vessels and nerve fibers (Dehao et al. 2015). It originates as a broad band from the transverse ligament and courses superolaterally to insert on the fovea capitis of the femoral head (Cerezal et al. 2010) (Fig. 21.1). Although it is relatively flat near its origin, it becomes thicker and more rounded as it approaches the femoral head. When the hip is flexed, adducted, and/or externally rotated, it becomes taut (Byrd and Jones 2004).

Histologically, the ligamentum teres has been proven to contain small vessels lined by fat and scattered nerve fibers (Dehao et al. 2015). These small vessels have little role in supplying the femoral head and may minimally nourish the substance of the ligamentum teres (Dehao et al. 2015). However, in a small percentage of the adult population (up to 30%), the ligamentum teres transmits a branch of the obturator artery, contributing to the femoral head blood supply (Anderson et al. 2001). Due to the scattered nerve fibers, the ligamentum teres plays a role in proprioception and fine motor coordination of the hip (Dehao et al. 2015), as well as nociception and painful symptoms when injured or torn.

21.2.3.1 Ligamentum Teres Tears

Ligamentum teres tears may be caused by acute trauma, congenital deformities, or chronic degeneration. Gray and Villar (1997) first described a three-part classification system for labral tears, including complete tears associated with dislocation or trauma, partial tears associated with a subacute event, and degenerative tears with associated joint pathology, such as osteoarthritis, chondral injury, or labral tears. Since the creation of this classification system, a study by Botser and colleagues demonstrated a much higher prevalence (about 50% of the population) with a more inclusive classification system that describes ligamentum injuries by degree of tear, including <50%, >50%, and 100% thickness tears (Botser et al. 2011).

As it may be the source of hip pain, it is important to assess the ligamentum teres in one's routine search pattern on hip MRI. The normal appearance on MRI is a hypointense band on all sequences, due to its fibrous nature and composition of tightly packed collagen bundles. Tears are most easily identified when complete, demonstrating absence when chronic and a redundant displaced band of tissue when acute. Other appearances of a torn ligamentum teres include thickened intermediate signal with degeneration or degenerative intra-substance tearing, irregularity of the fibers with fraying, and disrupted fibers or fluid signal intensity within a distorted ligament with partial tears (Blankenbaker et al. 2012) (Fig. 21.9). Although this may seem relatively simple, the ability to correctly identify ligamentum teres tears on MRI is limited, with sensitivities cited at 1.8–29% and false-positive rates up to 22% (Byrd and Jones 2004; Botser et al. 2011; Blankenbaker et al. 2012).

21.2.3.2 Normal Variants and Tear Mimics

To further complicate assessment of the already difficult-to-identify tears, there are several normal variants that can mimic ligamentum teres tears. Firstly, there may be congenital absence of the ligamentum teres, particularly in patients with a history of developmental dysplasia of the hip (DuBois and Omar 2010). Further, several normal variant plicae may persist in the hip after development. Two of these three plicae may

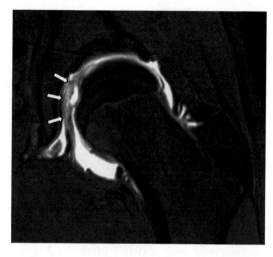

Fig. 21.9 13-year-old boy with left hip pain and concern for labral tear. Coronal fat-suppressed T1-W MR arthrographic image shows a high-grade partial-thickness tear of the ligamentum teres (*white arrows*). There is extensive irregularity of the ligament, greatest proximally near its insertion on the fovea, with hyperintense signal and contrast material extending through its fibers

mimic ligamentum teres pathology, namely, the ligamentous plicae, located within the acetabular fossa, and the neck plicae, found parallel to the inferior femoral neck near the transverse ligament (Bencardino et al. 2011). The ligamentous plicae are particularly problematic and may be confused with a partial-thickness longitudinal tear of the ligamentum teres as it courses parallel to the ligamentum teres from its base at the acetabular fossa (Bencardino et al. 2011) (Fig. 21.10).

Alternatively, an injured ligamentum teres with associated calcification may mimic an intra-articular body (Ebraheim et al. 1991). Lastly, the pectinofoveal fold, band-like tissue at the medial aspect of the hip joint extending from the proximal hip joint capsule inferolaterally to the femur, is a plica-like normal variant that may be confused for torn displaced ligamentum teres tissue. It is a smooth linear tissue identified in 95% of the normal population, with consistent origin from the joint capsule proximally and extension to or near the femur distally (Blankenbaker et al. 2009) (Fig. 21.5). Knowing the presence and appearance of these normal variants and potential confounding structures, or lack thereof, is important to avoid incorrect interpretation of a normal ligamentum teres.

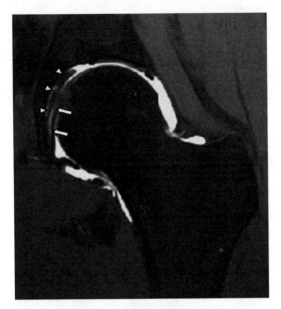

Fig. 21.10 Coronal fat-suppressed T1-W MR arthrographic image shows a linear band of hypointense tissue (*white arrowheads*) parallel to the ligamentum teres (*white arrows*), extending superolaterally from the acetabular fossa base to near the level of the fovea. This is a normal variant ligamentous plica, not to be mistaken for a partial-thickness or longitudinal tear of the ligamentum teres

21.3   Muscle and Soft Tissue Injuries and Mimics

Muscle and tendon injuries account for anywhere between 25% and 90% of injuries in athletes, both professional and recreational (Beiner and Jokl 2001; Ueblacker et al. 2015). Any of the muscles surrounding the hip may be injured, but the quadriceps, hamstring, and adductor muscles are the most commonly injured muscles of the hip and in the entire body (Armfield et al. 2006; Shelly et al. 2009). Acute injuries include tendon tears and avulsions, myotendinous strains, and muscle contusions. Edema is a main feature of acute muscle and tendon injuries on MRI but may also be seen with non-traumatic etiologies, such as normal exercise-induced muscle edema, denervation, and myositis (infectious or inflammatory). Attention to detail of the edema pattern, however, helps differentiate the type of injury and distinguish it from non-traumatic etiologies that can mimic an acute injury.

21.3.1   Tendon Tears and Avulsions

Acute tears and avulsions of tendons about the hip are less common than some of the other described injuries, such as strains and contusions, but are unique hip injuries and are important to recognize. These can be grouped into traumatic or degenerative categories. Acute traumatic injuries are result of extreme excessive force on the tendon or due to relatively normal forces applied to an abnormal or degenerated tendon. In children, the greatest weakness of the bone-tendon-muscle unit is at the unfused apophysis (Davis 2010), resulting in bony apophyseal avulsions.

Unlike children, adults are more likely to tear or avulse the tendon with similar injury mechanism. The result of complete tear or avulsion is tendon discontinuity from its bony attachment and a fluid-filled gap on T2-weighted images (Davis 2008) (Fig. 21.11). In the acute setting,

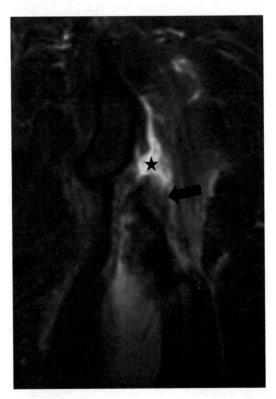

Fig. 21.11 45-year-old man with left buttock and hip pain. Coronal STIR MR image shows an acute complete avulsion of the left proximal common hamstring with an intervening fluid-filled gap (*star*), redundancy of the retracted tendon (*black arrow*), and associated surrounding edema and hemorrhage

bone marrow edema at the tendon's expected origin may also be present. It is important to differentiate these tears from tendinopathy (a thickened intermediate high signal tendon, not fluid signal) and from peritendinous bursae (a focal fluid collection adjacent to an intact continuous tendon). Because bursal fluid is linear or crescentic and associated with a nearby tendon, it may be easily mistaken for the fluid gap of a torn tendon. Examples of such bursae include the ischial bursa that overlies the proximal common hamstring tendon origin and the greater trochanteric bursa that overlies the gluteus medius tendon insertion.

The tendons that are more commonly avulse from their pelvic origins in adults during acute trauma or sporting injuries are those that are most commonly injured in general. These are the hamstring, quadriceps, and adductor tendons. Proximal common hamstring tendon tears or avulsions are relatively rare but are the most commonly described hip tendon avulsion in radiology and orthopedic literature (Fig. 21.11). These may be seen with the same forces that result in ischial avulsions in children, specifically forced flexion of the hip with an extended knee (such as in hurdling, splits, or kicking).

Even more infrequent, acute avulsions of the biceps femoris tendon may be seen (Fig. 21.12) and most commonly affect the direct head, given its primary function in initiation of hip flexion (Bordalo-Rodrigues and Rosenberg 2005). These injuries present with acute pain and a pop, followed by ecchymosis and swelling of the proximal anterior thigh. Adductor tendon or muscle avulsions are most commonly seen at the pubic origin and are more frequent in athletes who perform kicking motions where adduction may be resisted. This injury falls within the spectrum of sports hernias and athletic pubalgia, which is beyond the scope of this chapter.

Once an acute tendon tear or avulsion is identified, it is important to describe the presence and degree of tendon retraction because it affects surgical management. In general, retraction of >2 cm of any tendon avulsion may require surgical fixation. Specifically with the hamstring tendon origin, a three-tendon avul-

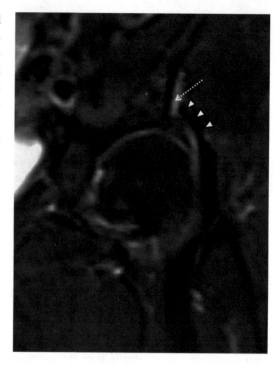

Fig. 21.12 67-year-old woman with left hip pain. Coronal STIR MR image shows a fluid-filled gap (*dotted arrow*) along the lateral acetabulum at the expected attachment of the indirect head of the rectus femoris tendon, which is slightly retracted (*arrowheads*). Avulsion of the direct head is more common than the indirect head shown here

sion regardless of degree of retraction requires urgent surgical repair to prevent future disability (Cohen et al. 2012).

Although the previously described tendon avulsions are rare, particularly in a healthy tendon, chronically injured or degenerated tendons may also be torn and should be appropriately recognized on imaging. Tendon degeneration may be due to overuse or sequela of a systemic process, such as rheumatoid arthritis, diabetes mellitus, chronic steroid use, or renal failure (Lecouvet et al. 2005). For example, tears at the greater trochanteric insertion of the gluteus medius and minimis tendons are relatively common in elderly patients and thought to be attritional (Stanton et al. 2012). These degenerative-type tears may be asymptomatic, but in the acute setting can produce pain and may be confused for "greater trochanteric pain syndrome." In the case of an acute retracted tear of a degenerated tendon, surgical fixation may still be the best treatment option. Thus, identification of the tear, measurement of tendon retraction, and note of muscle atrophy (indicating chronicity similar to rotator cuff muscles) are important descriptions to include.

Lastly, avulsion of the iliopsoas tendon from the lesser trochanter is another important tendon avulsion to recognize and accurately diagnose (Fig. 21.13). The appearance is similar to avulsion of the distal bicep tendon, with a fluid-filled gap and retracted distal tendon that may mimic a soft tissue mass, as well as bone marrow edema of the lesser trochanter (Lecouvet et al. 2005). Avulsion of this tendon has been described in case reports of older individuals (>60 years old) or in patients with underlying medical illness that predisposes to tendon weakness. However, careful analysis of the lesser trochanter is essential because an osseous tendon avulsion at this site is considered pathognomonic for an underlying pathologic lesion (Fig. 21.13), until proven otherwise.

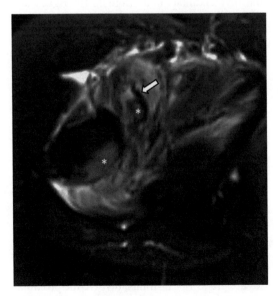

Fig. 21.13 66-year-old woman with severe progressive right hip pain. Axial fat-suppressed T2-W MR image shows a torn retracted iliopsoas tendon (*thick white arrow*) amidst extensive surrounding intramuscular edema. Careful analysis of the lesser trochanter reveals an underlying lesion and pathologic fracture of the trochanter (*asterisks*)

21.3.2 Myotendinous Strain

Myotendinous strains are an indirect stretch injury that causes fiber disruption of the muscle or myotendinous unit. Muscle strain is by far the commonest injury of the hip, accounting for up to 88% of hip injuries in elite soccer players (Ueblacker et al. 2015) and 59% of all hip injuries in a study of professional American football players (Feeley et al. 2008). Strains typically occur at the myotendinous junction, where the convergence of different tissues (muscle and tendon) is the weakest point of the bone-tendon-muscle unit. Additional anatomical and physiological characteristics that predispose specific muscles to strain include the following: (1) pennate muscle configuration, (2) biarticular myotendinous unit, (3) eccentric muscle contraction, and (4) high proportion of fast-twitch (type II) muscle fibers (Petersen and Holmich 2005; Thibodeau and Patton 2006). The rectus femoris and hamstring muscles fit each of these descriptions and are consequently the most commonly strained muscles of the hip and entire body (Shelly et al. 2009; Ueblacker et al. 2015).

Although often diagnosed clinically, MRI of muscle strains is quite useful for evaluation of strain severity and in guiding clinical treatment and return to play. These injuries are graded on MRI by feathery edema at the myotendinous junction (grade 1) (Fig. 21.14) and associated partial- (grade 2) or full-thickness (grade 3) tears. On axial images, this has a "bull's eye" appearance with a halo of high T2 (and possibly high T1) signal surrounding a central hypointense tendon (grade 1 and 2 injuries) (Fig. 21.15). Grade 2 and 3 injuries will demonstrate a fluid gap or hematoma, and those with complete tears often demonstrate retraction and resultant muscle enlargement (Shelly et al. 2009; McMahon et al. 2010). Fluid-sensitive sequences increase diagnostic sensitivity; however, T1-weighted sequences are equally important to identify loss of tissue planes and determine exact muscle and/or tendon involvement (De Smet and Best 2000). Chronic findings of muscle injury include hypointense scar at the site of injury (as early as 6 weeks after injury) and muscle atrophy with focal fatty replacement (Blankenbaker and Tuite 2010).

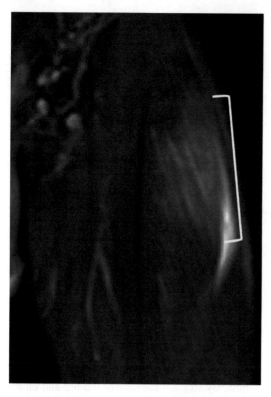

Fig. 21.14 19-year-old collegiate football player with painful palpable swelling in the left anterior thigh. Coronal STIR MR image shows feathery edema (*bracket*) following the pennate pattern of the rectus femoris muscle, consistent with a grade 1 strain

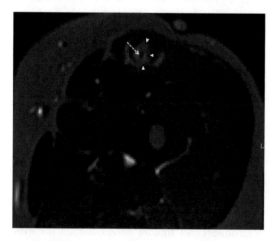

Fig. 21.15 16-year-old boy with left anterior thigh pain for 3–4 weeks, primarily when running or sprinting. Axial modified inversion recovery (MODIR) MR image shows the "bull's eye" sign of a strain of the rectus femoris tendon with a halo of high signal (*arrowheads*) surrounding the central hypointense tendon (*dashed arrow*)

As mentioned previously, the quadriceps, hamstring, and adductor muscles are most commonly strained. Given that these most commonly strained muscles are long muscles, a frequent pitfall is incompletely imaging the length of the muscle, excluding important information about the injury severity or extent. Thus, it is key to image the entire length of the muscle with both anatomy (T1-weighted or PD) and fluid-sensitive sequences. The rectus femoris tendon is the most central and superficial of the four quadriceps muscles. Proximally, it has two heads: the direct head originates from the anterior inferior iliac spine (AIIS) and indirect head from the anterolateral acetabular rim. The main functions of this muscle are to flex the hip and extend the knee. Therefore, it is most commonly injured with the hip hyperextended and knee flexed, such as in the backswing of kicking, or during sudden contraction of the rectus femoris, as when sprinting (Ouellette et al. 2006). Aside from rare avulsions that predominantly involve the direct head, the majority of rectus femoris strains involve the indirect head, particularly the deep muscular aspect of the proximal myotendinous unit (Bordalo-Rodrigues and Rosenberg 2005) (Fig. 21.14), with grade 2 strains being more common than grade 3. If an MR arthrogram is performed, contrast agent from the joint may transect the injured fibers due to the proximity and association with the hip joint capsule (Ouellette et al. 2006).

The hamstring is comprised of three myotendinous units, namely, the biceps femoris, semitendinosus, and semimembranosus, all of which originate from the ischial tuberosity and insert distally near the level of the knee. These muscles help in hip extension, knee flexion, and, most importantly, deceleration of knee extension by antagonizing the quadriceps muscle. Thus, the hamstring muscles are essential for most daily activities. The majority of acute hamstring injuries are grade 1 or 2 strains, involve the proximal myotendinous unit, and most commonly affect the biceps femoris muscle (De Smet and Best 2000; Silder et al. 2008). The intramuscular myotendinous junction is most often injured, rather than the proximal or distal attachment (De Smet and Best 2000). Focal hypointense signal or scar formation at the site of prior injury and atrophy of the injured biceps femoris muscle are often seen on follow-up imaging (Silder et al. 2008), contributing to the high prevalence of recurrent injury of this muscle group.

The adductor muscle group is comprised of the adductor longus, brevis, and magnus, as well as the pectineus and gracilis muscles. The adductor longus and brevis tendons originate from the superior pubic symphysis, where the longus has a larger footprint and the short adductor brevis tendon originates slightly posterolateral to the longus. Strains of this muscle group are most commonly seen in athletes who adduct or resist adduction of the leg most frequently, such as soccer, American football, and hockey players (Hölmich 2007; Feeley et al. 2008). These strains most commonly involve the proximal adductor longus myotendinous junction, with feathery intramuscular edema anterior to and within centimeters distal to the pubic symphysis (Koulouris 2008). A further discussion of chronic adductor dysfunction and athletic pubalgia is beyond the scope of this chapter but is an important source of groin pain in athletes.

21.3.3 Muscle Contusion

Acute muscle contusions most commonly occur at the anterior and lateral hip with contact sports, such as American football, rugby, soccer, lacrosse, and karate, and are often due to direct blows from an opponent's knee or helmet (Ryan et al. 1991). Contusions are caused by a crush injury of the muscle against the underlying firm immobile bone, predominantly affecting the deep muscle fibers. On clinical examination, there is often focal swelling and possibly a cutaneous hematoma at the site of injury. Contusion severity is classified clinically by loss of range of motion, such as limited extension of the knee with quadriceps contusions (Ryan et al. 1991).

The MRI appearance of contusions follows the underlying histological abnormality (Fig. 21.16). Focal, globular, or feathery intramuscular edema from extravasated blood, variable muscle fiber disruption, and reparative

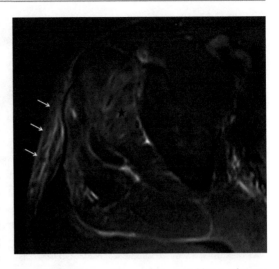

Fig. 21.16 24-year-old man with recent history of motor vehicle accident and persistent hip pain. Axial fat-suppressed T2-W MR image shows intramuscular hyperintense signal of the anterior gluteus minimis and medius muscles (*stars*) with overlying soft tissue edema (*arrows*), consistent with muscle and subcutaneous contusions

inflammatory cell-mediated edema is seen by 24 h after injury at the deep aspect of the muscle against the bone. The edema at the site of injury can appear somewhat mass-like due to an associated hematoma. Thus, signal characteristics should be carefully evaluated and correlated with the age of injury to accurately differentiate from a more ominous tumor. Acutely (<48 h), the T1 signal of a hematoma is isointense to muscle. Then, it becomes hyperintense on T1- and T2-weighted sequences in the subacute phase (<30 days) and eventually has a hypointense rim on all sequences in the chronic phase (Blankenbaker and Tuite 2010). The hematoma should decrease in size over 6–8 weeks. If it persists or enlarges, an underlying cause should be sought, such as a coagulopathy or an underlying hemorrhagic mass.

An important complication of direct muscle injury is myositis ossificans (Fig. 21.17). This is seen in up to 17% of direct trauma, particularly prevalent in the anterior compartment of the thigh. It is essential to accurately diagnose myositis ossificans because of its potential for misdiagnosis as a tumor on pathology. In the initial acute inflammatory and then subacute pseudotumoral stages, there

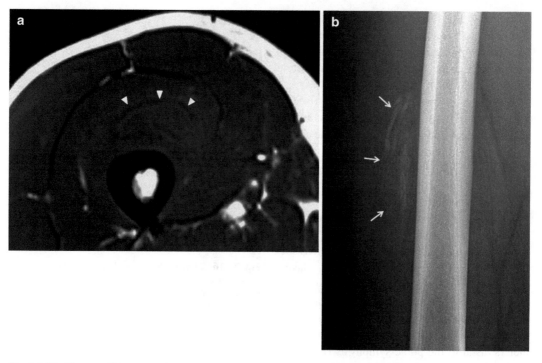

Fig. 21.17 15-year-old boy with femoral pain and history of trauma with contact of an opponent's helmet to his thigh while playing football. (**a**) Axial T1-W MR image of the anterior right proximal to mid-thigh shows a focal mass-like abnormality of the vastus intermedius muscle with a T1-hypointense rim (*arrowheads*). (**b**) Radiograph of the mid-femur shows developing peripheral ossification (*arrows*) confirming myositis ossificans as a result of prior muscle trauma and hematoma

is muscle enlargement, hyperintense T2 signal, and moderate surrounding edema/enhancement, due to degeneration and necrosis of the affected muscle. This occurs 1–2 weeks following injury and may mimic an abscess or tumor (Shelly et al. 2009). As the chronic mature stage ensues (as early as 2–4 weeks post injury), mesenchymal cells proliferate and peripheral calcification forms, resulting in a hypointense rim on MRI (Blankenbaker and Tuite 2010; Tyler and Saifuddin 2010). Again, this complication is one of the most important to recognize and accurately distinguish from a mass.

21.3.4 Pitfalls and Mimics of Acute Muscle and Tendon Injuries

The imaging patterns described above are helpful to identify acute injuries. Intramuscular and associated soft tissue edema may also be seen with non-traumatic causes and confused for injury, if not carefully scrutinized. Some of the causes include normal exercise-induced muscle edema, delayed-onset muscle soreness, denervation, and infectious or inflammatory myositis.

21.3.4.1 Exercise-Induced Muscle Edema and Delayed-Onset Muscle Soreness

An accumulation of extracellular water occurs normally during muscle exercise, which results in intramuscular T2-hyperintense signal on MRI and may be mistaken for strain, if imaged immediately following exertion. This typically resolves within minutes of rest (Counsel and Breidahl 2010). In those who are well trained, such as marathon runners, mild focal areas of T2 hyperintensity along the myotendinous junction, less prominent than strain or delayed-onset muscle soreness, may be seen and are believed to be a normal phenomenon from extreme exertion (Fleckenstein et al. 1989). Alternatively, strenuous activity in an otherwise sedentary individual may result in intramuscular and perifascial hyperintense T2 signal, which develops several days after activity and persists for days or weeks. This is known as delayed-onset muscle soreness (DOMS) and can be differentiated from strain by clinical history, where there is a delayed onset of symptoms as the name suggests (Fleckenstein et al. 1989).

21.3.4.2 Denervation

Denervation is another cause of diffuse high intramuscular signal, which can be seen within days of injury and be confused for muscle strain. Three distinct imaging features help distinguish acute or subacute denervation from strains, namely, a lack of perifascial edema (typical of strain), involvement of a group of muscles innervated by a single nerve, and nerve enlargement with hyperintense signal (Shelly et al. 2009). Patterns of denervation around the hip, common causes of entrapment or injury, and the expected affected muscle groups with signal change on MRI are described in Table 21.1. Although these are the expected patterns, one must realize that deviations from these

patterns may be due to aberrant or dual innervation, such as seen with the adductor brevis muscle (Petchprapa et al. 2010).

21.3.4.3 Myositis

Myositis, a broad term for infectious or other muscle inflammation, also results in muscle edema that may appear similar to traumatic muscle edema. Bacterial myositis is a result of direct spread from adjacent osteomyelitis or subcutaneous abscess (May et al. 2000). This manifests early on MRI as nonspecific muscle edema, progressing to intramuscular abscess later in its course. The key distinguishing feature is the associated osseous or subcutaneous infectious findings. Viral myositis also results in diffuse muscle edema, but without an associated infectious source to distinguish the cause, making history the most important differentiating feature for this process. Finally, idiopathic inflammatory myositides, including dermatomyositis and polymyositis, also produce diffuse muscle edema that can mimic traumatic muscle edema. On MRI, there is typically bilateral, symmetrical hyperintense T2 signal throughout the pelvic and thigh musculature (May et al. 2000) (Fig. 21.18), differentiating it from traumatic muscle edema.

Table 21.1 Neuropathies around the hip

Neuropathy	Entrapment	Muscle change on MRI
Femoral nerve Intrapelvic Distal	Iliac/psoas hematoma, injury At inguinal ligament	Iliopsoas Pectineus, sartorius, and quadriceps
Lateral femoral cutaneous nerve	At inguinal ligament Compressed (e.g., clothing)	None (sensory nerve)
Obturator nerve Anterior branch Posterior branch	Pelvic trauma, surgery, fascial adhesions from adductor brevis tendinopathy (athletes)	Adductor longus and gracilis Obturator externus and adductor magnus
Sciatic nerve	Iatrogenic (hip replacement), piriformis syndrome	Hamstrings and adductor magnus hamstring component
Superior gluteal nerve	Surgery (retraction)	Gluteus minimis and medius, tensor fascia lata

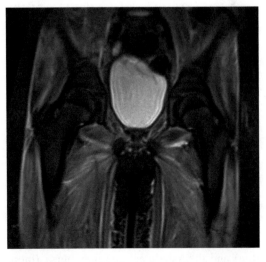

Fig. 21.18 9-year-old girl with progressive muscle weakness. Coronal STIR MR image shows diffuse bilateral symmetrical muscle edema throughout the pelvis and proximal thigh musculature, consistent with diffuse myositis

There are many causes of muscle edema that may mimic an acute muscle or tendon injury, a selection of which are described here. In general, the presence of perifascial edema and possibly associated subcutaneous edema favors a traumatic etiology (Counsel and Breidahl 2010).

21.3.5 Other Soft Tissue Normal Variants and Mimics

Bursal inflammation is a commonly diagnosed cause of hip pain. There are three main bursae of the hip, namely, the ischial bursa, iliopsoas bursa, and trochanteric bursa. As described previously, the ischial bursa overlies the proximal common hamstring tendon origin and may be confused for a tendon tear if not correctly identified.

The iliopsoas bursa is the largest bursa in the body, lying deep to the iliopsoas myotendinous junction and extending from the iliac fossa, beyond the anterior hip joint capsule, to its distal insertion on the lesser trochanter (Blankenbaker et al. 2006). This bursa, when filled with fluid, may indicate bursitis and cause for a patient's pain. However, one must take careful note of the presence of joint fluid because up to 15% of the general population have a normal communication between the hip joint capsule and the iliopsoas bursa (Varma et al. 1991) (Fig. 21.19). Therefore, fluid within the bursa may be an extension of hip joint fluid or arthrographic contrast agent when present, rather than a bursitis. Additionally, a rounded bursal fluid collection at the anterior hip should not be confused for a paralabral cyst. If pelvis imaging is equivocal, MR arthrogram may be beneficial to differentiate the two entities.

The greater trochanteric bursa overlies the posterior facet of the greater trochanter, near the attachment of the gluteus medius tendon insertion and vastus lateralis origin. Additional bursae in this region include the subgluteus medius bursa (deep to the gluteus medius tendon insertion) and the subgluteus minimis bursa (more anterior and deep to the gluteus minimis tendon insertion). Inflammation of these bursae is common and most often seen in middle-aged or

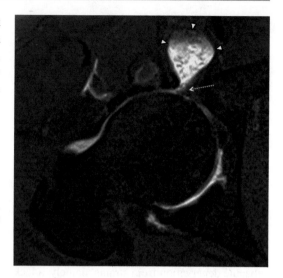

Fig. 21.19 44-year-old man with right hip pain. Axial fat-suppressed T1-W MR arthrographic image shows a distended iliopsoas bursa (*arrowheads*) containing debris, consistent with bursitis. However, it is noted that intra-articular contrast material fills the bursa and communicates with the hip joint space through a normal variant anterior communication (*dotted arrow*). Joint fluid or contrast material may be present due to this communication without presence of bursitis

older women, as well as those with obesity, trauma, and inflammatory arthritides (Hirji et al. 2011). While bursitis may be a cause of trochanteric pain, general peritrochanteric edema that is not a discrete fluid collection within the bursa may be seen in asymptomatic patients and should not be confused for bursitis (Blankenbaker et al. 2008).

21.4   Osseous Injuries and Mimics

Osseous injuries of the hip include a variety of fractures, including femoral head and neck fractures, fatigue and insufficiency fractures, and contusions. All these injuries have the potential to result in severe morbidity, which makes accurate diagnosis and differentiation from potential mimics essential. While acute traumatic fractures are important, most do not necessitate MRI. Rather, MRI is most useful for evaluation of suspected but radiographically occult fractures and "stress fractures."

21.4.1 Fatigue and Insufficiency Fractures

"Stress fracture" is a generalized term that includes two separate entities: fatigue and insufficiency fractures. The former is due to repetitive or abnormal stress on normal bone, and the latter are caused by normal stress on an abnormal bone. Fatigue and insufficiency fractures are common in the lower extremity, particularly in the proximal femur, because it is subjected to higher loading forces than other skeletal sites (Shane et al. 2014). Although these fractures are recognizable by characteristic MRI features, there are several non-traumatic causes of similar imaging findings that must be appropriately differentiated.

Fatigue fractures are most commonly seen in younger active individuals who participate in or are new to endurance athletics, such as long-distance running. These fractures occur most commonly at the inferomedial femoral neck where compressive trabeculae are receiving the most stress (referred to as a compressive-type fracture) (Lu et al. 2013; Sheehan et al. 2015). MRI reveals focal or diffuse bone marrow edema at the inferomedial femoral neck with or without a discrete linear T1-hypointense fracture line (Fig. 21.20). Opposite fatigue fractures are insufficiency fractures. These fractures occur in a number of locations around the hip, including at the femoral head, neck, and proximal lateral femoral diaphysis. They are most often found in elderly or osteoporotic individuals with abnormally weak bones that are injured by minimal or low-impact trauma.

At the femoral head, insufficiency fractures can be difficult to accurately diagnose, given their similarity to trauma-related subchondral fractures, as well as osteonecrosis. It is important to note, however, that these are three histopathologically distinct entities. Subchondral insufficiency fractures are typically located in the central or anterior femoral head and may occur with minimal trauma in older individuals (Figs. 21.7 and 21.21). On imaging, these fractures have been associated with concomitant cartilage loss, synovitis, and joint effusions, as well as greater trochanteric insertional tendinopathy (Hackney et al. 2015). MRI characteristics include a fracture line surrounded by

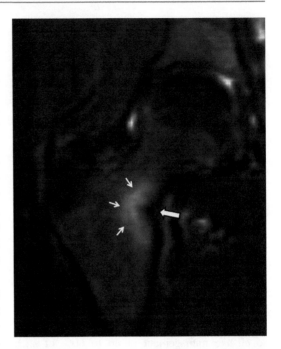

Fig. 21.20 26-year-old woman with history of hip pain. Coronal STIR MR image shows a fatigue fracture with focal bone marrow edema (*small white arrows*) and a small, incomplete transverse hypointense line (*thick arrow*) at the inferomedial femoral neck

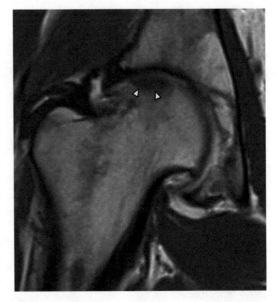

Fig. 21.21 44-year-old man with severe right hip pain. Coronal T1 MR image shows a subchondral convex hypointense line (*arrowheads*) at the superior femoral head with adjacent surrounding edema noted on fluid-sensitive images (Fig. 21.7), consistent with a subchondral insufficiency fracture

marrow edema (and contrast-enhancement) proximal and distal to the fracture line (Sheehan et al. 2015). The contour of the fracture line is typically described as parallel or convex (Hackney et al. 2015; Sheehan et al. 2015). These patterns, edema on either side of the fracture line, and the lack of a "double-line sign" (a bright T2 line of granulation tissue and an adjacent outer hypointense line of sclerotic bone) help differentiate it from its most commonly mistaken diagnosis of osteonecrosis.

Insufficiency fractures of the femoral neck are more commonly found at the lateral femoral neck (Fig. 21.22), where the tensile trabeculae extend more horizontally (hence, referred to as tensile-type fractures) (Lu et al. 2013; Sheehan et al. 2015). MRI is particularly helpful in these patients because these injuries are commonly radiographically occult in up to 44–85% of patients (Stiris and Lilleas 1997; Lee et al. 2004) and has been shown to change management in up to 60% of such patients (Lubovsky et al. 2005; Lee et al. 2004).

The third type of femoral insufficiency fracture identified in an older population is the atypical femur fracture, located at the lateral proximal femoral cortex. These fractures are associated with long-term bisphosphonate therapy as well as with other systemic illnesses, such as renal failure and corticosteroid use (Unnanuntana et al. 2013). On imaging, there is focal lateral proximal femoral cortical thickening (predominantly noted on radiographs) and associated focal marrow, endosteal, or periosteal edema on MRI (Sheehan et al. 2015). These fractures are located 60 mm distal to the greater trochanter on average, which helps differentiate it from mimics such as a prominent gluteal tubercle or third trochanter that measure an average of 3 mm distal to the trochanter (Maetani et al. 2015).

21.4.2 Contusions

Osseous contusions are another acute bony injury that could be confused for fracture or a more ominous osseous lesion, if not accurately recognized. Contusions are due to direct impact, often seen with contact sports such as American football, similar to

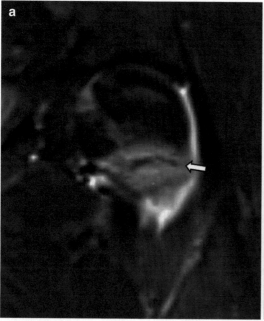
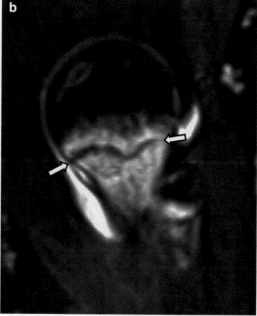

Fig. 21.22 60-year-old man with osteoporosis, renal failure, and hip pain. (**a**) Coronal STIR and (**b**) sagittal fat-suppressed T2-W MR images show extensive edema of the femoral neck with a central hypointense band, consistent with a fracture (*thick white arrows*). Given the position at the superolateral femoral neck and history of osteoporosis, this is consistent with an insufficiency (tensile-type) fracture of the femoral neck

muscle contusions. In these athletes, common locations include the iliac crests ("hip pointers") and proximal femoral diaphyses. The femoral neck and head are positioned in such a way that direct impact would be very difficult. Thus, femoral neck or head edema should not be related to a direct contusion. On MRI, there is a region of irregular bone marrow edema on fluid-sensitive sequences with or without associated hypointense T1 signal, depending on the severity of the edema. This edema may be similar in appearance to stress reaction. Therefore, patient history, physical examination (overlying ecchymosis), surrounding soft tissue edema, and location of the bone marrow edema are important differentiating features (Ladd et al. 2014).

21.4.3 Pitfalls and Mimics of Acute Osseous Injury

Bone marrow edema is the predominant finding of many of the aforementioned fractures and bone injuries. Similar edema patterns can be seen with a multitude of entities that may be confused for these traumatic osseous injuries, including bone tumors, infection, transient osteoporosis of the hip, and osteonecrosis.

21.4.3.1 Osteoid Osteomas

Bone tumors uncommonly produce significant bone marrow edema. However, for those that do, the diagnosis may be difficult on MRI. Osteoid osteomas are one benign bone tumor of the hip that may produce intramedullary edema that can mimic a traumatic injury (Fig. 21.23). Typically seen in adolescents and young adults, osteoid osteomas are most often found in the lower extremity, with 20–30% occurring in the proximal femur (Gaeta et al. 2004; Klontzas et al. 2015). The characteristic imaging features include a small central osteoid nidus surrounded by reactive sclerosis. When visible, the central nidus demonstrates intermediate to hyperintense signal on fluid-sensitive sequences. However, this nidus is often occult on MRI (Klontzas et al. 2015).

Intra-articular osteoid osteomas are particularly troublesome due to the lack of the classic reactive sclerosis and periosteal thickening, presenting with only the nonspecific findings of bone marrow edema, joint effusion and synovitis, and possibly peritumoral soft tissue edema (Gaeta et al. 2004) (Fig. 21.23). Klontzas and colleagues have proposed a "half-moon sign," as a characteristic feature of femoral neck osteoid osteomas. This sign is described as bone marrow

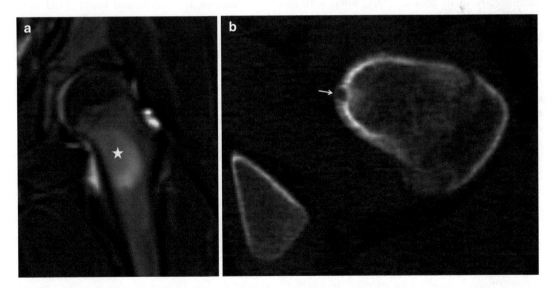

Fig. 21.23 9-year-old girl with left hip pain for 1 year. (**a**) Coronal STIR MR image shows edema throughout the inferomedial neck (*white star*) with an associated joint effusion. (**b**) Axial CT image confirms a small cortically based lucent nidus (*white arrow*), verifying an osteoid osteoma. Note that the nidus cannot be accurately identified on MRI

edema in the shape of a half-moon with the base along the cortex of the femoral neck. Although common in femoral neck osteoid osteomas, other pathology may infrequently demonstrate this sign as well (Klontzas et al. 2015). Thus, the patient's age, clinical symptoms, and additional imaging information, such as high- resolution CT for evaluation of a nidus, are most helpful in distinguishing this benign tumor from a traumatic etiology.

21.4.3.2 Septic Arthritis

Another concerning cause of bone marrow edema of the hip is septic arthritis. Although relatively rare, joint infections cause incredible morbidity and even mortality, if not diagnosed and treated promptly. The cause may be hematogenous spread from bacteremia or intravenous drug abuse or from direct spread from an adjacent infection (osteomyelitis or soft tissue abscess) or penetration (surgical/procedural or trauma). Other systemic risk factors include diabetes mellitus, rheumatoid arthritis, liver failure, and immunosuppression (Mathews et al. 2010). Given the overlap with other inflammatory and pain-producing etiologies, this diagnosis may not be clear clinically and may be radiographically occult early in its course. Thus, MRI, with its superior soft tissue contrast, is often used in the work-up of septic arthritis. MRI features are somewhat nonspecific but include joint effusion and synovitis, surrounding soft tissue inflammation, and bone marrow edema with or without erosions (Bierry et al. 2012). These findings may not be present until several days into the disease process, so identification of concerning features should be recognized and differentiated from a traumatic etiology promptly, and aspiration or surgical intervention should be pursued promptly to appropriately treat and preserve the joint.

21.4.3.3 Transient Osteoporosis of the Hip

Transient osteoporosis of the hip is yet another cause of bone marrow edema affecting the hip that may be mistaken for a traumatic etiology (Fig. 21.24). This self-limited process is characterized by acute onset, non-traumatic pain and bone

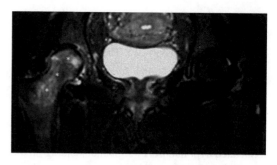

Fig. 21.24 Middle-aged woman with hip pain. Coronal STIR MR image of the pelvis shows marked diffuse edema (*asterisks*) throughout the right femoral head and neck without a hypointense fracture line, cartilage loss, or a significant joint effusion. These findings subsequently resolved with conservative treatment, confirming the diagnosis of transient osteoporosis of the hip

marrow edema of the femoral head and neck that may last up to 6–9 months (Hong et al. 2008; Korompilias et al. 2009). Typically affecting healthy middle-aged men and occasionally near-term gravid or postpartum women, the key feature in this process is its self-limited nature (Glockner et al. 1998; Korompilias et al. 2009). Many etiologies have been proposed, including a transient ischemic etiology, neurogenic origin, or prolonged bone repair, but the exact mechanism remains unknown.

Within 48 h of symptom onset, MRI may demonstrate florid bone marrow edema (diffuse T2-hyperintense and T1-hypointense signal) throughout the femoral head and neck, making it a valuable tool in identifying this process. Key features that separate it from a traumatic etiology, infection, or osteonecrosis (its most dreaded and similar differential diagnosis) include the following: no history of antecedent trauma, lack of associated subchondral imaging abnormalities, preserved joint space, and lack of surrounding soft tissue abnormality (Andrews 2000; Korompilias et al. 2009). Specifically, diffuse edema of the femoral head is believed to be a late finding of osteonecrosis and is not often seen without an associated subchondral band of T1-hypointense signal, unlike transient osteoporosis of the hip. Ultimately, this is a diagnosis of exclusion, and all other concerning causes, including stress fracture, osteonecrosis, and infection, should be carefully considered.

21.4.3.4   Osteonecrosis

Lastly, osteonecrosis may demonstrate bone marrow signal changes that could be confused for a traumatic etiology, specifically a femoral head subchondral insufficiency fracture (Fig. 21.25 compared to Figs. 21.7 and 21.21). The femoral head is one of the most susceptible locations in the body for osteonecrosis due to the limited vascular supply of the mature femoral head (Andrews 2000). The majority of patients afflicted with osteonecrosis have predisposing risk factors, including alcoholism, sickle cell disease, exogenous steroids, pancreatitis, trauma, infection, and caisson disease, among others (Andrews 2000; Korompilias et al. 2009). A missed diagnosis and delay in appropriate treatment may result in disease progression and significant morbidity with femoral head collapse and secondary osteoarthritis. Therefore, extra care in differentiating this process from other causes of femoral head or neck edema is warranted.

The MRI appearance is most commonly described as a geographic subchondral bone marrow signal abnormality, including band-like or linear T1-hypointensity. Associated bone marrow edema is often also present but is not diagnostic unless associated with the band-like subchondral signal abnormality and is less intense than transient osteoporosis of the hip (Hong et al. 2008) (Fig. 21.24). The "double-line sign" on T2-weighted images, described as a hypointense outer rim with inner rim of hyperintense granulation tissue, is pathognomonic for this process (Fig. 21.25). Subchondral collapse, which is often underestimated on MRI, is not seen until late in the disease process and is a sign of poor prognosis (Korompilias et al. 2009). The continuous linear hypointense signal abnormality with generally convex contour helps differentiate this entity from femoral head insufficiency fractures (Sheehan et al. 2015).

There are many causes of bone marrow edema of the hip, and careful consideration of the patterns described above will help to differentiate and diagnose the appropriate cause, leading to proper patient care.

> **Conclusion**
>
> Many anatomical structures, normal variants, and disease processes may mimic injuries of the hip on MRI. An understanding of the normal and abnormal appearance of hip anatomy, particularly the intra-articular, osseous, and surrounding soft tissue structures reviewed here, is vital to making an accurate assessment of hip.

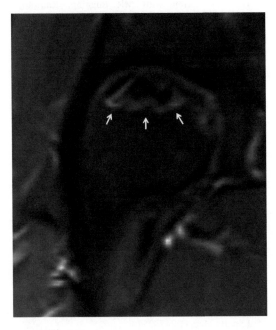

Fig. 21.25 59-year-old man with left hip pain. Coronal STIR MR image of the right hip shows a geographic region of abnormal bone marrow signal in the superior right femoral head with a "double-line sign" (*white arrows*). These features are classic for osteonecrosis. Note that there is little surrounding edema as would be seen with a subchondral insufficiency fracture

References

Anderson K, Strickland SM, Warren R (2001) Hip and groin injuries in athletes. Am J Sports Med 29:521–533

Andrews CL (2000) From the RSNA refresher courses. Evaluation of the marrow space in the adult hip. Radiographics 20:S27–S42

Armfield DR, Kim DH, Towers JD et al (2006) Sports-related muscle injury in the lower extremity. Clin Sports Med 25:803–842

Aydingöz U, Oztürk MH (2001) MR imaging of the acetabular labrum: a comparative study of both hips in 180 asymptomatic volunteers. Eur Radiol 11:567–574

Beiner JM, Jokl P (2001) Muscle contusion injuries: current treatment options. J Am Acad Orthop Surg 9:227–237

Bencardino JT, Kassarjian A, Vieira RL et al (2011) Synovial plicae of the hip: evaluation using MR arthrography in patients with hip pain. Skeletal Radiol 40:415–421

Bharam S (2006) Labral tears, extra-articular injuries, and hip arthroscopy in the athlete. Clin Sports Med 25:279–292

Bierry G, Huang AJ, Chang CY et al (2012) MRI findings of treated bacterial septic arthritis. Skeletal Radiol 41:1509–1516

Blankenbaker DG, De Smet AA, Keene JS (2006) Sonography of the iliopsoas tendon and injection of the iliopsoas bursa for diagnosis and management of the painful snapping hip. Skeletal Radiol 35:565–571

Blankenbaker DG, De Smet AA, Keene JS, Fine JP (2007) Classification and localization of acetabular labral tears. Skeletal Radiol 36:391–397

Blankenbaker DG, Ullrick SR, Davis KW (2008) Correlation of MRI findings with clinical findings of trochanteric pain syndrome. Skeletal Radiol 37:903–909

Blankenbaker DG, Davis KW, De Smet AA, Keene JS (2009) MRI appearance of the pectinofoveal fold. AJR Am J Roentgenol 192:93–95

Blankenbaker DG, Tuite MJ (2010) Temporal changes of muscle injury. Semin Musculoskelet Radiol 14:176–193

Blankenbaker DG, De Smet AA, Keene JS, Del Rio AM (2012) Imaging appearance of the normal and partially torn ligamentum teres on hip MR arthrography. AJR Am J Roentgenol 199:1093–1098

Bordalo-Rodrigues M, Rosenberg ZS (2005) MR imaging of the proximal rectus femoris musculotendinous unit. Magn Reson Imaging Clin N Am 13:717–725

Botser IB, Martin DE, Stout CE, Domb BG (2011) Tears of the ligamentum teres: prevalence in hip arthroscopy using 2 classification systems. Am J Sports Med 39(Suppl):117S–125S

Byrd JW, Jones KS (2004) Traumatic rupture of the ligamentum teres as a source of hip pain. Arthroscopy 20:385–391

Byrd JW (2012) Supraacetabular fossa. Radiology 265:648

Cerezal L, Kassarjian A, Canga A et al (2010) Anatomy, biomechanics, imaging, and management of ligamentum teres injuries. Radiographics 30:1637–1651

Cohen SB, Rangavajjula A, Vyas D, Bradley JP (2012) Functional results and outcomes after repair of proximal hamstring avulsions. Am J Sports Med 40:2092–2098

Cotten A, Boutry N, Demondion X, Paret C et al (1998) Acetabular labrum: MRI in asymptomatic volunteers. J Comput Assist Tomogr 22:1–7

Counsel P, Breidahl W (2010) Muscle injuries of the lower leg. Semin Musculoskelet Radiol 14:162–175

Czerny C, Hofmann S, Neuhold A et al (1996) Lesions of the acetabular labrum: accuracy of MR imaging and MR arthrography in detection and staging. Radiology 200:225–230

Davis KW (2008) Imaging of the hamstrings. Semin Musculoskelet Radiol 12:28–41

Davis KW (2010) Imaging pediatric sports injuries: lower extremity. Radiol Clin N Am 48:1213–1235

De Smet AA, Best TM (2000) MR imaging of the distribution and location of acute hamstring injuries in athletes. AJR Am J Roentgenol 174:393–399

Dietrich TJ, Suter A, Pfirrmann CW (2012) Supraacetabular fossa (pseudodefect of acetabular cartilage): frequency at MR arthrography and comparison of findings at MR arthrography and arthroscopy. Radiology 263:484–491

Dinauer PA, Flemming DJ, Murphy KP, Doukas WC (2007) Diagnosis of superior labral lesions: comparison of noncontrast MRI with indirect MR arthrography in unexercised shoulders. Skeletal Radiol 36:195–202

DuBois DF, Omar IM (2010) MR imaging of the hip: normal anatomic variants and imaging pitfalls. Magn Reson Imaging Clin N Am 18:663–674

Ebraheim NA, Savolaine ER, Fenton PJ, Jackson WT (1991) A calcified ligamentum teres mimicking entrapped intraarticular bony fragments in a patient with acetabular fracture. J Orthop Trauma 5:376–378

Feeley BT, Powell JW, Muller MS (2008) Hip injuries and labral tears in the national football league. Am J Sports Med 36:2187–2195

Fleckenstein JL, Weatherall PT, Parkey RW, Payne JA, Peshock RM (1989) Sports-related muscle injuries: evaluation with MR imaging. Radiology 172:793–798

Gaeta M, Minutoli F, Pandolfo I (2004) Magnetic resonance imaging findings of osteoid osteoma of the proximal femur. Eur Radiol 14:1582–1589

Glockner JF, Sundaram M, Pierron RL (1998) Radiologic case study. Transient migratory osteoporosis of the hip and knee. Orthopedics 21(600):594–596

Gray AJ, Villar RN (1997) The ligamentum teres of the hip: an arthroscopic classification of its pathology. Arthroscopy 13:575–578

Hackney LA, Lee MH, Joseph GB et al (2015) Subchondral insufficiency fractures of the femoral head: associated imaging findings and predictors of clinical progression. Eur Radiol. doi:10.1007/s00330-015-3967-x

Hirji Z, Hunjun JS, Choudur HN (2011) Imaging of the bursae. J Clin Imaging Sci 1:22

Hodler J, Yu JS, Goodwin D et al (1995) MR arthrography of the hip: improved imaging of the acetabular labrum with histologic correlation in cadavers. AJR Am J Roentgenol 165:887–891

Hölmich P (2007) Long-standing groin pain in sportspeople falls into three primary patterns, a "clinical entity" approach: a prospective study of 207 patients. Br J Sports Med 41:247–252

Hong RJ, Hughes TH, Gentili A, Chung CB (2008) Magnetic resonance imaging of the hip. J Magn Reson Imaging 27:435–445

Keene GS, Villar RN (1994) Arthroscopic anatomy of the hip: an in vivo study. Arthroscopy 10:392–399

Kim YT, Azuma H (1995) The nerve endings of the acetabular labrum. Clin Orthop Relat Res 320:176–181

Klontzas ME, Zibis AH, Karantanas AH (2015) Osteoid osteoma of the femoral neck: use of the half-moon sign in MRI diagnosis. AJR Am J Roentgenol 205:353–357

Korompilias AV, Karantanas AH, Lykissas MG, Beris AE (2009) Bone marrow edema syndrome. Skeletal Radiol 38:425–436

Koulouris G (2008) Imaging review of groin pain in elite athletes: an anatomic approach to imaging findings. AJR Am J Roentgenol 191:962–972

Ladd LM, Blankenbaker DG, Davis KW, Keene JS (2014) MRI of the hip: important injuries of the adult athlete. Curr Radiol Rep 2:1–19

Lecouvet FE, Vande Berg BC, Malghem J et al (1996) MR imaging of the acetabular labrum: variations in 200 asymptomatic hips. AJR Am J Roentgenol 167:1025–1028

Lecouvet FE, Demondion X, Leemrijse T et al (2005) Spontaneous rupture of the distal iliopsoas tendon: clinical and imaging findings, with anatomic correlations. Eur Radiol 15:2341–2346

Lee YP, Griffith JF, Antonio GE et al (2004) Early magnetic resonance imaging of radiographically occult osteoporotic fractures of the femoral neck. Hong Kong Med J 10:271–275

Lu Y, Wang L, Hao Y et al (2013) Analysis of trabecular distribution of the proximal femur in patients with fragility fractures. BMC Musculoskelet Disord 14:130. doi:10.1186/1471-2474-14-130

Lubovsky O, Liebergall M, Mattan Y et al (2005) Early diagnosis of occult hip fractures MRI versus CT scan. Injury 36:788–792

Maetani TH, Smith SE, Weissman BN (2015) Anatomic variants of the proximal lateral femoral cortex that mimic prefracture findings of atypical femoral fractures on conventional radiographs. In: Sonin A (ed). Scottsdale: Society of Skeletal Radiology 38th Annual Meeting March 8–11. Skeletal Radiol 44:1213–1233

Mathews CJ, Weston VC, Jones A et al (2010) Bacterial septic arthritis in adults. Lancet 375:846–855

May DA, Disler DG, Jones EA et al (2000) Abnormal signal intensity in skeletal muscle at MR imaging: patterns, pearls, and pitfalls. Radiographics 20:S295–S315

McCarthy J, Barsoum W, Puri L et al (2003) The role of hip arthroscopy in the elite athlete. Clin Orthop Relat Res 406:71–74

McMahon CJ, Wu JS, Eisenberg RL (2010) Muscle edema. AJR Am J Roentgenol 194:W284–W292

Mintz DN, Hooper T, Connell D et al (2005) Magnetic resonance imaging of the hip: detection of labral and chondral abnormalities using noncontrast imaging. Arthroscopy 21:385–393

Naraghi A, White LM (2015) MRI of labral and chondral lesions of the hip. AJR Am J Roentgenol 205: 479–490

Narvani AA, Tsiridis E, Kendall S, Chaudhuri R, Thomas P (2003) A preliminary report on prevalence of acetabular labrum tears in sports patients with groin pain. Knee Surg Sports Traumatol Arthrosc 11:403–408

Nguyen MS, Kheyfits V, Giordano BD, Dieudonne G, Monu JU (2013) Hip anatomic variants that may mimic abnormalities at MRI: labral variants. AJR Am J Roentgenol 201:W394–W400

Ouellette H, Thomas BJ, Nelson E, Torriani M (2006) MR imaging of rectus femoris origin injuries. Skeletal Radiol 35:665–672

Petchprapa CN, Rosenberg ZS, Sconfienza LM et al (2010) MR imaging of entrapment neuropathies of the lower extremity. Part 1. The pelvis and hip. Radiographics 30:983–1000

Petchprapa CN, Recht MP (2013) Imaging of chondral lesions including femoroacetabular impingement. Semin Musculoskelet Radiol 17:258–271

Petersen W, Petersen F, Tillmann B (2003) Structure and vascularization of the acetabular labrum with regard to the pathogenesis and healing of labral lesions. Arch Orthop Trauma Surg 123:283–288

Petersen J, Holmich P (2005) Evidence based prevention of hamstring injuries in sport. Br J Sports Med 39:319–323

Register B, Pennock AT, Ho CP et al (2012) Prevalence of abnormal hip findings in asymptomatic participants: a prospective, blinded study. Am J Sports Med 40:2720–2724

Ryan JB, Wheeler JH, Hopkinson WJ et al (1991) Quadriceps contusions. West Point update. Am J Sports Med 19:299–304

Schmerl M, Pollard H, Hoskins W (2005) Labral injuries of the hip: a review of diagnosis and management. J Manip Physiol Ther 28:632. doi:10.1016/j.jmpt. 2005.08.018

Schmid MR, Nötzli HP, Zanetti M et al (2003) Cartilage lesions in the hip: diagnostic effectiveness of MR arthrography. Radiology 226:382–386

Seldes RM, Tan V, Hunt J et al (2001) Anatomy, histologic features, and vascularity of the adult acetabular labrum. Clin Orthop Relat Res 382:232–240

Shane E, Burr D, Abrahamsen B et al (2014) Atypical subtrochanteric and diaphyseal femoral fractures: second report of a task force of the American Society for Bone and Mineral Research. J Bone Miner Res 29:1–23

Sheehan SE, Shyu JY, Weaver MJ et al (2015) Proximal femoral fractures: what the orthopedic surgeon wants to know. Radiographics 35:1563–1584

Shelly MJ, Hodnett PA, MacMahon PJ et al (2009) MR imaging of muscle injury. Magn Reson Imaging Clin N Am 17:757–773

Silder A, Heiderscheit BC, Thelen DG et al (2008) MR observations of long-term musculotendon remodeling following a hamstring strain injury. Skeletal Radiol 37:1101–1109

Smith TO, Hilton G, Toms AP et al (2010) The diagnostic accuracy of acetabular labral tears using magnetic resonance imaging and magnetic resonance arthrography: a meta-analysis. Eur Radiol 21:863–874

Stanton MC, Maloney MD, Dehaven KE, Giordano BD (2012) Acute traumatic tear of gluteus medius and minimus tendons in a patient without antecedent peritrochanteric hip pain. Geriatr Orthop Surg Rehabil 3:84–88

Stiris MG, Lilleas FG (1997) MR findings in cases of suspected impacted fracture of the femoral neck. Acta Radiol 38:863–866

Studler U, Kalberer F, Leunig M et al (2008) MR arthrography of the hip: differentiation between an anterior sublabral recess as a normal variant and a labral tear. Radiology 249:947–954

Sutter R, Zubler V, Hoffmann A et al (2014) Hip MRI: how useful is intraarticular contrast material for evaluating surgically proven lesions of the labrum and articular cartilage? AJR Am J Roentgenol 202: 160–169

Thibodeau GA, Patton KT (2006) Anatomy and physiology, 6th edn. Mosby Elsevier, St Louis

Thomas JD, Li Z, Agur AM, Robinson P (2013) Imaging of the acetabular labrum. Semin Musculoskelet Radiol 17:248–257

Tian CY, Wang JQ, Zheng ZZ, Ren AH (2014) 3.0 T conventional hip MR and hip MR arthrography for the acetabular labral tears confirmed by arthroscopy. Eur J Radiol 83:1822–1827

Tyler P, Saifuddin A (2010) The imaging of myositis ossificans. Semin Musculoskelet Radiol 14:201–216

Ueblacker P, Mueller-Wohlfahrt HW, Ekstrand J (2015) Epidemiological and clinical outcome comparison of indirect ('strain') versus direct ('contusion') anterior and posterior thigh muscle injuries in male elite football players: UEFA Elite League study of 2287 thigh injuries (2001-2013). Br J Sports Med. doi:10.1136/bjsports-2014-094285

Unnanuntana A, Saleh A, Mensah KA et al (2013) Atypical femoral fractures: what do we know about them?: AAOS Exhibit Selection. J Bone Joint Surg Am 95(e8):1–13. doi:10.2106/JBJS.L.00568

Varma DG, Richli WR, Charnsangavej C et al (1991) MR appearance of the distended iliopsoas bursa. AJR Am J Roentgenol 156:1025–1028

Wang BD, Tan KB, Young JLS (2015) Understanding the ligamentum teres of the hip: a histologic study. Acta Ortop Bras 23:29–33

Yen YM, Kocher MS (2010) Chondral lesions of the hip: microfracture and chondroplasty. Sports Med Arthrosc 18:83–89

Hip Injury: US Pitfalls

22

James Teh and David McKean

Contents

22.1	**Introduction**	415
22.2	**Pubic and Adductor-Related Groin Pain**	416
22.3	**Inguinal and Femoral Hernias**	416
22.4	**Hip Effusions and Synovitis**	418
22.5	**Labral Pathology**	419
22.6	**Iliopsoas Bursitis**	419
22.7	**Snapping Hip Syndrome**	419
22.8	**Trochanteric Pain Syndrome**	421
22.9	**Morel-Lavallée Lesions**	421
22.10	**Hamstring Injury**	421
22.11	**Rectus Femoris Injury**	423
Conclusion		423
References		424

J. Teh, BSc, MBBS, FRCP, FRCR (✉)
Department of Radiology, Nuffield Orthopaedic
Centre, Oxford University Hospitals NHS Trust,
Windmill Rd, Oxford OX3 7LD, UK
e-mail: jamesteh1@gmail.com

D. McKean, MA Hons, BM, BCh, FRCR
Department of Radiology, Stoke Mandeville Hospital,
Buckinghamshire Healthcare NHS Trust,
Mandeville Road, Buckinghamshire, Aylesbury HP21
8AL, UK
e-mail: David.Mckean@buckshealthcare.nhs.uk

Abbreviation

US   Ultrasound

22.1 Introduction

In patients with sports-related injuries around the hip, there are many potential causes to consider, and often, the cause of symptoms is multifactorial. Although ultrasound (US) imaging is an effective modality for evaluating the hip, the complex anatomy may prove challenging. A systematic protocol-driven approach should be used, taking careful consideration of the patient's symptoms and history. Certain technical aspects should always be considered when performing musculoskeletal US. Generally, when evaluating musculoskeletal structures, a high-frequency linear array probe should be used. However, in the hip, particularly in larger patients, a curvilinear probe with lower frequency and superior depth penetration may be required to obtain diagnostic images. Pertinent technical considerations relevant to musculoskeletal US imaging are described in Chap. 18.

Anisotropy is an artifact that occurs when the US beam is not perpendicular to an anatomical structure. It is more apparent in fibrillar structures such as ligaments and tendons, particularly when a linear probe is used to interrogate the structure in the longitudinal plane. The drop-off in signal may be misinterpreted as foci of tendon

© Springer International Publishing AG 2017
W.C.G. Peh (ed.), *Pitfalls in Musculoskeletal Radiology*, DOI 10.1007/978-3-319-53496-1_22

degeneration or partial tears. Confirming suspected pathology in orthogonal planes, increasing the gain, and repositioning the probe may be helpful. Compound scanning may also be useful to minimize this artifact. Comparison with the contralateral side, particularly if it is asymptomatic, is a simple and an effective technique to determine if an abnormality is present. The ultrasonographer should also be aware of the wide range of other artifacts inherent to US beam characteristics, velocity errors (refraction), attenuation errors (such as posterior acoustic shadowing or enhancement), or multiple echo paths, such as posterior reverberation or ring-down artifact (Feldman et al. 2009). For further information on US artifacts, also see Chap. 2.

22.2 Pubic and Adductor-Related Groin Pain

Groin pain is a common problem in athletes and is notorious for being difficult to evaluate. The wide range of pathology in numerous anatomical structures and high incidence of abnormal findings in asymptomatic subjects contribute to the difficulties in making an accurate diagnosis. The numerous terms used to describe groin injuries add further to the complexity. Different terms are often used to describe the same pathological processes, and the same term can have multiple interpretations (Weir et al. 2015). Pubic- and adductor-related groin pain may be caused by overload of the pubic symphysis, abnormality of the common aponeurosis of the rectus abdominis and adductor tendons, and parieto-abdominal weakness. Furthermore, pathologies affecting the adjacent structures such as the vertebral column, pelvis, and urogenital tract should also be considered (Balconi 2011).

US imaging examination should begin by scanning the lower rectus abdominis muscle in both transverse and longitudinal planes. Inferior to the pubic symphysis, a common aponeurosis is formed between the insertion of each rectus abdominis and each adductor longus tendon. In the groin, the transducer should be positioned obliquely along the adductor longus tendon with the hip in external rotation. In athletes with pubic-related groin pain, common findings include

hypoechoic swelling and anechoic clefts with cortical irregularity at the common aponeurosis (Robinson et al. 2011). Typically, no increased vascularity is demonstrated. Tears of the adductor longus are characterized by tendon retraction interposed with hypoechoic hemorrhage. Injuries of the pectineus muscle, gracilis muscle, or rectus abdominis insertion are less commonly encountered.

Pubic symphysis abnormalities may also be evident, including hypoechoic capsular distension, anechoic joint fluid, synovial hypertrophy with increased vascularity on Doppler US imaging, and cortical irregularity. A pitfall however is that cortical irregularity of the symphysis pubis may be physiological, related to unfused growth plates, which may persist until the mid-twenties (Robinson et al. 2011). Furthermore, chronic enthesopathic changes are common at the adductor insertion in many individuals, who may not be symptomatic. Close clinical correlation is therefore required to avoid overdiagnosis (Fig. 22.1). In view of the difficulties in diagnosis, radiographs and magnetic resonance imaging (MRI) are often performed in conjunction with US imaging. MRI findings commonly reported in athletes with adductor-related or symphyseal groin pain that may not be seen with US imaging include degenerative changes of the symphyseal joint and pubic bone marrow edema.

22.3 Inguinal and Femoral Hernias

Inguinal and femoral hernias should be considered in all patients presenting with groin pain. Imaging for hernias may be challenging, with US imaging of occult hernias having a reported sensitivity and specificity of 86% and 77%, respectively (Robinson et al. 2012). The identification of the Hesselbach triangle, formed by the lateral margin of the rectus abdominis, the inferior epigastric artery, and the inguinal ligament, is essential for the diagnosis of inguinal hernias, which may be indirect or direct (Jamadar et al. 2007). Indirect inguinal hernias are commoner than direct inguinal hernias. Indirect inguinal hernias are characterized by abnormal movement of

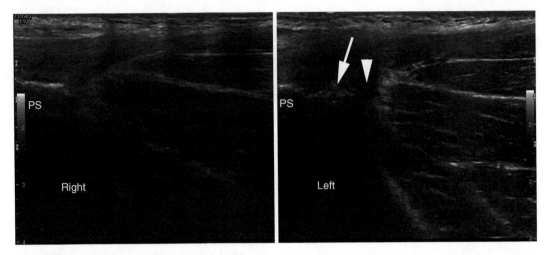

Fig. 22.1 Left adductor tendinosis with partial tear. Comparison US images of both groins. There is bony irregularity (*long arrow*) of the left pubic symphysis (*PS*) with a hypoechoic cleft (*arrowhead*) at the adductor insertion indicating a partial tear. The right groin is normal

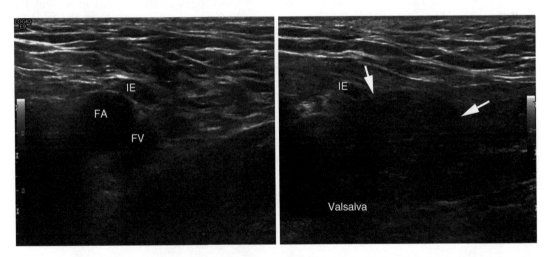

Fig. 22.2 Direct inguinal hernia. Axial US images through Hesselbach triangle show the femoral artery (*FA*), femoral vein (*FV*), and inferior epigastric artery (*IE*) in the relaxed state. With the Valsalva maneuver, there is a direct inguinal hernia (*arrows*) arising medial to the inferior epigastric vessels

intra-abdominal contents (fat, bowel, or a combination of both) through the deep inguinal ring into the inguinal canal. They occur lateral to the inferior epigastric artery and anterior to the spermatic cord in males. A large hernia may extend medially through the external or superficial inguinal ring into the scrotum or labia majora and may present as a groin mass. Direct inguinal hernias occur directly through Hesselbach triangle, medial to the inferior epigastric artery.

A major pitfall in the diagnosis of inguinal hernias is failure to document the presence of a hernia in two orthogonal planes (Jacobson et al. 2015).

On longitudinal views, with the Valsalva maneuver, the inguinal canal may move inferiorly, and direct herniation through the canal can be easily missed. Conversely, when assessing in the transverse plane, the normal movement of the intra-abdominal contents below the Hesselbach triangle with the Valsalva maneuver may simulate a direct inguinal hernia. Therefore, orthogonal views are essential to assess for hernias bulging in and out of the plane on Valsalva maneuvers (Fig. 22.2). A further pitfall in diagnosing inguinal hernias includes a spermatic cord lipoma. Assessment at the level of the deep inguinal ring is necessary to differentiate between a cord lipoma and a hernia, as a true direct inguinal hernia will extend from the abdominal cavity through this ring. With femoral hernias, there is abnormal movement of the intra-abdominal contents through the femoral canal medial to the femoral vein, which may be compressed.

A cyst of the canal of Nuck is a rare condition in female patients caused by a failure of complete obliteration of the canal of Nuck, an abnormal patent pouch of peritoneum extending anterior to the round ligament of the uterus into the labia majora (Park et al. 2014; Manjunatha et al. 2012). It is equivalent to a patent processus vaginalis in men, which may predispose to indirect inguinal hernia, hydrocele, and spermatic cord cyst. Typically, they present as a cystic mass lying superficial and medial to the femoral neurovascular bundle at the level of the superficial inguinal ring. There should be no communication with the peritoneum and no change with the Valsalva maneuver. The cyst may be confused with a distended iliopsoas bursa, which lies more laterally (Fig. 22.3).

22.4　Hip Effusions and Synovitis

There is a high prevalence of hip effusions in patients with painful hips (Bierma-Zeinstra et al. 2000), with a wide differential for hip effusions,

including traumatic, inflammatory, and infective causes. The area over the anterior femoral neck allows for the best assessment of the degree of joint effusion. Good technique is important to avoid misdiagnosis and inappropriate attempted aspiration. Normally, a hyperechoic area measuring up to 7 mm may be seen anterior to the femoral head and neck which represents the iliofemoral ligament and joint capsule (Robben et al. 1999; Weybright et al. 2012). If the US probe is not held in the perpendicular plane, this normal structure may appear hypoechoic due to anisotropy and be mistaken for a small effusion. In addition, internal rotation of the hip may result in the anterior joint capsule becoming convex and measuring greater than 7 mm.

It is important not to mistake the cartilage of the developing femoral head in a child for an effusion or synovitis (Fig. 22.4). Synovial hypertrophy may be difficult to differentiate from joint effusions. The presence of internal echoes, a lack of compressibility, or the presence of internal Doppler signal suggests synovitis. The differential for hip synovitis is very wide, and conditions such as infection, inflammatory arthropathy, and synovial proliferative disorders, such as pigmented villonodular synovitis, should be considered. In children, a major pitfall is the misdiagnosis of transient synovitis in cases of hip infection.

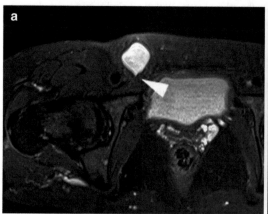
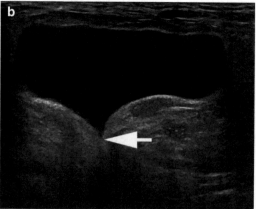

Fig. 22.3 Canal of Nuck cyst. (**a**) Axial STIR MR image shows a cystic structure arising medial to the femoral neurovascular bundle (*arrowhead*). This location differenti-ates the canal of Nuck cyst from an iliopsoas bursa. (**b**) Axial US image of the same patient shows the neck of the cystic structure (*arrow*)

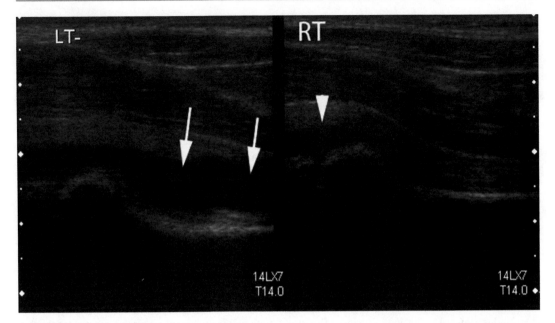

Fig. 22.4 Hip effusion in a child. Comparison longitudinal US images of the left and right hips. On the left (*LT*), there is a moderate hip effusion (*arrows*). On the right (*RT*), there is no effusion, but the articular cartilage (*arrowhead*) of the femoral head may mimic an effusion

22.5 Labral Pathology

Labral tears are a common cause of hip pain in athletes, often the result of femoroacetabular impingement. The anterior labrum can usually be visualized in the longitudinal plane, producing an image analogous to a sagittal MR image. Normally, the acetabular labrum appears as a hyperechoic compact triangular structure, owing to its composition of fibrocartilage. The anterior labrum is the most common site for labral pathology. Tears of the acetabular labrum are seen as irregular or linear hypoechoic fissures or clefts (Sofka et al. 2006). Finding of a paralabral cyst may also be helpful in confirming the presence of a labral tear. The diagnosis of labral tears on US imaging however is extremely challenging, and MR arthrography remains the gold standard for imaging (Fig. 22.5).

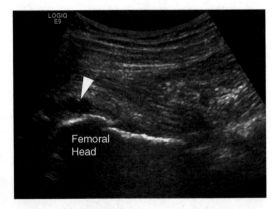

Fig. 22.5 Paralabral cyst. Longitudinal US image shows an anterior paralabral cyst (*arrowhead*) in a patient who was shown to have a labral tear on subsequent MRI

identified medial to the iliopsoas tendon at the level of the femoral head. A distended iliopsoas bursa may extend proximally along the psoas muscle into the abdomen and mimic a psoas abscess.

22.6 Iliopsoas Bursitis

The iliopsoas bursa is located medial and deep to the iliopsoas complex, where it passes over the ilium. The bursa may communicate with the hip joint in up to 15% of the population. This may be

22.7 Snapping Hip Syndrome

The snapping hip syndrome classically presents as a painful, palpable, and often audible snap caused during certain hip movements. Intra-articular and extra-articular causes have been described. Intra-articular causes include a labral tear, loose body, or chondral defects. Extra-articular causes are divided into internal and external causes. The former is caused by a snapping iliopsoas tendon and the latter by snapping iliotibial band and ischiofemoral impingement (Fang and Teh 2003; Bureau 2013). The snapping iliopsoas tendon affects predominantly young adults, especially women. Subjects who perform repeated hip abduction movements, such as ballet dancing, martial arts, and gymnastics, are at increased risk.

The iliopsoas complex is composed of several structures; abnormal movement of which may result in clicking and snapping. The most frequently reported mechanism is snapping of the psoas tendon on the superior pubic ramus after release of the medial fibers of the iliacus muscle (Deslandes et al. 2008). During flexion-abduction-external rotation of the hip, the medial fibers of the iliacus muscle become caught between the psoas tendon and the superior pubic ramus. On extension and adduction of the hip, these fibers abruptly release from this position, causing the psoas tendon to return suddenly against the superior pubic ramus, resulting in a snap. The probe should be placed in a transverse

oblique plane between the anteroinferior iliac spine and the superior pubic ramus to examine the iliopsoas musculotendinous complex. The movement of the psoas tendon and iliacus muscle is observed dynamically, while the patient executes a motion of flexion-abduction-external rotation, followed by extension and adduction of the hip. The main pitfall in imaging this condition is failure to perform the correct maneuvers to elicit the snap (Fig. 22.6).

The iliotibial band is a deep continuation of the deep fascia of the thigh, receiving insertions from the gluteus maximus and tensor fascia lata. It passes over the anterolateral aspect of the thigh and inserts onto the Gerdy tubercle on the anterolateral aspect of the proximal tibia. A transient subluxation of the junction between the iliotibial band and the anterior margin of the gluteus maximus muscle over the greater trochanter may result in an external snapping hip (Choi et al. 2002). To snap the tendon, the patient lies on the unaffected side. The hip is then adducted and extended, then moved into the flexed position. During the early phase of flexion, the iliotibial band and gluteus maximus are restrained transiently against the posterolateral aspect of the greater trochanter. As flexion continues, the

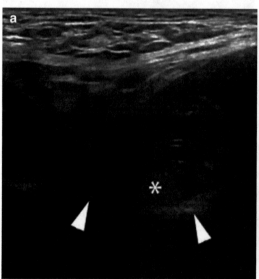
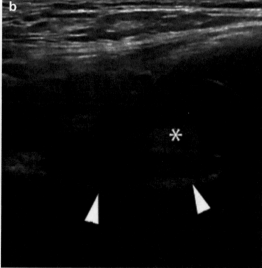

Fig. 22.6 Snapping iliopsoas tendon. (**a**) In the neutral position, US image shows that the psoas tendon (*asterisk*) lies against the iliac blade (*arrowheads*). (**b**) In flexion-abduction-external rotation, US image shows that the psoas tendon (*asterisk*) lies more centrally as the iliacus muscle is rotated medially

iliotibial band and gluteus maximus are suddenly released, moving forward abruptly over the anterior edge of the lateral facet of the greater trochanter, generating the snapping.

22.8 Trochanteric Pain Syndrome

Trochanteric pain syndrome is a term used to describe chronic pain over the region of the greater trochanter. It is most commonly found in middle-aged and elderly females but may be encountered as a sports injury. The pain has classically been attributed to trochanteric bursitis but more recently has been associated with gluteal tendinopathy (Kong et al. 2006). Failures to appreciate the bursal anatomy and identify gluteal tendinopathy are the main pitfalls in imaging this condition. Assessment of patients with trochanteric pain syndrome requires detailed knowledge of the underlying anatomy. The trochanteric bursa overlies the lateral and posterior aspect of the greater trochanter deep to the gluteus maximus. The subgluteus medius bursa lies deep to the gluteus medius tendon proximal to the greater trochanter, and the subgluteus minimus bursa lies between the gluteus minimus tendon and the anterior aspect of the greater trochanter (Pfirrmann et al. 2001) (Fig. 22.7). The gluteus minimus and gluteus medius tendons attach onto the anterior and lateral facets, respectively. Gluteal tendinosis is manifested by decreased and often heterogeneous echogenicity, often with tendon thickening. There is commonly enthesopathic change with slight bony irregularity of the insertion and small linear calcifications within the distal tendon. Increased Doppler US signal is rarely seen but may be helpful if present. Tears are evident as partial or complete thickness anechoic gaps within the tendon.

22.9 Morel-Lavallée Lesions

Morel-Lavallée lesions represent closed degloving shearing injuries, when the subcutaneous fatty tissue separates from the underlying fascia. This results in filling of the space with blood, fat, and lymphatic fluid, which may evolve into a hemo-

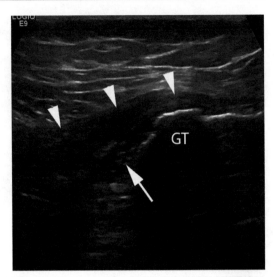

Fig. 22.7 Deep gluteus medius bursitis. Axial oblique US image shows a distended deep gluteus medius bursa lying deep to the gluteus medius tendon (*arrowheads*) which attaches to the greater trochanter (*GT*)

lymphatic mass (Neal et al. 2008). Typically, these occur over the greater trochanter. On US imaging, these lesions may be anechoic or hypoechoic and may contain septations. Internal debris, including fat globules, can give rise to echogenic foci. In the subacute period, they may have a lobulated contour but become flattened and better defined with time. US-guided aspiration may speed recovery and reduce the incidence of reaccumulation. A common pitfall is for these lesions to be misdiagnosed as soft tissue tumors (Fig. 22.8).

22.10 Hamstring Injury

A thorough knowledge of the anatomy of the posterior hip space is essential to interpret pathology in this region. The hamstring origin lies medially in the space between the posteromedial margin of the tip of the greater trochanter and the ischial tuberosity. The quadratus femoris muscle lies centrally, and deep to this is the obturator externus tendon. There are three hamstring muscles that arise from the ischial tuberosity from two tendons. The upper and lateral ischial tuberosity give rise to the semimembranosus tendon. The semitendinosus and biceps femoris originate from a conjoint

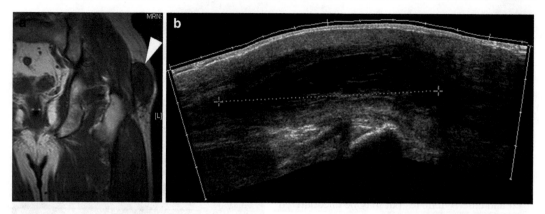

Fig. 22.8 Morel-Lavallée lesion of the hip mimicking a tumor. (**a**) Coronal T1-W MR image shows a heterogeneous mass (*arrowhead*) in the deep subcutaneous tissue.

(**b**) US image in the same patient shows a septated cystic lesion (*between cursors*) overlying the deep fascia

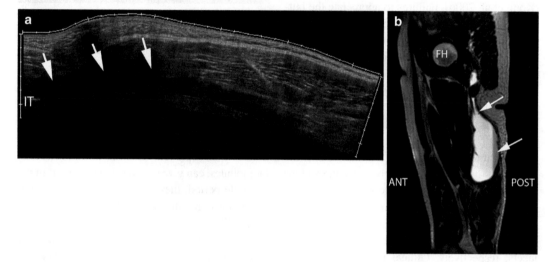

Fig. 22.9 Hamstring avulsion which was poorly assessed on US imaging. (**a**) Longitudinal US image shows a hamstring tendon avulsion with retraction (*arrows*). The full extent of injury is difficult to determine on US imaging.

(**b**) Sagittal T2-W MR image in the same patient shows a large layering hemorrhagic collection (*arrows*). The femoral head is shown (*FH*)

tendon from the lower aspect of the ischial tuberosity. The adductor magnus and the sacrotuberous ligament arise from the lower portion of the ischium. As the muscles are followed distally, the semimembranosus muscle becomes visible on the medial aspect of semitendinosus. Proximally, the semitendinosus is the larger muscle while distally, it is smaller. The biceps femoris muscle is the most lateral of the hamstrings and has a second short head that arises from the linea aspera. Examining the patient in the lateral decubitus position with the hip flexed often allows better evaluation.

Hamstring avulsions usually involve the tendon but not the bone in adults. Most avulsions involve the conjoint tendon (biceps femoris and semitendinosus muscles) and result in either complete or incomplete tearing of the semimembranosus. On US imaging, a major pitfall is the difficulty in determining the extent of hamstring injury, due to hemorrhage causing poor visualization (Fig. 22.9). In adolescents, the apophysis forms the weakest link in the musculotendinous unit, due to its incomplete ossification, resulting in osseous avulsions. Acute strains of the mid- and

Fig. 22.10 Rectus femoris musculotendinous injury resulting in pseudotumor. Longitudinal extended field-of-view US image shows retraction (*arrow*) of the rectus femoris muscle belly (*arrowheads*)

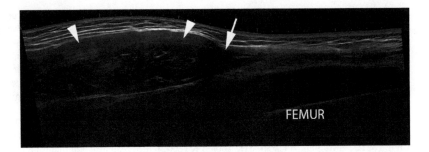

distal hamstring myotendinous complex are common athletic injuries. Partial tears of the hamstrings typically occur in the region of the myotendinous junction. On US imaging, there may be disorganization of the skeletal muscle architecture, with surrounding edema. Fluid and blood products dissecting along disrupted fibrils may create a feathered appearance.

22.11   Rectus Femoris Injury

For evaluation of the rectus femoris, assessment of both the straight and reflected heads is necessary. The iliac crest should be followed to the upper half of the anterior inferior iliac spine to where the straight head originates. The reflected head arises from a shallow concavity above the acetabulum and is the primary head. The two heads combine to form the conjoined tendon. This orientation results in the straight head being readily identified by its echogenic linear appearance, whereas the reflected head is typically identified by its anisotropic shadow, rather than being directly visualized. This may be misinterpreted as acoustic shadowing from calcification (Sarkar et al. 1996) or refraction of sound at the edge of a tendon tear. Scanning more laterally and medially angling the transducer may allow the reflected head to be more clearly identified. Rectus femoris tendinosis is manifested by altered echogenicity and thickening. In older patients, a tear of the rectus femoris musculotendinous junction or tendon may present as a soft tissue mass of the anterior thigh, without a significant history of trauma, and can mimic a soft tissue tumor clinically (Fig. 22.10).

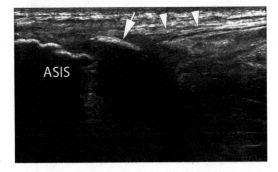

Fig. 22.11 Anterior superior iliac spine avulsion. Longitudinal US image shows a displaced bony fragment (*short arrow*) arising from the anterior superior iliac spine (*ASIS*) to which the sartorius tendon (*arrowheads*) attaches

Avulsion of the anterior inferior iliac spine occurs in adolescents as a result of a forceful contraction of the rectus femoris, as the hip extends and the knee is flexed. Males are more commonly affected, typically as a result of kicking sports such as football or running. Avulsions of the anterior superior iliac spine occur due to forceful hip extension with forceful contraction of the sartorius, typically during sprinting. Most avulsions are treated conservatively, but if there is displacement of more than 2 cm or the patient remains symptomatic, surgery may be indicated (Singer et al. 2014) (Fig. 22.11).

Conclusion

Sports-related hip pain may be difficult to assess clinically. Dynamic US imaging examination is an excellent tool for determining the cause of symptoms, but the operator must have a thorough knowledge of the anatomy and the numerous pitfalls.

References

Balconi G (2011) US in pubalgia. J Ultrasound 14: 157–166

Bierma-Zeinstra SM, Bohnen AM, Verhaar JA et al (2000) Sonography for hip joint effusion in adults with hip pain. Ann Rheum Dis 59:178–182

Bureau NJ (2013) Sonographic evaluation of snapping hip syndrome. J Ultrasound Med 32:895–900

Choi YS, Lee SM, Song BY, Paik SH, Yoon YK (2002) Dynamic sonography of external snapping hip syndrome. J Ultrasound Med 21:753–758

Deslandes M, Guillin R, Cardinal E et al (2008) The snapping iliopsoas tendon: new mechanisms using dynamic sonography. AJR Am J Roentgenol 190:576–581

Fang C, Teh J (2003) Imaging of the hip. Imaging 15:205–216

Feldman MK, Katyal S, Blackwood MS (2009) US artifacts. Radiographics 29:1179–1189

Jacobson JA, Khoury V, Brandon CJ (2015) Ultrasound of the groin: techniques, pathology, and pitfalls. AJR Am J Roentgenol 205:513–523

Jamadar DA, Jacobson JA, Morag Y et al (2007) Characteristic locations of inguinal region and anterior abdominal wall hernias: sonographic appearances and identification of clinical pitfalls. AJR Am J Roentgenol 188:1356–1364

Kong A, Van der Vliet A, Zadow S (2006) MRI and US of gluteal tendinopathy in greater trochanteric pain syndrome. Eur Radiol 17:1772–1783

Manjunatha Y, Beeregowda Y, Bhaskaran A (2012) Hydrocele of the canal of Nuck: imaging findings. Acta Radiol Short Rep 1(3). doi:10.1258/arsr.2012.110016

Neal C, Jacobson JA, Brandon C et al (2008) Sonography of Morel-Lavallée lesions. J Ultrasound Med 27:1077–1081

Park SJ, Lee HK, Hong HS et al (2014) Hydrocele of the canal of Nuck in a girl: ultrasound and MR appearance. Br J Radiol 77:243–244

Pfirrmann CWA, Chung CB, Theumann NH, Trudell DJ, Resnick D (2001) Greater trochanter of the hip: attachment of the abductor mechanism and a complex of three bursae – MR imaging and MR bursography in cadavers and MR imaging in asymptomatic volunteers. Radiology 221:469–477

Robben SGF, Lequin MH, Diepstraten AFM et al (1999) Anterior joint capsule of the normal hip and in children with transient synovitis: US study with anatomic and histologic correlation. Radiology 210:499–507

Robinson P, Bhat V, English B (2011) Imaging in the assessment and management of athletic pubalgia. Semin Musculoskelet Radiol 15:14–26

Robinson A, Light D, Kasim A, Nice C (2012) A systematic review and meta-analysis of the role of radiology in the diagnosis of occult inguinal hernia. Surg Endosc 27:11–18

Sarkar JS, Haddad FS, Crean SV, Brooks P (1996) Acute calcific tendinitis of the rectus femoris. J Bone Joint Surg Br 78:814–816

Singer G, Eberl R, Wegmann H et al (2014) Diagnosis and treatment of apophyseal injuries of the pelvis in adolescents. Semin Musculoskelet Radiol 18:498–504

Sofka CM, Adler RS, Danon MA (2006) Sonography of the acetabular labrum: visualization of labral injuries during intra-articular injections. J Ultrasound Med 25:1321–1326

Weir A, Brukner P, Delahunt E et al (2015) Doha agreement meeting on terminology and definitions in groin pain in athletes. Br J Sports Med 49:768–774

Weybright PN, Jacobson JA, Murry KH et al (2012) Limited effectiveness of sonography in revealing hip joint effusion: preliminary results in 21 adult patients with native and postoperative hips. AJR Am J Roentgenol 181:215–218

Redouane Kadi and Maryam Shahabpour

Contents

23.1	**Introduction**	425
23.2	**Anatomical Pitfalls**	426
23.2.1	Bone	426
23.2.2	Menisci	430
23.2.3	Other Anatomical Structures	444
23.3	**Technical Pitfalls**	446
23.3.1	Magic Angle Phenomenon	446
23.3.2	Truncation Artifact	446
23.3.3	Susceptibility Artifacts	446
23.3.4	Partial Volume Effect	448
23.3.5	Chemical Shift Artifact	448
23.3.6	Fat-Suppression Artifacts	448
23.3.7	Motion Artifacts	449
23.4	**Clinical Pitfalls**	449
23.4.1	Medial Knee Pain	450
23.4.2	Lateral Knee Pain	453
23.4.3	Anterior Knee Pain	456
23.4.4	Posterior Knee Pain	458
23.4.5	Knee Stiffness	459
Conclusion		467
References		467

R. Kadi, MD • M. Shahabpour, MD (✉)
Department of Diagnostic Radiology, University
Hospital of Brussels, Vrije Universiteit Brussel,
Laarbeeklaan 101, 1090 Brussels, Belgium
e-mail: redouane.kadi@gmail.com; maryam.
shahabpour@uzbrussel.be

Abbreviations

MRI   Magnetic resonance imaging

23.1 Introduction

Magnetic resonance imaging (MRI) is recognized as the imaging modality of choice for the assessment of chronic internal derangements of the knee. Accurate interpretation of MRI requires several prerequisites, including a precise knowledge of normal MRI anatomy and a good understanding of basic technical principles. These prerequisites help the understanding of the pathological conditions encountered in the area of interest. Anatomical variants are often incidental findings; knowledge and recognition of these variants are essential for an accurate analysis of MRI findings. Other potential pitfalls in the interpretation of MRI of the knee are from technical and clinical origins. Particular attention should be given to the anatomical variants and technical and clinical diagnostic pitfalls in order to avoid misinterpretations that may lead to unnecessary additional invasive investigations as diagnostic arthroscopy or lead to inappropriate therapeutic decisions as surgical procedures.

© Springer International Publishing AG 2017

W.C.G. Peh (ed.), *Pitfalls in Musculoskeletal Radiology*, DOI 10.1007/978-3-319-53496-1_23

23.2   Anatomical Pitfalls

23.2.1   Bone

23.2.1.1   Benign Hematopoietic Bone Marrow Hyperplasia

Small residual islands of red bone marrow or larger areas of bone marrow reconversion can be present in the metadiaphyseal region of the long bones (essentially in the distal femoral metaphysis) and are considered as being physiological (Fig. 23.1). They present with moderate signal hypointensity on T1- and T2-weighted MR images, higher than the muscle signal, and hyperintense signal on fat-suppressed T2-weighted images. They should not be confused with pathological bone marrow replacement (e.g., in lymphoma or other tumors) (Fig. 23.2). Contrary to benign hematopoietic marrow hyperplasia, those pathologies are characterized by very low signal intensity and an asymmetrical distribution with epiphyseal involvement. Benign hematopoietic marrow hyperplasia is most often idiopathic and can be observed not only in healthy subjects but also in obese females or in cases of increased hematopoietic demand created by relative hypoxemic states, such as decreased oxygen-carrying capacity (e.g., chronic anemia such as sickle cell disease and thalassemia), impaired oxygen delivery (e.g., smoking, high altitude, congenital heart disease), and increased oxygen demand (e.g., in athletes such as long-distance runners and free divers). It can be associated with chronic infection and cardiopathies or be iatrogenic (e.g., treatment with hematopoietic growth factors) (Chan et al. 2016).

23.2.1.2   Patella

The patella is the largest sesamoid bone in the human body. Several anatomical variants have been described, including variation in size such as *patella parva* (patellar hypoplasia) and *patella magna* (patellar hyperplasia). Variations in shape include "alpine hunter's cap," "pebble-like," and "half-moon"-shaped patella. To date, no correlation has been established between any

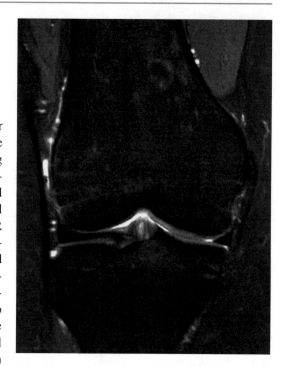

Fig. 23.1 Red bone marrow remnants. Coronal fat-suppressed PD-W MR image shows multiple small islands of residual red bone marrow of increased signal in the distal femur which is less pronounced in the proximal tibia

of these anatomical variants and chondromalacia or patellar instability. Different ossification and mineralization patterns can be encountered in the patella. The patella may present with irregular edges, an anterior discoid ossification (Fig. 23.3), or have multiple ossification centers. The ossification centers fuse during adolescence. The absence of fusion results in bipartite or multipartite patella.

Bipartite and multipartite patellas are characterized by the existence of one or more non-fused accessory ossification centers near the patella. Kavanagh et al. (2007) studied 400 knee MRI examinations and found the prevalence of bipartite patella to be 0.7%. Bipartite patella is often bilateral, more frequent in boys, and is more commonly seen than multipartite patella. The Saupe classification for bipartite patella is based on the position of the isolated

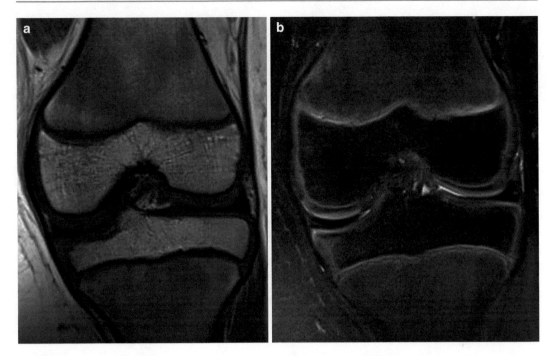

Fig. 23.2 Red bone marrow in a child. (**a**) Coronal T1-W and (**b**) fat-suppressed PD-W MR images show areas of red bone marrow of T1-hypointensity in the distal femoral diaphysis and proximal tibia with signal hyperintensity on the fat-suppressed PD-W image. Symmetrical distribution without epiphyseal involvement is present

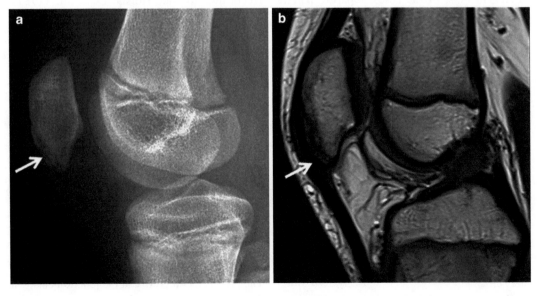

Fig. 23.3 Anterior discoid ossification of the patella. (**a**) Lateral radiograph and (**b**) sagittal T1-W MR image show heterogeneous appearance of the anteroinferior pole of the patella with irregular margins (*arrow*) corresponding to an anterior discoid ossification. The proximal attachment of the patellar tendon appears normal

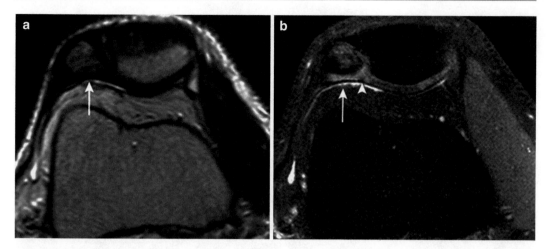

Fig. 23.4 Bipartite patella in a symptomatic patient. Axial PD-W MR images obtained (**a**) without and (**b**) with fat suppression show a type II non-fused lateral ossification center (*arrow*) in a bipartite patella. The presence of increased signal in the cartilaginous layer of the synchondrosis (*arrowhead*, **b**) and bone marrow edema in the accessory ossification center (*arrow*, **b**) suggests instability of this fragment that could explain the patient's symptoms. Bipartite patella differs from patellar fractures by its lateral localization and the absence of an associated cartilage tear

fragment: type I, at the patella lower pole (5%); type II, at the lateral margin (30%); and type III, the most common (75%), at the upper lateral pole. Although it presents as an incidental finding in most of the cases, bipartite patella may be symptomatic in some cases, inducing anterior knee pain. In these patients, bone marrow edema can be detected in both the ossification center and the adjacent patella along the margins of the synchondrosis, suggesting instability (Fig. 23.4). Differential diagnosis of bi- and multipartite patella includes marginal patellar fractures. However, bipartite patella differs by its lateral localization, its regular contours, and the preserved continuity of the overlying cartilage. Correlation with clinical history (acute onset of pain in fracture versus chronic knee pain in symptomatic bipartite or multipartite patella) is helpful for the differential diagnosis (Malghem et al. 1998; Kavanagh et al. 2007; Snoeckx et al. 2008; Kadi et al. 2015).

Dorsal defect of the patella is typically seen as a well-defined osteolytic lesion, which is generally located at the upper lateral part of the patella. On radiographs, the defect is radiolucent, has rounded contours, and is frequently delimited by a sclerotic border. According to Van Holsbeeck et al. (1987), abnormal constraints applied by the vastus lateralis muscle (which inserts at the superolateral aspect of the patella) could explain the pathophysiology of both dorsal defect of patella and bipartite patella. On MRI, a cortical defect filled by the cartilage is depicted at the superolateral pole of the patella, with an intact smooth cartilage surface covering the patella (Fig. 23.5). Patients are generally asymptomatic. Differential diagnoses include osteochondritis dissecans of the patella and, less commonly, Brodie abscess and bone tumors (Snoeckx et al. 2008; Vanhoenacker et al. 2016).

23.2.1.3 Distal Femoral Variants

The presence of a groove at the junction between the femoral condyle and the trochlea gives rise to an imprint on subchondral bone, which can

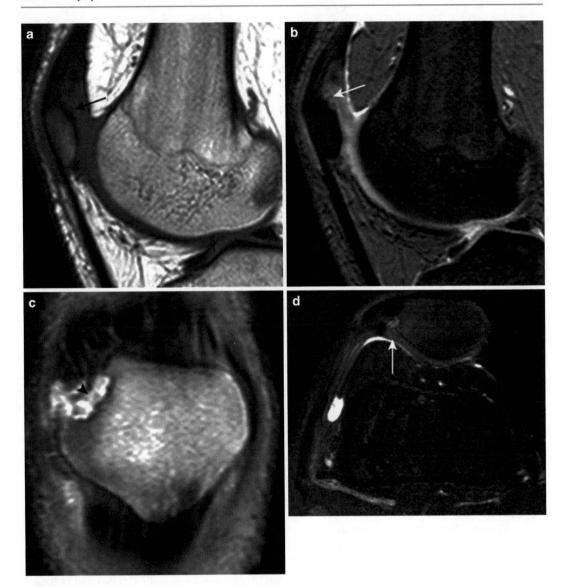

Fig. 23.5 Dorsal defect of patella. Sagittal (**a**) T1-W and (**b**) GRE T2*-W MR images show a well-defined bony defect (*arrow*) located in the superolateral portion of the patella. This is clearly visible on (**c**) coronal PD-W MR image (*arrowhead*). The cartilage covering the cortical defect is thickened on (**d**) axial fat-suppressed PD-W MR image (*arrow*)

simulate an osteochondral lesion. The groove can be identified at both femoral condyles. The overlying hyaline cartilage is continuous within the condylotrochlear groove (Herman and Beltran 1988; Shahabpour et al. 1991; Resnick and Kang 1997) (Fig. 23.6).

Cortical avulsive irregularity (also known as "cortical or subperiosteal desmoid" which incorrectly suggests that the lesion is of neoplastic origin) is a benign defect located along the posteromedial cortex of the distal femoral metaphysis in children and adolescents. Cortical

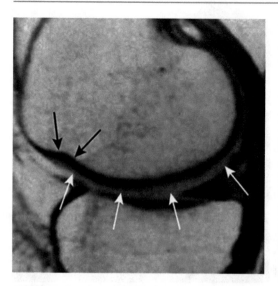

Fig. 23.6 Distal femoral groove. Sagittal PD-W MR image taken through the medial compartment shows a subchondral bone defect corresponding to a condylotrochlear groove (*black arrows*). This should not be confused with an osteochondral lesion. Normal overlying hyaline cartilage is continuous, even within the groove (*white arrows*)

avulsive irregularity is believed to result from chronic traction either of the medial head of the gastrocnemius muscle or of the insertion of the aponeurosis of the adductor magnus muscle at the posteromedial femoral condyle. MRI shows a well-delimited intracortical lesion with T1-hypointense and T2-hyperintense signal that may enhance after contrast injection and is surrounded by a hypointense rim (Fig. 23.7). The lesion should not be misinterpreted as an aggressive neoplastic lesion (Tyler et al. 2010; Vanhoenacker et al. 2016).

Other contour irregularities that have been described in children and adolescents (more often in boys) are multiple ossification centers generally located at the posterior femoral condyle (Fig. 23.8). These normal variants are common and should not be confused with early osteochondritis dissecans. The presence of an intact cartilaginous layer covering the bone defect and the absence of edema in the underlying bone marrow may be helpful

for the differential diagnosis (Gebarski and Hernandez 2005; Snoeckx et al. 2008; Jans et al. 2011).

23.2.1.4 Fabella and Cyamella

A fabella is a sesamoid ossicle typically located in the lateral side of the lateral gastrocnemius muscle/tendon (Fig. 23.9). According to Robertson et al. (2004), it is found in 11–13% of patients and is often bilateral. The fabella may be bipartite or tripartite. It should not be mistaken for a loose body (Snoeckx et al. 2008; Tyler et al. 2010). A cyamella, also called popliteal fabella, is an extremely rare sesamoid bone of the popliteus tendon. It is located near the proximal musculotendinous junction of the muscle, or even in the popliteal fossa. The cyamella must be differentiated from an intra-articular loose body or a heterotopic ossification of post-traumatic or iatrogenic origin (Akansel et al. 2006; Snoeckx et al. 2008).

23.2.2 Menisci

23.2.2.1 Morphological Variants

The discoid meniscus is the most common congenital anomaly of the meniscus, with reported prevalence in Western countries of 0.7–5.2% and with a much higher incidence, up to 16.6%, in the Asian patient population. Less frequently, the medial meniscus is involved (incidence 0.06–0.03%) and is found bilaterally in about 20% of the cases. Although often asymptomatic, it could be discovered in case of suspicion of meniscal tear. Patients could also present with pain, clicking, locking, or an audible snapping on flexion and extension of the knee. This is due to the shift of the discoid meniscus between the joint surfaces. Occasionally, it could present as simple discomfort. The discoid meniscus is often disk-shaped, explaining the term "discoid." According to the Watanabe classification

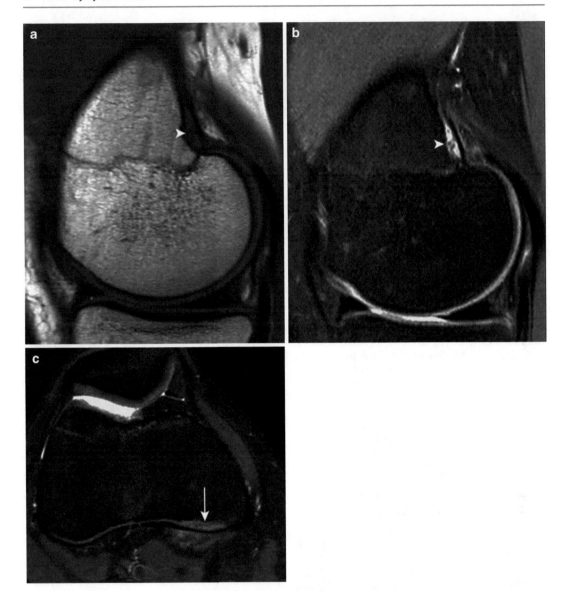

Fig. 23.7 Cortical avulsive irregularity of the distal femur in a 16-year-old adolescent. (**a**) Sagittal T1-W MR image shows the intracortical irregularity as a well-defined lesion with hypointense signal (*arrowhead*). The lesion is hyperintense on (**b**) sagittal and (**c**) axial fat-suppressed PD-W MR images (*arrowhead*, **b**; *arrow*, **c**). There is no periosteal reaction or associated mass in the overlying soft tissues

(Watanabe and Takeda 1974), the discoid meniscus can be subdivided into three types: type I, complete (round with a thick medial border, concave, and cup shaped); type II, incomplete (discoid anterior horn with larger apex extending toward the center, thin or smooth free edge and appearing as a too long meniscus triangle); and type III or Wrisberg ligament variant, in which the posterior meniscal attachment is absent, resulting in an unstable meniscus with hypermobility, causing a snapping knee syndrome.

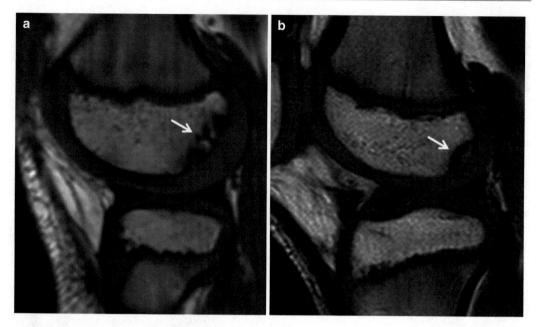

Fig. 23.8 Ossification centers of the femoral condyle. (**a**, **b**) Sagittal T1-W MR images in different patients show small subchondral bone defects (*arrow*) in the posterolateral aspect of the femoral condyle. In both patients, the overlying cartilage shows preserved thickness and outline as well as the absence of underlying bone marrow edema, which confirms an anatomical variant rather than a true osteochondral lesion

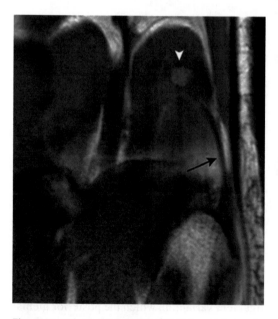

Fig. 23.9 Fabella. Coronal PD-W MR image shows the fabella (*arrowhead*) and a fabellofibular ligament (*arrow*), which is one of the components of the posterolateral corner ligaments that extends from the fabella to the fibular head. This sesamoid ossicle should not be mistaken for a loose bony fragment

On sagittal MR images, a discoid meniscus should be suspected if there is a continuity between the anterior and posterior horns in three or more contiguous images, or if the size between the free margin and the periphery of the body on coronal images exceeds 1.5 cm. On the mid-coronal MR images, the lateral discoid meniscus extends nearly to the intercondylar notch when it is complete, due to its abnormal width. The presence of intrasubstance degeneration with signal hyperintensity makes the discoid meniscus prone to tears. Because of its thickness and poor vascularization (associated, in some cases, with a thin capsular attachment), a discoid meniscus is exposed to a higher risk of tearing, compared to a normal meniscus (Rohren et al. 2001; Kim et al. 2006; Gill et al. 2014; Vanhoenacker et al. 2016) (Fig. 23.10).

A ring-shaped meniscus is a very rare congenital variant, most commonly involving the lateral meniscus. The anterior and posterior horns are connected by an inter-horn menis-

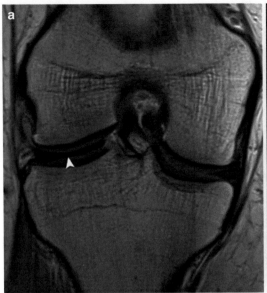
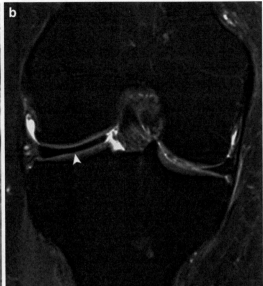

Fig. 23.10 Complete discoid lateral meniscus. Coronal PD-W MR images obtained (**a**) without and (**b**) with fat suppression taken through the middle horns of the menisci show a type I complete discoid meniscus. The middle portion of the lateral meniscus (*arrowhead*) is disk-shaped and extends through the whole lateral joint compartment

Table 23.1 Structures mimicking displaced meniscal fragments

Transverse (intermeniscal) ligament
Oblique meniscomeniscal ligaments
Anteromedial meniscofemoral ligament (AMMFL)
Fatty synovial folds
Vacuum phenomenon
Osteophytes
Intra-articular loose bodies
Ring meniscus

cal bridge between the meniscal roots, as described in the modified Watanabe classification of congenital meniscal abnormalities. This variant can mimic a medially displaced meniscal fragment from a bucket handle tear on coronal MR images (Kim et al. 2006; Nguyen et al. 2014) (Table 23.1).

The meniscus ossicle consists of an intrameniscal ossification. This rare variant is usually seen in the posterior horn of the medial meniscus and may be from a developmental, degenerative, or post-traumatic origin. The latter results from a

tibial avulsion associated with a longitudinal lesion of the meniscus. Standard radiographs show a bone fragment at the level of the posterior horn of the medial meniscus that can be mistaken for a loose body. MRI confirms the intra-articular location and may demonstrate a meniscal fissure. Meniscus ossicle shows central fat signal intensity on T1-weighted images, surrounded by a hypointense rim (Schnarkowski et al. 1995) (Fig. 23.11).

23.2.2.2 Pitfalls from Meniscal Origin (Table 23.2)

Meniscal flounce is a rare transient physiological condition indicating meniscus plasticity that can be seen in 0.2–0.3% of asymptomatic knees. It is secondary to flexion of the knee and redundancy of the free edge of the medial meniscus. It appears on sagittal MR images as a wavy S-shaped structure with folding or buckling of the inner edge of the meniscus, like a carpet that has a wrinkled edge, without any associated abnormal intrameniscal signal. On coronal MR images, it may simulate a truncated meniscus and mimic a radial

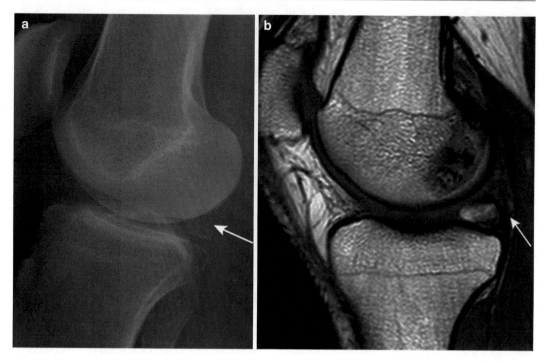

Fig. 23.11 Meniscal ossicle. (**a**) Lateral radiograph shows a bony fragment (*arrow*) at the posterior aspect of the tibiofemoral joint space. (**b**) Sagittal T1-W MR image shows the meniscal ossicle (*arrow*) located within the posterior horn of the medial meniscus, with fatty signal within the ossicle surrounded by a hypointense rim

Table 23.2 Meniscal pseudo-tears from anatomical origin

Meniscal flounce
Meniscal vascularization
Inferolateral genicular artery
Meniscocapsular attachment
Meniscal root and speckled meniscus
Transverse (intermeniscal) ligament
Oblique meniscomeniscal ligaments
Meniscofemoral ligament of Wrisberg
Popliteal tendon and recess

tear or degeneration. Its degree of distortion can change, with the meniscal location on the tibial plateau and the anatomical knee position in flexion or extension (Yu et al. 1997; Park et al. 2006; Nguyen et al. 2014) (Fig. 23.12).

In children, the presence of increased signal within the meniscus can correspond to normal blood vessels. This signal has been described in 82% of pediatric knees and should not be misinterpreted as mucinous or myxoid degeneration, like in adults. The MRI criteria for establishing the diagnosis of a meniscal tear are the same in children and adults. The most important criteria

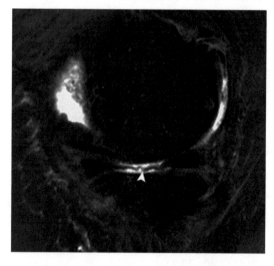

Fig. 23.12 Meniscal flounce. Sagittal fat-suppressed PD-W MR image taken through the medial meniscus shows a buckled appearance of the middle horn (*arrowhead*)

are increased intrameniscal signal that extends to the articular surface and abnormal meniscal morphology (King et al. 1996; Gill et al. 2014) (Fig. 23.13). In adults, vascularized tissue is confined to peripheral third of the meniscus.

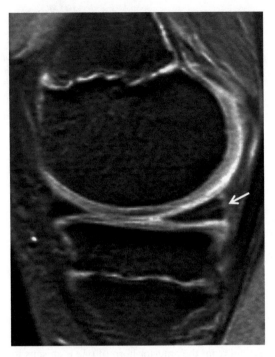

Fig. 23.13 Meniscal vascularization. Sagittal GRE MR image taken through the medial part of the tibiofemoral joint shows an area of linear hyperintensity (*arrow*), mimicking a meniscal tear, in the posterior horn of the medial meniscus. It corresponds to normal meniscus vascularization in children

23.2.2.3 Pitfalls Due to the Meniscal Attachments (Table 23.2)

The medial meniscus is closely attached to the knee capsule along its entire circumference. On peripheral sagittal MR images, the normal meniscocapsular attachment of the posterior horn of medial meniscus can generate an increased meniscal signal (intermediate on T2-weighted images) due to the presence of vessels in the peripheral border of the meniscus, known as the red zone. This increased signal can mimic meniscocapsular separation. The presence of small isolated T2-hyperintense fluid signal should not be misinterpreted as a meniscocapsular separation. On the contrary, abnormal T2-hyperintense signal (similar to fluid) detected between the meniscus and the capsule or within the peripheral zone of the meniscus, associated with irregular meniscal margins, an increased distance between medial collateral ligament and medial meniscus, and meniscal displacement from the tibia, indicates a meniscocapsular separation (Herman and Beltran 1988; Rubin et al. 1996; De Maeseneer et al. 2001, 2002; Bolog and Andreisek 2016; Vanhoenacker et al. 2016) (Fig. 23.14).

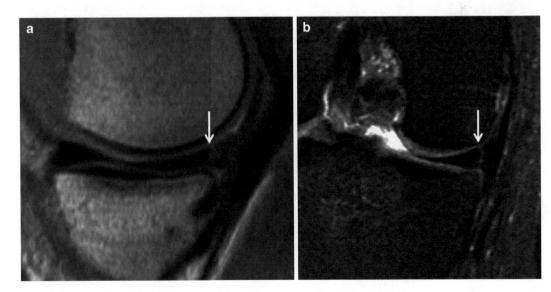

Fig. 23.14 Meniscocapsular separation. (**a**) Sagittal PD-W and (**b**) coronal fat-suppressed PD-W MR images show a thin vertical hyperintensity at the peripheral attachment of the medial meniscus (*arrows*) corresponding to a minor meniscocapsular separation without significant meniscal displacement. The lesion was not surgically repaired and healed spontaneously

The anterior and posterior roots attach the meniscus to the central tibial plateau. The intimate association between the anterior root of the lateral meniscus and the tibial attachment site of the anterior cruciate ligament (ACL) commonly results in a striated or comb-like appearance of the meniscal root with spots of increased signal on sagittal MR images, also known as the speckled appearance of the anterior horn of lateral meniscus (Fig. 23.15). In 2% of the population, an anomalous insertion of the medial meniscus parallels the ACL and can be mistaken for a meniscal tear. In addition, the anterior root of the medial meniscus can occasionally insert along the anterior margin of the tibia and mimic pathological subluxation (Shankman et al. 1997; Nguyen et al. 2014; Tan et al. 2014; Bolog and Andreisek 2016).

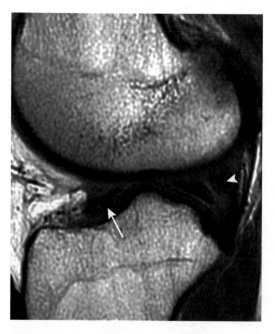

Fig. 23.15 Speckled meniscus. Sagittal T1-W MR image shows a striated anterior root of the lateral meniscus (*arrow*). This appearance results from the proximity of the distal fibers of the anterior cruciate ligament inserting near the anterior meniscal root. The posterior meniscofemoral ligament of Wrisberg is demonstrated close to its attachment on the posterolateral meniscus (*arrowhead*)

23.2.2.4 Pitfalls Due to Perimeniscal Ligaments (Tables 23.1 and 23.2)

The transverse (intermeniscal) ligament (also called the geniculate ligament, anterior meniscomeniscal ligament or intermeniscal ligament of Winslow) is a thin horizontal fibrous band that is present in 90% of cadaveric specimens and 83% of MRI studies (Fig. 23.16). It connects and stabilizes the anterior horns of the menisci. On sagittal MR images, this ligament may mimic an anterior meniscal root tear, a displaced meniscal fragment or a small intra-articular loose body. However, the transverse ligament can be recognized as it is visible on consecutive sagittal images (Marcheix et al. 2009; Nguyen et al. 2014) (Fig. 23.17).

In the literature, the prevalence of oblique meniscomeniscal ligaments ranges from 1% to 4%. The oblique meniscomeniscal ligaments extend from the anterior horn of one meniscus to the posterior horn of the opposite meniscus. They are named according to their anterior attachment site. The medial oblique meniscomeniscal ligament attaches the anterior horn of the medial meniscus to the posterior horn of the lateral meniscus (Fig. 23.18). The lateral oblique meniscomeniscal ligament attaches the anterior horn of the lateral meniscus to the posterior horn of the medial meniscus. These two ligaments cross the intercondylar notch running between the anterior and posterior cruciate ligaments. The oblique meniscomeniscal ligaments can mimic a bucket handle meniscal tear or a displaced meniscal fragment. Their extrasynovial course helps to differentiate them from a displaced meniscal fragment, especially when the meniscus is normal (Dervin and Paterson 1997; Sanders et al. 1999; Kim and Laor 2009; Claes and Pans 2011; Chan and Goldblatt 2012; Shahabpour et al. 2015; Kadi et al. 2016).

The meniscofemoral ligament connects the posterior horn of the lateral meniscus to the lateral surface of the medial femoral condyle. It splits into two bands at the level of the

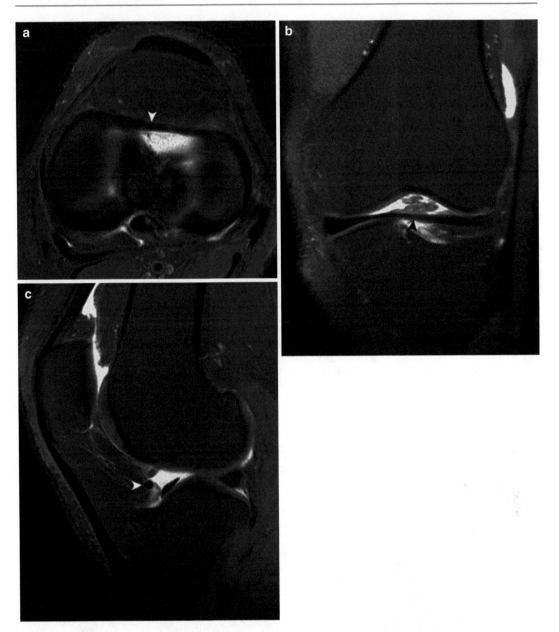

Fig. 23.16 Transverse (intermeniscal) ligament. (**a**) Axial, (**b**) coronal, and (**c**) sagittal fat-suppressed PD-W MR images show the transverse (geniculate) ligament (*arrowhead*) appearing as a hypointense linear band surrounded by fat and joint fluid. The ligament links the anterior horns of both menisci

posterior cruciate ligament. The most common is the posterior meniscofemoral ligament of Wrisberg, passing behind the posterior cruciate ligament (PCL) on sagittal MR images (Fig. 23.19). The anterior meniscofemoral ligament of Humphrey is less frequently found than the Wrisberg ligament and passes anterior to the PCL (Fig. 23.20). Close to the medial

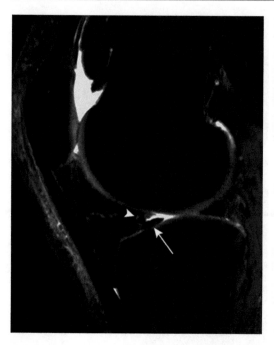

Fig. 23.17 Anterolateral meniscus pseudo-tear. Sagittal fat-suppressed PD-W MR image shows that the cross section of the transverse ligament (*arrowhead*) can mimic an anterior root tear of the lateral meniscus (*arrow*) or an intra-articular loose body

attachment on the posterior horn of the lateral meniscus, the posterior meniscofemoral ligament of Wrisberg may mimic a meniscal tear (Figs. 23.15 and 23.21). It may be directed obliquely, from the upper surface of the lateral meniscus toward its posterior and inferior portion, or vertically, parallel to the basis of the lateral meniscus. The absence of the zip sign (which is a form of meniscal tear progressing from the distal insertion of the Wrisberg ligament through the lateral meniscal wall on axial MR images) can confirm the absence of tear (Watanabe et al. 1989; Vahey et al. 1990; Mohankumar et al. 2014; Kadi et al. 2015; Shahabpour et al. 2015).

The anteromedial meniscofemoral ligament (AMMFL) is a rare variant of the anterior insertion of the medial meniscus, being found in 0.4% of patients in an arthroscopic study (Anderson et al. 2004). The AMMFL is rarer than the Wrisberg and Humphrey ligaments. It is a thin fibrous band running anterior to the whole length of the ACL and connects the anterior horn of the medial meniscus to the posterolateral wall of the

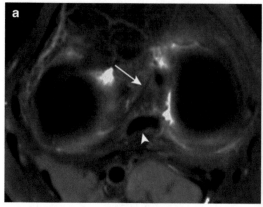

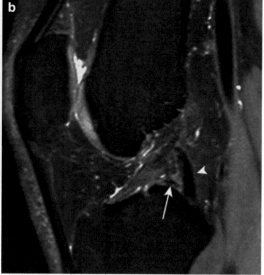

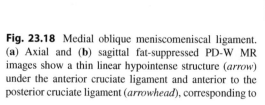

Fig. 23.18 Medial oblique meniscomeniscal ligament. (**a**) Axial and (**b**) sagittal fat-suppressed PD-W MR images show a thin linear hypointense structure (*arrow*) under the anterior cruciate ligament and anterior to the posterior cruciate ligament (*arrowhead*), corresponding to

the medial oblique meniscomeniscal ligament. Axial image shows the ligament extending from the anterior horn of the medial meniscus to the posterior horn of the lateral meniscus. This inconstant ligament should be differentiated from a displaced meniscal fragment

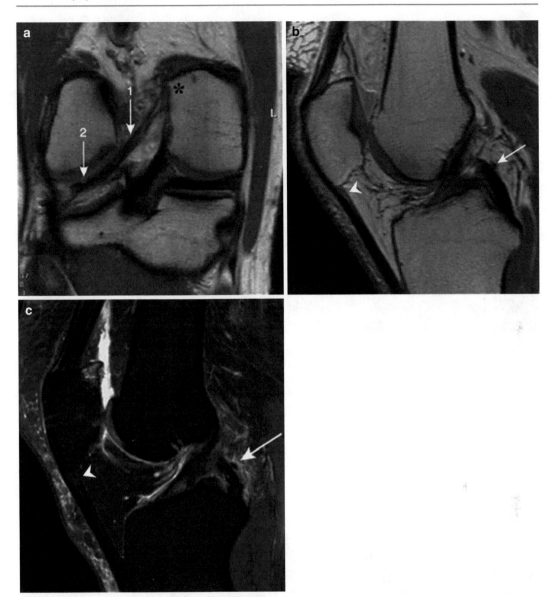

Fig. 23.19 Meniscofemoral ligament of Wrisberg. (**a**) Coronal PD-W MR image taken through the most posterior part of the femoral condyles shows the ligament of Wrisberg appearing as an oblique linear band (*1*) extending from the posterior horn of the lateral meniscus (*2*) to the posteromedial condyle (*asterisk*). Sagittal (**b**) PD-W and (**c**) fat-suppressed PD-W MR images show the Wrisberg ligament (*arrow*) behind the posterior cruciate ligament. Magic angle phenomenon is present in the proximal patellar tendon (*arrowhead*)

intercondylar notch. It can mimic a displaced meniscal fragment or simulate an infrapatellar plica (ligamentum mucosum). The infrapatellar plica extends from the apex of Hoffa fat pad instead of the medial meniscus (Anderson et al. 2004; Coulier and Himmer 2008) (Figs. 23.20 and 23.22). The rarest type of meniscofemoral ligament is the anterolateral meniscofemoral ligament (ALMFL) that is associated with a congenital absence of the ACL (Silva and Sampaio 2011).

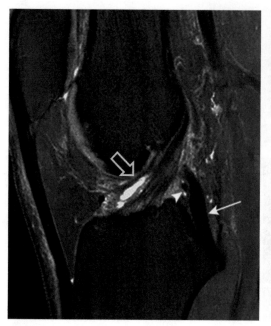

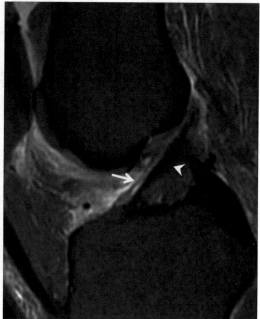

Fig. 23.20 Meniscofemoral ligament of Humphrey and anteromedial meniscofemoral ligament (AMMFL). Sagittal fat-suppressed PD-W MR image taken through the ACL shows the ligament of Humphrey (*arrowhead*) located anterior to the PCL (*arrow*). Another variant is seen on this image, a thin fibrous band running almost parallel and anterior to the ACL and arising from the transverse ligament in this case (*open arrow*). This band so-called the anteromedial meniscofemoral ligament (AMMFL) could simulate a longitudinal or partial tear of the ACL

Fig. 23.22 Anteromedial meniscofemoral ligament (AMMFL). Sagittal fat-suppressed PD-W MR image shows the anteromedial meniscofemoral ligament as a thin hypointense band (*arrow*) parallel to the anterior cruciate ligament (*arrowhead*). This ligament can be differentiated from the infrapatellar plica or ligamentum mucosum (which can similarly be parallel to the anterior cruciate ligament) by its distal attachment on the meniscus rather than on the patella

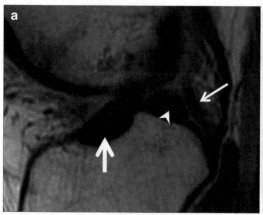

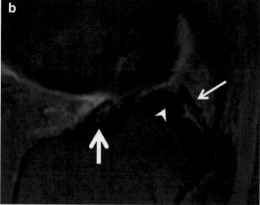

Fig. 23.21 Posterolateral meniscal pseudo-tear. Sagittal (**a**) PD-W and (**b**) fat-suppressed PD-W MR images show the posterior meniscofemoral ligament of Wrisberg (*thin arrow*) close to its attachment on the posterior root of the lateral meniscus (*arrowhead*). It may mimic a meniscal

tear on the midsagittal views. There was no zip sign on the axial views which can confirm the absence of tear. Note the magic angle phenomenon in the anterior horn of the lateral meniscus mimicking meniscal degeneration (*thick arrow*)

23.2.2.5   Pitfalls from Structures Adjacent to the Meniscus

Many structures adjacent to the meniscus may mimic meniscal tears (Table 23.2). A misleading

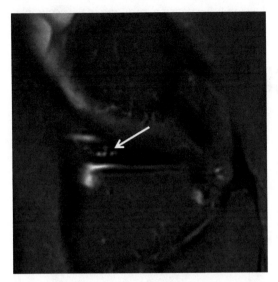

Fig. 23.23 Lateral inferior genicular artery. Sagittal fat-suppressed PD-WMR image shows small areas of hyperintense signal due to the lateral inferior genicular artery (*arrow*) which is located adjacent to the anterior horn of the lateral meniscus and can simulate a meniscal tear

appearance of lateral meniscal tear may also result from the presence of the genicular vessels, which are located in the fat between the peripheral portion of the lateral meniscus and the lateral collateral ligament. The lateral inferior genicular artery arises from the popliteal artery at the level of the tibiofemoral joint and courses anterolaterally to the genicular anastomosis. When the artery lies immediately adjacent to the anterior horn of the lateral meniscus, it can simulate a meniscal tear on sagittal MR images (Herman and Beltran 1988; Watanabe et al. 1989) (Fig. 23.23). This pitfall does not appear on coronal MR images. There is an intimate relationship between the posterior horn of the lateral meniscus and the popliteal tendon and recess (popliteal hiatus). The popliteal recess which lies close to the posterolateral meniscus may appear as an oblique thin band of hyperintense signal that separates the meniscus from the tendon and may be wrongly interpreted as a meniscal tear or meniscocapsular separation (Watanabe et al. 1989) (Fig. 23.24).

Some structures may mimic displaced meniscal fragments (Table 23.1). These include perimeniscal ligaments (i.e., transverse ligament, oblique meniscomeniscal ligaments, and antero-

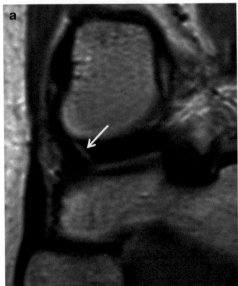
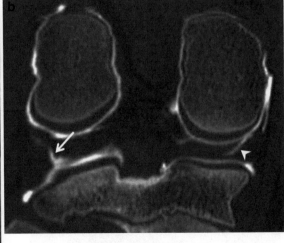

Fig. 23.24 Popliteal tendon and recess. Corresponding coronal (**a**) PD-W MR and (**b**) CT arthrographic images show the popliteal recess (*arrow*) between the popliteal tendon and the posterolateral portion of the lateral meniscus distended by native fluid on the (**a**) MR image and by injected contrast material on the (**b**) CT arthrographic image. The popliteal recess should not be confused with a peripheral meniscal tear. A meniscal tear (*arrowhead*) is detected at the posteromedial meniscus of the same patient on CT arthrogram

medial meniscofemoral ligament) that have been previously mentioned (see Sect. 21.2.2.4). A fatty synovial fold with T1-hyperintense signal may be detected adjacent to the central portion of the anterior horn of the medial meniscus and should not be interpreted as a displaced meniscal fragment or loose body (Fig. 23.25). Vacuum phenomenon can cause false images of displaced meniscal fragment or loose body, particularly on gradient-echo sequences (T2*-weighted images). This is a normal variant caused by negative pressure within the joint due to the position of the knee in full extension, resulting in the accumulation of gas. Intra-articular air interposed between

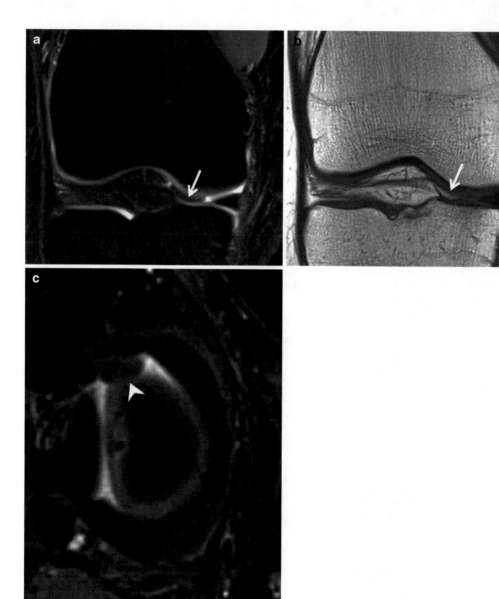

Fig. 23.25 Fatty synovial fold. MR images taken through the anterior horn of the medial meniscus show a fatty structure with hypointense signal on (**a**) coronal and (**c**) axial fat-suppressed PD-W MR images (*arrow*, a; *arrowhead*, c). This should not be interpreted as a displaced meniscal fragment or a loose body. The shape of the structure with hyperintense signal (*arrow*) on the (**b**) coronal T1-W MR image may help to identify the normal synovial fold (Courtesy of Prof. Bruno Vande Berg)

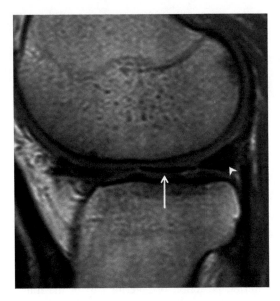

Fig. 23.26 Vacuum phenomenon. Sagittal T1-W MR image shows a horizontal linear structure (*arrow*) within the joint which has a lower signal intensity than the meniscus (*arrowhead*). This structure corresponds to gas accumulation which may mimic a displaced meniscal fragment or a loose body

the cartilage and meniscus can give rise to a horizontal hypointense linear structure within the joint. Correlation of the MRI findings with those of radiographs or computed tomography (CT) may be helpful, although the amount of gas necessary for the creation of these MRI findings is small enough in some cases to be undetectable on the radiographs (Shogry and Pope 1991) (Fig. 23.26).

In osteoarthritic knees, exuberant marginal osteophytes in the intercondylar notch may be difficult to differentiate from displaced meniscal fragments or loose bodies on coronal fat-suppressed MR images. The fat signal on T1-weighted images helps to identify and confirm the presence of marginal osteophytes (Fig. 23.27). Intra-articular loose bodies may also mimic displaced meniscal fragments and can be differentiated by the absence of an associated meniscal defect. Loose bodies and meniscal fragments may migrate toward the intercondylar notch and less frequently into the

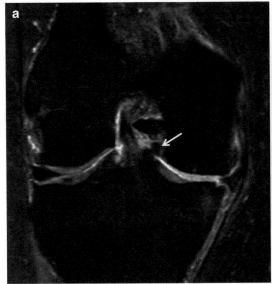
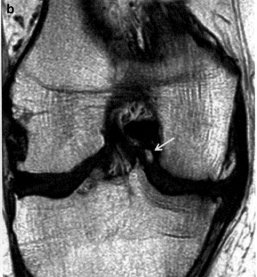

Fig. 23.27 Osteophytes in a patient with severe osteoarthritis and exuberant marginal osteophytes. (**a**) Coronal fat-suppressed PD-W MR image shows a small intercondylar structure (*arrow*) with hypointense signal which could be difficult to differentiate from a displaced meniscal fragment or loose body. The fat signal on (**b**) coronal T1-W MR image helps to identify and confirm the presence of an intercondylar osteophyte (Courtesy of Prof. Bruno Vande Berg)

perimeniscal recesses, whether between the capsule and the femoral condyles (superior meniscal recesses) or between the capsule and the tibial plateaus (inferior meniscal recesses). The precise displacement of free fragments is often underreported or disregarded. Moreover, these fragments may be difficult to identify at arthroscopy. Therefore, a correct description can provide crucial information for the surgeon (Vande Berg et al. 2005).

23.2.3 Other Anatomical Structures

23.2.3.1 Plica

The plica is a vestigial structure of the synovial membrane. The three most common are the suprapatellar, mediopatellar (Fig. 23.28), and infrapatellar plica. The infrapatellar plica is also known as the ligamentum mucosum and is the most common synovial plica in the knee. It is a remainder of the synovial fold between the medial and lateral compartments that occurs when the primitive embryologic intercompartment septum does not regress completely. The infrapatellar plica originates from the intercondylar notch and courses forward and downward

parallel to the ACL (intercondylar component) and then upward into the Hoffa fat pad (Hoffa fat component) to reach the lower pole of the patella. On midsagittal MR images, it appears as a thin curvilinear structure of signal hypointensity, which is better delineated in the presence of joint fluid (Kim et al. 1996; Kosarek and Helms 1999; Garcia-Valtuille et al. 2002; Tyler et al. 2010; Lee et al. 2012) (Fig. 23.29).

23.2.3.2 Hoffa Recess

The Hoffa recess is a synovial recess located along the posterior border of the infrapatellar Hoffa fat pad. On sagittal MR images, it can appear linear, pipelike, or globular, but is most often ovoid. In this plane, it can be located at the inferior, posterior, or anterior part of the transverse (intermeniscal) ligament, when both structures coexist. Identification of this recess is important as it has a connection with the joint cavity. Intra-articular loose bodies could be trapped in the recess and be overlooked at surgery (Aydingöz et al. 2005) (Fig. 23.30).

23.2.3.3 Muscle Variants

Variants of the gastrocnemius muscle are very rare. Most commonly, they are incidental findings.

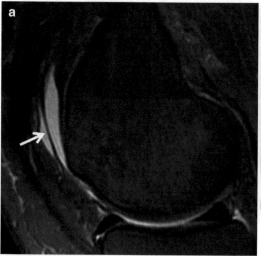
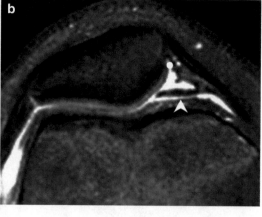

Fig. 23.28 Mediopatellar plica. (**a**) Sagittal and (**b**) axial fat-suppressed PD-W MR images from two different patients show a mediopatellar plica (*arrow*, **a**; *arrowhead*, **b**). A normal plica appears as a thin linear band with sig-

nal hypointensity (**a**). In **b**, the plica is too long and thickened, which can suggest a pathological plica in the medial plica syndrome

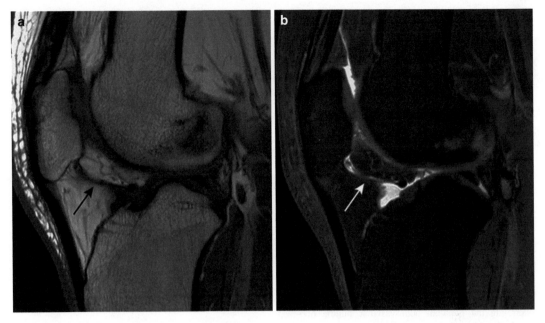

Fig. 23.29 Infrapatellar plica or ligamentum mucosum. Sagittal (**a**) T1-W and (**b**) fat-suppressed PD-W MR images show an infrapatellar plica (*arrow*) running from the transverse ligament in the Hoffa infrapatellar fat pad to the inferior pole of the patella; it is delineated by joint fluid

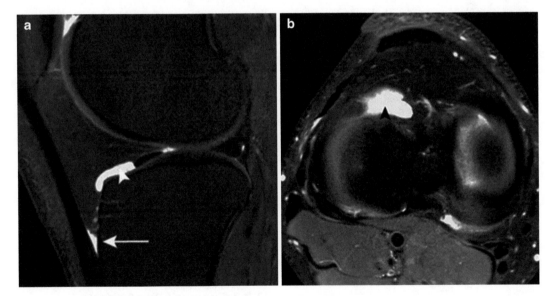

Fig. 23.30 Hoffa recess. (**a**) Sagittal and (**b**) axial fat-suppressed PD-W MR images show the Hoffa recess (*arrowhead*). It consists of a small hyperintense synovial fluid collection located along the posterior border of the Hoffa fat pad. A small fluid reaction is seen in the deep infrapatellar bursa (*arrow*, **a**)

The presence of an accessory bundle has been described at the medial and lateral heads of the gastrocnemius muscle. In some cases, these variants may cause a popliteal artery entrapment syndrome (Fig. 23.31). The accessory popliteal muscle, which can originate from the posterior part of the lateral femoral condyle or from the fabella, may be completely asymptomatic. This

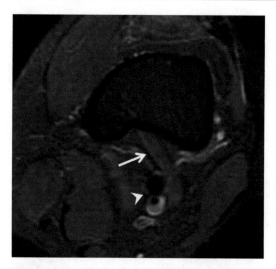

Fig. 23.31 Popliteal artery entrapment syndrome. Axial fat-suppressed PD-W MR image shows an aberrant origin of the lateral head of the gastrocnemius muscle (*arrow*), encircling the popliteal neurovascular bundle (*arrowhead*). Patients with this muscular variant may be asymptomatic or present with claudication

accessory muscle merges with the popliteal muscle at the posteromedial aspect of the tibia. The tensor fasciae suralis muscle is a very rare muscular variant, usually presenting as an asymptomatic popliteal mass. Recognizing this variant helps prevent unnecessary surgical exploration (Duc et al. 2004; Snoeckx et al. 2008).

23.3 Technical Pitfalls

This section covers interpretation errors due to technical artifacts (Table 23.3). For further information on MRI artifacts, also see Chap. 4.

23.3.1 Magic Angle Phenomenon

The magic angle phenomenon occurs on short TE (T1-weighted and proton density) images in fibers that are oriented 55° relative to the static magnetic field. This MRI artifact is a cause of hyperintense signal in the medial segment of the posterior horn of lateral meniscus or in the proximal attachment of the patellar tendon, mimicking tear or degeneration (Figs. 23.19 and 23.21). Imaging the knee joint in slight

Table 23.3 Meniscal pseudo-tears from technical origin

Magic angle phenomenon
Truncation artifact
Susceptibility artifacts
Partial volume effect
Chemical shift artifact
Fat-suppression artifacts
Motion artifacts

abduction can alter the orientation of the fibers in the posterolateral meniscus and eliminate this artifact. Using a TE of more than 37 milliseconds, comparison with T2-weighted images or repositioning of the patient may help identify or eliminate the magic angle artifact (Peterfy et al. 1994; Peh and Chan 2001; Singh et al. 2014; Tan et al. 2014).

23.3.2 Truncation Artifact

Truncation artifact occurs at high contrast boundaries, when there is a large difference in signal intensity between two interfaces, such as the articular cartilage and the menisci. It appears as a series of alternating parallel bands of bright and dark signal. This artifact is parallel to the meniscus borders, when a hyperintense line projects over a hypointense meniscus, mimicking a horizontal meniscal tear. It can also produce a laminar appearance in articular cartilage. This artifact results from inherent errors in the Fourier transformation method of image reconstruction and can be reduced by increasing the matrix size along the phase-encoding direction (Turner et al. 1991; Peh and Chan 2001; Rakow-Penner et al. 2008).

23.3.3 Susceptibility Artifacts

Magnetic susceptibility artifact arises in material being magnetized when exposed to the magnetic field, and it occurs at interfaces of structures having different magnetic susceptibility values (e.g., bone-soft tissue and air-soft tissue interfaces and any adjacent metallic implants). These artifacts can produce image distortion, signal loss, focal bright areas, and failure of fat suppression. The susceptibility effects are more severe in pulse sequences with a long echo time (due to a longer time for photons to diphase) and on gradient-echo images (due to the absence of the 180° refocusing pulse). The magnetic susceptibility artifact can be minimized by removing the metallic object if possible, optimizing patient positioning, switching orientation of frequency- and phase-encoding gradients, and using fast spin-echo sequences (Peh and Chan 2001; Chen et al. 2011; Tan et al.

2014). On the contrary, magnetic susceptibility artifacts can be an advantage in three-dimensional (3D) gradient-echo sequences. The increase of local magnetic field inhomogeneities in the subchondral bone can result in a better differentiation between bone and hyaline cartilage. This phenomenon, together with the decreased partial volume effect and chemical shift artifact, may allow a better analysis of the cartilage surfaces of the tibiofemoral joint (Fig. 23.32).

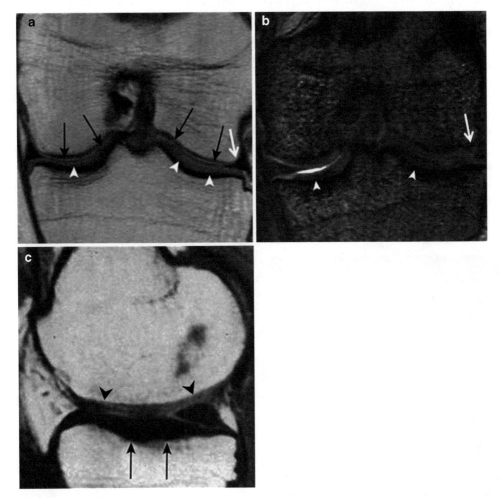

Fig. 23.32 Susceptibility artifacts, partial volume effect, and chemical shift artifact. Comparison of coronal MR images obtained with (**a**) PD-W FSE and (**b**) 3D DESS GRE sequences. On (**b**) 3D GRE sequence, the increased local magnetic field inhomogeneities in the subchondral bone result in a better differentiation between bone and hyaline cartilage (*arrowheads*). On (**a**) coronal and (**c**) sagittal PD-W MR images, chemical shift artifact produces an artificial thinning of the femoral cartilage surface and subchondral bone (*black arrows*, **a**; *black arrowheads*, **c**) associated with an apparent thickening of the tibial cartilage and subchondral bone (*arrowheads*, **a**; *black arrows*, **c**). With the (**b**) 3D GRE sequence, the chemical shift artifact is less pronounced. This advantage, combined with the decrease of partial volume effect (through the use of inframillimetric slices) and with the increase of magnetic susceptibility artifacts allows a better analysis of the two cartilaginous surfaces of the tibiofemoral joint, especially at the curved medial and lateral articular margins when the imaging plane is not perpendicular to the examined anatomic area (*white arrow*, **b** compared to **a**)

23.3.4 Partial Volume Effect

Large slice thickness and/or an inter-slice gap may result in problems due to partial volume effect that occurs when tissues with different MRI properties share the same voxel. At the proximal attachment of the anterior cruciate ligament, the presence of partial volume averaging can lead to a pseudo-medullary bone lesion of the lateral femoral condyle on midsagittal images (Fig. 23.33). This artifact can result in a hyperintense linear zone at the outer edge of the meniscus that may simulate a tear on peripheral sagittal MR images. Misinterpretation can be avoided by examining the coronal MR images. Partial volume averaging may occur in the evaluation of the cartilage at the medial and lateral margins of the tibiofemoral joint, when the imaging plane is not perpendicular to the examined anatomical area (Fig. 23.32). The volume averaging can be reduced by decreasing the field of view, slice thickness (2.5 mm to maximum 3 mm in classical 2D sequences and 0.5–1 mm with 3D sequences), and inter-slice gap. Compared with 1.5 T, 3 T MRI is preferred with the use of smaller slice thickness (with higher spatial resolution and faster imaging time) (Herman and Beltran 1988; Peh and Chan 2001; Tan et al. 2014).

23.3.5 Chemical Shift Artifact

Chemical shift artifact is due to the difference in resonance frequency of water and fat protons (e.g., at the interface between hyaline cartilage and underlying bone). In the tibiofemoral cartilage, this artifact can produce an artificial thickening or thinning of the cartilage surface which is perpendicular to the frequency-encoding direction (i.e., an artificially thinned femoral and thickened tibial cartilage and subchondral bone). This artifact is more severe in images obtained at higher field strengths. It may be reduced by switching the directions of the frequency- and phase-encoding gradients, by using fat suppression or by increasing the bandwidth. In 3D gradient-echo sequences, the chemical shift artifact is far less pronounced. This advantage, coupled with the decrease of partial volume effect (through the use of inframillimetric slices) and the increase of magnetic susceptibility artifacts (as mentioned above), results in a better differentiation between subchondral bone and hyaline cartilage and allows a better analysis of the two cartilaginous surfaces of the tibiofemoral joint (Shahabpour et al. 1997) (Fig. 23.32).

23.3.6 Fat-Suppression Artifacts

The use of fat suppression in fast spin-echo (FSE) or short tau inversion recovery (STIR) sequences increases the accuracy of meniscal tear detection and the visualization of bone or soft tissue edema. However, fat suppression is more susceptible to magnetic field and radio-frequency inhomogeneities. The magnetic field inhomogeneities result in a shift of resonance frequencies of lipid and water. Thus, in these areas, the fat suppression may be uneven, and the water signal may be suppressed instead of fat. This problem may be reduced by decreasing the field of view, proper centering over the area of interest, and the use of auto-shimming. Complete fat suppression needs

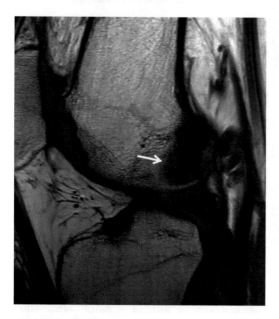

Fig. 23.33 Partial volume effect. Midsagittal T1-W MR image shows that at the proximal attachment of the anterior cruciate ligament on the lateral femoral condyle, the presence of partial volume averaging can lead to an image of bone marrow lesion with hypointense signal (*arrow*)

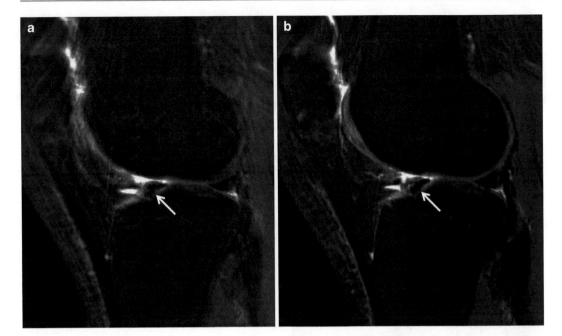

Fig. 23.34 Motion artifact from random patient movement. Sagittal fat-suppressed PD-W MR images obtained (**a**) during patient movement and (**b**) after patient immobilization. Motion artifact is characterized by parallel lines within the blurred MR image (**a**) and can lead to an area of linear hyperintensity in the anterior horn of the lateral meniscus (*arrow*, **a**). The meniscal pseudo-tear disappears after immobilization (*arrow*, **b**)

the radio-frequency pulse to be applied at exactly 90°. When the radio-frequency field is inhomogeneous, the pulse angles will be more or less than 90°, with resultant failure of fat suppression. Alternatively, the STIR technique, which is insensitive to magnetic inhomogeneity, may be used in place of fat-suppressed FSE T2-weighted sequences. But in practice, the knee joint is examined in the center of the magnet where the magnetic field is more homogeneous and the images are rarely disturbed by fat-suppression artifacts (Peh and Chan 2001; Tan et al. 2014).

23.3.7 Motion Artifacts

Motion is the most common MRI artifact and depends on the type of motion, speed and direction of the moving object, and the magnetic field strength. If a structure moves to different positions during image acquisition, the image appears blurred, and an intrameniscal signal resembling a tear may appear. Motion from random patient movement can be reduced by appropriate

immobilization, sedation, patient reassurance, and education. The periodic motion from vascular pulsation (especially the popliteal artery in the knee joint) may produce ghost artifacts (flow artifacts), which can be corrected or reduced by applying flow compensation, out-of-phase saturation pulse, increased number of signals acquired, and swapping the phase-encoding and frequency-encoding directions (Peh and Chan 2001; Tan et al. 2014) (Figs. 23.34 and 23.35).

23.4 Clinical Pitfalls

Some MRI findings are incidental, for example, asymptomatic medial meniscus signal abnormalities that do not correlate with the patient's symptoms and clinical findings. Medial meniscal pseudo-tears may also be incidental findings that are not symptomatic (i.e., not correlated with the patient's complaints). This section describes the different causes of knee pain (medial, lateral, anterior, and posterior) clinically mimicking a meniscal tear but without evidence of surgically significant

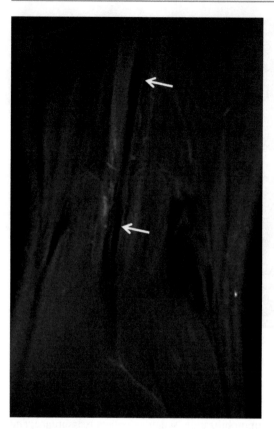

Fig. 23.35 Flow artifacts. Coronal fat-suppressed PD-W MR image shows vertical lines parallel to the popliteal artery (*arrows*) secondary to periodic motion from pulsation of the popliteal artery

meniscal tear on MRI. A stiff knee can be a clinical finding associated with knee pain in some of those pathologies. In some clinical conditions, where the knee appears clinically completely normal, knee pain could represent a referred pain from hip pathology. It is important for the radiologist to identify or recognize cases where an MRI finding, such as a meniscal signal abnormality, is incidental and not clinically relevant, in order to avoid unnecessary surgical treatment. Detection of an abnormality may reduce the detectability of another abnormality. Although additional findings are not always clinically significant, some abnormalities may have an impact on the treatment of the patient. To overcome the phenomenon of satisfaction of search, we recommend a systematic approach in the analysis of all intra- and extra-articular structures of the knee joint.

23.4.1 Medial Knee Pain

23.4.1.1 Fortuitous Meniscal Lesions

In the assessment of a chronic painful knee, some of the meniscal lesions are fortuitous findings, detected on MRI, while another joint pathology is present. The medial meniscal lesion could have spontaneously healed and become asymptomatic after a painful period, especially when the tear is horizontal or oblique without an unstable fragment. It is important to correlate the MR images to the clinical findings, before considering that a meniscal tear is surgically significant. According to Brunner et al. (1989), in a study of the MRI of professional basketball and collegiate football players, the meniscal tears were all asymptomatic. Reinig et al. (1991) showed that in asymptomatic college football players from a major team, a progression of meniscal degenerative changes, from grade 1 to grade 2 and from grade 2 to grade 3, after one single football season (Brunner et al. 1989; Reinig et al. 1991; De Smet et al. 1993; Shahabpour et al. 1997). If a stable meniscal lesion is overdiagnosed and surgically treated when it is unnecessary, the meniscal resection could have a harmful effect on the outcome of the tibiofemoral joint. The suppression of the protective role of the medial meniscus will favor the development of osteoarthritis or accelerate a prior osteoarthritis with cartilage degeneration, especially in patients with varus deformity. After arthroscopic resection of the meniscal tear, the knee complaints could transiently disappear, but the patient's cartilage and meniscus will further degenerate and may require total knee prosthesis on the long term (Fig. 23.36, Table 23.4).

23.4.1.2 Medial Knee Pain in Young Patients

The other causes of a painful medial compartment, especially in young patients, include osteochondrosis of the femoral condyles (and less frequently of the tibial condyles) and distal femoral exostosis (Fig. 23.37). Those could be ruled out by radiographs and MRI. Other etiologies to rule out in young patients are juvenile idiopathic arthritis (JIA), infectious arthritis, and early tumoral disease. Another disorder in the differen-

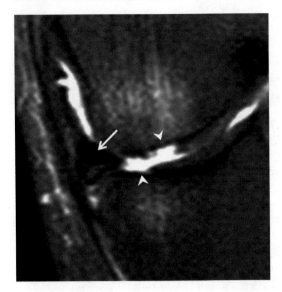

Fig. 23.36 Chondrolysis after partial medial meniscal resection. Coronal fat-suppressed T2-W MR image obtained 4 months after medial meniscal surgery shows a chondral abrasion with underlying bone marrow edema in the medial tibiofemoral compartment (*arrowheads*). There is no evidence of tear in the postoperative meniscal remnant (*arrow*). Cartilage damage may be secondary to the loss of meniscal tissue after partial or subtotal meniscectomy

tial diagnoses in children and young adults is chronic recurrent multifocal osteomyelitis (CRMO), characterized by nonbacterial osteomyelitis. The typical imaging findings of CRMO include osteolytic lesions in the metaphyses of long bones, adjacent to the growth plate, which are often present in a single symptomatic site, especially the knee joint (Fig. 23.38). Most cases undergo spontaneous resolution in several months. Making the right diagnosis could help minimize unnecessary biopsies, surgery, and antibiotic therapy (Jurik 2004; Gill et al. 2014) (Table 23.4).

23.4.1.3 Nontraumatic Medial Knee Pain

From a sports physician's perspective, in daily clinical practice, chondropathy or osteonecrosis of the medial tibiofemoral compartment can be extremely difficult to differentiate from a meniscal tear. A painful medial compartment from nontraumatic origin can be due to mechanical overload of the medial tibiofemoral compartment (e.g., in obesity, sports activities, and deformity of the lower limb

Table 23.4 Medial knee pain mimicking medial meniscal tear: causes

Medial knee pain	Causes
In young patients	Osteochondrosis of femoral and tibial condyle
	Distal femoral exostosis
	Juvenile idiopathic arthritis (JIA)
	Infection
	Tumor
	Chronic recurrent multifocal osteomyelitis (CRMO)
Nontraumatic	Mechanical overload of medial tibiofemoral compartment: Obesity, sport activity, genu varum
	Stress fracture of medial tibial plateau
	Insufficiency fracture (medial femoral or tibial condyle)
	Tibiofemoral/patellofemoral chondropathy
	Medial tibial and femoral osteochondral lesions/osteonecrosis
	Inflammatory disorders
	Gout
	Rheumatoid arthritis
	Psoriasis
	Microcrystalline arthropathy (chondrocalcinosis)
	Synovial pathologies
	Inflammatory synovitis (rheumatismal or septic origin)
	Osteochondromatosis/synovial chondromatosis
	Localized nodular synovitis or focal PVNS
	Cysts of cruciate ligaments
Traumatic	Fracture, MCL sprain, and sequels (Pellegrini-Stieda disease and Palmer syndrome)
	Patellar dislocation (with lesions of the medial retinaculum/patellar bone avulsion)

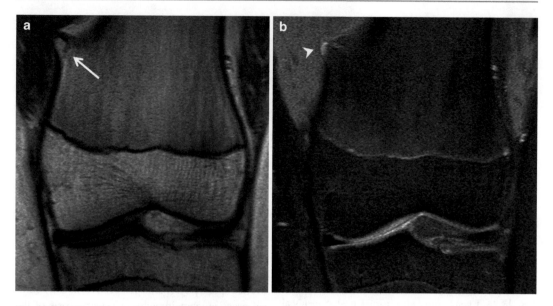

Fig. 23.37 Distal femoral exostosis in an adolescent. Coronal (**a**) PD-W and (**b**) fat-suppressed PD-W MR images show a focal contour deformity at the medial aspect of the distal femur. The small exostosis (*arrow*) is covered by a thin cartilage cap with hyperintense signal (*arrowhead*) and corresponds to a benign lesion. It can cause medial knee pain due to friction with the overlying vastus medialis muscle. This pathology should be ruled out in young patients with medial knee pain

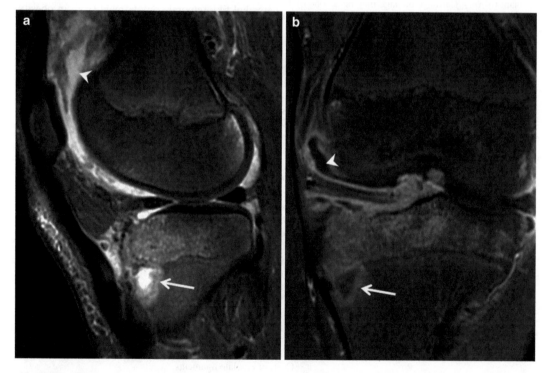

Fig. 23.38 Chronic recurrent multifocal osteomyelitis (CRMO) in an 11-year-old patient with a 3-month history of knee pain. (**a**) Sagittal fat-suppressed PD-W MR image shows an oval hyperintense lesion in the proximal tibial metaphysis adjacent to the physis (*arrow*) with surrounding bone marrow edema extending from the metaphysis to the epiphysis. Suprapatellar (*arrowhead*) and infrapatellar synovitis is detected. (**b**) Coronal contrast-enhanced fat-suppressed T1-W MR image shows peripheral enhancement (*arrow*) around the lesion. Synovitis is seen in the perimeniscal recesses (*arrowhead*)

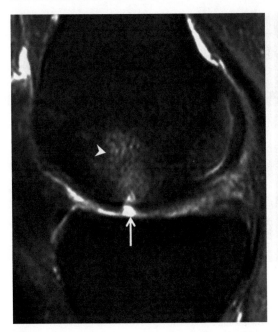

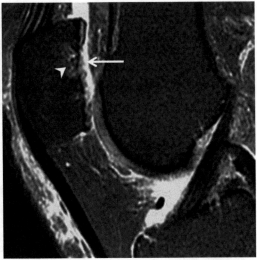

Fig. 23.40 Patellofemoral chondropathy. Sagittal fat-suppressed T2-W MR image shows signal hyperintensity and partial thickness cartilage loss (*arrow*) delineated by the reactive joint effusion. There is underlying subchondral bone marrow edema (*arrowhead*) which correlates with the patient's nontraumatic medial knee pain

Fig. 23.39 Tibiofemoral chondropathy. Sagittal fat-suppressed T2-W MR image shows signal hyperintensity in a deep cartilage defect (*arrow*) predominantly in the medial femoral condyle. There is associated bone marrow edema (*arrowhead*) in this patient who complained of medial knee pain

axis such as genu varum). These conditions can lead to a tibiofemoral chondropathy (Fig. 23.39) or stress fractures of the medial femoral or tibial condyle (and insufficiency fractures if the patient is osteoporotic). Patellofemoral chondropathy (Fig. 23.40) is frequently encountered between 30 and 40 years of age but, in most cases, are totally asymptomatic. The other causes include, on one hand, osteochondral lesions (Fig. 23.41) and osteonecrosis of femoral condyle or tibial plateau (Lecouvet et al. 2005) and, on the other hand, inflammatory disorders, which include gout; rheumatoid arthritis; psoriasis and microcrystalline arthropathy with chondrocalcinosis (Fig. 23.42); osteochondromatosis and synovial chondromatosis (Fig. 23.43); localized nodular synovitis or focal pigmented villonodular synovitis (PVNS), also called giant-cell tumor of the tendon sheath (Fig. 23.44); and cruciate ligaments cyst. MRI may be less sensitive and specific for the identification of calcifications, compared to radiographs. On MRI, meniscal calcifications can demonstrate hyperintense signal, which should not be mistaken for a meniscal tear. Comparison with radiographs helps to avoid this pitfall. Sometimes,

chondrocalcinosis can obscure a tear and result in a false-negative finding (Kaushik et al. 2001) (Table 23.4).

23.4.1.4   Traumatic Medial Knee Pain

The causes of post-traumatic medial pain include fractures and medial collateral ligament (MCL) sprain. MCL injuries can be complicated by Pellegrini-Stieda disease appearing months or years after knee injury and corresponding to ossifications along the proximal ligamentous attachment on the medial femoral condyle. Palmer syndrome is another outcome of MCL lesions appearing in the absence of early knee mobilization. It corresponds to an excessive retractile fibrous scarring of MCL after minor sprain (Fig. 23.45). Another post-traumatic etiology of medial knee pain is a patellar dislocation with rupture of the medial retinaculum and/or avulsion fracture of the medial border of the patella (Shahabpour et al. 1997) (Fig. 23.46, Table 23.4).

23.4.2   Lateral Knee Pain

Patients are frequently referred for lateral knee pain which can be due to different etiologies.

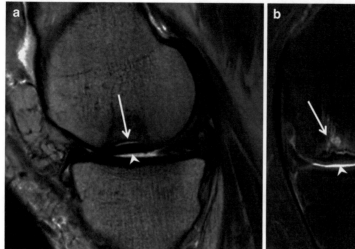

Fig. 23.41 Medial femoral osteochondral lesion. (**a**) Sagittal T2-W and (**b**) coronal fat-suppressed PD-W MR images show an osteochondral lesion in the weight-bearing surface of the medial femoral condyle (*arrow*). This is another cause of painful medial compartment in young adults. The lesion is covered by a thick cartilage layer (*arrowhead*) and outlined by underlying bone marrow edema

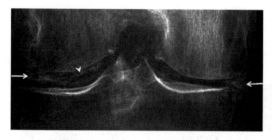

Fig. 23.42 Chondrocalcinosis/meniscocalcinosis. Antero posterior radiograph shows dense calcifications in both the menisci (*arrows*) and hyaline cartilage (*arrowhead*). Based on this image alone, one can diagnose only chondrocalcinosis, not pyrophosphate arthropathy

The onset of lateral knee pain may either be gradual over time or sudden following an injury. It may lead to sharp pain as well as restricted mobility and a wide variety of symptoms, simulating a lateral meniscal tear. There are many differential diagnoses of lateral knee pain ranging from articular pathology (chondropathy and lateral knee osteoarthritis, patellofemoral syndrome, proximal tibiofibular joint lesions,

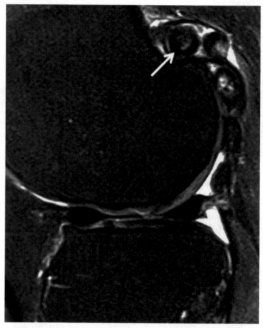

Fig. 23.43 Synovial chondromatosis. Sagittal fat-suppressed PD-W MR image shows multiple intra-articular round nodules with heterogeneous signal (*arrow*) suggestive of synovial chondromatosis

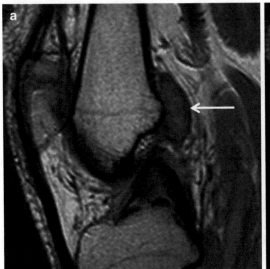

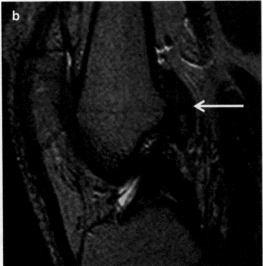

Fig. 23.44 Localized nodular synovitis (focal PVNS). Sagittal (**a**) PD-W and (**b**) T2-W MR images show a single nodular articular mass with hypointense signal (*arrow*). The very low signal on T2-weighted image cor-responds to high hemosiderin content. The patient presented with a stiff knee and extension deficit, in which the diagnosis was unclear despite two previous arthroscopic explorations

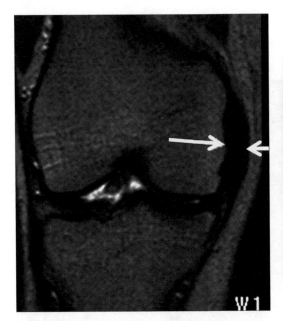

Fig. 23.45 Palmer syndrome. Coronal STIR MR image shows thickening of the proximal part of the MCL (*between arrows*) after a minor sprain. Excessive retractile fibrous scarring appeared a few weeks after the sprain due to prolonged immobilization. The patient presented with a stiff knee and deficit of flexion/extension movements with proximal pain (comparable to knife stabs). There was no ligamentous laxity or medial meniscal tear

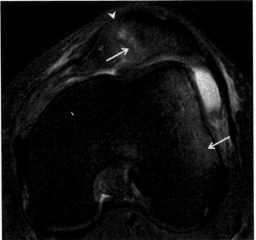

Fig. 23.46 Patellar dislocation. Axial fat-suppressed T2-W MR image shows typical MRI findings of transient patellar dislocation with bone bruises in the areas of impaction of the anterolateral femoral condyle and the medial patella (*arrows*) during spontaneous relocation of the patella. There is associated tear of the anterior aspect of the medial retinaculum (*arrowhead*). The trochlear groove is quite shallow in this patient presenting with trochlear dysplasia and medial knee pain

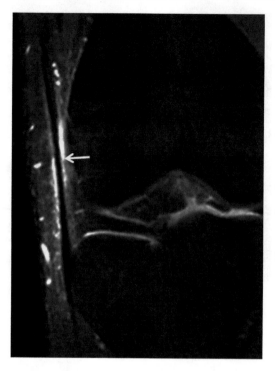

Fig. 23.47 Iliotibial band friction syndrome. Coronal fat-suppressed T2-W MR image shows soft tissue edema (*arrow*) around the iliotibial band which is slightly thickened. This is often clinically difficult to differentiate from a lateral meniscal tear

discoid lateral meniscus [Fig. 23.10]), musculo-tendinous tendinopathy and/or tears (especially the iliotibial band syndrome [Fig. 23.47] and biceps femoris or popliteal tendinopathy), and ligamentous disruption (lateral collateral ligament injury, injury of the posterolateral corner ligaments [Fig. 23.48]) that are frequently associated with PCL and ACL tears or an osseous origin (osteonecrosis [Fig. 23.49], complex regional pain syndrome, stress fracture, bone tumor) (Lecouvet et al. 2005). In daily clinical practice, as for the medial compartment, a chondropathy or an osteonecrosis of the lateral compartment can be extremely difficult to differentiate from a meniscal tear. Apart from the knee pathologies, lateral knee pain can also correspond to a referred pain resulting from L4 to L5 lumbar radiculopathy (Bozkurt and Dogan 2015; Chalès et al. 2016) (Table 23.5).

23.4.3 Anterior Knee Pain

Anterior knee pain is a common complaint in athletes and nonathletic patients. It may be

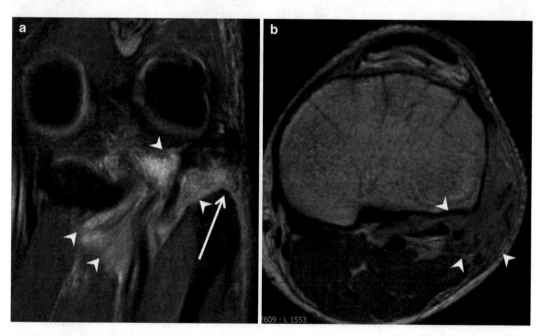

Fig. 23.48 Injury of posterolateral corner (PLC) ligaments. (**a**) Coronal fat-suppressed PD-W and (**b**) axial PD-W MR images performed 3 weeks after a severe soccer trauma show extensive edematous infiltration over the posterolateral corner (*arrowheads*) suggesting injury of the PLC ligaments. Distal detachment of the biceps tendon (*arrow*) and fabellofibular ligament was confirmed at surgical exploration

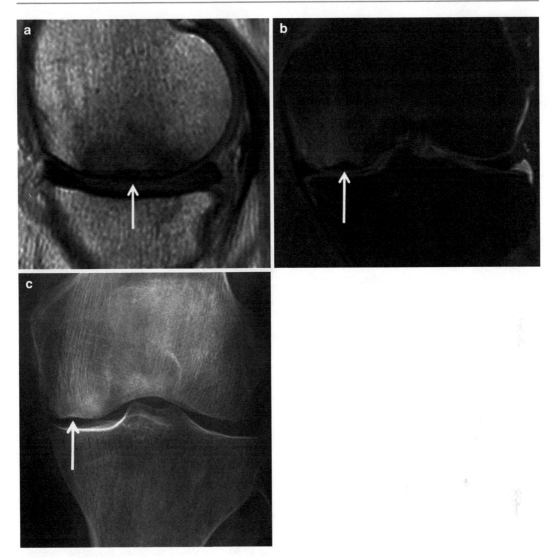

Fig. 23.49 Spontaneous osteonecrosis of the knee (SONK). (**a**) Sagittal T1-W and (**b**) coronal fat-suppressed T2-W MR images show an epiphyseal lesion with long anteroposterior extension in the medial femoral condyle (*arrow*). There is a subchondral area of T1-hypointense and T2-hypointense signal corresponding to an irreversible zone of osteonecrosis. (**c**) Anteroposterior radiograph shows inhomogeneous density with flattening of the subchondral bone in the medial femoral condyle (*arrow*)

caused by traumatic injuries but more often from repeated minor trauma and overuse. MRI is particularly important to confirm the diagnosis of lesions of the anterior compartment and to exclude other diagnoses such as tear of the anterior horn of the lateral meniscus, which is more frequent than the medial meniscus or a meniscal cyst arising from a lateral meniscal tear. Overuse injuries include chronic avulsion injuries of the tibial tuberosity or distal patellar pole, respectively, in Osgood-Schlatter (Fig. 23.50) and Sinding-Larsen-Johansson (Fig. 23.51) disease, patellar tendinopathy of the proximal attachment or jumper knee (Fig. 23.52), quadriceps tendinopathy, bipartite patella (Fig. 23.4), and stress fracture. In

Table 23.5 Lateral knee pain mimicking lateral meniscal tear: causes.

Lateral knee pain	Causes
Articular	Chondropathy and lateral knee osteoarthritis
	Patellofemoral syndrome
	Proximal tibiofibular joint lesions
	Discoid lateral meniscus
Musculotendinous	Iliotibial band syndrome (most frequent cause)
	Biceps femoris tendinopathy and/or tears
	Popliteal tendinopathy
Ligamentous	Lateral collateral ligament injury
	Injury of the posterolateral corner
	With/without PCL and ACL injuries
Osseous	Osteonecrosis
	Complex regional pain syndrome
	Stress fracture
	Bone tumor
Referred pain	L4–L5 radiculopathy

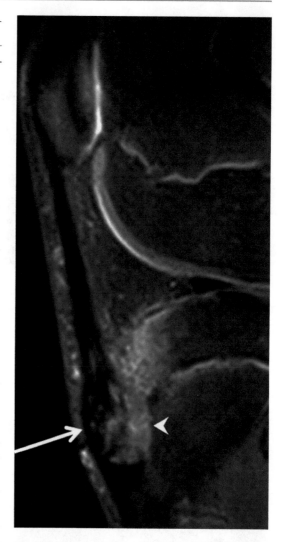

Fig. 23.50 Osgood-Schlatter disease. Sagittal fat-suppressed PD-W MR image of a young teenager shows hyperintense bone marrow edema within the anterior tibial tuberosity corresponding to an avulsed portion of the secondary ossification center (*arrowhead*). The distal attachment of the patellar tendon (*arrow*) is mildly thickened and demonstrates hyperintense signal in the deep fibers

trauma-related lesions, we find osteochondral injuries, bone bruising, and post-traumatic degenerative changes. The differential diagnoses of lesions from osseous origin include patellar and trochlear dysplasia, bone tumors, dorsal defect of the patella (Fig. 23.5), giant cell tumor, and osteosarcoma. Other causes that may lead to anterior knee pain include medial plica syndrome (Fig. 23.28) and prepatellar bursitis (Fig. 23.53) (Jackson 2001; Llopis and Padrón 2007) (Table 23.6).

23.4.4 Posterior Knee Pain

Posterior knee pain may be due to multiple etiologies, including lesions of bone and musculotendinous structures, ligaments, nerves, vessels, and bursae. It is most commonly caused by tendinopathies and muscle injuries, including hamstrings, gastrocnemius, and popliteus tendon/

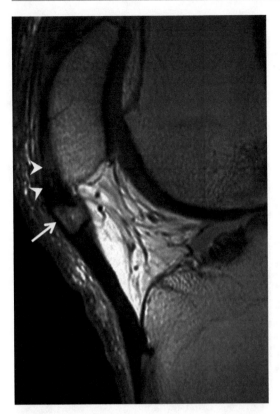

Fig. 23.51 Sinding-Larsen-Johansson disease. Sagittal PD-W MR image shows a chronic avulsion fracture at the inferior pole of the patella (*arrow*), embedded within the inferior patellar tendon, in a volleyball player. The patellar tendon attachment at the anterior aspect of the patella has inhomogeneous hyperintense signal proximal to the avulsed bone fragment (*arrowheads*)

muscle complexes. Other causes include injuries of the posterolateral and posteromedial corners, frequently associated with PCL and ACL injuries (Fig. 23.48). Cystic lesions can also cause posterior knee pain. The most commonly encountered is the classical Baker or popliteal cyst which is a distension of the common semimembranosus/medial gastrocnemius bursa that communicates with the knee joint (Fig. 23.54). Neurologic and vascular injuries are far less frequent causes of posterior knee pain. The common peroneal nerve

is most frequently entrapped by an extrinsic mass (e.g., muscle hematoma, ganglion, osteochondroma, or soft tissue tumors). Vascular injuries include popliteal artery entrapment syndrome (Fig. 23.31), aneurysm, and deep venous thrombosis. Posterior knee pain is rarely from an osseous origin as in severe osteoarthritis, tibial stress fracture, bone tumors (e.g., osteochondroma, osteosarcoma, chondroblastoma), synovial chondromatosis (Fig. 23.43), and PVNS (Fig. 23.55) or localized nodular synovitis (Muché and Lento 2004; English and Perret 2010) (Fig. 23.44, Table 23.7).

23.4.5 Knee Stiffness

Patients are sometimes referred to MRI for assessment of a painful stiff knee. Knee stiffness is characterized by a restricted knee motion which can be a source of significant disability for the patient, as it interferes with his daily activities. Recognition of the causes could have an important impact on therapeutic decisions. It could help to avoid unnecessary invasive therapy, such as manipulation under anesthesia or arthroscopic capsular release. The onset of knee stiffness may be acute or progressive. Flexion or extension can be limited from a few degrees to full stiffness with ankylosis. MRI is particularly helpful to determine the causes: post-traumatic, nontraumatic, or postoperative.

23.4.5.1 Post-traumatic Stiffness

The causes of post-traumatic stiffness include hemarthrosis (due to ACL rupture, peripheral capsuloligamentous tear, patellar dislocation, fracture, or osteochondral fracture); articular fluid effusion or hydrarthrosis and Baker cyst (associated with meniscal or pure chondral lesions), as well as minor sprain of the MCL with retractile scarring (Palmer syndrome) (Fig. 23.45); and

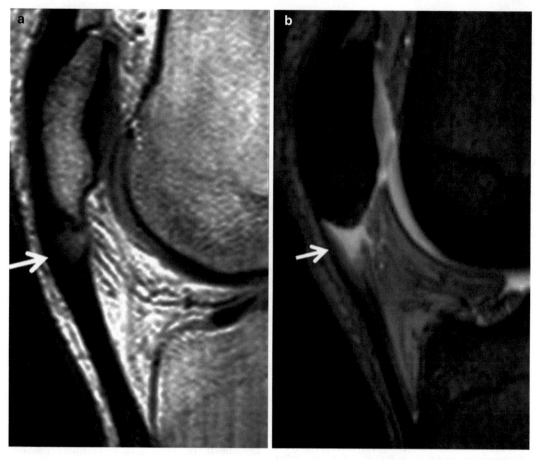

Fig. 23.52 Jumper knee. Sagittal (**a**) PD-W and (**b**) GRE T2*-W MR images of two different basketball players show slight thickening with hyperintense signal in the proximal attachment of the patellar tendon (*arrow*)

articular fibrous adhesions after prolonged immobilization (Table 23.8).

23.4.5.2 Nontraumatic Stiffness

Nontraumatic stiffness can be due to osseous pathology (complex regional pain syndrome or reflex sympathetic dystrophy, osteonecrosis (Fig. 23.49), malignant bone tumor) or be related to articular pathology (joint effusion, cartilaginous lesions, osteochondral lesions, synovial pathologies). In synovial disorders, the origin of the stiffness may be inflammatory (rheumatoid or septic). It can be caused by pathological plica (Fig. 23.28b), synovial chondromatosis (Fig. 23.43), PVNS (Fig. 23.55), lipoma arborescens (Fig. 23.56), or cruciate ligament cyst (Fig. 23.57, Table 23.8).

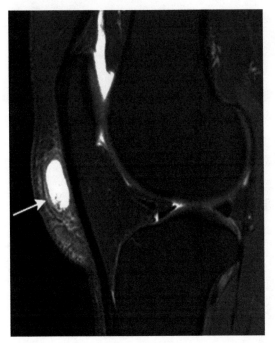

Table 23.6 Anterior knee pain mimicking meniscal tear: causes

Anterior knee pain	Causes
Overuse	Osgood-Schlatter disease
	Sinding-Larsen-Johansson disease
	Jumper knee
	Quadriceps tendinopathy
	Bipartite patella
	Stress fracture
Traumatic	Osteochondral injuries
	Bone bruising
	Post-traumatic degenerative changes
Other	Patellar and trochlear dysplasia
	Bone tumor
	Dorsal defect of patella
	Giant cell tumor
	Osteosarcoma
	Medial plica syndrome
	Prepatellar bursitis

Fig. 23.53 Prepatellar bursitis. Sagittal fat-suppressed PD-W MR image shows a small well-defined fluid collection anterior to the patellar tendon consistent with prepatellar bursitis (*arrow*). Such collections usually result from chronic friction or compression and are frequently associated with job activities performed by house cleaners, carpet layers, and others who work on their knees

23.4.5.3 Postoperative Stiffness

Loss of motion is a typical complication after surgery to the knee. It may be seen after meniscal repair. It more frequently develops after ACL reconstruction. A cyclops lesion (or localized anterior arthrofibrosis) is a nodule of fibrous tissue located within the intercondylar notch, anterior to the ACL graft. It can be due to repeated graft impingement that may result from a too anterior tibial tunnel (Fig. 23.58). A more diffuse arthrofibrosis with extensive scar tissue infiltration of the Hoffa fat pad together with postoperative adhesions can also develop after ACL graft impingement (Fig. 23.59). A too short or tense ACL graft due to a too posteriorly bored tibial tunnel will lead to a loss of extension (or flessum deformity) (Fig. 23.60).

After an ACL reconstruction using a portion of the patellar tendon (in bone-patellar tendon-bone graft [BPTB graft]), abnormalities of the donor site can be encountered, leading to a patella infera syndrome secondary to shortening of the patellar tendon (Fig. 23.61). Patellar entrapment syndrome is another complication of the BPTB graft, related to adherence of the patella to the adjacent infrapatellar fat (Fig. 23.62). Postoperative immobilization can be responsible for stiffness, as for preoperative prolonged immobilization (Harner et al. 1994; Gerbino 1998; McWilliams and Binns 2000; Papakonstantinou et al. 2003; Ehlinger et al. 2010) (Table 23.9).

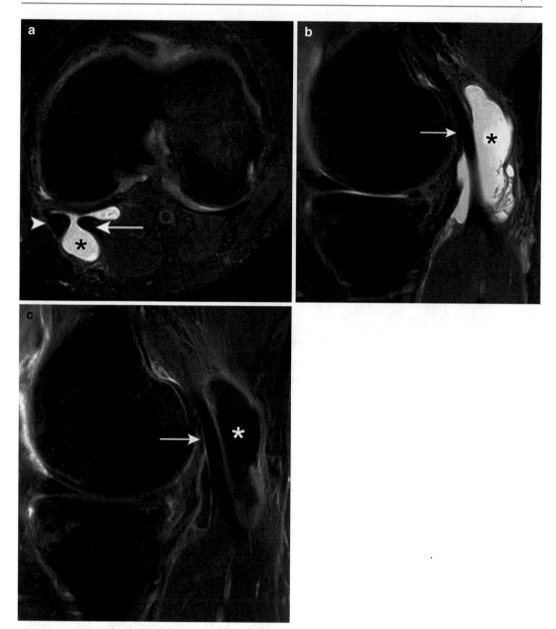

Fig. 23.54 Popliteal cyst (Baker cyst) in a patient complaining of painful posterior swelling in the popliteal fossa. (**a**) Axial and (**b**) sagittal fat-suppressed PD-W MR images show a popliteal cyst (*asterisk*) corresponding to a distension of the common bursa of the semimembranosus (*arrowhead*) and medial gastrocnemius (*arrow*) tendons. (**c**) Sagittal contrast-enhanced fat-suppressed T1-W MR image shows peripheral enhancement of the thickened synovium around the cyst

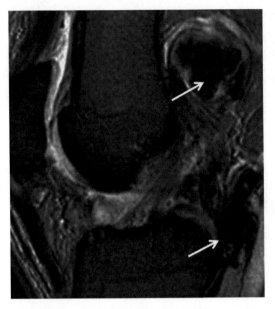

Fig. 23.55 PVNS in a patient with painful flexion/extension limitation of the knee. Sagittal GRE T2*-W MR image shows "blooming" of two hypointense posterior nodular areas (*arrows*). The nodules contain hemosiderin and present with signal hypointensity and appear larger than on spin-echo sequences. This is typical of PVNS

Table 23.7 Posterior knee pain mimicking meniscal tear: causes

Posterior knee pain	Causes
Tendinopathy/ muscular injuries	Hamstrings, gastrocnemius, popliteus tendon/muscle complexes
Ligamentous injuries	Posterolateral and posteromedial corners (with or without PCL and ACL injuries)
Cystic lesions	Popliteal or Baker cyst Ganglion cyst
Neurologic/vascular lesions	Common peroneal nerve Popliteal artery entrapment syndrome Aneurysm Deep venous thrombosis
Osseous	Osteoarthritis Tibial stress fracture Bone tumor Synovial chondromatosis PVNS or localized nodular synovitis

Table 23.8 Knee stiffness: causes

Knee stiffness	Causes
Traumatic	Hemarthrosis ACL rupture Peripheral capsuloligamentous tear Patellar dislocation Fracture/osteochondral fracture Hydrarthrosis/Baker cyst Meniscal tear Chondral lesion Palmer syndrome (minor sprain of MCL with retractile scarring) Fibrous adhesions post immobilization
Nontraumatic	Osseous pathology Complex regional pain syndrome Osteonecrosis Malignant bone tumor Articular pathology Joint effusion Cartilage lesions (osteoarthrosis) Osteochondral lesions Synovial pathologies Inflammatory synovitis (rheumatic diseases, infection) Pathological plica Osteochondromatosis/synovial Chondromatosis Pigmented villonodular Synovitis/localized nodular Synovitis Lipoma arborescens Cyst of cruciate ligaments

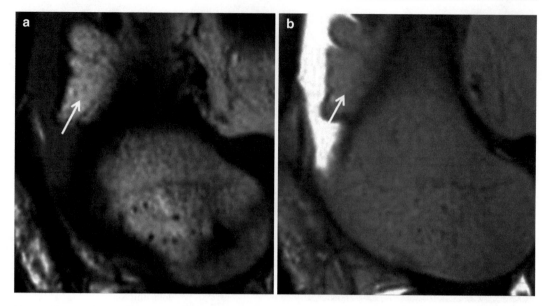

Fig. 23.56 Lipoma arborescens discovered in a nontraumatic stiff knee. Sagittal (**a**) T1-W and (**b**) T2-W MR images show a loculated hyperintense mass due to fatty proliferation of the synovium (*arrow*) with a signal identical to that of bone marrow. Note the frond-like, multiloculated papillary appearance of the intra-articular mass

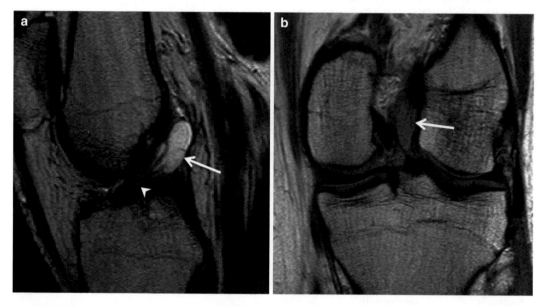

Fig. 23.57 Cyst of the anterior cruciate ligament in a patient with a painful extension deficit of the knee. (**a**) Sagittal T2-W and (**b**) coronal PD-W MR images show a focal oval hyperintense cystic structure within the anterior cruciate ligament and adjacent to it (*arrow*), displacing part of the fibers that are otherwise intact (*arrowhead*). ACL cysts may be asymptomatic incidental findings

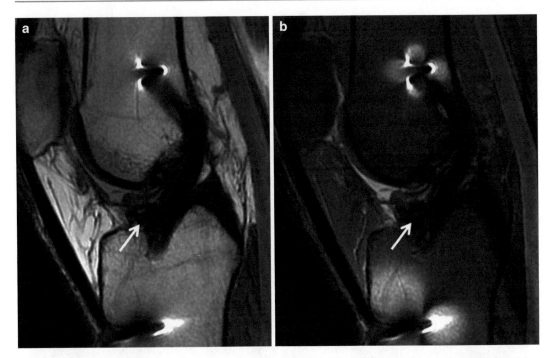

Fig. 23.58 Cyclops lesion (localized arthrofibrosis). Sagittal (**a**) PD-W and (**b**) fat-suppressed PD-W MR images show a nodular area of hypointense fibrous tissue in the fat anterior to the distal ACL graft, corresponding to a focal anterior arthrofibrosis or "cyclops" lesion (*arrow*). The patient complained of pain and postoperative knee stiffness. Focal arthrofibrosis is more common in patients with repeated intercondylar notch "roof impingement" in which ACL reconstruction is performed within 4 weeks of ACL tear, possibly due to ongoing inflammatory changes in the joint. Surgical resection for large symptomatic lesions is necessary

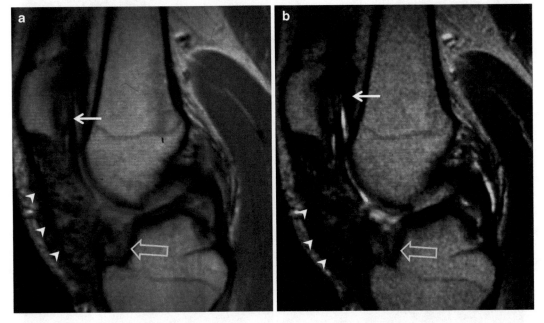

Fig. 23.59 Diffuse arthrofibrosis. Sagittal (**a**) PD-W and (**b**) T2-W MR images show a huge diffuse hypointense area of infiltration in the infrapatellar fat pad (*arrowheads*) with adhesions in the suprapatellar recess (*arrows*) due to a postoperative arthrofibrosis. This was responsible for the patient's disabling knee stiffness. Repeated ACL graft impingement due to too anterior positioning of the tibial tunnel (*open arrow*) resulted in a disruption of the graft (hypointense remnant in the enlarged tunnel on T2-W MR image) and diffuse arthrofibrosis

Fig. 23.60 Too posterior tibial tunnel. Sagittal PD-W MR image shows too posterior boring of the tibial graft tunnel (*arrow*) resulting in vertical orientation of the ACL graft (*arrowhead*) that led to a loss of extension (also called flessum deformity)

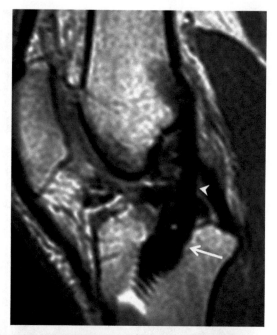

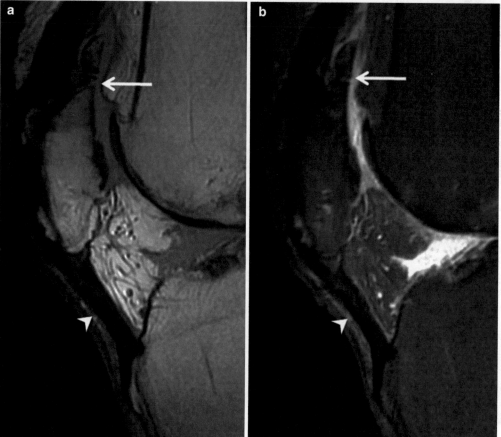

Fig. 23.61 Patella infera. Sagittal (**a**) PD-W and (**b**) fat-suppressed PD-W MR images show a patella infera syndrome with secondary shortening of the patellar tendon (*arrowhead*) after ACL reconstruction using a portion of the patellar tendon as donor site. Postoperative remodeling of the patella is seen anteriorly. The patient presented with signs of patellofemoral osteoarthrosis (*arrow*)

Fig. 23.62 Patellar entrapment syndrome. Sagittal T2-W MR image shows adherence of the patella and patellar tendon (*arrow*) to the adjacent infrapatellar fat pad as a complication of a bone-patellar tendon-bone ACL graft

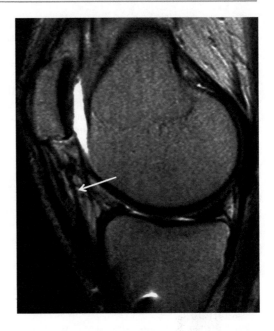

Table 23.9 Knee stiffness from postoperative origin

Meniscal repair
Anterior cruciate ligament reconstruction
Cyclops lesion (due to roof impingement of the ACL graft)
Arthrofibrosis/postoperative adhesions
Too short or stretched ACL graft
Patella infera (secondary to patellar tendon shortening after grafting)
Patellar entrapment syndrome
Prolonged immobilization

Conclusion

The knee is one of the most commonly examined joint in clinical practice of most MRI units. It is important to avoid pitfalls due to insufficient knowledge of anatomical variants and technical artifacts, to prevent interpretation errors and overdiagnosis that may lead to potentially harmful and unnecessary treatment. The radiologist should also consider age and clinical findings, as well as previous medical history and symptoms, before interpreting the images. He should use screening questionnaires to indicate the precise location and duration of the complaints, history of trauma, aggravating activities, underlying diseases, and previous surgery. He should also compare the findings with previous MRI and other imaging modalities (such as radiographs, CT, or ultrasound imaging); this can be extremely helpful for the correct diagnosis.

Of paramount importance, apart from common intra- and periarticular pathologies, is to look for and exclude the presence of other clinically atypical abnormalities (e.g., PVNS, gout, other crystal deposition diseases, ganglion cyst of the anterior cruciate ligament). To overcome the phenomenon of satisfaction of search, where detection of one abnormality may reduce the detectability of another abnormality, a systematic approach in the analysis of all intra- and extra-articular structures of the knee joint is recommended. It is probably appropriate to describe all MRI abnormalities within the radiological report, but to summarize only those findings which have a high probability of clinical significance in the conclusion of the report. Whenever MRI findings are equivocal, this should be clearly emphasized within the report.

References

Akansel G, Inan N, Sarisoy HT (2006) Popliteus muscle sesamoid bone (cyamella): appearance on radiographs, CT and MRI. Surg Radiol Anat 28:642–645

Anderson AF, Awh MH, Anderson CN (2004) The anterior meniscofemoral ligament of the medial meniscus: case series. Am J Sports Med 32:1035–1040

Aydingöz U, Oguz B, Aydingöz O et al (2005) Recesses along the posterior margin of the infrapatellar (Hoffa's) fat pad: prevalence and morphology on routine MR imaging of the knee. Eur Radiol 15:988–994

Bolog NV, Andreisek G (2016) Reporting knee meniscal tears: technical aspects, typical pitfalls and how to avoid them. Insights Imaging 7:385–398

Bozkurt M, Dogan M (2015) Lateral knee pain. In: Sports injuries. Springer, Berlin/Heidelberg

Brunner MC, Flower SP, Evancho AM et al (1989) MRI of the athletic knee: findings in asymptomatic professional basketball and collegiate football players. Invest Radiol 24:72–75

Chalès G, Albert J-D, Guillin R (2016) Douleurs latérales mécaniques du genou. Rev Rhum 83:138–143

Chan CM, Goldblatt JP (2012) Unilateral meniscomeniscal ligament. Orthopedics 35:e1815–e1817

Chan BY, Gill KG, Rebsamen SL, Nguyen JC (2016) MR imaging of pediatric bone marrow. Radiographics 36:1911–1930

Chen CA, Chen W, Goodman SB et al (2011) New MR imaging methods for metallic implants in the knee: artifact correction and clinical impact. J Magn Reson Imaging 33:1121–1127

Claes H, Pans S (2011) Oblique meniscomeniscal ligament: a potential pitfall in the diagnosis of knee injury. JBR-BTR 94:225

Coulier B, Himmer O (2008) Anteromedial meniscofemoral ligament of the knee: CT and MR features in 3 cases. JBR-BTR 91:240

De Maeseneer M, Shahabpour M, Van Roy F et al (2001) MR imaging of the medial collateral ligament bursa: findings in patients and anatomic data derived from cadavers. AJR Am J Roentgenol 177:911–917

De Maeseneer M, Shahabpour M, Vanderdood K et al (2002) Medial meniscocapsular separation: MR imaging criteria and diagnostic pitfalls. Eur J Radiol 41:242–252

De Smet AA, Norris MA, Yandow DR et al (1993) MR diagnosis of meniscal tears of the knee: importance of high signal in the meniscus that extends to the surface. AJR Am J Roentgenol 1993(161):101–107

Dervin GF, Paterson RS (1997) Oblique meniscomeniscal ligament of the knee. Arthroscopy 12:363–365

Duc SE, Wentz KU, Käch KP, Zollikofer CL (2004) First report of an accessory popliteal muscle: detection with MRI. Skeletal Radiol 33:429–431

Ehlinger M, Adam P, Bierry G et al (2010) Supra-patellar swelling and knee instability. Skeletal Radiol 39:1047–1048

English S, Perret D (2010) Posterior knee pain. Curr Rev Musculoskelet Med 3:3–10

Garcia-Valtuille R, Abascal F, Cerezal L et al (2002) Anatomy and MR imaging appearances of synovial plicae of the knee. Radiographics 22:775–784

Gebarski K, Hernandez RJ (2005) Stage-I osteochondritis dissecans versus normal variants of ossification in the knee in children. Pediatr Radiol 35:880–886

Gerbino PG 2nd (1998) An unusual presentation of locked knee. Orthopedics 21:362–364

Gill KG, Nemeth BA, Davis KW (2014) Magnetic resonance imaging of the pediatric knee. Magn Reson Imaging Clin N Am 22:743–763

Harner CD, Miller MD, Irrgang JJ (1994) Management of the stiff knee after trauma and ligament reconstruction. In: Siliski JM (ed) Traumatic disorders of the knee. Springer, New York

Herman LJ, Beltran J (1988) Pitfalls in MR imaging of the knee. Radiology 167:775–781

Jackson AM (2001) Anterior knee pain. J Bone Joint Surg Br 83:937–948

Jans LB, Jaremko JL, Ditchfield M, Verstraete KL (2011) Evolution of femoral condylar ossification at MR imaging: frequency and patient age distribution. Radiology 258:880–888

Jurik AG (2004) Chronic recurrent multifocal osteomyelitis. Semin Musculoskelet Radiol 8:243–253

Kadi R, Shahabpour M, De Maeseneer M (2015) Anatomie normale du genou en imagerie par résonance magnétique. EMC Radiologie et imagerie médicale musculosquelettique neurologique maxillofaciale 10:1–29

Kadi R, De Maeseneer M, Shahabpour M (2016) Normal variants, pitfalls and incidental findings in MRI of the knee. Feuill Radiol 56:387–403

Kaushik S, Erickson JK, Palmer WE et al (2001) Effect of chondrocalcinosis on the MR imaging of knee menisci. AJR Am J Roentgenol 177:905–909

Kavanagh EC, Zoga A, Omar I (2007) MRI findings in bipartite patella. Skeletal Radiol 36:209–214

Kim SJ, Min BH, Kim HK (1996) Arthroscopic anatomy of the infrapatellar plica. Arthroscopy 12:561–564

Kim YG, Ihn JC, Park SK, Kyung HS (2006) An arthroscopic analysis of lateral meniscal variants and a comparison with MRI findings. Knee Surg Sports Traumatol Arthrosc 14:20–26

Kim HK, Laor T (2009) Oblique meniscomeniscal ligament: a normal variant. Pediatr Radiol 39:634

King SJ, Carty HML, Brady O (1996) Magnetic resonance imaging of the knee injuries in children. Pediatr Radiol 26:287–290

Kosarek FJ, Helms CA (1999) The MR appearance of the infrapatellar plica. AJR Am J Roentgenol 172:481–484

Lecouvet FE, Malghem J, Maldague BE, Berg BCV (2005) MR imaging of epiphyseal lesions of the knee: current concepts, challenges, and controversies. Radiol Clin N Am 43:655–672

Lee YH, Song HT, Kim S et al (2012) Infrapatellar plica of the knee: revisited with MR arthrographies undertaken in the knee flexion position mimicking operative arthroscopic posture. Eur J Radiol 81:2783–2787

Llopis E, Padrón M (2007) Anterior knee pain. Eur J Radiol 62:27–43

Malghem J, Vande Berg B, Lebon C, Maldague B (1998) Imagerie ostéoarticulaire: pathologie locale. Flammarion Médecine-Sciences, Paris

Marcheix PS, Marcheix B, Siegler J et al (2009) The anterior intermeniscal ligament of the knee: an anatomic and MR study. Surg Radiol Anat 31:331–334

McWilliams TG, Binns MS (2000) A locked knee in extension: a complication of a degenerate knee with patella alta. J Bone Joint Surg Br 82:890

Mohankumar R, White LM, Naraghi A (2014) Pitfalls and pearls in MRI of the knee. AJR Am J Roentgenol 203:516–530

Muché JA, Lento PH (2004) Posterior knee pain and its causes: a clinician's guide to expediting diagnosis. Phys Sports Med 32:23–30

Nguyen JC, De Smet AA, Graf BK, Rosas HG (2014) MR imaging–based diagnosis and classification of meniscal tears. Radiographics 34:981–999

Papakonstantinou O, Chung CB, Chanchairujira K, Resnick DL (2003) Complications of anterior cruciate ligament reconstruction: MR imaging. Eur Radiol 13:1106–1117

Park JS, Ryu KN, Yoon KH (2006) Meniscal flounce on knee MRI: correlation with meniscal locations after positional changes. AJR Am J Roentgenol 187:364–370

Peh WCG, Chan JHM (2001) Artifacts in musculoskeletal magnetic resonance imaging: identification and correction. Skeletal Radiol 30:179–191

Peterfy CG, Janzen DL, Tirman PF et al (1994) "Magic-angle" phenomenon: a cause of increased signal in the normal lateral meniscus on short-TE MR images of the knee. AJR Am J Roentgenol 163:149–154

Rakow-Penner R, Gold G, Daniel B et al (2008) Reduction of truncation artifacts in rapid 3D articular cartilage imaging. J Magn Reson Imaging 27:860–865

Reinig JW, Mcdevitt ER, Ove PN (1991) Progression of meniscal degenerative changes in college football players: evaluation with MR imaging. Radiology 181:255–257

Resnick D, Kang HS (1997) Internal derangements of joints: emphasis on MR imaging. WB Saunders, Philadelphia

Robertson AI, Jones SC, Paes R, Chakrabarty G (2004) The fabella: a forgotten source of knee pain? Knee 11:243–245

Rohren EM, Kosarek FJ, Helms CA (2001) Discoid lateral meniscus and the frequency of meniscal tears. Skeletal Radiol 30:316–320

Rubin DA, Britton CA, Towers JD, Harner CD (1996) Are MR imaging signs of meniscocapsular separation valid? Radiology 201:829–836

Sanders TG, Linares RC, Lawhorn KW et al (1999) Oblique meniscomeniscal ligament: another potential pitfall for a meniscal tear anatomic description and appearance at MR imaging in three cases. Radiology 213:213–216

Schnarkowski P, Tirman PF, Fuchigami KD et al (1995) Meniscal ossicle: radiographic and MR imaging findings. Radiology 196:47–50

Shahabpour M, Osteaux M, Casteleyn PP (1991) The knee joint. In: Osteaux M, De Meirleir K, Shahabpour M (eds) MRI and spectroscopy in sports medicine. Springer, Berlin

Shahabpour M, Handelberg F, Casteleyn PP et al (1997) Imaging in sports medicine – knee. Eur J Radiol 26:23–45

Shahabpour M, Kadi R, De Maeseneer M (2015) Variantes et pièges en imagerie par résonance magnétique du genou. EMC Radiologie et imagerie médicale musculosquelettique neurologique maxillofaciale 10:1–13

Shankman S, Beltran J, Melamed E, Rosenberg ZS (1997) Anterior horn of the lateral meniscus: another potential pitfall in MR imaging of the knee. Radiology 204:181–184

Shogry ME, Pope TL Jr (1991) Vacuum phenomenon simulating meniscal or cartilaginous injury of the knee at MR imaging. Radiology 180:513–515

Silva A, Sampaio R (2011) Anterior lateral meniscofemoral ligament with congenital absence of the ACL. Knee Surg Sports Traumatol Arthrosc 19:192–195

Singh DR, Chin MSM, Peh WCG (2014) Artifacts in musculoskeletal MR imaging. Semin Musculoskelet Radiol 18:12–22

Snoeckx A, Vanhoenacker FM, Gielen JL et al (2008) Magnetic resonance imaging of variants of the knee. Singapore Med J 49:734–744

Tan HK, Bakri MM, Peh WCG (2014) Variants and pitfalls in MR imaging of knee injuries. Semin Musculoskelet Radiol 18:45–53

Turner DA, Rapoport MI, Erwin WD et al (1991) Truncation artifact: a potential pitfall in MR imaging of the menisci of the knee. Radiology 179:629–633

Tyler P, Datir A, Saifuddin A (2010) Magnetic resonance imaging of anatomical variations in the knee. Part 2: miscellaneous. Skeletal Radiol 39:1175–1186

Vahey TN, Bennett HT, Arrington LE et al (1990) MR imaging of the knee: pseudotear of the lateral meniscus caused by the meniscofemoral ligament. AJR Am J Roentgenol 154:1237–1239

Van Holsbeeck M, Vandamme B, Marchal G et al (1987) Dorsal defect of the patella: concept of its origin and relationship with bipartite and multipartite patella. Skeletal Radiol 16:304–311

Vande Berg BC, Malghem J, Poilvache P et al (2005) Meniscal tears with fragments displaced in notch and recesses of knee: MR imaging with arthroscopic comparison 1. Radiology 234:842–850

Vanhoenacker F, De Vos N, Van Dyck P (2016) Common mistakes and pitfalls in magnetic resonance imaging of the knee. J Belgian Soc Radiol 100:99. http://doi.org/10.5334/jbr-btr.1206

Watanabe M, Takeda S (1974) Arthroscopy of the knee joint. In: Helfet AJ (ed) Disorders of the knee. Lippincott, Philadelphia

Watanabe AT, Carter BC, Teitelbaum GP et al (1989) Normal variations in MR imaging of the knee: appearance and frequency. AJR Am J Roentgenol 153:341–344

Yu JS, Cosgarea AJ, Kaeding CC, Wilson D (1997) Meniscal flounce MR imaging. Radiology 203:513–515

Knee Injury: US Pitfalls

24

David McKean and James Teh

Contents

24.1   **Introduction** 471

24.2   **Extensor Mechanism Pathology** 471

24.3   **Sinding-Larsen-Johansson and Osgood-Schlatter Disease** 473

24.4   **Bursitis** 474

24.5   **Joint Effusions and Synovitis** 475

24.6   **Collateral Ligament Injury** 475

24.7   **Iliotibial Band Friction Syndrome** 476

24.8   **Meniscal Injuries** 477

Conclusion 477

References 477

Abbreviation

US   Ultrasound

D. McKean, MA Hons, BM, BCh, FRCR (✉)
Department of Radiology, Stoke Mandeville Hospital,
Buckinghamshire Healthcare NHS Trust,
Mandeville Road, Aylesbury, Buckinghamshire HP21
8AL, UK
e-mail: David.Mckean@buckshealthcare.nhs.uk

J. Teh, BSc, MBBS, FRCP, FRCR
Department of Radiology, Nuffield Orthopaedic
Centre, Oxford University Hospitals NHS Trust,
Windmill Rd, Oxford OX3 7LD, UK
e-mail: jamesteh1@gmail.com

24.1 Introduction

Ultrasound (US) imaging is a dynamic and effective technique for evaluating sports injuries around the knee. Correlation can be made with the patient's site of symptoms, and comparison can be made with the asymptomatic side. Although the internal structures of the knee, such as the cruciate ligaments, are not well evaluated, US imaging remains a very useful modality for assessing the extra-articular soft tissues which are commonly involved in overuse injuries. However, numerous pitfalls may be encountered, and a thorough understanding of the anatomy is required. Pertinent technical considerations relevant to musculoskeletal US imaging are described in Chap. 18. For further information on US artifacts, see Chap. 2.

24.2 Extensor Mechanism Pathology

The extensor mechanism of the knee consists of the quadriceps muscles, quadriceps tendon, patella, patellar retinaculum, and patellar tendon. Due to anisotropy, the appearance of the quadriceps and patellar tendons may vary as the angle of insonation changes, which can be mistaken for tendinopathy. Care should therefore be taken during US scanning to remain directly perpendicular to the tendon in both the transverse and longitudinal planes. Scanning with the knee in the flexed

© Springer International Publishing AG 2017
W.C.G. Peh (ed.), *Pitfalls in Musculoskeletal Radiology*, DOI 10.1007/978-3-319-53496-1_24

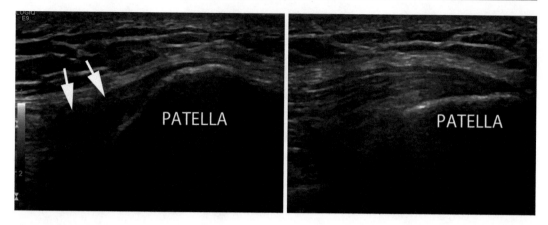

Fig. 24.1 Anisotropy of the quadriceps tendon mimicking tendinosis. Comparison US images of the right quadriceps tendon. On the *left* image, with the knee extended, there is a region of decreased echogenicity and loss of the fibrillar pattern in the distal tendon (*arrows*) suggestive of tendinosis. On the *right* image, with the knee flexed, the quadriceps tendon is stretched with return of the normal fibrillar pattern and echogenicity

position stretches the extensor mechanism and decreases the effects of anisotropy. Conversely, however, when using Doppler US imaging, it is important to ensure that the extensor tendons are not under tension, as this may decrease the amount of blood flow (Fig. 24.1).

The quadriceps tendon is a trilaminar structure with the superficial layer formed by the rectus femoris, the middle layer formed by the vastus medialis and vastus lateralis, and the deep layer formed by the vastus intermedius. On US imaging, the assessment of quadriceps tears can be difficult. Full-thickness tears involve all three layers, and partial tears may involve one or two layers. The quadriceps tendon is most often torn 1–2 cm from the patellar insertion. Full-thickness tears result in disruption of the tendon fibers with discontinuity and hypoechoic or mixed-echogenicity hemorrhage in the gap. On dynamic US scanning, there may be paradoxical motion of the torn tendon ends. The tendon ends may be retracted and have a wavy contour in the longitudinal plane, indicating laxity. With a partial tear, the abnormal segment of tendon is thickened or thinned but not discontinuous. A partial tear may be difficult to differentiate from severe tendinosis. Partial tears of the quadriceps may be missed, as remnant intact fibers may give the impression of tendon integrity. Flexing the knee stretches the tendon and increases the size of the gap in complete tears (Bianchi et al. 2006). The presence of scar tissue in the setting of chronic

injury may represent a potential pitfall in the assessment of partial versus complete quadriceps tears (La et al. 2003) (Fig. 24.2).

The patellar retinaculum is an important soft tissue stabilizer of the patellofemoral joint. It is composed of a medial and lateral component. With lateral patellar dislocations, the medial retinaculum may be injured or avulsed. Although magnetic resonance imaging (MRI) is the preferred imaging modality for assessing for lateral patellar dislocations, the diagnosis may be suggested on US imaging by disruption or avulsion of the medial retinaculum. The patellar tendon is readily assessed on US imaging and appears as a striated structure, which passes from the lower pole of the patella to the tibial tuberosity. Jumper knee or proximal patellar tendinosis typically affects individuals involved in sports that require repetitive contraction of the quadriceps muscle. On US imaging, the proximal patellar tendon is usually thickened with a central area of low echogenicity seen at the attachment of the posterior tendon to the patella. The anterior fibers that originate from the quadriceps tendon are less susceptible to injury. The presence of increased vascularity on Doppler US imaging interrogation is an important feature of tendinosis, with investigators showing good correlation between the presence of tendon neovascularity and pain (Zanetti et al. 2003). Calcification or dystrophic ossification may be seen in areas of chronic inflammation.

Fig. 24.2 Partial tear of the quadriceps tendon. (**a**) Extended field-of-view US image shows a defect in the quadriceps tendon (*arrow*) suggesting a full-thickness tear. (**b**) Sagittal fat-suppressed PD-W MR image in the same patient shows a partial tear of the quadriceps (*arrowhead*) with an intact deep layer (*arrow*)

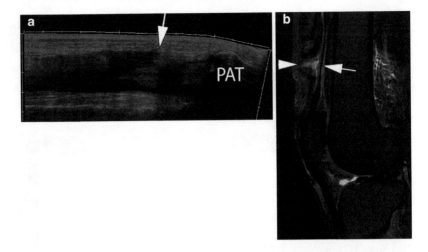

Fig. 24.3 Gouty infiltration of the extensor mechanism mimicking tendinosis. (**a**) Sagittal T1-W MR image shows a diffusely thickened extensor mechanism. (**b**) Extended field-of-view US image in the same patient shows a thickened heterogeneous extensor mechanism (*arrowheads*) with hyperechoic foci (*arrow*)

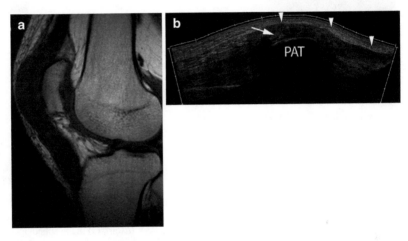

Intratendinous gouty infiltration of the extensor mechanism may simulate tendinosis and is a classic pitfall (Gililland et al. 2011). Typically, gouty involvement results in a mass-like swelling, which may be focal or diffuse. On US imaging, gouty tophi typically appear as clusters of hyperechoic heterogeneous areas with poorly defined contours, surrounded by an anechoic halo (de Ávila Fernandes et al. 2011) (Fig. 24.3).

24.3 Sinding-Larsen-Johansson and Osgood-Schlatter Disease

Sinding-Larsen-Johansson and Osgood-Schlatter disease are syndromes that occur in adolescence and are related to traction injuries at the immature osteotendinous junctions. Sinding-Larsen-Johansson disease occurs at the proximal tendon at its insertion to the patella, and Osgood-Schlatter disease affects the distal tendon at its insertion into the tibial tuberosity. The US imaging findings include irregularity and fragmentation at the insertion of the tendon, swelling of the unossified cartilage and overlying soft tissues, tendinosis, and overlying bursitis. Sinding-Larsen-Johansson disease may appear similar to jumper knee but occurs in adolescence, whereas jumper knee can occur at any age.

In children, the ossifying patella is weaker than the patellar tendon, so an acute traction injury may result in a patellar sleeve avulsion injury, which involves both the bone and cartilage at the inferior pole of the patella. The significance of the injury is that the sleeve of periosteum that is pulled off may continue to form bone, thus elongating or even duplicating the patella (Hunt

Fig. 24.4 Patellar
sleeve avulsion injury
mimicking Sinding-
Larsen-Johansson
disease. (**a**) US image
shows an avulsed bony
fragment at the inferior
pole of the patella
(*arrowheads*). (**b**)
Lateral radiograph of the
knee shows patellar
sleeve avulsion fracture
(*arrow*)

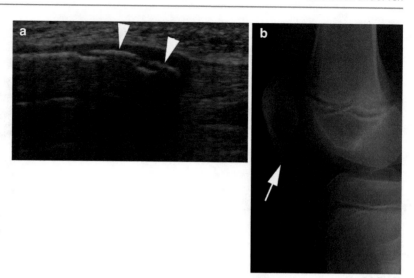

and Somashekar 2005). These injuries are therefore usually treated by surgical fixation. An
important mistake to avoid is diagnosing Sinding-
Larsen-Johansson disease in cases of patellar
sleeve avulsion (Fig. 24.4).

24.4   Bursitis

Bursitis adjacent to the patellar tendon may
involve the prepatellar bursae (clergyman knee)
or infrapatellar bursa (housemaid knee). US
imaging may demonstrate thickening of the bursal wall, a bursal effusion, and hypervascularity
on Doppler imaging. There may be no fluid present. Multiple echogenic foci may be evident,
representing areas of calcification. Morel-
Lavallée effusions result from trauma, causing
separation of subcutaneous tissue from the
underlying fascia with accumulation of blood,
lymph, and fat in the potential space. Around the
knee, these may be incorrectly diagnosed as bursitis, but usually the lesion lies outside the confines of a normal bursa (Borrero et al. 2008)
(Fig. 24.5). The pes anserine bursa is located at
the medial aspect of the knee (at the level of the
joint space) deep to the pes anserinus tendons at
the insertion of the conjoined tendons of sartorius, gracilis, and semitendinosus onto the
anteromedial proximal tibia. Pes anserine bursitis occurs as a result of overuse injury or may be

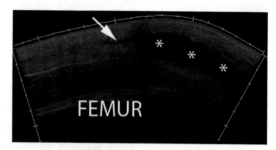

Fig. 24.5 Morel-Lavallée lesion of the knee mimicking
bursitis. Extended field-of-view US image shows fluid
(*asterisks*) in the subcutaneous tissues in the suprapatellar
region with shearing of the fat at the upper extent of the
lesion (*arrow*)

due to inflammatory arthropathy. US imaging
may reveal fluid within the bursa, thickening and
irregularity of the bursal wall, and surrounding
soft tissue edema. Pes anserine tendinosis may
be associated with bursitis.

Baker cysts are distensions of the
semimembranosus-gastrocnemius bursa and are
the commonest cause of posterior knee swelling.
US imaging demonstrates a typical "speech bubble" appearance as the cyst passes between the
medial head of the gastrocnemius and the semimembranosus tendons via a communication with
the knee joint. This typical configuration is important to identify, to help differentiate Baker cyst
from other posterior soft tissue masses or fluid
collections, such as meniscal cysts (Rutten et al.

1998). With large cysts, the origin may be difficult to delineate. There may be solid and cystic components to Baker cysts, and vascularity may be identifiable within the solid components. Since these cysts are in direct continuity with the knee, loose bodies such as cartilage or osteochondral bodies can traverse the one-way valve into the cyst. Acute rupture of a Baker cyst may present with sudden onset of calf pain. Fluid from the ruptured cyst may be seen tracking around the gastrocnemius muscle, and the deep veins should be assessed using Doppler US imaging to differentiate this from deep vein thrombosis. The semimembranosus tendon may simulate a Baker cyst as it curves anteriorly to attach to the posterior tibia, where anisotropy may make it hypoechoic (Jamadar et al. 2010) (Fig. 24.6).

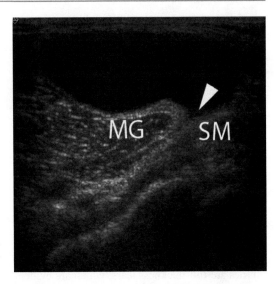

Fig. 24.6 Speech bubble appearance of Baker cyst. The speech bubble appearance should be identified whenever evaluating for Baker cyst on US imaging. The neck of the cyst (*arrowhead*) passes between the medial gastrocnemius (*MG*) and semimembranosus (*SM*) tendons

24.5   Joint Effusions and Synovitis

Effusions may be simple or complex, with associated synovial hypertrophy. An effusion may occur as a nonspecific response to a wide range of insults, including trauma, infection, inflammatory arthropathy, and degeneration. Generally, effusions are best detected in the suprapatellar pouch, but it may be helpful to scan the patient in flexion and extension, as joint fluid may displace into a more easily detectable location. Often, small effusions may only be detected in the medial or lateral recesses of the suprapatellar pouch. As in other joints, compression may be useful in distinguishing between effusion and synovitis. The presence of Doppler signal may allow synovitis to be distinguished from fluid. A major pitfall in the diagnosis of effusions is not to consider infection or inflammation, due to conditions such as pigmented villonodular synovitis as potential causes. Echogenic effusions suggest hemorrhage, while layering may occur with a lipohemarthrosis or settling of blood products. If a hemorrhagic effusion is seen, then radiographs are mandatory. Echogenic crystals within the synovium or along the articular cartilage may indicate crystal arthropathy such as calcium pyrophosphate deposition disease or gout (Fig. 24.7).

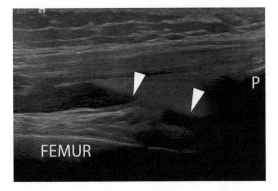

Fig. 24.7 Layering lipohemarthrosis. US image shows an echogenic layer of fat-containing fluid layering above a hypoechoic hemarthrosis. Arrowheads delineate the interface

24.6   Collateral Ligament Injury

The lateral collateral ligament (LCL) is comprised of the iliotibial band and the conjoint tendon, with the latter being formed by the confluence of the biceps femoris and fibular collateral ligament. The iliotibial band inserts onto Gerdy tubercle of the lateral tibial plateau. The LCL is part of the posterolateral corner, which also includes the popliteofibular ligament, the popliteus ligament, the arcuate ligament, and the posterolateral joint capsule. The medial collateral ligament has superficial and deep components. The superficial fibers attach proximally to the medial femoral condyle and distally to the medial aspect of the tibia. The deep fibers originate from the medial joint capsule and are attached to the medial meniscus.

Grade 1 injuries are sprains, which may be difficult to detect but fluid may been seen around the affected ligament. Grade 2 injuries are partial tears, which may be detected as thickening and loss of the normal ligament architecture. Hemorrhage and edema may surround the ligament but some fibers will remain intact. Grade 3 injuries are full-thickness tears, which are evident as discontinuity of the ligament with no intact fibers visible. Old ligament injuries often manifest as thickening of the ligament. On dynamic stressing, there may be joint widening. Pellegrini-Stieda lesions are focal areas of mineralization within the proximal portion of the medial collateral ligament, which occur following trauma. These appear as focal areas of echogenicity with posterior acoustic shadowing. A pitfall is to mistake these for acute avulsion injuries, which are uncommon and referred to as Stieda fractures (Fig. 24.8).

24.7 Iliotibial Band Friction Syndrome

Iliotibial band friction syndrome results from repetitive friction and abrasion of the iliotibial band across the lateral femoral condyle. This may result in bursal inflammation and iliotibial band tendinosis. It is usually seen in long-distance runners. On US imaging, there is thickening and loss of clarity of the iliotibial band, with fluid distension of the underlying bursa and increased vascularity. The US imaging findings can be misinterpreted as a partial tear of the iliotibial band (Bonaldi et al. 1998) (Fig. 24.9).

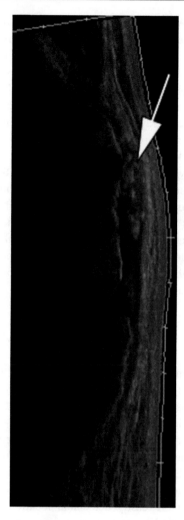

Fig. 24.8 Pellegrini-Stieda lesion. Extended field-of-view US image which has been rotated 90 degrees to depict a coronal plane scan of the medial collateral ligament. Echogenic calcified foci are present within the proximal ligament (*arrow*)

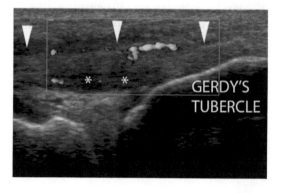

Fig. 24.9 Iliotibial band friction syndrome. Longitudinal US image shows thickening of the iliotibial band (*arrowheads*) with bursal thickening (*asterisks*) and increased vascularity

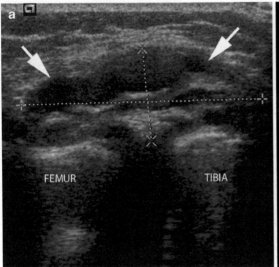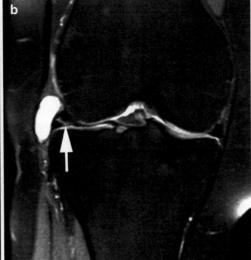

Fig. 24.10 Parameniscal cyst. (**a**) Longitudinal US image shows a cystic structure (*arrows*) intimately related to the lateral joint line. The underlying meniscus is poorly assessed. (**b**) Coronal fat-suppressed PD-W MR image in the same patient shows a lateral meniscal tear (*arrow*)

24.8   Meniscal Injuries

The normal meniscus has a homogeneous echotexture on US imaging and when visualized from the lateral aspect, has a triangular appearance. Meniscal tears appear as hypoechoic clefts within the body of the meniscus. A pitfall is that a cleft may be incorrectly diagnosed as a tear, as on US imaging, it is difficult to determine if a cleft truly extends to the articular surface. The sensitivity and specificity for the diagnosis of meniscal tears on US imaging range from 60% and 21% (Azzoni and Cabitza 2002) to 86% and 85% (Park et al. 2008), respectively. The general consensus is that meniscal tears cannot be accurately excluded based on US imaging findings alone; and if a meniscal tear is suspected, then MRI should be performed (Selby et al. 1987). Cysts appear as hypoechoic, fluid-filled, often loculated structures which may communicate with an underlying meniscal tear. A meniscal tear is more accurately diagnosed when associated with a parameniscal cyst (Fig. 24.10).

Conclusion

US imaging is an excellent technique for examining the superficial structures of the knee. Knowledge of the anatomy and the awareness of common pitfalls are crucial when performing US examinations. Comparison with the contralateral knee, the use of dynamic maneuvers and of Doppler imaging, and the judicious utilization of other imaging modalities such as MRI should ensure an accurate diagnosis.

References

Azzoni R, Cabitza P (2002) Is there a role for sonography in the diagnosis of tears of the knee menisci? J Clin Ultrasound 30:472–476

Bianchi S, Poletti PA, Martinoli C, Abdelwahab IF (2006) Ultrasound appearance of tendon tears. Part 2: lower extremity and myotendinous tears. Skeletal Radiol 35:63–77

Bonaldi VM, Chhem RK, García P et al (1998) Iliotibial band friction syndrome: sonographic findings. J Ultrasound Med 17:257–260

Borrero CG, Maxwell N, Kavanagh E (2008) MRI findings of prepatellar Morel-Lavallée effusions. Skeletal Radiol 37:451–455 de Ávila FE, Kubota ES, Sandim GB et al (2011) Ultrasound features of tophi in chronic tophaceous gout. Skeletal Radiol 40:309–315

Gililland JM, Webber NP, Jones KB et al (2011) Intratendinous tophaceous gout imitating patellar tendonitis in an athletic man. Orthopedics 34:223–223

Hunt DM, Somashekar N (2005) A review of sleeve fractures of the patella in children. Knee 12:3–7

Jamadar DA, Robertson BL, Jacobson JA et al (2010) Musculoskeletal sonography: important imaging pitfalls. AJR Am J Roentgenol 194:216–225

La S, Fessell DP, Femino JE et al (2003) Sonography of partial-thickness quadriceps tendon tears with surgical correlation. J Ultrasound Med 22:1323–1331

Park GY, Kim JM, Lee SM, Lee MY (2008) The value of ultrasonography in the detection of meniscal tears diagnosed by magnetic resonance imaging. Am J Phys Med Rehabil 87:14–20

Rutten MJ, Collins JM, van Kampen A, Jager GJ (1998) Meniscal cysts: detection with high-resolution sonography. AJR Am J Roentgenol 171:491–496

Selby B, Richardson ML, Nelson BD, Graney DO, Mack LA (1987) Sonography in the detection of meniscal injuries of the knee: evaluation in cadavers. AJR Am J Roentgenol 149:549–553

Zanetti M, Metzdorf A, Kundert HP et al (2003) Achilles tendons: clinical relevance of neovascularization diagnosed with power Doppler US. Radiology 227:556–560

Ankle and Foot Injuries: MRI Pitfalls

25

Yuko Kobashi, Yohei Munetomo, Akira Baba, Shinji Yamazoe, and Takuji Mogami

Contents

25.1	**Introduction**	479
25.2	**Anatomy of the Ankle Joint**	480
25.3	**Ankle Injuries**	480
25.4	**Lateral Ankle Pain**	481
25.4.1	Lateral Ligament Injuries	481
25.4.2	Bursitis of the Lateral Side	484
25.4.3	Peroneal Tendon Disorders	487
25.5	**Medial Ankle Pain**	493
25.5.1	Deltoid Ligament Tear	493
25.5.2	Flexor Hallucis Longus Disorders	496
25.5.3	Tibialis Posterior Tendonitis and Tear	497
25.5.4	Stress Fracture of the Medial Malleolus	498
25.6	**Dorsal Ankle Pain**	498
25.6.1	Anterior Inferior Tibiofibular Ligament Tear and Syndesmosis Injury	498
25.6.2	Footballer Ankle	499
25.6.3	Extensor Tendonitis and Tenosynovitis	500
25.7	**Posterior Ankle Pain**	500
25.7.1	Achilles Tendon Rupture	500
25.7.2	Achilles Tendinosis	500
25.8	**Mid- and Anterior Foot Pain**	501
25.8.1	Lisfranc Ligament Injury	501
25.8.2	Osteochondral Lesion of Talar Dome	502
25.8.3	Tarsal Coalition	505
Conclusion		508
References		508

Y. Kobashi, MD (✉) • Y. Munetomo, MD • A. Baba, MD
S. Yamazoe, MD • T. Mogami, MD
Department of Radiology, Tokyo Dental University,
Ichikawa General Hospital, 5-11-13 Sugano,
Ichikawa, Chiba 272-8513, Japan
e-mail: ykobashi@jikei.ac.jp

Abbreviations

AITFL   Anterior inferior tibiofibular ligament
ATFL   Anterior talofibular ligament
CFL   Calcaneofibular ligament
CT   Computed tomography
FHL   Flexor hallucis longus
MRI   Magnetic resonance imaging
PITFL   Posterior inferior tibiofibular ligament
PTFL   Posterior talofibular ligament

25.1 Introduction

Magnetic resonance imaging (MRI) is an excellent modality for assessment of sports and overuse injuries of the ankle and foot. However, the anatomy of this region is complex, with several bones, ligaments, and tendons being possibly injured. Ankle injuries can be categorized into five painful sites, namely, lateral, medial, dorsal, and posterior ankle and mid- and anterior foot. The most common trauma mechanism of ankle sprain is supination and adduction (inversion) of the plantar-flexed foot. The lateral collateral ligaments, especially the anterior talofibular ligament, are frequently involved. A severe inversion ankle sprain sometimes causes peroneal tendon disorder. Deltoid ligament injury can also occur with concomitant lateral ankle sprains, during fractures of the lateral malleolus, and in association with posterior tibial tendon pathology. Dorsal pain often means syndesmotic ligament injuries, which often occur in conjunction with other ankle injuries, including sprains and fractures. Achilles tendon injuries are the main cause of posterior pain. Midfoot sprains in athletes cause anterior pain and represent a lower-velocity injury, typically with no displacement or with only subtle diastases. Ankle sprain causes bony contusion between talar dome and tibial plafond and osteochondral lesion of talus. A good working knowledge of the appearances of normal anatomy, anatomical variants, and pathology is needed to avoid pitfalls in diagnosis.

25.2   Anatomy of the Ankle Joint

The ankle joint is formed by three bones, namely, the tibia and fibula of the lower leg and the talus of the foot. The tibia and fibula are bound together by strong tibiofibular ligaments, producing a bracket-shaped socket, which is known as a mortise. The talar body fits into the mortise formed by the bones of the lower leg. There are numerous ligaments in the ankle joint: anterior lateral ligaments include the anterior inferior tibiofibular ligament (AITFL) and anterior talofibular ligament (ATFL), and posterior lateral ligaments include the posterior inferior tibiofibular ligament (PITFL), calcaneofibular ligament (CFL), and posterior talofibular ligament (PTFL). Medial ligament consists of one medial collateral ligament (deltoid ligament) which extends from the medial malleolus to both talus and calcaneum. In addition, the joint capsule of ankle and the interosseous ligament (membrane) form the ankle mortise. Anatomy of the ankle joint ligaments is shown in Fig. 25.1. The ankle joint is a hinge-type joint, with movements possible in only one plane. Thus, plantar flexion and dorsiflexion are the only movements that occur at the ankle joint. Eversion and inversion are produced at the other joints of the foot, such as the subtalar joint. There are five tendons that extend from the lower leg to the foot. The tibialis posterior, flexor digitorum, and flexor hallucis longus tendons are present at the medial aspect of the ankle. The peroneus longus and brevis tendons are present at the lateral aspect of the ankle.

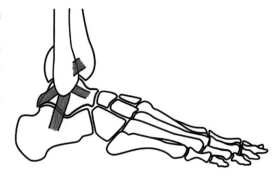

Fig. 25.1 Anatomy of lateral collateral ligaments. The ATFL extends from the anterior aspect of lateral malleolus to the lateral tubercle of talus. CFL is an extra-articular ligament which connects the inferior aspect of lateral malleolus to the tubercle on posterior and lateral aspect of calcaneus. PTFL is an intra-articular ligament and runs almost horizontally from the posterior aspect of lateral malleolus to the posterior surface of the talus

These tendons act during plantar flexion, inversion, and/or eversion of foot. The combination of hyperplantar flexion of ankle and inversion of subtalar joint causes severe ankle sprain and produces lateral ankle pain.

25.3   Ankle Injuries

Ankle sprain is one of the most common injuries among foot and ankle injuries. It is caused by frequent jumps, landings, cutting maneuvers, and contact with other players, all of which are inherent parts of the sport. It accounts for 10–15% of sport-related injuries (MacAuley 1999; Lynch 2002). There are two kinds of ankle sprain: inversion and eversion ankle sprain (Fig. 25.2). The inversion ankle sprain is the most common type of ankle sprain and occurs when the foot is inverted too much. ATFL is one of the most commonly involved ligaments in this type of sprain. The eversion ankle sprain is less common. When it occurs, the deltoid ligament is stretched too much. MRI is helpful in diagnosing foot and ankle injuries and can predict their prognosis. It is useful to categorize ankle injuries into five painful sites, namely, lateral, medial, dorsal, and posterior ankle and mid- and anterior foot, for the purpose of diagnosis on MRI.

25.4 Lateral Ankle Pain

25.4.1 Lateral Ligament Injuries

The most common trauma mechanism of ankle sprain is supination and adduction (inversion) of the plantar-flexed foot. Lateral collateral ligaments, especially the ATFL, AITFL, and CFL, are frequently involved. They may have lateral ankle pain with swollen soft tissue around lateral malleolus. Broström (1964) found that isolated, complete rupture of the ATFL was present in 65% of all ankle sprains. A combined injury involving the ATFL and the CFL occurred in 20% of his patients. PTFL and PITFL are less commonly injured.

25.4.1.1 ATFL Tear

The ATFL is about 2 cm long and extends from the anterior aspect of lateral malleolus to the lateral tubercle of talus. When the foot is in plantar flexion, the ligament courses parallel to the axis of the leg. The length of ATFL alters according to the position of the foot. If the foot is at a slight plantar-flexed position, the ATFL appears on MRI to be stretched, compared to the neutral (0°) position. If the foot is at a slight dorsiflexed position, the ATFL appears to be shortened, compared to the neutral (0°) position. The foot at the neutral (0°) position is the best one for evaluation of the ATFL (Fig. 25.3). Acute and chronic ATFL tears are different in their MRI findings. In addition, complete and partial ATFL tears are also

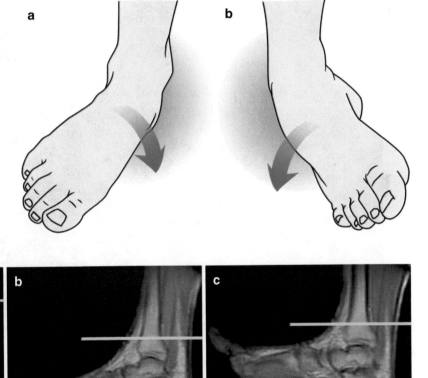

Fig. 25.2 Mechanism of ankle sprain. Diagram shows two kinds of ankle sprain: (**a**) eversion and (**b**) inversion. When a ligament is forced to stretch beyond its normal range, a sprain occurs. A severe sprain causes actual tearing of the fibers

Fig. 25.3 Length of ATFL changes with foot position. (**a**) If the foot is at slight plantarflexion position, the ATFL appears to be stretched compared to the one in the 0° position (*top row* in **d**). (**b**) The foot at the neutral (0°) position is best for evaluating the ATFL (*arrows*) (*middle row* in **d**). (**c**) If the foot is at slight dorsiflexion position, the ATFL appears to be shortened (*arrows*) compared to the 0° position (*bottom row* in **d**)

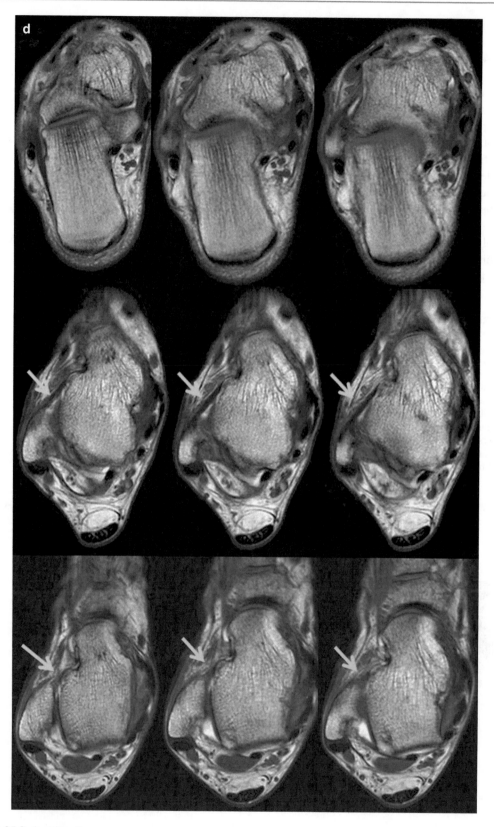

Fig. 25.3 (continued)

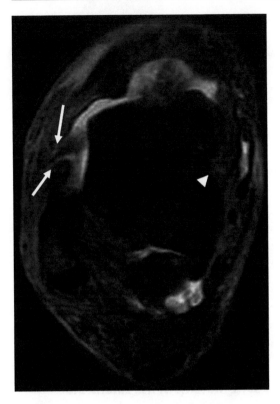

Fig. 25.4 Acute ATFL complete tear in a 27-year-old man. Axial STIR MR image shows complete tear of the ATFL at its midportion (*arrows*). Bone marrow edema due to a traction force from deltoid ligament is visualized in the medial aspect of talus (*arrowhead*). Fluid collection suggestive of hematoma around the ATFL is seen

different in their MRI findings. An acute ATFL complete tear shows swelling and signal hyperintensity with a gap in the ligament (Fig. 25.4). A localized fluid collection suggestive of hematoma is visible at the lateral malleolus. It is often difficult to detect a small ATFL gap on MRI. Obtaining an ankle MRI with 0° position may be useful to detect the ATFL gap.

An acute ATFL partial tear is seen as a swollen and hyperintense ATFL (Fig. 25.5). Caliber change of ATFL with clinical suspicion of tear may be visible. In a chronic ATFL complete tear, the ATFL is indistinct on MRI. A linear fibrotic hypointense structure may be visible at the lateral malleolus. A chronic ATFL partial tear shows a thinned ATFL without increased signal intensity. However, in patients who use their ankle intensively, e.g., athletes and those with history of several ankle sprains, we often see a thickened ATFL with fibrotic change of the ankle joint capsule on MRI. It is the result of chronic post-traumatic change of ATFL and other lateral collateral ligament tears. MRI findings of acute and chronic ATFL tears are listed in Table 25.1.

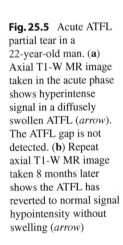

Fig. 25.5 Acute ATFL partial tear in a 22-year-old man. (**a**) Axial T1-W MR image taken in the acute phase shows hyperintense signal in a diffusely swollen ATFL (*arrow*). The ATFL gap is not detected. (**b**) Repeat axial T1-W MR image taken 8 months later shows the ATFL has reverted to normal signal hypointensity without swelling (*arrow*)

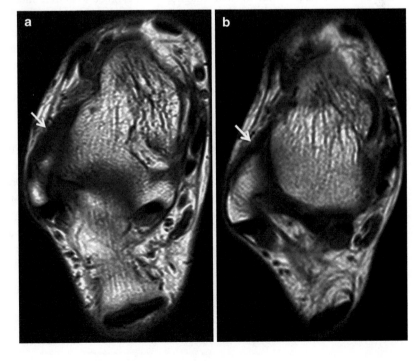

Table 25.1 Characteristic MRI findings of acute and chronic ATFL tears

	Acute	Chronic
Complete	Swollen ATFL stump Indistinct ATFL stump Hematoma around ATFL stump	Thinned or loss of ATFL Thickened ATFL and joint capsule No hematoma
Partial	Swollen ATFL with diffuse hyperintense signal Hematoma around ATFL	Thinned ATFL with caliber change No abnormal signal change of ATFL Thickened ATFL and joint capsule No hematoma

25.4.1.2 Avulsion Fracture of the Lateral Malleolus Tip

An avulsion fracture of the tip of the lateral malleolus is also caused by ankle sprain, following the same mechanism of the ATFL tear. Bony fragments of the avulsion fracture are big, and the fracture can be diagnosed easily on an ankle radiograph. On MRI, the bony fragment is attached to the ATFL and suggests that it is from the anterior tip of lateral malleolus. Therefore, this avulsion fracture is sometimes misdiagnosed as an ATFL tear.

25.4.1.3 CFL Tear

The CFL is a 2 cm long, extra-articular ligament which connects the inferior aspect of lateral malleolus to the tubercle on the posterior and lateral aspects of the calcaneus. It is in close contact with the medial peroneal sheath, but is not associated with either the ankle capsule or peroneal tendon sheath. The CFL acts primarily to stabilize the subtalar joint and limit inversion. On MRI, it is easy to detect the CFL on coronal images. CFL tear is also caused by ankle sprains but isolated CFL tear is rare. Therefore, CFL tear on MRI suggests a serious ankle sprain, and we need to

confirm ATFL and other lateral collateral ligament tears at the same time (Fig. 25.6). In addition, CFL tear may be complicated with a hematoma within the tarsal sinus. This may cause a tarsal sinus syndrome characterized by chronic pain at the lateral aspect of the ankle, if the hematoma is large and has filled the tarsal sinus. This associated injury should be looked out for.

25.4.1.4 PTFL Tear

The PTFL is an intra-articular ligament that runs almost horizontally from the posterior aspect of lateral malleolus to a posterior surface of the talus. The PTFL works as a joint stabilizer with the other lateral collateral ligaments. The PTFL is rarely torn in an ankle sprain because bony stability protects the ligament when the ankle is in dorsiflexion. One should be careful about diagnosis of PTFL tear, especially if it appears to be the sole structure injured.

25.4.2 Bursitis of the Lateral Side

There are numerous bursae in the foot and ankle (Fig. 25.7). Bursae are situated in various locations throughout joints where friction between tissues commonly occurs, and these bursae are designed to help reduce this friction and prevent pain. They are classified according to their location, namely, subcutaneous, subfascial, subtendinous, and submucosal (Resnick 1995; Hirji et al. 2011). Bursae can also be classified as communicating or non-communicating. When a bursa is located adjacent to a joint, the synovial membrane of the bursae may communicate with the joint (Farooki et al. 2002; Hirji et al. 2011). Repetitive movements, or prolonged and excessive pressure, are the most common causes of bursal inflammation. One of the most common bursitis of ankle and foot involves the retrocalcaneal bursa. It is situated between the calcaneus and the Achilles tendon and assists in decreasing friction during plantar flexion (Sutro 1966).

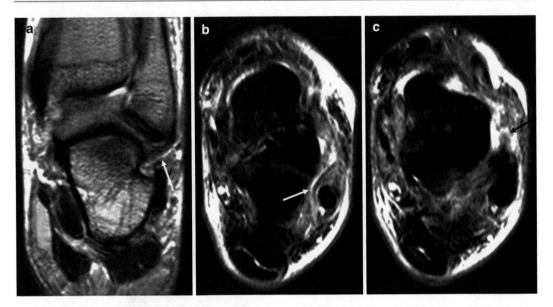

Fig. 25.6 CFL tear and ATFL tear in a 20-year-old man. (**a**) Coronal T2-W image shows a swollen and hyperintense CFL suggestive of partial tear (*arrow*). (**b**) Axial STIR MR image shows an abnormal wavy CFL (*arrow*). There is evidence of soft tissue swelling with hyperintense signal suggestive of hematoma along the CFL. (**c**) Axial STIR MR image taken at a more proximal level shows a complete tear of the ATFL (*arrow*)

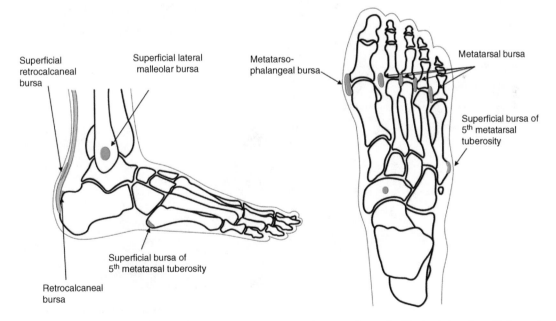

Fig. 25.7 Bursae at foot and ankle. Diagrams show the numerous bursae at foot and ankle that help reduce friction and prevent pain

Retrocalcaneal bursitis (Fig. 25.8) is caused by Achilles tendon disorders, such as Achilles tendinitis, tendinopathy, enthesopathy, and trauma, e.g., calcaneal fracture.

The superficial retrocalcaneal bursa lies between the Achilles tendon and overlying subcutaneous fat and is caused by poorly fitting shoes. *Seiza* (a traditional Japanese way of sitting straight) and sitting cross-legged may cause a superficial bursitis at level of the lateral malleolus (Fig. 25.9). Hence, Asian people sitting on the floor and Tatami mats are prone to this bursitis. In addition to superficial retrocalcaneal bursitis, superficial medial cuneiform bursitis can also result from poorly fitting shoes (Fig. 25.10). The metatarsal bursa is located at the base of the toes on the bottom of the foot. This bursa can be irritated when one metatarsal bone takes more load than the others. Metatarsal bursa at the first toe is particularly prevalent (Fig. 25.11). On MRI, a rounded fluid collection with a thickened wall is demonstrated at the anterior aspect of the lateral malleolus. The thick wall is enhanced following contrast administration. Treatment of bursitis is based mainly on conservative measures, such as rest, and nonsteroidal anti-inflammatory drugs (NSAIDs).

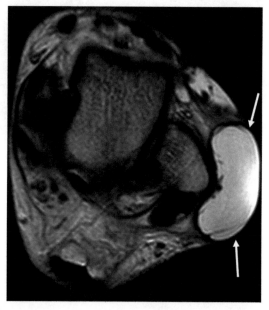

Fig. 25.9 Superficial lateral malleolar bursitis in a 40-year-old woman. Axial T2-W MR image shows an oval-shaped cystic lesion consistent with bursitis adjacent to the lateral malleolus (*arrows*)

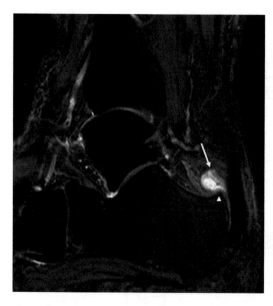

Fig. 25.8 Retrocalcaneal bursitis in a 30-year-old man. Sagittal fat-suppressed T2-W MR image shows an oval fluid collection that represents retrocalcaneal bursitis between calcaneus and Achilles tendon (*arrow*). Haglund deformity is also shown at superior posterior calcaneus (*arrowhead*)

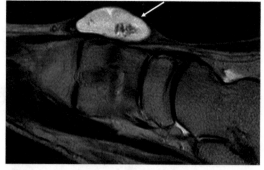

Fig. 25.10 Superficial medial cuneiform bursitis in a 30-year-old woman. Sagittal T2-W MR image shows a rounded cystic lesion consistent with superficial medial cuneiform bursitis adjacent to the dorsal cuneiform (*arrow*). Debris is present within the cystic mass

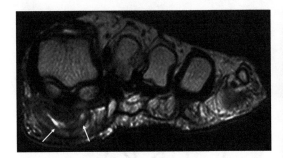

Fig. 25.11 Metatarsal bursitis of the first toe of a 38-year-old woman. Coronal T2-W MR image shows an area of band-like hyperintense signal with thick walls at the level of the first MTP joint (*arrow*). This lesion lies between the sesamoids and subcutaneous fat tissue

25.4.3 Peroneal Tendon Disorders

The peroneus longus and brevis tendons present at the lateral aspect of the ankle act during plantar flexion and eversion of the foot. A severe ankle sprain sometimes causes peroneal tendon disorder. Representative peroneal tendon disorders are peroneus brevis tendon tear, fifth metatarsal fracture, and dislocation of peroneal tendon. Similar symptoms are manifested by peroneus longus tendon inflammatory change.

25.4.3.1 Peroneus Brevis Tendon Tear

The peroneus brevis tendon arises at the level of the distal fibula, crosses behind the lateral malleolus, and connects to the base of the fifth metatarsal. Repetitive ankle motions in sports, such as jumping and running, and severe ankle sprain can lead to wear and tear (Fig. 25.12). Recently, some authors have reported that the superior peroneal retinaculum is partially torn from the posterior aspect of the fibula due to ankle sprain, making the peroneus brevis tendon somewhat unstable. This may result in inhibition of the tissue repair response, leading to subsequent tendon degeneration and tear (Sobel et al. 1991; Minoyama et al. 2002). Peroneus brevis tendon tear is usually visualized at level of lateral malleolus and typically forms a crescent-like shape on MRI.

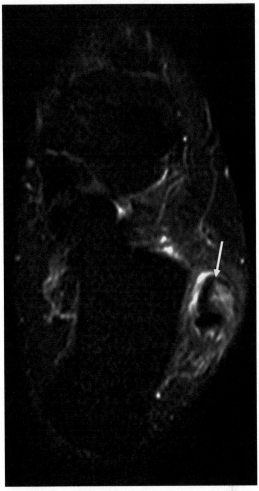

Fig. 25.12 Tear of peroneal brevis tendon in a 37-year-old woman who experienced pain at the lateral aspect of ankle while doing martial art. Axial STIR MR image shows a crescent-shaped peroneal brevis tendon indicative of tear (*arrow*). Hyperintense signal area around the peroneal brevis tendon consistent with hematoma is present

25.4.3.2 Avulsion Fracture of the Fifth Metatarsal

The peroneus brevis tendon connects to the base of the fifth metatarsal. Avulsion fracture of the fifth metatarsal is caused by forcible inversion of the foot in plantar flexion and may occur while stepping on a curb or climbing steps and sports, e.g., playing tennis and basketball. This fracture has many other names, such as tennis fracture,

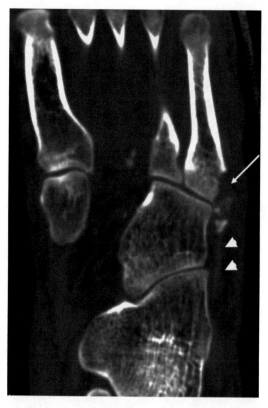

Fig. 25.13 Avulsion fracture of the fifth metatarsal in a 37-year-old man. Axial CT image of foot shows an avulsion fracture at the tip of the fifth metatarsal (*arrow*). The peroneus brevis tendon (*arrowheads*) attaches to the bony fragment of the fifth metatarsal

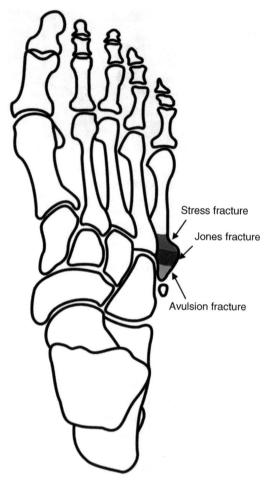

Fig. 25.14 Various kinds of fractures of the fifth metatarsal base. Diagram shows the three kinds of fracture at the fifth metatarsal base: avulsion fracture, Jones fracture, and stress fracture

pseudo-Jones fracture, and dancer fracture. In Japan, it is called geta fracture. Geta is a Japanese traditional shoe. Typically, elderly Japanese people who wear both geta and kimono suffer this fracture. Avulsion fractures account for more than 90% of fractures of the base of the fifth metatarsal. On radiograph and computed tomography (CT), small fractures of the tip of the proximal fifth metatarsal are oriented mostly transversely (Fig. 25.13). It usually does not reach the articular surface of the metatarsocuboid joint.

Differential diagnosis includes stress fracture of fifth metatarsal, Jones fracture, and disorder of

the os peroneum. Stress fracture, Jones fracture, and avulsion fracture of the fifth metatarsal present with similar symptoms but are located at different fracture sites at the fifth metatarsal (Fig. 25.14). Stress fracture of the fifth metatarsal occurs within 1.5 cm of the metadiaphyseal junction (i.e., distal to Jones fracture) (Fig. 25.15). Jones fracture is a horizontally oriented fracture and is present at the base of the fifth metatarsal,

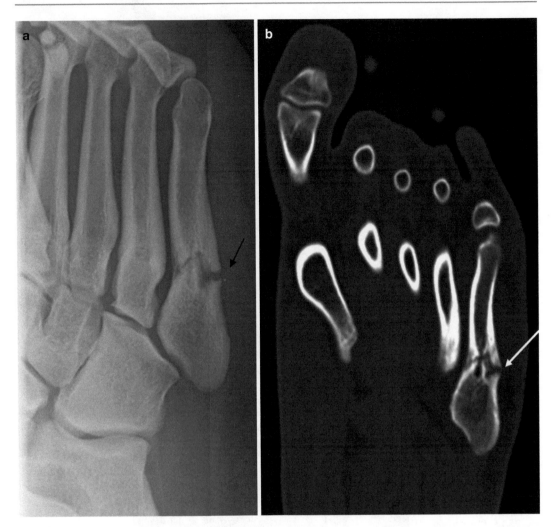

Fig. 25.15 A 17-year-old boy who plays football and developed lateral foot pain. (**a**) AP radiograph shows fracture at level of proximal diaphysis (*black arrow*) of the fifth metatarsal. (**b**) Axial CT image of the foot shows a fifth metatarsal fracture with slight callus formation (*white arrow*). Stress fracture of the fifth metatarsal is consistent from patient's history. This fracture is more distal in location than Jones and avulsion fractures

1.5–3 cm (about 2 cm) distal to the proximal tuberosity at the metadiaphyseal junction (Fig. 25.16). The fracture is believed to occur as a result of significant adduction force to the forefoot with the ankle in plantar flexion. Therefore, this fracture mechanism is different from that of the avulsion fracture of the fifth metatarsal.

25.4.3.3 Peroneal Tendon Subluxation

The tendons of the peroneal muscles pass together through a groove behind the lateral malleolus. The tendons are kept within the groove by a sheath that forms a tunnel around the tendons. The surface of this sheath is

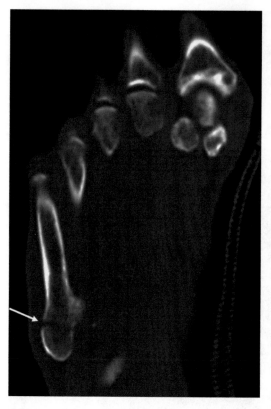

Fig. 25.16 Jones fracture in a 64-year-old man. Axial CT image of the foot shows a Jones fracture at the proximal metaphyseal area of fifth metatarsal (*arrow*)

reinforced by a ligamentous band called a retinaculum. In addition, there is a small fibrous cartilage called the fibrous ridge at the lateral aspect of the lateral malleolus (Figs. 25.17 and 25.18). The fibrous ridge behaves as a groyne against the peroneal tendons. Contracting the peroneal muscles makes the tendons glide in the

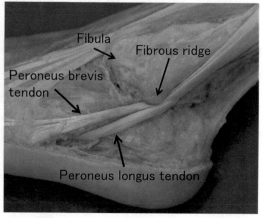

Fig. 25.17 Specimen photograph of the fibrous ridge. The fibrous ridge is a small fibrocartilage and is present at posterior and lateral aspect of lateral malleolus. It serves to prevent subluxation of peroneus longus and brevis tendons

Fig. 25.18 Comparison between (**a**) cadaver photograph and (**b**) axial T1-W MR image. The fibrous ridge is white in color on the cadaver image (**a**), but shows signal hypointensity on the MR image (**b**), consistent with fibrocartilage. Peroneus longus and brevis tendons are present behind the lateral malleolus

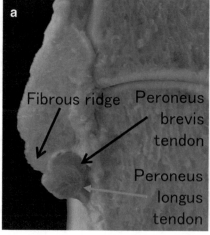
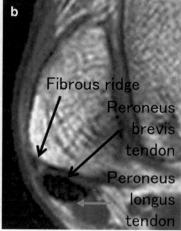

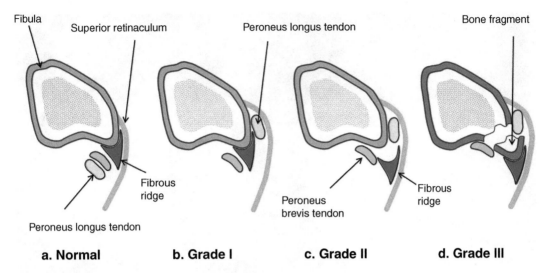

a. Normal   **b. Grade I**   **c. Grade II**   **d. Grade III**

Fig. 25.19 Diagram shows the classification of peroneus tendon subluxation (from Eckert and Davis). (**a**) Normal. (**b**) Grade I: Subluxation of peroneus longus tendon with retinaculum without laceration of fibrous ridge. (**c**) Grade II: Subluxation of peroneus longus tendon with laceration of both retinaculum and fibrous ridge. (**d**) Grade III: Subluxation of peroneus longus tendon with bony fragment attached to fibrous ridge

groove like a pulley. This pulley action points the foot downward (plantar flexion) and outward (eversion). The main cause of peroneal tendon subluxation is an ankle sprain. A sprain that injures the ligaments on the outer edge of the ankle can also damage the peroneal tendons. During the typical inversion ankle sprain, the foot rolls in. The forceful stretch of the peroneal muscle can rip the retinaculum and fibrous ridge that keeps the peroneal tendons positioned in the groove. As a result, the tendons can dislocate out of the groove. The tendons usually relocate by snapping back into place. The injury to the retinaculum and fibrous ridge may be overlooked initially, while treatment focuses on the injury to other ankle ligaments. This means that the subluxation may manifest much later, and it may not seem to be caused by the initial ankle sprain. If not corrected, this snapping of the tendons can become a chronic and recurring problem.

Eckert and Davis (1976) classified peroneal tendon subluxation into three grades: Grade I is only peroneus longus tendon subluxation without destroyed fibrous ridge; Grade II is the peroneus longus tendon subluxation with destroyed fibrous ridge; and Grade III corresponds to peroneus longus tendon subluxation with an avulsion fracture at the level of the fibrous ridge (Fig. 25.19). Combination of both peroneus longus and brevis subluxations is rare. On MRI, laceration and dislocation of the fibrous ridge with retinaculum are visible. Direct finding of peroneus longus subluxation may be difficult to demonstrate on routine MRI examination in the neutral position. However, in case of chronic peroneal tendon subluxation, some patients could dislocate their peroneus longus tendon by themselves. Then, the peroneus longus tendon and the lacerated fibrous ridge are detected at the lateral aspect of the lateral malleolus (Fig. 25.20). In acute peroneus longus tendon subluxation, bone marrow edema at the lateral

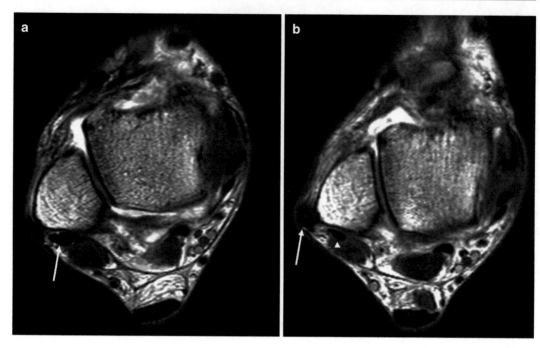

Fig. 25.20 Peroneus longus tendon subluxation: comparison between neutral position and dorsal position in a 23-year-old man. (**a**) Axial DESS image taken in the neutral position shows both peroneus longus and brevis tendons present behind the lateral malleolus (*arrow*). (**b**) Axial DESS image taken in the dorsal position shows that the peroneus longus tendon is dislocated to a dorsal position (*arrow*). The peroneus brevis tendon is not dislocated (*arrowhead*). The fibrous ridge is not detected on both (**a**) and (**b**) images

aspect of the lateral malleolus is present. It may suggest laceration of the fibrous ridge with both periosteum and retinaculum involvement, due to direct force from the peroneus longus tendon. A localized fluid collection called the pseudo-pouch may be visible at the lateral aspect of the lateral malleolus (Fig. 25.21). It is located between the lacerated periosteum and fibula.

25.4.3.4 Peroneus Longus Tendon Inflammatory Change

The peroneus longus tendon turns through a sharp angle to enter a fibro-osseous tunnel on the underside of the cuboid after passing posterior to the lateral malleolus. It inserts into the plantar surface of the first metatarsal (Fig. 25.22). Characteristic activities include marathon running or other sports which require repetitive use of the ankle. Patients usually present with pain around the back of the ankle. There is usually no history of a specific injury. Improper training or rapid increases in training can lead to peroneal inflammatory change, i.e., tendonitis or tendinosis. Patients who have a hindfoot varus posture may be more susceptible. This is because in these patients, the heel is slightly turned inward which requires the peroneal tendons to work harder. Their main job is to evert or turn the ankle to the outside, which fights against the varus position. The harder the tendons work, the more likely they are to develop peroneal inflammatory change.

There are two areas of inflammatory change: at level of the peroneal trochlea and the cuboid tunnel. These areas are narrow spaces that the peroneus longus tendon passes through, and the peroneus longus tendon usually rubs against the peroneal trochlea and the cuboid tunnel when in

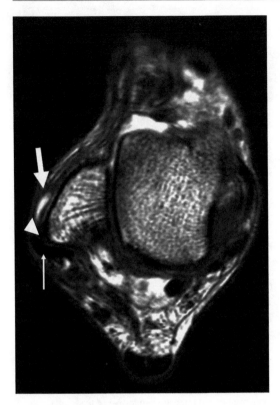

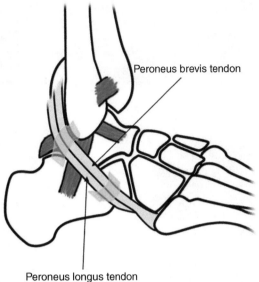

Peroneus brevis tendon

Peroneus longus tendon

Fig. 25.22 Diagram shows anatomy of the peroneus longus and brevis tendons. Peroneus longus and brevis tendon turn through a sharp angle to enter a fibro-osseous tunnel on the underside of the cuboid after passing posterior to the lateral malleolus. Superior retinaculum fixes both peroneus longus and brevis tendons in position

Fig. 25.21 Peroneus tendon subluxation at the dorsal position in a 17-year-old man. Axial DESS MR image taken in the dorsal position shows subluxation of peroneus longus tendon (*thin arrow*). Small hypointense structure consistent with the fibrous ridge is visualized between the peroneus longus tendon and lateral malleolus (*arrowhead*). Localized fluid collection suggestive of pseudopouch is demonstrated along the lateral malleolus (*thick arrow*)

action. MRI is useful for detection, showing hyperintense signal of the peroneus longus tendon with or without a fluid collection suggestive of tenosynovitis around it at the level of the peroneal trochlea (Figs. 25.23 and 25.24). Bone marrow edema at the peroneal trochlea may be seen. At level of the cuboid, an os peroneum may cause tear or degenerative change of the peroneus longus tendon (Fig. 25.25). The lateral longitudinal arch becomes flat due to dysfunction of peroneus longus tendon, and it may lead to early osteoarthritis of the ankle.

25.5 Medial Ankle Pain

Medial ankle pain is caused by deltoid ligament tear, disorder of tendons, e.g., flexor hallucis longus tendon and posterior tibialis tendon, and stress fracture of the medial malleolus.

25.5.1 Deltoid Ligament Tear

The deltoid ligament is a complex structure that spans from the medial malleolus to the navicular, talus, and calcaneus. It is responsible for stabilizing the medial side of the ankle to limit anterior, posterior, and lateral translation of the talus and to restrain talar abduction at the talocrural joint (Harper 1983). The deltoid ligament can be classified into superficial and deep layers. The superficial layer includes the tibiocalcaneal ligament, tibionavicular ligament, posterior

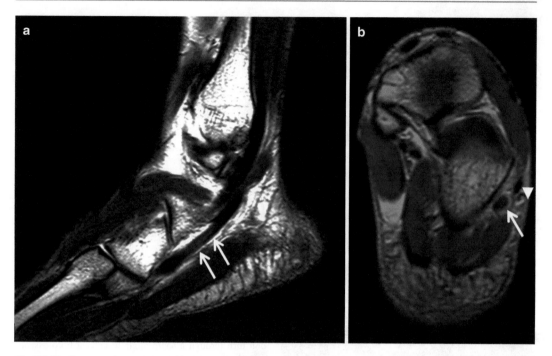

Fig. 25.23 Peroneus longus tendonitis at level of peroneal trochlea in a 16-year-old boy who developed pain at the lateral foot while playing tennis. (**a**) Sagittal DESS MR image shows hyperintense signal in the peroneus longus tendon (*arrows*). (**b**) Axial T1-W MR image shows the peroneus brevis tendon (*arrowhead*) has normal signal intensity but the peroneal longus tendon (*arrow*) shows increased signal intensity suggestive of tendonitis

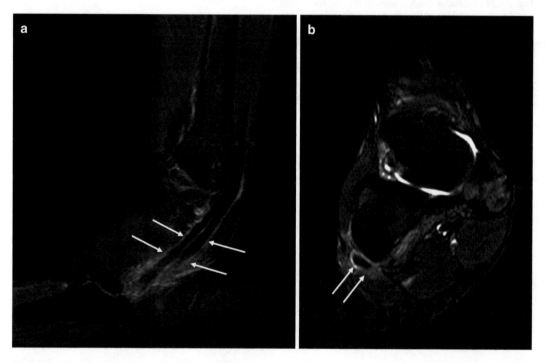

Fig. 25.24 Peroneus longus tenosynovitis at level of peroneal trachea in a 20-year-old man who had lateral foot pain while playing football. (**a**) Sagittal STIR MR image shows normal signal of the peroneus longus and brevis tendons surrounded by hyperintense signal fluid alongside the tendons (*arrows*). (**b**) Coronal STIR MR image shows the peroneus longus and brevis tendons are surrounded by hyperintense signal (*arrows*), consistent with tenosynovitis

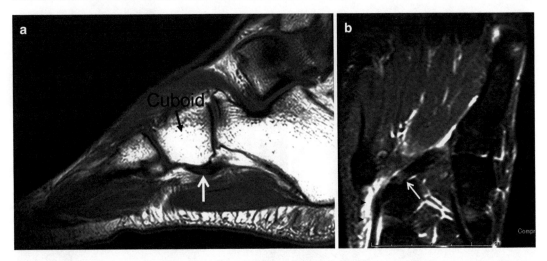

Fig. 25.25 Peroneus longus tendonitis at level of the cuboid in a 20-year-old man who had lateral foot pain while playing football. (**a**) Sagittal T1-W MR image shows hyperintense signal within the peroneus longus tendon suggestive of tendonitis (*arrow*). (**b**) Axial STIR MR image shows hyperintense signal (*arrowheads*) suggestive of fluid collection along the peroneus longus tendon. Both tenosynovitis and tendonitis (*arrow*) of the peroneus longus tendon are present

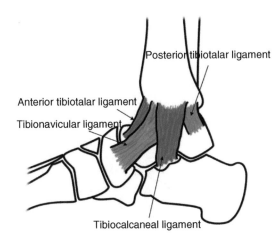

Fig. 25.26 Diagram shows anatomy of the deltoid ligament. The deltoid ligament has two layers: a superficial layer and a deep layer. The superficial layer includes the tibiocalcaneal ligament, tibionavicular ligament, posterior superficial tibiotalar ligament, and tibiospring ligament. The deep layer includes anterior tibiotalar ligament and posterior deep tibiotalar ligament

superficial tibiotalar ligament, and tibiospring ligament. The deep layer is intra-articular and is covered by synovium. It includes the anterior tibiotalar ligament and posterior deep tibiotalar ligament (Fig. 25.26).

Medial ankle sprains accounted for 5.1% of the ankle sprains reported by Watermann et al. (2010). Deltoid ligament injury can also occur with concomitant lateral ankle sprains, during fractures of the lateral malleolus, and in association with posterior tibial tendon pathology (Hintermann et al. 2004). In addition, overuse causes stress fracture of medial malleolus and flexor hallucis longus tendon pathology. It is rare to injure only the deltoid ligament. The lesion is frequently associated with other injuries to structures of the ankle, including the fibula, articular cartilage surfaces of talar dome, and syndesmosis. MRI is useful to detect deltoid ligament tear (Fig. 25.27). The deltoid tear is seen as a discontinuous ligament with signal hyperintensity. Swollen soft tissue is present around the medial malleolus. Most deltoid ligament injuries are treated conservatively. However, in patients who have chronic medial ankle instability, surgery to repair or to reconstruct the deltoid ligament may be necessary (Campbell et al. 2014). In some cases, deltoid ligament tear due to a severe lateral ankle sprain is associated with osteochondral lesion of the talar dome. In

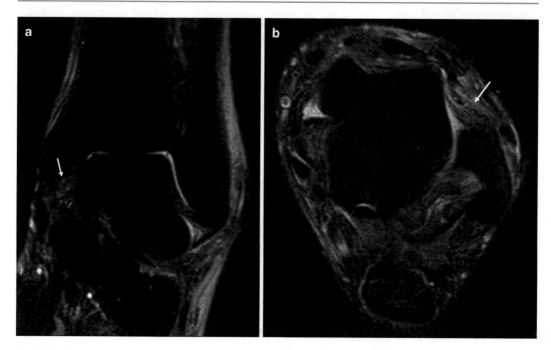

Fig. 25.27 Deltoid ligament tear in a 26-year-old man. (**a**) Coronal fat-suppressed T2-W MR image shows hyperintense signal in the deltoid ligament consistent with a tear (*arrow*).

(**b**) Axial fat-suppressed T2-W MR image shows swelling and signal hyperintensity in the ATFL consistent with a tear (*arrow*). Soft tissue swelling is seen around the ATFL tear

these cases, severe lateral ankle sprain causes bony collision between the medial aspect of the talar dome and the tibia. One should be aware of this associated bony injury.

25.5.2 Flexor Hallucis Longus Disorders

The flexor hallucis longus (FHL) muscle arises at the distal two-thirds of the posterior fibula, interosseous membrane, and adjacent intermuscular septum and connects to plantar surface of the base of the distal phalanx of the great toe (Fig. 25.28). The FHL passes through the posterior aspect of the fibro-osseous tunnel and plantar midfoot. This fibro-osseous tunnel is very narrow, so overuse may cause stenosing tenosynovitis of the FHL, FHL tear, and FHL tendonitis at level of the fibro-osseous tunnel. Stenosing tenosynovitis of the FHL is typical for ballet dancers who go from flat foot to the *en-pointe* position. Patients with stenosing tenosynovitis of the FHL have a swollen medial malleolus with pain and are not able to flex their great toe. On MRI, a

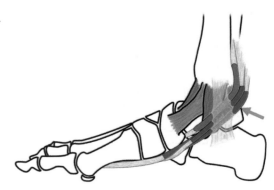

Fig. 25.28 Diagram shows anatomy of FHL. Flexor hallucis longus tendon (*red arrow*) turns through a sharp angle to enter a fibro-osseous tunnel at level of medial calcaneus after passing posterior to the medial malleolus. It then connects to the plantar surface of the base of the distal phalanx of the greater hallux. Flexor digitorum tendon and tibialis posterior tendon runs along the FHL at level of the medial malleolus

hypointense fibrotic structure is visible around the FHL at the level of the fibro-osseous membrane (Fig. 25.29). FHL tear or FHL tendonitis is rarely visualized in activities other than ballet dancing, in which extreme plantar flexion occurs.

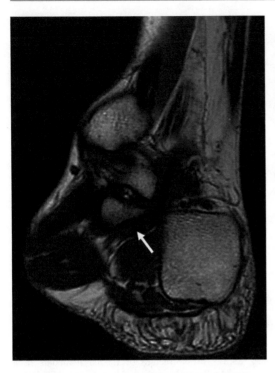

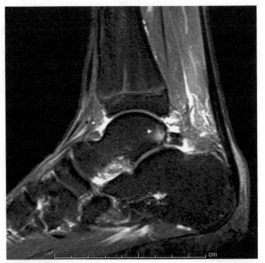

Fig. 25.30 Os trigonum in a 12-year-old boy who had hindfoot pain while playing football. Sagittal STIR MR image of the ankle shows a small bone consistent with an os trigonum adjacent to the posterior aspect of talus (*red arrow*). Bone marrow edema in both os trigonum and posterior aspect of talus (*arrowhead*) is seen. Hyperintense soft tissue swelling around the os trigonum is present

Fig. 25.29 Stenosing tenosynovitis of FHL in a 32-year-old female ballet dancer. Coronal T1-W MR image shows the FHL wrapped by intermediate signal intensity structure consistent with a fibrous tendon sheath (*arrow*) at level of fibro-osseous tunnel

Os trigonum is a bony ossicle of the foot and is estimated to be present in 7% of adults. The ossicle usually forms at 7–13 years of age and fuses with the talus in the majority of patients. If it does not, it persists as an os trigonum (Cerezal et al. 2003) (Fig. 25.30). The posterior ankle impingement (PAI) syndrome is one of the ankle impingement syndromes and occurs from repetitive ankle plantar flexion. PAI has been described in ballet dancers, football players, and other athletes who sustain repeated plantar flexion of the toes. For patients who have an os trigonum, pointing the toes downward can result in a "nutcracker injury," where the os trigonum is crushed together with adjacent soft tissues, and sometimes the FHL, between the ankle and calcaneus. The signs and symptoms of this disorder may include deep aching pain and swelling at the back of the ankle when pushing off the big toe or when doing plantar flexion of feet. MRI shows a flat-shaped FHL with signal hyperintensity between the os trigonum and talus. The os trigonum should not be

mistaken for a fracture fragment. If identified, it may be a cause of the patient's symptoms, particularly with FHL involvement in PAI.

25.5.3 Tibialis Posterior Tendonitis and Tear

The tibialis posterior muscle arises from the lateral part of the posterior surface of the tibia, medial two-thirds of the fibula, interosseous membrane, intermuscular septa, and deep fascia. The tendon passes behind the medial malleolus to attach to the bones that form the arch of the foot: the navicular, each cuneiform and cuboid, calcaneus, and second to fourth metatarsals. The tibialis posterior tendon produces inversion and plantar flexion of the foot at the ankle and is a medial ankle stabilizer. Tibialis posterior tendon tear is caused by too much force or repetition of tibialis posterior muscle contraction (Fig. 25.31). Patients with tibialis posterior tendonitis and tear may experience pain on the inside of their foot, ankle, and lower leg and may not be able to raise their heel during standing. The medial inner arch may become

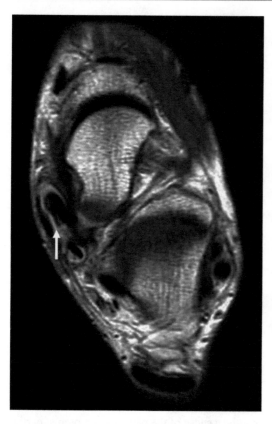

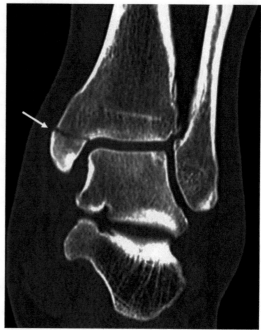

Fig. 25.32 Stress fracture of medial malleolus in a 16-year-old female basketball player. Coronal CT image of the ankle shows a horizontal fracture line at the medial malleolus (*arrow*)

Fig. 25.31 Partial tear of posterior tibialis tendon in a 40-year-old man who had pain while playing rugby. Axial PD-W MR image shows signal hyperintensity with indistinct margin at posterior aspect (*arrow*) of the posterior tibialis tendon, consistent with partial tear of the posterior tibialis tendon

flat, when compared to the normal side. MRI of tibialis posterior tendonitis and tear shows swelling and hyperintense signal with an indistinct margin. Fluid collection around the tibialis posterior tendon is also seen. In complete rupture of the tibialis posterior tendon, there is an empty space with absence of the tibialis posterior tendon.

25.5.4 Stress Fracture of the Medial Malleolus

The medial malleolus forms the support for the medial side of the ankle joint and is also the attachment site of the deltoid ligament. When the foot rolls inward, an isolated fracture of the

medial malleolus may occur, with a horizontal fracture usually visualized. In addition, repetitive force upon the medial malleolus can also result in stress fracture. A vertical fracture of the medial malleolus is often visible, but horizontal fracture of the medial malleolus is sometimes seen (Fig. 25.32). Patients present with pain at the medial aspect of the ankle. As the fracture line may be indistinct on radiographs when in the acute phase, CT and MRI are helpful for detection.

25.6 Dorsal Ankle Pain

25.6.1 Anterior Inferior Tibiofibular Ligament Tear and Syndesmosis Injury

The anterior inferior tibiofibular ligament (AITFL) is a triangular band of fibers located between the adjacent margins of the tibia and fibula, forming the anterior aspect of the syndesmosis. The syndesmosis is made up of the AITFL, interosseous ligament, and posterior inferior fibular ligament (PITFL). Syndesmotic ligament injuries often occur in conjunction with other ankle injuries, including sprains and fractures. If the syndesmosis is damaged, the ankle joint may become unstable. This is called "high ankle sprain." Syndesmosis injury occurs when the foot twists outward relative to the leg (external rotation injury), resulting in damage to the ligaments above the ankle joint (Fig. 25.33).

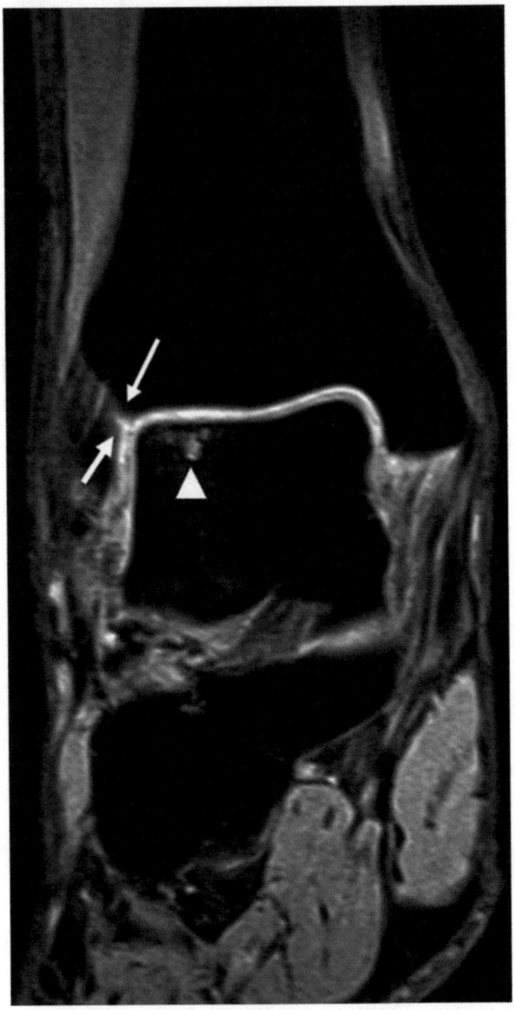

Patients have pain above the ankle and calf and inability to place weight on the leg. Stress radiographs are useful to detect instability. In a stress radiograph, the examiner will apply a force to the ankle to determine if the syndesmosis shifts. In addition, MRI can also be helpful in making the diagnosis. Syndesmosis injuries are repaired surgically using metal screws.

25.6.2 Footballer Ankle

Footballer ankle is a bony growth at the front of the ankle where the joint capsule attaches. The typical symptoms are pain across the front of the ankle when kicking a ball and dorsiflexion of the foot. In many cases, a hard lump appears on the front of the ankle which can be either a bone spur or sometimes the trapped ligament in between the bones on lateral radiograph (Fig. 25.34) and ankle CT. If the condition persists, surgical intervention may be necessary.

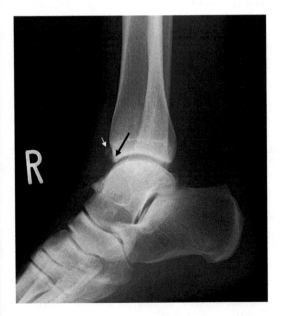

Fig. 25.33 Syndesmotic ligament tear in a 20-year-old man who had pain in the high ankle area with dorsiflexion. Coronal GRE MR image shows partial tear at the syndesmotic ligament (*arrows*). Osteochondral lesion is also seen at the lateral talar dome (*arrowhead*). Findings consistent with a severe ankle sprain

Fig. 25.34 Footballer ankle in a 20-year-old male football player. Lateral radiograph of the ankle shows spur formation at both anterior tip of the tibia (*black arrow*) and the talar neck (*arrowhead*). Bone fragment is seen in front of the tibial spur (*white arrow*). Collision between tibia and talar neck may cause the spur and bony fragment

25.6.3 Extensor Tendonitis and Tenosynovitis

Extensor tendonitis and tenosynovitis most commonly occur due to friction between the foot and shoe. It tends to affect people who spend long periods on their feet, walking or running on uneven surfaces or up and down hills, and who lace their shoes too tightly. People with high foot arches are more likely to have pressure at the top of their foot, and people with flat feet find their extensor tendons under more strain, both of which increase the chance of developing tendonitis. Presenting symptoms include dorsal foot pain, swelling, and/or bruising across the top of the foot. On MRI, extensor tendons show hyperintense signal with fluid collection.

25.7 Posterior Ankle Pain

25.7.1 Achilles Tendon Rupture

The Achilles tendon is the strongest and largest tendon in the body and connects the soleus and the two heads of the gastrocnemius muscles to the posterior aspect of the calcaneus. Achilles tendon rupture can occur at any age, but most often occurs in athletes and recreational athletes aged 30–50 years of age. It is commonly seen in football, running, basketball, tennis, and other sports which require a forceful push off with the foot. Some risk factors include increasing age; chronic or recurrent Achilles tendinosis; steroids; systemic conditions, e.g., gout, rheumatoid arthritis, and systemic lupus erythematosus; and quinolone antibiotics (Mazzone and McCue 2002). Patients have an acute onset of pain in the tendon initially, may notice an inability to stand on tiptoe, and have altered gait. A snap is heard as the tendon ruptures. The diagnosis may not be obvious initially. Radiographs show soft tissue swelling and obliteration of the pre-Achilles fat pad. MRI shows Achilles tendon rupture at a level 2–6 cm proximal to its insertion, which is a region of relative watershed hypovascularity.

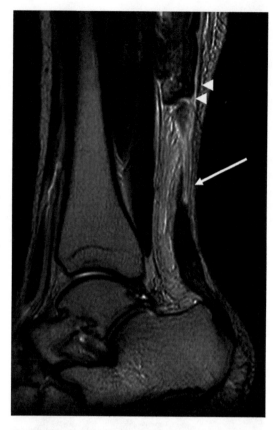

Fig. 25.35 Achilles tendon rupture in a 30-year-old female professional volleyball player. Sagittal T2-W MR image shows complete rupture of the Achilles tendon (*arrow*). Retraction of the Achilles tendon ends is shown (*arrowheads*)

Complete rupture shows retraction of tendon ends (Fig. 25.35). Partial tear of Achilles tendon shows hyperintense signal on fluid-sensitive MR sequences.

25.7.2 Achilles Tendinosis

Achilles tendinosis refers to degeneration of the Achilles tendon. This condition is common in athletes, runners, and patients who have calf tightness. Achilles tendinosis may occur in the middle of the tendon and at the point where the tendon connects to the calcaneus. The latter is called insertional Achilles tendinosis. Patients

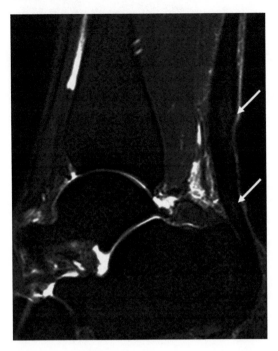

Fig. 25.36 Achilles tendinosis in a 32-year-old male runner. Sagittal fat-suppressed T2-W MR image shows a swollen and hyperintense Achilles tendon consistent with tendinosis (*arrows*)

have pain and/or tightness in the tendon behind the ankle. Most of the time, there is no trauma or injury, but rather a slow progression of pain. Many patients will notice a bump either in the tendon (mid-substance Achilles tendinosis) or right behind the calcaneus (insertional Achilles tendinosis). On radiographs, the Achilles tendon is swollen and thickened, and there may be bone spurs. MRI shows a hyperintense swollen tendon (Fig. 25.36). Reactive bone formation may be demonstrated within the Achilles tendon (Fig. 25.37). Treatment depends on the length and severity of the symptoms.

25.8 Mid- and Anterior Foot Pain

25.8.1 Lisfranc Ligament Injury

The Lisfranc ligament is a small and tough intraosseous ligament that connects the medial cuneiform and the base of the second metatarsal (Fig. 25.38). Midfoot sprains in athletes represent a lower-velocity injury, typically with no displacement or with

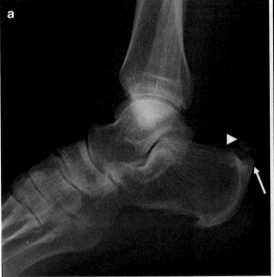
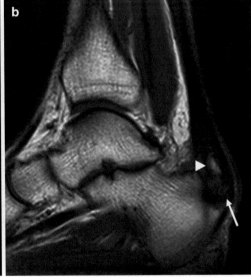

Fig. 25.37 Insertional Achilles tendinosis in a 40-year-old man. (a) Lateral ankle radiograph shows spur formation (*arrow*) and a loose body (*arrowhead*) at insertion of the Achilles tendon. (b) Sagittal PD-W MR image shows a swollen and hyperintense Achilles tendon at its insertion (*arrow*). The loose body (*arrowhead*) is seen within the Achilles tendon. These findings are consistent with insertional Achilles tendinosis

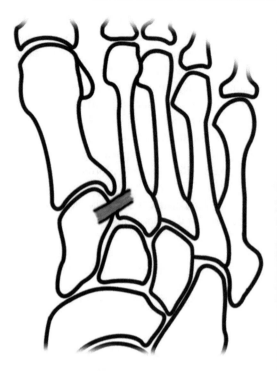

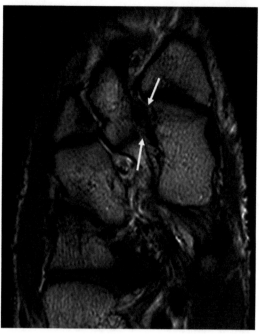

Fig. 25.39 Tear of Lisfranc ligament in a 23-year-old man. Axial T2-W MR image shows a Lisfranc tear at its midportion (*arrows*)

Fig. 25.38 Diagram shows anatomy of Lisfranc ligament. The Lisfranc ligament is a ligament which connects the superior-lateral surface of the medial cuneiform to the superior-medial surface of the base of the second metatarsal

only subtle diastases. Lisfranc ligament and Lisfranc joint have a role of maintaining a transverse arch of the midfoot. The Lisfranc joint forms a shallow arc between the medial base of the second metatarsal and the lateral margin of the distal medial cuneiform, a configuration that gives it little bony stabilization. The keystone of the transverse arch is the middle cuneiform which forms the focal point that supports the entire tarsometatarsal articulation. If the Lisfranc ligament and/or the Lisfranc joint are injured, the transverse arch will be flat (flat foot). Patients present with pain and swelling of midfoot, especially tarsometatarsal articulations, and instability when bearing weight.

Radiographs showing diastasis of the normal architecture confirm the presence of a severe sprain and possible dislocation. However, subtle midfoot sprains (diastasis of 1–5 mm) without fracture of the second metatarsal are difficult to diagnose on radiographs. MRI can prove very helpful for the evaluation of injuries to the

midfoot, particularly in the setting of normal radiographs. Specific injuries to the components of the Lisfranc ligament complex can be detected (Fig. 25.39). There are one to four Lisfranc ligaments on anatomical study, but most people have two Lisfranc ligaments (Hirano et al. 2013). Some of these Lisfranc ligaments can be detected on MRI. A missed diagnosis has serious consequences. An untreated midfoot sprain leads rapidly to osteoarthritis and flattening of the longitudinal arch, too. Treatment is usually surgical.

25.8.2 Osteochondral Lesion of Talar Dome

The talus has numerous articular surfaces, which account for more than 70% of the talus. The largest articular surface is the talar dome which forms the tibiotalar joint. The etiology of osteochondral lesion of the talar dome (OLT) is still debated, but is most often thought to be due to repetitive microtraumas associated with vascular impairment, causing progressive ankle pain and dysfunction in skeletally immature young adults. In addition, ankle sprain causing bony contusion between talar dome and tibial plafond may result in OLT. Symptoms include ankle pain at exercise, joint swelling, and instability during walking and even locking. Some patients are not symptomatic.

OLT is classically located in the medial aspect of the talar dome, while lateral and posterior involvement is less frequent. The osteochondral fragment of the OLT at the medial aspect is often semicircular in shape, while an osteochondral fragment at lateral aspect is wafer shaped. On the anteroposterior (AP) ankle radiograph, it is often possible to see a subchondral halo, a sign outlining the osteochondral fragment and subchondral cyst (Zanon et al. 2014). A radiograph with the ankle in 15° of internal rotation is particularly useful for investigating the superolateral corner of the talus given that in this position, it is free from fibular overlap. Stress radiographs are not of paramount importance for this lesion and may actually be impossible to perform in acute situations (Zanon et al. 2014).

CT gives precise information about the location and extent of the lesion, but does not allow assessment of the integrity of the cartilage. This information can instead be obtained using CT arthrography (CTA) or MRI. Although MRI has the advantage of being noninvasive, it does not allow precise evaluation of the depth of the osteochondral lesion whose edges are blurred by edema of the surrounding bone. Osteochondral fragments appear hypointense on T1-weighted images. On T2-weighted images, they have a very variable intensity, but they are always

characterized by a hyperintense line at their base, which is a sign of detachment (De Smet et al. 1990). Although, over the years, various classifications have been proposed using CT, MRI, or arthroscopy, Berndt and Harty's classification is still the most widely used (Berndt and Harty 1959; De Smet et al. 1990) (Table 25.2). Stage 2 has further been subclassified into 2A and 2B on both CT and MRI (Hepple et al. 1999; Ferkel et al. 2008) (Fig. 25.40). In stage 2A, CT shows a cystic lesion communicating to the talar dome surface, while on MRI, there is a cartilage injury with underlying fracture and surrounding bony edema. In stage 2B, CT shows an open articular surface lesion with overlying nondisplaced fragment, while MRI appearances are similar to stage 2A but without surrounding bone edema. MRI of the stages of OLT is illustrated (Figs. 25.41, 25.42, 25.43, 25.44, and 25.45).

Treatment of OLT is guided by the patient's age at the onset of symptoms, their severity, and the disease stage according to the Berndt and Harty classification. Stage 1 and stage 2 lesions

Table 25.2 Berndt and Harty classification of osteochondral lesions of the talus

Stage	Status
1	Small area of compression of the subchondral bone
2	Partially detached osteochondral fragment (flap)
3	Completely detached osteochondral fragment but undisplaced
4	Free osteochondral fragment

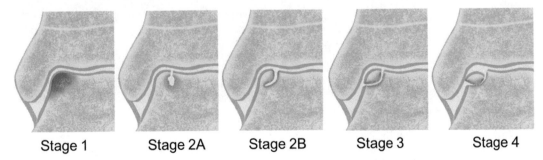

| Stage 1 | Stage 2A | Stage 2B | Stage 3 | Stage 4 |

Fig. 25.40 Diagram shows the classification of OLT. Stage 1: Small area of compression of the subchondral bone. Stage 2A: Partially detached osteochondral fragment (flap). 2B: Open articular surface lesion with overlying nondisplaced fragment. Stage 3: Completely detached but undisplaced osteochondral fragment. Stage 4: Free osteochondral fragment

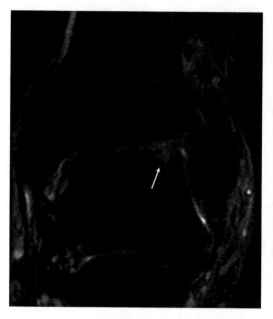

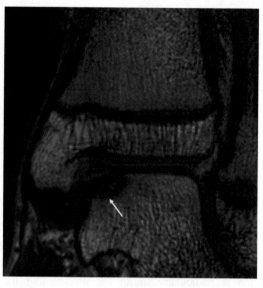

Fig. 25.43 OLT stage 2B in a 14-year-old boy who had ankle sprain. Coronal T1-W MR image shows a flap-like bony fragment at the medial aspect of talar dome (*arrow*)

Fig. 25.41 OLT stage 1 in a 20-year-old woman who had ankle sprain. Coronal STIR MR image shows faint signal hyperintensity consistent with bone contusion at the lateral talar dome (*arrow*)

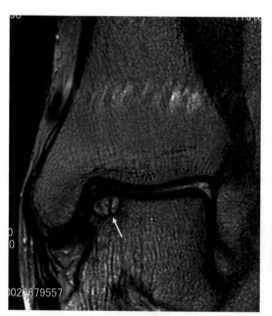

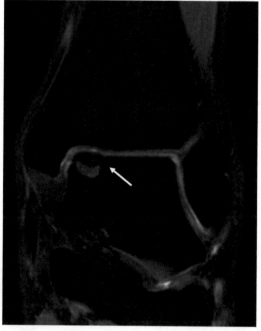

Fig. 25.42 OLT stage 2A in a 16-year-old girl who had ankle sprain. Coronal T2-W MR image shows a subchondral cyst at medial aspect of talar dome (*arrow*)

Fig. 25.44 OLT stage 3 in a 15-year-old girl who had ankle sprain. Coronal GRE T2*-W MR image shows a completely detached osteochondral fragment at the medial aspect of talar dome (*arrow*). Slight dislocation is seen

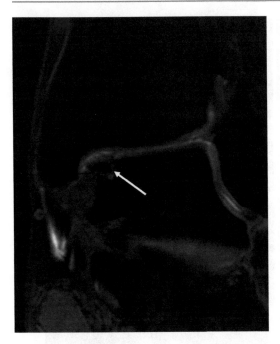

Fig. 25.45 OLT stage 4 in a 19-year-old man who had ankle sprain. Coronal GRE T2*-W MR image shows a free bony fragment with displacement at the medial aspect of the talar dome (*arrow*)

in teenagers are usually treated conservatively (Canale and Belding 1980). Indications for surgery are stage 3 or 4 lesions, failure of conservative treatment, detachment of the fragment, or decreased potential for revascularization. The general principle of surgical treatment is to recreate the cartilage or to refill the defect, restore the articular surface, and prevent the evolution toward osteoarthritis.

25.8.3 Tarsal Coalition

Tarsal coalition is a condition in which two or more tarsal bones have developed an abnormal union, resulting in restricted range of motion (Haendlmayer and Harris 2009). The prevalence of tarsal coalition has been estimated to range from less than 1% to 13% of the population, with 50% of the cases occurring bilaterally (Haendlmayer and Harris 2009; Kernbach 2010). Patients typically present with this condition in adolescence. There is a significant male predilection, with male to female ratio of 4:1 (Kaplan

2001). The two most common locations of tarsal coalition are the talocalcaneal and calcaneonavicular joints (Lyon et al. 2005; Haendlmayer and Harris 2009; Kernbach 2010; Suits and Oliver 2012). In Japan, tarsal coalitions between the navicular and medial cuneiform are called navicular-medial (or first) cuneiform coalition and are prominently encountered (Table 25.3). Tarsal coalitions are described based on the progressive morphology of the coalition, from fibrous (syndesmosis) to cartilaginous (synchondrosis) and finally to osseous (synostosis). A fibrous or cartilaginous coalition is considered an incomplete coalition, whereas an osseous union is a complete coalition. It refers to developmental fusion rather than fusion that is acquired secondary to conditions such as rheumatoid arthritis, trauma, or postsurgical. The types of tarsal coalitions are well depicted on MRI (Table 25.4).

25.8.3.1 Talocalcaneal Coalition

Talocalcaneal coalition (or subtalar coalition) is a coalition between the talus and calcaneus, usually involving the middle facet. Patients present with swelling and pain at the medial aspect of the ankle, during sports or walking. Lateral radiograph best shows the C-sign (complete posterior ring around the talus and sustentaculum tali) and talar beak sign (due to impaired subtalar movement). CT and MRI are both useful to show details of coalition (Fig. 25.4).

Table 25.3 Various types of tarsal coalition

1. Talocalcaneal coalition (−45%)
2. Calcaneonavicular coalition (−45%)
3. Navicular-medial (first) coalition: prominent in Japan, rare among Europeans
4. Cuboid navicular coalition: very rare in all over the world

Table 25.4 MRI signal appearances of tarsal coalition

Coalition	MRI findings
Osseous	Bone marrow signal
Fibrous	Hypointense signal on both T1- and T2-weighted images
Cartilaginous	Intermediate signal T2-weighted and STIR images with/without fluid signal

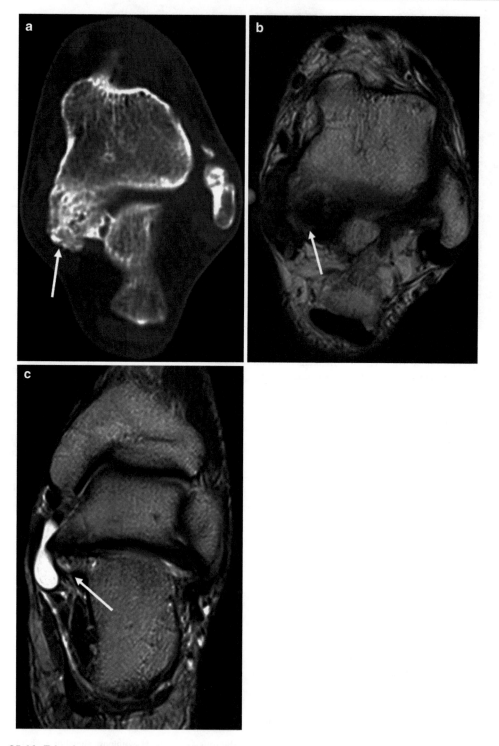

Fig. 25.46 Talocalcaneal coalition in a 30-year-old woman who had medial ankle pain after ankle sprain. (**a**) Axial CT image shows bone degenerative change associated with talocalcaneal coalition at the medial aspect of ankle (*arrow*). (**b**) Axial T1-W MR image shows hetero-geneous hypointense signal at the coalition (*arrow*). (**c**) The coalition extends from the sustentaculum tali (*arrow*) on the coronal T2-W MR image. Cystic lesion due to bursa formation is seen adjacent to the coalition

25.8.3.2 Calcaneonavicular Coalition

Calcaneonavicular coalition refers to connection between the posterolateral aspect of the navicular and the anterior process of calcaneus. Patients have lateral midfoot pain during physical activity. Oblique radiograph and CT are best to detect the anteater nose sign. Calcaneonavicular coalition is well depicted on MRI (Fig. 25.47).

25.8.3.3 Navicular-Medial Cuneiform Coalition

In navicular-medial cuneiform coalition, there is a coalition between the anterior aspect of navicular and the medial cuneiform. Patients have discomfort and fatigue when standing and wearing high heels. It is well seen on AP radiograph and cross-sectional imaging (Fig. 25.48).

25.8.3.4 Cuboid-Navicular Coalition

Cuboid-navicular coalition is extremely rare with less than ten reported cases to date (Awan and Graham 2015). This specific type of coalition has been reported as being asymptomatic, except at specific moments of stress and exercise. Though rare, one should be aware of the existence and appearances of tarsal coalitions so as to consider their diagnoses. Symptomatic coalitions may be treated conservatively with nonsteroidal anti-inflammatory drugs, casting, steroid injection, and orthotics; or can be treated surgically with excision.

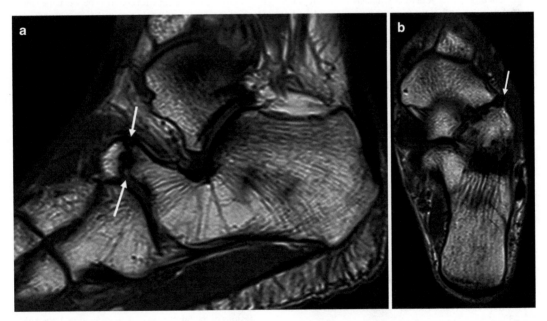

Fig. 25.47 Calcaneonavicular coalition in a 27-year-old woman who had ankle pain while running. (**a**) Sagittal T1-W MR image shows that the superior calcaneal head and navicular form an irregular articular surface (*arrows*). This is consistent with calcaneonavicular coalition. Elongation of superior calcaneal head is called anteater nose. (**b**) Axial T1-W MR image shows that the lateral aspect of the navicular connects to superior calcaneal head (*arrow*)

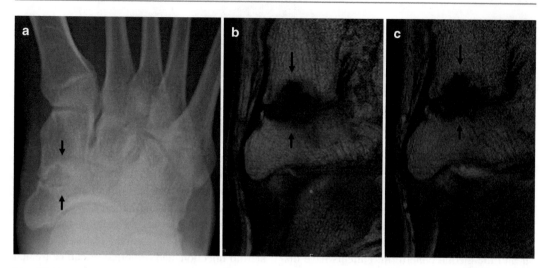

Fig. 25.48 Navicular-medial cuneiform coalition in a 30-year-old man who had pain at the dorsum of the foot while standing. (**a**) AP foot radiograph shows an irregular-shaped articular surface between the navicular and medial cuneiform (*arrows*). Both axial (**b**) T1-W and (**c**) T2-W MR images show articular surface irregularity with signal hypointensity consistent with coalition between the navicular and medial cuneiform (*arrows*)

Conclusion

MRI is an excellent modality for the assessment of injuries of the ankle and foot. Injuries can be categorized into five painful sites, namely, lateral, medial, dorsal, and posterior ankle and mid- and anterior foot. A good knowledge of the anatomy, anatomical variants, and various pitfalls, along with close clinical correlation, is essential for an accurate diagnosis.

References

Awan O, Graham JA (2015) The rare cuboid-navicular coalition presenting as chronic foot pain. Case Rep Radiol doi:10.1155/2015/625285, PMCID: PMC 4321666

Berndt A, Harty M (1959) Transchondral fractures (osteochondritis dissecans) of the talus. J Bone Joint Surg Am 41:988–1020

Broström L (1964) Sprained ankles I: anatomic lesions in recent sprains. Acta Chir Scand 128:483–495

Campbell KJ, Michalski MP, Wilson KJ et al (2014) The ligament anatomy of the deltoid complex of the ankle: a qualitative and quantitative anatomical study. J Bone Joint Surg Am 96:e62

Canale ST, Belding RH (1980) Osteochondral lesions of the talus. J Bone Joint Surg Am 62:97–102

Cerezal L, Abascal F, Canga A et al (2003) MR imaging of ankle impingement syndromes. AJR Am J Roentgenol 181:551–559

De Smet AA, Fisher DR, Burnstein MI et al (1990) Value of MR imaging in staging osteochondral lesions of the talus (osteochondritis dissecans): results in 14 patients. AJR Am J Roentgenol 154:555–558

Eckert WR, Davis EA Jr (1976) Acute rupture of the peroneal retinaculum. J Bone Joint Surg Am 58:670–672

Farooki S, Ashman C, Lee J et al (2002) Common bursae around the body: a review of normal anatomy and magnetic resonance imaging findings. Radiologist 9:209–211

Ferkel RD, Zanotti RM, Komenda GA et al (2008) Arthroscopic treatment of chronic osteochondral lesions of the talus: long-term results. Am J Sports Med 36:1750–1762

Haendlmayer KT, Harris NJ (2009) Flatfoot deformity: an overview. Orthop Trauma 23:395–403

Harper MC (1983) An anatomic study of the short oblique fracture of the distal fibula and ankle stability. Foot Ankle 4:23–29

Hepple S, Winson IG, Glew D (1999) Osteochondral lesions of the talus: a revised classification. Foot Ankle Int 20:789–793

Hintermann B, Valderrabano V, Boss A et al (2004) Medial ankle instability: an exploratory, prospective study of fifty-two cases. Am J Sports Med 32:183–190

Hirano T, Niki H, Beppu M (2013) Anatomical considerations for reconstruction of the Lisfranc ligament. J Orthop Sci 15:720–726

Hirji Z, Hunjun JS, Choudur HM (2011) Imaging of the bursae. J Clin Imaging Sci 1:22. doi:10.4103/2156-7514.80374

Kaplan P (2001) Musculoskeletal MRI. WB Saunders, Philadelphia

Kernbach KJ (2010) Tarsal coalitions: etiology, diagnosis, imaging, and stigmata. Clin Podiatr Med Surg 27:105–117

Lynch SA (2002) Assessment of the injured ankle in the athlete. J Athl Train 37:406–412

Lyon R, Liu XC, Cho SJ (2005) Effects of tarsal coalition resection on dynamic plantar pressures and electromyography of lower extremity muscles. Foot Ankle Surg 44:252–258

MacAuley D (1999) Ankle injuries: same joint, different sports. Med Sci Sports Exerc 31(7 suppl):409–411

Mazzone MF, McCue T (2002) Common conditions of the achilles tendon. Am Fam Physician 65:1805–1810

Minoyama O, Uahiyama E, Iwaso H (2002) Two cases of peroneus brevis tendon tear. Br J Sports Med 36:65–66

Resnick D (1995) Diagnosis of bone and joint disorders, 3rd edn. WB Saunders, Philadelphia

Sobel M, Bohne WHO, Markisz JA (1991) Cadaver correlation of peroneal tendon changes with magnetic resonance imaging. Foot Ankle 11:384–388

Suits JM, Oliver GD (2012) Bilateral tarsal coalition in national collegiate athletic association division I basketball player: a case report. J Athl Train 47:724–729

Sutro CJ (1966) The os calcis, the tendo-Achilles and the local bursae. Bull Hosp Jt Dis 27:76–89

Watermann BR, Belmont PJ Jr, Cameron KL et al (2010) Epidemiology of ankle sprain at the United States Military Academy. Am J Sports Med 38:797–803

Zanon G, Vico GD, Marllo M (2014) Osteochondritis dissecans of the talus. Joints 2:115–123

Ankle and Foot Injuries: US Pitfalls

26

Philip Yoong and James Teh

Contents

26.1	**Introduction**	511
26.2	**Achilles Tendon Lesions**	512
26.3	**Peroneal Tendon Lesions**	513
26.4	**Tibialis Posterior Tendinopathy**	514
26.5	**Spring Ligament Injury**	515
26.6	**Tibialis Anterior Injury**	516
26.7	**Lateral Ankle Ligament Injury**	516
26.8	**Ankle and Foot Effusions and Synovitis**	518
26.9	**Morton Neuroma**	519
26.10	**Plantar Plate Injury**	519
26.11	**Stress Fractures**	520
26.12	**Plantar Fascia Lesions**	520
	Conclusion	522
	References	522

Abbreviations

AP	Anteroposterior
ATFL	Anterior talofibular ligament
CFL	Calcaneofibular ligament
MRI	Magnetic resonance imaging
MTP	Metatarsophalangeal
US	Ultrasound

26.1 Introduction

Sports and overuse injuries of the ankle and foot are very common. The superficial nature of the soft tissue structures typically involved in injury enables ultrasound (US) to be used as an effective diagnostic and therapeutic tool. However, US imaging is entirely dependent on the skill and experience of the operator. Pertinent technical considerations relevant to musculoskeletal US imaging are described in Chap. 18. For further information on US artifacts, please refer to Chap. 2. In addition to technique, a high-quality examination requires knowledge of the appearances of both normal anatomy and pathology to avoid misdiagnosis. In this chapter, we discuss potential pitfalls in the US imaging of the ankle and foot.

P. Yoong, BSc, MBBS, MRCS, FRCR (✉)
Department of Radiology,
Royal Berkshire Hospital, Craven Road,
Reading RG1 5AN, UK
e-mail: philip.yoong@royalberkshire.nhs.uk

J. Teh, BSc, MBBS, FRCP, FRCR
Department of Radiology, Nuffield Orthopaedic
Centre, Oxford University Hospital NHS Trust,
Windmill Road, Oxford OX3 7LD, UK
e-mail: jamesteh1@gmail.com

© Springer International Publishing AG 2017
W.C.G. Peh (ed.), *Pitfalls in Musculoskeletal Radiology*, DOI 10.1007/978-3-319-53496-1_26

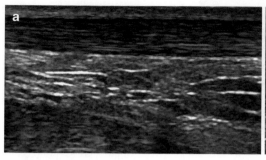
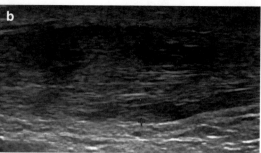

Fig. 26.1 US imaging of the Achilles tendon: normal and tendinopathic. (**a**) The normal Achilles tendon is thin and demonstrates the typical echogenic fibrillar pattern seen in normal tendons, whereas (**b**) in tendinopathy, the Achilles is thickened with areas of hypoechogenicity

26.2 Achilles Tendon Lesions

Compared to magnetic resonance imaging (MRI), US imaging assessment of the Achilles tendon has numerous advantages. US is accessible, quick to perform, and better tolerated by patients. In addition, comparison with the contralateral Achilles is easy to perform. US examination of the Achilles tendon should be performed in both the longitudinal and transverse planes. In the transverse plane, the normal Achilles tendon is concave or flat anteriorly and measures no more than 6 mm in anteroposterior (AP) dimension. In the longitudinal plane, the normal tendon has an echogenic fibrillar pattern in common with other tendons and lacks internal Doppler signal (Fig. 26.1). Extended field-of-view imaging enables an overview of the entire tendon to be presented.

The Achilles tendon is the most frequently injured tendon in the ankle and foot, with a range of pathology that includes paratendinitis, tendinopathy, and tearing (Schweitzer and Karasick 2000a). US imaging enables a comprehensive assessment for these conditions, as well as other injuries such as plantaris tendon rupture and medial gastrocnemius tearing which may mimic Achilles injury. Tendinopathy is easily demonstrated on US imaging as a thickened, hypoechoic tendon measuring in excess of 7 mm in the AP dimension. There is often increased Doppler signal within the affected tendon (Fig. 26.1). Tendinopathy is most commonly seen centered on the midportion of the tendon, away from the

insertion, but can also be centered on the calcaneal enthesis as well. Insertional tendinopathy is often associated with inflammation in the pre-Achilles (retrocalcaneal) bursa. Partial tears of the tendon may manifest as focal areas of altered echogenicity with tendon thickening but are difficult to distinguish from tendinopathy and should be diagnosed with caution.

Achilles tendon enlargement is not always due to tendinopathy. A rare pitfall is Achilles xanthoma which is a manifestation of familial hypercholesterolemia and most commonly presents as fusiform hypoechoic tendon enlargement (Bude et al. 1994). This can be difficult to distinguish from tendinopathy on US imaging, but the presence of more discrete areas of hypoechogenicity, less intratendinous Doppler signal, and similar findings in both Achilles tendons favor xanthoma.

Complete tears of the Achilles are easily diagnosed, and a gap between tendon ends filled with fluid and debris, visible retraction, and posterior acoustic shadowing in the region of a tear are typical findings. A possible pitfall is misinterpreting an intact plantaris tendon lying medial to the torn Achilles as some intact Achilles fibers: the conspicuity of the plantaris tendon is often increased by Achilles tears (Fig. 26.2). It is important to scan Achilles tears dynamically to evaluate the gap between the tendon ends. If the gap is more than 5 mm with the foot in the equinus position, surgery, as opposed to non-operative management, is advocated (Kotnis et al. 2006).

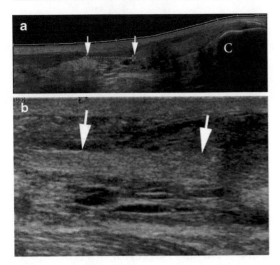

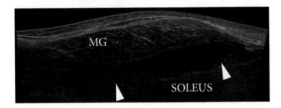

Fig. 26.2 Intact plantaris tendon in a complete Achilles rupture. (**a**) Extended field-of-view US image shows a retracted full-thickness Achilles tear (*small arrows*). (**b**) In the same patient, the plantaris tendon is seen adjacent to the defect between the retracted Achilles tendon ends (*large arrows*) which could be confused for intact Achilles fibers

Fig. 26.3 Medial gastrocnemius musculotendinous junction tear. There is an epimysial tear of the medial gastrocnemius muscle (*MG*) with a large hematoma (*arrowheads*) between the gastrocnemius and soleus muscles

With a normal Achilles tendon, another potential pitfall is not to consider injury of the plantaris tendon and the medial gastrocnemius musculotendinous junction as the cause of calf pain after injury. Both of these conditions are sometimes referred to as tennis leg, often interchangeably. Disruption of the normal muscular architecture of the distal medial gastrocnemius musculotendinous junction is easy to visualize on US imaging (Bianchi et al. 1998): fluid and retracted muscle are typically seen superficial to the echogenic fascial plane that separates the medial gastrocnemius from the underlying soleus muscle (Fig. 26.3).

The plantaris tendon lies medial to the distal Achilles tendon and passes up the calf between the medial head of gastrocnemius and soleus muscles. The tendon may tear in isolation and mimic Achilles injury: on US imaging, this can be seen as fluid in the plane between the soleus and medial head of gastrocnemius (Bianchi et al. 2011). The normal tendon is often difficult to visualize but normally is best seen as an echogenic focus lying adjacent to the medial aspect of the distal Achilles tendon.

26.3 Peroneal Tendon Lesions

The peroneus longus and brevis have a common tendon sheath posterior to the lateral malleolus (Bianchi et al. 2010). In this region, the two tendons can be distinguished by several features: the brevis lies underneath the longus and next to the bone (Brevis near Bone); longus is approximately three times larger in size (Longus is Larger), and the musculotendinous junction of brevis lies more distally than that of the longus. The relationship changes distal to the lateral malleolus as the tendons separate from each other. The brevis passes anterior to the longus and inserts onto the fifth metatarsal base, while the longus passes, inferiorly, under the cuboid and across the plantar aspect of the midfoot, to insert onto the medial cuneiform and first metatarsal base. With this anatomy in mind, an evaluation of the peroneal tendons should be performed in the axial plane, starting from proximal and posterior to the lateral malleolus. Careful dynamic adjustments of probe position must be made to avoid anisotropy as the tendons curve under the lateral malleolus.

The most frequently seen pathology of the peroneal tendons is tenosynovitis. This has a number of causes, such as overuse, inflammatory arthropathy, and trauma in the form of ankle sprains or fractures (Wang et al. 2005). A small amount of fluid in the peroneal tendon sheath is frequently seen in normal individuals and should not be mistaken for tenosynovitis. Increased Doppler signal, synovial thickening within the tendon sheath, as well as fluid that circumferentially surrounds the tendons suggest tenosynovitis. However, fluid in the peroneal tendon sheath may also be caused by a tear of the calcaneofibular ligament, through direct

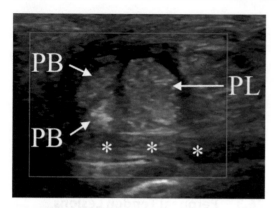

Fig. 26.4 Split tear of the peroneus brevis tendon. A hypoechoic cleft is seen dividing the peroneus brevis (*PB*) tendon. The adjacent peroneus longus (*PL*) tendon is also seen. The CFL is indicated by *asterisks*

communication with the ankle joint. It is therefore useful to examine the lateral ligaments before concluding that fluid in the peroneal tendon sheath is due to tenosynovitis.

Of the two tendons, the peroneus brevis is the more commonly injured due to its close apposition to the retromalleolar groove of the lateral malleolus deep to peroneus brevis. This may present as a U-shaped tendon or a longitudinal split into two portions which may or may not be separated by a peroneus longus tendon (Fig. 26.4). It is important not to confuse a split peroneus brevis tendon with an accessory peroneus quartus tendon. If present, this is seen posterior to the peroneus brevis and longus tendons behind the lateral malleolus. Peroneus longus tendinopathy and tenosynovitis can occur in the context of peroneus brevis pathology or in isolation. In isolation, peroneus longus may be irritated by an os peroneum (an accessory bone in the lateral and plantar aspect of the cuboid which lies within the peroneus longus tendon) or an enlarged peroneal tubercle (a bony prominence in the lateral calcaneus). It is therefore pertinent to look for these features if there is isolated peroneus longus pathology.

Painful os peroneum syndrome (POPS) describes a spectrum of disorders caused by chronic repetitive injury in patients who have an os peroneum (Sobel et al. 1994). POPS may be associated with a fracture of the os peroneum, with tenosynovitis or tendinosis. Peroneal tendon subluxation may occur as a result of peroneal

retinaculum injury, which may occur from an inversion injury of the ankle. The retinaculum itself may be torn or avulsed, typically from its fibular insertion. Subluxation may only be seen on dynamic US imaging, so if it is suspected clinically, the ultrasonographer should perform dynamic maneuvers of the ankle, particularly by placing the ankle in dorsiflexion and eversion. Sometimes the peroneal tendons may remain within the groove but reverse their positions, a condition referred to as "retromalleolar intrasheath dislocation."

26.4 Tibialis Posterior Tendinopathy

The tibialis posterior tendon forms in the lower leg and lies adjacent to the posteromedial aspect of the distal tibia, curves around the medial malleolus, and inserts predominantly onto the medial navicular. The main function of tibialis posterior is foot inversion and ankle plantar flexion. It also supports the medial arch of the foot, and dysfunction is the commonest cause of an acquired flatfoot deformity. Tibialis posterior tendon dysfunction is a common cause of medial-sided ankle pain and is particularly prevalent in the middle-aged female population. Dysfunction may manifest as tendinopathy, tearing, tenosynovitis, or a combination of these conditions (Schweitzer and Karasick 2000b).

The superficial nature of the tibialis posterior tendon enables US imaging to be highly useful in its assessment. Due to the curved nature of its course behind the medial malleolus to its navicular insertion, careful assessment in the axial plane is required. The normal tibialis posterior tendon appears hyperechoic and is approximately twice the size of the adjacent flexor digitorum longus (FDL) tendon (Bencardino et al. 2001) (Fig. 26.5). A loss of this echogenicity and normal size ratio between the tibialis posterior and FDL tendons is useful in the US imaging assessment of pathology. Most commonly, tibialis posterior tendinopathy manifests as an increase in size of the tendon with intrasubstance Doppler flow and loss of the normal tendon architecture with areas of

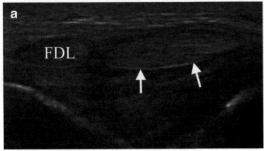

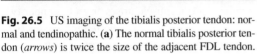

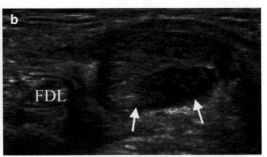

Fig. 26.5 US imaging of the tibialis posterior tendon: normal and tendinopathic. (**a**) The normal tibialis posterior tendon (*arrows*) is twice the size of the adjacent FDL tendon.

(**b**) A markedly enlarged tibialis posterior tendon (*arrows*) is more than twice the size of FDL and has areas of ill-defined hypoechogenicity within it, consistent with tendinopathy

hypoechogenicity and interstitial tearing (Fig. 26.5). Tendinopathy may also be seen as a reduction in the tendon size or atrophic tendinopathy. Complete rupture of the tendon reflects the end stage of the spectrum of tendinopathy and is relatively uncommon. Tendon retraction is uncommon in these cases.

As well as in the perimalleolar region, tendinopathy is also sometimes seen at the insertion of the tibialis posterior tendon onto the navicular bone. A potential pitfall in the assessment of the tendon insertion is that the distal tendon often appears enlarged and hypoechoic due to its complex insertion onto the navicular, cuneiforms, and second to fourth metatarsal bases. The presence of Doppler signal, pain on palpation, and fluid around the tendon insertion favors insertional tendinopathy. The presence of an os naviculare is associated with insertional tendinopathy. Care should be taken not to mistake an os naviculare for a fracture of the navicular (Fig. 26.6).

Tenosynovitis of the tibialis posterior may be seen in isolation, secondary to inflammatory arthropathy as well in the context of coexisting tendinopathy. A potential pitfall in the diagnosis of tenosynovitis is that a small amount of fluid is often found within the tibialis posterior tendon sheath below the medial malleolus. However, a volume of fluid that is more than the tendon it surrounds favors tenosynovitis. To avoid overdiagnosis, careful evaluation for associated synovial thickening and Doppler signal within the sheath should be performed.

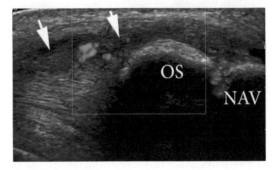

Fig. 26.6 Os naviculare. The os naviculare (*OS*) lies adjacent to the navicular (*NAV*) and should not be confused for a fracture. Note a thickened hypervascular tibialis posterior tendon insertion (*arrows*), consistent with tendinopathy

26.5 Spring Ligament Injury

The spring ligament supports the head of the talus and stabilizes the medial longitudinal arch of the foot. The proper name for the spring ligament is the plantar calcaneonavicular ligament. This is formed of three parts, namely, superomedial, inferoplantar longitudinal, and medioplantar oblique. The superomedial part is the most important for function and the largest and easiest to see on US imaging and MRI (Mansour et al. 2008). The superomedial portion of the spring ligament passes from the sustentaculum tali of the calcaneus to the dorsal aspect of the medial navicular. On US imaging, it is identified as an echogenic fibrillar structure between the medial head and neck of the talus and the overlying tibialis posterior tendon. A useful tip is to obtain a

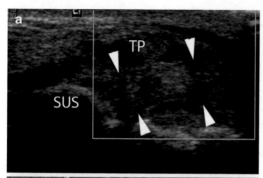

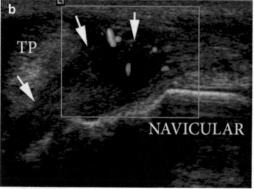

Fig. 26.7 Spring ligament tear. (**a**) Long-axis US image of the normal superomedial portion of the spring ligament (*arrowheads*), with the sustentaculum origin (*SUS*) and overlying tibialis posterior tendon (*TP*) shown. (**b**) There is a focally thickened, inflamed, and hypoechoic distal spring ligament (*arrows*), consistent with chronic tear and insufficiency

long axis view of the distal tibialis posterior tendon as it passes over the talar neck and rotate the distal probe superiorly, to take into account the more horizontal orientation of the underlying spring ligament (Fig. 26.7).

Spring ligament injury is strongly associated with tibialis posterior tendinopathy (Balen and Helms 2001). The normal spring ligament measures up to 7 mm in thickness. Injuries may manifest as a thickened hypoechoic ligament, atrophy, or discrete tearing with a fluid-filled gap (Fig. 26.7). A pitfall is not to assess the spring ligament when tibialis posterior tendinopathy is identified on US imaging. Isolated spring ligament injuries are very rare, and great caution is advised prior to diagnosing spring ligament injury when the tibialis posterior tendon is normal.

26.6 Tibialis Anterior Injury

Pathology of the anterior ankle tendons is infrequently encountered, compared to pathology in the medial and lateral tendons. Because of this, abnormalities of the tibialis anterior tendon are often overlooked in the context of dorsal ankle and midfoot pain. The tibialis anterior is the largest and most medial of the anterior ankle tendons. The tibialis anterior muscle arises from the upper two thirds of the lateral tibia; the tendon passes over the dorsum of the ankle and inserts into the medial aspect of the medial cuneiform and first metatarsal base. It acts to dorsiflex and invert the foot.

Distal tendinopathy/enthesopathy of the tibialis anterior tendon typically produces symptoms of medial midfoot pain. On US imaging, the tendon is hypoechoic and may be thickened with increased Doppler signal, with areas of bony irregularity at the medial cuneiform insertion. On MRI, signal change of the insertion and peritendinous edema are clearly demonstrated (Fig. 26.8). Tibialis anterior tendon tears are rare and often a delayed diagnosis, as intact extensor hallucis and digitorum longus tendons can maintain some active dorsiflexion of the foot. It often presents as a non-specific pain and a lump over the dorsum of the ankle. A tear is often seen as a bulbous hypoechoic swelling at the dorsal aspect of the distal lower and ankle, reflecting the retracted tendon end (Fig. 26.9).

26.7 Lateral Ankle Ligament Injury

Eighty-five percent of ankle sprains involve the lateral ligaments (Garrick 1977). Three ligaments form the lateral ankle ligament complex, namely, anterior talofibular ligament (ATFL), calcaneofibular ligament (CFL), and posterior talofibular ligament. The posterior talofibular ligament cannot be assessed on US imaging and is rarely injured. The ATFL runs from the anterior aspect of the lateral malleolus to the talar neck. The CFL runs from the inferior tip of the lateral malleolus posteroinferiorly

Fig. 26.8 Tibialis anterior insertional tendinopathy. (**a**) Axial and (**b**) coronal contrast-enhanced T1-W MR images of the foot show inflammation and thickening of the tibialis anterior insertion adjacent to the medial cuneiform (*arrows*)

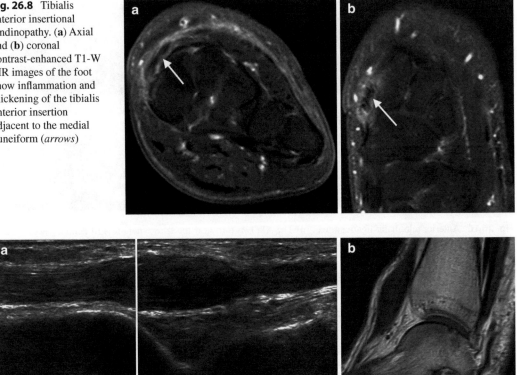

Fig. 26.9 Tibialis anterior tendon tear. (**a**) Longitudinal US image and (**b**) sagittal T1-W MR image of the dorsal ankle show a bulbous swelling of the tibialis anterior tendon, consistent with a tear

to a tubercle on the lateral calcaneum. The ATFL is the weakest of the ankle ligaments and is the first to tear with injury, followed by the CFL. Tears of both the ATFL and CFL indicate a more significant ligamentous injury and may result in instability.

Assessment of the ATFL is straightforward. The normal ligament is thin, hyperechoic, and overlies the normal anterolateral recess of the ankle joint, which may contain a small amount of normal fluid. An injured ligament may have a variety of appearances, depending on the severity and chronicity of the injury. The ATFL may be thickened, attenuated, and lax, demonstrating a partial defect or a complete defect with fluid extending from the joint into the adjacent soft tissues (Fig. 26.10). Avulsion fractures from the lateral malleolar or talar insertions may be seen. The injured CFL may show similar appearances but is more difficult to assess at its lateral malleolar insertion due to its concave course

(Fig. 26.11). The presence of fluid in the overlying peroneal tendon sheaths, as well as failure of the ligament to become taut with stressing, may indicate CFL tearing.

A potential pitfall is misdiagnosis of lateral ligament tears through poor visualization or anisotropy: this can be overcome with dynamic scanning. Stressing the ligaments during scanning can improve visualization and increase the conspicuity of tears. The ATFL is tensed through plantar flexion and internal rotation of the ankle and the CFL with dorsiflexion. It is important to recognize that more clinically significant sequelae of ankle sprains, such as occult fractures, talar osteochondral lesions, loose bodies, medial ligament disruption, and bone edema, are better assessed with MRI, and there should be low threshold for additional imaging, when clinically indicated.

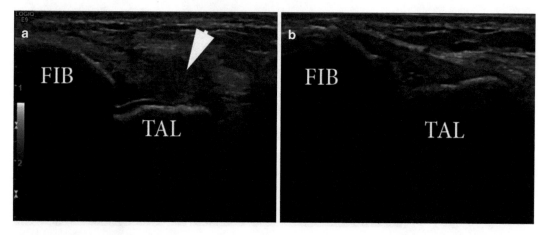

Fig. 26.10 Anterior talofibular ligament tear. (**a**) The ATFL is torn near the talus where it is ill-defined, swollen, and hypoechoic (*arrowhead*). (**b**) The normal ATFL is thin and taut and displays a hyperechoic fibrillar pattern

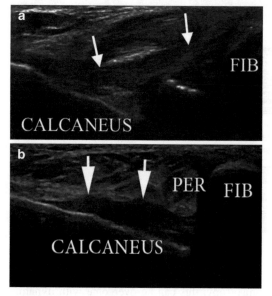

Fig. 26.11 Calcaneofibular ligament tear. (**a**) The normal CFL passes from the calcaneus to the fibula and displays a typical fibrillar echogenic pattern and is uniformly thin (*arrows*). (**b**) A chronic tear of the CFL (*arrows*) is irregular, thickened, and hypoechoic. The overlying peroneal tendons are shown (*PER*)

26.8 Ankle and Foot Effusions and Synovitis

Effusions and synovitis are commonly encountered in the joints of the foot and ankle. They are seen in a variety of conditions, such as inflammatory and degenerative arthropathy, trauma, and infection. In terms of US imaging technique, light probe pressure and ample US gel is essential to minimize any compression that reduces the visibility of effusions in the region of the probe and synovitis on Doppler interrogation. The major pitfall in evaluating the ankle and foot for synovitis and effusions is underdiagnosis through overcompression. Although they may be difficult to distinguish, effusions are uniformly hypoechoic and compressible, whereas synovitis demonstrates internal echoes, internal Doppler signal, and a lack of compressibility. Effusions and synovitis commonly coexist in inflamed joints.

As a rule, power Doppler is preferred to color Doppler in musculoskeletal US imaging as it is independent of direction and velocity of flow as well as angle of insonation, resulting in improved sensitivity in detecting low-flow pathology such as active synovitis (Teh 2006). In the ankle, effusions are most commonly seen in the anterior aspect of the joint, which is best imaged in the longitudinal plane between the distal tibia and talus (Fig. 26.12). Excessive plantar flexion may reduce the visibility of effusions: a neutral position of the ankle is advised. Synovitis may also be seen here but can often be demonstrated in the anterolateral recess of the ankle joint, best seen deep to the long axis of the ATFL (Fig. 26.13). In the metatarsophalangeal (MTP) joints, a small amount of joint fluid is seen in normal individuals, but synovitis is pathological. Evaluation is best performed using a dorsal and longitudinal approach.

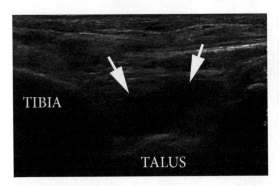

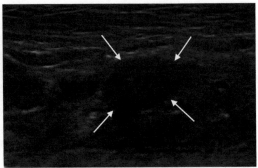

Fig. 26.12 Anterior ankle joint effusion. Longitudinal US image of the anterior ankle shows a moderate ankle joint effusion (*arrows*)

Fig. 26.14 Morton neuroma. Longitudinal US image of the second intermetatarsal space shows an ovoid hypoechoic nodule (*arrows*) typical of a Morton neuroma

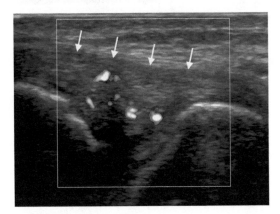

Fig. 26.13 Ankle joint synovitis. US image obtained along the long axis of the ATFL, which has a chronic partial tear with thickening (*arrows*). Synovitis with increased flow on color Doppler is seen in the underlying anterolateral recess of the ankle joint and adjacent ATFL

26.9   Morton Neuroma

Morton neuroma is an enlarged plantar digital nerve at the level of the metatarsal heads. Rather than a neuroma per se, it is composed of perineural fibrosis with elements of intermetatarsal bursitis and neural hypertrophy (Gentili et al. 2002). It is invariably only seen in the second and third intermetatarsal spaces with a strong female predominance (5:1). The symptoms are usually of pain and paresthesia under the forefoot, which may be worse on activity.

US imaging is best performed in the sagittal plane with the foot in the neutral position. The probe may be passed across each MTP joint into the metatarsal space either from a dorsal or plantar position, depending on operator preference. The conspicuity of Morton neuroma is usually increased through firm pressure into the space with the probe and a digit on the opposite side of the forefoot. The usual appearance of a Morton neuroma is of an ovoid hypoechoic nodule between the metatarsal heads. The size of the lesion is variable but is often more than 10 mm in diameter (Fig. 26.14). It is usually mildly but not completely compressible. There may be some fluid around the nodule reflecting intermetatarsal bursitis, and the intermetatarsal nerve may be seen to enter the mass.

There are several potential pitfalls when examining the foot for Morton neuromas. Firstly, a neuroma may be present but not be causing symptoms. This is especially seen in smaller neuromas, between 5 mm and 10 mm diameter. It is important to note whether compression of the intermetatarsal space reproduces the patient's symptoms. Secondly, a small amount of fluid can be seen within the intermetatarsal bursae in normal individuals. This fluid is completely compressible. Firm dynamic compression is therefore required to prevent misdiagnosis as a neuroma. Finally, it is extremely rare to find Morton neuromas in the first and fourth interspaces, and a diagnosis of neuroma should be made with great caution.

26.10   Plantar Plate Injury

Forced hyperextension of the MTP joint, particularly of the great toe, is common in athletes who use artificial pitches. This results in a capsuloligamentous injury of the first MTP joint plantar

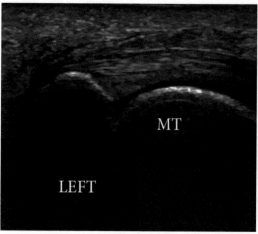
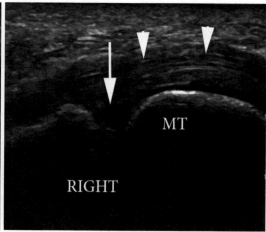
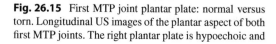

Fig. 26.15 First MTP joint plantar plate: normal versus torn. Longitudinal US images of the plantar aspect of both first MTP joints. The right plantar plate is hypoechoic and torn (*arrows*). The overlying flexor hallucis longus tendon is indicated (*arrowheads*). The left plantar plate is normal

plate, known as "turf toe" (Bowers and Martin 1976). The plantar plate extends from the base of the proximal phalanx and covers the cartilage of the undersurface of the metatarsal head. It acts to limit dorsiflexion and stabilizes the MTP joint. The medial and lateral sesamoids are embedded within the plantar plate which is thicker peripherally in the region of the sesamoids.

On US imaging, the plantar plate is best assessed in the longitudinal plane and is normally seen as a thin mildly hyperechoic band between the proximal phalanx and metatarsal, lying deep to the flexor hallucis longus in the midline and attached to the sesamoids medially and laterally. Injury may manifest as a hypoechoic thickened plantar plate or with focal discontinuity. Tears are typically seen at or near the distal attachment, and flexing the toe during dynamic scanning can increase the visibility of tears (Fig. 26.15). Common associations are synovitis, fluid in the flexor tendon sheath, and, with more severe injuries, proximal migration of the sesamoids. A potential pitfall is not to recall that the plantar plate is a relatively broad structure and may be focally injured medially, centrally, or laterally. Good US imaging technique requires longitudinal assessment in the plane of the medial and lateral sesamoids, as well as between them.

26.11 Stress Fractures

The first-line investigation for a suspected stress fracture should be radiographs (Teh et al. 2011). However, the sensitivity of radiographs for detecting early stress fractures is relatively poor, ranging from 15% to 56%. Therefore, if the radiograph is negative despite suggestive clinical features, then MRI should be performed. US imaging can detect cortical breaks and periosteal reactions but is not routinely used for the primary diagnosis of stress fractures. When examining patients with forefoot pain or metatarsalgia, an important pitfall is not to consider metatarsal stress fractures. A fracture line manifests as a focal cortical defect. The periosteal reaction associated with metatarsal stress fractures is demonstrated as irregular echogenic tissue adjacent to the metatarsal shaft, with posterior acoustic shadowing (Fig. 26.16).

26.12 Plantar Fascia Lesions

The plantar fascia is a thick fibrous band of tissue that connects the calcaneum to the metatarsal bases, supporting the medial and lateral arches of the foot. It is formed of three discrete bands and

Fig. 26.16 Metatarsal stress fracture. Longitudinal US image of the second metatarsal shows a stress fracture of the mid-shaft. A focal periosteal reaction (*arrow*) is seen

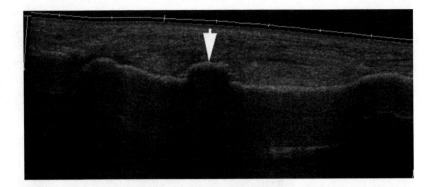

Fig. 26.17 Plantar fasciitis. Longitudinal US image shows a thickened hypoechoic plantar fascia at the calcaneal insertion (*arrow*). The more distal plantar fascia (*arrowheads*) is normal

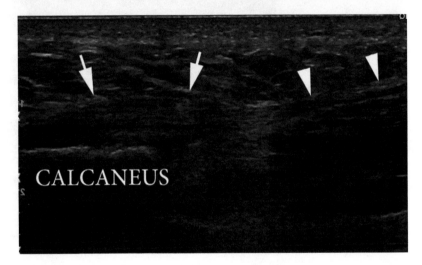

CALCANEUS

is narrow proximally and wider distally. The central band is the largest and most commonly affected by pathology. The central and lateral bands are attached to the calcaneus, whereas the medial cord is seen in the midfoot and is not clinically important. Three main conditions affect the plantar fascia, and it is necessary to recognize the clinical and US imaging features that distinguish them. Of these, fasciitis is much more frequent than tears and plantar fibroma (Theodorou et al. 2001).

Plantar fasciitis is a condition related to overuse and chronic repetitive low-grade injury through microtears. The typical patient is overweight and middle-aged and presents with heel pain that is worse on walking. A positive longitudinal US assessment shows a hypoechoic and thickened plantar fascia at the calcaneal insertion with focal tenderness on probe pressure.

The normal plantar fascia measures less than 5 mm in thickness (Fig. 26.17). Fascial inflammation can occasionally occur in the absence of fascial thickening; this can be difficult to see on US imaging and better visualized on MRI.

Fascial tears can be difficult to distinguish from plantar fasciitis as the appearance of tearing is similar to that of fasciitis, but there is usually a history of high-impact injury and forceful plantar flexion (Leach et al. 1978). In addition, the thickened fascia is often seen 2–4 cm away from the calcaneal insertion (Fig. 26.18). It is important to distinguish between the two conditions, as steroid injection is not considered an appropriate treatment for fascial rupture.

Plantar fibromatosis is similar to palmar fibromatosis and the conditions often coexist. On US imaging, there is nodular thickening of the plantar fascia. There may be increased vascularity on

Fig. 26.18 Plantar fascia tear. Longitudinal US image shows a thickened hypoechoic proximal plantar fascia (*arrows*) several centimeters away from the calcaneal insertion, in contrast to the insertional thickening typically seen in fasciitis. The more distal plantar fascia is normal

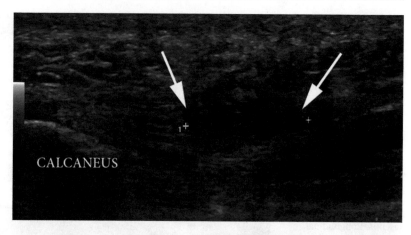

Fig. 26.19 Plantar fibromatosis. Longitudinal US image shows a nodular thickening of the midportion of the plantar fascia (*short arrows*) at the level of the metatarsal (*MT*) shaft. The adjacent plantar fascia (*long arrows*) is normal

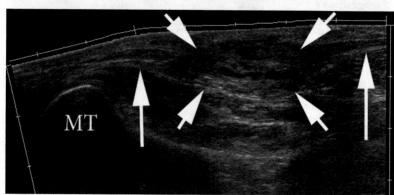

Doppler interrogation, particularly in larger lesions. In contrast to plantar fasciitis, it is commonly seen in the midportion of the plantar fascia at the level of the midfoot (Griffith et al. 2002) (Fig. 26.19). There is usually no history of trauma, and the fibromas are often multiple and bilateral, which can help distinguish them from a fascial tear (Griffith et al. 2002). Generally, these are considered "do not touch lesions," as injection or biopsy may lead to proliferation of tissue.

Conclusion

US imaging is an excellent modality for the assessment of sports injuries of the ankle and foot. A good knowledge of the anatomy, normal variations, and various pitfalls, along with close correlation, is essential for an accurate diagnosis.

References

Balen PF, Helms CA (2001) Association of posterior tibial tendon injury with spring ligament injury, sinus tarsi abnormality, and plantar fasciitis on MR imaging. AJR Am J Roentgenol 176:1137–4113

Bencardino JT, Rosenberg ZS, Serrano LF (2001) MR imaging of tendon abnormalities of the foot and ankle. Magn Reson Imaging Clin N Am 9:475–492

Bianchi S, Martinoli C, Abdelwahab IF, Derchi LE, Damiani S (1998) Sonographic evaluation of tears of the gastrocnemius medial head ("tennis leg"). J Ultrasound Med 17:157–162

Bianchi S, Delmi M, Molini L (2010) Ultrasound of peroneal tendons. Semin Musculoskelet Radiol 14:292–306

Bianchi S, Sailly M, Molini L (2011) Isolated tear of the plantaris tendon: ultrasound and MRI appearance. Skeletal Radiol 40:891–895

Bowers KD Jr, Martin RB (1976) Turf-toe: a shoe-surface related football injury. Med Sci Sports 8:81–83

Bude RO, Adler RS, Bassett DR (1994) Diagnosis of Achilles tendon xanthoma in patients with heterozygous familial hypercholesterolemia: MR vs sonography. AJR Am J Roentgenol 162:913–917

Garrick JG (1977) The frequency of injury, mechanism of injury, and epidemiology of ankle sprains. Am J Sports Med 5:241–242

Gentili A, Sorenson S, Masih S (2002) MR imaging of soft-tissue masses of the foot. Semin Musculoskelet Radiol 6:141–152

Griffith JF, Wong TY, Wong SM et al (2002) Sonography of plantar fibromatosis. AJR Am J Roentgenol 179:1167–1172

Kotnis R, David S, Handley R et al (2006) Dynamic ultrasound as a selection tool for reducing achilles tendon reruptures. Am J Sports Med 34:1395–1400

Leach R, Jones R, Silva T (1978) Rupture of the plantar fascia in athletes. J Bone Joint Surg Am 60:537–539

Mansour R, Teh J, Sharp RJ, Ostlere S (2008) Ultrasound assessment of the spring ligament complex. Eur Radiol 18:2670–2675

Schweitzer ME, Karasick D (2000a) MR imaging of disorders of the Achilles tendon. AJR Am J Roentgenol 175:613–625

Schweitzer ME, Karasick D (2000b) MR imaging of disorders of the posterior tibialis tendon. AJR Am J Roentgenol 175:627–635

Sobel M, Pavlov H, Geppert MJ et al (1994) Painful os peroneum syndrome: a spectrum of conditions responsible for plantar lateral foot pain. Foot Ankle Int 15:112–124

Teh J (2006) Applications of Doppler imaging in the musculoskeletal system. Curr Probl Diagn Radiol 35:22–34

Teh J, Suppiah R, Sharp R, Newton J (2011) Imaging in the assessment and management of overuse injuries in the foot and ankle. Semin Musculoskelet Radiol 15:101–114

Theodorou DJ, Theodorou SJ, Farooki S et al (2001) Disorders of the plantar aponeurosis: a spectrum of MR imaging findings. AJR Am J Roentgenol 176:97–104

Wang XT, Rosenberg ZS, Mechlin MB, Schweitzer ME (2005) Normal variants and diseases of the peroneal tendons and superior peroneal retinaculum: MR imaging features. Radiographics 25:587–602

Pediatric Trauma: Imaging Pitfalls

27

Timothy Cain and John Fitzgerald

Contents

27.1   Introduction 525

27.2   Imaging Techniques in Children 526

27.3   Pitfalls Due to Non-ossified Bone and
         Pattern of Growth 528

27.4   Pitfalls Due to Pliable Pediatric Bone 529

27.5   Pitfalls Related to the Growth Plates
         (Physes) 531

27.6   Pitfalls Related to Ossification of
         Epiphyses and Apophyses 533

27.7   Pitfalls Related to the Metaphysis 535

27.8   Pitfalls Due to Variations in
         Physeal Closure 536

27.9   Pitfalls Due to Vascularity 537

27.10 Agility/Coordination/Vulnerability
         Injuries 537

27.11 Pitfalls of Pediatric Spine Imaging 538

27.12 Miscellaneous Pediatric Injuries 540

27.13 Soft Tissues 541

27.14 Cooperation/Poor History 542

27.15 Trauma as the Presentation of
         Underlying Pediatric Conditions 542

27.16 Non-accidental Injury 543

Conclusion 544

References 545

Abbreviations

CT   Computed tomography
MRI   Magnetic resonance imaging
NAI   Non-accidental injury
US   Ultrasound

27.1   Introduction

There are many pitfalls in pediatric trauma radiology that occur because of the clinician's unfamiliarity with pediatric pattern of injury and assumption that children are just "little adults." Being aware of the developmental changes that occur in children and understanding the impact these changes have on the pattern of trauma assist in the prompt recognition of an injury and its significance. For the purposes of this discussion, pitfalls have been divided into categories that reflect the cause of the variation from common "adult trauma." Children will have varying amounts of non-ossified cartilage that can be injured. Also, the ligaments and tendons are relatively stronger than the more pliable bones.

The growth plates and non-united apophyses in children are associated with unique complications of trauma and can mimic fractures. Intra-articular disks and cartilage may be vascularized during growth, giving different imaging characteristics,

T. Cain, MBBS, MBA, FRANZCR, FAANMS (✉)
J. Fitzgerald, BSc, BMedSci, MBBS, FRANZCR
Department of Medical Imaging, The Royal
Children's Hospital Melbourne, 50 Flemington Road,
Parkville, VIC 3052, Australia
e-mail: Tim.Cain@rch.org.au; John.Fitzgerald@rch.org.au

compared to adults. While children are developing motor skills, they transition from immobile animals unable to fend for themselves through an awkward phase where suboptimal coordination and a desire to explore the world give an increased risk of injury. The development of their perception of the world around them will also influence their ability to describe their symptoms and cooperate with healthcare providers. Trauma can sometimes lead to identification of other pathologies; hence an understanding of conditions more common in children will reduce the risk of mistaking a significant mass or lesion as traumatic in etiology.

27.2 Imaging Techniques in Children

Radiographs remain the imaging investigation of choice in most circumstances. Orthogonal views are required, and images of the long bones should include both ends of the bone. However, if there are symptoms related to a joint, coned views of that joint are essential to accurately diagnose metaphyseal or epiphyseal injury. It is important that standard views are obtained, despite the fact children are sometimes incapable of cooperating

with the imaging procedure due to pain or lack of understanding. Careful and patient examination of a child will sometimes facilitate localizing the symptoms. This is important to avoid imaging requests such as "X-ray limb – unable to localize site of pain." Further clues as to the site of a bone or joint injury can be obtained by carefully reviewing the fat-muscle soft tissue planes. A fracture or significant local trauma will often cause edema within the subcutaneous fat that will help focus the attention of the radiologist to the bone close to the soft tissue swelling.

As with imaging of adult-type fractures, computed tomography (CT) can be invaluable when analyzing fractures that involve joints or the spine. In children, CT is also useful in complex fractures that involve growth plates, particularly when the fracture is in multiple planes. CT demonstrates the separate components of the fracture, allowing the orthopedic surgeon to understand the relationship of all fragments and plan the realignment and stabilization/fixation of the injury. For example, a comminuted Salter-Harris type IV fracture of the distal tibia with fragmentation of the tibial articular surface is well depicted on CT (Fig. 27.1). CT can also be useful during growth plate fracture healing, where bony

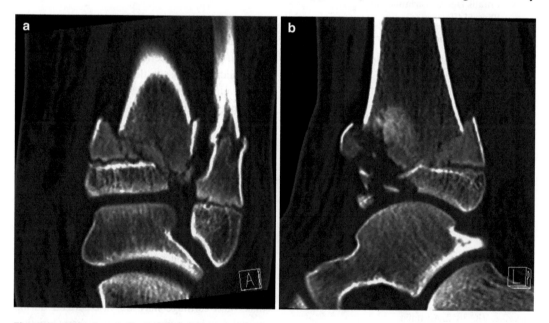

Fig. 27.1 Comminuted distal tibial Salter-Harris type IV fracture in a 15-year-old boy. (**a**) Coronal and (**b**) sagittal reformatted CT images of the left ankle show fragmentation of the articular surface and a distal fibula shaft fracture

bridges across the growth plate indicate damage to the physis and disruption to normal growth. Failure to recognize these changes in growth can cause long-term disability or predispose to degenerative joint changes.

It can be difficult to localize the site of injury requiring imaging when there is unobserved trauma and nonspecific clinical signs and symptoms. Radiographs may also be normal if the injury predominately involves the soft tissues or where the fracture is undisplaced, such as in toddler fracture of the tibia or a stress fracture. Magnetic resonance imaging (MRI), ultrasound (US) imaging, and bone scintigraphy are useful in children, particularly when the radiographs are normal. US imaging and MRI are preferred due to the absence of ionizing radiation. US is portable and provides real-time imaging suited to young children with limited ability to cooperate. It is particularly useful when there is possible injury to muscles or tendons or if a foreign body is suspected.

MRI requires a longer period of cooperation and is usually reserved for problem-solving or treatment planning. As with adult imaging, it is particularly useful for injuries involving a joint or the spine. Signal changes in the bone marrow may reveal sites of bone bruising where there is no macroscopic cortical fracture. Bone scintigraphy can be very useful in young patients where the radiographs are normal, particularly when the child presents with a limp of unknown etiology. While toddler fractures are the most common traumatic cause of a non-weight-bearing child, there are many times when the differential diagnosis is osteomyelitis or septic arthritis. As the origin of infection causing the limp may be in the spine (diskitis), foot, or anywhere in between, the ability of bone scintigraphy to easily screen the whole body is an advantage. Although the time required for nuclear medicine imaging may be similar to an MRI, the nuclear medicine gamma camera is less intimidating to young children and, in the authors' experience, has a much lower requirement for general anesthesia.

Young children pose additional challenges for successful motion-free imaging when they are too young to be able to cooperate with requests to keep still. The skill and patience of the medical imaging technologist is invaluable. This is particularly true when attempting to successfully obtain diagnostic images from young patients who are too young to understand the circumstances in which they find themselves; in pain and in a strange and unfamiliar environment. Time must be taken to gain the trust of the patient's parents (or carer) as a child will often adopt their anxiety. Preventing parental stress being relayed to the child may just require an explanation of the imaging requirements and reassurance that the imaging will be performed with as little additional pain to the patient as possible. On some occasions, the parent will need specific counseling on the impact of their emotions on their child's perception of the healthcare interaction and some guidance regarding their choice of words and nonverbal communications; this is preferable to having the parents leave the child. Educational play therapists (child life specialists) will greatly assist when greater cooperation is required for more complex imaging.

Radiographs can usually be obtained with minimal anxiety, particularly if a child-friendly environment is available and if the patient's parents or carers familiar to the patient are used to assist with patient positioning. Patience is required for successful positioning of the patient to allow standard views to be obtained. This is important to reduce the risk of poor radiographic technique being responsible for errors of interpretation. CT will often only require a few moments of absolute cooperation, but patience is still required for the patient not to be intimidated by the unfamiliar and complex-appearing equipment. MRI will require much greater patient preparation as well as the utilization of appropriate distraction techniques. The use of a "mock" or practice MRI will reduce the incidence of sedation and anesthesia, when used effectively. Nuclear medicine studies will involve the additional challenge of intravenous administration of a radiopharmaceutical, but there are many techniques available to minimize the distress associated with this intervention.

Oral sucrose, local anesthetic creams, ice packs, vibration devices, and distraction therapy all have their role in minimizing the distress associated with an intravenous injection, and age- appropriate techniques should be utilized routinely. Decorating medical equipment with child-friendly motifs will create a distraction that can also assist in placating an anxious child. The long-term importance of being sensitive to children's "imaging-associated anxiety" cannot be overemphasized, as fear generated by bad experiences can make future important health interventions much more complex. It is a mistake to think that it is all right to be forceful holding a child against his will and that it will always be forgotten. Appropriate explanation of a procedure and the use of distraction therapy, sedation, pain relief, or general anesthesia are important for the patient, their carers, and healthcare providers who wish to provide accurate and efficient patient services, as well as a safe and satisfying work environment for their staff.

27.3 Pitfalls Due to Non-ossified Bone and Pattern of Growth

Ossification of bones begins *in utero*, but many bones are mostly cartilage at birth, and some will not be ossified until early childhood or reach skeletal maturation until the second or third decade of life. Trauma to the neonatal musculo-

skeletal system is uncommon but is a recognized complication of difficult deliveries. Fractures of the clavicles occur as a complication of shoulder dystocia, but injuries to the humerus or femur can occur, depending on the presenting limb. Ribs can be but are rarely fractured during delivery (Bhat et al. 1994; Bulloch et al. 2000).

On radiographs, it can be difficult to differentiate between fractures of cartilaginous bone and dislocation of a joint, when the injury is to the cartilaginous bone of a neonate. Recognition of the injury partly relies on the knowledge that the ligaments and tendons are stronger than the forming bone, so it is more likely to suffer a fracture than a dislocation. Figure 27.2 demonstrates an injury first interpreted as a dislocation but recognized and confirmed later as a fracture of the proximal tibia. The initial image shows malalignment of the knee, but careful examination of the soft tissues shows that the patella tendon attaches normally to the cartilaginous proximal tibia which is aligned normally with the femoral articular cartilage. Images obtained during healing show that the fracture in the tibia was distal to the growth plate and through the non-ossified diaphyseal cartilage.

Neonates and infants are not able to generate sufficient force to injure themselves, so injuries occur due to accidents (e.g., motor vehicle, dropped by carer) or non-accidental injury (NAI).

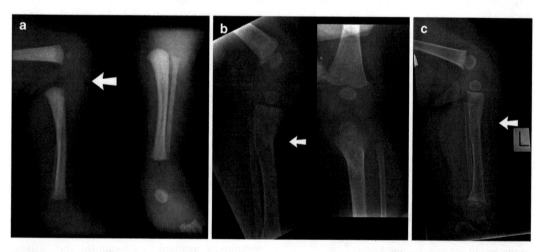

Fig. 27.2 (a) Lateral and AP radiographs of the tibia taken at presentation on the day of birth show a fracture of the proximal tibia. Note the normal attachment of the patella tendon to the cartilaginous proximal tibia (*arrow*).

Subsequent radiographs taken at (b) day 83 and (c) at 9 months. The two most recent lateral radiographs also show significant post-injury remodeling at the site of the fracture (*arrow*) that can occur in growing bones

Other congenital conditions such as osteogenesis imperfecta and metabolic bone disease that predispose the bones to fracture should also be considered when reviewing skeletal trauma in neonates, infants, and young children.

27.4   Pitfalls Due to Pliable Pediatric Bone

Certain subtle patterns of fracture occur specifically in the pediatric population because the bone is more pliable than adult bones and will undergo a greater degree of plastic deformation before fracturing. The most classic of these is the greenstick fracture, which produces discontinuity of part of the bony cortex, but the fracture is incomplete, and part of the bone maintains integrity of its periosteum and cortical outline. However, there are micro-fractures associated with the deformity, which can sometimes be subtle (Fig. 27.3).

Torus or buckle fractures represent a variant of the incomplete greenstick fractures associated with relatively soft and pliable bone. The buckle injury is seen in the metaphysis where the cortical bone is thin. They occur as a result of compression forces that disrupt the normal trabecular pattern of the peripheral medullary bone and cause micro-fractures in the cortex without significant periosteal

disruption. There is a variable contour irregularity on only one side of a bone that can be easily overlooked and may only be visible on one projection of a pair of orthogonal radiographic images. The cortical buckle is usually associated with a subtle change in the contour of the adjacent bony trabeculae where a focal curve or wave can be seen in the alignment of the medullary trabeculae.

On some occasions, a subtle torus fracture may only be recognized retrospectively on a follow-up radiograph as a subtle band of sclerosis across the metaphysis or diametaphysis that represents the osteoblastic activity associated with fracture healing (Fig. 27.4). This is different to the growth arrest lines associated with systemic illness or immobilization. It is important to differentiate a greenstick fracture with a buckled cortex together with a cortical break from a torus fracture; the latter is considered more stable with treatment often involving a shorter period of less rigid immobilization. Figure 27.5 demonstrates what appears to be a torus fracture of the distal radius in a child who suffered non-accidental injury (NAI), but the presence of an associated longitudinal component indicates a significant cortical breach and a greenstick fracture.

Plastic bowing fractures are another variant of incomplete fractures that do not have a discrete break in the cortical bone. These fractures may only be visible in one projection and can be overlooked

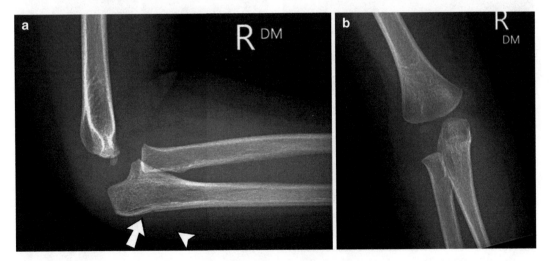

Fig. 27.3 (a) Lateral and (b) AP radiographs of the proximal ulna of a 28-month-old boy show cortical irregularity (*arrow*) as well as focal change in the clarity of the subcutaneous fat-muscle interface due to edema (*arrowhead*) associated with the proximal ulna greenstick fracture

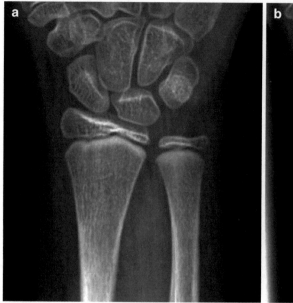

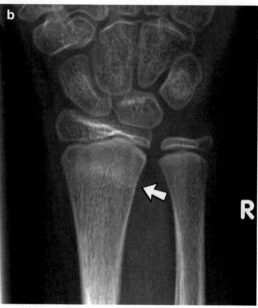

Fig. 27.4 PA radiograph of the distal radius of an 11-year-old girl taken (**a**) at time of injury when the lateral radiograph was considered normal and (**b**) 1 month after injury which shows a band of sclerosis from a healing torus fracture (*arrow*)

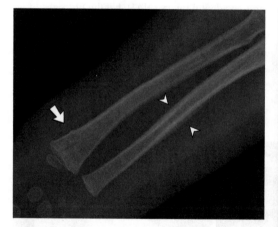

Fig. 27.5 Radiograph of the forearm of a 17-month-old girl shows a torus fracture and longitudinal greenstick fracture of the metaphyseal cortex (*arrow*) together with localized periosteal new bone over the midshaft of the ulnar from previous non-accidental injury (*arrowheads*)

as a normal variant, if not carefully reviewed. They are most commonly seen in the forearm bones with increased curvature of one of the long bones but without a discrete cortical break or evidence of dislocation (Fig. 27.6). The bowing seen in the lower legs in young children (tibial bowing) is a different entity and not considered a result of trauma.

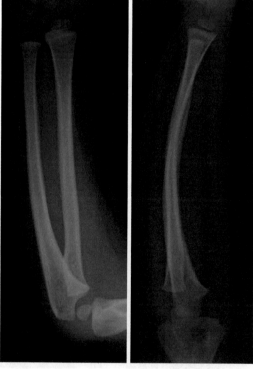

Fig. 27.6 AP and lateral radiographs of the forearm of a 4-year-old boy shows plastic bowing fracture of radius on only the lateral view

27.5 Pitfalls Related to the Growth Plates (Physes)

Growth plates found at both ends of long bones and one end of short bones represent sites of bone growth, particularly responsible for increasing length. The growth plate is made up of resting cartilage on the epiphyseal side, but the diaphyseal side of the growth plate has a zone of proliferating cartilage which is calcified in the metaphysis and grows toward the diaphysis. The bony margins of the growth plate on the epiphyseal and diaphyseal sides of the growth plate gradually become flatter and undulating as the epiphysis approaches skeletal maturity. These roughly parallel lines of calcification define the growth plate.

Fractures through growth plates are a common injury of long bones in children, and the Salter-Harris classification is used as an effective method to describe the type of injury. It is important to identify fractures that involve the physis due to the impact on growth of the bone. Fractures that damage most of the growth plate can result in reduced longitudinal growth and relative bone shortening (Fig. 27.7). This is significant if it involves only one of the paired forearm or lower leg bones or if the growth disruption causes a limp. Damage to only part of the growth plate is more common and can result in asymmetrical growth of the bone, causing angulation of the adjacent articular surface and an increased incidence of joint symptoms in the future.

Salter-Harris type I fractures can be difficult to diagnose and can present as a diagnostic dilemma. Injuries to the ankle causing soft tissue swelling over the lateral malleolus will often cause the radiologist to wonder whether the distal fibular growth plate is slightly widened. A similar dilemma can present with injuries to the wrist and with the distal ulnar growth plate. In both these situations, the growth plate is relatively small, and it is hard to assess the relationship of the undulating parallel lines of the bony margins of the physis. If there is no malalignment, then the patient can be treated symptomatically and reviewed with reassurance that Salter-Harris type I fractures generally have a good prognosis. Slipped upper femoral epiphysis (slipped femoral capital epiphysis) is a variation of a Salter-Harris type I fracture that has long-term complications if missed. To avoid missing this "chronic" fracture, orthogonal radiographs of the femoral heads are required, and careful review of the alignment of the bony margins of the diaphyseal and epiphyseal sides of the growth plate is necessary.

An obvious fracture that involves the growth plate is not a diagnostic dilemma, and clinicians managing these should know when to ask for additional imaging in order to plan treatment appropriately. Not recognizing physeal bars that indicate focal growth plate arrest is a pitfall of interpretation that can be minimized by awareness and appropriate cross-sectional imaging, when the radiographs are inconclusive. A localized physeal bar can be surgically resected, with fat, Silastic, or other materials interposed to prevent bone bridge formation. Alternative methods of treatment include performing an epiphysiodesis of the contralateral or ipsilateral growth plates.

Most growth plates are disk-like and lie mostly in one plane, making them easy to image and recognize. When the growth plate has a more complex shape, its appearance can be misinterpreted as a fracture. This is particularly true for the proximal humerus and, to a lesser degree, the proximal tibia. Looking for the parallel lines of the growth plate and being aware of the normal appearance will avoid this error of interpretation. When the growth plate lies in a plane that is not perpendicular to the long axis of the long bone, it can be difficult to profile on standard imaging of the long bones. This is particularly true for the growth centers around the elbow joint. The complex arrangement can be confusing for radiologists unfamiliar with the pattern and order of ossification. Figure 27.8 demonstrates a fracture of the lateral condyle of the distal humerus that is only clearly seen on the oblique view.

Apophyses have a similar appearance to epiphyses but are found at sites of attachment of muscles/tendons and do not contribute to increase in length of a long bone. Medial epicondyle avulsion fractures of the distal humerus are associated with dislocation of the elbow, and the

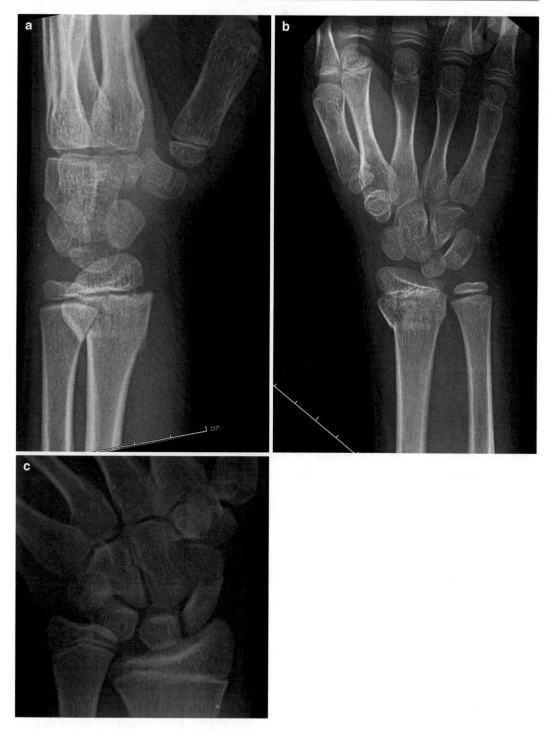

Fig. 27.7 (**a**) Lateral and (**b**) AP radiographs of a 12-year-old boy taken at the time of original injury show a distal radius fracture with growth plate involvement. (**c**) PA radiograph of the same boy taken when aged 16 years shows asymmetrical growth of the radius and ulna due to post-traumatic premature growth plate closure

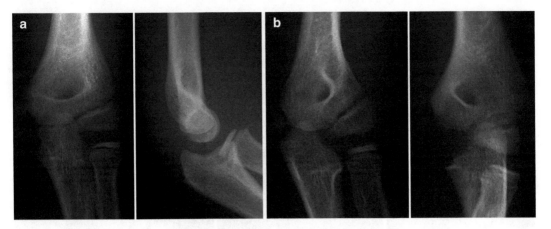

Fig. 27.8 (**a, b**) Radiographs of the distal humerus show a fracture of the lateral condyle that is only seen on the (**b**) internal oblique view

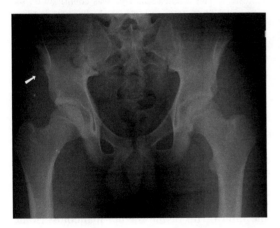

Fig. 27.9 AP radiograph shows an avulsion fracture of anterior inferior iliac spine (*arrow*) in a 15-year-old male sprinter

displaced medial epicondyle can be easily over-looked if it is not searched for. The problem can be exacerbated by the often suboptimal images obtained from a child with a painful dislocated elbow that is difficult to position for standard radiographic projections.

Avulsion fractures of the anterior inferior iliac spines can present with "hip pain," requiring careful review of the bony pelvis adjacent to the hip joint for the injury to not be overlooked. Initially, the displacement is often minimal, and the injury may only be detected after a period of ongoing pain (Fig. 27.9). The fifth metatarsal base apophysis has a typical appearance, with the long axis of the apophysis parallel to the long

axis of the fifth metatarsal. Fractures of the fifth metatarsal base are characteristically perpendicular to the long axis of the metatarsal. The patella can also have anterior and inferior apophyses that can be mistaken for sleeve fractures. Careful attention to the presence or absence of parallel lines of the normal apophysis, or the hallmarks of a fracture being ill defined or angular margins and the associated clinical findings will often allow an astute clinician to differentiate between a normal variant and a localized injury.

27.6 Pitfalls Related to Ossification of Epiphyses and Apophyses

During development of the epiphyses, the changing appearance presents a number of stages which may be potentially confused with traumatic injury. Typically, the epiphysis has a smooth contour defined on radiographs by a continuous, initially ovoid line of bone. Sometimes, the epiphysis can have more than one center of ossification and appear bifid or even as an apparent conglomeration of small ossification centers. At the very outset of epiphyseal development, the site of the secondary ossification center may be transiently seen as a focus of T2 hyperintensity within the cartilage, referred to as the pre-ossification center, before the development of epiphyseal bone. Most frequently seen in the

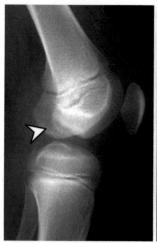 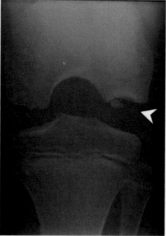 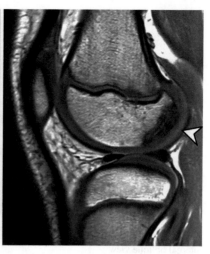

Fig. 27.10 Initial (**a**) lateral and (**b**) AP knee radiographs in a 10-year-old boy show an ossific body (*arrowheads*) separate from the remainder of the lateral condyle, which is particularly conspicuous on the intercondylar view. The corticated ovoid appearance and typical posterior location indicate variant ossification. This was confirmed on the (**c**) sagittal T1-W MR image which shows intact cartilage (*arrowhead*) between these accessory ossification centers and the femoral epiphysis

humeral trochlea and distal femur, these can develop at any site where ossification is occurring within cartilage and should not be mistaken for injury to the cartilage. In general, these can be recognized by the small ovoid appearance at a typical site and by recognizing the age of the developing ossification center.

Accessory ossification centers can present further dilemmas, once they begin to ossify. In particular, it can be difficult to distinguish an unfused accessory ossification center from a fracture, such as at the tip of the fibula or margin of the glenoid. In some cases, the rounded and corticated appearance of an accessory ossification center will be clear on radiographs, but there may be a question of whether the ossification center has been displaced following an injury through the non-ossified cartilage. Distinguishing accessory ossification centers from osteochondral injury in the distal femur has been discussed in the literature. Accessory ossification centers typically lie posteriorly in the femoral condyles, while osteochondral defects are most frequently seen in the most inferior aspect, especially where they abut the tibial spines. At other locations where the distinction is less clear, MRI may be necessary to assess whether the suspect areas of bone show features

of intervening fracture, or are connected by intact cartilage indicating variant ossification (Fig. 27.10).

The foot is a common site of injury and secondary ossification centers. These can be difficult to differentiate from fractures, particularly those forming adjacent to the distal fibula and the inferior tip of the medial malleolus. Some of these will remain non-united, to become the os subfibulare adjacent to the distal fibula and the os subtibiale adjacent to the medial malleolus of the distal tibia. It is often speculated and sometimes proven that the small bone "fragments" masquerading as non-united secondary ossification centers are the result of previous trauma (Pill et al. 2013). When the bone fragment margins appear well defined and smooth or the adjacent epiphysis is still mostly cartilaginous and immature, a normal variant should be considered (Fig. 27.11). The presence of localized soft tissue swelling and point tenderness from injury to the adjacent ligaments can make it difficult to make a definitive diagnosis. Ongoing symptoms, such as ankle joint instability, may be the only finding that allows the correct diagnosis to be made. Other common sites where an apophysis or non-united

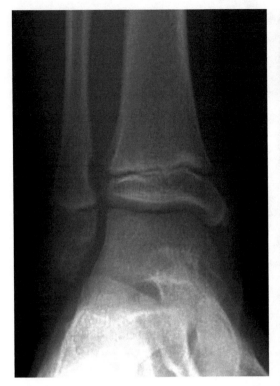

Fig. 27.11 AP radiograph of the right ankle of an 8-year-old girl shows smooth and corticated secondary ossification centers adjacent to the medial and lateral malleolus

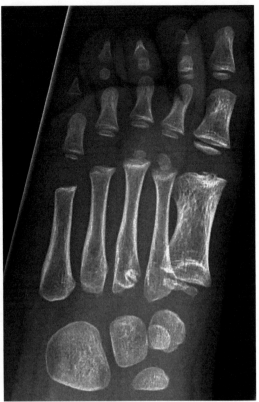

Fig. 27.12 Oblique radiograph of the foot shows a cleft in the base of the third metatarsal that appears as a result of variant non-epiphyseal ossification. The smooth margins aid differentiation from a fracture

secondary ossification center may be mistaken for bone injury are the navicular, scapula, acetabulum, ischial tuberosity, and the femoral greater and lesser trochanters.

There are a large number of variations in the appearances of epiphyses, apophyses, and synchondroses, particularly early in their development. Generally, variants will be symmetrical and be accompanied by similar variations in adjacent or similar ossification centers. However, asymmetrical development is not unusual and should be considered. For example, a cleft in the base of the third metatarsal represents variant non-epiphyseal growth rather than a fracture (Ogden et al. 1994) (Fig. 27.12). Texts devoted to these variations are an essential resource for even experienced musculoskeletal radiologists. Review of these references is preferable to routine imaging of contralateral limbs for comparison and minimizes radiation exposure.

27.7 Pitfalls Related to the Metaphysis

The concept of bone growth occurring at the growth plate is commonly understood, but it can easily be forgotten that there is considerable remodeling of the bone formed at the metaphysis of long bones. The metaphysis is wider than the diaphysis, especially for the long bones of the upper and lower limbs. As the bone initially formed at the physis comes to form part of the diaphysis, there is resorption of subperiosteal bone and laying down of endosteal bone, which results in the thicker and stronger cortex of the diaphysis of a mature skeleton. Remodeling of the subcortical bone at the metaphysis results in a wide variation in appearance of the metaphyseal margins of the growth plate. When this marginal metaphyseal bone is "pointed," it may be mistaken for a classic metaphyseal lesion (corner fracture), and if it is "squared off," it may be mistaken for a buckle fracture. The absence of cortical breaks and the often similar appearance of other metaphyses will aid differentiation from classic metaphyseal lesions. The absence of disruption to adjacent trabeculae will allow differentiation from buckle fractures.

This metabolically active area around the circumference of the metaphysis can be seen, especially early in development, as a thin stripe of hyperintense signal on proton density or T2-weighted MRI in a subperiosteal location, extending from the growth plate and tapering toward the diaphysis. Referred to as the "metaphyseal stripe" (Laor and Jaramillo 2009), this appears linear when imaged along the bone, or as a circumferential rim in cross section. It will generally enhance brightly with contrast agent administration and should not be mistaken for injury or other pathology.

27.8 Pitfalls Due to Variations in Physeal Closure

Around the time of growth plate closure, a further phenomenon can be seen in adolescent patients that can mimic fracture. It is not infrequent that small areas of the physis narrow and begin to close earlier than the remainder. This results in localized stress and a striation of marrow edema extending typically into the metaphysis, sometimes also into the epiphysis from the focus of early closure. This appearance of edema is referred to as a "focus of periphyseal edema" or FOPE (Zbojniewicz and Laor 2012) and commonly encountered around the knee (Fig. 27.13). These are not of clinical significance, if small and occurring close to the time of normal growth plate closure, but the edema can mimic trabecular fracture in some cases.

Perhaps the growth plate responsible for the most consternation around the time of closure is the ischiopubic synchondrosis joining the

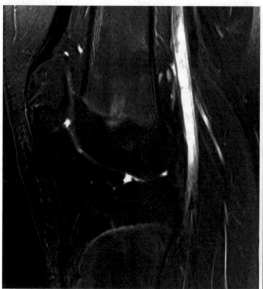 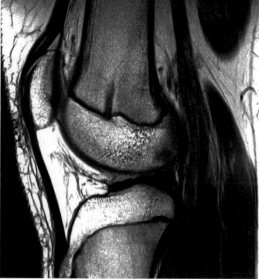

Fig. 27.13 Focus of periphyseal edema (FOPE). Sagittal (**a**) fat-suppressed T2-W and (**b**) PD-W MR images of the knee in an active 13-year-old boy show focal marrow edema around a small focus of early growth plate closure in the distal femur. The edema extends more into the metaphysis than the epiphysis

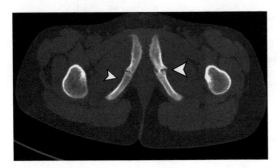

Fig. 27.14 Axial CT image taken following trauma shows unfused ischiopubic synchondroses bilaterally. The left synchondrosis has been fractured (*larger arrowhead*), and a very subtle buckle fracture is identified in the right ischium (*smaller arrowhead*) a short distance posterior to the right synchondrosis

inferior pubic ramus to the ischium. Fusion here is very variable, though typically occurring before or early in puberty, and asymmetry is the rule rather than the exception. The unique feature of the ischiopubic synchondrosis is that it may frequently enlarge just prior to closure, presumably due to mechanical stresses. Generally, this is asymptomatic and considered normal development. However, the appearances on radiographs can be striking due to the asymmetry and can mimic a healing fracture or expansile lucent lesion. When symptomatic, this is considered to represent an osteochondrosis, which has been referred to as van Neck-Odelberg disease. More rarely, other pathologies can be present, including fracture (Fig. 27.14). However, it should be borne in mind that most frequently, enlargement of this synchondrosis prior to closure is a normal developmental variant.

27.9 Pitfalls Due to Vascularity

Prominent vascularity in musculoskeletal structures can be more conspicuous in the pediatric population than in adults, due to the metabolic demands of growth. As an example, pediatric knee MRI can show higher signal within the sub-

stance of the menisci, related to increased extent of the "vascular zone," and instances have been reported where this has been misinterpreted as a meniscal tear (Takeda et al. 1998). MR arthrography has been suggested to clarify difficult cases, but, in general, this should not be necessary if the normal range of pediatric appearance is borne in mind, particularly with the improved resolution of modern MRI systems. A related phenomenon can be observed in pediatric spinal MRI, where the epidural venous plexus and small veins around the spinous processes can be more conspicuous than usually seen in adults. Hyperintense signal related to these vascular structures can mimic ligamentous injuries, particularly with partial volume effects on sagittal images of the cervical spine. Awareness of this mimic and review of multiple image planes are therefore important.

27.10 Agility/Coordination/ Vulnerability Injuries

Attaining effective control of an increasingly capable musculoskeletal system is one of the tasks of childhood. Children can appear clumsy while learning to walk, run, jump, and tumble as their muscles and bones develop strength, and their central nervous system acquires the ability to adequately coordinate their actions. Falling and tripping is part of the process by which children learn to become more coordinated and to use their increasingly versatile limbs effectively. Consequently, they often present for medical care with injuries to the limbs sustained during a failure of adequate musculoskeletal coordination. Fractures of the distal forearm and the distal humerus are the most common injuries sustained by children, followed by injuries to the ankles and lower limb long bones. Recognizing common patterns of injuries and the circumstances of the injury can be useful in differentiating genuine accidental trauma from NAI; the latter commonly having an implausible explanation for the injury.

Toddler fractures occur when a torsional force is applied to the tibia, usually by having the foot relatively fixed as the body turns. The fracture occurs while the child is developing coordination and before the bone has reached full weight-bearing strength. The fracture is frequently minimally displaced due to largely intact periosteum, and the oblique line of the fracture may result in the fracture line not being visible on routine radiographs. Repeat imaging at 5–10 days may demonstrate fracture margins due to the initial bone resorption phase of fracture healing or only demonstrate periosteal new bone formation as the radiological sign of bone injury. The fracture may be diagnosed with bone scintigraphy or MRI, as nontraumatic causes of a limp may be considered if the initial radiograph is considered normal. A similar fracture can occur in the femur of walking children but is much less common.

27.11 Pitfalls of Pediatric Spine Imaging

The pattern of cervical spine injury is different in children compared to adults. The head of a child is disproportionately large, and their neck muscles are weaker compared to adults; both factors compounding the challenge of maintaining control of the head and preventing injury. In addition, the vertebral bodies have a larger proportion of more pliable cartilage, and the articular facet joints are more horizontally orientated. The immature vertebral bodies can have an irregular and almost wedge-shaped appearance, mimicking a vertebral crush fracture.

The relative mobility of the vertebral segments will also often give rise to minor malalignment in the cervical spine, referred to as "pseudo-subluxation." This is a subtle malalignment that is most commonly seen in the upper cervical spine at the C2-3 and C3-4 levels, with the superior vertebra anteriorly displaced relative to the vertebra below. This anterior subluxation is less than 4 mm, and the posterior arches should remain well aligned. Specifically, in pseudo-subluxation, the posterior arch of C2 vertebra should not be seen more than 2 mm anterior to

the "Swischuk line" between the C1 and C3 posterior arches (Swischuk 1977). This phenomenon can be seen on both horizontal ray supine and erect lateral radiographs of the cervical spine.

Prevertebral soft tissue prominence can vary significantly with respiration and swallowing, especially in infants. While it is a recognized sign of spine trauma, it is important to remember that it may be present due to the timing of the radiograph. In some cases, it can be absent, despite significant spine injury. Cervical rotatory subluxation is a phenomenon which is rare in adults and can be difficult to distinguish from rotation due to muscular spasm alone. The atlantoaxial joint is held in a relatively fixed rotation to one side or the other, due to a fixed subluxation of the lateral articular surfaces. It is more readily diagnosed when severe and usually associated with a transverse ligament injury. Definitive diagnosis requires imaging to exclude unstable fractures, followed by separate imaging sequences with careful left and right rotation of the head (Fig. 27.15), typically with CT, in order to show the presence of fixed relationship of the C1 and C2 lateral masses and a fixed degree of rotation of C1 on C2 vertebrae.

The dens of the C2 vertebra has a varied pattern of ossification, and an accessory ossification center may appear to represent a fracture before skeletal maturity. An incidental os odontoideum will have well-defined bony margins, and no other signs of traumatic injury. Ancillary imaging findings such as soft tissue swelling or MRI evidence of bone marrow edema and ligamentous disruption may be required to confidently differentiate a normal variation from a significant spinal column injury. It should be remembered that fractures can occur through synchondroses (Fassett et al. 2006), and this should be considered if there is any widening of a synchondrosis or if there are any associated signs of spinal column or spinal cord injury. Similarly, the variable pattern of the synchondroses present during ossification of the C2 vertebral body can present problems for clinicians wishing to exclude significant bony trauma.

Cervical spine injuries during childhood are more commonly found in the upper cervical

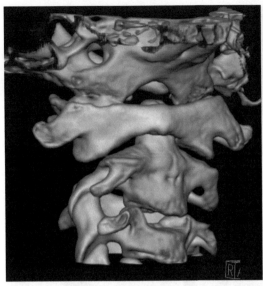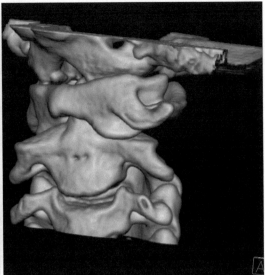

Fig. 27.15 Rotational subluxation in the cervical spine generally occurs as a consequence of trauma, subluxing one of the C1–C2 lateral articulations and producing relatively fixed rotation of C1 on C2. This can be difficult to distinguish from muscular spasm or poor positioning. Sequential CT imaging with left and then right rotation of the head may be necessary to demonstrate the limitation of rotation at the C1-C2 level

spine, with the relative frequency of upper spine injuries reducing with age as the spine reaches skeletal maturity. There is also a higher incidence of craniocervical disruption and spinal cord injury without radiological (radiographic or CT) abnormality – also known as SCIWORA. Craniocervical disruption is difficult to detect due to the relative width of the articular cartilage and the possibility that the subluxation is reduced with clinical stabilization of the cervical spine during initial emergency room treatment. The spinal column made of bone, cartilage, and ligaments is paradoxically more pliable and able to resist tension forces to a greater degree than the soft tissues of the spinal cord and nerve roots. Radiographs and CT of the spinal column can appear normal despite spinal cord disruption (Fig. 27.16). This emphasizes the importance of clinical correlation and MRI in the assessment of spinal cord injury in children.

The Chance fracture is another spinal injury that is more common in children in whom the interspinous ligaments are relatively stronger than the bone. The horizontal (axial plane) distraction fracture through the spinous process and posterior elements extends anteriorly into the vertebral body

as a compression injury. The flexion-distraction injury is frequently associated with intra-abdominal injuries and although the fracture is unstable due to its disruption of all vertebral columns, it is not often associated with neurological symptoms. It most commonly occurs as a consequence of a patient wearing a lap-sash seat belt in a motor vehicle accident. The fracture may be subtle and can be overlooked; it is most easily identified on sagittal plane imaging.

An incidental finding that may be confused for an acute injury is a limbus vertebra. This entity is caused by herniation of the nucleus pulposus of an intervertebral disk between the ring apophysis and the vertebral body prior to fusion of the ring apophysis at skeletal maturity. It is considered likely to be a result of previous trauma and is most commonly seen at the anterosuperior endplate of a lumbar vertebra, but it can occur laterally or posteriorly and may be seen in the thoracic spine. The triangular bone fragment and the defect in the vertebral body usually have corticated margins, which aid in the differentiation from an acute vertebral fracture for those unfamiliar with the appearance or when the location

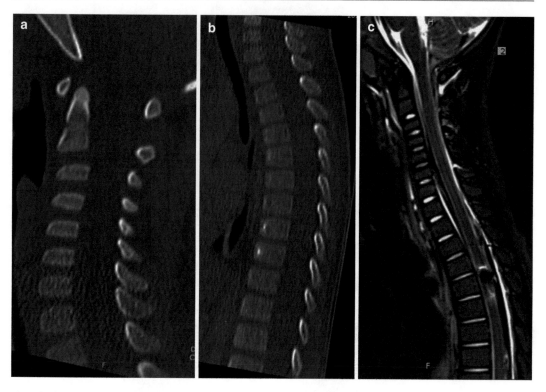

Fig. 27.16 A 3-year-old boy injured in a motor vehicle accident. Sagittal CT images of the (**a**) cervical and (**b**) thoracic spine show no bony abnormality compared with the (**c**) sagittal T2-W MR image which shows a transected spinal cord at T5 level

is uncommon. They are usually asymptomatic, the exception being posterior ring apophysis lesions that may cause nerve root compression (Yen et al. 2009).

27.12 Miscellaneous Pediatric Injuries

Ligament and tendon injuries are much less common than bony injury in children as they are relatively stronger than the bony skeleton. Bone contusions suggestive of ligamentous injury may be demonstrated on MRI, without evidence of the ligamentous injury usually found in adults with the same constellation of bone marrow changes, particularly around the knee. Tibial spine fractures occur with increased frequency in children compared to adults due to the relative weakness of the bone compared to the anterior cruciate ligament (Mitchell et al. 2015).

Radial head subluxation is an injury that is associated with normal or near-normal elbow radiographs without a joint effusion. The injury is most commonly caused by traction on the arm of a young child, often by a carer lifting a child by their arm; hence the name "nursemaid elbow" was given. The radial head is held in position relatively loosely by the immature annular ligament, facilitating subluxation with minor force. The subluxation is often reduced during radiography, if the positioning for the diagnostic imaging includes flexion of the elbow for the lateral elbow image and supination or pronation of the wrist for the anteroposterior (AP) image.

Children do get stress fractures despite the bones of children generally being more pliable until skeletal maturity, and these are particularly seen during adolescence. Repetitive stress injuries in children and adolescents have similar distribution and causation as in adults. In addition to sports and other repetitive use injuries, children

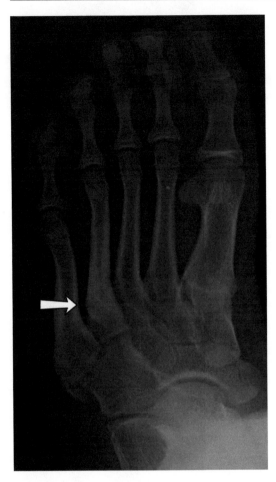

Fig. 27.17 Stress fracture of the fourth metatarsal in a 14-year-old boy with a past history of calcaneo-varus (club) foot. Oblique radiograph of the foot shows a stress fracture of the fourth metatarsal (*arrow*)

with gait disorders and congenital abnormalities are prone to stress fractures associated with the abnormal load bearing, particularly of the feet (Fig. 27.17).

27.13 Soft Tissues

Inflammation of a bursa may present after minor trauma and require clinical correlation to differentiate idiopathic inflammatory causes from infection and repetitive/overuse injuries. Common sites include the femoral greater trochanter, olecranon process, knee (prepatellar), supraspinatus, and calcaneum. Vascular malfor-

mations may come to clinical attention after local trauma. Those that have associated skin pigmentation may not be a diagnostic dilemma, but some lymphatic malformations may present as a lump after minor trauma. Lymphatic malformations usually present as slow-growing painless lumps but can present after trauma due to intralesional hemorrhage. The large cystic or multicystic lesion should not be confused with a muscle hematoma but may require MRI to fully define the extent of the lesion. Vascular malformations presenting as soft tissue lumps after minor trauma are usually more likely to require differentiation from a soft tissue tumor than a traumatic hematoma, if the preexisting nature of the abnormality was not recognized.

Foreign bodies can also cause a diagnostic dilemma, when the symptoms appear to be related to an unobserved period of physical activity. An easily identifiable skin entry point may not be apparent, and an abscess does not always form soon after the injury. If the foreign body is radiolucent, US imaging will often be required to assist diagnosis and localization. When examining soft tissues for foreign bodies using US, it is important that sufficient transducer coupling gel is used in the region of interest to allow the angle of insonation to be varied during the examination. This will facilitate the detection of small foreign bodies that can only be seen when the US beam is perpendicular to the foreign body.

Complex regional pain syndrome (CRPS) type I has previously been known as reflex sympathetic dystrophy and Sudeck atrophy. It is a poorly understood condition, probably originating from the sympathetic nervous system, which results in pain that occurs days or up to months after a sometimes minor episode of trauma. The symptoms are usually worse than the clinical findings, which include pain, swelling, skin atrophy, and extreme sensitivity to touch. The radiological findings are often subtle or absent but include patchy osteoporosis. MRI can show quite striking but generally patchy marrow edema, and care must be taken to differentiate this pattern of hyperintense T2 marrow signal from a fracture.

Bone scintigraphy in patients with CRPS type I often shows an abnormal pattern of activity on the blood flow, blood pool, and delayed scan images. The pattern of uptake can vary during disease evolution; in adults, there is typically increased activity in the affected region on all three phases of the bone scintiscan at presentation, changing to decreased activity on all three phases when long standing. However, children most commonly present with a vasospastic form of CRPS where the blood flow, blood pool, and delayed scintiscan activity are reduced, generally within the affected limb at the time of presentation (Low et al. 2007). This pattern of radiopharmaceutical distribution can also be seen with non-weight-bearing, particularly if there is effective immobilization of a limb, such as with application of a splint and use of crutches.

27.14 Cooperation/Poor History

Children are not always able to accurately convey the nature of their symptoms and some complaints are only appreciated after a period of time. This can mean that there is a delay between the onset of symptoms and the recognition of the symptoms. As children are often falling over or bumping into things, trauma can sometimes be attributed as the cause of symptoms when it is not, or the temporal relationship of the symptoms to the trauma may be ignored. Clinicians must be aware of the possibility that unrecognized trauma may be a cause of symptoms. Limb symptoms caused by osteomyelitis may be inappropriately attributed to an undisplaced fracture when patients present with normal radiographs and equivocal laboratory markers of infection. Bone scintigraphy and MRI are particularly useful in identifying bone marrow abnormalities that are not demonstrated on radiographs in patients who have unexplained symptoms.

Juvenile idiopathic arthritis can also present as a diagnostic dilemma to clinicians who forget that children may also be afflicted with joint inflammation. This is most commonly a transient reactive (post-viral) arthritis and is most common in the hip but can affect almost any synovial joint. More debilitating inflammatory arthritis can also present after what is interpreted as bone, joint, or soft tissue trauma. The relapsing/intermittent nature of the presentation and the absence of objective clinical signs can make the diagnosis difficult. US imaging and MRI may show evidence of synovial thickening and/or inflammation, or a joint effusion. Bone scintigraphy may show increased synovial blood pool activity and delayed uptake involving both sides of the joint but it often shows no focal abnormality. As the joint symptoms can be transient and the radiographs normal, the symptoms may not be recognized as a primary inflammatory arthritis, until many episodes have been reported or many joints involved.

Children with lower limb pathology due to trauma or inflammation will often present with nonspecific symptoms that are difficult to localize. A limp may be due to pathology anywhere in the lower limb or lumbar spine. Symptoms apparently arising from the knee can require extension of the radiological survey proximally to include the hip and or distally to include the ankle joints and foot, if the initial knee examination is normal.

27.15 Trauma as the Presentation of Underlying Pediatric Conditions

In many instances, a child will present after trauma, but while the trauma is the cause for the presentation, the more important diagnosis is of an underlying condition. Children can present with pathological fractures not only due to focal bone lesions but also due to bone dysplasias and other systemic conditions. Osteogenesis imperfecta may be diagnosed antenatally, as intrauterine fractures are identified by US imaging, but more commonly after presentation with fractures that occur with relatively minor trauma. The connective tissue disorder is commonly associated with other clinical features such as blue sclera and "loose" joints which can be an aid to diagnosis of the milder forms. Osteogenesis imperfecta can present with unusual patterns of fracture or evidence of fractures of different ages – the major differential in such cases is NAI – and it is not infrequent that one must consider both these possibilities at the first such presentation. NAI is an important topic in its own right, discussed below in Sect. 27.16.

The role of vitamin D deficiency in bone weakness in the general population is controversial (Clark et al. 2006), although vitamin D-resistant rickets and other recognized abnormalities of the calcium metabolic pathways are important considerations in the differential diagnosis of bones prone to fracture or curvature. The diagnosis of bone dysplasias and metabolic bone diseases used to rely heavily on the radiological findings, but genetic and histopathological markers now give more accurate diagnosis and at an earlier stage of clinical presentation. Children with gracile and osteopenic bones due to cerebral palsy and other neuromuscular disorders are also prone to bone fractures.

Pathological fractures in children most commonly occur through benign tumors, tumor-like lesions, bone abnormalities due to underlying metabolic disease or infection, and only rarely through metastatic lesions (De Mattos et al. 2012). The most common lesion found is unicameral bone cyst. Malignant sarcomas may be identified as a consequence of minor trauma but are usually easily identified as primary bone tumors on radiographs at presentation. Some pediatric musculoskeletal sarcomas can present as soft tissue masses requiring US imaging or MRI for differentiation from a hematoma.

27.16 Non-accidental Injury

Non-accidental injury (NAI) is a condition that reflects the vulnerability of children to trauma inflicted intentionally by others and is the form of child abuse/neglect that requires radiological assessment. Very young children are especially vulnerable, as they are unable to escape from their attacker and are prone to skull, rib, and metaphyseal injuries. Defense-type forearm fractures can be seen in older children. Although there are some fractures commonly seen in children who have been the subject of NAI, virtually any fracture can be seen as an inflicted injury.

The key role for the radiologist reviewing the images is to recognize fractures with high specificity for NAI, identify injuries with more than one point of trauma (e.g., nonadjacent rib fractures), describe injuries that have different ages, and assess whether the pattern of injury matches the offered explanation. Figure 27.5 demonstrates fractures of different ages in the one limb; this requires explanation for at least two episodes of trauma. Figure 27.18 shows a typical metaphyseal injury received during a shaking injury and how the injury to the ossifying cartilage and periosteum may not be evident on radiographs until there is calcifying callus. It is not the radiologist who must decide who inflicted the injury or why it happened, but he/she does have to assess whether the explanation provided with the clinical history is consistent with the radiological findings. They may also be asked to offer likely mechanisms of injury and approximate age of the injuries. Familiarity with the common injuries of birth trauma can be very useful when dealing with the radiological assessment of possible NAI.

Determining the age of fractures is difficult and not always possible to the degree requested by lawyers or the justice system. It is important to recognize the limitations of fracture age estimation and not feel obliged to make an estimation that would not survive scientific scrutiny or aggressive cross examination in a court of law. Another pitfall in describing injuries associated with NAI is to feel obliged to make a diagnosis of an inflicted injury when there is insufficient evidence. Radiological investigation is only one component in the assessment of child abuse which can have radiologically occult soft tissue injuries or neglect as more definitive evidence.

Injury to the periosteum of a long bone can result in subperiosteal hemorrhage which elevates the periosteum from the cortical bone. The healing process often involves formation of periosteal new bone. This subperiosteal ossification can also be seen associated with bone tumor, infection, and metabolic bone disease but are accompanied by other radiological findings. However, infants often demonstrate periosteal new bone that is physiological and not associated with focal bone trauma. The features which help differentiate physiological subperiosteal

Fig. 27.18 Non-accidental injury. AP radiographs of the right knee show a classic metaphyseal fracture obtained at the time of presentation (*left image*) and obtained 10 days later (*right image*). The later image (*right*) shows extensive changes to the metaphysis associated with disruption of the immature bone adjacent to the growth plate

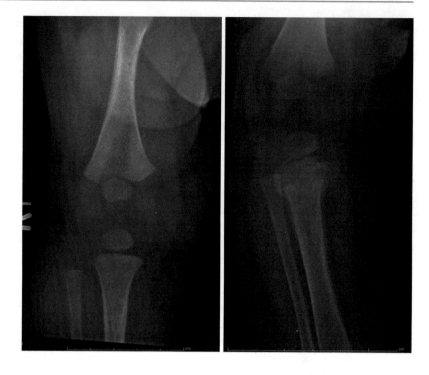

ossification from traumatic periosteal injury are that the physiological new bone is smooth, symmetrical, and extends the length of the diaphysis of upper and lower limb long bones. It can be seen in about a third of infants aged 1–4 months (Kwon et al. 2002). Traumatic periosteal injury is more likely to be asymmetrical, undulating, and associated with other signs of local bone injury, especially classic metaphyseal lesions (Figs. 27.5 and 27.18).

Conclusion

Imaging in pediatric trauma presents a number of challenges for the general radiologist. In the broadest terms, some features of true injury may not be noticed because in some circumstances, the injuries are different and more subtle than in the adult population. Familiarity with these subtle features, and understanding the reasons for these different patterns of injury, is critical to interpretation of pediatric trauma imaging. As a second broad area, many aspects of normal pediatric appearance can mimic the expected appearance of trauma in an adult, in many cases, due

to incomplete or variant ossification on radiographs or CT or due to areas of high signal on MRI in locations not seen in the adult population. A third broad class of pitfalls in pediatric trauma are those cases where a traumatic injury is correctly recognized as such, but atypical features are present which indicate an important underlying condition, such as a pathological fracture due to a lesion, e.g., osteogenesis imperfecta or, perhaps even more importantly, NAI. Failure by the radiologist to recognize such features can have catastrophic consequences, particularly in the case of NAI. Instances where the suspicion is raised inappropriately can also have significant consequences for the child and family.

The final class of pitfalls faced by the general radiologist is not related to interpretation but occur even before the images are obtained – the challenge of imaging in children differs significantly from adults. This relates not only to choice of modality and minimizing radiation exposure, but understanding how the imaging algorithm may differ in pediatric injury and obtaining quality imaging despite difficulties with cooperation. Careful clinical assessment and good communication with referrers is required to best target imaging, for choice of modality, as well as for interpretation of findings. In all circumstances, upset and anxiety for both patients and parents should be minimized. With skilled staff and, ideally, a well-designed environment, imaging can be performed with the least possible need for sedation or forcible immobilization. Awareness of these areas of difference and potential pitfalls, and care and attention to performing best imaging, is vital to providing best diagnosis and doing so while dealing most gently with pediatric patients and their parents.

References

Bhat BV, Kumar A, Oumachigui A (1994) Bone injuries during delivery. Indian J Pediatr 61:401–405

Bulloch B, Schubert CJ, Brophy PD et al (2000) Cause and clinical characteristics of rib fractures in infants. Pediatrics 105:e48

Clark EM, Tobias JH, Ness AR (2006) Association between bone density and fractures in children. Pediatrics 117:e291–e297

De Mattos CBR, Binitie O, Dormans JP (2012) Instructional review: oncology pathological fractures in children. Bone Joint Res 1:272–280

Fassett DR, McCall T, Brockmeyer DL (2006) Odontoid synchondrosis fractures in children. Neurosurg Focus 20:E7

Kwon DS, Spevak MR, Fletcher K, Kleinman PK (2002) Physiologic subperiosteal new bone formation: prevalence, distribution, and thickness in neonates and infants. AJR Am J Roentgenol 179:985–988

Laor T, Jaramillo D (2009) MR imaging insights into skeletal maturation: what is normal? Radiology 250:28–38

Low AK, Ward K, Wines AP (2007) Pediatric complex regional pain syndrome. J Pediatr Orthop 27:567–572

Mitchell JJ, Sjostrom R, Mansour AA et al (2015) Incidence of meniscal injury and chondral pathology in anterior tibial spine fractures of children. J Pediatr Orthop 35:130–135

Ogden JA, Ganey TM, Light TR et al (1994) Ossification and pseudoepiphysis formation in the "nonepiphyseal" end of bones of the hands and feet. Skeletal Radiol 23:3–13

Pill SG, Hatch M, Linton JM, Davidson RS (2013) Chronic symptomatic os subfibulare in children. J Bone Joint Surg Am 95:e115(1–6). doi:10.2106/JBJS.L.00847

Swischuk LE (1977) Anterior displacement of C2 in children: physiologic or pathologic? Radiology 122:759–763

Takeda Y, Ikata T, Yoshida S et al (1998) MRI high-signal intensity in the menisci of asymptomatic children. J Bone Joint Surg Br 80:463–467

Yen CH, Chan SK, Ho YF, Mak KH (2009) Posterior lumbar apophyseal ring fractures in adolescents: a report of four cases. J Orthop Surg (Hong Kong) 17:85–89

Zbojniewicz AM, Laor T (2012) Focal periphyseal edema (FOPE) zone on MRI of the adolescent knee: a potentially painful manifestation of physiologic physeal fusion? AJR Am J Roentgenol 197:998–1004

Musculoskeletal Soft Tissue Tumors: CT and MRI Pitfalls

28

Richard W. Whitehouse and Anand Kirwadi

Contents

28.1	Introduction	547
28.2	Imaging Techniques	548
28.3	Clinical Features of Malignant Soft Tissue Tumors	548
28.4	Imaging Features of Soft Tissue Tumors (Benign or Malignant)	549
28.5	Tumors and Masses with Characteristic Imaging Appearances	555
28.5.1	Benign Masses	556
28.5.2	Malignant Tumors	568
28.6	Conditions Associated with Multiple Soft Tissue Masses	574
28.6.1	Neurofibromatosis Type 1	574
28.6.2	Neurofibromatosis Type 2 and Schwannomatosis	574
28.6.3	Maffuci Syndrome	574
28.6.4	Mazabraud Syndrome	574
28.6.5	Familial Polyposis Coli	576
28.6.6	Dercum Disease	577
28.6.7	Metastatic Disease	577
Conclusion		578
References		579

R.W. Whitehouse, MBChB, MD, FRCR (✉)
A. Kirwadi, MBBS, FRCS, FRCR
Department of Diagnostic Radiology,
University of Manchester Medical School,
Manchester Royal Infirmary, Oxford Road,
Manchester M13 9WL, UK
e-mail: Richard.Whitehouse@cmft.nhs.uk;
anand.kirwadi@cmft.nhs.uk

Abbreviations

CT   Computed tomography
MRI   Magnetic resonance imaging

28.1 Introduction

Computed tomography (CT) is rarely used for the routine assessment of soft tissue masses, as magnetic resonance imaging (MRI) has greater sensitivity and specificity with no ionizing radiation burden. Occasionally, patients with claustrophobia or other contraindication to MRI may undergo CT. CT is also valuable for demonstrating calcification or ossification in a lesion, though an appropriate radiograph may suffice.

The most serious pitfall in the interpretation of the imaging of a soft tissue mass is to ascribe benignity to the appearances of what transpires to be a malignant tumor. This error derives from a failure to appreciate the lack of specificity of many of the imaging features of soft tissue tumors (Patel et al. 2015). The World Health Organization (WHO) recommends that "soft tissue masses that do not demonstrate tumor-specific features on MR images should be considered indeterminate and biopsy should always be obtained to exclude malignancy" (Fletcher et al. 2002). Despite this long-standing recommendation, inappropriate surgery for presumed benign soft tissue masses still occurs.

Soft tissue sarcomas are rare but more common than bone sarcomas. Despite this, there appears to be much greater awareness of the imaging features of bone sarcomas among radiologists, perhaps because of the easily appreciated radiographic features of the latter that have been known and taught for many decades. These features do not transcribe to soft tissue sarcomas – a well-defined sclerotic margin, for example, is reassuring in a bone tumor, but a well-defined pseudocapsule is of little value in excluding a soft tissue sarcoma.

28.2   Imaging Techniques

The interpretation of imaging appearances may be influenced by the chosen scan parameters and imaging technique. For CT, artifacts from beam hardening, movement, and reconstruction algorithms can significantly affect measured CT numbers. Conversely, dual energy CT can characterize sodium urate in gouty tophi.

On MRI, susceptibility and chemical shift artifacts that are particularly prominent on gradient-echo T2-weighted sequences can be intrusive and lead to misinterpretation. Orthopedic metalwork will create large regions of surrounding artifact that can mimic or obscure a soft tissue mass. We have seen soft tissue extension of a chondrosarcoma arising in the proximal femur obscured by artifact from an adjacent hip replacement. Modified MRI sequences by using wide bandwidth and high image matrices, avoiding gradient-echo sequences, repeating sequences with phase- and frequency-encoding directions swapped, and using STIR rather than fat suppression will all reduce the influence of this artifact.

Fat suppression MRI techniques can be inconsistent across a field of view, particularly in the periphery of the image and at irregular air/tissue boundaries such as the limbs. STIR sequences, being insensitive to magnetic field inhomogeneities, produce more uniform fat suppression but cannot be used for contrast-enhanced imaging and may also produce less marked fat suppression. Fat-suppressed T1-weighted sequences will emphasize contrast enhancement, but identical plane pre- and post-contrast-enhanced sequences should be performed as hemorrhage may mimic enhancement on fat-suppressed T1-weighted MR images.

The use of oil capsules taped to the skin at sites of suspected pathology, while valuable in confirming that the region of interest has been scanned, can distort the adjacent tissues and also create signal intensity artifacts within adjacent tissue. We have seen a small subcutaneous sarcoma recurrence overlooked due to this. We advise that oil capsule markers be taped *lightly* to the skin around a region of interest, rather than directly over it. Where the upper limb has been scanned in the "superman" position, with the fingertips entering the scanner above the head, this is anatomically equivalent to entering the scanner feet first. If this is not correctly entered into the scan parameters, then the image side markers will be transposed.

28.3   Clinical Features of Malignant Soft Tissue Tumors

The clinical features of a soft tissue mass that should alert the clinician to the possibility of a malignancy are any of the following:

- Size greater than 5 cm diameter
- Pain
- Enlarging mass
- Fixed
- Located deep to the deep fascia

The presence of any one of these features should result in referral for further investigation, which may include an MRI of the mass. The reporting radiologist's role is to confirm the presence of a mass; document its size; describe its location and its relationship to the deep fascia, neurovascular structures, and closest joint; confirm it is solitary; and describe the imaging features of the mass itself. If these conform to a specific lesion, then a diagnosis can be offered; but nonspecific or atypical features should precipitate referral to a sarcoma service for consideration of biopsy. The radiologist should be aware of the limitations of the clinical features, the absence of which does not exclude a sarcoma.

Size > 5 cm   This is an arbitrary size criterion. Most benign soft tissue tumors are smaller than

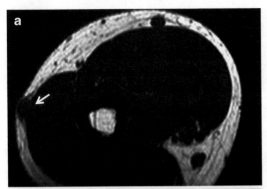

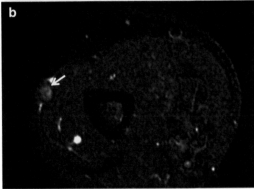

Fig. 28.1 Myofibroblastic sarcoma with nonspecific imaging features. Axial (**a**) T1-W and (**b**) fat-suppressed PD-W MR images of a subcentimeter subcutaneous soft tissue tumor in the midarm (*arrows*). Histology showed a myofibroblastic sarcoma

5 cm in diameter, while malignant tumors will (eventually) exceed this. All malignant soft tissue tumors will however have previously been, or may still be, less than 5 cm in diameter and may not exceed this diameter for months or years (Fig. 28.1). The prognosis is significantly worsened for larger tumors; diagnosis made when still less than 5 cm in diameter therefore has the potential to improve prognosis as well as reduce the morbidity of surgery and/or radiotherapy (Grimer 2006).

Pain Soft tissue sarcomas are commonly painless but can be painful, involve adjacent neurovascular structures or have inflammatory features, and be tender to palpation.

Enlarging mass The rate of enlargement of a soft tissue sarcoma can appear misleadingly slow. A tumor 5 mm in diameter with a malignant rate of growth, e.g., doubling in tumor volume in 6 months, will then be 6.3 mm in diameter, which is an almost imperceptible change. This tumor will not be 5 cm in diameter until more than 4 years later. If there is serial imaging, it is imperative that direct comparison and accurate measurements in three dimensions are made, with any detectable enlargement being treated with suspicion.

Fixed This is a clinical feature, but involvement of adjacent structures may be demonstrated on imaging.

Deep to the deep fascia Tumors deep to the deep fascia tend to be larger at presentation, with a higher probability of being malignant. Soft tissue sarcomas can, however, also arise in superficial tissues.

Analysis of the MRI characteristics of benign and malignant soft tissue masses has shown that absence of hypointense signal on T2-weighted images, mean diameter greater than 33 mm, and inhomogeneous signal on T1-weighted images gave the highest sensitivity for malignancy, while the highest specificity was achieved for evidence of necrosis, bone or neurovascular involvement, metastases, and mean diameter greater than 66 mm (De Schepper et al. 1992). A more recent study analyzing superficial versus deep location, size (< or ≥50 mm), and signal heterogeneity on T2-weighted images confirmed all these as significant (Chung et al. 2012). However, multiple logistic regression analysis showed depth of lesion was not helpful, possibly because deeper lesions are larger at presentation. Even so, best use of T2-weighted signal heterogeneity, size, and depth still gave an accuracy of only 77%, reinforcing the nonspecific imaging appearances of many soft tissue sarcomas.

28.4 Imaging Features of Soft Tissue Tumors (Benign or Malignant)

Smooth, well-defined margins This is a nonspecific feature. Most uncomplicated benign soft tissue masses will have smooth, well-defined margins, but many sarcomas are also smooth and well-defined, particularly when small.

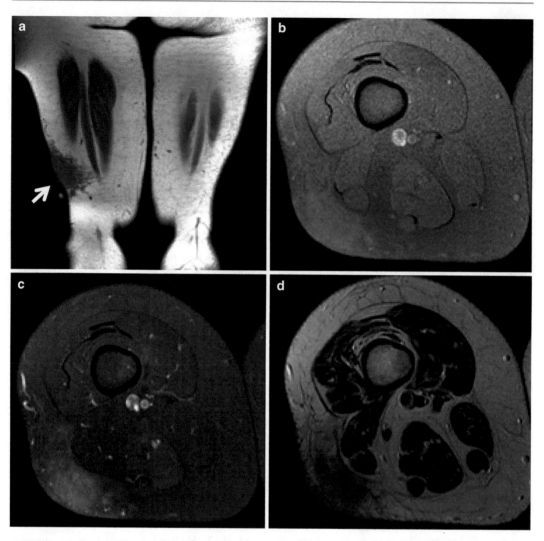

Fig. 28.2 Sarcoma mimicking an inflammatory mass. (**a**) Coronal T1-W, (**b**) axial fat-suppressed T1-W, (**c**) axial contrast-enhanced fat-suppressed T1-W, and (**d**) axial T2-W MR images show an indistinctly marginated but enhancing lesion in the subcutaneous fat of the posterolateral thigh (*arrow*). Although suggestive of an inflammatory lesion, this was a sarcoma

Indistinct, infiltrative, inflammatory margins or surrounding edema These are best considered to be nonspecific features seen in some sarcomas, soft tissue metastases, benign vascular tumors, fibromatosis, abscesses, hematomas, and inflammatory masses (Fig. 28.2).

Cystic Having an inner wall of synovium is required to define a cyst, differentiating it from a ganglion that has no synovial lining. On imaging, a uniloculate, thin-walled lesion containing fluid can be considered to be a cyst or a ganglion, if it is in an appropriate location. The MRI characteristics of fluid, being T2-hyperintense and T1-hypointense, are not, however, diagnostic. These may be mimicked by myxoid lesions and tumor necrosis. MRI interpretation of suspected cysts can be improved by windowing the images to maximize the gray scale across the suspected cyst, rather than allowing it to be bright beyond the window width of the image on T2-weighted images. Any heterogeneity of signal in the lesion will then be appreciated and raise the concern that the lesion is complex or solid. Confirmation of a cyst, if there is concern, requires a contrast-enhanced MRI or ultrasound (US) imaging. Hemorrhage or fibrinoid/proteinaceous material in cysts or bursae may create complex imaging

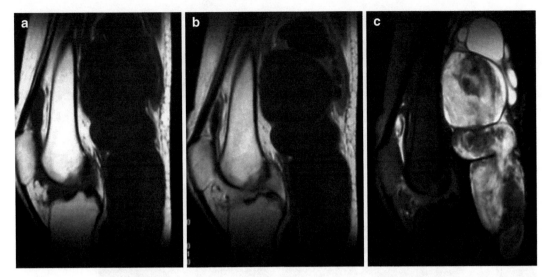

Fig. 28.3 Large popliteal (Baker) cyst in a patient with rheumatoid arthritis. (**a**) Sagittal T1-W MR image shows a large lobulated heterogeneous mass in the popliteal fossa. (**b**) After contrast administration, only a thin peripheral wall enhances. Note enhancing synovial thickening in the suprapatellar pouch. (**c**) Sagittal fat-suppressed PD-W MR image shows that the heterogeneous content is due to fibrinoid detritus

appearances, suggesting a malignant tumor. Contrast enhancement limited to a thin surrounding capsule and relevant clinical history, such as rheumatoid arthritis, may be helpful (Fig. 28.3).

Lobulated and loculated structures There may be fibrous septa separating lobulations of a solid soft tissue tumor, which may be mistaken for septa between loculations of a cystic lesion (Fig. 28.4). This pitfall is a reiteration of the need to differentiate solid from cystic by manipulating the image window, adding contrast enhancement, or US imaging assessment.

Hemorrhagic Spontaneous soft tissue hemorrhage should be considered unusual, and a cause therefore needs to be sought. The commonest predisposing cause is anticoagulation. Clotting studies may be appropriate. In the absence of a clinical cause, the presumed hematoma should be imaged. Hemorrhage can be confirmed by the signal characteristics of altered blood (Fig. 28.5), but careful review of the full extent of the lesion on matched pre- and post-contrast-enhanced T1-weighted sequences is recommended to identify any underlying enhancing tumor nodule (Kontogeorgakos et al. 2010). As hemorrhage may be relatively T1-hyperintense, it will look even more hyperintense on fat-suppressed T1-weighted images – this

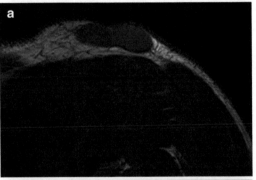

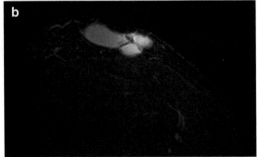

Fig. 28.4 Sarcoma mimicking a benign cystic lesion. (**a**) Coronal T1-W MR image of a 2 cm long-axis subcutaneous mass in the shoulder region shows homogeneous signal intensity in a bilobed lesion, with surrounding thin higher signal intensity wall and septum. (**b**) Fat-suppressed T2-W MR image also shows homogeneous hyperintense signal content with thin hypointense septations. Although a multiloculated benign cystic lesion was diagnosed, subsequent US imaging demonstrated a solid mass. Biopsy confirmed a sarcoma

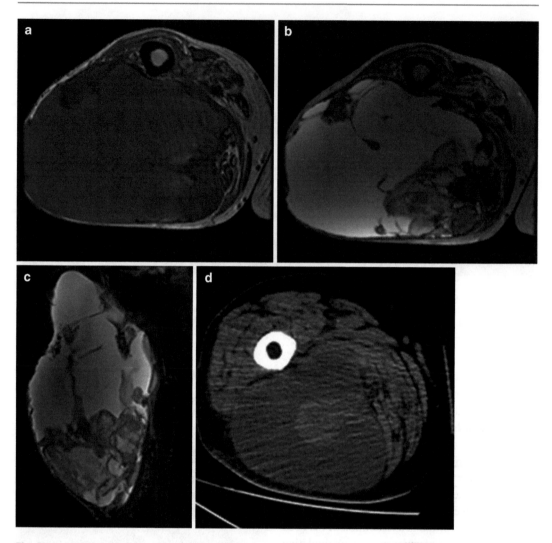

Fig. 28.5 Hemorrhagic sarcoma mimicking hematoma. (a) Axial T1-W, (b) axial T2-W, and (c) coronal fat-suppressed T2-W images show a large heterogeneous lesion with large regions of homogeneous T1-intermediate signal content, consistent with hematoma. (d) Axial unen-hanced CT image confirms a hyperdense area of bleeding within the central part of the lesion. Biopsy of the heterogeneous portion of the lesion confirmed a hemorrhagic sarcoma

can be mistaken for enhancement. We therefore recommend performing pre- and post-contrast-enhanced T1-weighted MRI using the same sequence. Follow-up scanning to confirm resolution may also be appropriate.

Necrotic Tumor necrosis is an important feature in a soft tissue mass, significantly increasing the probability of a malignancy. Necrosis tends to be central, resulting in regions of non-enhancing T1-hypointense and T2-hyperintense signal, with irregular, relatively indistinct margins to the surrounding viable tumor. The latter will enhance with contrast administration and help in targeting the suitable areas for image-guided biopsy.

Lipomatous Recognition of fat on MRI requires demonstration of hyperintense signal on T1-weighted, plus hypointense signal on fat-suppressed or STIR sequences. It is a potential pitfall to rely on only two of these three imaging sequence characteristics. It may also be difficult to correlate the spatial location of the relevant signal if the three sequences are not in the same slice location and the lesion is heterogeneous.

Myxoid Although described above in cystic lesions, differentiation of myxoid from cystic is of such importance that it bears repeating here. Myxoid material occurs in both benign and malignant tumors. The benign intramuscular myxoma can be mistaken for a cyst as it has very uniform hypointense signal on T1-weighted and very hyperintense uniform signal contents on T2-weighted MR sequences. Myxoid material in malignant soft tissue sarcomas also shows these signal characteristics. US scanning or contrast-enhanced MRI is appropriate to confirm or refute apparently cystic lesions (Murphey et al. 2002).

Mineralization The presence of mineralization in a lesion may be overlooked on MRI. Performing a radiograph should always be considered to identify the presence of calcification or ossification in a soft tissue mass and to characterize its appearance. CT is more sensitive in documenting the early peripheral calcification seen in myositis ossificans.

Lesion location Some lesions arise in characteristic locations, such as the subscapular location of elastofibromata. Location alone is not sufficient criterion for diagnosis, but may help inform a differential diagnosis, particularly in certain benign tumors.

Benign tumor location

- Hand and wrist: ganglion, giant cell tumor of the tendon sheath, accessory/anomalous muscles
- Elbow: biceps paratenon inflammation, biceps pseudotumor from tendon rupture, epitrochlear lymph node
- Shoulder: bursal collections, subscapular location of elastofibroma dorsi, fibromatosis
- Chest wall: costochondral calcifications/inflammation, intercostal nerve sheath tumor
- Paraspinal: lymphadenopathy, neurogenic tumors, extramedullary hematopoiesis (Fig. 28.6)
- Abdominal wall: hernia, rectus sheath hematoma, desmoid (fibromatosis)

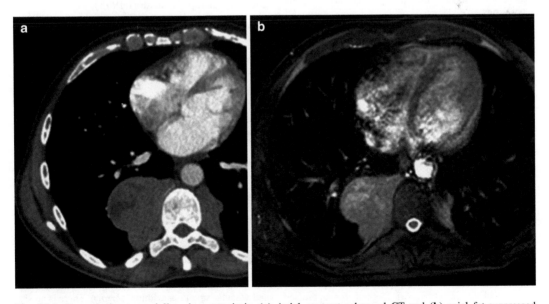

Fig. 28.6 Paraspinal extramedullary hematopoiesis. (**a**) Axial contrast-enhanced CT and (**b**) axial fat-suppressed PD-W MR images show paraspinal soft tissue masses of extramedullary hematopoiesis

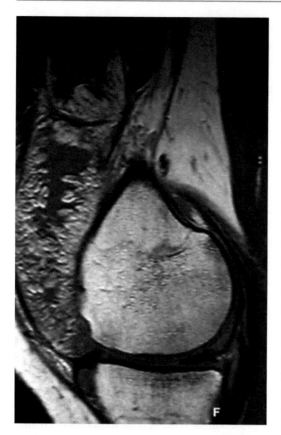

Fig. 28.7 Lipoma arborescens. Sagittal T1-W MR image shows fronded synovial lipomatous hypertrophy in a patient with psoriatic arthropathy. Diagnosis is lipoma arborescens

- Hip/pelvis/groin: bursa, hernia, lymph node, synovial osteochondromatosis
- Knee: bursa, ganglion, popliteal lymph node
- Ankle: ganglion, accessory muscles (soleus, peroneus quartus)
- Foot: tophaceous gout, plantar fibroma, intermetatarsal bursa, Morton neuroma
- Intra-articular: pigmented villonodular synovitis, lipoma arborescens (Fig. 28.7), tuberculosis (Fig. 28.8)

Malignant tumor location

Sarcomas may occur anywhere but are most common in the lower limbs. The age of the patient may influence the likely histological diagnosis of sarcoma. Most sarcomas occur in patients older than 50 years of age, with patients older than 65 years of age most commonly having undifferentiated sarcoma, leiomyosarcoma, or liposarcoma. Synovial sarcoma is commoner in patients between 15 and 45 years of age and rhabdomyosarcoma and fibrosarcoma in children under the age of 5 years. Malignant peripheral nerve sheath tumor is commonest in those aged 16–25 years old, arising particularly in patients with neurofibromatosis. There is some variation in likely tumor type with anatomical location in each age group (Kransdorf 1995).

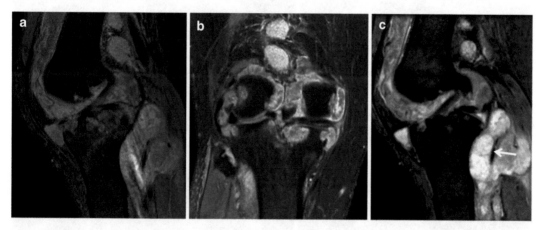

Fig. 28.8 Grossly destructive knee monoarthropathy due to tuberculosis infection. (**a**) Sagittal fat-suppressed PD-W, (**b**) coronal fat-suppressed PD-W, and (**c**) sagittal GRE T2*-W MR images show hypointense signal at the edges of the distended joint cavity on the GRE sequence due to chemical shift artifact at the margins of the lesion and vascular structures within it (*arrow*). There is no significant hemosiderin "blooming" artifact. This was proven to be tuberculous infection, and not PVNS

28.5 Tumors and Masses with Characteristic Imaging Appearances

A less serious but commoner pitfall is to diagnose malignancy in what transpires to be a benign lesion, when the lesion has features that can lead to a specific correct diagnosis. The radiologist should, in any case, ensure that there is an appropriate referral pathway for suspected malignant soft tissue tumors, in order that unnecessarily wide surgical excision is not performed without secondary review and confirmatory histology from biopsy. There are many benign lesions that have characteristic appearances (Arkun and Argin 2014). The following list of conditions and their descriptions are not comprehensive. Rare conditions may have very characteristic imaging appearances with which one is unfamiliar. It is a pitfall to ascribe an unusual appearance to an atypical form of a common condition, without considering this possibility. Many nonspecific soft tissue masses will transpire to be benign, but biopsy is still required to confirm the diagnosis (Fig. 28.9).

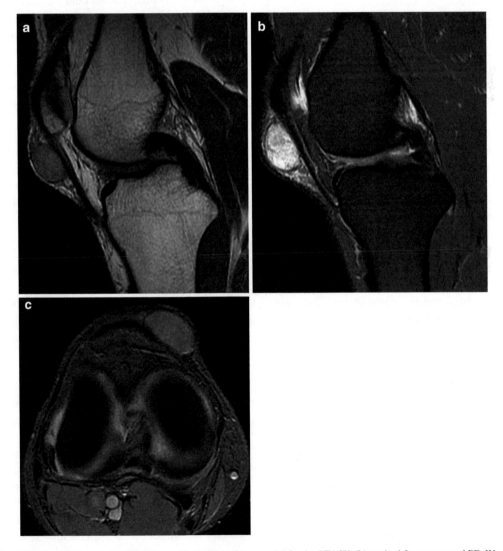

Fig. 28.9 Angioleiomyoma with nonspecific imaging features. (**a**) Sagittal T1-W, (**b**) sagittal fat-suppressed PD-W, and (**c**) axial GRE T2*-W MR images show a nonspecific soft tissue mass. Histological diagnosis was angioleiomyoma

28.5.1 Benign Masses

28.5.1.1 Ganglion/Bursa/Cyst

Ganglia are not included in the WHO classification of soft tissue tumors as they are not true neoplasms. Ganglia are most commonly encountered in the hand, wrist, and feet. These usually arise from joint capsules, bursae, ligaments, tendons, or subchondral bone (Siegel 2001). Their etiology remains controversial: many theories have been proposed, including development from synovial rests deposited at embryogenesis, proliferation and metaplasia of mesenchymal cells, degeneration of connective tissue owing to chronic trauma, and origination from the articular capsule (Malghem et al. 1998).

Clinical symptoms include palpable swelling with or without pain and secondary compression effect on the neurovascular structures and adjacent tissues. Radiographs are usually unremarkable in these situations; rarely a long-standing lesion may demonstrate benign cortical changes. US imaging is the modality of choice for superficial lesions. These appear uniformly hypoechoic with posterior acoustic enhancement. For deeper lesions, MRI is the preferred modality. These lesions are typically round or ovoid and can either be uni- or multiloculated, with a smooth or slightly lobulated contour, and are usually in close proximity to a joint or tendon. On MRI, ganglia tend to be iso- to hypointense on T1-weighted and hyperintense on T2-weighted MR images, and demonstrate a thin rim of contrast enhancement, with or without thin hypointense enhancing septa (Kim et al. 2004). It is important to evaluate these lesions with either contrast-enhanced MRI or with US imaging to confirm they are purely cystic in nature. Otherwise, they can be confused with myxoid lesions which can demonstrate similar findings on unenhanced MRI.

28.5.1.2 Pigmented Villonodular Synovitis

Pigmented villonodular synovitis (PVNS) is a benign, hypertrophic synovial process characterized by villous, nodular, and villonodular proliferation with pigmentation from hemosiderin. The knee, followed by the hip joint, is the most common location for PVNS. A localized extra-articular form of PVNS occurs in tendon sheaths – giant cell tumor of the tendon sheath (GCTTS) and other extra-articular sites. Over 75% of these lesions are localized/unifocal and the infrapatellar region is the commonest site (Murphey et al. 2008).

Radiographic features are nonspecific and radiographs may appear normal. The diffuse intra-articular form of PVNS often demonstrates a joint effusion and extrinsic erosion of bone on both sides of the joint, but the joint space is unaffected. The localized forms of disease usually reveal only a soft tissue mass. CT depicts these lesions as diffuse thickening of the tissue about the joint. On MRI, these lesions show hypo- to isointense signal on all pulse sequences. Use of gradient-echo pulse sequences helps to confirm the presence of hemosiderin, which appears as a prominent "blooming" of hypointense signal due to magnetic susceptibility artifact (Fig. 28.10). The "blooming" artifact that is typically seen in PVNS can also be seen in synovial hemangioma and hemophiliac arthropathy (Murphey et al. 2008), while T2-hypointense signal may also be seen in rheumatoid nodules, fibromatosis, and osteochondromatosis. Not all forms of nodular synovitis are pigmented; consequently, susceptibility artifact may not be present (Huang et al. 2003). Disease location and extent should be accurately identified, as these features are important both for diagnosis and to guide treatment.

28.5.1.3 Accessory Muscle

Within the appendicular skeleton, multiple accessory, supernumerary, and anomalous muscles have been described in the literature. It is important to recognize these, as they can mimic soft tissue tumors. MRI is considered to be the examination of choice for diagnosing accessory muscles, delineating their relationship to adjacent neurovascular structures, and will help in differentiating them from soft tissue tumors. Accessory muscles are isointense to skeletal muscle on all pulse sequences and typically attach by muscular

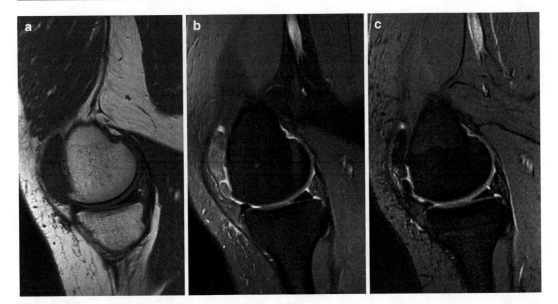

Fig. 28.10 Focal pigmented villonodular synovitis. Sagittal (**a**) T1-W, (**b**) fat-suppressed PD-W and (**c**) GRE T2*-W MR images of focal pigmented villonodular syno- vitis in the knee joint. Note the hypointense signal due to susceptibility artifact from hemosiderin deposition on the GRE image

or tendinous insertions. Although they are most often asymptomatic and identified as incidental findings, accessory muscles have been implicated as a source of clinical symptoms. When symptomatic, most often they present as a palpable mass or secondary to compression effect on the neighboring neurovascular structures (Sookur et al. 2008) (Fig. 28.11). Hence, it is essential to have knowledge of normal muscle anatomy, in particular being aware of spaces where muscles should not normally exist.

28.5.1.4 Myositis Ossificans

Myositis ossificans most commonly develops as a post-traumatic phenomenon, whereby heterotopic ossification develops in striated muscle. It may also develop in collagenous structures such as fasciae, aponeuroses, tendons, and ligaments. Characteristically, the ossification is predominantly peripherally situated around an inflammatory soft tissue mass but may also conform to the outline of the affected muscle fibers. The lesion develops ossification with time and may initially appear as a nonspecific soft tissue mass. CT scanning to demonstrate the developing peripheral

ossification may confirm the diagnosis. Ossification and calcification in malignant soft tissue tumors, by contrast, tends to be central. An extremely rare inherited condition, formerly termed myositis ossificans progressiva or myositis ossificans congenita, has been renamed fibrodysplasia ossificans progressiva, in which similar masses of ossifying connective tissue develop after minimal trauma; this condition is associated with bone dysplasia, having characteristically short thumbs and great toes (Tyler and Saifuddin 2010).

28.5.1.5 Elastofibroma

Elastofibroma is a relatively uncommon benign soft tissue pseudotumor, typically located around the inferior angle of the scapula deep to the serratus anterior. Usually, it presents as a longstanding swelling with discomfort and intermittent pain. It is most common in elderly male patients (Chandrasekar et al. 2008). The other locations of elastofibroma are the greater trochanter, deltoid muscle, ischial tuberosity, breast, foot, stomach, mediastinum, orbits, cornea, and oral mucosa (Kapff et al. 1987). It can be

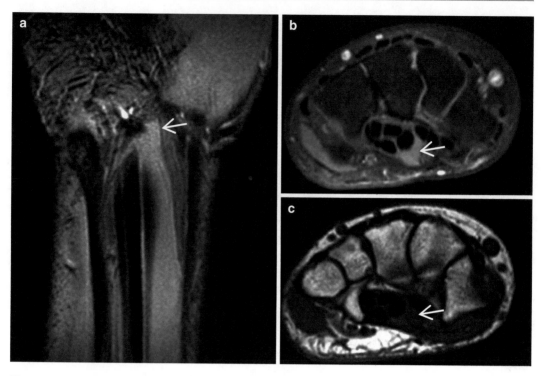

Fig. 28.11 Anomalous flexor digitorum superficialis muscle. (**a**) Coronal GRE T2*-W, (**b**) axial fat-suppressed PD-W, and (**c**) axial T1-W MR images show an anomalous muscle belly extending along flexor digitorum super-ficialis into the carpal tunnel. The anomalous muscle (*arrows*) shows the same signal intensity as normal muscle on all sequences

bilateral in up to 13% of patients (Chandrasekar et al. 2008).

On US imaging, elastofibroma consists of arrays of linear strands against an echogenic background (Ozpolat et al. 2008). Although CT is not routinely used for diagnosis, elastofibroma can be seen as incidental lesions on CT examinations performed for other clinical indications, appearing as ill-defined lesions with attenuation characters similar to a mixture of muscle fibers and fat (Onishi et al. 2011). MRI reveals a lenticular unencapsulated, poorly defined, soft tissue mass with signal characteristics of skeletal muscle attenuation interspersed with strands of fat attenuation (Naylor et al. 1996) (Fig. 28.12). Given the typical location and imaging appearance, image-guided biopsy is not routinely warranted. This lesion is not routinely surgically resected.

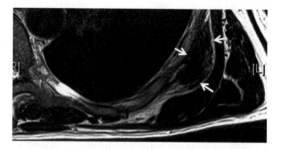

Fig. 28.12 Elastofibroma. Axial T2-W MR image taken through the left shoulder girdle shows an elastofibroma in a typical location (*arrows*), deep to serratus anterior muscle

28.5.1.6 Depositional Diseases

Tophaceous gout, tophaceous pseudogout, amyloidoma, and tendon xanthoma are all deposition diseases that may form soft tissue masses. Tophaceous gout characteristically forms soft tissue masses of sodium urate in juxta-articular

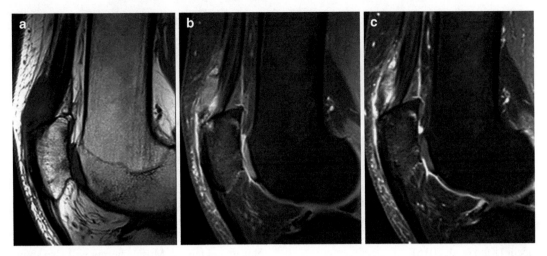

Fig. 28.13 Tophaceous gout. Soft tissue mass projecting from the quadriceps tendon. Sagittal (**a**) T1-W, (**b**) fat-suppressed PD-W, and (**c**) contrast-enhanced fat-suppressed T1-W MR images show a heterogeneously enhancing mass. As malignant tumors arising from tendons are rare, deposition disease should be considered. This was tophaceous gout

locations (Fig. 28.13). They may be relatively dense but are not commonly heavily mineralized (Yu et al. 1997). Juxta-articular bone erosions are usually present. Dual energy CT can characterize the deposits. Tophaceous pseudogout is due to deposits of calcium pyrophosphate salts and is consequently of calcific density on CT and radiography. Large masses of pseudogout may mimic a soft tissue tumor (Havitcioglu et al. 2003). Amyloidoma is a rare cutaneous deposit of amyloid, not usually associated with systemic amyloidosis (Pasternak et al. 2007). Tendon xanthoma is deposition of cholesterol and triglycerides in tendons in patients with hyperlipidemia. Large deposits may be seen in the Achilles tendon, and characteristically, these are bilateral. In contrast, malignant tumor developing in tendon is rare.

28.5.1.7 Benign Fatty Tumors

Benign fatty tumors are the commonest soft tissue tumors but can vary widely in appearance (Bancroft et al. 2006). The majority are composed of mature adipose tissue with homogeneous sequence-appropriate fat signal on MRI and fat density on CT. These lipomas can be further classified as superficial or deep and single or multiple. There are variants of lipoma including angiolipoma, myoli-

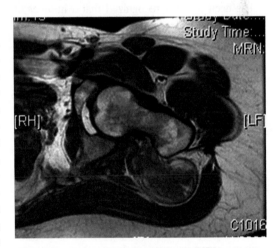

Fig. 28.14 Hibernoma. Axial T1-W MR image of the hip shows a mixed lipomatous and soft tissue tumor posterior to the greater trochanter. Biopsy confirmed a hibernoma

poma, chondroid lipoma, lipoblastoma, and pleomorphic lipoma. There are lipomatous tumors of specific sites, e.g., intra- and intermuscular lipoma; lipomatosis of nerve or of tendon sheath or joint; and infiltrating lipomas such as diffuse lipomatosis, symmetric lipomatosis, and adiposis dolorosa; and there are benign tumors of brown fat (or hibernomas) (Goldblum et al. 2013b) (Fig. 28.14).

These variants contain or are associated with non-fatty soft tissue components that will alter their imaging appearances. Lipomatous tumors of nerves may be due to local somatic mutations of PIK3CA (see Sect. 28.5.1.9 below).

28.5.1.8 Pilomatricoma

Pilomatricoma (or calcifying epithelioma of Malherbe) is a benign tumor of the hair follicle, commonest on the face and neck. It is usually heavily calcified. The superficial location and calcification on radiograph or CT is suggestive. The MRI signal characteristics are very variable. Rarely, malignant pilomatrix carcinoma can occur (Kato et al. 2016).

28.5.1.9 Soft Tissue Overgrowth Conditions

It has been recently recognized that a number of apparently diverse soft tissue overgrowth conditions that may present as soft tissue tumors are due to local somatic mutations of the PIK3CA gene. These include lipofibromatous hamartoma of nerve (Fig. 28.15), macrodystrophia lipomatosa and other more extensive limb overgrowth syndromes, cystic hygroma, and the Klippel-Trenaunay syndrome. Recognition of the condition and its genetic etiology, which can be confirmed on biopsy specimens from the lesion, is important, as medical therapy targeting the affected mTOR metabolic pathway is now available (Keppler-Noreuil et al. 2014).

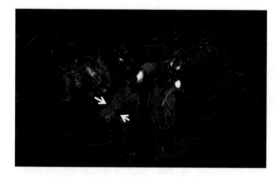

Fig. 28.15 Lipofibromatous hamartoma. Axial fat-suppressed T2-W MR image taken through the pelvis. The right hip is overgrown and osteoarthritic. The sciatic nerve (*arrows*) is markedly expanded with thickened fascicles and intervening fatty septa, due to a PIK3CA somatic mutation. Diagnosis is lipofibromatous hamartoma

28.5.1.10 Post-traumatic Muscle Lesions

Muscle tears, musculotendinous junction tears, and muscle avulsions are usually obvious by their clinical presentation. Late presentation may cause uncertainty. Although a palpable defect may be evident at the site of the tear, the muscle adjacent to the tear may "bunch up" and form a palpable mass (Fig. 28.16). On MR imaging, the muscle defect may contain fat and/or fibrosis (Anderson et al. 2005). The bunched-up muscle shows signal intensities identical to normal muscle on all sequences. It may also show marked contour change, if scanned with the muscle both relaxed and tensed. Muscle hernia will also show these features (Boutin et al. 2002). Post-radiotherapy muscle signal change may also simulate a mass. Characteristically, this will have a well-defined straight margin corresponding to the radiation field.

28.5.1.11 Abscess/Myositis/ Inflammatory Masses

Soft tissue infections may produce masses with solid-appearing imaging characteristics, before central liquefaction results in an abscess. Intramuscular infection can cause large ramifying collections with heterogeneous imaging appearances (Figs. 28.17 and 28.18). Tuberculous infection may extend through small perforations in the fascial planes to form larger collections on each side. The lack of clinical inflammatory response in tuberculous infection causes "cold abscesses," potentially mimicking soft tissue tumor. Immunocompromised patients may also form cold abscesses from unusual infecting organisms (Gaskill et al. 2010). Cat scratch fever, or subacute regional lymphadenitis, is caused by *Bartonella henselae*. The organism is commonly carried by cats and transferred by scratches or bites, typically on the hands, and can consequently result in characteristic inflammation of the epitrochlear lymph node at the elbow (Fig. 28.19) and other infections in the forearm or hand. Mononucleosis and secondary syphilis are also associated with epitrochlear lymphadenopathy. Maduramycosis (Madura foot) is uncommon, but has a characteristic MRI appearance of hypointense rings around a hyperin-

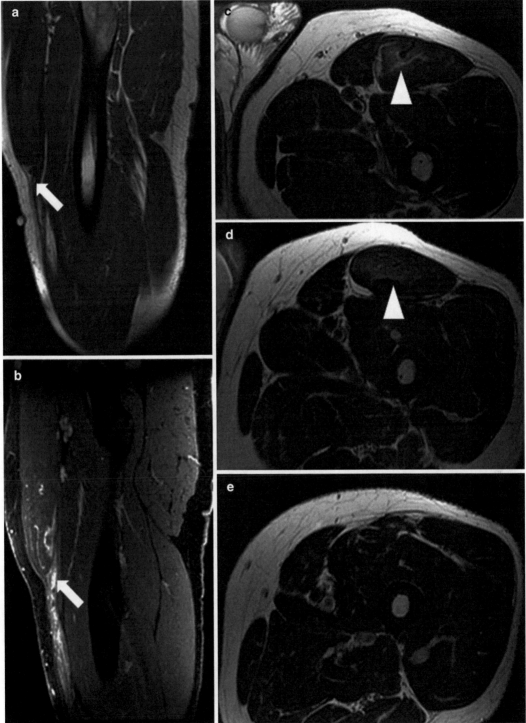

Fig. 28.16 Rectus femoris muscle tear. Sagittal (**a**) T1-W and (**b**) fat-suppressed PD-W MR images show the bulky muscle retracted into the proximal thigh (*arrows*). (**c–e**) Axial T2-W MR images show (**c, d**) hyperintense signal in the muscle (*arrowheads*) around the musculotendinous junction in the upper thigh with (**e**) deficient muscle distally

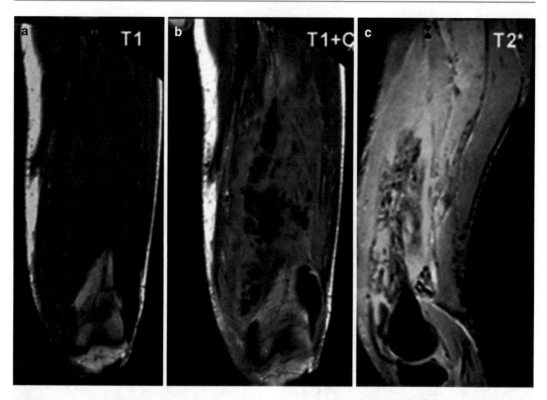

Fig. 28.17 Intramuscular abscesses. (**a**) Coronal T1-W, (**b**) coronal contrast-enhanced T1-W, and (**c**) sagittal GRE T2*-W MR images of the thigh show a ramifying collection with enhancing walls and septations throughout the vastus intermedius. The unenhanced T1-W image shows a "penumbra sign" of hyperintense signal in the walls and septa. This is approximately 50% sensitive and 98% specific for abscess formation (McGuinness et al. 2007)

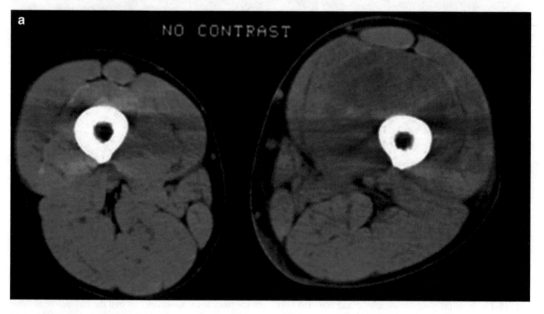

Fig. 28.18 Intramuscular abscesses. Axial (**a**) pre- and (**b**) post-contrast-enhanced CT images show low-density expansion of the left vastus intermedius with peripheral contrast enhancement in the intramuscular abscess (also demonstrated in Fig. 28.17)

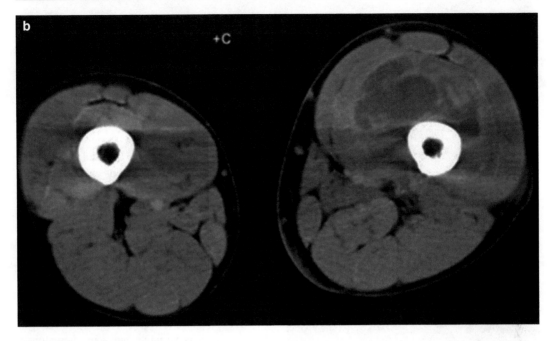

Fig. 28.18 (continued)

tense area but containing a hypointense "dot" in the middle, due to fungal hyphae in the abscess cavities (Fig. 28.20) (Jain et al. 2012).

28.5.1.12 Myonecrosis

Myonecrosis may produce a soft tissue swelling with mass-like appearances (Delaney-Sathy et al. 2000; Kattapuram et al. 2005). It can occur in sickle cell crisis, diabetic myonecrosis, compartment syndrome, crush injury, severe ischemia, intra-arterial chemotherapy, and rhabdomyolysis (May et al. 2000). Knowledge of the patient's history is therefore crucial. Dense peripheral calcification may form around post-traumatic myonecrosis, giving a characteristic radiographic appearance of calcific myonecrosis (Dhillon et al. 2004). This persists indefinitely, but the calcific wall may rupture, allowing the central fluid contents to form a new adjacent swelling (Fig. 28.21).

28.5.1.13 Hemangioma

Although hemangiomas are common tumors in infancy and childhood, they can occur in any age group (Kransdorf 1995). The terminologies used by various specialist and general radiologists can be confusing. The International Society for the Study of Vascular Anomalies (ISSVA) classification system has been widely accepted by various subspecialists who care for patients with these malformations. This system provides a comprehensive approach, based on histopathology, clinical course, and treatment (Vilanova et al. 2004). Slow flow malformations tend to demonstrate phleboliths on radiographs which represent focal dystrophic areas of calcification within a thrombus. On US imaging evaluation, it may be difficult to accurately elicit the vascular flow, as these generally tend to have very slow flow through them. However, these will be compressible on US probe palpation. Occasionally, periosteal reaction, cortical and medullary changes, and overgrowth can be seen affecting the adjacent bones (Kransdorf and Murphey 2006). MRI has an important role in diagnosing, characterizing, and determining the vascular malformations. Hemangiomas may be well-circumscribed or have poorly defined margins, with varying amounts of hyperintense T1 signal owing to either reactive fat overgrowth or hemorrhage (Kransdorf and Murphey 2006). Areas of slow flow typically have T2-hyperintense signal, while rapid flow can demonstrate a signal

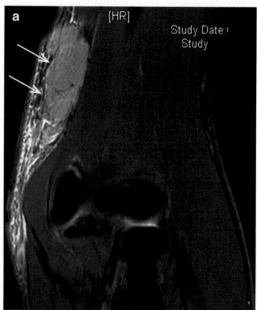

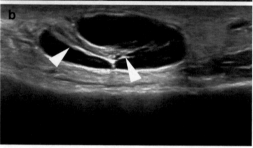

Fig. 28.19 Inflamed epitrochlear lymph node due to cat scratch fever. (**a**) Coronal fat-suppressed PD-W MR image shows a lobulated intermediate signal intensity soft tissue mass (*arrows*) in the subcutaneous fat proximal to the medial epicondyle of the humerus, at the expected location of the epitrochlear lymph node. There is fluid signal in the adjacent fat. (**b**) US image more clearly shows a fatty hilum (*arrowheads*) within the subcutaneous mass, confirming a lymph node. There was a history of recent cat scratch to the hand

void on images obtained with a non-flow-sensitive sequence. The T1- and T2-hypointense foci are due to phleboliths within these lesions.

28.5.1.14 Hematoma and Hemophiliac Pseudotumor

Soft tissue pseudotumor may be due to chronic organizing hematoma in patients with hemo-

philia (Park and Ryu 2004). Spontaneous hematoma should be viewed with suspicion. Current treatment with anticoagulants is the commonest cause. Evidence of an unrecognized clotting disorder should be sought and the possibility of an underlying hemorrhagic sarcoma considered (Sreenivas et al. 2004). Pre- and post-contrast-enhanced MRI using the same T1-weighted sequence should therefore be used to look for focal regions of enhancement indicative of a focus of tumor, although some foci of enhancement can be seen in organizing hematomas due to fibrovascular tissue forming in the hematoma. Biopsy of these regions or follow-up scanning until the lesion resolves is suggested.

Fat-suppressed T1-weighted MR sequences may show hyperintense signal from methemoglobin, which can be mistaken for enhancement. The time course of signal changes in hematomas is variable, but acute hematomas (up to 1 week) are usually of similar or lower signal intensity than muscle on both T1- and T2-weighted MRI. Subacute hematomas (1 week to 3 months) are usually more hyperintense than muscle on both T1- and T2-weighted sequences, often with a more hyperintense internal rim on T1-weighted images. Chronic hematomas are also usually hyperintense on both sequences but may develop a hypointense rim of hemosiderin and/or fibrosis. Very chronic hematomas (years) may be hypointense on T2-weighted images. If there is persisting uncertainty, follow-up to confirm resolution of the hematoma is advised.

28.5.1.15 Aneurysm

Although occasionally presenting as a soft tissue mass, either clinically or on imaging, the location arising from an artery is characteristic. MRI artifact from blood flow and pulsation, a layered appearance due to lining thrombus of varying ages, and a history of local trauma should be recognized.

28.5.1.16 Morel-Lavallée Lesion

The Morel-Lavallée lesion is a post-traumatic lesion, arising as a consequence of a shearing

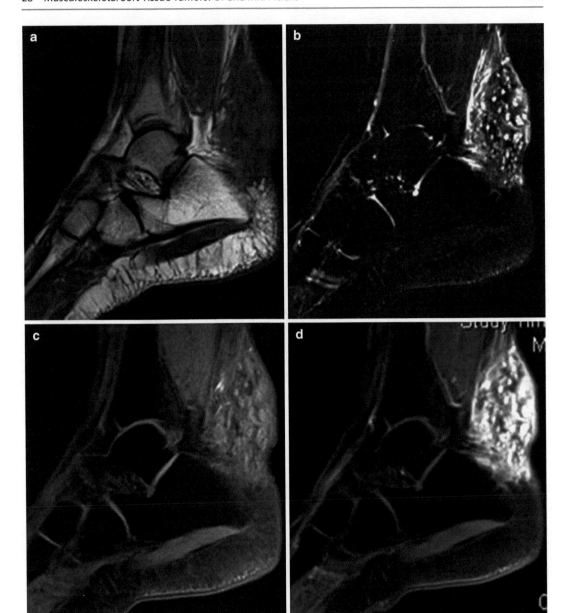

Fig. 28.20 Madura foot (or maduramycosis). Sagittal (**a**) T1-W, (**b**) fat-suppressed T2-W, (**c**) fat-suppressed T1-W, and (**d**) contrast-enhanced fat-suppressed T1-W MR images of the foot show an unusual indistinctly marginated mass containing multiple hypointense rings. Some of the rings contain a central hypointense signal "dot." This is characteristic of maduramycosis (Courtesy of Dr. R. Mehan, Bolton Hospitals NHS Foundation Trust, UK)

injury through the subcutaneous fat, usually close to the deep fascia. Commonest around the pelvis and lateral side of the thigh, the contents are usually fluid – serous or blood, sometimes containing globules of fat, with the expected signal characteristics of fat in fluid on MRI (Fig. 28.22) and equivalent densities on CT (Mellado and Bencardino 2005). This is a closed degloving injury that may take years to resolve.

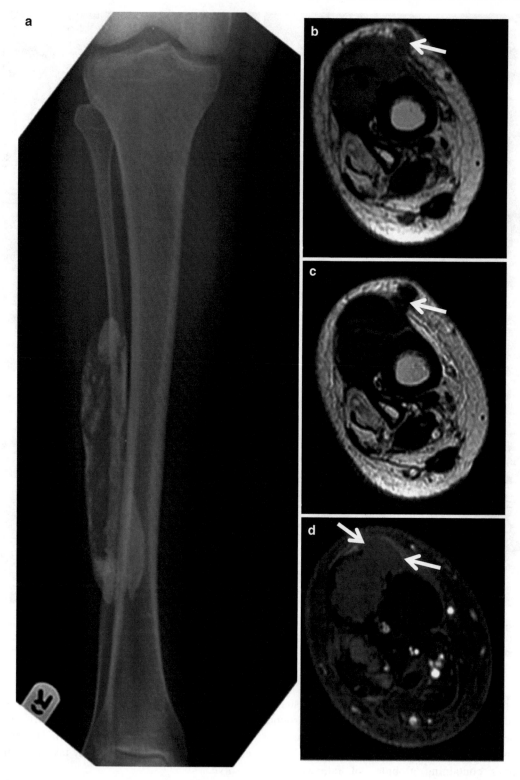

Fig. 28.21 Calcific myonecrosis. (a) AP radiograph shows a large peripherally calcified mass of calcific myonecrosis in the calf. Axial (b) T1-W, (c) T2-W, and (d) fat-suppressed PD-W MR images show the lesion to have central intermediate signal on T1-W but hypointense signal on T2-W MR images. The new focal swelling the patient complained of was subsequently shown to be due to rupture and leakage of the contents anteriorly (*arrows*)

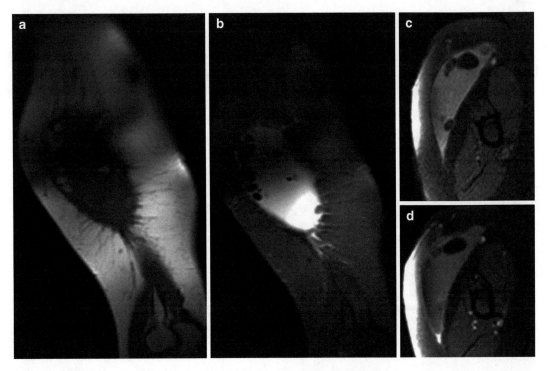

Fig. 28.22 Morel-Lavallée lesion. Sagittal (**a**) T1-W and (**b**) fat-suppressed PD-W, and (**c**, **d**) axial fat-suppressed PD-W MR images taken through a shearing injury of subcutaneous fat of the arm show fluid and multiple fat globules. This is typical of a Morel-Lavallée lesion

28.5.1.17 Tumoral Calcinosis

Tumoral calcinosis is a primary familial condition, most commonly found in Africa. Soft tissue masses of heavily mineralized bursal collections develop in juxta-articular locations, commonest over the greater trochanter and then at other extensor sides of joints, particularly the elbow, shoulder, foot, and wrist. Secondary tumoral calcinosis is dystrophic or metabolic calcification, such as may occur in renal osteodystrophy, connective tissue diseases, hypercalcemia from metabolic or endocrine causes, and other conditions. Secondary tumoral calcinosis is better named after its cause, such as calcinosis of renal failure. The "milk of calcium" suspension in bursal fluid may sediment out to create density layers on CT and signal intensity layers on MRI. The MRI appearances are of hypointense masses on T1-weighted images, with heterogeneous signal on T2-weighted images. Radiographs to demonstrate the degree and appearance of the calcification are valuable (Olsen and Chew 2006; Chaabane et al. 2008).

28.5.1.18 Aggressive Fibromatosis

Fibromatosis refers to a group of tumors comprising benign fibrous tissue composed of uniform cells surrounded and separated by abundant collagen, considered as intermediate lesions (Goldblum et al. 2013a). They are classified as either deep or superficial. Deep (musculoaponeurotic) fibromatosis is also commonly referred to as extra-abdominal desmoid tumor (Goodwin et al. 2007). The tumors are usually intermuscular although muscle invasion is common (Fig. 28.23).

Most often, US imaging is performed for initial evaluation of the soft tissue lesions. However, US imaging features are nonspecific in fibromatosis (Otero et al. 2015). MRI is the most important modality for initial diagnoses, surgical staging, and follow-up. Fibromatosis normally demonstrates heterogeneous signal intensity on T2- weighted images, reflecting the variable quantities and distribution of myofibroblasts, extracellular collagen, and myxoid matrix; it is these appearances that raise suspi-

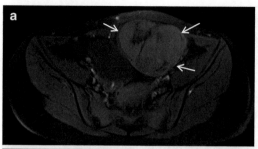

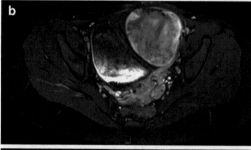

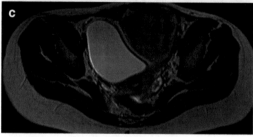

Fig. 28.23 Aggressive fibromatosis (or desmoid tumor). Axial (**a**) unenhanced fat-suppressed T1-W, (**b**) contrast-enhanced fat-suppressed T1-W, and (**c**) T2-W MR images show a tumor in the left rectus abdominus muscle (*arrows*) of a young adult female patient. The location, age of the patient, and heterogeneous regions of hypointense signal on T1-W and T2-W images all favor diagnosis of desmoid tumor

cion for the diagnosis of fibromatosis (Lee et al. 2006). Areas of linear signal void on all sequences are said to be characteristic of, but not specific for, aggressive fibromatosis and are likely to correspond to dense collagen (Goodwin et al. 2007). In the early stage, lesions are more cellular and, as a result, are predominantly T2-hyperintense (Fig. 28.24). At later stages, there is an increase in collagen deposition and therefore decrease in extracellular space, resulting in a decrease in T2 signal intensity (Fig. 28.25). This pattern is also seen in lesions as they respond to treatment; due to progressive

collagen deposition, there is a corresponding reduction in tumor signal intensity.

Lesions display moderate to marked enhancement with gadolinium contrast agents, other than the hypointense collagen bundles which do not enhance (Otero et al. 2015). The infiltration along the fascia is described as a "fascial tail" and can be seen in approximately 80% of cases (Dinauer et al. 2007). Other infiltrative lesions such as malignant fibrous histiocytoma, fibrosarcoma, lymphoma, and densely calcified masses need to be considered in the differential diagnosis. In practice, the wide variation in MRI signal characteristics that may be displayed by fibromatosis can make diagnosis uncertain.

28.5.2 Malignant Tumors

While many soft tissue malignancies have non-specific appearances, some may show diagnostic features. These lesions are described in this section.

28.5.2.1 Atypical Lipomatous Tumor

Atypical lipomatous tumor (ALT) and low-grade liposarcoma are currently considered to be the same lesion. These tumors contain a high proportion of lipomatous tissue, with its characteristic imaging density on CT and signal intensities on MRI. There may however be a greater degree of septation (Fig. 28.26) with increased amounts of nonfatty soft tissue compared to a typical lipoma (Fig. 28.27). Lesions greater than 10 cm in diameter and deep to the deep fascia are best considered to be ALT/low-grade liposarcoma, however homogeneously lipomatous they appear. These tumors may display increased MDM2 gene amplification, allowing diagnostic confirmation from biopsy tissue.

28.5.2.2 Liposarcoma

Higher grades of liposarcoma may still have some discernable lipomatous content. Careful correlation of T1-weighted, T2-weighted, and fat-suppressed MR images may identify the fat content, allowing an imaging diagnosis of liposarcoma to be made.

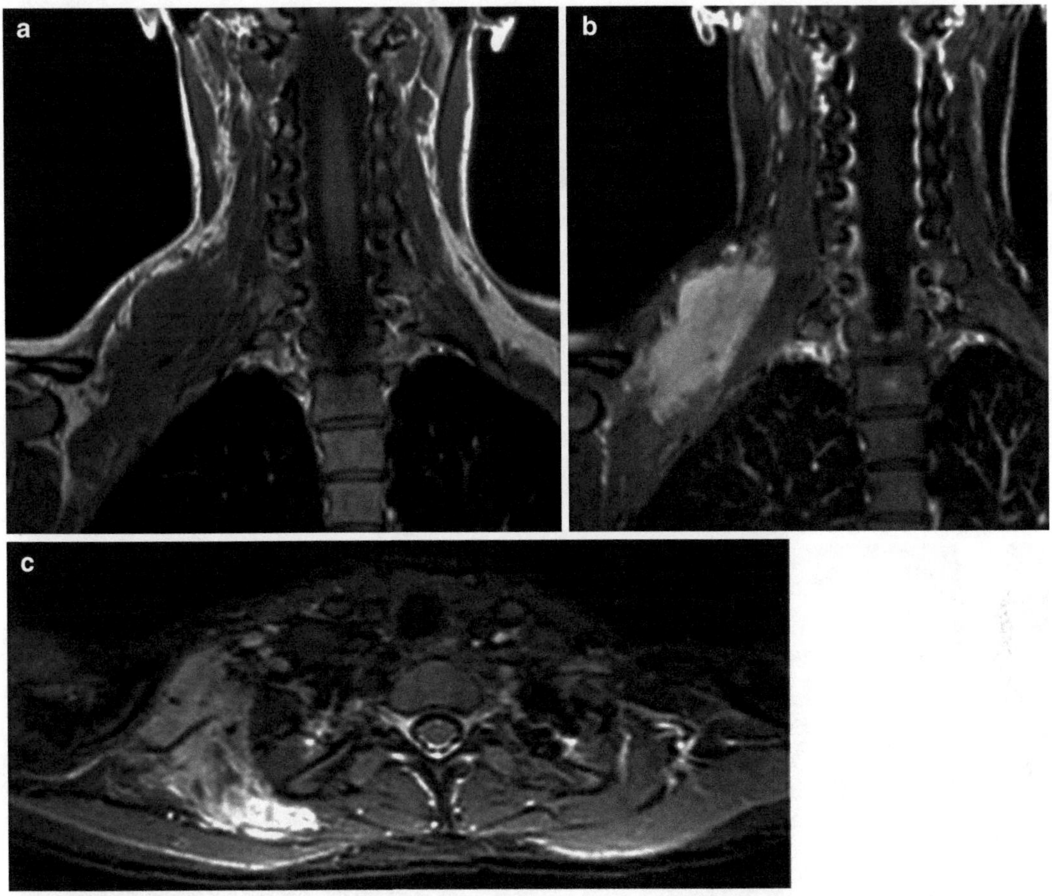

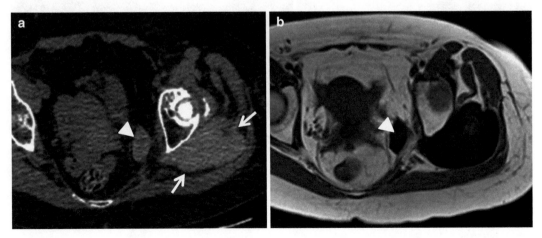

Fig. 28.24 Cellular fibromatosis. Coronal (**a**) T1-W, (**b**) contrast-enhanced fat-suppressed T1-W, and (**c**) axial contrast-enhanced T1-W MR images show cellular fibro-matosis at the right shoulder girdle, with infiltration into the musculature

Fig. 28.25 Mature fibromatosis. (**a**) Axial unenhanced CT image shows a mass with higher density than muscle, immediately posterior to the left hip (*arrows*). This mass is of hypointense signal on axial (**b**) T1-W, (**c**) T2-W, and (**d**) fat-suppressed PD-W MR images. There is a separate nodule in the pelvis (*arrowhead*)

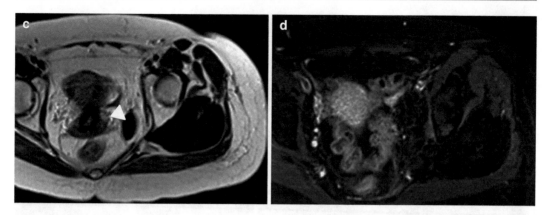

Fig. 28.25 (continued)

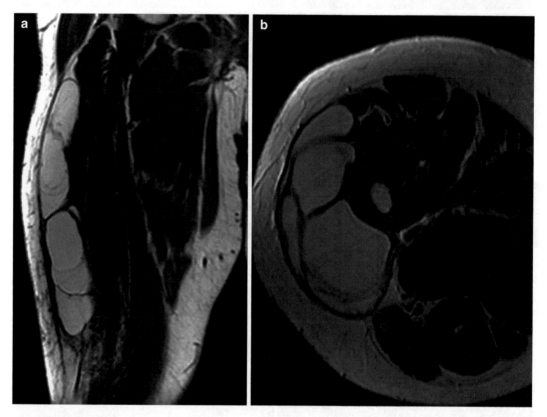

Fig. 28.26 Recurrent atypical lipomatous tumor/low-grade liposarcoma. (**a**) Coronal T1-W and (**b**) axial T-W MR images of a recurrent atypical lipomatous tumor/low-grade liposarcoma show multiple septations but homogeneous fat signal in the tumor lobulations

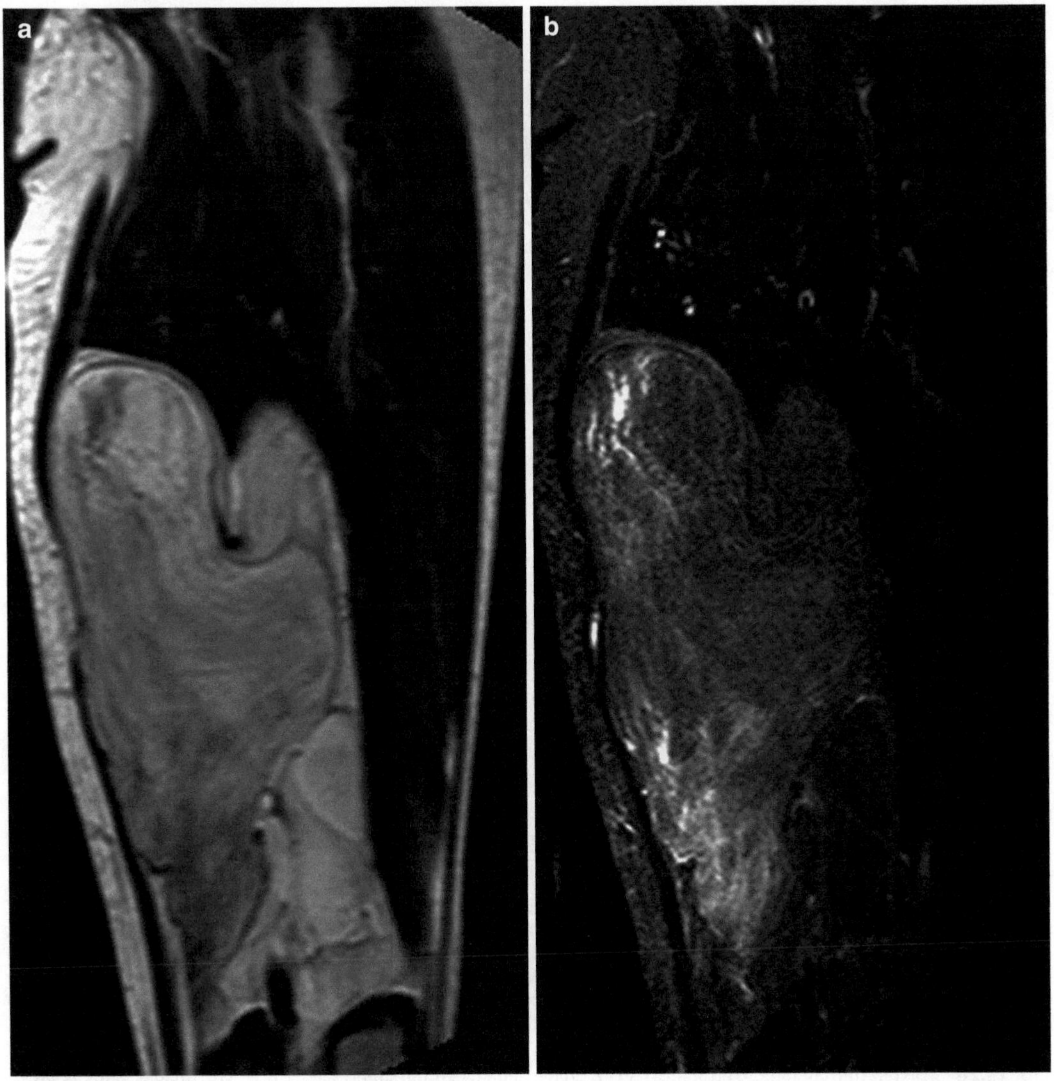

Fig. 28.27 Atypical lipomatous tumor/low-grade liposarcoma. (**a**) Coronal T1-W MR image of the posterior thigh shows a large predominantly fatty lesion containing strands and inhomogeneous indistinct regions of lower signal intensity. (**b**) Corresponding coronal fat-suppressed T2-W MR image shows fat suppression in the lesion but with strands and inhomogeneous indistinct regions of signal hyperintensity corresponding to the T1-hypointense regions. This was an atypical lipomatous tumor/low-grade liposarcoma

28.5.2.3 Myxoid Liposarcoma

The typical appearances of myxoid tissue may be identifiable. If fat can also be identified in the lesion, then a diagnosis of myxoid liposarcoma can be suggested (Fig. 28.28). In the absence of any discernable fat content, myxofibrosarcoma is more likely, particularly in elderly patients (Sung et al. 2000).

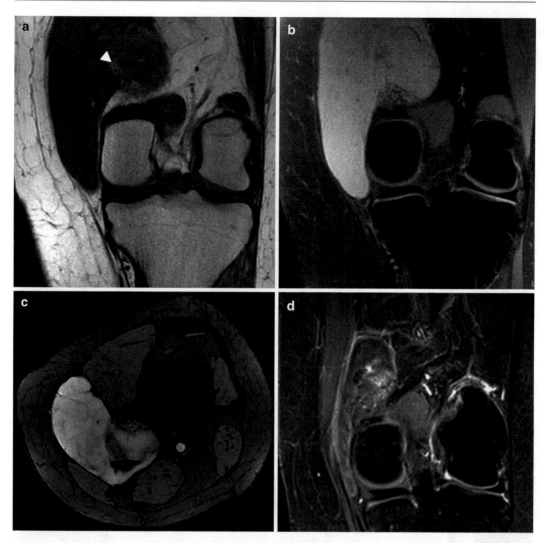

Fig. 28.28 Myxoid liposarcoma. Coronal (**a**) T1-W and (**b**) fat-suppressed PD-W MR images show a relatively homogeneous superficial, "cyst-like" appearance. This region shows greater heterogeneity on (**c**) axial GRE T2*-W and some enhancement on (**d**) coronal contrast-enhanced fat-suppressed T1-W MR images. This is myxoid material. The deeper component shows some patchy hyperintense signal on the T1-W image (*arrowhead*), which shows fat suppression, hence representing a fat-containing region

28.5.2.4 Synovial Sarcoma

Synovial sarcoma is a misnomer, as it does not arise from synovium, but has a histological appearance reminiscent of synovial cells and also tends to arise near (but not within) joints. This tumor also occurs over a wide age range and so may be seen relatively more often in younger patients. Characteristically the tumor has cystic components and may also contain calcifications, resulting in heterogeneous signal on MRI (Fig. 28.29).

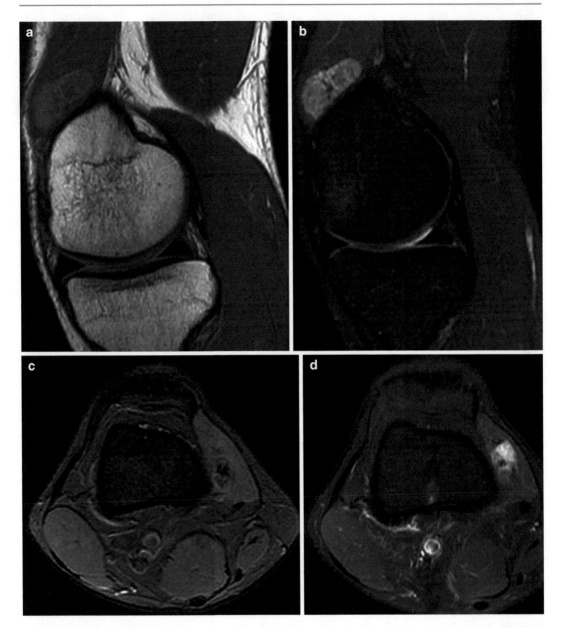

Fig. 28.29 Synovial sarcoma. Sagittal (**a**) T1-W and (**b**) fat-suppressed PD-W and axial (**c**) GRE T2*-W and (**d**) contrast-enhanced fat-suppressed T1-W MR images show an intramuscular soft tissue mass containing focal hypointense areas, consistent with calcifications. Although small, this lesion is deep to the deep fascia, contains calcifications, and is close to an articulation. Histology confirmed a synovial sarcoma

28.5.2.5 Malignant Peripheral Nerve Sheath Tumor

Nerve sheath tumors characteristically have the nerve of origin passing through them, giving rise to a "comet tail sign." Fifty percent of malignant peripheral nerve sheath tumors (MPNSTs) arise in patients with neurofibromatosis. Any enlarging neurofibroma in a patient with this condition should therefore be treated with suspicion (Fig. 28.30).

28.5.2.6 Extra-Nodal Lymphoma

Lymphoma may arise *de novo* in non-nodal sites. Such extra-nodal disease characteristically shows uniform intermediate signal intensity on T2-weighted images and homogeneous contrast enhancement (Fig. 28.31). Lymphoma may infiltrate into bone and muscle, often with remarkably little disruption to the bone cortex and/or muscle architecture (Chun et al. 2010). This appearance is also seen in small round blue cell tumors, e.g., rhabdomyosarcoma, Ewing's sarcoma, and primitive neuroectodermal tumor.

28.5.2.7 Primary Bone Tumors Arising *De Novo* in Soft Tissue

Primary bone tumors arising *de novo* in soft tissue, such as osteosarcoma and chondrosarcoma, are rare tumors. The radiographic appearance of ossification or calcification is similar to that seen in the same tumor types of bony origin and may suggest the diagnosis.

28.6 Conditions Associated with Multiple Soft Tissue Masses

28.6.1 Neurofibromatosis Type 1

Neurofibromatosis type 1 (NF1) is characterized by multiple focal neurofibromata and bone dysplasia. The latter is associated with a surrounding rind of neurofibromatous periosteum, cutaneous lesions such as café au lait spots, and superficial plexiform neurofibromatous lesions. The disease can be mosaic, segmental, or generalized. The neurofibromata may be predominantly superficial but can also involve all the major nerves, with masses of neurofibromata replacing all the spinal nerve roots, plexus and major nerve trunks (the spinal phenotype of NF1).

28.6.2 Neurofibromatosis Type 2 and Schwannomatosis

Intracranial and intraspinal tumors as well as peripheral schwannomas occur in these conditions, which are genetically distinct from NF1. Schwannomatosis is also genetically distinct from both NF1 and NF2. Patients with NF1 and NF2 have an increased risk of malignant diseases, not just MPNST.

28.6.3 Maffuci Syndrome

Angelo Maffuci first described the syndrome, multiple enchondromas and hemangiomas, in 1881. This became more widely recognized following a report by Carleton et al. in 1942, in which the authors reported two new cases. Pathologically, Maffucci syndrome is classified as a mesodermal dysplasia, manifesting as a combination of enchondromatosis and hemangiomatosis (Lewis and Ketcham 1973). The hand is most frequently involved (88%), followed by the foot (61%), lower leg (59%), femur (53%), humerus (42%), forearm (41%), pelvis (21%), and vertebrae (10%). Both bone and soft tissue lesions can undergo malignant transformation. Chondrosarcoma is the most frequently encountered malignant tumor in these patients. Other tumors have also been described, including angiosarcoma and fibrosarcoma (Foreman et al. 2013). Radiographs demonstrate multiple enchondromas in the bones and phleboliths due to slow flow arteriovenous (AV) malformations in the soft tissues. US imaging does not have a significant role in diagnosis but is used to aid targeted biopsy of the extraosseous soft tissue component. MRI is indicated for surveillance, monitoring for malignant transformation indicated by the myxoid change and directing the relevant areas for biopsy.

28.6.4 Mazabraud Syndrome

Henschen et al. first described an association between fibrous dysplasia and soft tissue myxomas in 1926. This became well-established in the medical literature, only after it was reported by Mazabraud et al. in 1967. Although the etiology

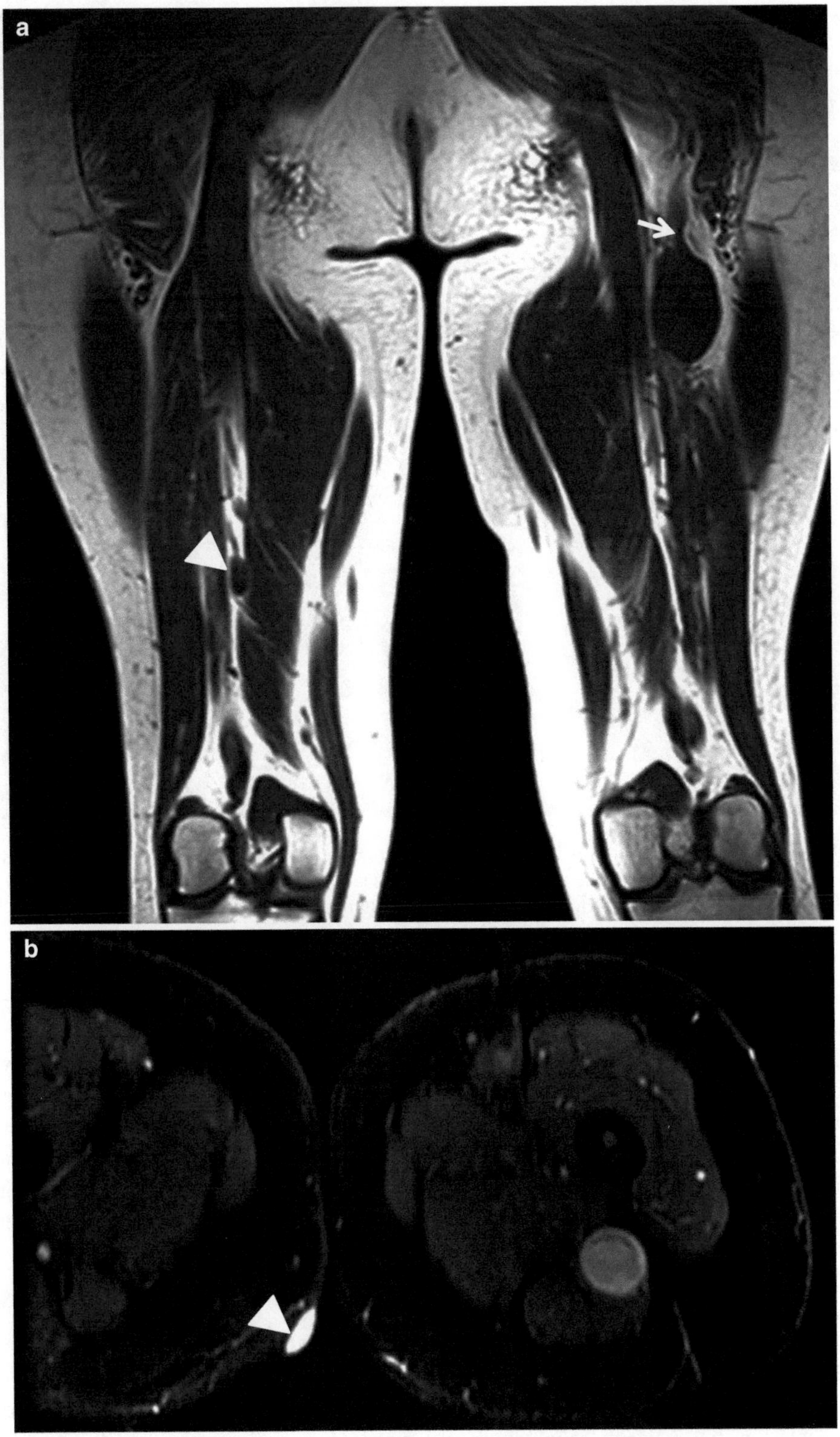

Fig. 28.30 Malignant peripheral nerve sheath tumor (MPNST) in a patient with neurofibromatosis type 1. (**a**) Coronal T1-W and (**b**) axial fat-suppressed PD-W MR images of the thighs show a mass in the left sciatic nerve with a "comet tail" seen superiorly (*arrow*) and several other neurofibromata (*arrowheads*)

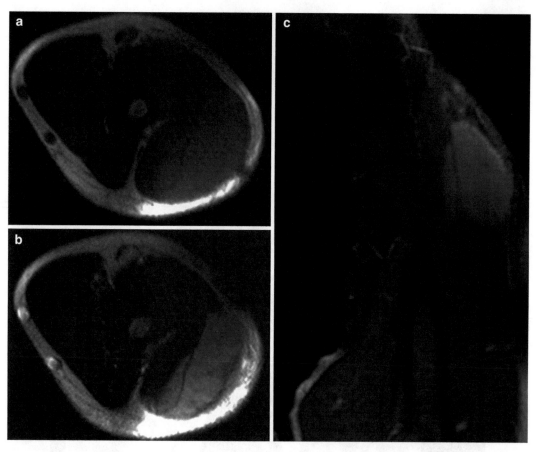

Fig. 28.31 (**a**) Axial T1-W, (**b**) axial T2-W, and (**c**) coronal fat-suppressed PD-W MR images of the midarm show a mass infiltrating the triceps muscle which is very homogeneous in signal intensity on all sequences and infiltrates across the musculotendinous junction without distortion. This is typical (although not diagnostic) of small round blue cell tumor. The diagnosis was lymphoma

of Mazabraud syndrome is unknown, many theories have been put forward to explain the link between fibrous dysplasia and soft tissue myxomas, including a common histogenetic origin, a shared abnormality in tissue metabolism, or a genetic predisposition. The fibrous dysplasia tends to be polyostotic in nature in Mazabraud syndrome. In subtle cases, CT can be used to confirm the presence of ground glass matrix within the fibrous dysplasia. With regard to myxomas, radiographs normally show a fairly nonspecific and poorly defined soft tissue mass. On CT, there is usually a homogeneous well-circumscribed lesion. US imaging demonstrates a well-defined hypoechoic lesion, the majority of which show small fluid-filled spaces which conglomerate to form a microcystic pattern. On MRI, the myxomas appear as a well-defined T1-hypointense and T2-hyperintense lesions (Fig. 28.32), with an absence of perilesional edema (Jonelle et al. 2014). There is heterogeneous contrast enhancement. Heterogeneous enhancement is useful to distinguish myxomas from more homogeneous cystic lesions such as bursae, ganglia, and even abscesses (Iwasko et al. 2002).

28.6.5 Familial Polyposis Coli

The term "desmoid" originates from the Greek word "desmos," meaning band- or tendon-like, and was first applied in 1838. Desmoid tumors

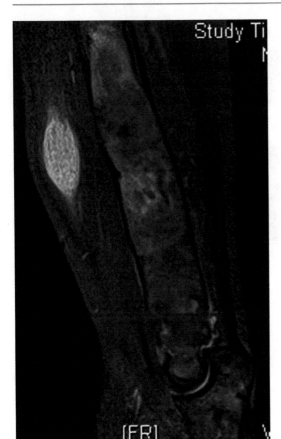

Fig. 28.32 Mazabraud syndrome. Sagittal fat-suppressed PD-W MR image of the distal arm shows fibrous dysplasia expanding the humerus and a myxoma in the biceps muscle

are rare (0.03% of all neoplasms), histologically benign proliferations of stromal cells, but may grow locally aggressive (Escobar et al. 2011). A small fraction of these are associated with Gardner syndrome and mutations of the familial adenomatous polyposis (FAP) gene. In patients with familial adenomatous polyposis, 9–18% of patients develop desmoid tumors. Most of these tumors are situated within the mesentery of the small bowel (Teo et al. 2005). These can develop anywhere in body site, but the abdominal wall and soft tissues of the extremities, shoulder, neck, and chest wall are the most commonly involved sites (Escobar et al. 2011).

Desmoid tumors are classified as intra- or extra-abdominal types, but the histological findings in these lesions are similar. MRI is the modality of choice for imaging these tumors. The MRI features of desmoid tumors show wide variability, depending on the stage at which they are imaged. MRI features include a soft tissue mass with heterogeneous signal intensity approximating that of fat on T2-weighted images and that of skeletal muscle on T1-weighted images (Quinn et al. 1991). Malignant tumors tend to have areas of signal intensity that are greater than that of fat on T2-weighted images. CT is not routinely used for diagnosis. The CT appearance of desmoid tumors varies, depending on their composition. Lesions may appear hypo-, iso-, or hyperintense, when compared with the attenuation of muscles. However, CT is also used to perform image-guided biopsies.

28.6.6 Dercum Disease

Dercum disease (or adiposis dolorosa) was first described by Roux and Vitaut in 1901. This disease classically presents as multiple, painful, fatty superficial lesions. Women are more commonly affected, with presumed autosomal dominant with incomplete penetrance. Histologically, these can appear as normal lipomas, inflammatory changes, or angiolipoma-like features. Radiographs and CT normally do not have a role in diagnosis. On US imaging, these lesions are most commonly superficial, less than 2 cm in diameter, and may appear more hyperechoic than the adjacent fat. The long axis of these lesions is to be parallel to the skin surface (Schaffer et al. 2014). They may not demonstrate increased vascularity (Tins et al. 2013). On MRI, they are nodular with increased fluid signal. Larger lesions were more inhomogeneous on MRI. No contrast enhancement is present.

28.6.7 Metastatic Disease

Soft tissue metastases have been reported to arise most commonly from carcinomas of the lung, kidney, and colon. There are also case reports in

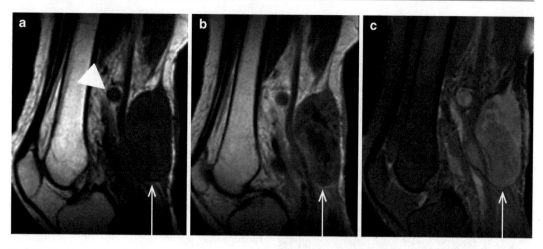

Fig. 28.33 Metastasis mimicking a malignant peripheral nerve sheath tumor. Sagittal (**a**) T1-W, (**b**) contrast-enhanced T1-W, and (**c**) fat-suppressed PD-W MR images show a large tumor (*arrows*) in the popliteal fossa with a "comet tail" superiorly and inferiorly. However, this is a metastatic deposit of squamous carcinoma. There is a separate nodal metastasis in the upper popliteal fossa (*arrowhead*). The patient has epidermolysis bullosa, which predisposes to squamous carcinoma

the literature that have reported soft tissue metastasis from less likely primary sources including the breast, prostate, and thyroid. Rarely, myeloma, lymphoma, melanoma, astrocytoma, chondroblastoma, and primary sarcoma have been reported to metastasize to the soft tissue (Damron and Heiner 2000). Metastases at nodal sites should suggest a peripheral primary tumor (Fig. 28.33). As most of these are solitary lesions, they are often considered to be soft tissue sarcomas clinically. Ossification within colonic metastases, typically mucinous adenocarcinomas, has been reported frequently, including in the abdominal wall and psoas muscles (Stabler 1995). Most often, the imaging features are nonspecific in nature. Radiographs may demonstrate a soft tissue lesion. On US imaging, these may appear mixed echogenic with variable neovascularity. These lesions are often discovered incidentally on CT examinations. On MRI, these have poorly defined margins, hypointense signal on T1-weighted sequences, variably hyperintense signal on T2-weighted sequences, and enhance heterogeneously. Surrounding edema is a common feature. Patients with known or suspected malignant disease may, however, coincidentally have any of the benign or malignant soft tissue

masses detailed in this chapter, requiring the same analysis of clinical features and imaging appearances as in patients without known malignancy (Ulaner et al. 2013a, b).

Conclusion

An increased awareness of the nonspecific imaging appearances of many malignant soft tissue masses is required. A low threshold for recommending referral to a sarcoma service for consideration of biopsy is suggested. The age of the patient, location of the mass, clinical presentation, and preexisting pathologies must all be taken into consideration, along with the imaging appearances. The possibility of multiple lesions should be considered. Further imaging should also be performed where appropriate so that where possible, the characteristic appearances that allow a confident specific diagnosis to be made can be demonstrated. Previous imaging, where performed, should be retrieved and compared to assess previous imaging appearances and rate of growth. A specific diagnosis should only be offered when the imaging appearances are pathognomonic with no atypical features.

Where this is not achieved, the diagnosis of a nonspecific or indeterminate soft tissue mass is made (Wu and Hochman 2009). The referring clinician must be informed, so as to facilitate urgent referral to a soft tissue sarcoma service for biopsy.

References

Anderson SE, Hertel R, Johnston JO et al (2005) Latissimus dorsi tendinosis and tear: imaging features of a pseudotumor of the upper limb in five patients. AJR Am J Roentgenol 185:1145–1151

Arkun R, Argin M (2014) Pitfalls in MR imaging of musculoskeletal tumors. Semin Musculoskelet Radiol 18:63–78

Bancroft LW, Kransdorf MJ, Peterson JJ, O'Connor MI (2006) Benign fatty tumors: classification, clinical course, imaging appearance, and treatment. Skeletal Radiol 35:719–733

Boutin RD, Fritz RC, Steinbach LS (2002) Imaging of sports-related muscle injuries. Radiol Clin N Am 40:333–362

Chaabane S, Chelli-Bouaziz M, Jelassi H et al (2008) Idiopathic tumoral calcinosis. Acta Orthop Belg 74:837–845

Chandrasekar CR, Grimer RJ, Carter SR et al (2008) Elastofibroma dorsi: an uncommon benign pseudotumor. Sarcoma. doi:10.1155/2008/756565

Chun CW, Jee WH, Park HJ et al (2010) MRI features of skeletal muscle lymphoma. AJR Am J Roentgenol 195:1355–1360

Chung WJ, Chung HW, Shin MJ et al (2012) MRI to differentiate benign from malignant soft-tissue tumors of the extremities: a simplified systematic imaging approach using depth, size and heterogeneity of signal intensity. Br J Radiol 85:e831–e836

Damron TA, Heiner J (2000) Distant soft tissue metastases: a series of 30 new patients and 91 cases from the literature. Ann Surg Oncol 7:526–534

De Schepper AM, Ramon FA, Degryse HR (1992) Statistical analysis of MRI parameters predicting malignancy in 141 soft tissue masses. Rofo 156:587–591

Delaney-Sathy LO, Fessel DP, Jacobson JA et al (2000) Sonography of diabetic muscle infarction with MR imaging, CT, and pathologic correlation. AJR Am J Roentgenol 174:165–169

Dhillon M, Davies AM, Benham J et al (2004) Calcific myonecrosis: a report of ten new cases with an emphasis on MR imaging. Eur Radiol 14:1974–1979

Dinauer PA, Brixey CJ, Moncur JT et al (2007) Pathologic and MR imaging features of benign fibrous soft-tissue tumors in adults. Radiographics 27:173–187

Escobar C, Munker R, Thomas JO et al (2011) Update on desmoid tumors. Ann Oncol 23:562–569

Fletcher CD, Unni KK, Mertens F (eds) (2002) WHO classification of tumors: pathology and genetics of tumors of soft tissue and bone. IARC, Lyon

Foreman KL, Kransdorf MJ, O'Connor MI, Krishna M (2013) AIRP best cases in radiologic-pathologic correlation: maffucci syndrome. Radiographics 33:861–868

Gaskill T, Payne D, Brigman B (2010) Cryptococcal abscess imitating a soft-tissue sarcoma in an immunocompetent host: a case report. J Bone Joint Surg Am 92:1890–1893

Goldblum JR, Folpe AL, Weiss SW (2013a) Benign fibroblastic/myofibroblastic proliferations, including superficial fibromatosis. In: Enzinger and Weiss's soft tissue tumors, 6th edn. Elsevier Saunders, Philadelphia

Goldblum JR, Folpe AL, Weiss SW (2013b) Benign lipomatous tumors. In: Enzinger and Weiss's soft tissue tumors, 6th edn. Elsevier Saunders, Philadelphia

Goodwin RW, O'Donnell P, Saifuddin A (2007) MRI appearances of common benign soft-tissue tumors. Clin Radiol 62:843–853

Grimer RJ (2006) Size matters for sarcomas. Ann R Coll Surg Engl 88:519–524

Havitcioglu H, Tatari H, Baran O et al (2003) Calcium pyrophosphate dihydrate crystal deposition disease mimicking malignant soft tissue tumor. Knee Surg Sports Traumatol Arthrosc 11:263–266

Huang GS, Lee CH, Chan WP et al (2003) Localized nodular synovitis of the knee: MR imaging appearance and clinical correlates in 21 patients. AJR Am J Roentgenol 181:539–543

Iwasko N, Steinbach LS, Disler D et al (2002) Imaging findings in Mazabraud's syndrome: seven new cases. Skeletal Radiol 31:81–87

Jain V, Makwana GE, Bahri N et al (2012) The "dot in circle" sign on MRI in maduramycosis: a characteristic finding. J Clin Imaging Sci 2:66

Jonelle M, Petscavage-Thomas JM, Walker EA et al (2014) Soft-tissue myxomatous lesions: review of salient imaging features with pathologic comparison. Radiographics 34:964–980

Kapff PD, Hocken DB, Simpson RHW (1987) Elastofibroma of the hand. J Bone Joint Surg Br 69:468–469

Kato H, Kanematsu M, Watanabe H et al (2016) MR imaging findings of pilomatricomas: a radiological-pathological correlation. Acta Radiol 57:726–732

Kattapuram TM, Suri R, Rosol MS et al (2005) Idiopathic and diabetic skeletal muscle necrosis: evaluation by magnetic resonance imaging. Skeletal Radiol 34:203–209

Keppler-Noreuil KM, Sapp JC, Lindhurst MJ et al (2014) Clinical delineation and natural history of the PIK3CA-related overgrowth spectrum. Am J Med Genet A 164:1713–1733

Kim JY, Jung SA, Sung MS et al (2004) Extra-articular soft tissue ganglion cyst around the knee: focus on the associated findings. Eur Radiol 14:106–111

Kontogeorgakos VA, Martinez S, Dodd L, Brigman BE (2010) Extremity soft tissue sarcoma presented as hematomas. Arch Orthop Trauma Surg 130:1209–1214

Kransdorf MJ (1995) Benign soft-tissue tumors in a large referral population: distribution of specific diagnoses by age, sex, and location. AJR Am J Roentgenol 164:395–402

Kransdorf MJ, Murphey MD (2006) Vascular and lymphatic tumors. In: Imaging of soft tissue tumors, 2nd edn. Lippincott, Williams & Wilkins, Philadelphia

Lee JC, Thomas JM, Phillips S et al (2006) Aggressive fibromatosis: MRI features with pathologic correlation. AJR Am J Roentgenol 186:247–254

Lewis RJ, Ketcham AS (1973) Maffucci's syndrome: functional and neoplastic significance—case report and review of the literature. J Bone Joint Surg Am 55:1465–1479

Malghem J, Vande Berg BC, Lebon C et al (1998) Ganglion cysts of the knee: articular communication revealed by delayed radiography and CT after arthrography. AJR Am J Roentgenol 170:1579–1583

May DA, Disler DG, Jones EA et al (2000) Abnormal signal intensity in skeletal muscle at MR imaging: patterns, pearls, and pitfalls. Radiographics 20:S295–S315

McGuinness B, Wilson N, Doyle AJ (2007) The "penumbra sign" on T1-weighted MRI for differentiating musculoskeletal infection from tumor. Skeletal Radiol 36:417–421

Mellado JM, Bencardino JT (2005) Morel-Lavallée lesion: review with emphasis on MR imaging. Magn Reson Imaging Clin N Am 13:775–782

Murphey MD, McRae GA, Fanburg-Smith JC et al (2002) Imaging of soft tissue myxoma with emphasis on CT and MRI and comparison of radiologic and pathological findings. Radiology 225:215–224

Murphey MD, Rhee JH, Lewis RB et al (2008) Pigmented villonodular synovitis: radiologic-pathologic correlation. Radiographics 28:1493–1518

Naylor MF, Nascimento AG, Sherrick AD, McLeod RA (1996) Elastofibroma dorsi: radiologic findings in 12 patients. AJR Am J Roentgenol 167:683–687

Olsen KM, Chew FS (2006) Tumoral calcinosis: pearls, polemics, and alternative possibilities. Radiographics 26:871–885

Onishi Y, Kitajima K, Senda M et al (2011) FDG PET/CT imaging of elastofibroma dorsi. Skeletal Radiol 40:849–853

Otero S, Moskovic EC, Strauss DC et al (2015) Desmoid-type fibromatosis. Clin Radiol 70:1038–1045

Ozpolat B, Yazkan R, Yilmazer D et al (2008) Elastofibroma dorsi: report of a case with diagnostic features. J Ultrasound Med 27:287–291

Park JS, Ryu KN (2004) Hemophilic pseudotumor involving the musculoskeletal system: spectrum of radiologic findings. AJR Am J Roentgenol 183:55–61

Pasternak S, Wright BA, Walsh N (2007) Soft tissue amyloidoma of the extremities: report of a case and review of the literature. Am J Dermatopathol 29:152–155

Patel A, Davies AM, James SL (2015) Imaging of extremity soft tissue masses: pitfalls in diagnosis. Br J Hosp Med 76:344–352

Quinn SF, Erickson SJ, Dee PM et al (1991) MR imaging in fibromatosis: results in 26 patients with pathologic correlation. AJR Am J Roentgenol 156:539–542

Schaffer PR, Hale CS, Meehan SA, Shupack JL, Ramachandran S (2014) Adiposis dolorosa. Dermatol Online J 20(12) pii: 13030/qt1st6x3dm

Siegel MJ (2001) Magnetic resonance imaging of musculoskeletal soft tissue masses. Radiol Clin N Am 39:701–720

Sookur PA, Naraghi AM, Bleakney RR et al (2008) Accessory muscles: anatomy, symptoms, and radiologic evaluation. Radiographics 28:481–499

Sreenivas M, Nihal A, Ettles DF (2004) Chronic hematoma or soft-tissue neoplasm? A diagnostic dilemma. Arch Orthop Trauma Surg 124:495–497

Stabler J (1995) Case report: ossifying metastases from carcinoma of the large bowel demonstrated by bone scintigraphy. Clin Radiol 50:730–731

Sung MS, Kang HS, Suh JS et al (2000) Myxoid liposarcoma: appearance at MR imaging with histologic correlation. Radiographics 20:1007–1019

Teo HEL, Peh WCG, Shek TWH (2005) Case 84: desmoid tumor of the abdominal wall. Radiology 236:81–84

Tins BJ, Matthews C, Haddaway M et al (2013) Adiposis dolorosa (Dercum's disease): MRI and ultrasound appearances. Clin Radiol 68:1047–1053

Tyler P, Saifuddin A (2010) The imaging of myositis ossificans. Semin Musculoskelet Radiol 14:201–216

Ulaner G, Hwang S, Landa J et al (2013a) Musculoskeletal tumors and tumor-like conditions: common and avoidable pitfalls at imaging in patients with known or suspected cancer. Int Orthop 37:871–876

Ulaner G, Hwang S, Landa J et al (2013b) Musculoskeletal tumors and tumor-like conditions: common and avoidable pitfalls at imaging in patients with known or suspected cancer. Part B: malignant mimics of benign tumors. Int Orthop 37:877–882

Vilanova JC, Barcelo J, Smirniotopoulos JG et al (2004) Hemangioma from head to toe: MR imaging with pathologic correlation. Radiographics 24:367–385

Wu JS, Hochman MG (2009) Soft-tissue tumors and tumorlike lesions: a systematic imaging approach. Radiology 253:297–316

Yu JS, Chung C, Recht M et al (1997) MR imaging of tophaceous gout. AJR Am J Roentgenol 168:523–527

Esther H.Y. Hung and James F. Griffith

Contents

29.1	**Introduction**	581
29.2	**Ultrasound Imaging of Soft Tissue Masses: General Principles**	582
29.3	**Hematoma and Hemorrhagic Solid Soft Tissue Neoplasm: Mimics**	584
29.4	**Non-tumoral Conditions Which May Mimic Tumors**	585
29.4.1	Healing Muscle Tear	585
29.4.2	Delayed Onset Muscle Soreness	588
29.4.3	Anomalous Muscles	589
29.4.4	Diabetic Muscle Infarction	589
29.5	**Common Tumors that Mimic Other Common Tumors**	589
29.5.1	Slow-Flow Vascular Malformation	589
29.5.2	Atypical Appearing Lipoma	591
29.5.3	Nerve Sheath Tumor Versus Vascular Leiomyoma	591
29.5.4	Atypical Nerve Sheath Tumors	592
Conclusion		594
References		594

E.H.Y. Hung, MBChB, FRCR
J.F. Griffith, MD, MRCP, FRCR (✉)
Department of Imaging and Interventional Radiology,
The Chinese University of Hong Kong, Prince of
Wales Hospital, Hong Kong, SAR, China
e-mail: hunghiuyee@yahoo.com.hk;
hhy707@ha.org.hk; griffith@cuhk.edu.hk

Abbreviation

US   Ultrasound

29.1 Introduction

Soft tissue tumor is a common clinical entity with a benign-malignant ratio of approximately 100:1 (Hung et al. 2014). The vast majority of soft issue tumors is located in the subcutaneous tissue layer, is small to medium-sized, and presents as a readily palpable lump. It is often not possible to make a definitive diagnosis on the nature of the mass based on clinical grounds alone, and more importantly, it is often not possible to convincingly exclude malignancy. As such, many soft tissue tumors are referred for imaging assessment soon after clinical presentation. Since the mid-1990s, high-resolution ultrasound (US) has been increasingly used as the first-line investigation to evaluate soft tissue tumors (Bureau et al. 1998; Fornage 1999; Hwang and Adler 2005; Chiou et al. 2007; McNally 2011). The application of high-resolution US imaging in the evaluation of soft tissue tumor has now extended far beyond differentiating whether a mass is solid or cystic.

29.2 Ultrasound Imaging of Soft Tissue Masses: General Principles

With the affinity to accurately discriminate tissue layers, high spatial and moderate contrast resolution, real-time imaging capability, the ability to evaluate lesion compressibility, and determine vascular flow as well as directly relate the US imaging findings to the clinical symptoms, high-resolution US is an ideal imaging modality to initially evaluate most soft tissue lumps and bumps. It can help to (1) confirm the presence of a tumor; (2) determine its anatomical location, extent, and its relationship to the investing fascia, neurovascular bundle, and other tissues; (3) allow recognition of a specific tumor type in most cases; and (4) determine with greater clarity the need for percutaneous biopsy or additional imaging such as magnetic resonance imaging (MRI) or clinical follow-up.

Routine US-guided biopsy of all soft tissue tumors is neither practical nor cost-effective and increases the likelihood of patient anxiety and inadvertent harm. Such a policy is not warranted given that the US imaging appearances of most tissue tumors are sufficiently specific to allow one to make a definitive or near-definitive diagnosis based on US imaging alone. The US imaging appearances of most of the common soft tissue masses have been described (Fornage and Tassin 1991; Paltiel et al. 2000; Bedi and Davidson 2001; Ahuja et al. 2003; Choong 2004; Inampudi et al. 2004; Middleton et al. 2004; Reynolds et al. 2004; Chiou et al. 2009; Dubois and Alison 2010; Kim et al. 2010; Paunipagar et al. 2010; Haun et al. 2011; Kubiena et al. 2013; Yuan et al. 2012; Griffith 2014). US imaging diagnosis of soft tissue tumors is formulated not just on the basis of one or two US imaging signs. Instead, the US imaging diagnosis is based on a spectrum of clinical and imaging features (Table 29.1) and afforded different diagnostic weighting depending on the particular clinical context. In most cases, this will allow a definitive or near-definitive diagnosis to be made without the need for percutaneous biopsy or fine needle aspiration for cytology (FNAC).

Table 29.1 (**a**) Pertinent clinical factors that should be considered during US imaging of a soft tissue mass. (**b**) US imaging factors that should be specifically considered

(a) Pertinent clinical questions to ask
How long has the mass been present for?
Is the mass growing, static in size, or becoming smaller?
Is the mass painful or tender?
Is there more than one mass?
Has there been an injury to this area?
Is there a known malignancy?

	(b) US imaging considerations
Location	Truncal, proximal, or distal appendicular location Dermal, subcutaneous, fascial, subfascial, intermuscular, intramuscular, submuscular, juxtacortical, periosteal, arising from joint, subungual
Appearances	Mass-like, infiltrative, or intrinsic swelling Size, shape, well-defined or ill-defined, lobulation, track, encapsulation, internal echogenicity, internal architecture (linear echoes, laminated or whorled pattern, linear bands, clefts, speckles, moving echoes, comet pain artifacts, calcification (mild, moderate, or heavy), cystic areas, septae, acoustic transmission)
Consistency	Compressible soft, firm, or hard
Color Doppler imaging	Presence or absence of hyperemia, degree of hyperemia, peripheral or central pattern or mixed, organized or chaotic vascular pattern, arterial, venous or cavernous.
Surrounding soft tissues	Relationship to skin, subcutaneous tissues, investing fascia, muscle, bone, tendon, tendon sheath, nerves, joints, muscle fascia Edema, swelling and hyperemia of surrounding soft tissues Tissue atrophy

In a 12-year retrospective review of 714 superficial soft tissue tumors that underwent US imaging examination in our hospital, 35% of tumors underwent surgical excision or percutaneous biopsy, and a correct specific US imaging diagnosis had been made in 77% of these excised tumors (Hung et al. 2014). In clinical practice, the diagnostic capability of US imaging is likely to be higher than 77%, since the study design is negatively biased, given that those tumors with nonspecific appearances were more likely to undergo surgical excision or biopsy for clarification. Clinical follow-up of those cases without histological confirmation showed that not a solitary malignant tumor was missed or misdiagnosed over that time period. Regarding differentiation of benign from malignant, US imaging correctly identified 16 of 17 malignant tumors and 695 of 697 benign tumors, according to histopathological confirmation and clinical follow-up. The sensitivity and specificity of US imaging in identifying malignancy for superficial soft tissue tumors was 94.1% and 99.7%, respectively. One dermatofibrosarcoma protuberans was misdiagnosed as a nerve sheath tumor in the cohort with pathology. Two suspected metastases were shown to be benign on subsequent follow-up in the cohort without pathology. These were the only three cases in which US imaging was incorrect in distinguishing malignant from benign.

A golden caveat to follow when performing US imaging of musculoskeletal tumors is to not label a tumor as benign, unless one can put a specific label on that tumor, based on the US imaging appearances or duration. In other words, one can correctly label a tumor as benign if one can say, based on the clinical and US imaging appearances, that it is, for example, a nerve sheath tumor, lipoma, fibromatosis, or giant cell tumor of tendon sheath. Also tumors which have been present for a long time (i.e., for more than a year) without change in clinical size or appearance can be happily labeled as benign without a specific diagnosis, provided there are no aggressive features such as infiltration on US examination, and it is reasonable to continue following up these tumors clinically without histological confirmation.

The presence of rapid clinical growth, a known primary tumor, a medium-sized to large tumor, deep tumor location, and moderate to severe intra-tumoral hyperemia should all raise the suspicion of a malignant soft tissue tumor. These are all suggestive but not absolute criteria of tumor aggressiveness. Over and above these criteria, however,

Table 29.2 Features suspicious of malignant superficial soft tissue masses

Rapid clinical growth
Known primary tumor
Moderate to large tumor size
Moderate to severe intra-tumoral hyperemia
Absence of recognized US imaging features of specific benign tumor type (e.g., lipoma, nerve sheath tumor)

the single most important criteria for diagnosis of a malignant tumor is lack of similarity with the recognized US imaging appearances of any benign soft tissue tumor. In other words, if a tumor does not look like any recognized benign soft tissue tumor and particularly if it has additional suspicious features (e.g., large size, rapid growth, deep location, chaotic-type hyperemia), this should prompt one to consider a malignant tumor (Table 29.2). One can readily appreciate, therefore, the importance of knowing the range of US imaging appearances of benign soft tissue tumors.

Radiologists need to be aware of the level of certainty with which specific diagnoses can be made, based on the US imaging appearances and clinical presentation. A large number of the patients who present with a soft tissue lump are concerned about the possibility of malignancy. Immediate reassurance at the time of US examination greatly alleviates this anxiety. Such reassurance can, however, only be provided if the attending radiologist is able to make a specific diagnosis based on US imaging appearances alone. The radiologist should be familiar with the specific tumor types that can be diagnosed with a quite high level of certainty on US imaging and recognize that even with these particular tumors, pitfalls may occasionally arise in that these tumors may present with atypical US imaging appearances.

Following US examination, one should undertake percutaneous biopsy or recommend excisional biopsy only for those selected tumors in which one is both (1) unsure of the diagnosis and (2) have a moderate to high suspicion of malignancy. For those tumors in which one is unsure and have a low index of suspicion, one can either follow up with repeat US imaging or proceed to additional imaging. The remainder of this chapter will focus on (1) hematoma and hemorrhagic solid soft tissue neoplasms which have a propensity for mimicking each other, (2) nontumoral conditions which may mimic tumors on US imaging, and (3) US imaging appearances of some common tumors that can mimic those of other common tumors.

29.3 Hematoma and Hemorrhagic Solid Soft Tissue Neoplasm: Mimics

Distinguishing between hematoma and hemorrhagic soft tissue tumor is sometimes not clear-cut. Firstly, trauma may induce bleeding in a previously unrecognized soft tissue neoplasm, leading to the misdiagnosis of a hematoma. Alternatively, the disorganized and abnormal vasculature of soft tissue neoplasm can result in

either spontaneous hemorrhage or bleeding during physiological activity. A large hemorrhagic component is a recognized feature of many soft tissue sarcomas such as angiosarcoma, synovial sarcoma, epitheloid sarcoma, rhabdomyosarcoma, and malignant fibrous histiocytoma (Niimi et al. 2006) (Fig. 29.1). Secondly, particularly in patients with a coagulopathy or those on anticoagulant or antiplatelet therapy, hematoma can occur during physiological physical exertion or even during a trivial event such as coughing or sneezing. Intramuscular hematoma can also rarely occur *de novo* in the absence of any recognizable trauma or risk factors. Absence of a specific precipitating cause should not fully negate the possibility of soft tissue hematoma.

Organizing hematoma can mimic a hemorrhagic soft tissue neoplasm through progressive growth over a few weeks or months. Hematoma organizes through fibroblastic proliferation and endothelial cell ingrowth into the periphery of the blood clot, with removal of necrotic cellular elements by

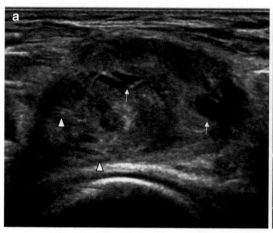
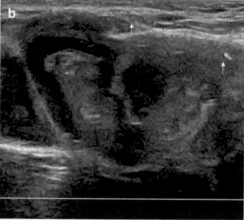
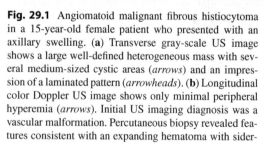

Fig. 29.1 Angiomatoid malignant fibrous histiocytoma in a 15-year-old female patient who presented with an axillary swelling. (**a**) Transverse gray-scale US image shows a large well-defined heterogeneous mass with several medium-sized cystic areas (*arrows*) and an impression of a laminated pattern (*arrowheads*). (**b**) Longitudinal color Doppler US image shows only minimal peripheral hyperemia (*arrows*). Initial US imaging diagnosis was a vascular malformation. Percutaneous biopsy revealed features consistent with an expanding hematoma with sider-

ophagic aggregates and iron encrustation. There was no evidence of malignancy. (**c**) Axial GRE MR image shows a well-defined heterogeneous mass with areas of hemosiderin deposition (*arrows*) suggestive of chronic blood product deposition. Contrast-enhanced MRI (not shown) shows no intrinsic enhancement. MRI diagnosis was an expanding hematoma. (**d**) Follow-up gray-scale US image after 1 month shows mild interval increase in tumor size. Surgical excision revealed an angiomatoid malignant fibrous histiocytoma

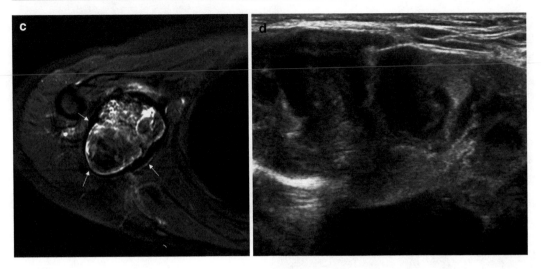

Fig. 29.1 (continued)

phagocytosis and reabsorption of serous elements. The formation of a fibrous capsule around the hematoma limits subsequent vascular ingrowth and hence absorption. If further bleeding occurs deep to the fibrous capsule, the hematoma can expand and simulate a growing soft tissue tumor such as a sarcoma (Reid 1980; Ryu et al. 2011).

The imaging features of organizing hematoma and hemorrhagic soft tissue neoplasm can overlap considerably (Imaizumi et al. 2002; Taïeb et al. 2009; Ryu et al. 2011; Carra et al. 2014). The imaging appearances of a hematoma vary with chronicity. Fresh hematoma typically presents as a well-defined mass hyperechoic to adjacent muscle, with a multi-laminated whorled appearance, containing small cystic areas and minimal or no marginal hyperemia. The degree and maturity of marginal hyperemia increases as the hematoma organizes. Both peripheral and central vascularity may be seen on color Doppler US imaging in a well-organized hematoma (Fig. 29.2), making differentiation from soft tissue sarcoma difficult, especially when the hematoma is large.

A history of past trauma, a slowly evolving mass, involvement of the more superficial tissues, and a location overlying a bony prominence have all been identified as features that can help differentiating tumor from organizing hematoma (Okada et al. 2001 ; Hung et al. 2014); though in some circumstances, some or all of these features can be absent. One needs to be aware of the US imaging appearances of hematoma and consider it as a differential in certain soft tissue masses. Usually, close follow-up US imaging to assure regression is sufficient though occasionally, particularly with suspected expanding hematoma, tissue confirmation via biopsy may be necessary. In addition, gradient-echo T2-weighted MRI can help confirm the presence of hemosiderin.

29.4 Non-tumoral Conditions Which May Mimic Tumors

29.4.1 Healing Muscle Tear

Occasionally, muscle tears can occur in the absence of any specific injury. Reparative healing of such tears can simulate a soft tissue sarcoma (Walker et al. 2013). MRI or positron emission tomography (PET) imaging shows contrast enhancement or metabolic activity, respectively, due to ongoing muscle repair which may add to confusion through simulation of a malignant tumor (Fig. 29.3). These lesions will appear on

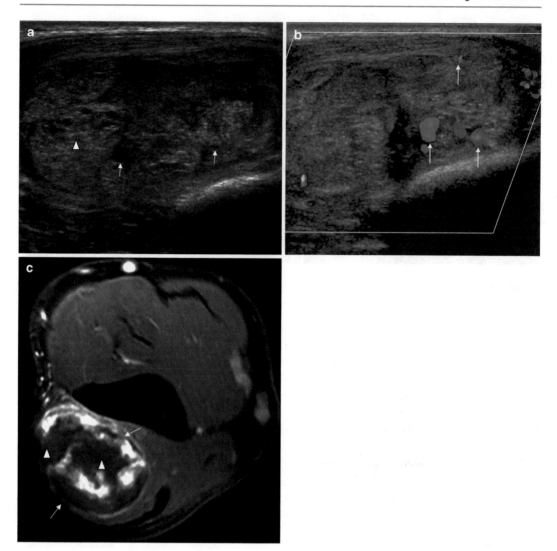

Fig. 29.2 Organizing hematoma in a 47-year-old man who presented with a slow-growing mass in the arm. (**a**) Longitudinal gray-scale US image shows a well-defined intramuscular echogenic mass with small cystic areas (*arrows*) and a mildly laminated pattern (*arrowhead*). (**b**) Color Doppler US image shows the presence of mild peripheral and intrinsic vascularity (*arrows*). A spontaneous hematoma was considered as likely diagnosis on US imaging though the appearances were suspicious enough to warrant further investigation. (**c**) Axial contrast-enhanced fat-suppressed T1-W MR image shows a moderately-enhancing tumor (*arrows*) with large areas devoid of enhancement (*arrowheads*). No hemosiderin was evident. A soft tissue sarcoma was suspected. US-guided biopsy revealed an organizing hematoma

US imaging as irregular hyperechoic masses with marginal hyperemia and edema. One can get the impression of the mass (due to healing tear) communicating with, rather than displacing the adjacent muscle (Fig. 29.3). The original muscle architecture is often discernible within the mass. Usually, no discrete tear is present. As always, being aware of this entity and correlating the clinical history and US imaging findings help one to make this diagnosis. US imaging is particularly helpful, as it usually allows one to appreciate the underlying, albeit altered, muscle architecture more readily than with other imaging modalities and has the dynamic component where one may be able to see the healing muscle tear move with muscle contraction.

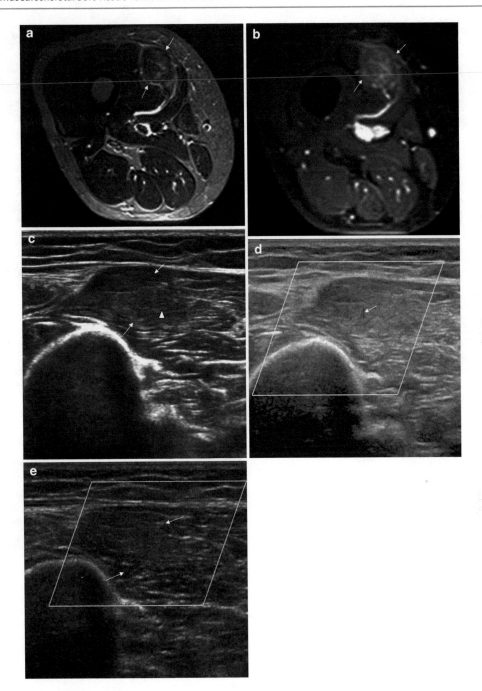

Fig. 29.3 Muscle tear in a 61-year-old woman who presented with a 1-month history of a painful medial thigh swelling. There was no history of trauma. (**a**) Axial fat-suppressed T2-W MR image shows a hyperintense mass (*arrows*) within the vastus medialis muscle. (**b**) Axial contrast-enhanced fat-suppressed T1-W MR image shows the intramuscular lesion to be hyperemic with moderate contrast enhancement (*arrows*). (**c**) Transverse gray-scale US image shows an ill-defined medium-sized swelling (*arrows*) within the vastus medialis with some preserva-tion of the internal muscular architecture (*arrowhead*). (**d**) Axial color Doppler US image shows minimal intrinsic hyperemia (*arrow*). A muscle tear was considered, but the lesion was still sufficiently suspicious to warrant a biopsy. US-guided biopsy revealed focal infiltration of skeletal muscle by benign-appearing fibroblastic tissue. (**e**) Follow-up transverse gray-scale US image taken 2 month later shows moderate resolution of the vastus medialis lesion with reduced muscle swelling (*arrows*). Overall appearances were compatible with a healing muscle tear

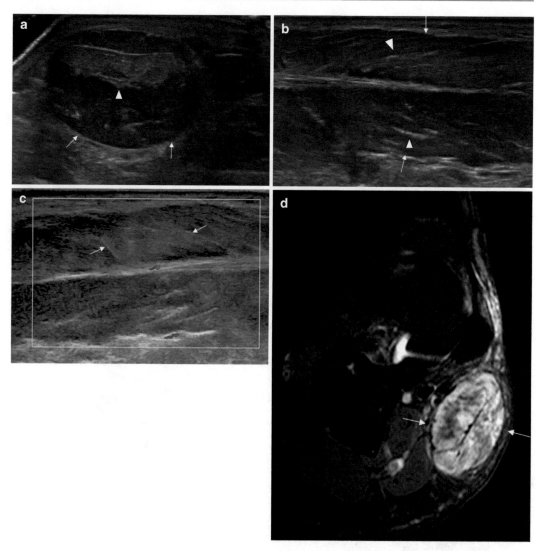

Fig. 29.4 Delayed onset of muscle soreness (DOMS) in a 55-year-old man who presented with painful medial foot swelling 1 day after strenous exercise. (**a**) Transverse gray-scale US image shows severe diffuse swelling of the abductor hallucis longus muscle (*arrows*) with ill-defined hyperechoic areas (*arrowhead*). (**b**) Longitudinal gray-scale US image shows diffuse muscle swelling (*arrows*) without a discrete muscle tear. Note the preservation of the normal muscular fibrillary pattern (*arrowheads*). (**c**) Longitudinal color Doppler US image shows moderate diffuse muscle hyperemia (*arrows*). (**d**) Coronal fat-suppressed T2-W MR image shows severe diffuse swelling and edema of the adductor hallucis longus muscle (*arrows*). The entire muscle appears hyperintense

29.4.2 Delayed Onset Muscle Soreness

Another pseudotumor of muscle one may encounter is delayed onset muscle soreness (DOMS). DOMS presents 12–24 h after unaccustomed strenuous exercise. This history of vigorous unaccustomed exercise must be present to make a diagnosis of DOMS. One or more than one muscle can be affected. On US imaging, the affected muscles are diffusely swollen with areas of geographical hyperechogenicity, preserved muscle architecture, no calcification, and mild to moderate hyperemia. No discrete

muscle tear is evident. Considerable soft tissue edema around the swollen muscles may
be present. The typical clinical presentation
and appreciation of muscle echotexture usually
allows differentiation of this entity from soft tissue tumors (Fig. 29.4). The muscle swelling and
edema gradually settles over the ensuing weeks
with no residual sequelae.

29.4.3 Anomalous Muscles

Although common in the musculoskeletal system, anomalous or hypertrophied muscles hardly
ever cause difficulty with regard to simulating
sarcoma, as they will show the typical unmistak-
able US imaging (or MRI) appearances and shape
of skeletal muscle.

29.4.4 Diabetic Muscle Infarction

Diabetic muscle infarction typically gives rise to
a focal ill-defined swelling and hypoechogenicity
within muscle, which may be misinterpreted as a
muscle metastatic deposit or a sarcoma (Baker et al.
2012). The intrinsic muscle architecture is usually
visible, though disrupted, within this edematous or
mass-like area. One may see surrounding muscle
or subcutaneous edema. Intralesional hemorrhage,
fluid collection, or gas may occur, if a large muscle area is infarcted. Initially, the affected area is
hypovascular relative to the surrounding muscle
but later become hyperemic. The typical patient
is middle-aged to elderly, with poorly controlled
diabetes mellitus associated with nephropathy,
neuropathy, retinopathy, and arteriopathy, who
presents with an acute onset of muscle pain and
swelling. This pain subsides after about a week,
at which stage a clinically palpable muscle mass
may be present, simulating a sarcoma (Fig. 29.5).
The diagnosis is made by recognizing the typical US imaging appearances in a suitably at risk
patient. Serial US examination can help confirm
the diagnosis, with progressive peripheral hyperemia, clearer delineation, and slow regression of
the area of infarcted muscle.

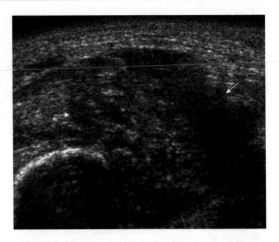

Fig. 29.5 Diabetic muscle infarction in a 35-year-old
man with diabetic nephropathy who presented with gradual onset of thigh swelling over a few days. Transverse
gray-scale US image shows an ill-defined localized swelling within the vastus intermedius and vastus medialis
muscles (*arrows*). Moderate to severe hyperemia is demonstrated on color Doppler US imaging (not shown). In
this clinical context, the appearances are consistent with
diabetic muscle infarction. The lesion gradually resolved
after 2 months

29.5 Common Tumors that Mimic Other Common Tumors

29.5.1 Slow-Flow Vascular Malformation

The US imaging accuracy for making a diagnosis of a slow-flow vascular malformation is
high, when one sees the typical appearances of
a hypervascular mass with large dilated vascular channels and phleboliths. In our experience,
the sensitivity and specificity of US imaging in
making a firm diagnosis of a subcutaneous vascular malformation is 73% and 98%, respectively
(Hung et al. 2014). Most errors occur when the
vascular malformations are capillary or venous
cavernous in type. Capillary vascular malformations are mainly comprised of echogenic connective tissue stroma, which histologically contains
many small capillaries too small to be resolved
on US imaging. These capillary-type vascular
malformations are sometimes misdiagnosed as
lipoma (Fig. 29.6).

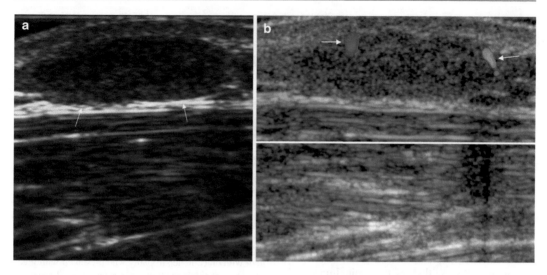

Fig. 29.6 Slow-flow vascular malformation with predominant stromal pattern in a 49-year-old man who presented with a subcutaneous soft tissue leg mass. (**a**) Longitudinal gray-scale US image shows a well-defined partially compressible hypoechoic mass (*arrows*) in the subcutaneous layer without deep extension. (**b**) Longitudinal color Doppler US image shows mild intrinsic hyperemia (*arrows*). The initial US imaging diagnosis was a subcutaneous angiolipoma. Subsequent histology revealed a capillary-type vascular malformation

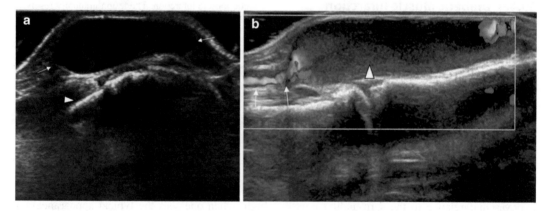

Fig. 29.7 Venous vascular malformation in a 55-year-old woman who presented with dorsal foot swelling, with fluctuation in size over the past couple of years. (**a**) Longitudinal gray-scale US image shows a well-defined cystic mass (*arrows*) overlying the tarsometatarsal junction. Posterior acoustic enhancement is present (*arrowhead*). (**b**) Longitudinal color Doppler US image shows a vessel (*arrows*) supplying the lesion and moving echoes (*arrowhead*) within the lesion on real-time imaging, all consistent with a slow-flow vascular malformation. The lesion was proven pathologically to be a venous vascular malformation. Slow-flow venous vascular malformations may sometimes mimic a cystic lesion such as a ganglion cyst or other cystic-type masses such as a myxoma

Cavernous-type venous vascular malformation may manifest as a dilated cystic-type space or spaces without detectable vascularity on color Doppler US imaging. These lesions are sometimes misdiagnosed as ganglion cysts. Very slow intravascular flow is often more readily appreciable on real-time gray-scale US than on color Doppler imaging. Slow vascular flow is seen on gray-scale US imaging as slow moving echoes or speckles due to red cell aggregation (Fig. 29.7). To observe this gray-scale effect, hold the transducer steady over the lesion with minimal transducer pressure and look carefully for any moving echoes within the cystic component of the lesion. Also, the majority of ganglia are anechoic and noncompressible, while the cavernous spaces of slow-flow vascular malformations tend to be more echo-poor rather than anechoic and are often compressible.

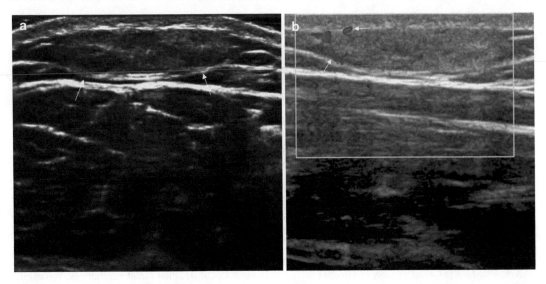

Fig. 29.8 Angiolipoma in a 51-year-old man who presented with 3-year history of arm swelling. (**a**) Longitudinal gray-scale US image shows a well-defined, slightly heterogeneous, partially compressible echogenic subcutaneous mass (*arrows*). (**b**) Longitudinal color Doppler US image shows mild peripheral hyperemia (*arrows*). The differential diagnoses were a slow-flow capillary-type vascular malformation or angiolipoma. Subsequent histology confirmed angiolipoma

29.5.2 Atypical Appearing Lipoma

In our experience, the accuracy of US imaging in diagnosing superficial lipoma is high with a sensitivity and specificity of 95% and 94%, respectively (Hung et al. 2014). This high level of accuracy applies particularly to superficial lipoma but also to a lesser degree, subfascial lipoma. The diagnosis of lipoma is based on a constellation of findings, including a well-encapsulated oblong compressible mass with fine linear striations parallel to the skin and with an echogenicity similar to fat. However, the echogenicity of lipoma is variable, depending on the degree of cellularity, fat-water content, as well as atypical features such as fat necrosis, fibrosis, and calcification. A small number of lipomas may be more hypoechoic than usual, without the obvious typical thin linear striations running parallel to the skin surface. In retrospect, even for these tumors, the US imaging appearances of lipoma are still usually present, though more subtle than one usually encounters. These more atypical superficial lipomas may be misdiagnosed as slow-flow vascular malformations or epidermoid cysts (Fig. 29.8).

29.5.3 Nerve Sheath Tumor Versus Vascular Leiomyoma

Both of these tumors occur adjacent to the neurovascular bundle and are therefore open to misinterpretation. The classical US imaging appearance of a nerve sheath tumor with thickening of the entering and exiting nerves is not invariably present in nerve sheath tumor arising from small peripheral nerves. In this instance, the US imaging description of a small well-defined hypoechoic mass with internal hypoechoic areas, mild acoustic enhancement, and moderate hyperemia could well apply to either a nerve sheath tumor or a vascular leiomyoma (Fig. 29.9). Both these lesions occur along neurovascular bundles, further adding to the confusion. Nerve sheath tumors arising from small peripheral nerves and vascular leiomyomas may therefore be mistaken for one another. The main distinguishing feature recognized to date is that vascular leiomyomas tend to have intrinsic linear vessels converging to a single point in the tumor on color Doppler US imaging. This is known as "vascular convergence" (Park et al. 2012).

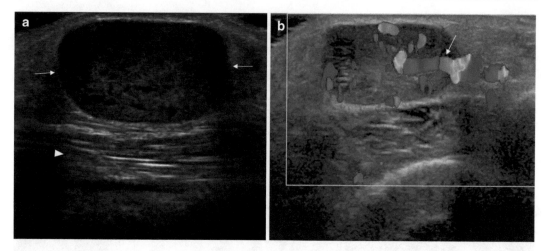

Fig. 29.9 Vascular leiomyoma in a 46-year-old patient who presented with a 6-month history of a lump in the leg. (a) Transverse gray-scale US image shows a well-defined hypoechoic mass (*arrows*) with mild internal heterogeneity and posterior enhancement (*arrowhead*) in the antero- lateral aspect of the lower leg. (b) Transverse color Doppler US image shows moderate intrinsic vascularity that converges to a single point eccentrically (*arrow*). The lesion was initially considered to be a nerve sheath tumor but was later proven to be a vascular leiomyoma

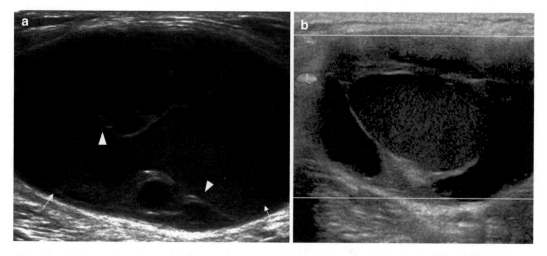

Fig. 29.10 Ancient schwannoma in a 56-year-old woman who presented with an enlarging arm mass. (a) Transverse gray-scale US image shows a cystic lesion (*arrows*) with a few internal septations (*arrowheads*) close to the median nerve. (b) Color Doppler US image shows no significant intrinsic vascularity. Ancient schwannoma with a completely cystic component can sometimes be difficult to differentiate from other cystic lesions such as a ganglion cyst, especially when it is arising from a small nerve, so that there is no visible entering or exiting nerve

29.5.4 Atypical Nerve Sheath Tumors

A small percentage of nerve tumors can either show no internal vascularity on color Doppler US imaging or else possess a purely cystic component as in "ancient schwannoma." Appearances of both of these tumor types are open to misinterpretation. Nerve sheath tumor without apparent vascularity may be misdiagnosed as a fibroma or granuloma on US imaging. Alternatively, purely or partially cystic nerve sheath tumors may be diagnosed as ganglia or myxoma (Fig. 29.10). The clue to the correct diagnosis in both these instances is demonstrable continuity with the parent nerve. The differentiation may be difficult if no entering or exiting nerve can be identified. Cystic degeneration is more commonly seen in schwannoma but can also occur in neurofibroma. Diffuse neurofibroma, which is mostly sporadic, has a 10% association with neurofibromatosis and is a recognized US imaging pitfall. Diffuse neurofibroma appears as diffuse echogenic thickening of the skin, subcutaneous tissue, or muscles, with mild to moderate hyperemia, and may be misdiagnosed as angiolipoma, soft tissue infection, or edema (Figs. 29.11 and 29.12).

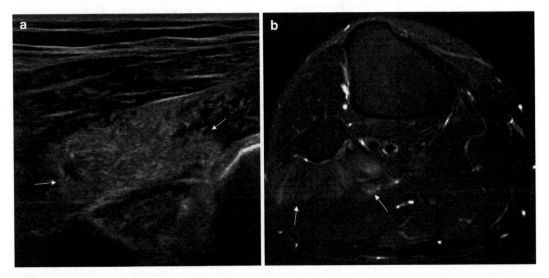

Fig. 29.11 Diffuse neurofibroma in a 45-year-old man who presented with nonspecific calf discomfort. (**a**) Transverse gray-scale US image shows a poorly-defined hyperechoic area (*arrows*) within the soleus muscle laterally. No discrete mass is present on US imaging. Note the abrupt transition between normal-looking hypoechoic muscle and the hyperechoic lesion. (**b**) Axial fat-suppressed T2-W MR image shows an infiltrative area of T2 hyperintensity (*arrows*) in the posterior compartment of the leg. The initial differential diagnosis was muscle edema due to a focal myositis. US-guided biopsy revealed a diffuse neurofibroma

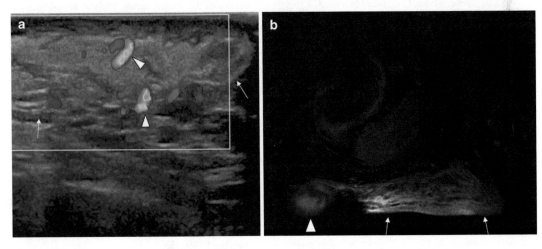

Fig. 29.12 Diffuse neurofibroma in a 17-year-old patient with neurofibromatosis. (**a**) Transverse US image shows a poorly-defined hyperechoic subcutaneous soft tissue thickening (*arrows*) over the posterolateral chest wall with moderate hyperemia (*arrowheads*). The lesion was initially diagnosed as angiolipoma but on biopsy was shown to be a diffuse neurofibroma. (**b**) Axial contrast-enhanced digital subtraction T1-W MR image shows reticular-like enhancement (*arrows*) in the subcutaneous tissue with a more discrete nodular mass (*arrowhead*) more medially. This abnormality was due to diffuse neurofibroma

Conclusion

As radiologists become more familiar with the varied appearances of soft tissue masses, US imaging is becoming more accurate at allowing a specific diagnosis of most soft tissue masses, and particularly superficial soft tissue tumors, based on the US imaging appearances alone. Being able to provide a specific label to a soft tissue tumor greatly optimizes the clinical efficiency of US imaging. Similarly, awareness of both the common and varied US imaging appearances of benign soft tissue tumors allows one to isolate with greatly clarity, the likelihood of a more sinister lesion which does not fit into a recognizable benign tumor pattern and which warrants either further investigation, biopsy, or imaging follow-up. In this chapter, we have presented some of the common pitfalls and mimics of soft tissue tumors that one may encounter during US imaging in routine clinical practice.

References

Ahuja A, Richards P, Wong K et al (2003) Accuracy of high-resolution sonography compared with magnetic resonance imaging in the diagnosis of head and neck venous vascular malformations. Clin Radiol 58:869–875

Baker J, Demertzis J, Rhodes N et al (2012) Diabetic musculoskeletal complications and their imaging mimics. Radiographics 32:1959–1974

Bedi D, Davidson D (2001) Plantar fibromatosis: most common sonographic appearance and variations. J Clin Ultrasound 29:499–505

Bureau N, Cardinal E, Chhem R (1998) Ultrasound of soft tissue masses. Semin Musculoskelet Radiol 2:283–298

Carra B, Bui-Mansfield L, O'Brien S et al (2014) Sonography of musculoskeletal soft-tissue masses: techniques, pearls, and pitfalls. AJR Am J Roentgenol 202:1281–1290

Chiou H, Chou Y, Chiou S et al (2007) High-resolution ultrasonography in superficial soft tissue tumors. J Med Ultrasound 15:152–174

Chiou H, Chou Y, Chiu S et al (2009) Differentiation of benign and malignant superficial soft-tissue masses using grayscale and color Doppler ultrasonography. J Chin Med Assoc 72:307–315

Choong K (2004) Sonographic appearance of subcutaneous angiolipomas. J Ultrasound Med 23:715–717

Dubois J, Alison M (2010) Vascular anomalies: what a radiologist needs to know. Pediatr Radiol 40:895–905

Fornage B, Tassin G (1991) Sonographic appearances of superficial soft tissue lipomas. J Clin Ultrasound 19:215–220

Fornage B (1999) Soft tissue masses: the underutilization of sonography. Semin Musculoskelet Radiol 3:115–133

Griffith J (2014) Soft tissue and bone tumors. In: Diagnostic ultrasound. Musculoskeletal, 1st edn. Elsevier/Amirsys, Philadelphia

Haun D, Cho J, Kettner N (2011) Symptomatic plantar fibroma with a unique sonographic appearance. J Clin Ultrasound 40:112–114

Hung E, Griffith J, Hung Ng A et al (2014) Ultrasound of musculoskeletal soft-tissue tumors superficial to the investing fascia. AJR Am J Roentgenol 202:W532–W540

Hwang S, Adler R (2005) Sonographic evaluation of the musculoskeletal soft tissue masses. Ultrasound Q 21:259–270

Imaizumi S, Morita T, Ogose A et al (2002) Soft tissue sarcoma mimicking chronic hematoma: value of magnetic resonance imaging in differential diagnosis. J Orthop Sci 7:33–37

Inampudi P, Jacobson J, Fessell D et al (2004) Soft-tissue lipomas: accuracy of sonography in diagnosis with pathologic correlation. Radiology 233:763–767

Kim H, Kim S, Lee S et al (2010) Subcutaneous epidermal inclusion cysts: ultrasound (US) and MR imaging findings. Skeletal Radiol 40:1415–1419

Kubiena H, Entner T, Schmidt M et al (2013) Peripheral neural sheath tumors (PNST)–what a radiologist should know. Eur J Radiol 82:51–55

McNally E (2011) The development and clinical applications of musculoskeletal ultrasound. Skeletal Radiol 401:223–1231

Middleton W, Patel V, Teefey S et al (2004) Giant cell tumors of the tendon sheath: analysis of sonographic findings. AJR Am J Roentgenol 183:337–339

Niimi R, Matsumine A, Kusuzaki K et al (2006) Soft-tissue sarcoma mimicking large haematoma: a report of two cases and review of the literature. J Orthop Surg (Hong Kong) 14:90–95

Okada K, Sugiyama T, Kato H (2001) Chronic expanding hematoma mimicking soft tissue neoplasm. J Clin Oncol 19:2971–2972

Paltiel H, Burrows P, Kozakewich H et al (2000) Soft-tissue vascular anomalies: utility of US for diagnosis. Radiology 214:747–754

Park H, Kim S, Lee S et al (2012) Sonographic appearances of soft tissue angioleiomyomas: differences from other circumscribed soft tissue hypervascular tumors. J Ultrasound Med 31:1589–1595

Paunipagar B, Griffith J, Rasalkar D et al (2010) Ultrasound features of deep-seated lipomas. Insights Imaging 1:149–153

Reid J (1980) Chronic expanding hematomas. A clinico-pathologic entity. JAMA 244:2441–2442

Reynolds D, Jacobson J, Inampudi P et al (2004) Sonographic characteristics of peripheral nerve sheath tumors. AJR Am J Roentgenol 182:741–744

Ryu J, Jin W, Kim G (2011) Sonographic appearances of small organizing hematomas and thrombi mimicking superficial soft tissue tumors. J Ultrasound Med 30:1431–1436

Taïeb S, Penel N, Vanseymortier L et al (2009) Soft tissue sarcomas or intramuscular haematomas? Eur J Radiol 72:44–49

Walker E, Brian P, Longo V et al (2013) Dilemmas in distinguishing between tumor and the posttraumatic lesion with surgical or pathologic correlation. Clin Sports Med 32:559–576

Yuan W, Hsu H, Lai Y et al (2012) Differences in sonographic features of ruptured and unruptured epidermal cysts. J Ultrasound Med 31:265–272

Bone Tumors: Radiographic Pitfalls

30

Sumer N. Shikhare, Niraj Dubey,
and Wilfred C.G. Peh

Contents

30.1	**Introduction**	597
30.2	**Classification**	598
30.3	**Pseudo-Lesions**	598
30.3.1	Humerus	598
30.3.2	Supratrochlear Foramen	598
30.3.3	Radial Tuberosity	598
30.3.4	Hip (Ward Triangle)	599
30.3.5	Calcaneus	600
30.4	**Congenital and Anatomical Variants**	600
30.4.1	Synovial Herniation Pit in the Proximal Femur	600
30.4.2	Supracondylar Process of the Humerus	600
30.4.3	Soleal Line	602
30.4.4	Nail-Patella Syndrome	602
30.5	**Inflammation and Infection**	602
30.5.1	Subchondral Cyst	602
30.5.2	Gout	603
30.5.3	Bone Infection	604
30.6	**Metabolic Causes**	606
30.6.1	Brown Tumor	606
30.6.2	Skeletal Amyloidosis	607
30.7	**Traumatic Causes**	608
30.7.1	Stress Fracture	608
30.7.2	Myositis Ossificans	608
30.7.3	Healed Avulsion Fracture	609
30.7.4	Radiation Changes	610
30.7.5	Bone Graft Donor Site	611
30.8	**Miscellaneous Lesions**	611
30.8.1	Melorheostosis	611
30.8.2	Osteonecrosis	612
30.8.3	Fibrous Dysplasia	612
30.8.4	Paget Disease	613
30.8.5	Unicameral (Simple) Bone Cyst	614
30.8.6	Bizarre Parosteal Osteochondromatous Proliferation (Nora Lesion)	615
30.8.7	Osteopoikilosis	615
	Conclusion	618
	References	618

S.N. Shikhare, DNB, MMed, FRCR (✉)
N. Dubey, MD, FRCR • W.C.G. Peh, MD, FRCPE, FRCPG, FRCR
Department of Diagnostic Radiology, Khoo Teck Puat Hospital, 90 Yishun Central, Singapore 768828, Republic of Singapore
e-mail: Nrupendra.shikhare.sumer@alexandrahealth.com.sg; Dubey.niraj@alexandrahealth.com.sg; Wilfred.peh@alexandrahealth.com.sg

30.1 Introduction

Focal bone lesions can be identified quite commonly as incidental findings on radiographs. While some of these lesions are true bone tumors, others are potential pitfalls mimicking bone tumors on radiographs. These lesions include pseudo-lesions, normal anatomical variants, and other benign osseous lesions which, if identified, correctly require no further work-up. It is imperative for a radiologist to be familiar with the characteristic radiographic appearance of these bone tumor mimics, allowing differentiation between them and true bone tumors, and thus avoid potential misdiagnosis. The aim of this chapter is to review bone tumor mimics and discuss clinical

© Springer International Publishing AG 2017
W.C.G. Peh (ed.), *Pitfalls in Musculoskeletal Radiology*, DOI 10.1007/978-3-319-53496-1_30

and key imaging features that can help differentiate these lesions from true bone tumors.

30.2 Classification

Based on the radiographic appearances, bone tumor mimics can be broadly categorized as pseudo-lesions, congenital/anatomical variants, infection/inflammatory processes, metabolic causes, traumatic causes, and miscellaneous causes.

30.3 Pseudo-Lesions

Pseudo-lesions are normal anatomical structures which, on routine radiographs, may appear as relatively ill-defined or partly circumscribed radiolucent areas mimicking bone tumors. The common sites include greater tuberosity of the humerus, supratrochlear foramen, radial tuberosity, neck of femur, and calcaneum. If correctly identified, further investigation or diagnostic work-up of these pseudo-lesions is not required, and interventions such as biopsy can be avoided (Gould et al. 2007).

30.3.1 Humerus

A humerus pseudo-lesion is seen as a radiolucent area in the humeral head on shoulder radiographs performed for shoulder-related symptoms. The area appears relatively radiolucent, probably due to increased fat and decreased bone trabeculae in the region. On radiographs, the usual location of this pseudo-lesion is the superolateral aspect of the humeral head, and it has a sharp inferior border demarcating it from adjacent marrow (Fig. 30.1). This demarcating border represents the line of fusion between the greater tuberosity apophysis and the humeral shaft (Resnick and Cone 1984; Mhuircheartaigh et al. 2014). This apparent radiolucent area is a potential diagnostic pitfall on radiographs and, if one is unaware, has the likelihood of being misdiagnosed as a giant cell tumor, chondroblastoma, or metastasis.

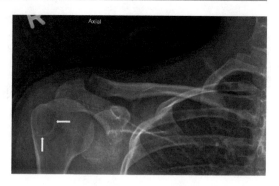

Fig. 30.1 Humeral pseudocyst in a 40-year-old man presenting with right shoulder pain. Frontal radiograph of the shoulder shows a round to oval normal area of radiolucency in the greater tuberosity (*arrows*) of the right humerus

30.3.2 Supratrochlear Foramen

The olecranon and the coronoid fossa are separated by a thin plate of bone, which may be very thin or in some cases becomes perforated to give rise to a supratrochlear foramen. Hence, on radiographs, a supratrochlear foramen may appear as an osteolytic defect (Fig. 30.2) and may be erroneously misinterpreted as a primary or secondary bone tumor. Thus, an awareness of this entity and its characteristic location is required to avoid potential misinterpretation (De Wilde et al. 2004; Nayak et al. 2009).

30.3.3 Radial Tuberosity

On lateral projections of the elbow joint, the radial tuberosity is imaged en face and is seen as an ovoid radiolucent lesion (Fig. 30.3). To the unwary, it can be misdiagnosed as an osteolytic bone tumor such as giant cell tumor, metastasis, or osteochondroma. An osteochondroma can appear radiolucent if imaged *en face*; however, the orthogonal view is confirmatory. Similarly, on frontal projections, the radial tuberosity becomes clear, and the apparent radiolucency disappears. Hence, it is important to review orthogonal projections to avoid potential misdiagnosis (Mhuircheartaigh et al. 2014).

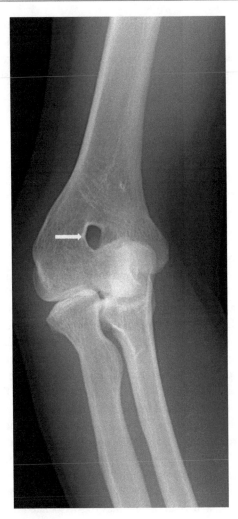

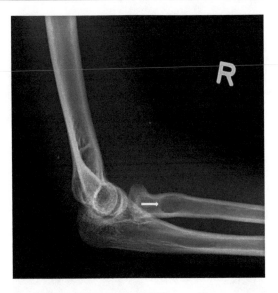

Fig. 30.3 Radial tuberosity in a 35-year-old man presenting with elbow pain. Lateral radiograph of the right elbow shows an oval area of radiolucency in the radial tuberosity (*arrow*), which disappears on the frontal radiograph

Fig. 30.2 Supratrochlear foramen in a 45-year-old woman with history of fall. Frontal radiograph of the elbow shows a round area of radiolucency in the interepicondylar region of distal humerus in keeping with normal supratrochlear foramen (*arrow*)

30.3.4 Hip (Ward Triangle)

The Ward triangle is seen as a focal area of radiolucency in the region of neck of the femur, at the junction of the principle compressive, secondary compressive, and primary tensile trabeculae (Fig. 30.4). The location and radiographic appearance of this apparent triangle is quite characteristic and, if one is unacquainted, may be misinterpreted as an osteolytic bone tumor (Mhuircheartaigh et al. 2014).

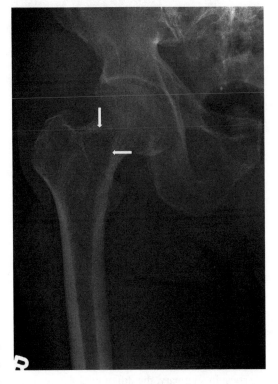

Fig. 30.4 Ward triangle in a 63-year-old man presenting with right hip pain. Frontal radiograph of the right hip shows a triangular area of radiolucency in the femoral neck (*arrows*)

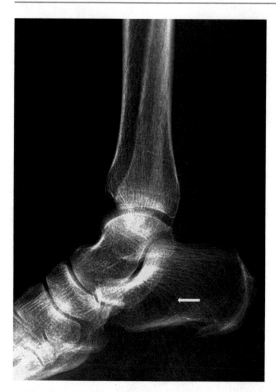

Fig. 30.5 Calcaneal pseudocyst in a 50-year-old man presenting with heel pain. Lateral radiograph of the heel shows an oval area of relative radiolucency and is seen in the anterior-inferior calcaneus (*arrow*) with prominent trabeculation and ill-defined margins

30.3.5 Calcaneus

Another common site for an apparent radiolucency, mimicking a bone tumor, is the anteroinferior aspect of the calcaneal facet (Gould et al. 2007) (Fig. 30.5). Radiologists should be familiar with this entity and inspect this area carefully, as this location is associated with characteristic bone tumors such as chondroblastoma and intraosseous lipoma. Chondroblastomas usually demonstrate ring- and arc-like chondral calcifications, and an intraosseous lipoma usually develops central dystrophic calcification due to necrosis. Both lesions tend to have well-defined sclerotic margins (Mhuircheartaigh et al. 2014).

Thus, in summary, the differential diagnosis of pseudo-lesions usually includes radiolucent bone tumors such as giant cell tumor, chondroblastoma, intraosseous lipoma, and metastasis. Findings such as intralesional calcification, sclerotic or irregular margins, cortical disruption, and periosteal reaction favor true bone tumors rather than a pseudo-lesion. Pseudo-lesions can be easily differentiated from true bone tumors, based on their characteristic location and radiographic appearances.

30.4 Congenital and Anatomical Variants

30.4.1 Synovial Herniation Pit in the Proximal Femur

Synovial herniation pits are small well-defined subcortical osseous defects that occur on the anterosuperior aspect of the proximal femoral neck. A pit may be a normal variant or may represent herniation of synovium into the cortical defect. It usually occurs in up to 5% of adults (Gould et al. 2007). The characteristic radiographic appearance is that of a well-defined round or oval radiolucency surrounded by thin zone of sclerosis seen in the anterosuperior aspect of the proximal femoral neck (Mhuircheartaigh et al. 2014) (Fig. 30.6). Classically, these lesions measure less than 1 cm in diameter but may reach up to 2–3 cm in greatest diameter (Nokes et al. 1989). The majority are asymptomatic and detected incidentally and are only rarely symptomatic. In some cases, a herniation pit may be associated with femoro-acetabular impingement (Kavanagh et al. 2011). Radiographically, it may mimic an osteoid osteoma. However, the characteristic location, radiographic appearance, and absent relevant clinical history help rule out this entity. In addition, lack of periosteal reaction and surrounding reactive bone formation also helps to rule out the diagnosis of osteoid osteoma (Pitt et al. 1982).

30.4.2 Supracondylar Process of the Humerus

The supracondylar process of the humerus is also known as the supracondyloid, epicondylar, epicondylic, and supraepitrochlear process. It is a small bony spur arising and extending downward from the anteromedial surface of the humerus

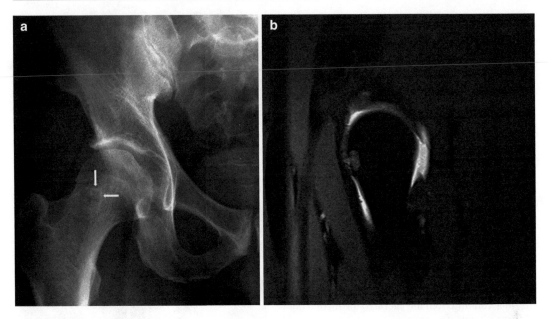

Fig. 30.6 Synovial herniation pit in a 54-year-old man presenting with right hip pain. (**a**) Frontal radiograph shows a well-defined radiolucency with sclerotic margins (*arrows*) at the superolateral aspect of the right femoral neck. (**b**) Sagittal fat-suppressed T2-W MR image in the same patient confirms a small focus of hyperintense signal at the femoral neck with no surrounding edema

Fig. 30.7 Supracondylar process of the humerus in a 34-year-old man presenting with right elbow pain. (**a**) Frontal and (**b**) lateral radiographs of the elbow show a bony outgrowth at the anteromedial aspect of the distal humerus (*arrow*)

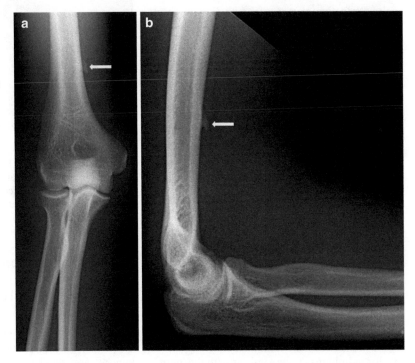

(Fig. 30.7). It usually originates approximately 5–7 cm cranial to the medial epicondyle. The process ends in a roughened point which occasionally may give rise to a ligament (the ligament of Struthers) continuing up to the medial epicondyle, creating a tunnel where the median nerve and brachial artery may get entrapped. Considering that it is a bony spur, some may wrongly diagnose it as a distal humeral osteochondroma. However, the distinguishing feature of an osteochondroma is that it characteristically projects away from the joint, whereas a supracondylar process points toward the elbow joint (Curtis et al. 1977).

30.4.3 Soleal Line

An unusually prominent soleal line can form at the attachment of the soleus along the posterior aspect of the tibia (Mhuircheartaigh et al. 2014). The soleal line usually begins 1–2 cm below the fibular facet and ends between the upper and middle thirds of the bone (Mysorekar and Nandedkar 1983). A prominent soleal line is seen as an area of cortical thickening on the posterior aspect of upper third of the tibia, running from the lateral to the medial borders (Fig. 30.8). It is better appreciated on lateral radiographs and may closely mimic periostitis secondary to a bone tumor such as an osteoid osteoma or parosteal osteosarcoma or benign conditions such as infection or stress fracture (Levine et al. 1976; Mhuircheartaigh et al. 2014).

30.4.4 Nail-Patella Syndrome

Nail-patella syndrome (NPS) is a rare hereditary disorder known by many other names, such as hereditary onycho-osteodysplasia (HOOD) and Fong disease (Mankin 2009). It is characterized by the tetrad of aplastic or hypoplastic nail, patella hypoplasia or aplasia, elbow dysplasia, and iliac horns. The presence of iliac horns is considered pathognomonic (Fong 1946), and finding of patellar and nail abnormalities is the cardinal features for diagnosis (West and Louis 2015). Iliac horns are usually bilateral, are seen as osseous projections projecting dorsolaterally from the posterior iliac bone (Fig. 30.9), and may closely mimic an osteochondroma on pelvic radiographs (West and Louis 2015). It is imperative for radiologists to be familiar with this entity and correlate with other associated radiographic abnormalities such as hypoplastic or aplastic patella (Fig. 30.9) or elbow dysplasia, thus avoiding misdiagnosis.

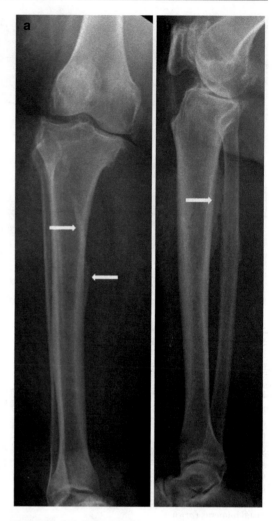

Fig. 30.8 Soleal line in a 61-year-old woman presenting with right leg cellulitis. (**a**) Frontal and (**b**) lateral radiographs of the tibia show linear cortical thickening (*arrows*) along the proximal tibia, extending lateral to medial along the posterior cortex. This corresponds to an enthesophyte from the attachment of the soleus

30.5 Inflammation and Infection

30.5.1 Subchondral Cyst

Subchondral cysts are also known as synovial cysts, subarticular pseudocysts, necrotic pseudocysts, and geodes. These are not true cysts, as they are not lined by epithelium, and are usually associated with osteoarthritis (OA) (Beaman and Peterson 2007). The postulated mechanisms include (1) increased intra-articular pressure

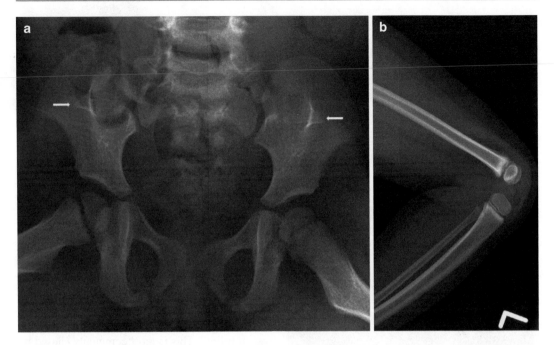

Fig. 30.9 Nail-patella syndrome. (**a**) Frontal radiograph of the pelvis in a child shows bilateral triangular osseous excrescences from the posterior aspect of the iliac bones in keeping with iliac horns (*arrows*). (**b**) Lateral radiograph of the knee of the same child shows absence of the patella

forcing synovial fluid through damaged articular cartilage, with subsequent subchondral cyst formation (Freud 1940), and (2) cystic necrosis in the subchondral bone secondary to underlying impaction fracture and vascular insufficiency (Rhaney and Lamb 1955). OA commonly affects weight-bearing joints such as the hips, knees, and lumbar and cervical spine. Radiographically, subchondral cysts are seen as well-defined osteolytic lesions with a thin sclerotic rim at the subarticular surface of the weight-bearing joint (Fig. 30.10). Other degenerative changes which can be seen on radiographs include reduced joint space, subchondral sclerosis, and marginal osteophytes. These radiographic findings help differentiate a subchondral cyst from subchondral (epiphyseal) osteolytic bone tumors such as giant cell tumor, chondroblastoma, and metastasis.

30.5.2 Gout

Gout is the commonest inflammatory and crystalline arthropathy affecting men (Agudelo and Wise 2001; Girish et al. 2013). The characteristic feature

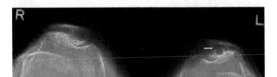

Fig. 30.10 Subchondral cyst in a 70-year-old man presenting with left knee pain. Skyline patellar radiograph shows a subarticular radiolucent lesion with a sclerotic rim (*arrow*) at the left patella. There is associated narrowing of the patellofemoral joint and osteophytosis, consistent with degenerative osteoarthritis

is hyperuricemia leading to deposition of monosodium urate crystals, resulting in acute episodes of inflammation and related symptoms. In the long term, the arthropathy results in articular and periarticular inflammatory changes (Girish et al. 2013). The characteristic site for gout involvement is the first metatarsophalangeal joint of the foot. Other joints may be affected as well, such as the interphalangeal joints of the hands and feet along with the tarsal bones. On radiographs, in chronic cases, gouty arthritis may manifest as marginal erosions near a joint and have overhanging margins with sclerotic borders, giving a punched-out appearance, or may present as an intraosseous osteolytic

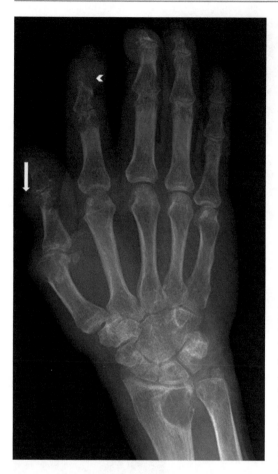

Fig. 30.11 Gout in a 48-year-old man presenting with wrist pain. Frontal radiograph of the hand shows a well-defined subarticular radiolucent lesion with sclerotic margins in the right distal radius. There are also punched-out erosions (*arrowhead*) and soft tissue densities due to tophi (*arrow*) involving the small bones of hand, typical of gout

lesion (Jacobson et al. 2008) (Fig. 30.11). To an inexperienced observer, the erosions may mimic an aggressive bone tumor, but the characteristic location, sclerotic margins, and associated hyperdense soft tissue swelling help in reaching the diagnosis of gout. Other clues to look for are the clinical features and serum uric acid levels which are usually elevated, helping to confirm the diagnosis of gout.

30.5.3 Bone Infection

30.5.3.1 Osteomyelitis
Osteomyelitis (OM) is usually caused by hematogenous spread of infection. Other modes include

spread from adjacent soft tissue or direct inoculation. It commonly affects the metaphyseal regions of tubular bones in children. In adults, however, it commonly involves the spine, pelvis, and small bones. Radiographically visible osseous findings in acute OM are osteoporosis, permeative bone erosion, and trabecular destruction, followed by cortical erosion and periostitis in advanced cases (Tehranzadeh et al. 2001) (Fig. 30.12). These findings can closely mimic an aggressive bone tumor such as osteosarcoma and Ewing sarcoma in children and metastasis and chondrosarcoma in adults. An appropriate clinical history and laboratory investigations help to reach correct diagnosis.

30.5.3.2 Brodie Abscess
In the subacute or chronic stage, some young patients may develop an intraosseous abscess known as Brodie abscess, also referred to as "cystic osteomyelitis." This is most commonly caused by *Staphylococcus aureus*. Brodie abscess frequently affects the long bone metaphysis, particularly the proximal or distal tibial metaphysis. In some instances, it may extend into the epiphysis, crossing the physeal plate. On radiographs, these lesions are seen as a well-defined round to oval osteolytic lesion with dense surrounding sclerosis and may have associated mild periosteal reaction (Gould et al. 2007; Pineda et al. 2009) (Fig. 30.13). This can pose as a potential diagnostic pitfall mimicking bone tumors such as osteoid osteoma, osteosarcoma, and Ewing sarcoma. An epiphyseal-located abscess can mimic chondroblastoma, giant cell tumor, and Langerhans cell histiocytosis.

Computed tomography (CT) usually shows cortical thickening and sinus tracts. Magnetic resonance imaging (MRI) characteristically demonstrates a "target sign" produced by four concentric layers of tissue. The center is composed of necrotic tissue which is hypointense on T1-weighted images and hyperintense on T2-weighted images. The adjacent layer of granulation tissue demonstrates intermediate signal (isointense to muscle) on both T1- and T2-weighted images. The next sclerotic or fibrotic layer shows very low signal intensity on T1- and T2-weighted images. The outermost rim of edema shows signal hypointensity

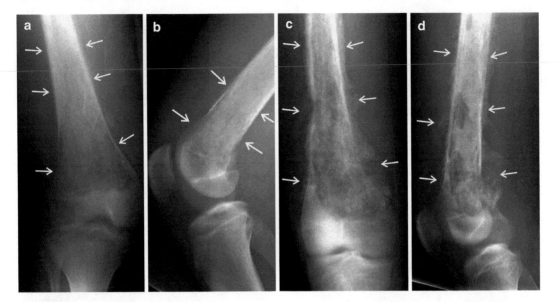

Fig. 30.12 15-year-old boy with neglected osteomyelitis of the right distal femur. Initial (**a**) frontal and (**b**) lateral radiographs show mottled appearance of the distal femoral diametaphysis with associated aggressive-appearing periostitis (*arrows*). The preliminary diagnosis was possible Ewing sarcoma. One month later, after surgical debridement and initiation of intravenous antibiotics, repeat (**c**) frontal and (**d**) lateral radiographs show mixed sclerotic and osteolytic appearance of the femoral lesion with associated extensive periostitis, consistent with known chronic osteomyelitis but mimicking osteosarcoma. The diagnosis of osteomyelitis (*Staphylococcus aureus*) was confirmed by blood cultures and biopsy/aspiration (Reproduced with permission from: Taljanovic and Hoover (2015))

on T1-weighted images and signal hyperintensity on T2-weighted images (Gould et al. 2007). The radiographic findings in osteomyelitis may be nonspecific and may mimic bone tumors, as stated above. Hence, advanced imaging and bone biopsy are often necessary to confirm the diagnosis and to identify the causative organism (Hatzenbuehler and Pulling 2011). However, the significance of a proper history cannot be overemphasized, since this may channel the management in an optimal direction.

30.5.3.3 Tuberculosis Osteomyelitis

Tuberculosis (TB) OM is most prevalent in underdeveloped countries and is characteristically insidious in onset and indolent in manifestation. It most commonly spreads by the hematogenous route, generally from the lung. No skeletal area is immune. It is usually monostotic, but multifocal involvement is not infrequent. TB OM commonly affects the proximal long bones, short tubular bones, carpal and tarsal bones (especially the calcaneum), and flat bones such as the ribs and iliac bones. Radiographically, TB OM is a great mimicker and may have varied appearances, including osteolysis with little or no reactive change, erosions, minimal periosteal reaction, and soft tissue swelling (Fig. 30.14), mimicking primary bone tumors and metastases.

Spina ventosa, also known as tuberculous dactylitis, is a form of TB OM affecting short tubular bones. It has characteristic radiographic findings in the form of fusiform expansion of the diaphysis, cyst-like bone destruction, periosteal thickening, and surrounding soft tissue swelling (Fig. 30.15). It commonly affects short tubular bones of the hands and feet (Shikhare et al. 2011). This needs to be differentiated from bone tumors commonly affecting tubular bones such as enchondroma. The appropriate clinical background and characteristic radiographic appearances help in reaching the correct diagnosis.

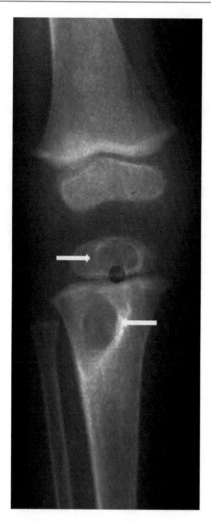

Fig. 30.13 Brodie abscess in a child presenting with fever and knee pain. Frontal radiograph of the right knee shows radiolucent lesions with sclerotic borders in the proximal tibial epiphysis and metaphysis (*arrows*)

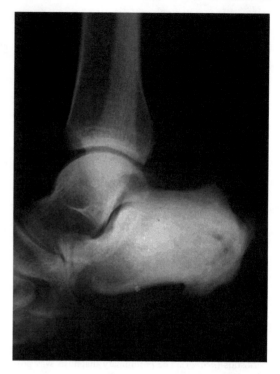

Fig. 30.14 Tuberculous osteomyelitis in a young man presenting with fever and heel pain. Lateral ankle radiograph shows an area of sclerosis with few osteolytic foci involving the calcaneus

30.6 Metabolic Causes

30.6.1 Brown Tumor

Brown tumors (osteoclastomas) are benign osteolytic lesions found in less than 5% of patients with primary and secondary hyperparathyroidism. It is usually seen in untreated long-standing hyperparathyroidism, the incidence of which has decreased in recent times due to early diagnosis (Mhuircheartaigh et al. 2014). The underlying mechanism is increased bone turnover due to elevated levels of parathyroid hormone. The

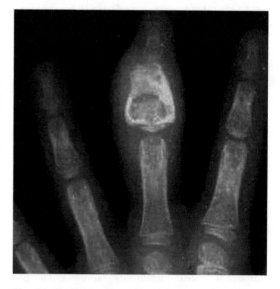

Fig. 30.15 Tuberculous dactylitis in a young female patient presenting with soft tissue swelling involving the middle finger. Frontal radiograph of the fingers shows an expansile radiolucent lesion with sclerosis and soft tissue swelling involving the middle phalanx of the middle finger

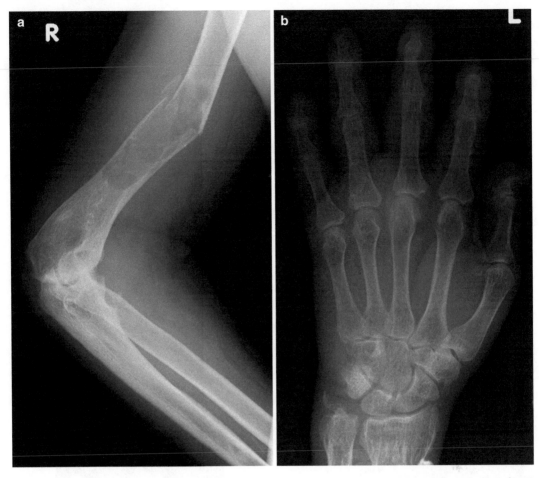

Fig. 30.16 Secondary hyperparathyroidism in a 45-year-old man with known chronic renal failure and history of fall. (**a**) Lateral radiograph of the right elbow joint shows a well-defined radiolucent lesion with narrow zone of transition involving the distal metaphysis of the right humerus. There is associated pathological fracture. (**b**) Frontal radiograph of the right hand of the same patient shows diffuse osteopenia, subperiosteal bone erosion, and cortical tunneling involving middle phalanges and acro-osteolysis, characteristic for hyperparathyroidism

commonest site for brown tumor is long bones, but it may also affect the ribs and jaws. Radiographically, a brown tumor is seen as a well-defined expanded osteolytic lesion with internal septation or sclerosis. It may present with a pathological fracture (Fig. 30.16). In adults, it may mimic osteolytic bone tumors such as plasmacytoma and metastasis. The clue to the diagnosis is the clinical background and appropriate laboratory data (Gould et al. 2007). Another helpful clue is that posttreatment brown tumors reossify and radiographically demonstrate increase in density (Agarwal et al. 2002).

30.6.2 Skeletal Amyloidosis

Systemic amyloidosis can affect various anatomical sites in varied forms. In the skeletal system, amyloidosis may present as an expanded osteolytic lesion with areas of sclerosis, giving an aggressive pattern, and thus simulates a primary or secondary bone tumor (Fig. 30.17). The common sites include the pelvis, hip, and shoulder. A prospective radiographic diagnosis of skeletal amyloidosis is quite impossible, and the diagnosis is usually made after biopsy (Kim et al. 2011).

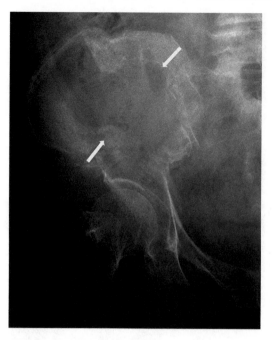

Fig. 30.17 Amyloidosis in a 60-year-old woman with history of fall. Frontal radiograph of the pelvis shows a large radiolucent lesion with ill-defined margins involving the body of the right iliac bone (*arrows*) with associated pathological fracture

30.7 Traumatic Causes

30.7.1 Stress Fracture

Stress fractures may occur in a normal bone secondary to excessive repetitive force, known as fatigue fracture, or in an abnormal bone after normal stress, known as insufficiency fracture, such as in osteoporosis or Paget disease. Common sites include the posterior tibia, metatarsals, and tarsals (Krestan et al. 2011). Initial radiographs may not reveal stress fractures, which are better demonstrated on MRI or technetium (Tc)-99 m pyrophosphate bone scintigraphy (Mhuircheartaigh et al. 2014). At the time of initial presentation, stress fractures are visible radiographically in only 10–25% of cases (Gould et al. 2007) and usually demonstrate a fracture line that is perpendicular to the cortex. This is better seen on CT. At a later stage, a stress fracture may develop periosteal reaction (Fig. 30.18) with cortical resorption and can mimic an osteoid osteoma or an aggressive bone tumor such as osteosarcoma (Stacy and

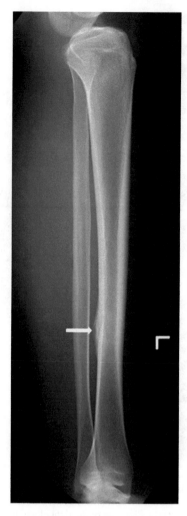

Fig. 30.18 Stress fracture in a 38-year-old man who developed left lower limb pain while playing football. Lateral radiograph of the tibia shows smooth continuous cortical thickening (*arrows*) along the posterior aspect of the tibia mimicking a bone tumor such as osteoid osteoma

Kapur 2011; Mhuircheartaigh et al. 2014). The radiographic features which favor the diagnosis of stress fracture and rule out other entities include the classic location, presence of a fracture line, absence of soft tissue mass, and signs of healing on follow-up studies. Additionally, the clinical history is often definitive.

30.7.2 Myositis Ossificans

Myositis ossificans is an inflammatory pseudotumor, whereby heterotopic ossification occurs in skeletal muscle as a post-traumatic phenomenon (Mhuircheartaigh et al. 2014). It most commonly occurs following trauma, comprising 60–75% of all cases. However, in many cases (40%), the patient may not remember the traumatic episode. Myositis ossificans may also be associated with other conditions such as paraplegia, burns, immobility, and tetanus (Gould et al. 2007). Post-traumatic myositis ossificans commonly occurs in the proximal muscle groups of the upper and lower extremities. Clinically, patients may be asymptomatic or may present with localized pain, swelling, and a palpable mass 4–5 days after injury (Mhuircheartaigh et al. 2014). It may be accompanied by an elevated erythrocyte sedimentation rate and alkaline phosphatase (Parikh et al. 2002).

Initially, radiographs may be normal or may show a nonspecific soft tissue mass. Later, usually 3–8 weeks after the onset, ossification begins at the periphery and progresses centrally. Subsequently, the central region, too, develops dense osteoid matrix and, months later, forms a dense osteoid mass (Fig. 30.19). Radiographically, myositis ossificans may mimic a juxtacortical or parosteal osteosarcoma. The clue to the diagnosis of myositis ossificans is a radiolucent cleft between the lesion and the adjacent cortex and dense peripheral ossification, in contrast to parosteal osteosarcoma which is denser centrally (Gould et al. 2007; Mhuircheartaigh et al. 2014). CT helps confirm the diagnosis by showing peripheral ossification and a lucent cleft. MRI is quite nonspecific in the diagnosis of myositis ossificans, and the appearance varies, depending on the stage of development. Radiologists should be aware of the characteristic radiographic appearance of this entity, as misdiagnosis may lead to unnecessary intervention such as biopsy, which may further add to the confusion, as it is difficult to differentiate myositis ossificans from an osteosarcoma, even on histology [Klapsinou et al. 2012].

30.7.3 Healed Avulsion Fracture

Avulsion injuries are common among athletes, football, and baseball players. These usually occur at the sites of ligamentous or tendinous insertions, with common locations being the pelvis, knee,

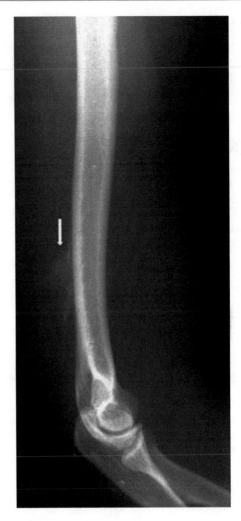

Fig. 30.19 Myositis ossificans in a 34-year-old man presenting with elbow pain and previous history of trauma. Lateral elbow radiograph shows a large nonspecific heterogeneous partially calcified mass (*arrow*) along the posterior aspect of the distal humerus. There is no periosteal or cortical abnormality or underlying bone erosion

ankle, foot, shoulder, and elbow (Brandser et al. 1995; Gould et al. 2007). Avulsion injuries are more common in adolescents, as these locations are inherently weak due to unfused or incompletely fused apophyses. Avulsion fractures may occur acutely after a single traumatic episode or may result from repetitive microtrauma (Tehranzadeh 1987; Gould et al. 2007). On radiographs, an avulsion fracture is seen as an area of cortical disruption with a faint osseous density adjacent to the injured bone, where a tendon or ligament inserts. The healing stage of an avulsion fracture may put

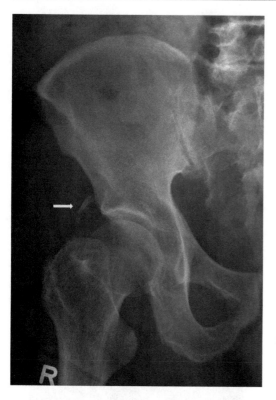

Fig. 30.20 Healed avulsion fractures in a 49-year-old man presenting with right hip pain. Frontal radiograph of the pelvis shows a healed avulsion fracture at the anterior superior iliac spine (*arrow*)

a radiologist in a diagnostic dilemma, as it may appear osteolytic and aggressive. An ossified protuberant mass adjacent to the sites of avulsion injuries may resemble an infectious process or even a bone tumor such as osteochondroma (Gould et al. 2007) (Fig. 30.20). Clinical history of trauma, characteristic location (enthesis and adjacent to apophysis), and characteristic radiographic appearance help in avoiding misdiagnosis.

30.7.4 Radiation Changes

Radiation therapy damages osteoblasts, resulting in decreased production of the bone matrix. Radiographically, it manifests as osteopenia usually seen about 1 year after irradiation (Bluemke et al. 1994). Vascular damage causes bone atrophy followed by repair, with deposition of bone on unresorbed trabeculae (Mitchell and Logan

1998). Radiographs obtained 2–3 years postradiation demonstrate heterogeneous, mottled bone density with focal areas of increased density, osteopenia, and coarse trabeculation (Fig. 30.21). These radiation-induced bone changes are often referred to as radiation osteitis or radiation necrosis. Specific radiographic appearances vary with the radiation site (Bluemke et al. 1994). The bone changes can look like Paget disease, except that bone expansion is not present in cases of radiation osteitis. Radiographically, the differential diagnosis of radiation osteitis includes radiation-induced sarcoma, recurrent neoplasm, and infection (Paling and Herdt 1980). The aspects favoring diagnosis of radiation osteitis include appropriate clinical background, bone changes confined to the field of radiation, absence of soft tissue mass, no bone erosion, and interval stability of the bone changes. Moreover, compared to radiation-induced sarcoma, bone changes in radiation osteitis occur quite early after the therapy (Bluemke et al. 1994; Mitchell and Logan 1998).

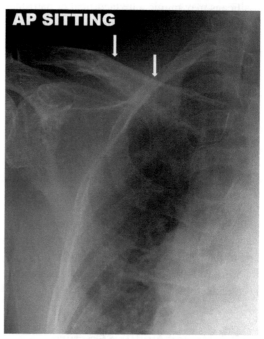

Fig. 30.21 Radiation changes in a 57-year-old woman with history of radiation therapy for right breast carcinoma. Frontal chest radiograph shows cortical thickening and coarse trabecular pattern involving the right clavicle (*arrows*) in keeping with postradiation changes

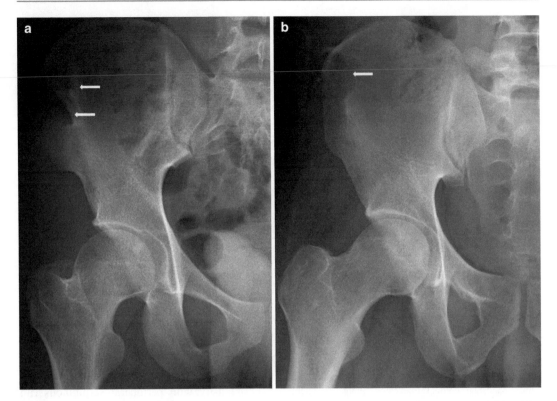

Fig. 30.22 Bone graft donor sites. (**a, b**) Frontal radiographs of pelvis show a bone defect in the region of right iliac crest – a characteristic bone graft donor site (*arrows*)

30.7.5 Bone Graft Donor Site

Bone graft donor sites, commonly the iliac bone, may appear as an irregular osteolytic bone defect, with or without sclerotic borders (Fig. 30.22). If not correlated clinically and historically, it may act as potential diagnostic pitfall mimicking an aggressive primary or secondary bone tumor. Hence, the characteristic location and appropriate clinical background help in achieving the correct diagnosis (Mhuircheartaigh et al. 2014).

30.8 Miscellaneous Lesions

30.8.1 Melorheostosis

Melorheostosis is a rare sclerosing bone dysplasia also known as Leri disease (Leri and Joanny 1922). The name melorheostosis is derived from the Greek words "melos" meaning limb and "rhein" meaning flow, due to the characteristic

appearance of flowing hyperostosis. Patients are often asymptomatic or may present with limb stiffness or pain (Bansal 2008). It may be associated with soft tissue hemangiomas and neurofibromas (Mhuircheartaigh et al. 2014). Melorheostosis generally affects the appendicular skeleton, most commonly the long bones of the upper and lower extremities. It can affect tubular bones in the hands and feet as well. Axial skeleton involvement is quite rare (Bansal 2008). It may be monostotic, monomelic, or polyostotic (Greenspan and Azouz 1999).

Radiologically, melorheostosis may present with five patterns: classic, osteoma like, myositis ossificans like, osteopathia striata like, and mixed (Bansal 2008). On radiographs, melorheostosis is characteristically seen as irregular linear bands of increased sclerosis along the outer bony cortex, often described as "dripping candle wax" appearance, or may present with endosteal cortical thickening with intramedullary extension (Fig. 30.23). It commonly affects the diaphysis of long bones.

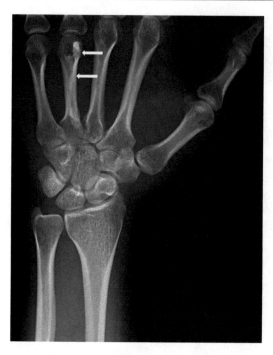

Fig. 30.23 Melorheostosis in a 37-year-old man presenting with wrist pain. Frontal radiograph of the left hand shows endosteal cortical thickening along the lateral aspect of the fourth metacarpal (*arrows*)

There is clear demarcation between the normal and the affected bone. Radiographically, the differential diagnosis includes bone tumors such as osteoma, parosteal osteosarcoma, and sclerotic bone metastasis. Hence, radiologists must be aware of the characteristic radiographic appearance of melorheostosis, avoiding misdiagnosis, and further imaging or intervention (Sureka et al. 2014). On MRI, melorheostosis shows signal hypointensity on all pulse sequences and may show increased activity on Tc-99 m pyrophosphate bone scintigraphy (Mhuircheartaigh et al. 2014).

30.8.2 Osteonecrosis

Ischemic bone necrosis occurs due to reduced or complete loss of blood supply to bone. It is caused by a variety of causes, the commonest being idiopathic, trauma, corticosteroids, and alcoholism. The usual sites of osteonecrosis include the femoral head, humeral head, femoral metadiaphysis, tibial metadiaphysis, scaphoid, lunate,

and talus. The patients with osteonecrosis are usually asymptomatic but may present with pain and reduced range of motion. On radiographs, the initial finding may be a focal area of bone sclerosis with surrounding osteopenia. The characteristic radiographic appearance, however, is patchy serpiginous areas of sclerosis and lucency. When it involves the epiphysis, it can result in subchondral bone collapse and secondary osteoarthritis. In the metadiaphyseal region, the rim of sclerosis has characteristic serpentine or undulating appearance (Fig. 30.24). Bone infarcts in the metadiaphyseal region of long bones may mimic an enchondroma and chondrosarcoma. The radiographic clues favoring osteonecrosis, rather than enchondroma or chondrosarcoma, include lack of central calcification, endosteal scalloping, and bone erosion. MRI is regarded as the most sensitive and specific modality for detection of bone infarcts. Early-stage osteonecrosis demonstrates nonspecific marrow edema, while in later stage, it characteristically shows central area of signal hyperintensity with peripheral serpiginous rim of signal hypointensity on non-fat-suppressed T2-weighted images (Mhuircheartaigh et al. 2014; Murphey et al. 2014).

30.8.3 Fibrous Dysplasia

Fibrous dysplasia is a non-inherited developmental bone disease wherein normal marrow and cancellous bone are replaced by immature bone and fibrous stroma due to abnormal differentiation of osteoblasts. It forms less than 2.5% of all primary bone lesions and may be seen in children or adults. Fibrous dysplasia can be either monostotic or polyostotic. It may be associated with McCune-Albright syndrome or Mazabraud syndrome. Common sites include the ribs, tibia, proximal femur, pelvis, skull, and humerus. Radiographically, fibrous dysplasia lesions typically are well defined, expansile, and intramedullary and may be associated with cortical thinning and endosteal scalloping (Fitzpatrick et al. 2004). As the lesion is composed of fibrous tissue, the matrix may appear ground glass in appearance. It may have a cystic component and internal

Fig. 30.24 Bone infarcts in a 45-year-old man, who was on steroids for systemic lupus erythematosus, presenting with bilateral lower limb pain. Frontal radiograph of both distal femurs shows a centrally located mixed lucent-sclerotic lesion with calcified serpiginous margins. There is no endosteal scalloping. Findings are characteristic for bone infarcts

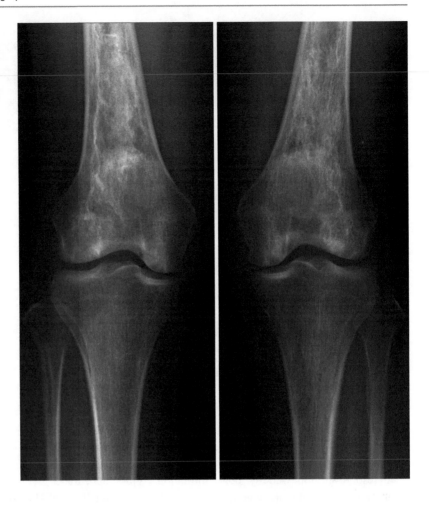

septations. Due to softening, the long bones may become bowed, a classic appearance being the "shepherd crook" deformity of the femur.

Patients may present with a pathological fracture. Differential considerations include unicameral bone cyst, enchondroma, aneurysmal bone cyst, myeloma, or metastatic disease, depending on patient age and lesion location. However, characteristic radiographic features such as central location within metadiaphysis, sclerotic borders, ground-glass matrix, and no cortical erosion or periosteal reaction (Fig. 30.25) help differentiate fibrous dysplasia from the above-listed possibilities. If the patient is asymptomatic and the lesion has characteristic radiographic appearances, no further imaging is required (Gould et al. 2007). MRI usually shows areas of hypointense signal on T1- and T2-weighted images. The cystic component demonstrates hyperintense sig-

nal on T2-weighted images. The lesion shows variable enhancement with a non-enhancing cystic component (Azouz 2002; Shah et al. 2005).

30.8.4 Paget Disease

Paget disease, also known as osteitis deformans, is a chronic bone disorder characterized by excessive abnormal remodeling of bone. Sir James Paget described the condition in 1877 (Paget 1877). It affects approximately 3–4% of individuals older than 40 years of age. Clinically, patients with Paget disease are usually asymptomatic and are often first diagnosed as an incidental finding on radiographs obtained for other reasons. Symptomatic patients usually present with pain and tenderness, bowing deformities, kyphotic deformity, pathological fractures, or

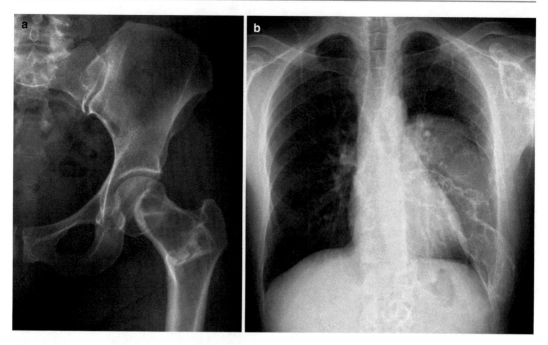

Fig. 30.25 Fibrous dysplasia. (**a**) Frontal radiograph of the pelvis of a 48-year-old woman shows a well-defined radiolucent lesion with thick sclerotic rim and ground-glass matrix in the left femur neck. (**b**) Frontal chest radiograph of a 39-year-old man shows expansile radiolucent lesions involving multiple ribs and scapula on the left side

symptoms due to malignant transformation. Paget disease is considered to progress through various phases of activity, starting from focal bone resorption, followed by bone formation resulting in abnormal bone remodeling (Resnick 2002). Classically, three phases are recognized: first is the lytic phase, wherein osteoclastic resorption predominates; followed by the mixed phase, comprising of osteoclastic and predominantly osteoblastic activity; and lastly, the blastic phase, dominated by osteoblastic activity (Mirra et al. 1995). Paget disease most commonly affects the lumbar spine, pelvic bone, sacrum, femur, and cranium. Less common sites include the cervical and thoracic spine, humerus, and scapula. Polyostotic presentation is more common than monostotic (Theodorou et al. 2011).

Among the imaging modalities, radiography is quite specific in diagnosing Paget disease of bone. The role of CT, bone scintigraphy, and MRI is to confirm the radiographic diagnosis and evaluate complications associated with Paget disease such as pathological fracture or malignant transformation. In the osteolytic phase, particu-larly in the long bones, radiographs show an area of lucency which may appear wedge shaped in the metadiaphyseal region giving a "blade of grass appearance" (Fig. 30.26). This is quite characteristic and should not be confused with primary or secondary osteolytic bone malignancy. In later stages, the affected bones may demonstrate osteolytic-sclerotic or purely sclerotic lesions due to osteoblastic activity, mimicking sclerotic bone tumors (Theodorou et al. 2011). The radiographic features which favor the diagnosis of Paget disease and help avoid misdiagnosis include lamellar cortical thickening, coarse trabecular pattern, and bone enlargement (Fig. 30.27).

30.8.5 Unicameral (Simple) Bone Cyst

Unicameral or simple bone cyst is a relatively common bone lesion usually seen in the proximal humerus or proximal femur in the immature skeleton. It is usually seen in children in the first and second decades of life. It consists of a

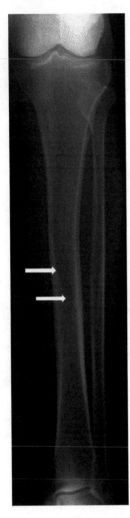

reaction, or soft tissue component. If complicated by a fracture, a dependent fractured bone fragment may be seen in the unilocular cavity giving a "fallen fragment sign" appearance (Fig. 30.28). Radiographically, it may mimic osteolytic bone tumors such as non-ossifying fibroma, primary bone tumor, or metastasis. However, the characteristic location, radiographic appearance, and age at presentation help in reaching a correct diagnosis (Hammoud et al. 2005).

30.8.6 Bizarre Parosteal Osteochondromatous Proliferation (Nora Lesion)

Bizarre parosteal osteochondromatous proliferation (BPOP), also known as Nora lesion, is a rare lesion. The lesion is more common in the 20–30 years age group. It commonly affects the middle and proximal phalanges and the metacarpal or metatarsal bones. On radiographs, the lesion is seen as an exophytic outgrowth from the cortical surface of the bones of the hands and feet (Fig. 30.29). Owing to its parosteal location and occasional rapid growth, it may be mistaken for a neoplastic process such as osteochondroma or parosteal osteosarcoma. However, its characteristic location in the small tubular bones of hands and feet and lack of continuity of this lesion with the medullary canal help distinguish it from malignant lesions (Gruber et al. 2008).

Fig. 30.26 Early Paget disease in a 56-year-old man who presented with left lower limb pain. Frontal radiograph of the tibia shows a subtle area of radiolucency involving the proximal metadiaphysis of left tibia giving the "blade of grass appearance" (*arrows*)

30.8.7 Osteopoikilosis

unilocular cavity in the bone, filled with fluid and lined by a fibrous membrane. It is commonly seen in the metaphysis of a long bone and migrates into the diaphysis with age. Clinically, simple bone cysts are asymptomatic and, hence, are often discovered incidentally when patients present with complications such as pathological fracture. On radiographs, they characteristically appear as a well-defined osteolytic lesion with narrow zone of transition and sclerotic margins, located centrally in the metaphyseal region of long bone. The cyst is not associated with cortical erosion, periosteal

Osteopoikilosis, also known as osteopathia condensans disseminata, or "spotted bone disease," is a disorder of endochondral bone maturation. It may occur sporadically or may have an autosomal dominant inheritance. There is no gender predilection. The entity is asymptomatic and usually diagnosed incidentally on radiographs. The sites commonly involved are small bones of hand and foot, carpal and tarsal bones, pelvis, and epimetaphyseal regions of the long bones. On radiographs, they present as numerous, 2–10 mm round to oval radiodensities

Fig. 30.27 (a) Paget disease in a 63-year-old man presenting with back pain. Lateral radiograph of the lumbar spine shows thickening of the endplates and coarse trabecular pattern involving L4 vertebral body (*arrows*). (b) Bone scintiscan of the same patient shows solitary diffuse increased uptake in the L4 vertebral body

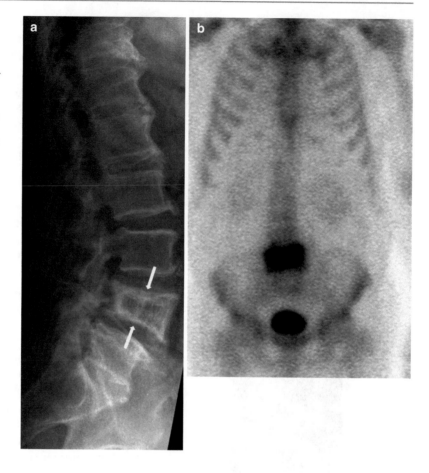

distributed symmetrically in the periarticular regions and epimetaphyseal regions of long bone (Fig. 30.30). These radiodensities represent multiple enostosis. The radiographic appearance of osteopoikilosis is characteristic and should not be confused with osteoblastic bone metastases, thus avoiding unnecessary investigations. Features which favor the diagnosis of osteopoikilosis include symmetrical distribution of lesions, epiphyseal and metaphyseal involvement, and uniform size of the radiodense foci (Khot et al. 2005).

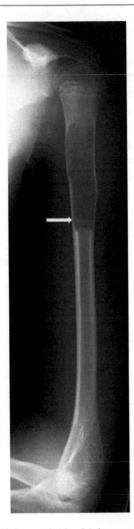

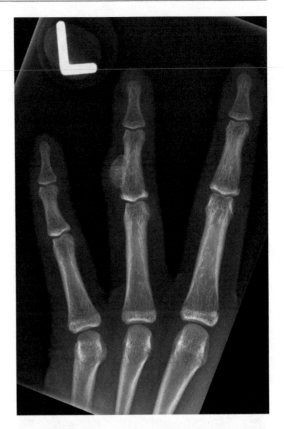

Fig. 30.29 Bizarre parosteal osteochondromatous proliferation (BPOP) in a 25-year-old woman with soft tissue swelling of the left ring finger. Frontal radiograph of the left finger shows an ossified lesion attached to the middle phalanx of left index finger without alteration of the underlying cortex

Fig. 30.28 Unicameral (simple) bone cyst of a young male patient with history of fall and left shoulder pain. Frontal radiograph of the left humerus shows a well-defined radiolucent lesion in the proximal metadiaphysis region with pathological fracture and fallen fragment sign (*arrow*), characteristic for simple bone cyst

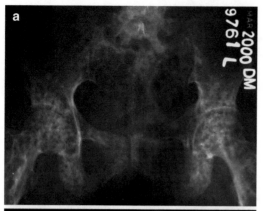

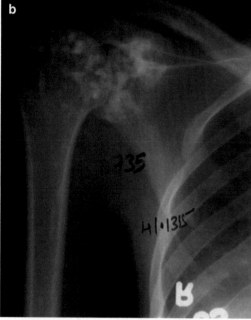

Fig. 30.30 Osteopoikilosis. (**a**) Frontal radiograph of the pelvis shows numerous discrete sclerotic foci in a symmetric periarticular distribution at the hips and sacroiliac joints. (**b**) Frontal radiograph of the right shoulder shows multiple small discrete periarticular sclerotic lesions involving the humerus and scapula

Conclusion

Radiographs remain the mainstay for evaluating musculoskeletal pathologies. However, on numerous occasions, a radiologist may come across normal anatomical variants and nonneoplastic bone lesions that may mimic bone tumors and pose a diagnostic pitfall. These diagnostic pitfalls can be avoided with a good understanding of the normal anatomy, anatomical variants, and characteristic radiographic appearance and location of the nonneoplastic

pathologies. Radiologists should also be aware of distinguishing features between a true bone tumor and tumor mimic, to avoid unnecessary additional imaging and procedures. Emphasis should also be given to clinical correlation, as traumatic, inflammatory, and metabolic bone pathologies can be easily diagnosed on radiographs alone, based on a proper history and evaluation of biochemical parameters. While a scrupulous approach combined with an experienced understanding of bone tumor mimics will maximize diagnostic accuracy, a good report should also be able to guide clinicians in deciding which lesions are "do not touch" entities and which need further work-up, thus helping reduce patient anxiety and limiting cost.

References

Agarwal G, Mishra SK, Kar DK et al (2002) Recovery pattern of patients with osteitis fibrosa cystica in primary hyperparathyroidism after successful parathyroidectomy. Surgery 132:1075–1085

Agudelo CA, Wise CM (2001) Gout: diagnosis, pathogenesis, and clinical manifestations. Curr Opin Rheumatol 13:234–239

Azouz EM (2002) Magnetic resonance imaging of benign bone lesions: cysts and tumors. Top Magn Reson Imaging 13:219–229

Bansal A (2008) The dripping candle wax sign. Radiology 246:638–640

Beaman FD, Peterson JJ (2007) MR imaging of cysts, ganglia, and bursae about the knee. Radiol Clin N Am 45:969–982

Bluemke DA, Fishman EK, Scott WW Jr (1994) Skeletal complications of radiation therapy. Radiographics 14:111–121

Brandser EA, El-Koury GY, Kathol MH (1995) Adolescent hamstring avulsions that simulate tumors. Emerg Radiol 2:273–278

Curtis JA, O'Hara AE, Carpenter GG (1977) Spurs of the mandible and supracondylar process of the humerus in Cornelia de Lange syndrome. AJR Am J Roentgenol 129:156–158

De Wilde V, De Maeseneer M, Lenchik L et al (2004) Normal osseous variants presenting as cystic or lucent areas on radiography and CT imaging: a pictorial overview. Eur J Radiol 51:77–84

Fitzpatrick KA, Taljanovic MS, Speer DP et al (2004) Imaging findings of fibrous dysplasia with histopathologic and intraoperative correlation. AJR Am J Roentgenol 182:1389–1398

Fong EE (1946) Iliac horns (symmetrical bilateral central posterior iliac processes). Radiology 47:517

Freud E (1940) The pathological significance of intraarticular pressure. Edinburgh Med J 47:192

Girish G, Glazebrook KN, Jacobson JA (2013) Advanced imaging in gout. AJR Am J Roentgenol 201:515–525

Gould CF, Ly JQ, Lattin GE Jr et al (2007) Bone tumor mimics: avoiding misdiagnosis. Curr Probl Diagn Radiol 36:124–141

Greenspan A, Azouz EM (1999) Bone dysplasia series: melorheostosis – review and update. Can Assoc Radiol J 50:324–330

Gruber G, Giessauf C, Leithner A et al (2008) Bizarre parosteal osteochondromatous proliferation (Nora lesion): a report of 3 cases and a review of the literature. Can J Surg 51:486–489

Hammoud S, Weber K, McCarthy EF (2005) Unicameral bone cysts of the pelvis: a study of 16 cases. Iowa Orthop J 25:69–74

Hatzenbuehler J, Pulling TJ (2011) Diagnosis and management of osteomyelitis. Am Fam Physician 84:1027–1033

Jacobson JA, Girish G, Jiang Y, Sabb BJ (2008) Radiographic evaluation of arthritis: degenerative joint disease and variations. Radiology 248:737–747

Kavanagh EC, Read P, Carty F et al (2011) Three-dimensional magnetic resonance imaging analysis of hip morphology in the assessment of femoral acetabular impingement. Clin Radiol 66:742–747

Khot R, Sikarwar JS, Gupta RP, Sharma GL (2005) Osteopoikilosis: a case report. Indian J Radiol Imaging 15:453–454

Kim SY, Park JS, Ryu KN et al (2011) Various tumor-mimicking lesions in the musculoskeletal system: causes and diagnostic approach. Korean J Radiol 12:220–231

Klapsinou E, Despoina P, Dimitra D (2012) Cytologic findings and potential pitfalls in proliferative myositis and myositis ossificans diagnosed by fine needle aspiration cytology: report of four cases and review of the literature. Diagn Cytopathol 40:239–244

Krestan CR, Nemec U, Nemec S (2011) Imaging of insufficiency fractures. Semin Musculoskelet Radiol 15:198–207

Leri A, Joanny JP (1922) Une affection non de'critedes os: hyperostose "en coule'e" surtoute lalongueur d'un membreou "me'lorhe'ostose". Bull Mem Soc Med Hop Paris 46:1141–1145

Levine AH, Pais MJ, Berinson H, Amenta PS (1976) The soleal line: a cause of tibial pseudoperiostitis. Radiology 119:79–81

Mankin H (2009) Nail-patella syndrome: hereditary onycho-osteodysplasia. In: Mankin H (ed) Pathophysiology of orthopaedic diseases. American Academy of Orthopaedic Surgeons, Rosemont

Mhuircheartaigh JN, Lin YC, Wu JS (2014) Bone tumor mimickers: a pictorial essay. Indian J Radiol Imaging 24:225–236

Mirra JM, Brien EW, Tehranzadeh J (1995) Paget's disease of bone: review with emphasis on radiologic features – part I. Skeletal Radiol 24:163–171

Mitchell MJ, Logan PM (1998) Radiation-induced changes in bone. Radiographics 18:1125–1136

Murphey MD, Foreman KL, Klassen-Fischer MK et al (2014) From the radiologic pathology archives.

Imaging of osteonecrosis: radiologic-pathologic correlation. Radiographics 34:1003–1028

Mysorekar VR, Nandedkar AN (1983) The soleal line. Anat Rec 206:447–451

Nayak SR, Das S, Krishnamurthy A et al (2009) Supratrochlear foramen of the humerus: an anatomico-radiological study with clinical implications. Ups J Med Sci 114:90–94

Nokes SR, Vogler JB, Spritzer CE et al (1989) Herniation pits of the femoral neck: appearance at MR imaging. Radiology 172:231–234

Paget J (1877) On a form of chronic inflammation of bones (osteitis deformans). Med Chir Trans (Lond) 60:37–64

Paling MR, Herdt JR (1980) Radiation osteitis: a problem of recognition. Radiology 137:339–342

Parikh J, Hyare H, Saifuddin A (2002) The imaging features of post-traumatic myositis ossificans, with emphasis on MRI. Clin Radiol 57:1058–1066

Pineda C, Espinosa R, Pena A (2009) Radiographic imaging in osteomyelitis: the role of plain radiography, computed tomography, ultrasonography, magnetic resonance imaging, and scintigraphy. Semin Plast Surg 23:80–89

Pitt MJ, Graham AR, Shipman JH, Birkby W (1982) Herniation pit of the femoral neck. AJR Am J Roentgenol 138:1115–1121

Resnick D, Cone RO 3rd (1984) The nature of humeral pseudocysts. Radiology 150:27–28

Resnick D (2002) Paget's disease. In: Resnick D (ed) Diagnosis of bone and joint disorders, 4th edn. Saunders, Philadelphia

Rhaney K, Lamb DW (1955) The cysts of osteoarthritis of the hip: a radiologic and pathologic study. J Bone Joint Surg Br 37:663–875

Shah ZK, Peh WCG, Koh WL, Shek TWH (2005) Magnetic resonance imaging appearances of fibrous dysplasia. Br J Radiol 78:1104–1115

Shikhare SN, Singh DR, Shimpi TR, Peh WCG (2011) Tuberculous osteomyelitis and spondylodiscitis. Semin Musculoskelet Radiol 15:446–458

Stacy GS, Kapur A (2011) Mimics of bone and soft tissue neoplasms. Radiol Clin N Am 49:1261–1286

Sureka B, Mittal MK, Udhaya K et al (2014) Melorheostosis: two atypical cases. Indian J Radiol Imaging 24:192–195

Taljanovic MS, Hoover K (2015) Musculoskeletal system. In: Peh WCG (ed) Pitfalls in diagnostic imaging. Springer, Berlin/Heidelberg

Tehranzadeh J (1987) The spectrum of avulsion and avulsion-like injuries of the musculoskeletal system. Radiographics 7:945–974

Tehranzadeh J, Wong E, Wang F, Sadighpour M (2001) Imaging of osteomyelitis in the mature skeleton. Radiol Clin North Am 39:223–250

Theodorou DJ, Theodorou SJ, Kakitsubata Y (2011) Imaging of Paget disease of bone and its musculoskeletal complications: review. AJR Am J Roentgenol 196:S64–S75

West JA, Louis TH (2015) Radiographic findings in the nail-patella syndrome. Proc (Bayl Univ Med Cent) 28:334–336

Remide Arkun and Mehmet Argin

Contents

31.1	**Introduction**	621
31.2	**Normal Hematopoietic Bone Marrow**	622
31.3	**Melorheostosis**	623
31.4	**Traumatic Disorders**	624
31.4.1	Stress Fracture	624
31.4.2	Avulsion Fracture	627
31.5	**Erdheim-Chester Disease**	629
31.6	**Nora Lesion (Bizarre Parosteal Osteochondromatous Proliferation)**	630
31.7	**Fibrous Dysplasia**	630
31.8	**Fibroxanthoma**	633
31.9	**Unicameral (Simple) Bone Cyst**	633
31.10	**Aneurysmal Bone Cyst**	636
31.11	**Juxta-Articular Bone Cyst/Geode**	636
31.12	**Hydatid Disease**	637
31.13	**Hemophilic Pseudotumor**	640
31.14	**Paget Disease**	643
Conclusion		644
References		644

R. Arkun, MD (✉) • M. Argin, MD
Department of Radiology, Ege University Medical
School, 35100, Bornova/Izmir, Turkey
e-mail: rarkun@yahoo.com; remide.arkun@ege.edu.
tr; margin35@yahoo.com

Abbreviations

CT	Computed tomography
MRI	Magnetic resonance imaging

31.1 Introduction

Bone tumors are a relatively infrequent finding in musculoskeletal radiology, and malignant bone tumors are far less common than benign ones. The incidence of bone sarcoma is estimated to be 0.2% of the overall human tumor burden. A wide range of musculoskeletal tumors and tumor-like conditions may be encountered when patients undergo radiological examinations. The imaging features of certain normal, reactive, benign neoplastic, inflammatory, traumatic, and degenerative processes in the musculoskeletal system may mimic malignant tumors. Misinterpretation of the imaging findings can lead to inappropriate clinical management of the patient. Tumor-like lesions also can show similar imaging findings to benign and malignant bone tumors. Radiography is accepted as the single most valuable imaging modality in the diagnosis of bone lesions. Although the differential diagnosis of primary bone tumor remains based on their radiographic appearances, evaluation of bone tumors involves a multimodality approach, and cross-sectional imaging has extraordinarily improved the ability to characterize tumors.

© Springer International Publishing AG 2017

W.C.G. Peh (ed.), *Pitfalls in Musculoskeletal Radiology*, DOI 10.1007/978-3-319-53496-1_31

Magnetic resonance imaging (MRI) is the most sensitive and accurate imaging technique for evaluation of musculoskeletal tumors. MRI demonstrates the depth, size, and local extent of tumors. Published opinions regarding the value of MRI in characterizing the pathological nature of musculoskeletal masses and discriminating between benign and malignant lesions are divergent, with different papers showing that specificity values of MRI range from 76% to 90%. There are also opposing reports that MRI has low specificity in differentiation between benign and malignant masses, and most lesions demonstrate a nonspecific appearance. Besides benign and malignant bone tumors, there are numerous non-tumoral entities which have similar morphologic and signal changes and can mimic the imaging findings of bone tumors.

A large number of these lesions clearly have the characteristic findings of nonneoplastic entities and do not need further workup. The remainder of non-tumoral and tumor-like lesions needs management that includes close collaboration with orthopedic oncologists and further investigation such as biopsy or surgery. In the evaluation of bone tumors with MRI, the radiologist should be familiar with the imaging findings of non-tumoral and tumor-like lesions which will cause confusion. This chapter aims to highlight some pitfalls, including normal variants, congenital and traumatic disorders, and tumor-like disease of bone, which may mimic MRI findings of bone tumors.

31.2   Normal Hematopoietic Bone Marrow

Bone marrow is one of the largest organs in the body, after the osseous skeleton, skin, and body fat, and the marrow cavity of the skeleton contains both fat and hematopoietic cells. The normal composition and distribution of bone marrow change with age and affect the MRI signal appearances of marrow. Because metastatic and primary hematologic malignancies commonly involve the bone marrow, knowledge of the normal distribution of red and yellow marrow and variances is of primary necessity for correct interpretation. On gross examination, bone marrow appears red (hematopoietic marrow) or yellow (fatty marrow), depending on its predominant components. Normal red marrow has lower signal intensity than that of fat and generally equal or higher signal intensity than that of skeletal muscle on T1-weighted MR images. Normal yellow marrow has similar signal intensity to subcutaneous fat on T1-weighted MR images and appears darker on T2-weighted MR images obtained with fat suppression. On fat-suppressed T2-weighted MRI, the signal intensity of normal red marrow is higher than that of yellow marrow and is often similar to or slightly higher than that of skeletal muscle (Vogler and Murphy 1988; Hwang and Panicek 2007).

At birth, hematopoietic marrow is present throughout the entire skeleton, but various regions of hematopoietic marrow then start converting to fatty marrow. The transition occurs over two decades in a predictable sequence, beginning in the periphery of the skeleton and extending in a symmetrical centripetal manner into the central skeleton and from diaphyseal to metaphyseal regions in the long bones. Following attainment of an adult pattern, the fractional balance of red and yellow marrow contained within axial and proximal long bones may slowly change with advancing age (Vogler and Murphy 1988; Hwang and Panicek 2007; Howe et al. 2013). This appearance is usually appreciated on shoulder and hip MRI examinations. Although the distal appendicular skeleton usually has a uniform distribution of yellow marrow in adults, increased residual red marrow can be seen within the distal femur in knee MRI of patients who are heavy smokers, marathoners, and obese females of menstruating age. Knowledge of the typical distribution of residual red marrow in adults and the signal characteristics of normal red marrow should allow the avoidance of misdiagnosis.

The signal intensity, morphology, and distribution of marrow also can help to distinguish such normal variations from marrow lesions (Fig. 31.1). Marrow metastases usually have lower signal intensity than that of muscle and tend to be more rounded with sharply defined borders, whereas foci of red marrow also can often be recognized by their poorly defined

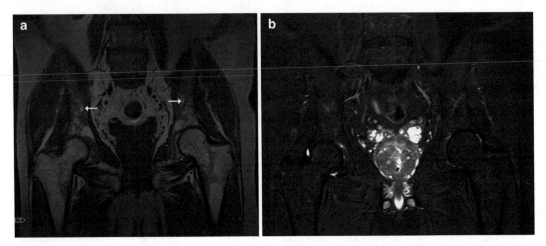

Fig. 31.1 Bone marrow reconversion in a 66-year-old man who is a heavy smoker. (**a**) Coronal T1-W MR image of the pelvis shows heterogeneous intermediate to hypointense signal in both iliac bones with focal hyperintense residue fatty marrow (*arrows*). There is a similar appearance in the L4 and L5 vertebral bodies. Note patchy intermediate signal changes due to residual red marrow on both medial aspects of the femoral neck. (**b**) The corresponding coronal STIR MR image of the pelvis shows diffuse, slightly more hyperintense signal than that of skeletal muscle in the L4 and L5 vertebral bodies and both iliac bones. There is no abnormal focal signal hyperintensity to suggest tumoral infiltration

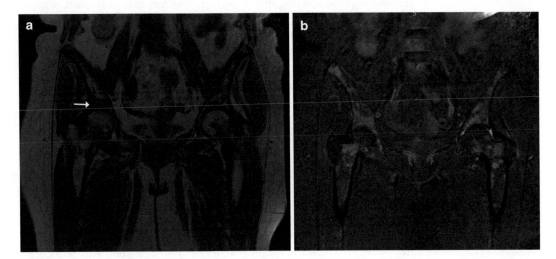

Fig. 31.2 Breast carcinoma metastases in a 55-year-old woman. (**a**) Coronal T1-W MR image of the pelvis shows areas of heterogeneous hypointense signal in both iliac bones and femoral necks. Signal intensity is lower than that of the muscle at the right acetabular roof (*arrow*). (**b**) The corresponding coronal STIR MR image of the pelvis shows heterogeneous hyperintense signal in both iliac bones. There are also rounded hyperintense foci in both femoral necks

feathery margins that interdigitate with fatty marrow on T1-weighted MR images, as well as by its asymmetrical distribution. On fluid-sensitive MRI sequences, metastatic lesions have higher signal intensity than that of normal hematopoietic red marrow (Howe et al. 2013; Arkun and Argin 2014) (Fig. 31.2).

31.3 Melorheostosis

Melorheostosis is an uncommon, nonhereditary, benign, sclerosing mesodermal disease that affects the skeleton and adjacent soft tissues, with an incidence of 0.9 cases per million. Appendicular skeleton involvement is more common than the axial skeleton. The periosteal hyperostosis along the cortex of long bones, resembling the dripping or flowing of candle wax, gives the condition its name, which is derived from Greek. Besides bone changes, para-articular soft tissue masses, intra-articular extensions, and spinal involvement have been described. Cross-sectional imaging techniques are useful to reveal manifestation of the disease and allow differentiation from other disease and malignancy. The characteristic radiographic appearance is that of flowing cortical hyperostosis along one side of the shaft of the long bone resembling "melting wax flowing down the side of a candle." However, it can be seen as an osteoma-like appearance or can be seen together with complete bony obliteration of bone marrow, bony overgrowth, or paraosseous soft tissue ossifications.

On MRI, due to cortical hyperostosis, signal hypointensity is seen on all pulse sequences, with encroachment on marrow space resulting from endosteal involvement. Intramedullary focal signal hyperintensity on T2-weighted MR images is a very rare finding. If there is a para-articular soft tissue mass, the MRI appearance of a soft tissue mass is variable, and heterogeneous signal intensity due to mineralized areas, fat-containing areas, and fibrovascular tissue may be seen (Fig. 31.3). This can mimic parosteal osteosarcoma, and computed tomography (CT) is helpful to demonstrate the cleft in between the bone and the soft tissue mass (Azouz and Greenspan 2005; Suresh et al. 2010).

31.4 Traumatic Disorders

31.4.1 Stress Fracture

Bone marrow edema may result from a variety of nonneoplastic disorders. Although stress fracture is one of the common causes of bone marrow edema, it is a diagnostic challenge in skeletal imaging. The term "stress fracture" refers to the failure of the skeleton to withstand submaximal forces over time. Two forms of stress fracture have been defined, namely, fatigue fracture which occurs in normal bone placed under the stress of a new or abnormal activity and insufficiency fractures which are the result of normal activities on bones of abnormal or deficient bone mineral (Fayad et al. 2005; Wall and Feller 2006; Arkun and Argin 2014). However, in the literature, the term stress fracture has generally been used, instead of fatigue fracture (Arkun and Argin 2014).

Although radiography is the first imaging technique for bone lesions, stress fractures are usually not visible radiographically at the time of initial presentation. Radiographs are positive in only 10–25% of cases at the initial presentation; and 2–12 weeks after injury, radiographs can be still normal in up to 33–50% of cases. If a stress fracture is visible on radiographs, cortical resorption, periosteal reaction, cortical thickening, endosteal sclerosis, and sclerotic line perpendicular to the trabeculae are typical imaging findings. For a patient who has extremity pain, with or without swelling and tenderness, and does not have a clear history of trauma or chronic overuse type of activity and normal radiographs, there is necessity for another imaging technique.

MRI typically shows periosteal and bone marrow edema without a visible fracture line in the early phase of the disease. There may be a variable degree of surrounding soft tissue edema. Enhancement of the marrow and surrounding soft tissues may be seen after contrast administration, mimicking other disease such as infection or tumor (Fig. 31.4). A hypointense fracture line, which is seen as a linear area of hypointense signal, with surrounding ill-defined T2-hyperintense signal (edema) on fluid-sensitive sequences, allows an accurate diagnosis of stress fractures (Fayad et al. 2005; Gould et al. 2007; Arkun and Argin 2014). Stacy and Dixon (2007) stated that the edema associated with stress fracture is frequently much more pronounced on fat-suppressed T2-weighted images than on T1-weighted MR images and is often ill-defined, particularly on T1-weighted images. In contrast, a well-defined hypointense rounded lesion is usually evident on T1-weighted images in patients with a neoplasm.

Insufficiency fractures occur more commonly in the elderly and, in particular, patients with

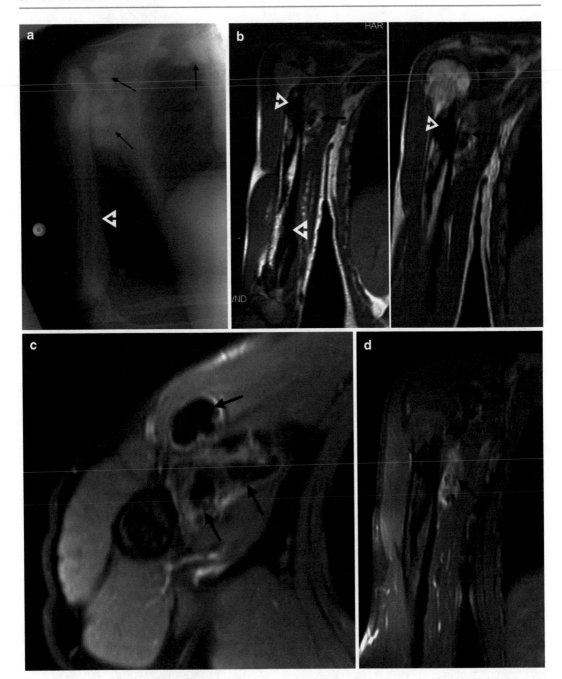

Fig. 31.3 Melorheostosis in a 40-year-old woman with right shoulder pain. (**a**) Right humerus radiograph, including the shoulder joint and right hemithorax, shows flowing cortical hyperostosis along the medial shaft of the humerus (*open arrow*). There is also paraosseous soft tissue ossification in the right axilla and parasternal region (*arrows*). (**b**) Contiguous coronal T1-W MR images of the humerus show markedly hypointense flowing cortical hyperostosis (*open arrows*) and a heterogeneous irregular mass adjacent to the proximal metaphysis of the humerus (*black arrows*). The lesion has areas of signal void due to mineralization. (**c**) Axial fat-suppressed T2-W MR image shows markedly hypointense intramedullary involvement and a heterogeneous irregular mass adjacent to the bone (*arrows*). Note that there is no continuity between the cortical bone and the soft tissue mass. (**d**) Coronal contrast-enhanced fat-suppressed T1-W MR image shows enhancement of the soft tissue mass (*arrow*)

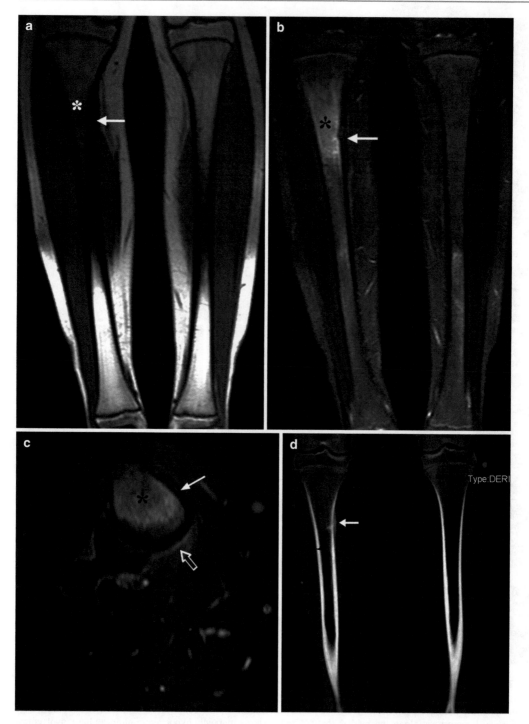

Fig. 31.4 Stress fracture in a 13-year-old boy with right leg pain. (**a**) Coronal T1-W MR image of the lower extremities shows an area of hypointense bone marrow signal in the proximal metaphysis of the right tibia (*black asterisk*) and cortical thickening at the medial cortex of the right tibia (*white arrow*). (**b**) The corresponding coronal fat-suppressed T2-W MR image shows an area of hyperintense signal due to bone marrow edema (*black asterisk*) and cortical thickening due to periosteal reaction (*arrow*). (**c**) Axial contrast-enhanced fat-suppressed T1-W MR image shows enhancement of the bone marrow (*black asterisk*), periosteal reaction (*arrow*), and soft tissue edema (*open arrow*). (**d**) The fracture line (*black curved arrow*) with solitary periosteal reaction (*white arrow*) is better delineated on the coronal reformatted CT image

cancer. These patients can be detected inciden-tally during MRI or CT examinations which are performed for other reasons. Several pathological conditions which include postmenopausal osteo-porosis, corticosteroid-induced osteoporosis, radiation therapy, rheumatoid arthritis, Paget dis-ease of bone, renal osteodystrophy, and long-standing bed rest may decrease bone resistance and predispose the development of insufficiency fractures (Fayad et al. 2005; Cabarrus et al. 2008; Arkun and Argin 2014). The most common loca-tions are the pelvic girdle including the sacrum, proximal femur, and vertebral bodies, particu-larly the lumbar and lower thoracic spine. Patients typically present with acute pain, depending on the site of the fracture. Because of the nonspe-cific clinical presentation, imaging has an impor-tant role in the detection and diagnosis of insufficiency fractures.

Frequently, these fractures are radiographi-cally occult, and some of these fractures, in par-ticular sacral insufficiency fractures, are relatively underdiagnosed. If an insufficiency fracture is visible on radiographs, common findings include a sclerotic band or line, bone expansion, and exu-berant callus. The lytic fracture line or cortical break is rarely observed. If the radiologist is not aware of this appearance, particularly in setting of existing malignant disease, insufficiency frac-ture may be misdiagnosed as bone metastasis (Cabarrus et al. 2008; Krestan et al. 2011). Sacral insufficiency fractures can be associated with insufficiency fractures of the pubic rami and parasymphyseal region. Early diagnosis is best made with bone scintigraphy or MRI. Although bone scintigraphy is highly sensitive, it relies on accurate interpretation of the uptake pattern, and atypical uptake patterns may be difficult to inter-pret. In bilateral sacral insufficiency fractures, H-shaped (Honda sign) increased activity or the combination of concomitant sacral and parasym-physeal uptake is considered a typical finding of insufficiency fractures (Campbell and Fajarda 2008; Krestan et al. 2011).

MRI is as sensitive as bone scintigraphy but is of higher specificity, both in isolating the exact anatomical location and in distinguishing frac-tures from tumors or infection. Moreover, MRI is the most sensitive imaging technique in the early stage of insufficiency fracture (Cabarrus et al. 2008; Campbell and Fajardo 2008; Krestan et al. 2011). MRI shows hypointense signal on T1-weighted images and hyperintense signal on T2-weighted images. In the sacrum, linear bands are seen within the sacral ala and body, with the bands being parallel to the sacroiliac joints (Fig. 31.5). Although on MRI, signal hyperinten-sity and a hypointense fracture line within the area of edema are characteristic findings, a hypointense fracture line is not seen in 7% of cases. The benefit of Gadolinium-based contrast agent administration is controversial and is not commonly applied. Radiologists should be famil-iar with imaging findings of insufficiency frac-tures because malignant lesions are frequently suspected in patients who have undergone radia-tion therapy and chemotherapy of the pelvis (Cabarrus et al. 2008; Lyders et al. 2010). It has been reported that ill-defined signal hypointen-sity on T1-weighted images is significantly more likely to represent insufficiency fractures, while adjacent muscle signal abnormality reflects path-ological fracture (Campbell and Fajardo 2008). Occasionally, MRI can be confusing, especially if a fracture line is not evident, and correlative CT or follow-up imaging may be useful (Cabarrus et al. 2008; Lyders et al. 2010).

31.4.2 Avulsion Fracture

An avulsion fracture is one that occurs when a joint capsule, ligament, or muscle insertion or its origin is pulled off from the bone as a result of a sprain, dislocation, or strong contracture of the muscle against resistance. As the soft tissue is pulled away from the bone, a bony fragment (or fragments) remains attached to the soft tissue. It is usually seen among athletes and most commonly occurs at the pelvis, shoulder, elbow, knee, ankle, and foot. In a basic avulsion fracture, radiographs of the site reveal that a small piece of bone has been torn away. Physical findings, symptoms, the patient's age, and biomechanical analysis of the accident can collectively raise the suspicion of an avulsion fracture, and conventional radiography

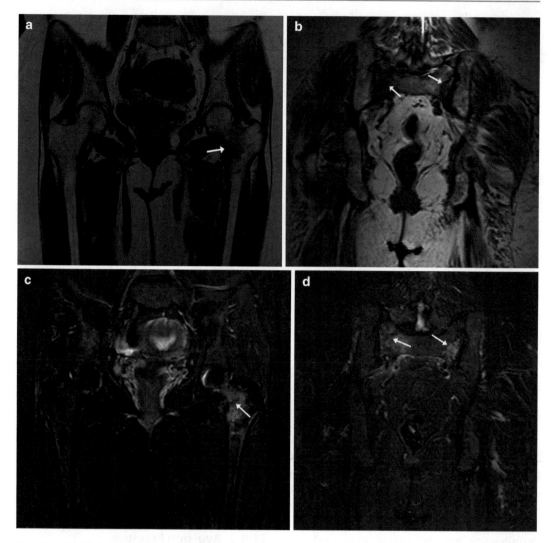

Fig. 31.5 Multiple insufficiency fractures in a 75-year-old woman. (**a, b**) Contiguous coronal T1-W MR images of the pelvis show an area of signal hypointensity in the left femoral neck (*arrow* in **a**) and right sacral ala (*arrow* in **b**) and a hypointense linear band that is located in the left sacral ala (*arrow*). (**c, d**) Contiguous coronal STIR MR images of the pelvis show hypointense fracture lines surrounded by bone marrow edema adjacent to the medial cortex of the left femoral neck (*arrow* in **c**) and within the sacral ala bilaterally (*arrows* in **d**)

can confirm the diagnosis, especially in long bones. In adolescents, because of inherent weakness of the apophysis, avulsion fracture is seen together with musculotendinous junction injuries. In the pelvis, avulsion injuries usually occur before closure of the apophysis as a result of trauma. Among six sites, the ischial tuberosity is the most common site for pelvic avulsion injury.

A clinical history of sudden onset of severe pain at the site of avulsion is common in acute injury. Diagnosis can be achieved by clinical examination together with radiographs, and MRI or CT, as determined by availability. In case of a displaced fracture fragment, this is seen at the origin or insertion of a muscle or tendon. If an apophyseal avulsion is non-displaced or when the apophysis is unossified, radiographs can be negative. MRI will show hematoma, bone marrow edema, and periosteal stripping at the tendinous attachment sites (Stevens et al. 1999) (Fig. 31.6). In the healing phase, avulsion fractures can have an aggressive appearance with a protuberant mass and resemble an infectious or malignant process. Young adults with pelvic

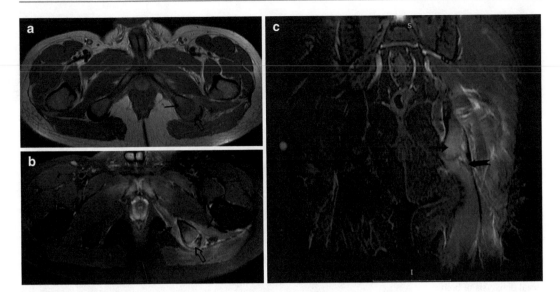

Fig. 31.6 Avulsion fracture in a 22-year-old male soldier who had pain in his left hip with walking difficulty. (**a**) Axial T1-W MR image of the pelvis shows an area of hypointense signal in the left ischium (*black arrow*) and hyperintense signal and separation of ischial tuberosity (*open black arrow*). (**b**) The corresponding axial fat-suppressed T2-W MR image shows muscle edema in the quadratus femoris and obturator internus muscles (*black arrows*). There is also hyperintense signal due to hematoma at the ischial tuberosity (*open black arrow*). (**c**) Coronal fat-suppressed T2-W MR image shows bone marrow edema in the ischium (*arrow*) and an area of signal hyperintensity due to musculotendinous junction injury at the proximal insertion of hamstrings (*closed arrow*) and extensive hamstring muscle edema

avulsion injuries can especially be mistaken as having a malignant tumor due to an aggressive appearance caused by exuberant bone marrow and soft tissue edema. CT will nicely identify any present bone fragments and delineate findings associated with healing (Gould et al. 2007; Arkun and Argin 2014).

31.5 Erdheim-Chester Disease

Erdheim-Chester disease (ECD) is a rare non-familiar disorder, first described by Jakob Erdheim and William Chester in 1930 as "lipid granulomatosis". Until now, approximately 500 cases had been reported in the literature. The clinical manifestations of ECD are nonspecific and depend on the affected organ. It may be asymptomatic, clinically indolent, or, sometimes, life threatening. Bone involvement is almost universal in ECD (96% of cases), and more than 50% of cases have at least one site of associated extra-skeletal involvement, such as the kidney, skin, central nervous system, or heart. Patients may have bone pain, frequently juxta-articular at the knees and ankles. In long bones, ECD is characterized by bilateral symmetrical sclerosis of the diametaphyseal regions of long bones and infiltration of foamy lipid-laden histiocytes. This may be difficult to diagnose because it is rarely seen and has a broad spectrum of clinical manifestations.

The diagnosis is based on radiological findings of striking patchy medullary sclerosis in the diametaphyseal region, which is mostly confined to the appendicular skeleton in a symmetrical fashion. Radiographs show bilateral and symmetrical cortical osteosclerosis of the diaphyseal and metaphyseal regions of the long bones, with a clear-cut limit between the involved portion of the bone and the epiphyseal region, which is usually spared. Rarely, these alterations may be associated with periostitis and endosteal thickening. On MRI, skeletal involvement consists of extensive replacement of the fatty marrow by hypointense signal on T1-weighted images, heterogeneous signal on T2-weighted/STIR images, and enhancement after gadolinium injection (Fig. 31.7). MRI is useful to evaluate the extent of medullary bone disease and

Fig. 31.7 Erdheim-Chester disease proven by bone biopsy in a 60-year-old woman who had bilateral knee pain. (**a**) Coronal T1-W MR image of the lower extremities shows extensive replacement of fatty marrow with areas of signal hypointensity bilaterally. Note that the distal epiphyses of both tibias are spared. (**b**) The corresponding coronal STIR MR image shows symmetrical heterogeneous signal hypointensity with cystic changes at the distal diaphysis of both tibias

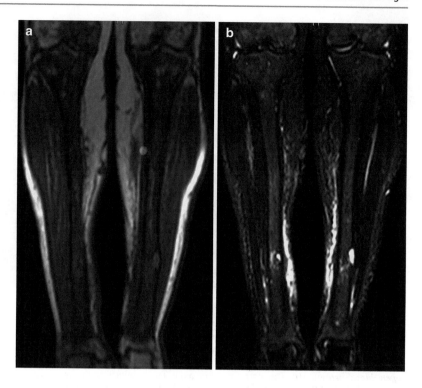

diagnose the presence of associated osteonecrosis. Partial epiphyseal involvement can be seen on MRI. Symmetrical involvement almost excludes diseases such as osteomyelitis, Paget disease, lymphoma, and sclerotic sarcoidosis (Eyigor et al. 2005; Dion et al. 2006; Antunes et al. 2014).

31.6 Nora Lesion (Bizarre Parosteal Osteochondromatous Proliferation)

This entity is also known as bizarre parosteal osteochondromatous proliferation (BPOP) and may be mistaken for a surface or central osteosarcoma in the peripheral skeleton or in the long bones. Even if it is considered a reactive process, chromosomal abnormalities have been described, suggesting the possibility of a neoplasm. There is no gender predominance, and it is more common in the second and third decades of life. Although the classical location is on the surfaces of the small bones of hand and feet, 25% of cases are located in long bones, especially the radius and humerus. Radiographically, there is a heterotopic, well-defined calcified or ossified mass

attached to cortical surface of bone. The mass can be pedunculated or sessile. There is no continuity between the lesion and cortex and medulla of host bone and no contact with the growth plate. On MRI, Nora lesion shows variable signal intensity on T1-weigheted images. It may show hyperintense signal on fluid-sensitive sequences and/or edema in the bone marrow and surrounding soft tissues and mild heterogeneous enhancement after gadolinium injection (Fig. 31.8). CT is more helpful than MRI in providing a better delineation of the relationship between the lesion and the host bone (Dhondt et al. 2006; Kershen et al. 2012; Rapppaort et al. 2014; Olvi et al. 2015b).

31.7 Fibrous Dysplasia

Rather than being a true neoplasm, fibrous dysplasia (FD) is a developmental anatomy of bone in which the normal medullary space is replaced by fibro-osseous tissue and small spicules of woven bone. FD may present in either monostotic (70–85%) or polyostotic (15–30%) forms. Although any bone within the skeleton can be affected, the tibia, proximal femur, pelvis, ribs,

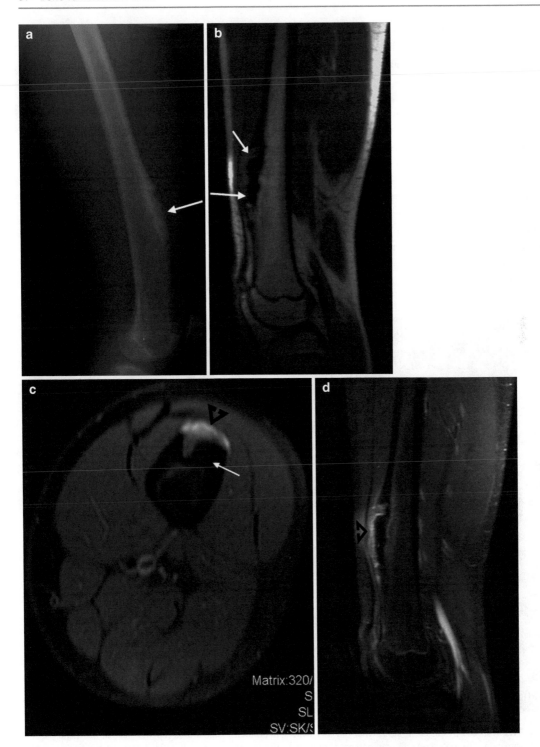

Fig. 31.8 Nora lesion in a 16-year-old boy with distal left thigh pain. (**a**) Left femur radiograph shows a sessile protuberant ossified mass attached to the anterior cortex of the left femur (*arrow*). (**b**) Sagittal T1-W MR image of the femur shows a sessile protuberant hypointense mass with a soft tissue component which has intermediate signal intensity located in the distal diaphysis of the femur (*arrows*). (**c**) Axial fat-suppressed T2-W MR image shows an ossified mass attached to the anterior cortex (*white arrow*) with a hyperintense soft tissue component (*open black arrow*) due to cartilage component. There is no continuity in between the lesion and medullary bone. (**d**) There is marked peripheral enhancement of the lesion on the sagittal contrast-enhanced fat-suppressed T1-W MR image (*open black arrow*)

and skull are the most common locations. It is usually located in the metadiaphysis, and radiographically, the most characteristic finding is a "ground-glass" radiolucent appearance within the bone. Other classical radiological findings include mild bony expansion with or without sclerosis, cortical thinning, and endosteal scalloping. Epiphyseal involvement is unusual, particularly before closure of the growth plate. Cortical destruction, soft tissue component, and any type of periosteal reaction are not seen, if there is no fracture. When the radiological appearance is typical and the patient is asymptomatic, further imaging is unnecessary. CT and MRI will show a solid heterogeneous lesion with possible cystic components.

On MR imaging, FD has signal hypointensity on T1-weighted images and variable signal intensity due to T2-weighted images. Lesions tend to be relatively homogeneous, unless complicated by fracture or secondary aneurysmal bone cyst. A peripheral hypointense rim corresponds to marginal sclerosis on radiographs. As the lesion matures, foci of hypointense signal appear that corresponds histologically to hypercellular fibrous tissue and hemosiderin deposits. This heterogeneous signal intensity and prominent bony expansion may simulate malignancy (Fig. 31.9). After gadolinium administration, variable enhancement can be seen, due to cystic and solid parts of the lesion. Adjacent marrow edema is generally absent in uncomplicated lesions.

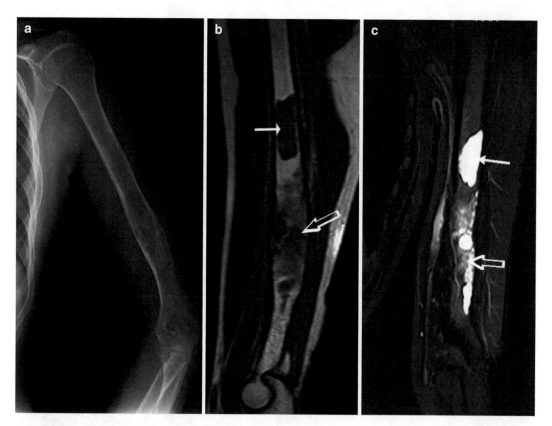

Fig. 31.9 Fibrous dysplasia in an 18-year-old girl with left arm pain. (**a**) Left humerus radiograph shows an expansile osteolytic lesion with well-defined margins, cortical thinning, and characteristic "ground-glass" appearance at the distal diaphyseal region. (**b**) Sagittal T1-W MR image shows different imaging findings in the humerus. There is bony expansion and heterogeneous hypointense signal area (*open arrow*) at the distal part of the lesion and a well-defined hypointense lesion at the proximal part of the lesion (*arrow*) (**c**) Coronal STIR MR image shows the lesion to have heterogeneous intermediate signal (*open arrow*) and cystic changes (*arrow*) with well-defined hypointense margins

Differential considerations may include unicameral bone cyst, non-ossifying fibroma (NOF), enchondroma, eosinophilic granuloma, aneurysmal bone cyst, myeloma, or metastatic disease, depending on location, patient age, and imaging appearances. Fibrous dysplasia may rarely undergo malignant transformation, with reported prevalence of 0.5% (Smith and Kransdorf 2000; Alyas et al. 2007; Arkun and Argin 2014).

31.8 Fibroxanthoma

The term "fibroxanthoma" is a common definition encompassing non-ossifying fibroma (NOF), fibrous cortical defect (FCD), and benign fibrous histiocytoma (BFH). All these lesions are a histologically identical benign fibrous neoplasm in the metaphysis of growing bones. It is one of the most frequent tumor-like lesions of bone and is more frequent in males (60%) than in females (40%). The historical division between FCD and NOF has been defined by size and natural history. FCDs are small metaphyseal cortical defects that disappear spontaneously (most common), whereas NOFs persist over time and may demonstrate interval growth into adulthood. It is located in the metaphyseal or metadiaphyseal area of long bones, and the most common locations are the distal femur and distal or proximal tibia, usually at the posteromedial surface. The long axis of the lesion is usually parallel to that of the host bone.

Radiographic findings of fibroxanthoma are typical and are seen as an eccentric ovoid osteolytic lesion of the metaphysis (or diametaphysis) arising close to the physeal plate, with a scalloped contour and well-demarcated sclerotic margins. Larger and multiple lesions can create confusion, when they are found incidentally on MRI which have been obtained for another reason in cancer patients. On MRI, NOF has hypointense and heterogeneous signal intensity on T1- and T2-weighted images related to its fibrous content, with a well-limited scalloped contour (Fig. 31.10). Areas of hyperintense signal due to microfractures or occult fractures may be seen on fat-suppressed T2-weighted images, and there is intense enhancement after gadolinium injection (Smith and Kransdorf 2000; Alyas et al. 2007; Arkun and Argin 2014).

31.9 Unicameral (Simple) Bone Cyst

Unicameral (or simple) bone cyst is an intramedullary, usually unilocular, cystic cavity filled with serous or serosanguineous fluid and lined by a membrane of variable thickness. Unicameral bone cyst is mostly seen in the first decades of life, which accounts for 80% of cases. The most common locations are the metaphysis of proximal humerus, proximal femur, and proximal tibia. The ilium, calcaneus, and talus are often affected in older patients. There is a centrally and symmetrically expanded osteolytic lesion with well-defined margins located at the metaphysis of long bones on radiographs. Epiphyseal involvement is uncommon. A multilocular or trabeculated appearance may be seen, due to prominent endosteal bony ridges in the inner cortical wall. When unicameral bone cyst is complicated by fracture, there may be small "fallen fragment" sign that has migrated and found floating in the fluid. There is no periosteal reaction except at sites of fracture.

Uncomplicated unicameral bone cysts have hypointense signal on T1-weighted images and hyperintense signal on T2-weighted MR images. Lesions that have a pathological fracture have heterogeneous signal intensities on both T1- and T2-weighted images, because of bleeding within the cyst. After gadolinium injection, they demonstrate enhancement with focal thick peripheral, heterogeneous, or subcortical patterns (Fig. 31.11). Septations within the lesions may be observed on MRI which may not be visualized on radiographs. Uncomplicated lesions are diagnosed easily on MRI. Lesions complicated by pathological fractures may reveal areas of heterogeneous signal and irregular enhancement patterns after the contrast administration. Differential considerations may include aneurysmal bone cyst, fibrous dysplasia, NOF, eosinophilic granuloma, and enchondroma (Mascard et al. 2015; Olvi et al. 2015a).

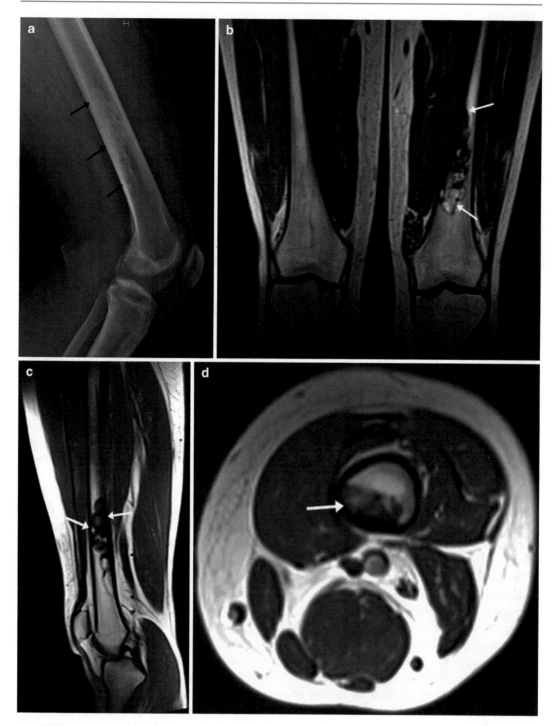

Fig. 31.10 Non-ossifying fibroma in a 17-year-old girl. (a) Left femur radiograph shows a lobulated intramedullary ossified lesion at the distal metadiaphyseal area of the bone (*arrows*). (b) Coronal, (c) sagittal, and (d) axial T1-W MR images show that the lesion has lobulated margins and heterogeneous signal intensity and the relationship of the lesion with the posterior endosteal cortex (*arrows*)

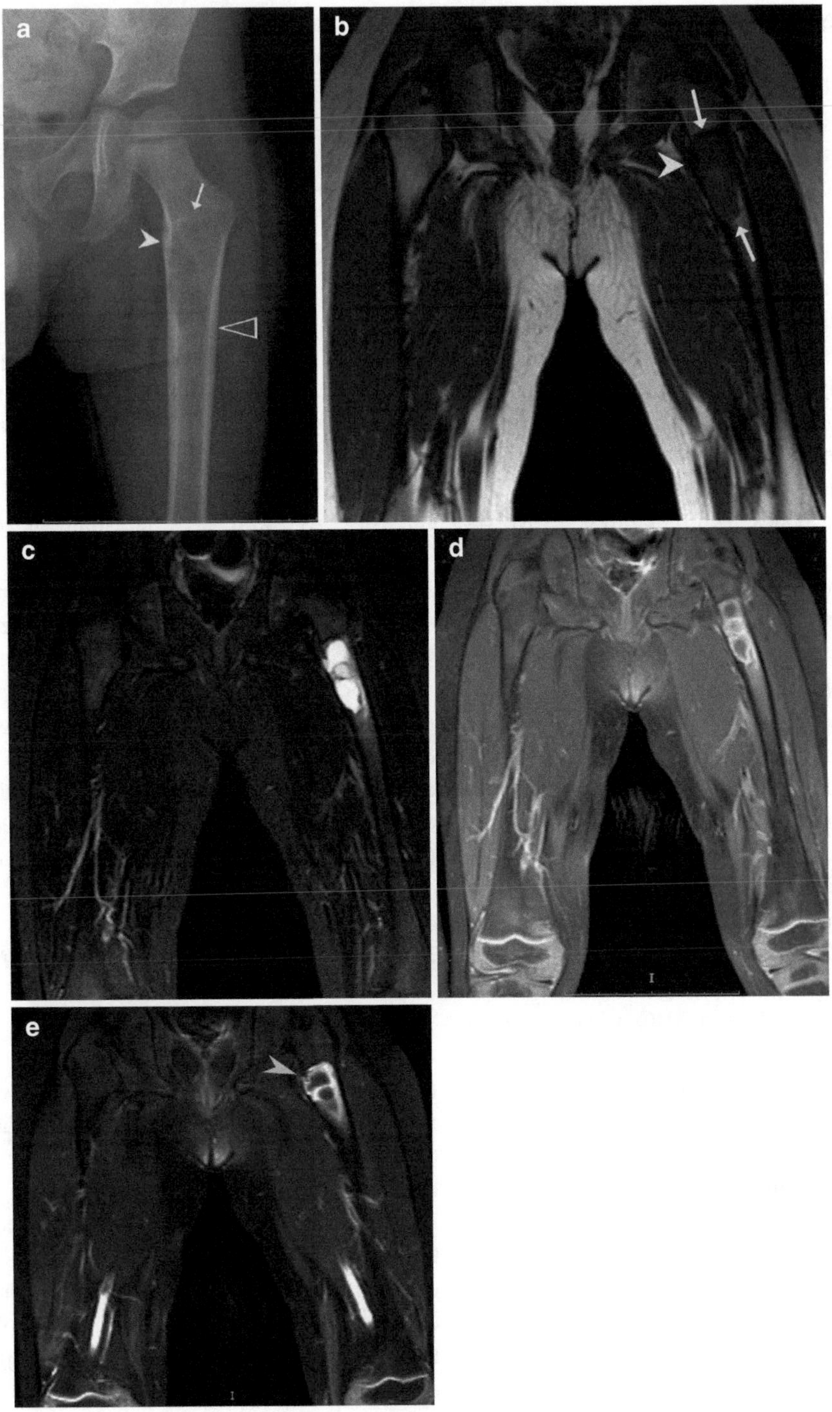

Fig. 31.11 Unicameral bone cyst in a 4-year-old boy with left hip pain after a fall. (**a**) Left femur radiograph shows a well-defined (*arrow*), slightly expanded osteolytic lesion with cortical thickening at the medial cortex (*closed arrowhead*) and solitary periosteal reaction at the lateral aspect of the left femoral proximal metadiaphyseal region (*open arrowhead*). (**b**) Coronal T1-W MR images show a slightly expanded heterogeneously hypointense lesion with well- defined margins (*arrows*) located at the femoral proximal metadiaphyseal region. There is also cortical irregularity at the medial aspect of femoral shaft (*arrowhead*). (**c**) This lesion has heterogeneously hypointense signal with thin sep- tations on the corresponding coronal fat-suppressed T1-W MR image. (**d**, **e**) Contiguous coronal contrast-enhanced fat- suppressed T1-W MR images show septal enhancement. There is also a fracture at the medial cortex (*arrowhead*)

31.10 Aneurysmal Bone Cyst

Aneurysmal bone cyst (ABC) is an intramedullary eccentric metaphyseal and rapidly expansible benign osteolytic lesion with multiloculated blood-filled cystic cavities. There are various forms of ABC: the commonest form is primary ABC which accounts for 70% of cases. The others are secondary ABC (associated with another lesion such as osteoblastoma, chondroblastoma, giant cell tumor, and fibrous dysplasia), solid ABC or giant cell reparative granuloma, and soft tissue ABC. Although ABC may affect any age group, 75–90% of cases occur before the age of 20 years. Although ABC can involve any part of skeleton, long bones with metaphyseal involvement, spine, and pelvis are the most common locations. The distal femur, tibia, humerus, and fibula are the most involved long bones. In the spine, the posterior elements are usually affected.

Radiographs show purely osteolytic, eccentric, aggressive expansile ballooning with a soap bubble pattern, internal trabeculae, and rapid progression, without periosteal reaction. When there is a cortical break, the lesion usually forms a thin sclerotic rim of ossification due to periosteal new bone formation. ABC may cross joints and involve an adjacent bone. CT and MRI are helpful to make differentiation in between ABC and unicameral bone cyst. Although "fluid-fluid" levels were first described in ABC, it can occur in many other lesions such as telangiectatic osteosarcoma (OS), giant cell tumor, chondroblastoma, and metastasis. CT is less sensitive than MRI and reveals a lesion with a thin surrounding shell of bone. A thin shell of soft tissue attenuation, representing the fibrous periosteum, can also been seen (Mascard et al. 2015; Olvi et al. 2015a). CT shows fluid-fluid levels about one-third of lesions. In complex regions, such as the spine and pelvis, CT is helpful to provide a lesion map and planning possible instrumentations. MRI confirms the entirely cystic nature of the lesion, with internal septations and fluid-fluid levels on T2-weighted images. There is enhancement at the cyst walls and internal septae. Primary ABCs have thin septae and minimal or no solid component (Fig. 31.12), whereas secondary ABCs tend to have nodular septae and a larger

solid component on MRI. Differential diagnosis includes unicameral bone cyst, giant cell tumor, osteoblastoma, hydatid disease, and telangiectatic OS (Chen et al. 2005; Remotti and Feldman 2012).

Telangiectatic OS was described by Gaylord as a "malignant bone aneurysm" in 1903. This subtype of osteosarcoma is primarily (>90%) composed of multiple aneurysmal dilated cavities that contain blood, with high-grade sarcomatous cells in the peripheral rim and septations around these spaces. Telangiectatic OS may be confused with ABC, both radiologically and pathologically (Remotti and Feldman 2012). MRI demonstrates predominantly signal hyperintensity as well as fluid-fluid levels on T2-weighted images. Murphey et al. (2003) showed that 52% of cases showed hyperintense signal on T1-weighted images. In telangiectatic OS, there is thick nodular solid tissue surrounding the cystic spaces. This finding is especially prominent after contrast administration (Fig. 31.13). Telangiectatic OS has also a more aggressive growth pattern than ABC, with cortical destruction together with a soft tissue mass (Murphy et al. 2003; Olvi et al. 2015a, b, c, d).

31.11 Juxta-Articular Bone Cyst/ Geode

A juxta-articular bone cyst is an intraosseous nonneoplastic subchondral cystic lesion which is not related to joint pathology. If there is association with degenerative arthritis, the lesion is defined as subchondral pseudocyst or geode which is a well-defined osteolytic lesion adjacent to the periarticular surface. A geode is one of the common differential diagnoses of an osteolytic epiphyseal lesion. This is originally a geological term referring to rounded formations in igneous and sedimentary rocks. Geodes and juxta-articular bone cysts have similar radiological findings except for the presence of osteoarthritis in the former. Geodes can vary in size and are often multiple. Size greater than 2 cm is an unusual finding. On MRI, there is a well-defined round T1-hypointense and T2-hyperintense lesion which may be surrounded by bone marrow

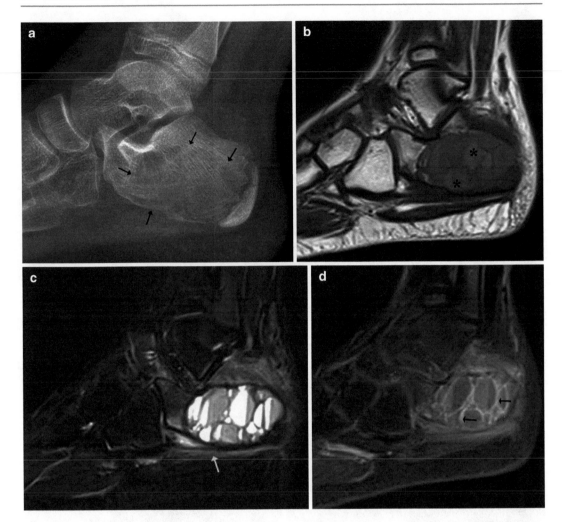

Fig. 31.12 Aneurysmal bone cyst in a 12-year-old boy with left heel pain. (**a**) Lateral radiograph of the left calcaneus shows an osteolytic lesion with loss of bony trabeculation and cortical thinning at the plantar aspect of calcaneus (*arrows*). (**b**) Sagittal T1-W MR image shows a slightly expansile, heterogeneously hypointense lesion within the medullary cavity. The lesion has hypointense well-defined borders and hyperintense blood level components (*black asterisks*). (**c**) The corresponding sagittal STIR MR image shows multiple fluid-fluid levels with thin hypointense septations. The lesion has well-defined hypointense sclerotic margins with minimal soft tissue edema on the plantar aspect of the calcaneus (*arrow*). There is no cortical destruction. (**d**) Thin septal enhancement is seen on sagittal contrast-enhanced fat-suppressed T1-W MR image (*arrows*)

edema and is located in the subchondral bone (Fig. 31.14). Communication of the geode with the joint space is not commonly seen (Arkun and Argin 2014; Olvi et al. 2015c).

31.12 Hydatid Disease

Human echinococcosis is a zoonotic infection. There are four different organisms which may lead to echinococcosis in humans. Hydatid dis-

ease (HD), caused by *Echinococcosis granulosus,* is a widespread infestation in the Mediterranean region, Central Asia, South America, South Europe, and Australia. Osseous hydatid disease and muscular hydatidosis are rare, accounting for 0.5–2.5% and 0.5–4%, respectively, of all hydatidosis cases, even in endemic areas. Dogs and other carnivores are definitive hosts; while sheep and other ruminants are intermediate hosts. Humans are secondarily infected by ingestion of food or water contaminated by feces of the dog

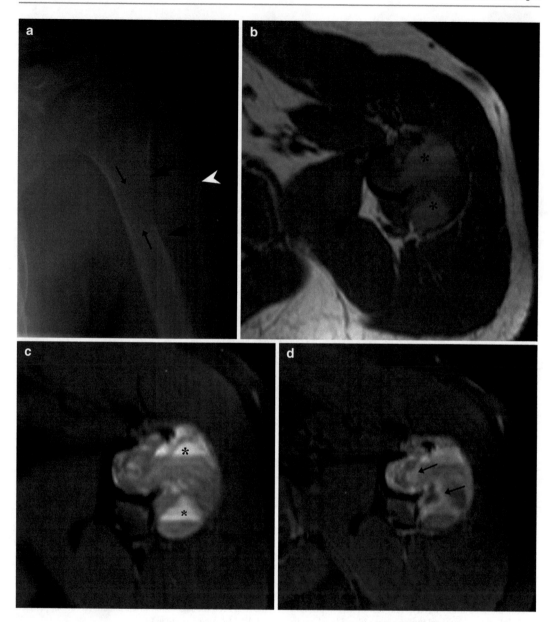

Fig. 31.13 Telangiectatic osteosarcoma in a 25-year-old man with left arm pain and swelling. (**a**) Left humerus radiograph shows an ill-defined intramedullary osteolytic lesion (*thin black arrows*) with cortical destruction (*thick black arrows*) and a soft tissue mass (*white arrowhead*) located at the proximal metaphysic of the humerus. (**b**) Axial T1-W MR image shows an expansile intramedullary bone lesion with cortical destruction. The lesion itself is hypointense with areas of hyperintense signal representing hemorrhage (*black asterisks*). The corresponding (**c**) fat-suppressed T2-W and (**d**) contrast-enhanced fat-suppressed T1-W MR images show multiple fluid-fluid levels and thick irregular septal enhancement (*arrows*)

containing the parasite eggs. After ingestion, the embryos are released from the eggs, transverse the intestinal mucosa, and are disseminated systemically via venous and lymphatic channels. Most of the embryos lodge in the hepatic capillaries, while some pass through capillary sieve and lodge in the lungs and other organs (Polat et al. 2003). Hydatid cyst has three layers, namely, endocyst-germinal layer, ectocyst-laminated membrane, and pericyst. The inner or germinal layer produces the laminated membrane and the scolices that represent the larval stage. Scolices

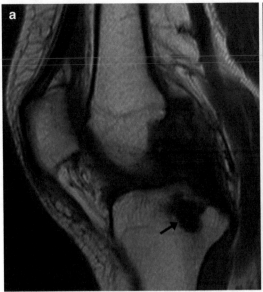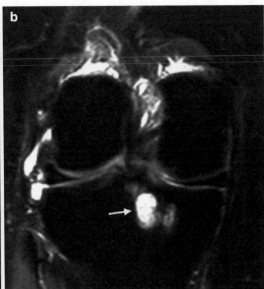

Fig. 31.14 Geode in a 34-year-old woman with right knee pain. (**a**) Sagittal T1-W MR image shows a well-defined hypointense lesion located at the proximal tibial epiphysis (*black arrow*). Posterior cruciate ligament shows thickening with heterogeneous intermediate signal intensity due to myxoid degeneration. (**b**) Coronal fat-suppressed T2-W MR image shows a well-defined, round hyperintense lesion located at the subchondral bone (*white arrow*). Articular cartilage is intact and there is no communication with the joint space

are also produced by the brood capsule, which are small spheres of disrupted germinal membrane. These may remain attached to the germinal membrane, but free-floating brood capsules and scolices form a white sediment known as hydatid sand. Clinically, lesions in bones may present with pain, pathological fracture, secondary infection, deformity, or neurovascular symptoms due to compression (Arkun and Dirim Mete 2011).

Hydatid disease in bones occurs mostly in richly vascularized areas such as vertebrae and long bones. The spine is the most common location, accounting for about 50% of osseous hydatidosis, followed by the pelvis and hip, femur, tibia, ribs, and scapula. Imaging findings are variable, according to stage of the disease. In early stage of the disease, due to microvesicular infiltration into medulla of the bone, embryos reach the medullary cavity. Osteolytic and inflammatory changes without bone expansion occur, which mimics any kind of nonspecific or specific osteomyelitis (e.g., tuberculosis or actinomycosis). Because there are no connective tissue barriers in bone, daughter cysts develop and extend into the bone, with infiltration and replacement of the medulla. Lacking the constraints of this external layer, the cyst progressively enlarges, filling the

medullary cavity to a variable extent. Bone erosion and destruction may lead to almost complete osteolysis, bone may distort, and on occasion, its radiological appearance may be confused with ABC, giant cell tumor, myeloma, atypical osteomyelitis, cystic metastases, and fibrous dysplasia. In time, with the erosion of cortex, the lesion extends into the surrounding soft tissues. In the later stage, the disease appears as a well-defined multiloculated osteolytic lesion. Periosteal reaction and sclerosis are uncommon. Direct spread from adjacent skeletal sites such as joint cavity can be seen, especially in juxta-articular lesions.

CT and MRI are useful imaging techniques to show extension of the disease. The CT appearances of bone lesions are similar to those demonstrated on radiographs. However, CT contributes to a better evaluation of extension within the bone, with a clear demarcation of the lesion. MRI provides excellent definition of the lesion size and extension, with its multiplanar imaging capability. On MRI, in case of bone involvement, unilocular or multilocular expansile osteolytic lesion with irregular boundaries shows medium to hyperintense signal on T1-weighted images and hyperintense signal on T2- weighted images. Multiple daughter cysts embedded in a large cystic lesion also can be detected. Extension of the cyst into adjacent soft tissues and marrow changes are best evaluated with MRI (Figs. 31.15 and 31.16). Bone tumors, tumor-like lesions, and specific and nonspecific infections should be considered in the differential diagnosis. Radiological, laboratory, and clinical findings combined with strong element of suspicion are the key for diagnosis (Arkun 2004; Arkun and Dirim Mete 2011; Ratnaparkhi et al. 2014).

31.13 Hemophilic Pseudotumor

Hemophilia represents a hereditary defect in coagulation. The characteristic clinical presentation of hemophilia is bleeding tendency. Hemophilic pseudotumors are chronic, organized, and encapsulated cystic masses that result from recurrent bleeding in extra-articular musculoskeletal systems. The three forms of pseudotumor are intraosseous, subperiosteal (or cortical),

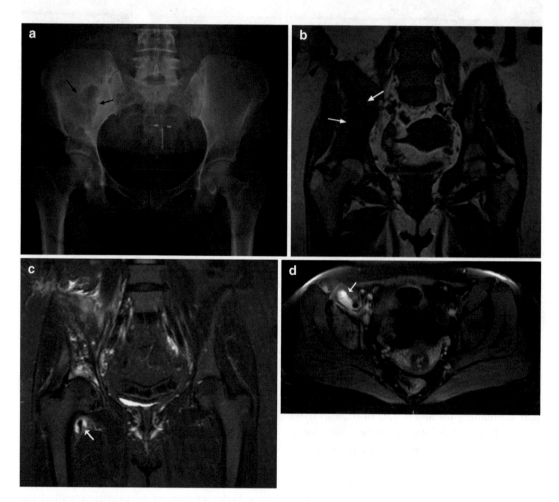

Fig. 31.15 Hydatid disease in a 40-year-old woman who had incomplete surgery 6 months ago. (**a**) Pelvic radiograph shows a well-defined geographic osteolytic lesion in the right iliac bone (*arrows*). (**b**) Coronal T1-W MR image shows an area of heterogeneous signal hyperintensity with cortical destruction in the right iliac bone (*white arrows*). There is a hypointense irregular mass-like lesion (*black arrowhead*) adjacent to the right superior iliac spine in the subcutaneous fat due to prior operation. (**c**)

Coronal STIR MR image shows heterogeneously hyperintense signal changes in the right iliac bone. There is also a round hyperintense soft tissue mass which has central area of signal void adjacent to the medial aspect of the right femoral neck (*white arrow*) and postoperative changes in the right iliopsoas muscle and subcutaneous fat. (**d**) Axial fat-suppressed T2-W MR image shows a daughter cyst in the iliopsoas bursa (*white arrow*) with hyperintense signal

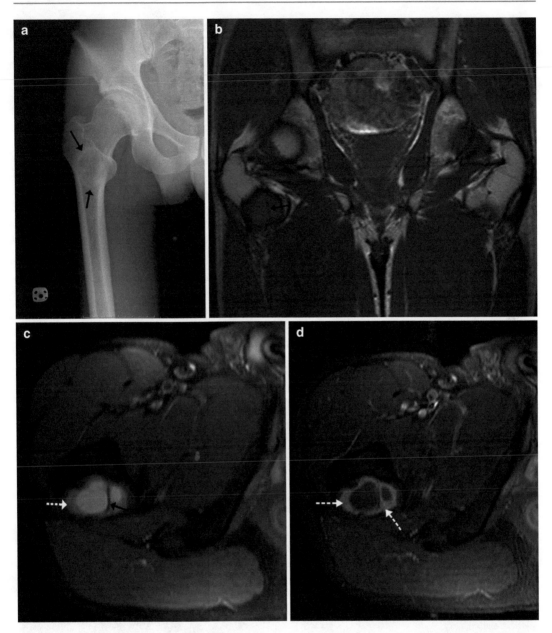

Fig. 31.16 Hydatid disease in a 32-year-old man. (**a**) Right femur radiograph shows a well-defined, slightly osteolytic lesion with sclerotic rim in the lesser trochanter. (**b**) Coronal T1-W MR image shows a tumor-like lesion which has well-defined borders and a hypointense rim in the lesser trochanter of the right femur. There is intermediate signal intensity inside the lesion with thin septae (*arrow*). (**c**) Axial fat-suppressed T2-W MR image shows the multicystic nature of the lesion. The central part of the lesion which is hyperintense with thick hypointense septae (*black arrow*) is surrounded by intermediate signal intensity (*dotted white arrow*). (**d**) The corresponding axial contrast-enhanced fat-suppressed T1-W MR image shows thick peripheral and septal enhancement (*dotted arrows*). This appearance is similar to soft tissue hydatid disease

and soft tissue. The intraosseous form is most common in the femur, pelvic bones, tibia, and hand bones; these lesions can be variably sized. The pseudotumor is usually well demarcated, but it may also be bubbly and destructive. Intraosseous pseudotumors may simulate primary and secondary bone neoplasms (giant cell tumor, desmoplastic fibroma, plasmacytoma, metastasis), tumor-like lesions (unicameral bone cyst, ABC, brown tumor), and even infection or parasitic disease (echinococcosis) because of the pseudotumor's aggressive appearance.

Radiographs, ultrasound imaging, CT, and MRI each play an important role in diagnosis, characterization, and management of pseudotumor. On radiography, intraosseous pseudotumors produce a well-defined, unilobular, or multilobular, expanded osteolytic lesion of variable size. Osseous pseudotumors occur in any portion of the tubular bones, including the metadiaphysis or epiphysis, and have ventral or eccentric epicenters. They may show endosteal scalloping, cortical thinning, or thickening, as well as peripheral sclerosis. Pseudotumors may be quite destructive and completely replace segments of the bone. Repetitive bleeding into soft tissue that is not resolved and replaced by fibrous tissue causes joint contractures and soft tissue pseudotumors.

MRI is the best imaging technique to detect soft tissue pseudotumor. On MRI, a heterogeneous signal in pseudotumors on both T1-weighted and T2-weighted images reflect blood products in various stages of evolution. A peripheral rim of signal hypointensity on all sequences is consistent with the fibrous capsule or hemosiderin (Arkun and Argin 2014) (Fig. 31.17). The diagnosis of an osseous hemophilic pseudotumor relies, in particular, on the knowledge of the underlying bleeding dyscrasia. The radiologist should be aware of the imaging characteristics of this rare complication of hemophilia, in order to avoid misinterpretation of the lesion as a tumoral or infectious

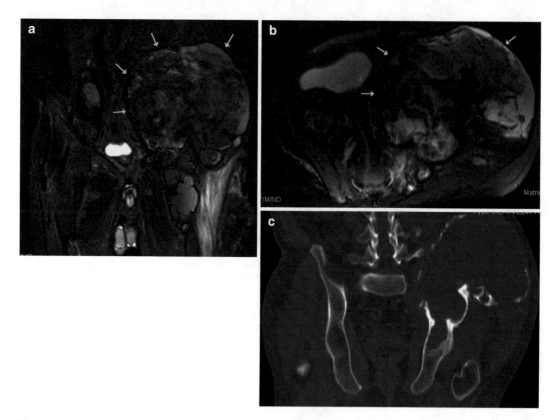

Fig. 31.17 Hemophilic pseudotumor in a 62-year-old man with known hemophilia. (**a**) Coronal and (**b**) axial STIR MR images show a large expansile lesion in the left iliac bone. This lesion has heterogeneous signal intensity with peripheral hypointense rim (*arrows*). (**c**) Coronal reformatted CT image shows a large expansile osteolytic lesion with cortical thinning

lesion, because of the high risk of a preoperative biopsy. Furthermore, cross-sectional imaging is useful in defining the local extent of the lesions, needed for a safe surgical excision of the lesion (Geyskens et al. 2004).

31.14 Paget Disease

Paget disease (PD) is a chronic disorder that can result in enlarged and misshapen bones. This is due to a disturbance in bone modeling and remodeling, resulting from an increase in osteo-

blastic and osteoclastic activity. The etiology of the condition remains unproven. The overall prevalence of PD is 3–3.7% and increases with age. Pelvic bones, spine, and femur are the most common locations, and 25% of cases are monostotic. Macroscopically and radiologically, PD goes through three phases, namely, an initial, often short-lived, osteolytic phase; an intermediate mixed phase; and a subsequent chronic, and usually quiescent, sclerotic phase. These phases may exist in the same bone. PD usually produces specific features on radiographs (Fig. 31.18a). Characteristic radiographical findings such as

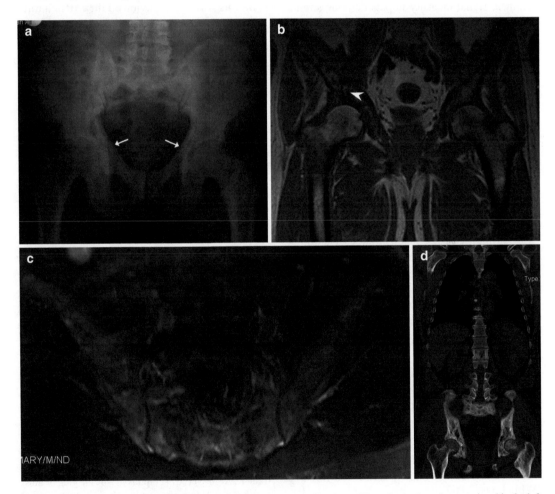

Fig. 31.18 Paget disease in a 67-year-old man. (**a**) Pelvis radiograph shows classical findings of Paget disease such as enlargement of pelvic bones, increased bone density with coarse trabeculation, bilateral hip joint space narrowing, thickening of iliopectineal lines (*arrows*), and heterogeneous increased density in the left femoral head. (**b**) Coronal T1-W MR image shows that the lesion is heterogeneously hypointense with trabecular thickening (*arrowhead*) and maintained yellow marrow (*asterisk*) in the

right iliac bone. There is also hypointense signal in the left iliac bone and signal hypointensity with coarse trabeculation in the left femoral head and neck. (**c**) Axial fat-suppressed T2-W MR image shows intermediate and heterogeneous hypointense signal in both iliac bones and sacrum. (**d**) Coronal reformatted CT image shows trabecular coarsening, cortical thickening, and osseous expansion in the pelvic bone. Similar imaging findings are seen in the L1 vertebral body (*arrow*)

bone expansion, coarsened and disorganized trabecular thickening, and splitting of the cortex are seen, except in the initial phase of the disease. On bone scintigraphy, PD produces an increased uptake with characteristic distribution of the disease giving rise to characteristic scintigraphic appearances. However, the polyostotic and atypical monostotic forms of PD can cause confusion in cancer patients (Olvi et al. 2015d; Theodorou et al. 2011).

MRI findings of PD in bone are variable and heterogeneous. Signal intensity depends on the phase of the disease. The most common pattern is dominant signal intensity in pagetic bone similar to that of fat, due to long-standing disease. In the early phase of the disease, there is T1-hypointense signal and T2-hyperintense signal, which probably corresponds to granulation tissue, hypervascularity, and edema. In the late phase, there is signal hypointensity on both T1- and T2-weighted MR images, suggesting the presence of compact bone or fibrous tissue (Fig. 31.18). It should be remembered that PD is a cortical bone disease and the preservation of fatty marrow signal in pagetic bone generally excludes metastatic disease or tumoral infiltration of marrow. There is usually no contrast enhancement in PD disease.

In difficult cases, CT conspicuously exhibits the classic findings of Paget disease that include osteolysis, trabecular coarsening, cortical thickening, and osseous expansion (Whitehouse 2002; Arkun and Argin 2014; Olvi et al. 2015a, b, c, d) (Fig. 31.18d). Soft tissue masses may rarely develop adjacent to Paget disease of bone. These may be due to unmineralized pagetic osteoid, but extraskeletal hematopoiesis has also been described in Paget disease in the paraspinal region. The MRI appearances of parafemoral, parahumeral, and paratibial masses of pagetic osteoid have also been described with a "pseudosarcomatous" appearance. This entity may be misdiagnosed as parosteal osteosarcoma (Whitehouse 2002).

Conclusion

Bone tumors are a relatively infrequent finding in musculoskeletal radiology, and malignant bone tumors are far less common than benign ones. A wide range of musculoskeletal tumors and tumor-like conditions may be encountered when patients undergo radiological examinations. The imaging features of certain normal, reactive, benign, inflammatory, traumatic, and degenerative processes as well as the tumor-like lesions in the musculoskeletal system may mimic malignant tumors. Although MRI is a powerful medical imaging method that has been used extensively in the evaluation of musculoskeletal tumors, non-tumoral or tumor-like lesions can have similar imaging findings. We have reviewed the MRI characteristics of non-tumoral bone lesions which are located in the marrow cavity and cortical bone and which may be misinterpreted as sarcoma. Knowledge of these conditions, combined with recognition of the pattern of abnormal signal intensity and additional clues that may be present on the MRI and correlation with findings from other imaging studies and with the clinical history, frequently helps one narrow the differential diagnosis sufficiently to make the correct diagnosis, or determine whether biopsy is necessary or appropriate.

References

Alyas F, James SL, Davies AM, Saifuddin A (2007) The role of MR imaging in the diagnostic characterisation of appendicular bone tumours and tumour-like conditions. Eur Radiol 17:2675–2686

Antunes C, Graca B, Donato P (2014) Thoracic, abdominal and musculoskeletal involvement in Erdheim-Chester disease: CT, MR and PET imaging findings. Insights Imaging 5:473–482

Arkun R (2004) Parasitic and fungal disease of bones and joints. Semin Musculoskelet Radiol 8:231–242

Arkun R, Dirim Mete B (2011) Musculoskeletal hydatid disease. Semin Musculoskelet Radiol 15:527–540

Arkun R, Argin M (2014) Pitfalls in MR imaging of musculoskeletal tumors. Semin Musculoskelet Radiol 18:63–78

Azouz M, Greenspan A (2005) Melorheostosis. Orphanet Encyclopedia:1–3

Cabarrus MC, Ambekar A, Lu Y, Link TM (2008) MRI and CT of insufficiency fractures of the pelvis and the proximal femur. AJR Am J Roentgenol 191:995–1001

Campbell SE, Fajardo RS (2008) Imaging of stress injuries of the pelvis. Semin Musculoskelet Radiol 12:62–71

Chen LK, Chen HY, Perng HL et al (2005) Imaging features and review literature of aneurysmal bone cyst. Chin J Radiol 30:269–275

Dhondt E, Oudenhoven L, Khan S et al (2006) Nora's lesion, a distinct radiological entity? Skeletal Radiol 35:497–502

Dion E, Graef C, Miquel A et al (2006) Bone involvement in Erdheim-Chester disease: imaging findings including periostitis and partial epiphyseal involvement. Radiology 238:632–639

Eyigor S, Kirazli Y, Memis A, Basdemir G (2005) Erdheim-Chester disease: the effect of bisphosphonate treatment-a case report. Arch Phys Med Rehabil 86:1053–1057

Fayad LM, Kamel IR, Kawamoto S et al (2005) Distinguishing stress fractures from pathologic fractures: a multimodality approach. Skeletal Radiol 34:245–259

Geyskens W, Vanhoenacker FM, van der Zijden T, Peerlinck K (2004) MR imaging of intra-osseous hemophilic pseudotumor: case report and review of the literature. JBR–BTR 87:289–293

Gould CF, Ly JQ, Lattin GE Jr, Beall DP, Sutcliffe JB III (2007) Bone tumor mimics: avoiding misdiagnosis. Curr Probl Diagn Radiol 36:124–141

Howe BM, Johnson GB, Wenger DE (2013) Current concepts in MRI of focal and diffuse malignancy of bone marrow. Semin Musculoskelet Radiol 17:137–144

Hwang S, Panicek DM (2007) Magnetic resonance imaging of bone marrow in oncology, part 1. Skeletal Radiol 36:913–920

Krestan CR, Nemec U, Nemec S (2011) Imaging of insufficiency fractures. Semin Musculoskelet Radiol 15:198–207

Kershen LM, Schucany WG, Gilbert NF (2012) Nora's lesion: bizarre parosteal osteochondromatous proliferation of the tibia. Proc (Bayl Univ Med Cent) 25:369–371

Lyders EM, Whitlow CT, Baker MD, Morris PP (2010) Imaging and treatment of sacral insufficiency fractures. AJNR Am J Neuroradiol 31:201–210

Mascard E, Gomez-Brouchet A, Lambot K (2015) Bone cysts: unicameral and aneurysmal bone cyst. Orthop Traumatol Surg Res 101(1 Suppl):S119–S127

Murphey MD, Jaovisidha S, Temple HT et al (2003) Telangiectatic osteosarcoma: radiologic-pathologic comparison. Radiology 229:545–553

Olvi LG, Lembo GM, Velan O, Santini-Araujo E (2015a) Simple bone cyst. In: Santini-Araujo E, Kalil RK, Bertoni F, Park YK (eds) Tumors and tumor-like lesions of bone, 1st edn. Springer, London

Olvi LG, Gonzalez ML, Santini-Araujo E (2015b) Bizzare parosteal osteochondromatous proliferation. In: Santini-Araujo E, Kalil RK, Bertoni F, Park YK (eds) Tumors and tumor-like lesions of bone, 1st edn. Springer, London

Olvi LG, Lembo GM, Velan O, Santini-Araujo E (2015c) Juxta-articular bone cyst. In: Santini-Araujo E, Kalil RK, Bertoni F, Park YK (eds) Tumors and tumor-like lesions of bone, 1st edn. Springer, London

Olvi LG, Gonzalez ML, Santini-Araujo E (2015d) Paget's disease of bone and sarcoma complicating Paget's disease. In: Santini-Araujo E, Kalil RK, Bertoni F, Park YK (eds) Tumors and tumor -like lesions of bone, 1st edn. Springer-Verlag, London

Polat P, Kantarci M, Alper F, Suma S et al (2003) Hydatid disease from head to toe. Radiographics 23:475–494

Rappaport A, Moermans A, Delvaux S (2014) Nora's lesion or bizarre parosteal osteochondromatous proliferation: a rare and relatively unknown entity. JBR-BTR 97:100–102

Ratnaparkhi CR, Mitra KR, Kulkarni A et al (2014) Primary musculoskeletal hydatid mimicking a neoplasm. J Case Rep 4:424–427

Remotti F, Feldman F (2012) Nonneoplastic lesions that simulate primary tumors of bone. Arch Pathol Lab Med 136:772–788

Smith S, Kransdorf MJ (2000) Primary musculoskeletal tumors of fibrous origin. Semin Musculoskelet Radiol 4:73–88

Stacy GS, Dixon LB (2007) Pitfalls in MR image interpretation prompting referrals to an orthopedic oncology clinic. Radiographics 27:805–828

Stevens MA, El-Khoury GY, Kathol MH, Brandser EA, Chow S (1999) Imaging features of avulsion injury. Radiographics 19:655–672

Suresh S, Muthukumar T, Saifuddin A (2010) Classical and unusual imaging appearances of melorheostosis. Clin Imaging 65:593–600

Theodorou DJ, Theodorou SJ, Kakitsubata Y (2011) Imaging of Paget disease of bone and its musculoskeletal complications: review. AJR Am J Roentgenol 196:S64–S75

Vogler JB III, Murphy WA (1988) Bone marrow imaging. Radiology 168:679–693

Wall J, Feller JF (2006) Imaging of stress fractures in runners. Clin Sports Med 25:781–802

Whitehouse R (2002) Paget's disease of bone. Semin Musculoskelet Radiol 6:313–322

Musculoskeletal Tumors Following Treatment: Imaging Pitfalls

32

Wouter C.J. Huysse, Lennart B. Jans, and Filip M. Vanhoenacker

Contents

32.1 **Introduction** 647

32.2 **Posttreatment Lesions of Bone Mimicking Tumor Recurrence** 648
32.2.1 Postoperative Bone Marrow Edema 648
32.2.2 Periosteal Reaction 648
32.2.3 Hematopoiesis 649
32.2.4 Post-radiotherapy Changes 650

32.3 **Posttreatment Lesions of Soft Tissues Mimicking Tumors** 657
32.3.1 Soft Tissue Edema and Inflammation 657
32.3.2 Seroma and Abscess 657
32.3.3 Hematoma 659
32.3.4 Fat Necrosis 659
32.3.5 Scar Tissue Formation 663
32.3.6 Amputation Neuroma 663
32.3.7 Reactive Lymph Nodes 665
32.3.8 Varicose Vein 666

32.4 **Reconstructive Surgery** 667

32.5 **Recommendations for Posttreatment Imaging** 668
32.5.1 Multidisciplinary Discussion 668
32.5.2 Standardized Use of Imaging Protocols 668

Conclusion 669

References 669

Abbreviations

CT   Computed tomography
MRI   Magnetic resonance imaging

32.1 Introduction

The main goal of imaging after treatment of a musculoskeletal tumor is to detect residual tumor and/or tumor recurrence as early as possible. It is particularly challenging for the radiologist to distinguish residual tumor or local recurrence from other posttreatment changes. After treatment of a soft tissue tumor, many pseudotumoral conditions may have a nodular appearance and thus present the radiologist with a diagnostic dilemma. After treatment of bone tumors, although the imaging findings are much more specific, also in this scenario, changes induced by previous therapy may mimic tumor recurrence. This chapter aims to give an overview of the imaging pitfalls that may occur when performing imaging after treatment of a musculoskeletal tumor.

W.C.J. Huysse, MD (✉) • L.B. Jans, MD, PhD
Department of Radiology, Ghent University Hospital, De Pintelaan 185, Gent, Belgium
e-mail: Wouter.Huysse@ugent.be; Lennart.jans@ugent.be

F.M. Vanhoenacker, MD, PhD
Department of Radiology, Ghent University Hospital, De Pintelaan 185, Gent, Belgium

Department of Radiology, University Hospital Antwerp, Wilrijkstraat, 10, B-2650 Edegem, Belgium

General Hospital Sint-Maarten Duffel-Mechelen, Rooienberg 25, B-2570 Duffel, Belgium
e-mail: filip.vanhoenacker@telenet.be

© Springer International Publishing AG 2017
W.C.G. Peh (ed.), *Pitfalls in Musculoskeletal Radiology*, DOI 10.1007/978-3-319-53496-1_32

32.2 Posttreatment Lesions of Bone Mimicking Tumor Recurrence

32.2.1 Postoperative Bone Marrow Edema

On magnetic resonance imaging (MRI), postoperative bone marrow edema can be seen as a diffuse, ill-defined T2-hyperintense area within the bone and is a normal finding after surgery or radiotherapy of a bone lesion. Bone marrow edema will typically enhance mildly after contrast administration, as it represents an inflammatory process. The lack of both sharp margins and significant enhancement make it easy to differentiate bone marrow edema from tumor recurrence.

32.2.2 Periosteal Reaction

Whenever a disruption of the periosteum occurs, periosteal reaction is commonly seen. At the site of an extensive osseous defect created after tumor resection, the abrupt interruption of the thickened periosteum may mimic a Codman triangle, which is the hallmark of primary bone tumors. A similar image can be seen at the interface between the healthy bone and the bone that has been treated with extracorporeal irradiation. As the periosteum of the treated segment has been destroyed along with any other viable cells, the periosteal reaction of the adjacent healthy bone may display an abrupt-ending Codman-like appearance. Careful follow-up with radiographs or MRI is needed in these cases to help differentiate it from recurrent tumor (Fig. 32.1).

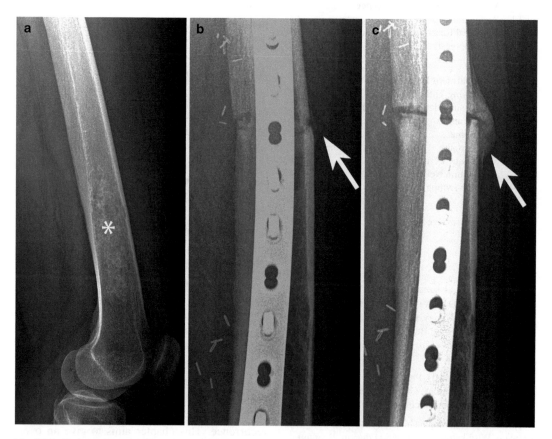

Fig. 32.1 Periosteal reaction after extracorporeal irradiation of chondrosarcoma. (**a**) Preoperative lateral radiograph shows a grade II chondrosacroma (*asterisk*). (**b**) Magnified lateral radiograph taken at 2 months after extracorporeal irradiation shows periosteal reaction developing only on the viable proximal side of the osteotomy (*arrow*). This might be misinterpreted as a Codman triangle. (**c**) Enlarged lateral radiograph taken at 6 months shows normal periosteal reaction (*arrow*)

32.2.3 Hematopoiesis

If malignant tumors are treated with chemotherapy and/or radiotherapy, secondary reactivation of bone marrow may occur. This may result even early on in hypointense signal intensity on T1-weighted and hyperintense signal on T2-weighted MR images, due to transient bone marrow edema (van Kaick and Delorme 2008). After 2–4 weeks, these changes regress, only to reappear during successive chemotherapy cycles. This may result in a mottled aspect of the bone, especially of the vertebral bodies. If additional growth factors are administered, this pattern becomes even more confusing. This hypointense signal on T1-weighted images is, however, always more intense than that of muscle or the intervertebral disk due to the high fatty content. This feature is best demonstrated on T1-weighted images, obtained in phase and out of phase, where the pockets of hematopoietic cells lose signal intensity as opposed to tumor recurrence or metastatic lesions (Fig. 32.2). Even without previous systemic treatment, pockets of active hematopoietic cells may persist in the appendicular skeleton, often having a nodular appearance, with hyperintense signal on fluid-sensitive and hypointense signal on T1-weighted sequences. Here too, the hypointense signal on T1-weighted images is always more intense than that of muscle and decreases markedly on out-of-phase T1-weighted images.

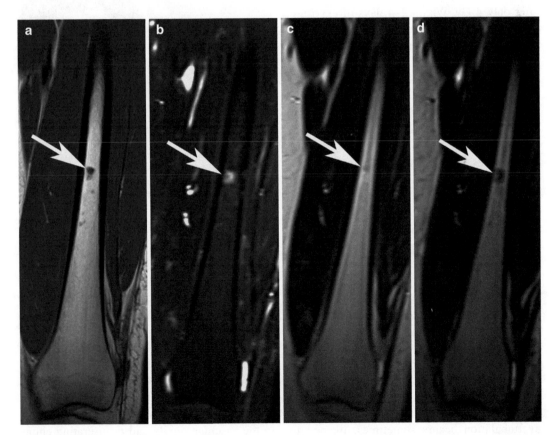

Fig. 32.2 Pocket of active hematopoietic cells in a 37-year-old woman who underwent irradiation after resection of a fibromyxoid sarcoma. Coronal (**a**) T1-W, (**b**) fat-suppressed T2-W, (**c**) in-phase T2-W, and (**d**) opposed-phase T2-W MR images show a T1-hypointense and T2-hyperintense nodule (*arrow*) in the femoral diaphysis. Hypointense signal on the opposed-phase image is indicative for a mixture of fat and fluid as seen in red bone marrow

32.2.4 Post-radiotherapy Changes

Irradiation of the bone, be it direct or as part of the radiation field of a non-osseous target, may cause significant changes in its microscopic and macroscopic structure, especially in pediatric patients. It is important to recognize the skeletal complications of radiotherapy as they can cause diagnostic errors, and some are associated with significant morbidity.

32.2.4.1 Immature Skeleton

In the immature long bone, the chondrocytes in the epiphyseal growth plate are the most radiosensitive area (Williams and Davies 2006). Microscopic changes in growth plate chondrocytes can be seen with radiation doses as low as 3 Grays (Gy), and growth retardation may occur after only 4 Gy. Within 2–4 days of exposure, chondrocytes in the zone of provisional calcification swell, degenerate, and fragment with a resulting decrease in their overall number (Dawson 1968). There is usually recovery up to 12 Gy, but with increased exposure, more severe cellular damage occurs (Dalinka and Mazzeo 1985). Changes may be delayed for 6 months or longer following exposure, and it is not clear whether these are secondary to vascular or cellular damage or a combination of both. Metaphyseal sclerosis, fraying, and growth plate widening (Fig. 32.3), resembling rickets, can be seen 1–2 months following long bone irradiation and may return to normal by 6 months. A dense metaphyseal band may also appear temporarily after treatment. Absence of these metaphyseal changes may indicate sterilization of cartilage cells and, more significantly, resultant limb shortening. The growing diaphysis is relatively less sensitive to irradiation, but endosteal new bone formation is impaired more than periosteal new bone formation (Dawson 1968).

Narrowing of the diaphyseal diameter or overtubulation occurs sometimes, likened to the changes seen in osteogenesis imperfecta.

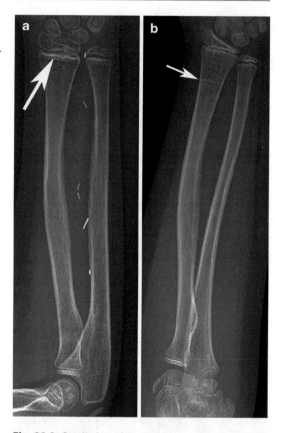

Fig. 32.3 Irradiation of the left forearm in a 9-year-old girl with Ewing sarcoma of the radius. (**a**) Radiograph taken 6 months after radiotherapy shows slightly irregular growth plate and metaphyseal sclerosis (*arrow*). (**b**) Radiograph taken 24 months after radiotherapy shows a dense metaphyseal band in the radius (*arrow*) and narrowing of the ulnar diaphysis

As a result, the bone is more susceptible to fracture. Slipped upper epiphysis in both the femur and the humerus have been described after pelvic or shoulder irradiation, with the former being the more common. This is a late effect, occurring 1–8 years after treatment and most often in children who received radiotherapy before the age of 4 years (Silverman et al. 1981). This post-radiotherapy complication is thought to occur secondary to radiation injury to the vascular supply and proliferating chondroblasts in the growth plate, leading to

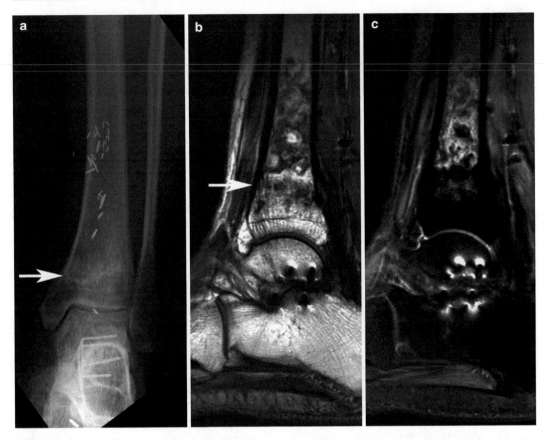

Fig. 32.4 Bone infarction 15 years after radiotherapy following excision of rhabdomyosarcoma in a 30-year-old woman. (**a**) Anteroposterior radiograph and sagittal (**b**) T1-W and (**c**) fat-suppressed T2-W MR images show avascular necrosis secondary to radiotherapy. An insufficiency fracture has developed (*arrows*) below the necrotic area

structural weakness (Eifel et al. 1995). Avascular necrosis (Fig. 32.4) may also occur secondary to therapeutic irradiation, between 1 and 8 years after treatment (Libshitz and Edeiken 1981). Chemotherapy and steroids may have a synergistic effect in these patients, but their exact role is not known because many patients receive both.

Growth of flat bones such as the ribs, ilium, and facial bones is also affected by radiotherapy which can give rise to severe hypoplasia and significant cosmetic and functional deformity. This in turn may have profound psychological effects. Spinal changes secondary to irradiation of the spine occur following doses of 10–20 Gy (Neuhauser et al. 1952). Horizontal lines of increased density are present parallel to the vertebral endplates (Fig. 32.5), and occasionally, a "bone within a bone" appearance may be seen 9–12 months after treatment. These changes are not confined to the radiation field and are thought to be related to a general effect on bone growth, similar to growth arrest lines in the long bones. Following doses of 20–30 Gy, irregularity and scalloping of the vertebral endplates (Fig. 32.6) are seen in the irradiated area, and vertebral body height is decreased. Scoliosis occurs as a result of asymmetrical vertebral

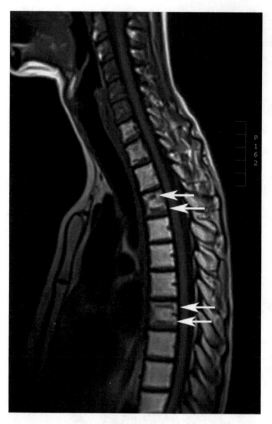

Fig. 32.5 Sequelae of radiotherapy treatment for Hodgkin lymphoma of the spine. Sagittal T1-W MR image of the thoracic shows horizontal lines of increased density parallel to the vertebral endplates (*arrows*) that have arisen after radiotherapy

growth and is concave to the side of the radiation port (Fig. 32.7). This is a combination of the direct effects of radiation on bone growth and secondary effects of scarring and fibrosis in the adjacent soft tissues, which also restricts growth. Even when the entire vertebral body is irradiated, deformity can still occur, but asymmetrical irradiation is associated with more frequent and severe deformity (Gawade et al. 2014).

32.2.4.2 Mature Skeleton

The effects of radiation on the mature bone also vary according to the absorbed dose and other factors such as beam energy and fractionation. Irradiation causes damage to osteoblasts, resulting in decreased production of bone matrix and unopposed resorption by osteoclasts. The osteo-

blasts may be killed, either immediately or delayed, or cell division may be affected. The threshold for these changes is believed to be 30 Gy, with cell death occurring at 50 Gy. The bony changes can be regarded as a spectrum ranging from mild osteopenia to osteonecrosis (Fig. 32.8). Due to the slow turnover of the mature bone, radiographic changes only appear after approximately 1 year. In the course of 2–3 years, the initial osteopenia progresses to mottled areas of coarse trabeculation, osteopenia, and increased bone density, as repair occurs with the deposition of the bone on unresorbed trabeculae.

If more extensive damage occurs in the bone, the terms radiation osteonecrosis or osteoradionecrosis are used. These imply greater damage to the bone resulting in cell death and, in turn, more severe changes on imaging. Most authors believe that the changes described result from the combined effects of radiation on osteoblasts complicated by late vascular changes (Dalinka and Mazzeo 1985). The bony changes resemble those in Paget disease (Fig. 32.9), except that unlike Paget disease, bony expansion does not occur. If there is bony destruction, periosteal new bone formation or a soft tissue mass, infection, and malignancy must be considered, bearing in mind that the latent period for development of a radiation-induced sarcoma is approximately 10 years. Uncomplicated radiation osteitis is not typically accompanied by a soft tissue mass and is confined to the radiation field, and imaging appearances are stable over time. Structural weakness of the radiation-damaged bone means that it is susceptible to acute fracture formation following only minor trauma. More common are the insufficiency-type stress fractures (Figs. 32.4 and 32.10) that may be difficult to identify on radiographs, particularly in complex anatomical sites such as the pelvis. CT can be helpful in confirming the fractures and excluding true bone destruction and soft tissue extension that would suggest infection or malignant transformation.

32.2.4.3 Fatty Replacement of Bone Marrow and Recovery

The hematopoietic elements of bone marrow are extremely radiosensitive. Recovery is dose dependent and usually occurs with doses below

Fig. 32.6 Sequelae of radiotherapy for rhabdomyosarcoma in an immature spine. (**a**) Anteroposterior radiograph shows scoliosis resulting from irradiation of the right side of the lumbar spine at the age of 3 years. (**b**) Focal lateral radiograph of the spine shows horizontal lines of increased density parallel to the vertebral endplates (*arrow*) and scalloping of the vertebral endplates

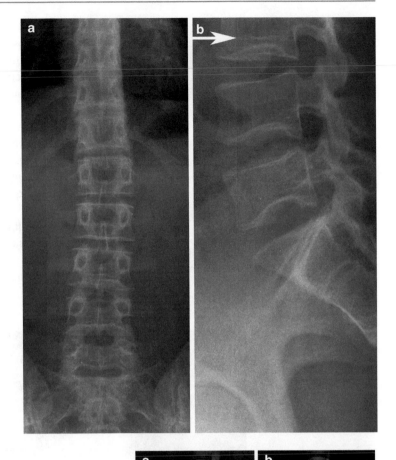

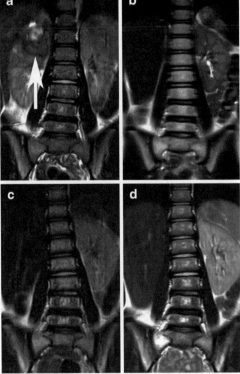

Fig. 32.7 Effects of radiotherapy on bone marrow in a 6-year-old boy who underwent irradiation for a right renal nephroblastoma. (**a**) Coronal T2-W MR image shows no scoliosis and normal signal intensity of bone marrow before resection and irradiation of the nephroblastoma in the right kidney (*arrow*). (**b**) Coronal T1-W MR image taken at 6 months shows marked signal hyperintensity of bone marrow due to fatty replacement 6 months after irradiation. (**c**) Coronal T2-W MR image taken at 18 months shows repopulation by hematopoietic cells resulting in a mottled pattern of signal change. (**d**) Coronal T2-W MR image taken 24 months after irradiation shows almost normal signal intensity of bone marrow but with development of scoliosis

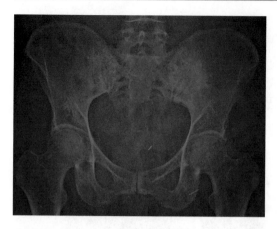

Fig. 32.8 Radiation-induced osteonecrosis of the sacrum in a 62-year-old woman with uterine leiomyosarcoma. Radiograph shows radiation osteonecrosis of the sacrum with coarse trabeculation and increased density of the bone

30 Gy. Above 50 Gy, the effects are usually irreversible (Casamassima et al. 1989). Irradiation of the bone containing red marrow results in replacement of hematopoietic elements with adipocytes. The earliest change is a transient increase in signal intensity on fluid-sensitive sequences, which probably represents acute marrow edema, necrosis, and hemorrhage (Stevens et al. 1990; Sugimura et al. 1994). After this, there is a fatty replacement of the irradiated marrow with a consequent increase in signal intensity on T1-weighted sequences. Radiation-induced changes are confined precisely to the radiation field, characteristically showing a sharp "cutoff" at the edge of the radiotherapy portal (Fig. 32.11). A progressive decrease in signal intensity on T1-weighted sequences denotes vertebral marrow

Fig. 32.9 Effects of radiotherapy on mature bone in a 35-year-old man with malignant peripheral nerve sheath tumor. (**a**) Anteroposterior radiograph shows cortical thickening and coarse trabeculae after radiotherapy which resemble the changes seen in Paget disease. Coronal (**b**) T1-W and (**c**) fat-suppressed T2-W MR images show the thickened cortex with cystic lucencies and the heterogeneous signal changes in the medullary cavity, which also resemble those seen in Paget disease

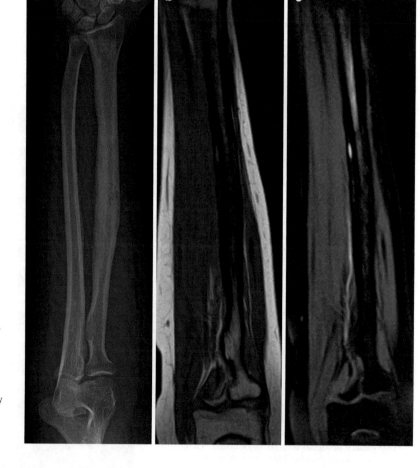

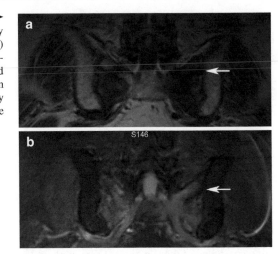

Fig. 32.10 Radiation osteonecrosis with insufficiency fracture of the pelvis in a 79-year-old woman. Coronal (**a**) T1-W and (**b**) STIR MR images show a sharply but irregularly delineated area of T1-hypointense and T2-hyperintense signal in the right wing of the sacrum indicative of radiation osteonecrosis. The markedly hypointense line (*arrows*) indicates an insufficiency-type stress fracture in the left sacral ala

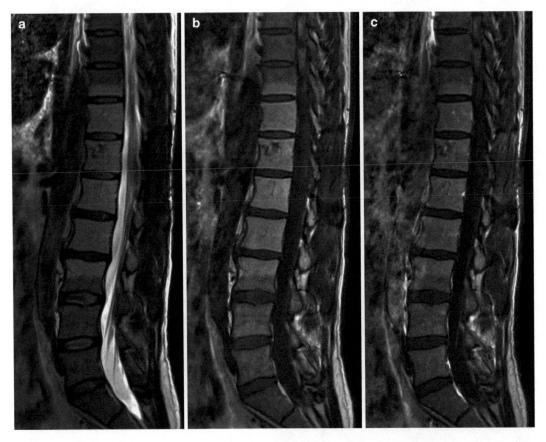

Fig. 32.11 Sharp "cutoff" edge of the radiotherapy portal in a 47-year-old man who underwent irradiation after subtotal resection of hemangiopericytoma of the back. Sagittal (**a**) T2-W, (**b**) T1-W, and (**c**) contrast-enhanced T1-W MR images show sharp edges of fatty transformation of bone marrow that demarcate the boundaries of the radiation field

recovery and repopulation by hematopoietic cells (Fig. 32.7). The likelihood of marrow reconversion decreases with an increased radiation dose but may be enhanced by granulocyte colony-stimulating factor. A mottled or band-like pattern of signal change during the recovery period may be seen (Cavenagh et al. 1995).

32.2.4.4 Malignant Transformation

Postradiation sarcomas of the bone are rare, accounting for approximately 1.5% of all bone sarcomas. The reported incidence is thought to range between 0.1% and 0.2% of breast cancer survivors but may actually be higher, due to longer survival of these patients (Kim et al. 1978; Weatherby et al. 1981). The latent period for the development of postradiation sarcomas ranges from 4 to 55 years, with an average of 12 years

(Wiklund et al. 1991). The latency period is not different in the immature skeleton, but a higher prevalence is to be expected in children, as the immature skeleton is more susceptible to radiation-induced malignant transformation, and the period over which they are at risk is longer.

Approximately one-third of postradiation sarcomas arise in preexisting lesions such as giant cell tumor, bone lymphoma, osteosarcoma, or round cell tumors such as Ewing sarcoma. They usually develop in areas where the dose has been sufficient to cause cell mutation but not complete sterilization. For this reason, postradiation sarcomas tend to occur in the periphery of the radiation field, arising at some distance from the primary tumor (Fig. 32.12). Osteosarcoma and spindle cell sarcoma (fibrosarcoma and pleomorphic undifferentiated sarcoma) account for more

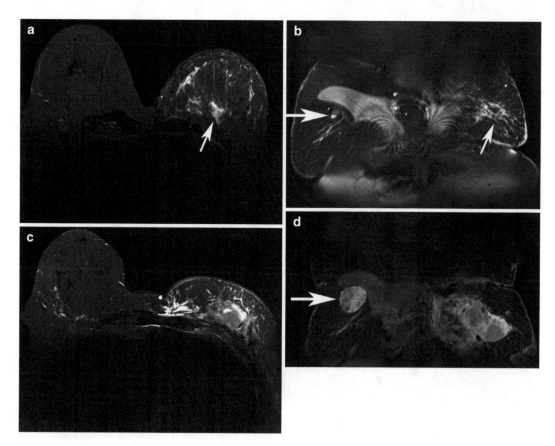

Fig. 32.12 Radiation-induced malignancy in a 72-year-old woman 12 years after radiation therapy for breast cancer. (a) Axial fat-suppressed T2-W and (b) coronal contrast-enhanced fat-suppressed T1-W MR images show radiation-induced fibrosis (*small arrow*) in the left breast 12 years after radiotherapy. Note the normal lymph node in the right pectoral region (*large arrow* in b). (c) Axial fat-suppressed T2-W and (d) coronal contrast-enhanced fat-suppressed T1-W MR images taken after a 2-year interval show development of postradiation angiosarcoma in the left breast with malignant spread to the right axillary lymph node (*large arrow* in d)

than 90% of radiation-induced sarcomas. Chondrosarcomas account for less than 10% of the total (Smith 1987).

The imaging features of these induced sarcomas are similar to primary sarcomas, although the malignant osteoid formation in radiation-induced osteosarcomas tends to be denser. Coexisting radiation changes in the surrounding bone and soft tissues are present in more than 50% of patients and are an important clue toward the diagnosis. However, differentiating radiation changes from malignant transformation can be difficult on radiography. The bony architecture may be greatly distorted by the coexisting ghost of the original lesion and radiation bone changes. Relative lack of change on serial radiographs favors radiation change. On the other hand, pain, presence of a soft tissue mass, and increasing osteolysis favor the diagnosis of recurrent tumor or radiation-associated sarcoma.

If, as is frequently the case, there is a long latent period, previous imaging may not be available for comparison. MRI is particularly useful in this situation. The absence of true bone destruction, soft tissue mass, and lack of enhancement after injection of gadolinium chelate suggest that there is no tumor present. Conversely, bone destruction, soft tissue mass, and active enhancement are suggestive of tumor. Most primary tumors, including giant cell tumor of the bone and sarcoma, will tend to recur within 5 years of initial treatment with radiotherapy. Therefore, the longer the period over 5 years between treatment and development of an aggressive tumor, the more likely the tumor is to be radiation associated.

32.3 Posttreatment Lesions of Soft Tissues Mimicking Tumors

32.3.1 Soft Tissue Edema and Inflammation

Any surgery of the soft tissues will result in some form of inflammation, so soft tissue edema is to be expected at the surgical site. This edema will result in a diffuse hyperintense signal on water-sensitive sequences. The signal is diffuse and

may involve all structures adjacent to the site of surgery, including subcutaneous fat and the adjacent muscles. As this edema represents an inflammatory process, some form of contrast enhancement will occur (Fig. 32.13). Contrary to what is expected, however, the presence of soft tissue edema on imaging in the first few months after treatment is much more prevalent after radiotherapy (up to 80%) (Fig. 32.14) than it is after surgery (approximately 20–25%) (Shapeero et al. 2009, 2011).

32.3.2 Seroma and Abscess

Formation of a seroma is possible after any type of surgery but is more likely to form after a more extensive procedure. Especially after the resection of a large amount of soft tissue, as is often the cases in the surgical treatment of malignant soft tissue tumors, perfect closure of the different tissue layers in the operated region cannot always be achieved. Fluid collects in these defects to form a seroma (Davies et al. 2004). This process starts immediately after surgery, but it may take several weeks to become noticeable. A seroma is more likely to develop if postoperative extracorporeal radiotherapy is administered and even more so after brachytherapy. According to the literature, 26–56% of patients develop a seroma after extracorporeal radiotherapy and up to 75% after a combination of extracorporeal and brachytherapy (Shapeero et al. 2011).

On MRI, a seroma typically demonstrates hyperintense signal on fluid-sensitive sequences and has a rather ovoid shape, which mimics tumor remnant or recurrence. This resemblance becomes even more striking, if residual blood components or cellular debris accumulate in the fluid, making it slightly less intense on T2-weighted images and more isointense to the muscle on T1-weighted images. Contrast administration is particularly helpful, as the seroma will not enhance centrally. Subtle rim enhancement may be seen (Figs. 32.14 and 32.15). Ultrasound (US) imaging is the best modality to differentiate these entities from tumor recurrence, but cellular debris in the seroma may cause confusion. On follow-up examinations every 4–6 months, a seroma tends to decrease in size and disappear

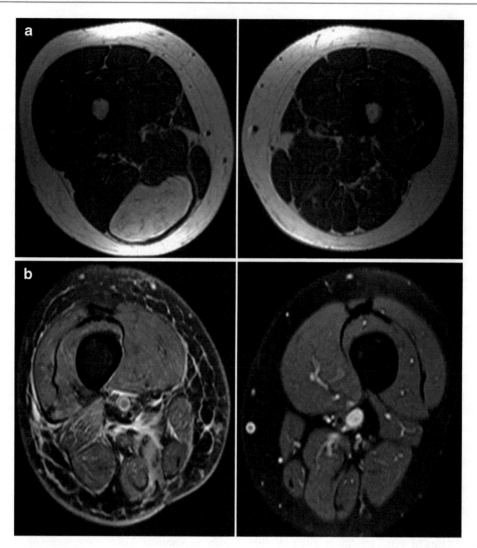

Fig. 32.13 Inflammatory changes after resection of an atypical lipomatous tumor. (**a**) Axial T1-W MR image obtained before treatment shows a large fatty tumor in the right hamstring compartment. (**b**) Axial contrast-enhanced fat-suppressed T1-W MR image obtained 3 months after tumor resection shows extensive soft tissue edema in the subcutaneous fat, in between the muscles, and to a lesser extent, in the hamstring and adductor muscles

over 2–3 years, although this is variable, and some may persist over an extended period of time (Kransdorf and Murphey 2006). An initial increase in size may be seen within the first 4–6 weeks following surgery.

When the rim enhancement becomes more pronounced and extends into the surrounding tissues, a secondary infection of a seroma or an abscess should be suspected (Fig. 32.16). As the enhancing rim can be wide and the enhancement itself can be very fast and intense, an abscess can mimic tumor recurrence. Diagnosis of infection after excision of bone and soft tissue tumors is challenging because of highly variable clinical symptoms (Kapoor and Thiyam 2015). If there is a high probability of infection based on clinical evidence and imaging findings, a trial with antibacterial agents can help confirm the diagnosis; but in previously irradiated tissue or in the presence of orthopedic hardware, this therapy may be unsuccessful, necessitating surgical intervention for both the final diagnosis and the treatment.

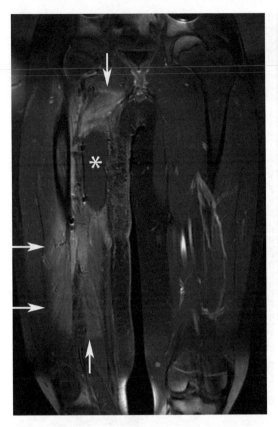

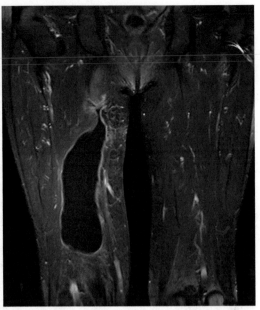

Fig. 32.15 Large fluid-filled cavity in a 55-year-old woman who underwent removal of a large grade 2 liposarcoma. Coronal contrast-enhanced fat-suppressed T1-W MR image obtained 3 months after surgery excision shows that the cavity has filled up with fluid. The homogeneous signal and the subtly enhancing rim are indicative of a seroma

Fig. 32.14 Effect of radiotherapy on soft tissues after marginal resection of myxoid fibrosarcoma. Coronal contrast-enhanced fat-suppressed T1-W MR image shows that similar to the bone, the reactive changes demarcating the boundaries of the radiation field are very sharp (*arrows*). Note the presence of a seroma (*asterisk*) in the operated area

32.3.3 Hematoma

At the site of surgery, hemorrhage may lead to the formation of a nodular-shaped hematoma. Differentiation from tumor can be made as a hematoma will show a hyperintense signal on T1-weighted images. In addition, a hematoma will not enhance after contrast administration (Fig. 32.17). However, be aware that spectral fat suppression, which is often used after contrast administration, can give rise to a higher relative signal in fluid with high-protein content and can be mistaken for contrast enhancement in a solid tumor. Ideally, either a subtraction technique is used or a fat-suppressed pulse sequence is acquired before and after contrast administration

to differentiate between true enhancement, implying a solid tumor and possible tumor recurrence and a relative increase in signal intensity due to the application of spectral fat suppression (Fig. 32.18). In selected cases, such as in tumors with myxoid features, distinction may be especially difficult as the tumor recurrence is not expected to show much enhancement either. In these cases, reevaluating after 3–4 months might provide an answer as most seromas seem to resolve in 3–18 months (Poon-Chue et al. 1999). Although this time is variable and they may persist for an extended period of time.

32.3.4 Fat Necrosis

Fat necrosis occurs when fat is broken down into fatty acids and glycerol, typically occurring in subcutaneous tissue after trauma or postoperatively. Fat necrosis may have a nodular appearance (Chan et al. 2003). There is commonly a

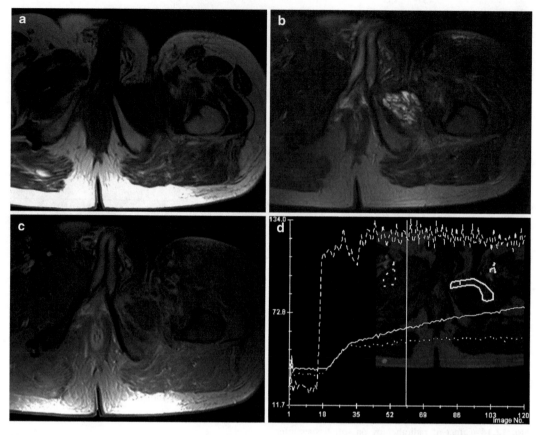

Fig. 32.16 Postoperative abscess after resection of a pleomorphic sarcoma in a 62-year-old man. Axial (**a**) T1-W, (**b**) fat-suppressed T2-W, and (**c**) contrast-enhanced fat-suppressed T1-W MR images show an ill-defined lesion that is T1-hypointense, heterogeneously T2-hyperintense, and has pronounced enhancement extending into the surrounding tissues. (**d**) Time-intensity curve (TIC) generated after dynamic contrast-enhanced MRI shows that the rim displays moderately fast enhancement in the first-pass phase and continuing enhancement in the later phase, indicating a lesion with high vascularity and a large interstitial volume. This is compatible with an abscess but does not, in itself, exclude tumor recurrence. Note the fatty replacement of bone marrow in the femur and the ischial tuberosity

prolonged time between the trauma and the recognition of a soft tissue mass. Most patients present with a firm non-tender lump, typically in areas of bone prominence where the overlying soft tissues are more prone to undergo non-lacerating compressive force. The nodule resolves spontaneously in weeks or up to 6 months, sometimes leaving atrophy of the subcutaneous tissues, resulting in a local depression (Tsai et al. 1997). US imaging is often sufficient for diagnosis, particularly when fat necrosis shows a characteristic appearance of a

hyperechoic nodule in the subcutaneous tissues with fuzzy margins and little vascularity on color Doppler US imaging. Fat necrosis presenting with a hypoechoic appearance or with a hypoechoic halo surrounding a hyperechoic nodule has also been documented (Walsh et al. 2008). The variability in appearance likely reflects the stage of evolution and the severity of associated hemorrhage, particularly in posttraumatic cases.

On MRI, fat necrosis can be depicted as abnormal linear signal intensity in the subcutaneous

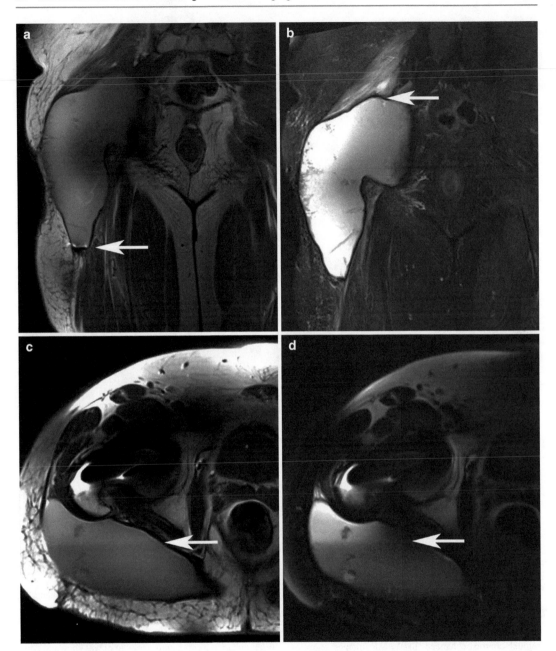

Fig. 32.17 Recurrent hemorrhage after resection of an extraskeletal myxoid chondrosarcoma in a 45-year-old man. Coronal (**a**) T1-W and (**b**) STIR MR images show a large T1- and T2-hyperintense fluid collection indicating a protein-rich content with susceptibility artifacts in the inferior extent due to hemosiderin accumulation (*arrow* in **a**) and a marked hypointense rim that is also caused by iron deposition (*arrow* in **b**). Axial (**c**) T1-W and (**d**) fat-suppressed T2-W MR images show the fluid-fluid level between protein-rich plasma on top and cellular blood components on the bottom (*arrows*) is indicative of a chronic liquefied hematoma

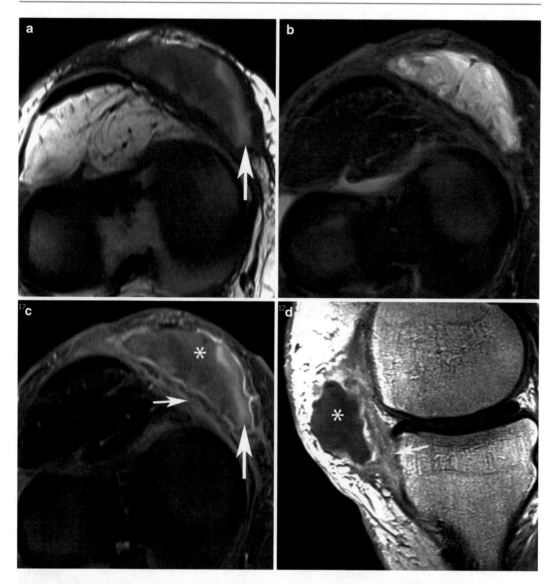

Fig. 32.18 Hematoma and residual tumor after intralesional resection of pleomorphic sarcoma in a 76-year-old woman. (**a**) Axial T1-W, (**b**) axial fat-suppressed T2-W, and (**c**) axial contrast-enhanced fat-suppressed and (**d**) sagittal contrast-enhanced T1-W MR images show an inhomogeneous moderately hyperintense mass with an area of marked signal hyperintensity (*large arrow* in **a**, **c**) corresponding to a hematoma with blood components in various states of decomposition. The central part (*asterisk* in **c**, **d**) does not enhance but a relative increase in signal intensity is observed with spectral fat suppression. The thick-enhancing rim (*small arrow* in **c**) was shown to contain residual malignant tissue after resection

tissues (Tsai et al. 1997), with capsulated areas that are hypointense on T1-weighted images and of mixed hyperintensity and hypointensity on T2-weighted images, representing a mixture of glycerol and regular interstitial fluid or transudate from the surrounding tissues. More commonly, however, it presents as a lobulated area in the sub-cutaneous fat that is surrounded by hypointense septations and has T1- and T2-signal hyperintensity (Canteli et al. 1996) (Fig. 32.19). On fat-suppressed images, the glycerol will lose signal intensity. Contrast enhancement of the rim may be either present (Chan et al. 2003) or absent (Lopez et al. 1997).

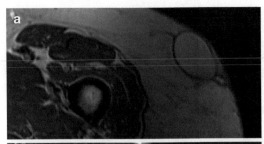
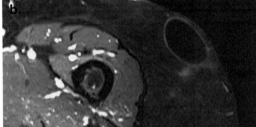
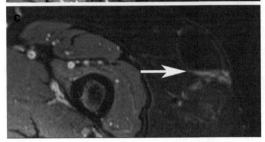

Fig. 32.19 Fat necrosis after prolonged tumor surgery in a 36-year-old man. Axial (**a**) T1-W, (**b**) contrast-enhanced fat-suppressed T1-W, and (**c**) fat-suppressed T2-W MR images show a cystic lesion filled with fatty fluid (glycerol) in the proximal thigh due to fatty necrosis of the subcutaneous fat after resection and extracorporeal irradiation of a tibial chondrosarcoma. There is complete suppression of signal intensity on the fat-suppressed T2-W MR image except for a small amount of transudate (*arrow* in **c**)

32.3.5 Scar Tissue Formation

After surgery, formation of granulation tissue is to be expected along the surgical planes. At an early stage, this is typically hyperintense on fluid-sensitive sequences and hypointense on T1-weighted images but can be differentiated from tumor recurrence by its linear and strand-like aspect. However, if the primary tumor displays a strand-like pattern of growth, such as is the case in aggressive fibromatosis or an angiosarcoma, differentiation becomes very difficult on imaging. Furthermore, the granulation tissue can present in a more nodular fashion, espe-

cially after extensive surgery, increasing the resemblance to tumor recurrence even more (Fig. 32.20). Even the enhancement pattern on dynamic contrast-enhanced MRI, the fluorodeoxyglucose (FDG) uptake on positron emission tomography (PET)-CT, and other quantitative imaging parameters of active granulation tissue can be indistinguishable from that of tumor recurrence. For this reason, follow-up imaging is not advised in the first 6–8 weeks after surgery.

At a later stage, the confusing inflammatory characteristics of active granulation tissue disappear, leaving only hypointense strands (Fig. 32.21). These too can still be misinterpreted as tumor recurrence in aggressive fibromatosis, but normal scar tissue lacks the nodular contrast-enhancing foci of an active desmoid tumor. Another distinguishing property of postoperative scar tissue is the presence of small blooming artifacts along its course caused by microscopic metallic fragments left behind by the surgical instruments. This feature can, however, be present in recurrent pigmented nodular synovitis and giant cell tumor of tendon sheath, so accurate knowledge of the primary tumor is mandatory when interpreting postoperative imaging.

32.3.6 Amputation Neuroma

When large nerves are damaged (e.g., after lower-limb resection), a proliferation of axons, Schwann cells, endoneurial cells, and perineurial cells in a dense collagenous matrix with surrounding fibroblasts may develop at the proximal end of the severed or amputated nerve. This phenomenon is known as amputation neuroma, false neuroma, or pseudoneuroma. These have a "bulbous-end" morphology (Figs. 32.22 and 32.23), in continuity with the normal nerve proximally. They arise 1–12 months after transection or injury and are variable in size (Murphey et al. 1999). At high-resolution US imaging, the neuroma appears homogeneously hypoechoic, sometimes with small hyperechoic internal bands. No degenerative or necrotic pseudocystic foci are found. Duplex

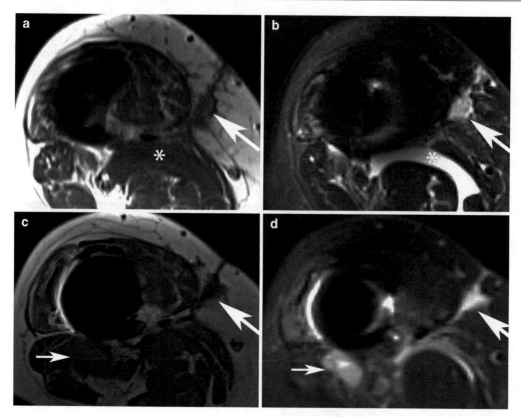

Fig. 32.20 Scar tissue or recurrent aggressive fibromatosis? Axial (**a**) T1-W and (**b**) STIR MR images obtained 6 months after surgery show a T1-hypointense and T2-hyperintense spiculated mass (*arrows*) in the surgical scar. Although tumor recurrence cannot be excluded, both the patient and the oncologic surgeon decide to wait. There is a seroma in the operated area (*asterisk*). Axial (**c**) T1-W and (**d**) STIR MR images obtained 9 months after surgery show an unchanged spiculated mass (*arrows*) proving it is normal scar tissue. The patient had recurrent aggressive fibromatosis posterior to the femur (*small arrows*)

Fig. 32.21 Scar tissue after resection of aggressive fibromatosis. (**a**) Axial T1-W and (**b**) sagittal contrast-enhanced fat-suppressed T1-W MR images show lack of nodular contrast-enhancing foci, indicative of normal scar tissue and not of active desmoid tumor (*arrow* in **a**). There are small blooming artifacts along the course of the scar caused by microscopic metallic fragments left behind by surgical instruments (*arrow* in **b**)

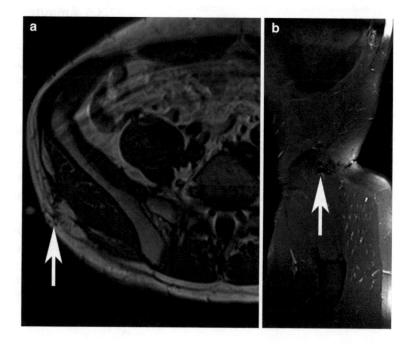

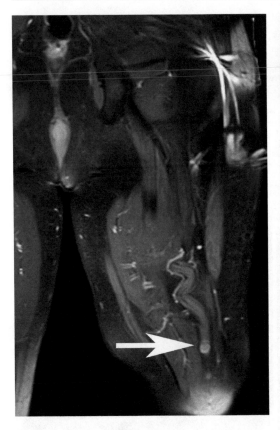

Fig. 32.22 Amputation neuroma of the left sciatic nerve in 46-year-old man. Coronal contrast-enhanced fat-suppressed T1-W MR image shows enlargement of the left sciatic nerve proximal to the site of amputation. There is "bulbous-end" morphology of the nerve at the amputation site (*arrow*) and absence of significant enhancement of the sciatic nerve

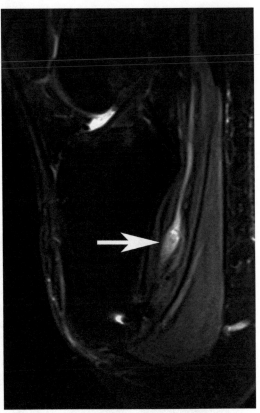

Fig. 32.23 Amputation neuroma of the right tibial nerve in 46-year-old man. Sagittal fat-suppressed T2-W MR image shows signal hyperintensity but no enlargement of the tibial nerve proximal to the site of amputation. "Bulbous-end" morphology of the nerve at the amputation site (*arrow*) is seen

high-resolution US imaging usually does not show any perfusion. These characteristics should allow traumatic neuromas to be distinguished from other causes of amputation stump pain, including recurrent malignant tumor, abscess, bursitis, and foreign bodies (Li et al. 2008). Traumatic neuromas typically have intermediate signal intensity (similar to that of muscle) on T1-weighted MR images and intermediate to hyperintense signal on T2-weighted images. The absence of a target sign may be helpful in differentiating amputation neuroma from a true neurogenic tumor (Ahlawat et al. 2016). Enhancement after intravenous gadolinium chelate injection, when present, is variable and nonspecific (Abreu et al. 2013).

32.3.7 Reactive Lymph Nodes

Lymph nodes will react when surgery is performed in the parts of the body that they drain. This results in an increase in size and may be confused with tumor recurrence or local spread. From a morphologic point of view, only a frank interruption of the capsule of a lymph node and infiltration of the surrounding tissue are unambiguous signs of tumor invasion. In a setting of primary osteosarcoma or chondrosarcoma, ossifications or calcifications on CT, or US imaging in a suspicious lymph node are highly suggestive of metastatic invasion. However, after treatment or with a prior history of chronic low-grade infection, these findings are much less specific (Frija et al. 2005).

As the presence of any nodular structure in an area previously treated for a tumor or soft tissue lesion is suspicious, absolute size and the ratio between long and short axis are semiologic parameters that cannot be used to exclude malignancy. The presence of a fatty center, easily identifiable on most imaging modalities, indicates that the nodular lesion is not a tumor recurrence or metastasis (Fig. 32.24). However, its absence can by no means be interpreted as proof of malignancy. The same can be said about the presence

or absence of the typical Doppler US imaging pattern of hilar blood vessels seen in normal lymph nodes.

32.3.8 Varicose Vein

After surgery, distended veins are often seen as small nodular structures that are hyperintense on fluid-sensitive sequences and located in the periphery of the operated area. These are rarely a source

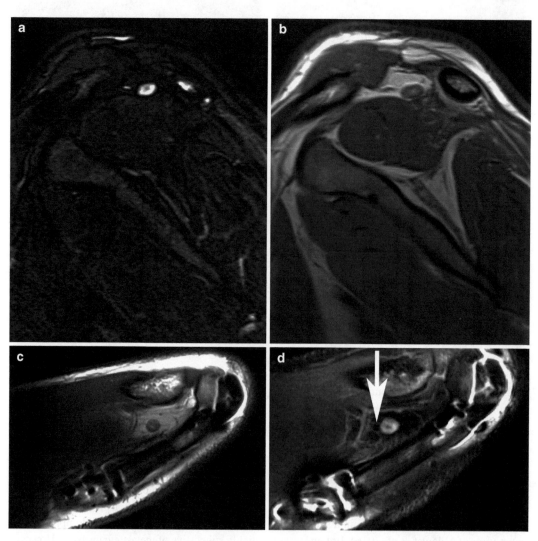

Fig. 32.24 Lymph node in an atypical location after resection of grade 2 chondrosarcoma in a 17-year-old patient. Oblique sagittal (**a**) STIR and (**b**) T1-W and axial (**c**) T1-W and (**d**) contrast-enhanced fat-suppressed T1-W MR images show a central fatty hilum indicating that the nodular lesion is not a tumor recurrence. Note the small blood vessels entering the hilum (*arrow*). This was a histologically proven lymph node in an atypical location after resection of an osteochondroma of the scapular spine that underwent malignant transformation

of confusion in posttreatment imaging of bone and soft tissue tumors, as the efferent and afferent blood vessels are easily visualized. However, if these are lacking or the varicose dilatation is disproportionately large, some confusion may occur. Moreover, if dynamic contrast-enhanced MRI is performed to further characterize an unexpected finding, the time-intensity curve will demonstrate a high initial enhancement with subsequent washout, an enhancement pattern that is generally associated with malignant lesions and possible tumor recurrence. In these cases, US imaging is ideally suited to demonstrate the vascular nature of the lesion and the associated vein (Fig. 32.25).

32.4 Reconstructive Surgery

The extensive tissue resection required to achieve adequate surgical margins in oncological surgery often requires soft tissue reconstructive surgery. Myocutaneous flaps are used in more than two-thirds of extremity sarcoma surgeries. Myocutaneous flaps contain both muscle and overlying skin and can be either rotational flaps, covering the soft tissue defect and preserving the native neurovascular supply via a pedicle, or free flaps which are completely detached, placed into the soft tissue defect, and reanastomosed

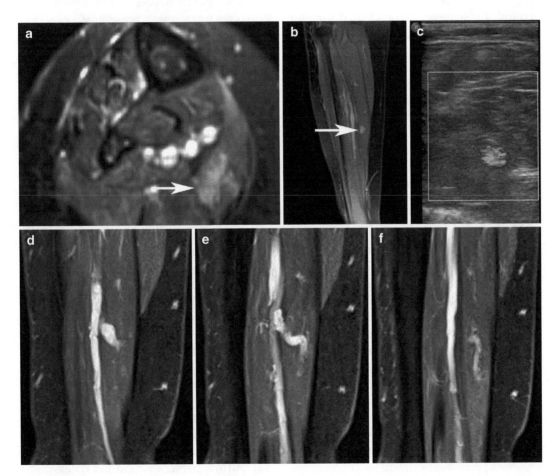

Fig. 32.25 Localized varicose vein in a 68-year-old woman. (**a**) Axial fat-suppressed T2-W and (**b**) coronal contrast-enhanced fat-suppressed T1-W MR images obtained 12 months after resection of a myxoid liposarcoma show an elongated moderately hyperintense nodule (*arrow* in **a**) enhancing after I.V. Gadolinium administration (*arrow* in **b**). There was no obvious connection to the surrounding veins. (**c**) Color Doppler US image shows no solid mass and only a varicose vein. (**d**–**f**) Consecutive fat-suppressed T2-W MR images taken 3 months later confirm the varicose vein. A longer segment of the blood vessel now shows distention, and a clear connection to the nearby vein is visible

using a microvascular technique (Garner et al. 2011). The appearance of myocutaneous flaps varies over time, showing initially signal hyperintensity on T2-weighted images, which returns to something similar to the signal intensity of the surrounding muscle in one-third of cases in 5 to 21 months. All flaps show subsequent atrophy of the muscular component with progressive fatty replacement (Fox et al. 2006). The appearance of a myocutaneous flap is quite typical, so it seldom poses a diagnostic problem. The only exception is the possible confusion between the fatty content in the flap and tumor recurrence of a primarily fatty tumor such as an atypical lipomatous tumor. The distinction can be made over time, as an atrophied flap will not increase in size.

32.5 Recommendations for Posttreatment Imaging

Some guidelines for posttreatment imaging to avoid misinterpretation of posttreatment changes as residual tumor or tumor recurrence are briefly discussed in this section.

32.5.1 Multidisciplinary Discussion

Many tertiary care medical centers have multidisciplinary teams of specialized health practitioners and physicians in the hope of advancing long-term outcomes in cancer patients through coordinated collaboration. Specifically, in bone and soft tissue tumors, a multidisciplinary team ideally includes medical oncologists, radiation oncologists, orthopedic oncology surgeons, musculoskeletal pathologists, and musculoskeletal radiologists (Garner and Kransdorf 2016). The challenge of distinguishing posttreatment change may be minimized, considering the patient's clinical history, treatment regime (e.g., surgical procedure, radio- and/or chemotherapy), and accurate knowledge of the primary tumor. Previous imaging studies should be available for comparison.

32.5.2 Standardized Use of Imaging Protocols

The standardized use of imaging protocols and fixed intervals for posttreatment imaging is recommended. The specific type of imaging for follow-up to check for local recurrence should depend on the site of the original tumor (osseous versus soft tissue) as well as the type of therapy used, all taking into account the presence or absence of hardware (Roberts et al. 2016). US imaging may be useful as a cost-effective screening tool for follow-up of superficially located soft tissue tumors. US imaging can accurately detect recurrent vascular tumors or differentiate cystic lesions, such as seromas, hematomas, or incidental findings such as synovial cyst, from recurrent solid tumor. FDG-PET/CT has emerged as a powerful tool for evaluating local recurrence, particularly in case of suboptimal cross-sectional imaging due to large amounts of metal, but the mainstay to evaluate for recurrent soft tissue tumors is MRI.

Vanel et al. (1987) suggested an algorithm for following up soft tissue tumors postoperatively. This algorithm starts with fat-suppressed T2-weighted imaging or a STIR sequence. Signal hypointensity or diffuse signal hyperintensity on T2-weighted images excludes tumor recurrence in 99% of patients. If a mass is present on T2-weighted images, it should be followed by T1-weighted sequences with and without contrast agent administration. This procedure generally distinguishes hematoma and seroma from tumor or inflammation. If necessary, this procedure can be followed by dynamic contrast-enhanced imaging, which further helps to differentiate tumors from inflammation and scar tissue (Vanel et al. 1998). Unfortunately, this protocol will not always yield the high level of diagnostic accuracy mentioned in the original article.

The American College of Radiology (Roberts et al. 2016) recommends local and systemic surveillance every 3 months for 2 years, every 4 months for the next 2 years, every 6 months for the fifth year, and then annually for years 5–10 in high-risk soft tissue sarcoma patients. This group is defined as patients with extremity tumors over 5 cm in diameter and with trunk or retroperitoneal tumors of any size. For detection of metastasis to non-pulmonary sites, F-18 FDG-PET/CT has recently been shown to be superior to bone scintigraphy and anatomical imaging (Iagaru et al. 2006; Qureshi et al. 2012).

Diffusion-weighted imaging (DWI) with apparent diffusion coefficient (ADC) mapping is able to depict the restriction in Brownian motion of water molecules in lesions with high cellularity by persistence of hyperintensity at progressively higher B values, with corresponding low signals on the ADC map. Although DWI has proven helpful in assessing the response to neoadjuvant treatment in malignant bone and soft tissue tumors, few have reported on the use in posttreatment settings (Baur et al. 2001; Fayad et al. 2012; Del Grande et al. 2014). The largest study on the topic found that comparison of ADC values could distinguish recurrence from postoperative hematomas or scar (Del Grande et al. 2014). Unfortunately, there is no standardization for DWI protocols with ADC mapping across institutions, hindering the ability to establish reliable cutoff ADC values. In addition to the lack of standardization, Subhawong et al. (2014) describe other important pitfalls to consider when using DWI, including greater susceptibility artifacts at tissue boundaries with 3 T, low sensitivity of DWI to sclerotic bone lesions due to normal hypointensity of background marrow, overlap of low ADC values between tumor and benign hematoma or fat, and DWI neoplastic mimickers, such as abscess.

The abovementioned algorithm is not relevant after treatment of locally non-aggressive benign bone and soft tissue tumors. In most cases, no further follow-up is warranted. Conventional radiographs may suffice in the follow-up of cystic bone lesions treated with bone grafts or cement, especially in the peripheral skeleton.

Conclusion

In both malignant and benign tumors, regular follow-up imaging is required to discover local recurrence at an early stage. Interpretation of posttreatment images can be complicated by posttreatment changes. Distinguishing between recurrent tumor and these changes in the affected area not only requires familiarity with the primary tumor but also accurate knowledge of the changes that are to be expected after both local and systemic treatment using different imaging modalities. Furthermore, meticulous comparison with previous examinations, both pre- and posttreatment, is mandatory to provide the diagnostic accuracy required for optimal patient management. In this chapter, we hope to have provided an overview of the imaging pitfalls due to posttreatment changes and how to distinguish these from local tumor recurrence.

References

Abreu E, Aubert S, Wavreille G et al (2013) Peripheral tumor and tumor-like neurogenic lesions. Eur J Radiol 82:38–50

Ahlawat S, Belzberg AJ, Montgomery E, Fayad LM (2016) MRI features of peripheral traumatic neuromas. Eur Radiol 26:1204–1212

Baur A, Huber A, Arbogast S et al (2001) Diffusion-weighted imaging of tumor recurrences and posttherapeutical soft-tissue changes in humans. Eur Radiol 11:828–833

Canteli B, Saez F, de los Rios A, Alvarez C (1996) Fat necrosis. Skeletal Radiol 25:305–307

Casamassima F, Ruggiero C, Caramella D et al (1989) Hematopoietic bone marrow recovery after radiation therapy: MRI evaluation. Blood 73:1677–1681

Cavenagh EC, Weinberger E, Shaw DW et al (1995) Hematopoietic marrow regeneration in pediatric patients undergoing spinal irradiation: MR depiction. Am J Neuroradiol 16:461–467

Chan LP, Gee R, Keogh C, Munk PL (2003) Imaging features of fat necrosis. AJR Am J Roentgenol 181:955–959

Dalinka MK, Mazzeo VP (1985) Complications of radiation therapy. Crit Rev Diagn Imaging 23:235–267

Davies AM, Hall AD, Strouhal PD et al (2004) The MR imaging appearances and natural history of seromas following excision of soft tissue tumours. Eur Radiol 14:1196–1202

Dawson WB (1968) Growth impairment following radiotherapy in childhood. Clin Radiol 19:241–256

Del Grande F, Subhawong T, Weber K et al (2014) Detection of soft-tissue sarcoma recurrence: added value of functional MR imaging techniques at 3.0 T. Radiology 271:499–511

Eifel PJ, Donaldson SS, Thomas PR (1995) Response of growing bone to irradiation: a proposed late effects scoring system. Int J Radiat Oncol Biol Phys 31:1301–1307

Fayad LM, Jacobs MA, Wang X et al (2012) Musculoskeletal tumors: how to use anatomic, functional, and metabolic MR techniques. Radiology 265:340–356

Fox MG, Bancroft LW, Peterson JJ et al (2006) MRI appearance of myocutaneous flaps commonly used in orthopedic reconstructive surgery. AJR Am J Roentgenol 187:800–806

Frija J, Bourrier P, Zagdanski AM, de Kerviler E (2005) Diagnosis of a malignant lymph node (Le diagnostic d'un ganglion tumoral). J Radiol 86(2 Pt 1):113–125

Garner HW, Kransdorf MJ, Peterson JJ (2011) Posttherapy imaging of musculoskeletal neoplasms. Radiol Clin N Am 49(1307–23):vii

Garner HW, Kransdorf MJ (2016) Musculoskeletal sarcoma: update on imaging of the post-treatment patient. Can Assoc Radiol J 67:12–20

Gawade PL, Hudson MM, Kaste SC et al (2014) A systematic review of selected musculoskeletal late effects in survivors of childhood cancer. Curr Pediatr Rev 10:249–262

Iagaru A, Quon A, McDougall IR, Gambhir SS (2006) F-18 FDG PET/CT evaluation of osseous and soft tissue sarcomas. Clin Nucl Med 31:754–760

Kapoor SK, Thiyam R (2015) Management of infection following reconstruction in bone tumors. J Clin Orthop Trauma 6:244–251

Kim JH, Chu FC, Woodard HQ et al (1978) Radiation-induced soft-tissue and bone sarcoma. Radiology 129:501–508

Kransdorf MJ, Murphey MD (2006) Soft tissue tumors: post-treatment imaging. Radiol Clin N Am 44:463–472

Li CS, Huang GS, Wu HD et al (2008) Differentiation of soft tissue benign and malignant peripheral nerve sheath tumors with magnetic resonance imaging. Clin Imaging 32:121–127

Libshitz HI, Edeiken BS (1981) Radiotherapy changes of the pediatric hip. AJR Am J Roentgenol 137:585–588

Lopez JA, Saez F, Alejandro Larena J et al (1997) MRI diagnosis and follow-up of subcutaneous fat necrosis. J Magn Reson Imaging 7:929–932

Murphey MD, Smith WS, Smith SE et al (1999) From the archives of the AFIP. Imaging of musculoskeletal neurogenic tumors: radiologic-pathologic correlation. Radiographics 19:1253–1280

Neuhauser EBD, Wittenborg MH, Berman CZ, Cohen J (1952) Irradiation effects of roentgen therapy on the growing spine. Radiology 59:637–650

Poon-Chue A, Menendez L, Gerstner MM et al (1999) MRI evaluation of post-operative seromas in extremity soft tissue sarcomas. Skeletal Radiol 28:279–282

Qureshi YA, Huddy JR, Miller JD et al (2012) Unplanned excision of soft tissue sarcoma results in increased rates of local recurrence despite full further oncological treatment. Ann Surg Oncol 19:871–877

Roberts CC, Kransdorf MJ, Beaman FD et al (2016) ACR appropriateness criteria follow-up of malignant or aggressive musculoskeletal tumors. J Am Coll Radiol 13:389–400

Shapeero LG, De Visschere PJL, Verstraete KL et al (2009) Post-treatment complications of soft tissue tumours. Eur J Radiol 69:209–221

Shapeero LG, Poffyn B, Visschere D et al (2011) Complications of bone tumors after multimodal therapy. Eur J Radiol 77:51–67

Silverman CL, Thomas PR, McAlister WH et al (1981) Slipped femoral capital epiphyses in irradiated children: dose, volume and age relationships. Int J Radiat Oncol Biol Phys 7:1357–1363

Smith J (1987) Postradiation sarcoma of bone in Hodgkin disease. Skeletal Radiol 16:524–532

Stevens SK, Moore SG, Kaplan ID (1990) Early and late bone-marrow changes after irradiation: MR evaluation. AJR Am J Roentgenol 154:745–750

Subhawong TK, Jacobs MA, Fayad LM (2014) Insights into quantitative diffusion-weighted MRI for musculoskeletal tumor imaging. AJR Am J Roentgenol 203:560–572

Sugimura H, Kisanuki A, Tamura S, Kihara Y, Watanabe K, Sumiyoshi A (1994) Magnetic resonance imaging of bone marrow changes after irradiation. Invest Radiol 29:35–41

Tsai TS, Evans HA, Donnelly LF et al (1997) Fat necrosis after trauma: a benign cause of palpable lumps in children. AJR Am J Roentgenol 169:1623–1626

van Kaick G, Delorme S (2008) Therapy-induced effects in normal tissue (Therapieinduzierte Effekte am Normalgewebe). Radiologe 48:871–880

Vanel D, Lacombe MJ, Couanet D et al (1987) Musculoskeletal tumors: follow-up with MR imaging after treatment with surgery and radiation therapy. Radiology 164:243–245

Vanel D, Shapeero LG, Tardivon A et al (1998) Dynamic contrast-enhanced MRI with subtraction of aggressive soft tissue tumors after resection. Skeletal Radiol 27:505–510

Walsh M, Jacobson JA, Kim SM et al (2008) Sonography of fat necrosis involving the extremity and torso with magnetic resonance imaging and histologic correlation. J Ultrasound Med 27:1751–1757

Weatherby RP, Dahlin DC, Ivins JC (1981) Postradiation sarcoma of bone: review of 78 Mayo Clinic cases. Mayo Clin Proc 56:294–306

Wiklund TA, Blomqvist CP, Raty J et al (1991) Postirradiation sarcoma. Analysis of a nationwide cancer registry material. Cancer 68:524–531

Williams HJ, Davies AM (2006) The effect of X-rays on bone: a pictorial review. Eur Radiol 16:619–633

Musculoskeletal Infection: Imaging Pitfalls

33

Nuttaya Pattamapaspong

Contents

33.1	**Introduction**	671
33.2	**Soft Tissue Infection and Mimics**	672
33.2.1	Superficial Soft Tissue Infection	672
33.2.2	Necrotizing Fasciitis	673
33.2.3	Pyomyositis	674
33.2.4	Bursitis and Tenosynovitis	678
33.3	**Septic Arthritis**	679
33.3.1	Challenges in the Diagnosis of Septic Arthritis	679
33.3.2	Rice Bodies	681
33.4	**Osteomyelitis and Mimics**	682
33.4.1	Acute Osteomyelitis	682
33.4.2	Subacute and Chronic Osteomyelitis	683
33.4.3	Skin Sinus with Malignant Transformation	686
33.4.4	Hematogenous Osteomyelitis	686
33.4.5	Post-traumatic Osteomyelitis	687
33.4.6	Noninfectious Osteomyelitis	687
33.5	**Unrecognized Retained Foreign Bodies**	689
33.6	**Diabetic Pedal Infection**	690
	Conclusion	693
	References	693

N. Pattamapaspong, MD
Department of Radiology, Faculty of Medicine,
Chiang Mai University,
110 Intawaroros Road, Chiang Mai 50200, Thailand
e-mail: nuttaya@gmail.com

Abbreviations

CT — Computed tomography
MRI — Magnetic resonance imaging

33.1 Introduction

Early diagnosis of musculoskeletal infection leads to timely appropriate treatment and prevention of severe complications. The mechanism of infection includes hematogenous spread, extension from contiguous infection, and penetrating injuries. Subsequently, infection can cause tissue destruction, abscess formation, and reaction of the surrounding tissue. All these changes, combined with the reparative process, affect imaging features. Disease severity is variable, depending on the location affected, virulence of the pathogen, and host immune response. In musculoskeletal infections, imaging studies play an important role in diagnosis, evaluation of the extent, and localization of target areas for intervention.

Diagnosis of musculoskeletal infection can be challenging, since clinical and imaging features can mimic other entities such as autoimmune inflammatory diseases, tumors, or traumatic injuries. Symptoms may range from mild extremity discomfort to severe febrile illness with necrosis of the limb. Even with clinical presentations of infection, imaging studies may under- or overestimate the severity and extent of the disease. This chapter highlights common pitfalls in the interpretation of images of musculoskeletal infections organized into three broad sections, namely, soft tissue infection, septic arthritis, and osteomyelitis. Problems in the diagnosis of unrecognized retained foreign bodies and diabetic pedal infection are also discussed.

33.2 Soft Tissue Infection and Mimics

33.2.1 Superficial Soft Tissue Infection

The entire soft tissue structure comprises the skin, subcutaneous tissue, superficial fascia, deep fascia, muscle, bursa, and tendon sheath. The main superficial soft tissue infections include dermatitis, cellulitis (infection of subcutaneous tissue), and superficial fasciitis (Fig. 33.1). Infections involving tissue deeper than the deep fascia are considered deep soft tissue infections. Because most superficial soft tissue infections are diagnosed clinically, imaging studies are usually not required. Imaging studies are necessary when initial medical treatment has failed or deeper tissue infection is suspected. Complications such as thrombophlebitis and deeper soft tissue infection may prolong the course of disease.

Mycetoma is a chronic granulomatous infection caused by fungi or actinomycetes. The disease commonly affects the skin and subcutaneous tissue but may involve deeper structures. Patients present with painless subcutaneous nodules or masses which are clinically similar to rheumatoid nodules, gout, or skin tumors. Mycetoma can present as an ill-defined mass or nodules with a characteristic "dot-in-circle" sign. On T2-weighted magnetic resonance imaging (MRI), the "dot-in-circle" sign is seen as a small round hyperintense lesion surrounded by a hypointense circle with a central hypointense dot (Fig. 33.2). Histologically, the hyperintense area represents granulomatous inflammation, the hypointense circle is fibrous stroma, and the central dot is a grain of fungus or bacterial organisms (Sarris et al. 2003).

Early-stage malignant T-cell lymphoma of the subcutaneous tissue may mimic cellulitis, both clinically and radiologically. Classic presentation of the disease starts with erythematous skin, followed by infiltrative or indurated plaque, mass formation, and involvement of the deep visceral organs (Ruzek and Wenger 2004). Suspicions should be raised when there is a failure of response to antibiotic treatment. In the later stages, nodular or infiltrative mass-like lesions can be detected by computed tomography (CT) and MRI (Kim et al. 2004) (Fig. 33.3).

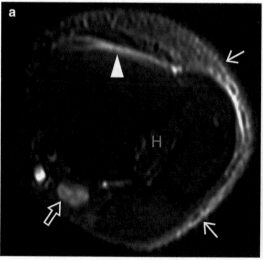
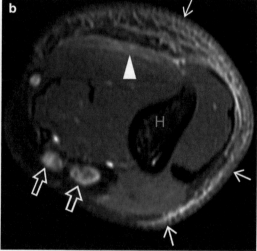

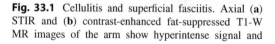

Fig. 33.1 Cellulitis and superficial fasciitis. Axial (**a**) STIR and (**b**) contrast-enhanced fat-suppressed T1-W MR images of the arm show hyperintense signal and enhancement of the subcutaneous tissue (*arrows*) and superficial fascia (*arrowheads*). Note the enlarged lymph nodes (*open arrows*) [*H* humerus]

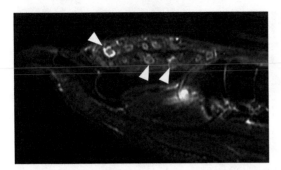

Fig. 33.2 Mycetoma in a 47-year-old woman who had a mass on the dorsum of her foot for 1 year. Sagittal fat-suppressed T2-W MR image shows a "dot-in-circle" sign (*arrowheads*) which indicates a central hypointense signal of grains of microorganism surrounded by hyperintense signal granulomatous inflammation and hypointense signal fibrous circle. Tissue biopsy revealed actinomycotic mycetoma

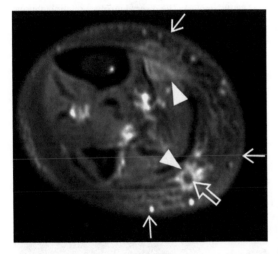

Fig. 33.3 Malignant T-cell lymphoma of the subcutaneous tissue in a patient presenting with skin swelling and redness for 2 weeks. Axial contrast-enhanced fat-suppressed T1-W MR image of the leg shows thickening and enhancement of the subcutaneous tissue (*arrows*) similar to that of cellulitis. Mass-like lesions (*arrowheads*) are the key findings of lymphoma. Note thrombosis of the superficial vein (*open arrow*)

33.2.2 Necrotizing Fasciitis

Necrotizing fasciitis is a potentially life-threatening condition leading to extensive necrosis of the deep fascia. The deep fascia is a dense connective tissue consisting of peripheral and intermuscular layers. The peripheral layer attaches to the epimysium of the outer surface of muscle, while the intermuscular layer extends between muscles and divides them into various compartments. Necrotizing fasciitis is the most severe form of soft tissue infection which requires early recognition and urgent adequate debridement.

Necrotizing fasciitis is a clinical diagnosis. Clinical findings include skin necrosis, crepitus, and hypotension. Pain and underlying tissue damage often extends beyond the apparent skin inflammation (Malghem et al. 2013). The disease is typically unilateral, focal, and rapidly progressive. The area of necrotizing fasciitis tends to be painful in the early stages but become painless in more advanced stages (Chaudhry et al. 2015). MRI is the best modality for the detection of fascial necrosis and perifascial fluid which are seen as signal hyperintensity of the deep fascia on either T2-weighted or short tau inversion recovery (STIR) MR images. Necrotizing fasciitis can be excluded if there is absence of the T2-hyperintense signal along the fascia. In severely ill patients, CT may be the preferred modality because of its wide availability, rapid acquisition, and high sensitivity to fascial gas (Fig. 33.4). Presence of gas along the fascia is highly specific, but it is not usually present. Gas can be demonstrated as areas of signal void along the fasciae on T2-weighted MR images, but detection of gas is better on gradient-echo images.

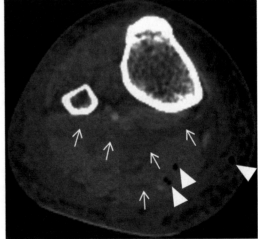

Fig. 33.4 Necrotizing fasciitis in a 51-year-old woman who presented with fever and limb swelling for 4 days. Axial contrast-enhanced CT image shows perifascial fluid (*arrows*) and soft tissue gas (*arrowheads*)

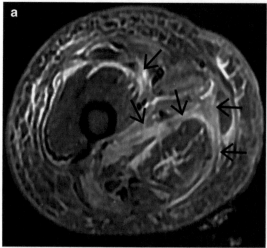

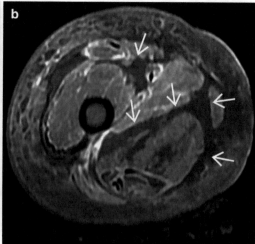

Fig. 33.5 Necrotizing fasciitis in a 57-year-old woman who presented with fever and thigh pain for 3 days. (**a**) Axial STIR MR image shows thickening and signal hyperintensity of the intermuscular fascia (*black arrows*).

(**b**) Axial contrast-enhanced fat-suppressed T1-W MR image shows fluid along the non-enhancing necrotic fascia (*white arrows*). The disease involves multiple muscle compartments

Distinguishing necrotic from non-necrotic fasciae is crucial in surgical planning, in order to avoid unnecessary debridement. Apart from the detection of gas, MRI features of necrotic fascia include significant thickening of the abnormal signal intensity of the fascia on T2-weighted images (greater than 3 mm) and focal or diffuse non-enhancing fascia. Necrotizing fasciitis tends to involve intermuscular fascia in multiple compartments (Kim et al. 2011) (Fig. 33.5). Hyperintense signal intensity of the deep fascia on T2-weighted images can be due to a number of diagnoses, such as muscle injury, venous congestion, lymphedema, neoplastic disease, and other deep-seated infections. Other noninfectious fasciitis such as eosinophilic fasciitis, paraneoplastic fasciitis, and graft-versus-host disease can result in a thickened and enhanced fascia which can mimic necrotizing fasciitis (Chaudhry et al. 2015). Severe cellulitis can produce edema of the peripheral layer and the outer portion of intermuscular layer of deep fascia. T2-signal hyperintensity of the adjacent muscle may occur, but this is considered to be a reactive change because of adjacent fascial inflammation rather than infection of the muscle itself (Ali et al. 2014) (Fig. 33.6).

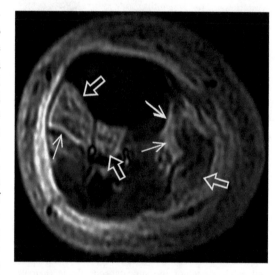

Fig. 33.6 Reactive muscle edema in necrotizing fasciitis. Axial STIR MR image of the leg shows hyperintense signal along the fascia (*arrows*) and reactive muscle edema (*open arrows*)

33.2.3 Pyomyositis

Pyomyositis is an infection of skeletal muscle which commonly occurs in the large muscles of the pelvic girdle and lower extremities (Bickels

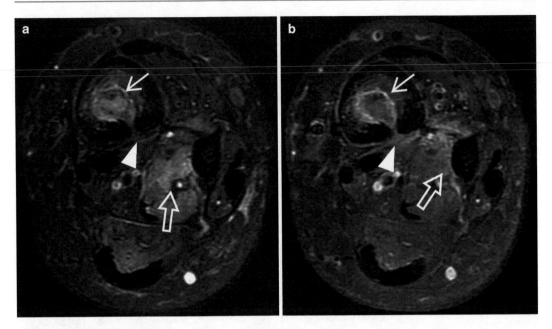

Fig. 33.7 Early stages of pyomyositis spreading from the adjacent osteomyelitis. (**a**) Axial fat-suppressed T2-W and (**b**) contrast-enhanced fat-suppressed T1-W MR images show hyperintensity of the muscle with muscle enhancement (*open arrows*). Note the osteomyelitis in the tibia (*arrows*) and spread of infection via the sinus tract (*arrowheads*)

et al. 2002). The disease process starts with diffuse muscle inflammation, with subsequent tissue liquefaction and abscess formation. Pyomyositis can be initiated by hematogenous spread from a remote site or direct extension from adjacent infection. In early stages, muscle is enlarged, showing diffuse hyperintense signal on T2-weighted MRI and contrast enhancement (Fig. 33.7). Other muscle diseases, such as autoimmune myositis, subacute muscle denervation, and damage due to radiation therapy, can show similar abnormalities and can be distinguished from pyomyositis, based on clinical history and the extent of the lesion. Lymphoma insinuating into the muscle fibers can present as diffuse muscular enlargement with preservation of muscle shape and intermuscular fat planes, simulating early pyomyositis (Ruzek and Wenger 2004).

In the later stages, tissue necrosis leads to abscess formation. With adequate host response, the abscess is walled off by thick fibrovascular tissue. On MRI, the wall of a well-formed abscess is hyperintense on T1-weighted images and hypointense on T2-weighted images, owing to the presence of thick fibrous tissue, blood products, bacterial or macrophage sequestration of iron, and free radicals (Fleckenstein et al. 1991) (Fig. 33.8a–c). The signal intensity of central necrotic tissue is variable, depending on protein content and hemorrhage. A well-formed abscess can present with a mass-like appearance, mimicking a necrotic or cystic tumor. In contrast to necrotic tumors, the inner wall of abscesses is smooth, while the wall of a necrotic tumor has a nodular or mass-like appearance. An abscess may appear as a mass in the transverse plane but usually maintains a normal fusiform shape in the longitudinal plane (Stacy and Dixon 2007) (Fig. 33.8d). Foci of gas within the fluid collection strongly suggest pyomyositis (Fig. 33.9). Stranding and enhancement of the adjacent fascia and subcutaneous tissue favor the diagnosis of pyomyositis (Gordon et al. 1995). However, changes in adjacent soft tissue

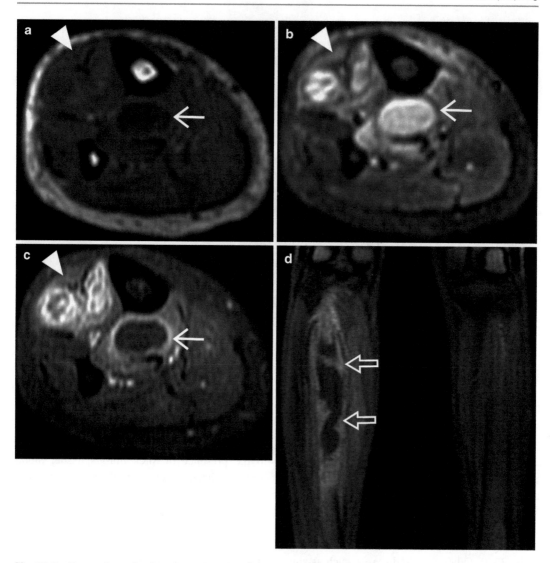

Fig. 33.8 Abscess formation in pyomyositis of the leg. Axial (**a**) T1-W, (**b**) fat-suppressed T2-W, and (**c**) contrast-enhanced fat-suppressed T1-W MR images show a well-formed abscess (*arrows*). The smooth wall of the abscess is T1-hyperintense and T2-hypointense and enhances. Note the early stage of abscess with muscle enhancement (*arrowheads*). (**d**) The abscess presents a fusiform shape along the muscle in the coronal plane (*open arrows*)

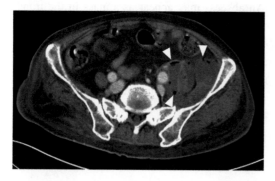

Fig. 33.9 Gas within abscesses. Axial contrast-enhanced CT image shows left iliopsoas abscesses containing gas bubbles (*arrowheads*)

may be minimal in granulomatous infection and immunosuppressed patients (Stacy and Kapur 2011).

Diabetic muscle infarction may result in edema, signal abnormality, and enhancement of muscle and may be mistaken for pyomyositis (Fig. 33.10). The disease can be unilateral or bilateral, and there is usually multifocal involvement (Baker et al. 2012). The history and biochemical markers lead to the diagnosis of diabetic muscle infarction. Patients present with acute painful swelling of the affected extremity, combined with severe target

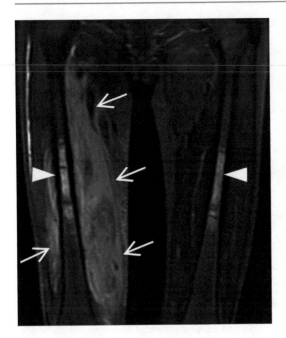

Fig. 33.10 Diabetic muscle infarction in a 28-year-old woman who presented with right thigh pain for 1 week. Coronal STIR image of the thighs shows hyperintense signal in the muscles (*arrows*). Hyperintense signal in the bone marrow of the femur represents early stage of bone marrow infarction (*arrowheads*). The patient was afebrile and her symptoms improved without antibiotic treatment

organ diseases such as retinopathy, nephropathy, and neuropathy as a result of poorly controlled diabetes mellitus. Fever or leukocytosis does not usually present in cases of diabetic muscle infarction (Jelinek et al. 1999). Adjacent bone infarction may occur (Chatha et al. 2005).

Heterotopic bone formation is important in the differential diagnosis of abscesses, especially in paralyzed patients. Early bone formation is seen as hyperintense signal on T2-weighted MR images and rim enhancement, similar to abscesses (Ledermann et al. 2002b) (Fig. 33.11). Peripheral amorphous calcification presenting at the third or fourth weeks helps in arriving at an accurate diagnosis (Ma et al. 1995). Use of gradient-echo images to detect blooming artifacts and supporting evidence of calcification on radiographs or CT also aids in an accurate diagnosis. Distribution of lesions around joints, commonly around the hip, in the absence of surrounding tissue infection, is another clue to diagnosis.

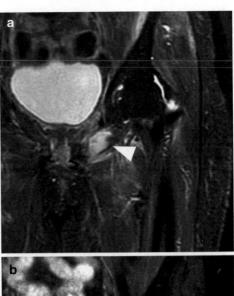

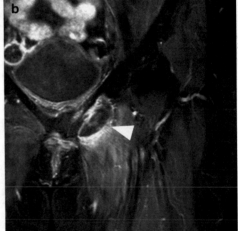

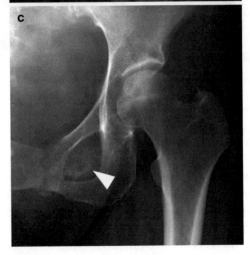

Fig. 33.11 Heterotopic bone formation. (**a**) Coronal fat-suppressed T2-W MR image of the right hip shows an area of muscle hyperintensity (*arrowhead*). (**b**) Rim enhancement is present on the contrast-enhanced fat-suppressed T1-W MR image (*arrowhead*). (**c**) Follow-up radiograph at 6 weeks shows heterotopic bone formation (*arrowhead*)

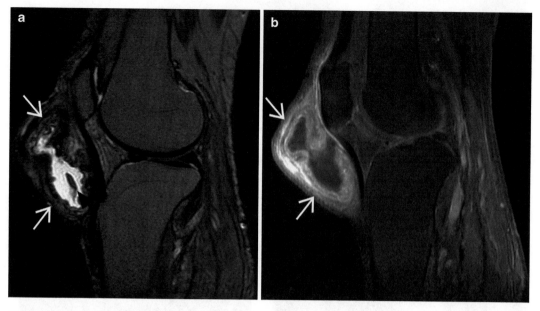

Fig. 33.12 Infrapatellar bursitis in a 49-year-old woman. (**a**) Sagittal T2-W MR image shows a bursa with a thickened synovium (*white arrows*) and debris (*black arrows*).

(**b**) Sagittal contrast-enhanced fat-suppressed T1-W MR image shows enhancement of the synovium (*white arrows*). Aspirated bursal fluid grew *S. aureus*

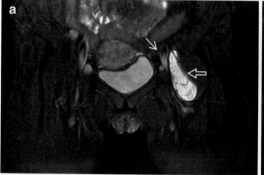
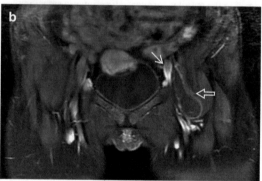

Fig. 33.13 Iliopsoas bursitis. Coronal (**a**) STIR and (**b**) contrast-enhanced fat-suppressed T1-W MR images obtained anterior to the hip joint show a left iliopsoas bur-

sitis. The enlarged bursa is seen as a rim-enhancing cystic mass (*open arrows*) in the inguinal region near the femoral artery (*arrows*)

33.2.4 Bursitis and Tenosynovitis

Bursitis and tenosynovitis, especially when due to granulomatous infection, can present clinically as a mass mimicking a soft tissue tumor. The characteristic imaging finding of bursitis is a distended cystic structure, accompanied by synovial hypertrophy and enhancement (Fig. 33.12). The bursa and tendon sheath, which contain loose bodies, blood product, or debris, may produce a more complex appearance which may be mistaken for neoplasm. Familiarity with locations of bursae is useful. Infectious bursitis and tenosynovitis are

indistinguishable from those of inflammatory arthritis on imaging alone.

The iliopsoas bursa lies between the iliopsoas tendon and anterior aspect of the hip. Communication with the underlying hip joint is common (Wunderbaldinger et al. 2002). Fluid from the hip joint may decompress through the hip capsule into the bursa, forming an inguinal mass. Painful enlarged iliopsoas bursitis can be misdiagnosed as a femoral artery aneurysm or pseudoaneurysm or an inguinal hernia (Ghazizadeh et al. 2014) (Fig. 33.13). In bursae connected to joints, gas

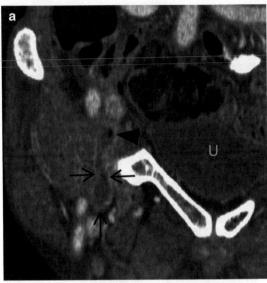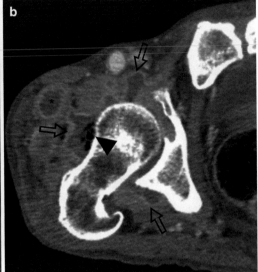

Fig. 33.14 Gas-containing bursitis and septic arthritis in a 63-year-old man. (**a**) Coronal contrast-enhanced CT image shows iliopsoas bursitis with a rim-enhancing wall (*arrows*) and gas bubble (*arrowhead*). (**b**) Axial CT image of the hip joint shows intra-articular gas (*arrowhead*), joint effusion (*open arrows*), and para-articular abscess (***). Aspirated joint fluid grew *E. coli* [*U urinary bladder*]

bubbles resulting from the vacuum phenomenon can migrate from the joint space to bursae, simulating gas-containing abscesses (Coulier and Cloots 2003). Diagnosis should be based on the patient's clinical condition. In abscesses, surrounding inflammatory change and a rim-enhancing wall should be evident (Fig. 33.14).

33.3 Septic Arthritis

33.3.1 Challenges in the Diagnosis of Septic Arthritis

Infection of the joint may be primary from the spread of infection via the subsynovial artery or secondary infection from osteomyelitis. Without proper treatment, septic arthritis can cause cartilage and bone destruction, leading to permanent joint damage. Disruption of the adjacent joint capsule and tendon results in malalignment, spreading of infectious contents into surrounding soft tissue structures, and formation of para-articular abscesses. On radiographs, the early findings include juxta-articular osteoporosis, loss of subchondral bone plate, effusion, and soft tissue swelling. The other causes which lead to regional osteoporosis, such as disuse osteoporosis, transient osteoporosis, and reflex sympathetic dystrophy, may simulate septic arthritis. Destruction of subchondral bone plate and bone erosions are eventually observed in septic arthritis but not in regional osteoporosis (Fig. 33.15).

Ultrasound (US) imaging is a good modality for the detection of effusion, particularly in the shoulder and hip joints, which may be difficult to detect by physical examination (Bierma-Zeinstra et al. 2000; Zubler et al. 2011). Many US imaging signs that suggest infected fluid include peripheral hyperemia, internal debris, and septation, but diagnosis remains based on joint effusion analysis and culture (Margaretten et al. 2007). The presence of clear anechoic effusion does not exclude infection (Carra et al. 2014). Joint effusion is common, but absence of effusion can occur, particularly in the small joints of hands and feet (Karchevsky et al. 2004).

MRI features of septic arthritis include synovial thickening and enhancement, perisynovial edema, joint effusion, cartilage loss, and bone marrow changes. Septic arthritis can induce edematous changes in the adjacent bone without osteomyelitis. Reactive edematous change can be observed on T2-weighted images, but the signal intensity remains normal or faintly hypointense on T1-weighted images. Obvious signal changes in the bone marrow on T1-weighted images along

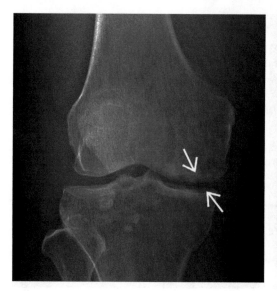

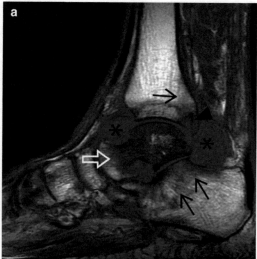

Fig. 33.15 Septic arthritis with bone erosions in a 57-year-old man who presented with fever and knee pain for 1 week. Radiograph of the knee shows loss of subchondral bone plate and bone erosions (*arrows*)

with bone marrow enhancement indicate osteomyelitis (Toledano et al. 2011) (Fig. 33.16). However, distinguishing between reactive bone marrow edema and associated osteomyelitis is sometimes difficult.

Several clinical and imaging features of septic arthritis overlap with inflammatory arthritis, especially in cases of low virulence infection. Although monoarticular involvement is common, approximately 15% of patients with septic arthritis present with multiple joint involvement (Dubost et al. 1993). On the other hand, inflammatory arthritis can initially present as a monoarticular disease. In a study comparing MRI features of tuberculous arthritis and rheumatoid arthritis, Choi et al. (2009) found that synovitis in tuberculous arthritis tends to

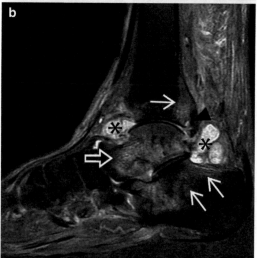

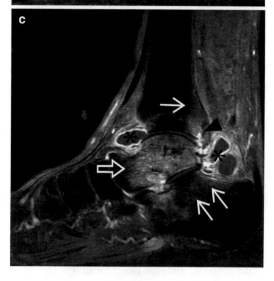

Fig. 33.16 Septic arthritis with osteomyelitis in a 65-year-old man. Sagittal (**a**) T1-W, (**b**) fat-suppressed T2-W, and (**c**) contrast-enhanced fat-suppressed T1-W MR images of the ankle show obvious signal abnormality of the talus on both T1- and T2-weighted images with enhancement (*open arrows*), indicating osteomyelitis. Note ankle joint effusion (*) and bone erosion (*arrowheads*). Areas of faint T2-signal abnormality in the distal tibia and calcaneus (*arrows*) are compatible with reactive bone marrow edema. Biopsy of the talus revealed osteomyelitis and culture revealed *P. aeruginosa*

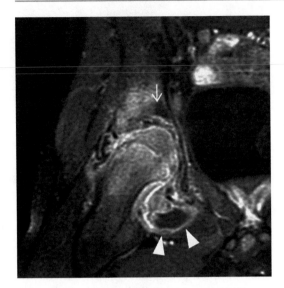

Fig. 33.17 Tuberculous arthritis in a 17-year-old girl with right hip pain. Coronal contrast-enhanced fat-suppressed T1-W MR image of the right hip shows an intraosseous abscess in the acetabulum (*arrow*) with thin and smooth synovitis (*arrowheads*)

be smooth and thin, while in rheumatoid arthritis, it is thick and irregular. Large rim-enhancing bone erosions and extra-articular fluid collection are more frequently found in tuberculous arthritis (Fig. 33.17). The difficulty in diagnosis of septic arthritis occurs when infection is superimposed on a damaged joint. The clinical and radiological abnormality of septic joints can be hidden by the preexisting joint diseases. Suspicion should be raised if rapid destruction is confined to one joint and the symptoms are unresponsive to the treatment of pre-existing joint disease (Ashrani et al. 2008).

33.3.2 Rice Bodies

Rice bodies consist of fibrin, collagen, mononuclear cells, and dystrophic calcification forming nodules that resemble rice grains (Cheung et al. 1980; Popert 1985; Li-Yu et al. 2002) (Fig. 33.18). They are associated with chronic synovitis of joints, bursae, or tendon sheaths. Rice bodies are commonly described in chronic infection due to *Mycobacterium spp.* and fungus (Schasfoort et al. 1999; Lee et al. 2004; Jeong et al. 2013) but can be found in chronic inflammatory joint diseases such as rheumatoid

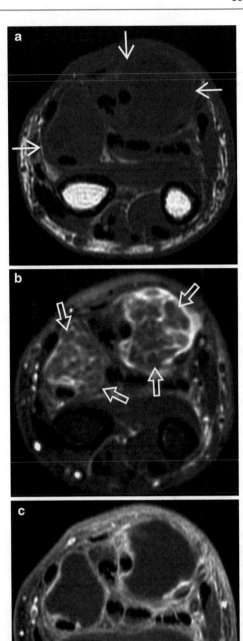

Fig. 33.18 Rice bodies in a tuberculous tenosynovitis. Axial (**a**) T1-W, (**b**) fat-suppressed T2-W, and (**c**) contrast-enhanced fat-suppressed T1-W MR images of the forearm show effusion in the flexor tendon sheath (*arrows*). Rice bodies are seen as T2-hypointense nodules resembling grains of rice (*open arrows*), imperceptible on T1-weighted images, and are not enhanced in the contrast-enhanced images

arthritis and seronegative arthropathies (Popert et al. 1982). The MRI appearance of rice bodies may mimic that of synovial chondromatosis. Both are hypointense on T2-weighted images; but on T1-weighted images, rice bodies are almost imperceptible or faintly visualized, while signal intensity of synovial chondromatosis is mildly hyperintense (Griffith et al. 1996; Chen et al. 2002; Lee et al. 2004). Both are not enhanced on contrast-enhanced MR images.

33.4   Osteomyelitis and Mimics

33.4.1 Acute Osteomyelitis

Bone changes related to infection depend on the anatomy of affected bone and the degree of bone destruction or repair. Osteomyelitis may take up to 2 weeks to be visualized on radiographs because at least 30–50% of the bone needs to be destroyed first (Ardran 1951; Mellado Santos 2006). In children, the lesion can initially occur in the cartilaginous epiphysis, which can only be diagnosed on MRI (Yoo et al. 2014). On radiographs, permeative or moth-eaten osteolytic lesions, cortical destruction, and periosteal reaction in acute osteomyelitis may simulate the changes in bone tumor

and tumorlike conditions such as Ewing sarcoma, eosinophilic granuloma, and skeletal metastasis. Presence of intraosseous or soft tissue abscesses is the key feature of osteomyelitis; however, loculated fluid collection in the setting of fracture may simulate the features of abscesses (Bohndorf 2004). Although seldom present, fat globules in the bone, subperiosteum, or soft tissue are suggestive of osteomyelitis (Figs. 33.19 and 33.20). Destruction of bone marrow cavities and increased intramedullary pressure from infection produce lipocyte necrosis, fat release, and formation of fat globules (Davies et al. 2005).

Ewing sarcoma can mimic osteomyelitis, with the presenting symptoms of infection such as fever, localized bone pain, leukocytosis, and elevated inflammatory markers. Radiographic findings of aggressive intramedullary bone destruction and variable degrees of periosteal reaction could indicate either osteomyelitis or Ewing sarcoma. If an extraosseous mass is not present, MRI of both entities shows infiltrative bone marrow lesion, cortical destruction, and periosteal reaction. On MR images, margins of the bone lesion in osteomyelitis tend to be hazy with a wide transition zone, in contrast to the sharp and well-defined margins of Ewing sarcoma (Henninger et al. 2013) (Fig. 33.20). Eosinophilic granuloma usually has a very similar appearance to osteomyelitis, being seen as an

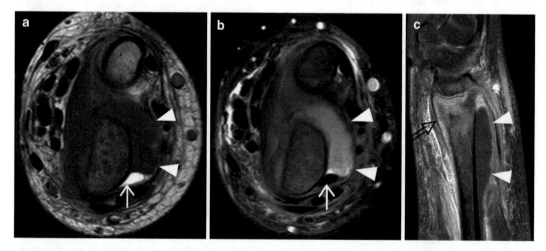

Fig. 33.19 Subperiosteal abscess and fat globule in acute osteomyelitis of the radius in a 13-year-old boy. Axial (**a**) T1-W and (**b**) fat-suppressed T2-W MR images show subperiosteal abscess (*arrowheads*) and fat globules (*arrows*).

(**c**) Sagittal contrast-enhanced fat-suppressed T1-W MR image of the radius shows enhancement of the bone marrow in the distal radius (*open arrows*) and subperiosteal abscess (*arrowheads*)

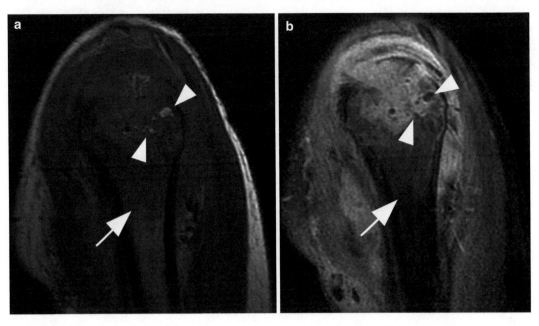

Fig. 33.20 Osteomyelitis in a 22-year-old woman. Sagittal (**a**) T1-W and (**b**) fat-suppressed T2-W MR images of the humerus show intraosseous fat globules (*arrowheads*) and blurring of the lesion margins (*arrows*)

aggressive osteolytic lesion with poorly defined borders and periosteal reaction. A lesion that is centered in the diaphysis favors eosinophilic granuloma over osteomyelitis (Pugmire et al. 2014).

33.4.2 Subacute and Chronic Osteomyelitis

Incompletely healed acute osteomyelitis may progress to subacute and chronic osteomyelitis. Clinically, osteomyelitis can be classified as subacute if the duration of illness is longer than weeks and chronic if more than 3 months (Peltola and Paakkonen 2014). However, a clear distinction between the stages of osteomyelitis using imaging features is not always possible. The role of imaging studies is to establish the diagnosis and to detect areas of residual active infection. Osseous sclerosis, thickened cortex, and periosteal bone formation are the common features of osteomyelitis. Reliable signs of active infection include intraosseous abscesses, sequestra, and sinus formation (Bohndorf 2004). Chronic skin sinuses may become malignant.

Brodie abscess consists of a central area of suppuration and necrosis which is walled off by granulation tissue and has a fibrous capsule, with imaging findings of a sclerotic margin and surrounding bone marrow edema. This usually occurs in the metaphyseal region. The differential diagnosis includes benign bone tumors such as unicameral bone cyst and enchondroma. In contrast to bone tumors, presence of patchy osteosclerosis of the surrounding bone on radiographs is the key finding indicating reactive bone change in osteomyelitis (Fig. 33.21a). In Brodie abscess, there may be a tunnel connecting to the adjacent physeal plate (Fig. 33.21). On T1-weighted MR images, the vascularized granulation tissue in the wall of an abscess presents with T1-hyperintensity – also called a penumbra sign (Fig. 33.22). The hyperintense T1 signal could be due to the high protein content of the granulation tissue or free paramagnetic radicals produced by activated macrophages (Davies and Grimer 2005). The penumbra sign is highly specific to abscesses, although it is not always present. If present, it is a useful feature to differentiate an abscess from a bone tumor (McGuinness et al. 2007). However, this sign has

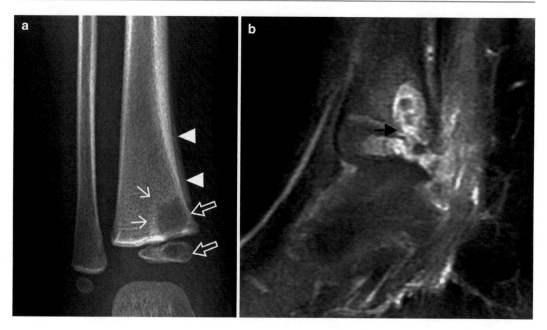

Fig. 33.21 Brodie abscess with a tunnel. (**a**) Radiograph shows Brodie abscesses in the metaphysis and epiphysis (*open arrows*) of the tibia. Note the reactive osteosclerosis (*white arrows*) around the Brodie abscess and periosteal reaction (*arrowheads*). (**b**) Sagittal contrast-enhanced fat-suppressed T1-W MR image shows spread of infection from the metaphysis to epiphysis via a tunnel (*black arrows*)

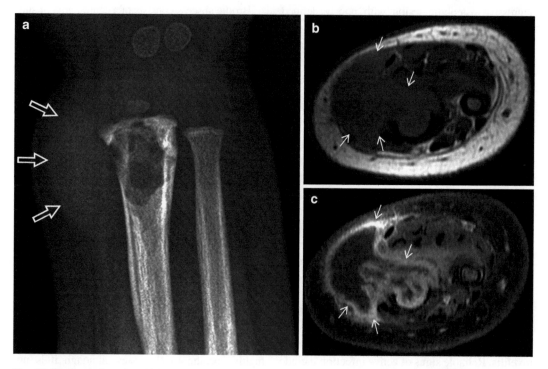

Fig. 33.22 Penumbra sign. Tuberculous osteomyelitis developing in a 1-year-old girl who presented with wrist swelling for 1 month. (**a**) Radiograph of the wrist shows bone destruction in the radius with associated soft tissue mass (*open arrows*). (**b**) Axial T1-W MR image of the wrist shows hyperintense signal in the wall of the intraosseous and soft tissue abscesses compatible with penumbra sign (*arrows*). (**c**) Axial contrast-enhanced fat-suppressed T1-W MR image shows that the wall of the abscess is enhanced (*arrows*)

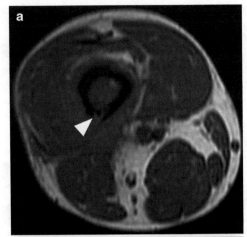

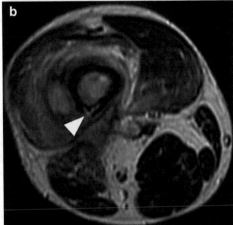

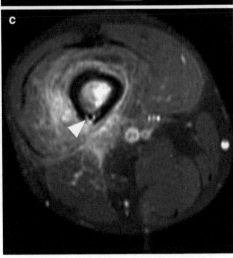

Fig. 33.23 Sequestrum in osteomyelitis. Axial (**a**) T1-W, (**b**) T2-W, and (**c**) contrast-enhanced fat-suppressed T1-W MR images of the thigh show sequestrum (*arrowheads*) which is markedly hypointense on all MRI pulse sequences. Note the cortical bone destruction, abnormal signal intensity of the bone marrow, and surrounding soft tissue inflammation in osteomyelitis

been reported in low-grade chondrosarcoma, eosinophilic granuloma, cystic bone lesions following curettage, and intraosseous ganglion cyst (Grey et al. 1998; Davies and Grimer 2005). The penumbra sign is also observed in soft tissue abscesses (McGuinness et al. 2007). In children, when intraosseous abscesses occur in the epiphysis, the lucent lesion leads to differential diagnoses including chondroblastoma, enchondroma, and eosinophilic granuloma.

Osteomyelitis and osteoid osteoma share some similar imaging features. Both osteomyelitis and osteoid osteoma can present with sclerotic margins and extensive bone and soft tissue edema. The nidus of osteoid osteoma can be mineralized and demonstrates markedly hypointense signal on all MRI pulse sequences, similar to sequestrum in osteomyelitis (Fig. 33.23). Extensive periosteal new bone formation is common in osteoid osteoma, whereas in infection, cortical destruction is predominant. The central nidus of osteoid osteoma demonstrates intense enhancement in the arterial phase on gadolinium administration, with early washout (Liu et al. 2003). On CT, radiating radiolucent grooves surrounding the osteoid osteoma nidus or vascular groove sign help in distinguishing osteoid osteoma from osteomyelitis (Liu et al. 2011) (Fig. 33.24).

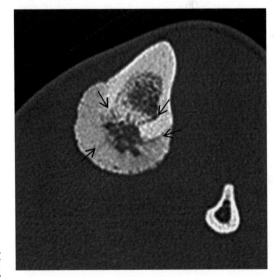

Fig. 33.24 Vascular groove sign in osteoid osteoma. Axial CT image of the leg shows cortical bone thickening and radiating radiolucent grooves (*arrows*) surrounding the osteoid osteoma nidus

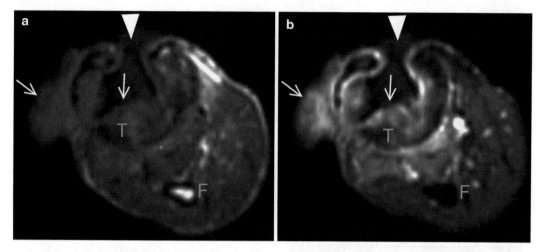

Fig. 33.25 Squamous cell carcinoma arising from the sinus tract in a 53-year-old man who presented with a post-traumatic draining sinus for 20 years. Axial (**a**) T1-W and (**b**) contrast-enhanced fat-suppressed T1-W MR images show an enhancing mass (*arrows*) in the bone cavity and around the sinus tract (*arrowheads*) [*T tibia, F fibula*]

33.4.3 Skin Sinus with Malignant Transformation

With chronic skin sinuses, malignant tumors, mainly squamous cell carcinoma, can arise from chronic osteomyelitis (McGrory et al. 1999). Typically, the risk of malignant tumor occurs when there has been a history of sinus draining over a period of 10 years (Saglik et al. 2001). Suspicion should be raised with associated clinical evidence of pain, hemorrhage, increased drainage, foul odor from the sinus tract, mass, and lymphadenopathy (Altay et al. 2004). Radiographs may show new osteolytic changes in the affected area; however, serial radiographs may appear unchanged (Saglik et al. 2001). MRI and CT can demonstrate formation of masses in the sinus tract (Fig. 33.25).

33.4.4 Hematogenous Osteomyelitis

Hematogenous osteomyelitis, particularly granulomatous infection, shares features with metastasis or multiple myeloma by presenting as multiple bone

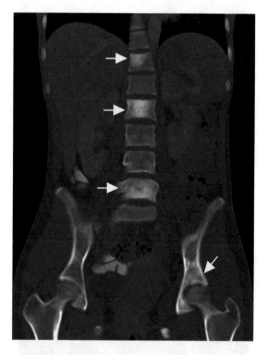

Fig. 33.26 Hematogenous osteomyelitis in a 25-year-old woman who presented with prolonged fever. Coronal CT image shows multiple osteosclerotic lesions in the vertebrae and pelvic bones (*arrows*). Tissue culture revealed nontuberculous mycobacteria

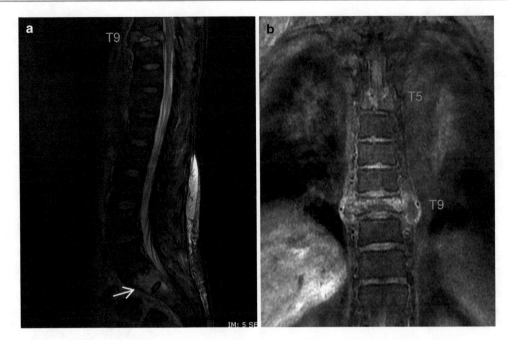

Fig. 33.27 Hematogenous osteomyelitis in a 59-year-old woman who presented with back pain and weakness for 2 weeks. (**a**) Sagittal fat-suppressed T2-W MR image of the lower thoracic and lumbar spine shows hyperintense lesions in the sacrum (*arrow*) and collapse of the vertebral body at T9 level resulting in spinal cord compression. (**b**) Coronal contrast-enhanced fat-suppressed T1-W MR image shows an abscess around the T9 level and signal abnormality in the vertebral body at T5 level. Bone biopsy revealed osteomyelitis

lesions occurring more frequently in the axial skeleton. Osteomyelitis can present with either osteolytic or sclerotic lesions (Fig. 33.26). Detection of abscesses either in the bone, subperiosteum, or soft tissue leads to correct diagnosis (Fig. 33.27).

33.4.5 Post-traumatic Osteomyelitis

Detection of osteomyelitis may be extremely difficult in a bone that has been altered by traumatic injury and the healing process. Radiographic features of the healing process, including bone resorption, periosteal reaction, cortical thickening, and bone sclerosis, resemble the changes evident in osteomyelitis. Serial radiographs can demonstrate the subtle changes, but sensitivity and specificity are reported to be only 14% and 70%, respectively. On MRI, signal changes of the bone marrow related to post-traumatic fibrovascular tissue can persist for up to

approximately 12 months (Kaim et al. 2002). Cystic accumulations of sterile fluid can be observed in the fracture for several years after the injury. Cystic inclusions are sharply demarcated with an absence of enhancement or surrounding bone marrow edema (Bohndorf 2004). The appearances in post-traumatic osteomyelitis are similar to those in non-violated bones. Presence of a sequestrum, fistula, or abscess indicates active osteomyelitis (Fig. 33.28).

33.4.6 Noninfectious Osteomyelitis

Noninfectious osteoarticular inflammatory conditions including chronic recurrent multiple focal osteomyelitis (CRMO) and synovitis, acne, pustulosis, hyperostosis, and osteitis (SAPHO) syndromes share several features with infection. Although etiology of the diseases remains unclear, several studies support the hypothesis that the disease is related to autoimmune and genetic factors (Leone et al. 2015). CRMO is a noninfectious osteomyelitis affecting children and adolescents, commonly involving metaphysis of long bones and medial clavicles. Radiographs show an osteolytic lesion in the initial stages, followed by progressive osteosclerosis and hyperostosis. Bone marrow edema, periosteal new bone formation and adjacent soft tissue inflammation can be seen on MRI (Fig. 33.29). Unlike infectious osteomyelitis,

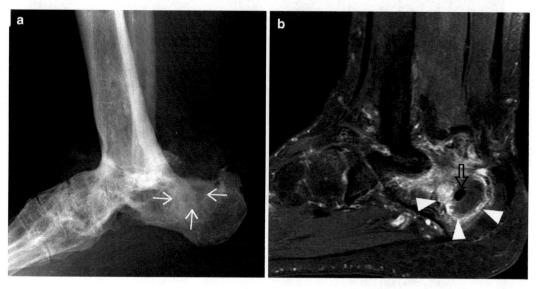

Fig. 33.28 Post-traumatic osteomyelitis with abscess in a 57-year-old man with a previous history of a complex fracture of the foot and ankle who presented with a draining sinus at the heel. (**a**) Lateral radiograph shows an osteolytic lesion with sclerotic border in the calcaneus (*arrows*). Note the surgical fusion of the ankle and subtalar joints. (**b**) Sagittal contrast-enhanced fat-suppressed T1-W MR image shows an intraosseous abscess in the calcaneus (*arrowheads*). A gas bubble (*open arrow*) indicates a connection between the abscess and skin sinus

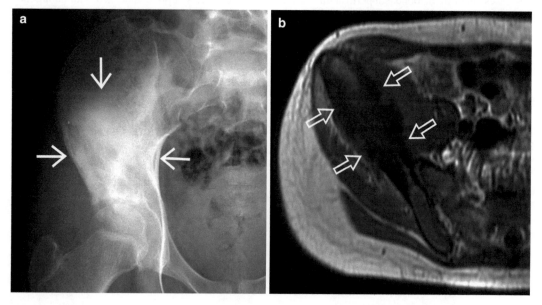

Fig. 33.29 Chronic recurrent multifocal osteomyelitis in a 14-year-old girl who presented with hip pain for the past year. (**a**) Radiograph of the pelvis shows an osteosclerotic lesion in the right ilium (*arrows*). Axial (**b**) T1-W, (**c**) STIR, and (**d**) contrast-enhanced fat-suppressed T1-W MR images show hyperostosis of the ilium with enhancement of the surrounding soft tissue (*open arrows*) indicating adjacent soft tissue inflammation. No abscess is detected

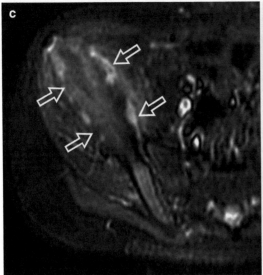
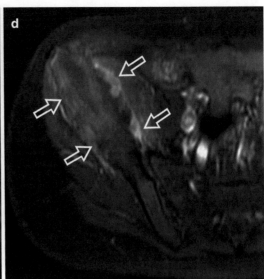

Fig. 33.29 (continued)

abscesses, cloacae, and sequestra do not form (Khanna et al. 2009). SAPHO occurs in adults and commonly involves the anterior chest wall and axial skeleton. Although skin lesions are described as a component of SAPHO syndrome, the absence of concurrent skin lesions is not uncommon. Skin lesions may occur before or after the onset of osteoarticular lesions, generally within a 2-year interval, but delayed presentation of as long as 20 years has been reported (Kahn et al. 1991; Hayem et al. 1999). Noninfectious osteomyelitis is a diagnosis of exclusion, requiring biopsy to rule out infectious osteomyelitis and malignancy.

33.5   Unrecognized Retained Foreign Bodies

After suffering a penetrating injury, pain, swelling, and the resultant wound are usually followed by a period of improvement. Subsequently, unrecognized retained foreign bodies result in repeated soft tissue infection leading to chronic pain, discharge, and soft tissue masses. Clinical and imaging features vary according to the composition of the foreign body, depth of

penetration, and affected tissue. Clinical presentation may be delayed for several months or years after the penetrating injury.

Radiography can detect radiopaque foreign bodies, but the sensitivity decreases when they are located in complex bony structures owing to the chance that foreign bodies are obscured by bones (Pattamapaspong et al. 2013). US imaging is a valuable modality for the detection of a foreign body in soft tissue. However, foreign bodies, which are generally echogenic, can be difficult to visualize if embedded in a tendon or close to a bone (Bray et al. 1995). Surrounding inflammation helps in the detection of foreign bodies; however, it is inconsistently present and can be completely absent (Fig. 33.30). Detection of foreign bodies by MRI and CT can be exceedingly difficult if a penetrating injury is unsuspected. Surrounding inflammation is sometimes large, simulating the appearance of soft tissue tumors. On MRI, a foreign body can present as a central signal void surrounded by an area of inflammation or abscess (Monu et al. 1995) (Fig. 33.31). Foreign bodies containing gas and metal may produce magnetic susceptibility artifact.

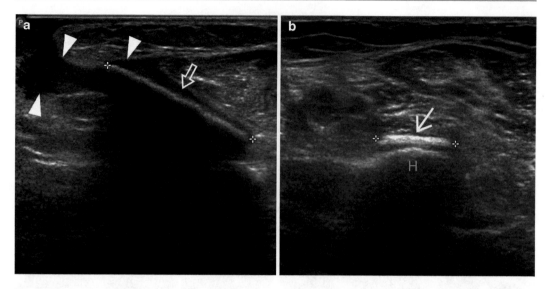

Fig. 33.30 Retained wooden foreign bodies in a 43-year-old women who presented with arm pain 9 months after a penetrating injury. (**a**) US image of the arm shows an echogenic wooden foreign body (*open arrow*) with surrounding abscess and a sinus tract (*arrowheads*). (**b**) US image of another foreign body in the same arm (*arrows*) shows absence of inflammatory response. The severity of inflammation surrounding these two foreign bodies was different [*H humerus*]

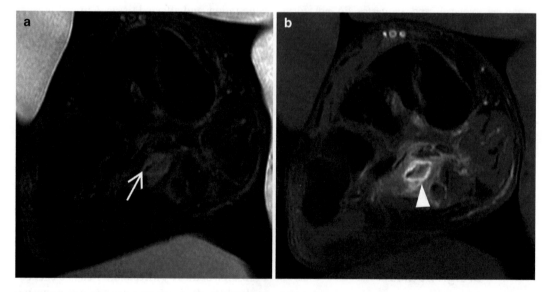

Fig. 33.31 Retained wooden foreign bodies in a 65-year-old man with a history of a penetrating injury of the foot which occurred 1 year ago. Coronal (**a**) fat-suppressed T2-W and (**b**) contrast-enhanced fat-suppressed T1-W MR images of the foot show a signal void foreign body (*arrow*) surrounded by a rim-enhancing abscess (*arrowhead*)

33.6   Diabetic Pedal Infection

Diabetic foot problems are mostly the combination of vasculopathy, neuropathy, and infection, which can affect the skin, soft tissue, joint, and bone. Radiography is the initial study, providing details of bone destruction, soft tissue gas, retained foreign bodies, and detailed information regarding prior surgical intervention. MRI has the highest accuracy in the detection of soft tissue infection and osteomyelitis. Before performing MRI, the foot should be examined clinically, and an external marker should be positioned over the ulcer. To achieve homogeneous fat suppression and high spatial resolution, the study should focus on the specific location in question and obtain as thin sections as possible. A large field of view covering the entire foot should be avoided. If there are no contraindications, imaging after administration of intravenous gadolinium chelate is useful in the detection of nonviable tissue and also in differentiating cellulitis from edematous subcutaneous tissue related to diabetic vasculopathy and neuropathy (Russell et al. 2008).

Changes in the biomechanics in the diabetic foot lead to skin callus formation at the weight-bearing and friction sites, commonly near metatarsal heads. On MRI, skin calluses demonstrate focal subcutaneous lesions with signal hypointensity on T1-weighted images and hypointense to intermediate signal on T2-weighted images (Fig. 33.32). Enhancement of calluses may mimic cellulitis, but the location of lesions and lack of adjacent inflammatory subcutaneous fat stranding should aid in the diagnosis (Chatha et al. 2005). In contrast to skin calluses, ulceration and cellulitis are seen as areas of hyperintense signal intensity on T2-weighted images. However, persistent weight-bearing and microtrauma can result in callus breakdown, ulceration, and eventually cellulitis.

With progression of infection, deeper soft tissue infection, septic arthritis, and osteomyelitis

can occur. Diabetic pedal osteomyelitis is a distinct form of osteomyelitis which is almost invariably associated with a contiguous ulcer or soft tissue abscess (Baker et al. 2012). The key imaging feature of osteomyelitis is bone marrow signal changes adjacent to the ulcer or soft tissue infection (Craig et al. 1997) (Fig. 33.33). The bone marrow changes are shown as signal hypointensity on T1-weighted images, signal hyperintensity on T2-weighted images, and contrast enhancement. Locations of osteomyelitis are mostly related to bone protuberances and pressure points of the foot, including the first and fifth metatarsal bones, first distal phalanx, calcaneum, and malleoli (Ledermann et al. 2002a).

Neuropathic osteoarthropathy may mimic infection. In the early stages, neuropathic osteoarthropathy presents with soft tissue swelling and skin redness, mimicking soft tissue infection. Decreased sensation may not occur at this stage and radiographs of the foot remain normal. MRI features of the early neuropathic osteoarthropathy include bone marrow signal changes and enhancement around joints without adjacent ulcers (Fig. 33.34). The midfoot region around the Lisfranc and Chopart joints are commonly involved (Ledermann and Morrison 2005). Muscular denervation in the subacute phase is seen as diffuse signal hyperintensity on T2-weighted images which can be mistaken for soft tissue edema or infection. In denervation, the muscle size reduces, accompanied by fat replacement (Fleckenstein et al. 1993) (Fig. 33.35). In more advanced stages, foot deformity leads to

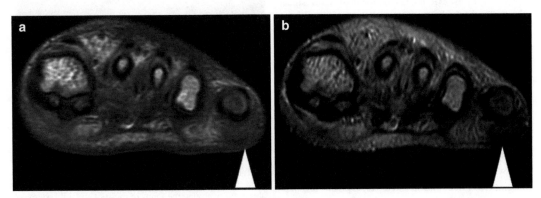

Fig. 33.32 Skin callus. Coronal (**a**) T1-W and (**b**) T2-W MR images of the foot show hypointense skin callus (*arrowheads*) without surrounding inflammation

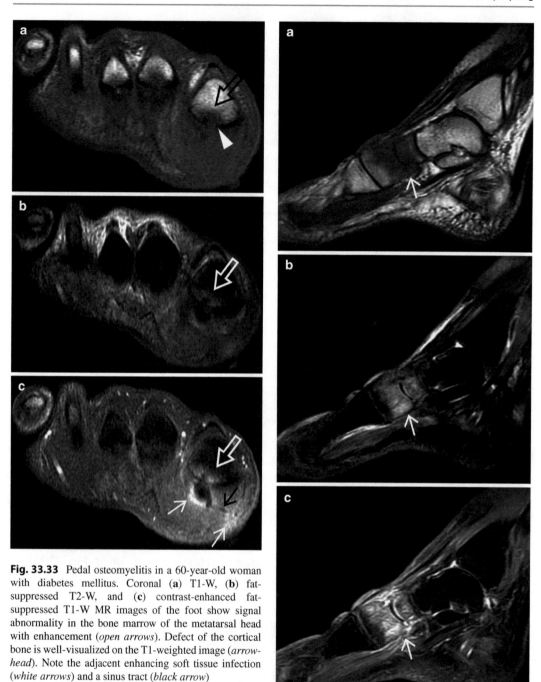

Fig. 33.33 Pedal osteomyelitis in a 60-year-old woman with diabetes mellitus. Coronal (**a**) T1-W, (**b**) fat-suppressed T2-W, and (**c**) contrast-enhanced fat-suppressed T1-W MR images of the foot show signal abnormality in the bone marrow of the metatarsal head with enhancement (*open arrows*). Defect of the cortical bone is well-visualized on the T1-weighted image (*arrowhead*). Note the adjacent enhancing soft tissue infection (*white arrows*) and a sinus tract (*black arrow*)

abnormal pressure distribution, skin ulcers, and subsequently osteomyelitis.

When osteomyelitis coexists with neuropathic osteoarthropathy, delineation of the extension of the disease may be difficult. On radiographs, poorly marginated bone and cortical disruption are not usually present in neuropathic arthropathy unless infection has become superimposed. MRI signal

Fig. 33.34 Early neuropathic osteoarthropathy in a 50-year-old woman with diabetes mellitus who presented with a foot swelling but no skin ulcer. Sagittal (**a**) T1-W, (**b**) fat-suppressed T2-W, and (**c**) contrast-enhanced fat-suppressed T1-W MR images show bone marrow signal abnormality around the joints of midfoot and mild edema of the adjacent soft tissue (*arrows*). Her symptoms improved with casting and no antibiotic treatment was required

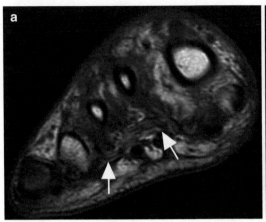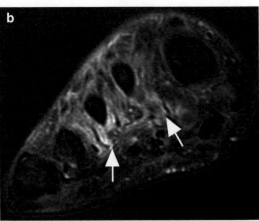

Fig. 33.35 Muscle denervation in a 57-year-old man with diabetes mellitus. (**a**) Coronal T1-W MR image shows reduction of muscle bulk. (**b**) Coronal fat-suppressed T2-W MR image shows signal hyperintensity in muscles of the foot (*arrows*)

changes of bone marrow and cortical disruption at the location of ulcer or soft tissue abscess remain the key findings of infected neuropathic osteoarthropathy. Reactive bone marrow edema can occur adjacent to the site of soft tissue infection, but T1-weighted marrow signal approximates to that of normal marrow signal intensity, and the cortical bone is preserved. On the serial MR images, progression of bone erosions and loss of subchondral bone cysts favor the diagnosis of superimposed infection (Ledermann and Morrison 2005).

Conclusion

Imaging features of musculoskeletal infection are related to structural damage, host response, and the reparative process. A key feature of infection is the formation of abscesses. Infection commonly spreads from a tissue compartment to the adjacent compartment. The patterns are extremely varied and can mimic other diseases. Radiologists should aim to recognize these patterns in order to avoid pitfalls in interpretation.

References

Ali SZ, Srinivasan S, Peh WCG (2014) MRI in necrotizing fasciitis of the extremities. Br J Radiol 87(1033):20130560. doi:10.1259/bjr.20130560

Altay M, Arikan M, Yildiz Y, Saglik Y (2004) Squamous cell carcinoma arising in chronic osteomyelitis in foot and ankle. Foot Ankle Int 25:805–809

Ardran GM (1951) Bone destruction not demonstrable by radiography. Br J Radiol 24:107–109

Ashrani AA, Key NS, Soucie JM et al (2008) Septic arthritis in males with haemophilia. Haemophilia 14: 494–503

Baker JC, Demertzis JL, Rhodes NG et al (2012) Diabetic musculoskeletal complications and their imaging mimics. Radiographics 32:1959–1974

Bickels J, Ben-Sira L, Kessler A, Wientroub S (2002) Primary pyomyositis. J Bone Joint Surg Am 84:2277–2286

Bierma-Zeinstra SM, Bohnen AM, Verhaar JA et al (2000) Sonography for hip joint effusion in adults with hip pain. Ann Rheum Dis 59:178–182

Bohndorf K (2004) Infection of the appendicular skeleton. Eur Radiol 14(Suppl 3):E53–E63

Bray PW, Mahoney JL, Campbell JP (1995) Sensitivity and specificity of ultrasound in the diagnosis of foreign bodies in the hand. J Hand Surg Am 20:661–666

Carra BJ, Bui-Mansfield LT, O'Brien SD, Chen DC (2014) Sonography of musculoskeletal soft-tissue masses: techniques, pearls, and pitfalls. AJR Am J Roentgenol 202:1281–1290

Chatha DS, Cunningham PM, Schweitzer ME (2005) MR imaging of the diabetic foot: diagnostic challenges. Radiol Clin N Am 43:747–59, ix.

Chaudhry AA, Baker KS, Gould ES, Gupta R (2015) Necrotizing fasciitis and its mimics: what radiologists need to know. AJR Am J Roentgenol 204:128–139

Chen A, Wong LY, Sheu CY, Chen BF (2002) Distinguishing multiple rice body formation in chronic subacromial-subdeltoid bursitis from synovial chondromatosis. Skeletal Radiol 31:119–121

Cheung HS, Ryan LM, Kozin F, McCarty DJ (1980) Synovial origins of rice bodies in joint fluid. Arthritis Rheum 23:72–76

Choi JA, Koh SH, Hong SH et al (2009) Rheumatoid arthritis and tuberculous arthritis: differentiating MRI features. AJR Am J Roentgenol 193:1347–1353

Coulier B, Cloots V (2003) Atypical retroperitoneal extension of iliopsoas bursitis. Skeletal Radiol 32: 298–301

Craig JG, Amin MB, Wu K et al (1997) Osteomyelitis of the diabetic foot: MR imaging-pathologic correlation. Radiology 203:849–855

Davies AM, Grimer R (2005) The penumbra sign in subacute osteomyelitis. Eur Radiol 15:1268–1270

Davies AM, Hughes DE, Grimer RJ (2005) Intramedullary and extramedullary fat globules on magnetic resonance imaging as a diagnostic sign for osteomyelitis. Eur Radiol 15:2194–2199

Dubost JJ, Fis I, Denis P et al (1993) Polyarticular septic arthritis. Medicine 72:296–310

Fleckenstein JL, Burns DK, Murphy FK et al (1991) Differential diagnosis of bacterial myositis in AIDS: evaluation with MR imaging. Radiology 179:653–658

Fleckenstein JL, Watumull D, Conner KE et al (1993) Denervated human skeletal muscle: MR imaging evaluation. Radiology 187:213–218

Ghazizadeh S, Foss EW, Didier R et al (2014) Musculoskeletal pitfalls and pseudotumours in the pelvis: a pictorial review for body imagers. Br J Radiol 87(1042):20140243. doi:10.1259/bjr.20140243

Gordon BA, Martinez S, Collins AJ (1995) Pyomyositis: characteristics at CT and MR imaging. Radiology 197:279–286

Grey AC, Davies AM, Mangham DC et al (1998) The 'penumbra sign' on T1-weighted MR imaging in subacute osteomyelitis: frequency, cause and significance. Clin Radiol 53:587–592

Griffith JF, Peh WCG, Evans NS et al (1996) Multiple rice body formation in chronic subacromial/subdeltoid bursitis: MR appearances. Clin Radiol 51:511–514

Hayem G, Bouchaud-Chabot A, Benali K et al (1999) SAPHO syndrome: a long-term follow-up study of 120 cases. Semin Arthritis Rheum 29:159–171

Henninger B, Glodny B, Rudisch A et al (2013) Ewing sarcoma versus osteomyelitis: differential diagnosis with magnetic resonance imaging. Skeletal Radiol 42:1097–1104

Jelinek JS, Murphey MD, Aboulafia AJ et al (1999) Muscle infarction in patients with diabetes mellitus: MR imaging findings. Radiology 211:241–247

Jeong YM, Cho HY, Lee SW et al (2013) Candida septic arthritis with rice body formation: a case report and review of literature. Korean J Radiol 14:465–469

Kahn MF, Bouvier M, Palazzo E et al (1991) Sternoclavicular pustulotic osteitis (SAPHO). 20-year interval between skin and bone lesions. J Rheumatol 18:1104–1108

Kaim AH, Gross T, von Schulthess GK (2002) Imaging of chronic posttraumatic osteomyelitis. Eur Radiol 12:1193–1202

Karchevsky M, Schweitzer ME, Morrison WB, Parellada JA (2004) MRI findings of septic arthritis and associated osteomyelitis in adults. AJR Am J Roentgenol 182:119–122

Khanna G, Sato TS, Ferguson P (2009) Imaging of chronic recurrent multifocal osteomyelitis. Radiographics 1159–1177

Kim EY, Kim SS, Ryoo JW et al (2004) Primary peripheral T-cell lymphoma of the face other than mycosis fungoides. Computed tomography and magnetic resonance findings. J Comput Assist Tomogr 28: 670–675

Kim KT, Kim YJ, Won Lee J et al (2011) Can necrotizing infectious fasciitis be differentiated from nonnecrotizing infectious fasciitis with MR imaging? Radiology 259:816–824

Ledermann HP, Morrison WB, Schweitzer ME (2002a) MR image analysis of pedal osteomyelitis: distribution, patterns of spread, and frequency of associated ulceration and septic arthritis. Radiology 223: 747–755

Ledermann HP, Schweitzer ME, Morrison WB (2002b) Pelvic heterotopic ossification: MR imaging characteristics. Radiology 222:189–195

Ledermann HP, Morrison WB (2005) Differential diagnosis of pedal osteomyelitis and diabetic neuroarthropathy: MR imaging. Semin Musculoskelet Radiol 9:272–283

Lee EY, Rubin DA, Brown DM (2004) Recurrent *Mycobacterium marinum* tenosynovitis of the wrist mimicking extraarticular synovial chondromatosis on MR images. Skeletal Radiol 33:405–408

Leone A, Cassar-Pullicino VN, Casale R et al (2015) The SAPHO syndrome revisited with an emphasis on spinal manifestations. Skeletal Radiol 44:9–24

Liu PT, Chivers FS, Roberts CC et al (2003) Imaging of osteoid osteoma with dynamic gadolinium-enhanced MR imaging. Radiology 227:691–700

Liu PT, Kujak JL, Roberts CC, de Chadarevian JP (2011) The vascular groove sign: a new CT finding associated with osteoid osteomas. AJR Am J Roentgenol 196:168–173

Li-Yu J, Clayburne GM, Sieck MS et al (2002) Calcium apatite crystals in synovial fluid rice bodies. Ann Rheum Dis 61:387–390

Ma LD, Frassica FJ, Scott WW Jr et al (1995) Differentiation of benign and malignant musculoskeletal tumors: potential pitfalls with MR imaging. Radiographics 15:349–366

Malghem J, Lecouvet FE, Omoumi P et al (2013) Necrotizing fasciitis: contribution and limitations of diagnostic imaging. Joint Bone Spine 80:146–154

Margaretten ME, Kohlwes J, Moore D, Bent S (2007) Does this adult patient have septic arthritis? JAMA 297:1478–1488

McGrory JE, Pritchard DJ, Unni KK et al (1999) Malignant lesions arising in chronic osteomyelitis. Clin Orthop Relat Res 362:181–189

McGuinness B, Wilson N, Doyle AJ (2007) The "penumbra sign" on T1-weighted MRI for differentiating musculoskeletal infection from tumour. Skeletal Radiol 36:417–421

Mellado Santos JM (2006) Diagnostic imaging of pediatric hematogenous osteomyelitis: lessons learned from a multi-modality approach. Eur Radiol 16:2109–2119

Monu JU, McManus CM, Ward WG et al (1995) Soft-tissue masses caused by long-standing foreign bodies in the extremities: MR imaging findings. AJR Am J Roentgenol 165:395–397

Pattamapaspong N, Srisuwan T, Sivasomboon C et al (2013) Accuracy of radiography, computed tomography and magnetic resonance imaging in diagnosing foreign bodies in the foot. Radiol Med 118:303–310

Peltola H, Paakkonen M (2014) Acute osteomyelitis in children. New Engl J Med 370:352–360

Popert AJ, Scott DL, Wainwright AC et al (1982) Frequency of occurrence, mode of development, and significance or rice bodies in rheumatoid joints. Ann Rheum Dis 41:109–117

Popert J (1985) Rice-bodies, synovial debris, and joint lavage. Br J Rheumatol 24:1–2

Pugmire BS, Shailam R, Gee MS (2014) Role of MRI in the diagnosis and treatment of osteomyelitis in pediatric patients. World J Radiol 6:530–537

Russell JM, Peterson JJ, Bancroft LW. MR imaging of the diabetic foot. Magn Reson Imaging Clin N Am. 2008;16:59–70, vi.

Ruzek KA, Wenger DE (2004) The multiple faces of lymphoma of the musculoskeletal system. Skeletal Radiol 33:1–8

Saglik Y, Arikan M, Altay M, Yildiz Y (2001) Squamous cell carcinoma arising in chronic osteomyelitis. Int Orthop 25:389–391

Sarris I, Berendt AR, Athanasous N, Ostlere SJ (2003) MRI of mycetoma of the foot: two cases demonstrating the dot-in-circle sign. Skeletal Radiol 32:179–183

Schasfoort RA, Marck KW, Houtman PM (1999) Histoplasmosis of the wrist. J Hand Surg Br 24:625–627

Stacy GS, Dixon LB (2007) Pitfalls in MR image interpretation prompting referrals to an orthopedic oncology clinic. Radiographics 27:805–26; discussion 827–808.

Stacy GS, Kapur A (2011) Mimics of bone and soft tissue neoplasms. Radiol Clin N Am 49:1261–86, vii.

Toledano TR, Fatone EA, Weis A, Cotten A, Beltran J (2011) MRI evaluation of bone marrow changes in the diabetic foot: a practical approach. Semin Musculoskelet Radiol 15:257–268

Wunderbaldinger P, Bremer C, Schellenberger E, Cejna M, Turetschek K, Kainberger F (2002) Imaging features of iliopsoas bursitis. Eur Radiol 12:409–415

Yoo WJ, Choi IH, Yun YH et al (2014) Primary epiphyseal osteomyelitis caused by mycobacterium species in otherwise healthy toddlers. J Bone Joint Surg Am 96(17):e145. doi:10.2106/JBJS.M.01186

Zubler V, Mamisch-Saupe N, Pfirrmann CW, Jost B, Zanetti M (2011) Detection and quantification of glenohumeral joint effusion: reliability of ultrasound. Eur Radiol 21:1858–1864

Inflammatory Arthritides: Imaging Pitfalls

34

Paul Felloni, Neal Larkman, Rares Dunca, and Anne Cotten

Contents

34.1 **Introduction** 697

34.2 **Axial Spondyloarthritis: Sacroiliitis?** 697
34.2.1 Diagnosis 697
34.2.2 Mimics and Pitfalls 698

34.3 **Axial Spondyloarthritis: Spine Involvement?** 702
34.3.1 Diagnosis 702
34.3.2 Mimics and Pitfalls 704

34.4 **Peripheral Spondyloarthritis** 706
34.4.1 Diagnosis 706
34.4.2 Mimics and Pitfalls 707

34.5 **Rheumatoid Arthritis** 709
34.5.1 Diagnosis 709
34.5.2 Mimics and Pitfalls 709

Conclusion 710

References 710

Abbreviations

BME Bone marrow edema
CT Computed tomography
MRI Magnetic resonance imaging

P. Felloni, MD • N. Larkman, MD • R. Dunca, MD
A. Cotten, MD, PhD (✉)
Service de Radiologie et Imagerie
Musculosquelettique, Centre de consultations et
d'imagerie de l'appareil locomoteur (CCIAL),
Rue du professeur Emile Laine, CHRU de Lille,
59037 Lille, France
e-mail: anne.cotten@chru-lille.fr

RA Rheumatoid arthritis
SpA Spondyloarthritis
US Ultrasound

34.1 Introduction

Inflammatory arthritides represents a heterogeneous group of inflammatory disorders characterized by chronic inflammation of joints. Since their early diagnosis and treatment have been recognized as essential for the improvement of patients' clinical outcome, imaging has been increasingly used in clinical practice. As a consequence, depiction of early and therefore subtle imaging signs of inflammatory arthritis exposes the radiologist to diagnostic pitfalls and in particular, to false positives. The aim of this chapter is to present the main imaging pitfalls that may be encountered in daily practice when faced with a clinical suspicion of inflammatory arthritides. Therefore, this chapter will be focused on the main joints affected early in these disorders (i.e., sacroiliac, spine, and peripheral joints).

34.2 Axial Spondyloarthritis: Sacroiliitis?

34.2.1 Diagnosis

The sacroiliac joints are nearly always affected in spondyloarthritis (SpA), with sacroiliitis usually

© Springer International Publishing AG 2017
W.C.G. Peh (ed.), *Pitfalls in Musculoskeletal Radiology*, DOI 10.1007/978-3-319-53496-1_34

being the initial manifestation. Erosions and sub-chondral sclerosis can be detected by radiographs, but it often takes 6–8 years before sacroiliitis is detectable on radiographs (Mau et al. 1987; Bennett et al. 2008). Computed tomography (CT) may depict subtle structural lesions more accurately, but it has the same limitations as radiographs, as these imaging modalities can detect only the structural damage of the joints resulting from inflammation and not the active inflammation itself. This is why new Assessment of Spondyloarthritis International Society (ASAS) criteria have been defined to help identify patients with early axial SpA (Rudwaleit et al. 2009a, b, c). In patients younger than 45 years with low back pain for more than 3 months, the imaging arm of these criteria requires the presence of sacroiliitis either on radiographs, which defines the ankylosing spondylitis patients, or active inflammation on magnetic resonance imaging (MRI), which defines the non-radiographic axial SpA group (Rudwaleit et al. 2009a, b). According to these criteria, bone marrow edema (BME) is regarded as essential for the definition of active sacroiliitis on MRI (Rudwaleit et al. 2009a, b).

As a consequence, MRI is nowadays frequently and widely performed for diagnostic purposes. At an early stage of the disease, BME may be uni- or bilateral, focal, multifocal, or diffuse. It is usually seen on both sides of the joint but unilateral involvement is possible. It tends to predominate on the iliac side, but a sacral predominance is also possible. It may be isolated or associated with other inflammatory or structural damage, these additional features improving diagnostic certainty. Subtle early MRI features of sacroiliitis require differentiation from other disorders that may be accompanied by BME.

34.2.2 Mimics and Pitfalls

34.2.2.1 Red Bone Marrow and Ossifying Cartilage

Particularly in young patients, BME has to be differentiated from red bone marrow and ossifying cartilage, for which signal intensity is usually less intense on fat-suppressed T2-weighted images and the distribution bilateral and more uniform (Fig. 34.1). Residual areas can also be seen along the lateral aspects of the distal sacrum. Irregularities

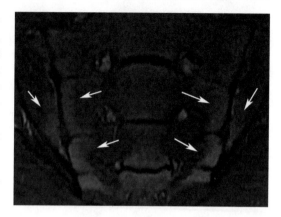

Fig. 34.1 Oblique coronal fat-suppressed T2-W MR image shows bilateral hyperintense subchondral areas related to the presence of red bone marrow or ossifying cartilage (*arrows*)

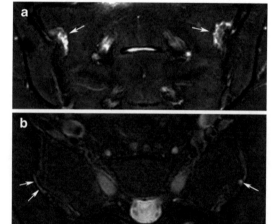

Fig. 34.2 Vessels (*arrows*) in the transitional area of the sacroiliac joints mimicking BME on the (**a**) oblique coronal fat-suppressed T2-W MR image is easily recognized on (**b**) oblique axial fat-suppressed T2-W MR image

of the sacroiliac joint surfaces can also be demonstrated until 16–18 years of age, due to the immaturity of the ossification process (Bollow et al. 1997; Sheybani et al. 2013).

34.2.2.2 Vessels

Vessels which are abundant in the transitional area between the cartilaginous and the ligamentous joints (Egund and Jurik 2014) can be misleading on the oblique coronal sections when the latter involve this area, mimicking synovitis or BME (Fig. 34.2). However, they are easily recognized on the oblique axial images, which are particularly useful in any doubtful cases.

34.2.2.3   Tiny Lesions

Since small foci of subchondral BME are sometimes seen in healthy volunteers (Weber et al.
2013), a size criterion has been proposed to
increase the specificity of this sign for the diagnosis of active sacroiliitis (Rudwaleit et al. 2009a, b).
If there is only one edematous lesion seen on a
single slice, that lesion must be present on one of
the adjacent slices (Fig. 34.3). If there is more
than one lesion on a single slice, one slice may be
sufficient. In summary, the lesion must be large
enough and is not significant when alone/isolated
and small-sized. The use of this definition should
allow most of the nonsignificant small edematous
areas that can be encountered in the subchondral
bone marrow to be eliminated (Fig. 34.4).

34.2.2.4   Mechanical Overload

It is also fundamental to analyze the location of
BME; as in the sacroiliac joints, mechanical overload is usually concentrated in a precise region, i.e.,
the anterior part of the middle third of the joint.

This is why degenerative changes and osteitis condensans ilii are located or predominate in this region
(Olivieri et al. 1996; Shibata et al. 2002). One
should keep in mind that the most anterior oblique
coronal sections involve this region. As a consequence, abnormal signal intensities of the subchondral bone marrow (edema, sclerosis, fat, or erosions)
at this sole location, sometimes even on two or three
adjacent slices, are not relevant for the diagnosis of
sacroiliitis (Fig. 34.5). Axial sections will easily
confirm the anterior location of these features, often
triangular in shape, sometimes with some bony proliferation at the articular margins and often bilateral
in distribution (Fig. 34.6). These changes related to
mechanical stress, of which topography is the key
discriminating factor, represent the main pitfall
when reading MRI of the sacroiliac joints. In contrast, presence of BME in the other parts of the joint
not involved by mechanical loading such as the
proximal or distal third of the joint, or its posterior
part, is highly suggestive of SpA, if the previously
described criteria of size are respected.

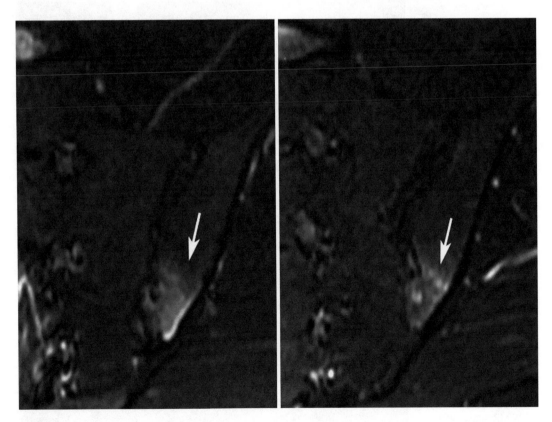

Fig. 34.3 Two consecutive oblique coronal fat-suppressed T2-W MR images show sacroiliitis with subchondral BME
(*arrows*)

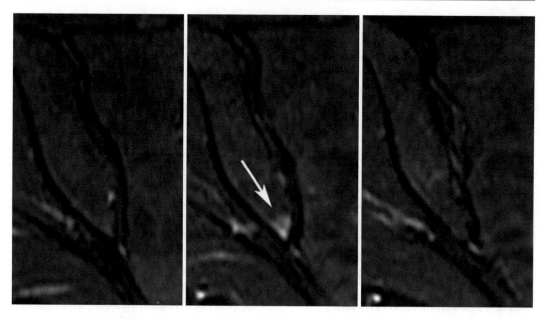

Fig. 34.4 Area of isolated subchondral BME (*arrow*) seen in only one out of three contiguous oblique coronal fat-suppressed T2-W MR images

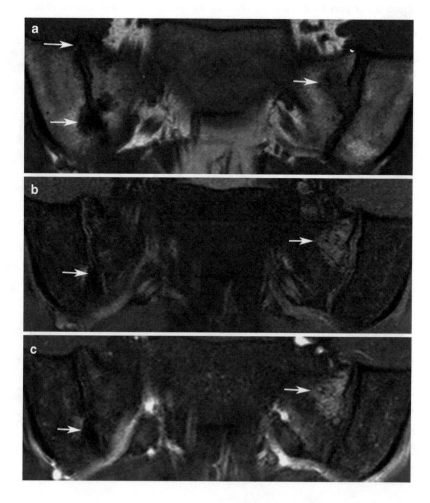

Fig. 34.5 Oblique coronal (**a**) T1-W, (**b**) fat-suppressed T2-W, and (**c**) contrast-enhanced fat-suppressed T1-W MR images show subchondral mechanical changes (*arrows*) of both sacroiliac joints

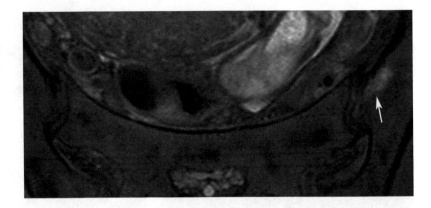

Fig. 34.6 Oblique axial fat-suppressed T2-W MR image shows subchondral mechanical changes predominating at the anterior part of both sacroiliac joints, particularly at the left side (*arrow*)

34.2.2.5 Anatomical Variants

Several anatomical variants (e.g., accessory sacroiliac joint, iliosacral complex, semicircular defects) can be misleading on coronal images, particularly when they are associated with edema related to microtrauma or degenerative changes. Once again, axial sections are also particularly helpful for their recognition.

34.2.2.6 Sacral Fracture

Bone insufficiency fractures in a sagittal plane have to be kept in mind when BME is mainly located on the sacral side (Peh et al. 1996; Ahovuo et al. 2004) (Fig. 34.7). The hypointense fracture line may sometimes be difficult to identify on MR images, being embedded in the adjacent edema. However, the age of the patient is typically different, and the edema tends to predominate in the sacral wing with a relative preservation of the subchondral bone marrow, in contrast to sacroiliitis.

34.2.2.7 Septic Sacroiliitis

Clinical and biological symptoms are often suggestive of an infectious process, although spondylodiskitis is usually evoked. Septic sacroiliitis is typically unilateral. It is usually associated with a joint effusion and extensive BME and periarticular soft tissue changes, including abscess (Stürzenbecher et al. 2000) (Fig. 34.8).

34.2.2.8 Tumors

Infrequently, BME associated with tumors (such as osteoid osteoma whose nidus may be undetectable on MRI) (Llauger et al. 2000) or tumoral bone marrow infiltration such as in lymphoma (Bereau et al. 2011) can be misleading. Analysis of the

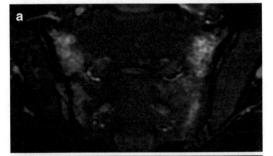

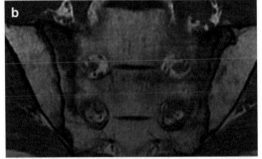

Fig. 34.7 Oblique coronal (**a**) fat-suppressed T2-W and (**b**) T1-W MR images show bilateral insufficiency fractures of the sacrum

topography of these abnormal signal intensity changes, located or extending far away from the joint space and/or depiction of extension into the adjacent soft tissues, may suggest the correct diagnosis.

34.2.2.9 Hyperparathyroidism

Bilateral subchondral bone resorption of the sacroiliac joints may be seen in hyperparathyroidism, either in its primary or secondary form, mimicking sacroiliitis (Bywaters et al. 1963). However, suggestive features include unusually intense and extensive subchondral bone resorption, only minimal cartilage surface irregularity

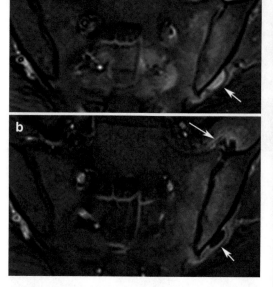

Fig. 34.8 Oblique coronal (**a**) fat-suppressed T2-W and (**b**) contrast-enhanced T1-W MR images show left infectious sacroiliitis (*arrows*)

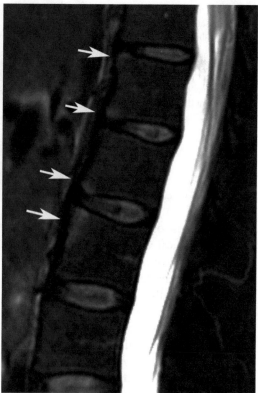

Fig. 34.10 Sagittal fat-suppressed T2-W MR image of the thoracolumbar junction shows four anterior inflammatory corners of the vertebral bodies suggesting SpA (*arrows*)

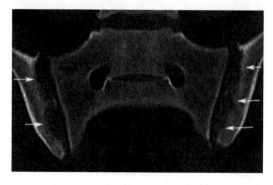

Fig. 34.9 Oblique coronal CT image shows hyperparathyroidism with bilateral extensive subchondral bone resorption of the iliac side of both SI joints (*arrows*)

(Tuite 2008), absent or minimal BME, and no evolution toward ankylosis (Fig. 34.9).

34.3   Axial Spondyloarthritis: Spine Involvement?

34.3.1 Diagnosis

The spine is also frequently involved in SpA. On radiographs, the initial features typically start at the thoracolumbar junction, particularly at the anterior corners of the vertebral bodies, as this is a region rich in entheses (annulus fibrosus, deep fibers of the anterior longitudinal ligament). The Romanus lesion refers to marginal bone resorption or erosion of the anterior vertebral corners due to osteitis and enthesitis, which is responsible for squaring of the vertebral bodies. The healing of the inflammatory changes may result in sclerosis and bone proliferation along the peripheral fibers of the annulus fibrosus and the deep fibers of the anterior longitudinal ligament. Posterior arch involvement on radiographs cannot be identified until late in the disease.

MRI can again be particularly useful for the depiction of early features. Inflammatory anterior corners of the thoracolumbar vertebral bodies are particularly well demonstrated. The presence of at least three of them in a patient younger than 45 years of age is considered to be very suggestive of SpA (Weber et al. 2009) (Fig. 34.10).

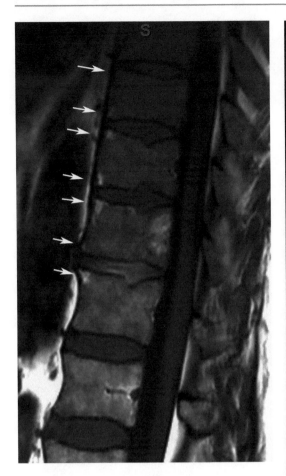

Fig. 34.11 Sagittal T1-W MR image of the thoracic spine shows several anterior fatty corners of the vertebral bodies (*arrows*) suggesting SpA

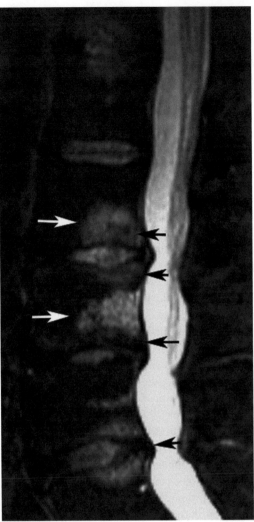

Fig. 34.12 Sagittal fat-suppressed T2-W MR image of the lumbar spine shows several Andersson lesions characterized by chronic inflammatory changes of vertebral endplates. There is well-limited BME (*white arrows*) and sclerosis of endplates (*black arrows*)

They are triangular in shape or demonstrate a more vertical distribution along the anterior cortical bone. Fatty vertebral corner can also be demonstrated (Fig. 34.11). Their diagnostic usefulness for SpA is significant when at least five are present (Hermann et al. 2012). Sometimes, BME is very extensive, with involvement of nearly the entire vertebral body. There may also be associated squaring but its assessment can be quite subjective. Less frequently, these inflammatory changes involve the posterior corners, the lateral edge, and/or the vertebral endplates. Andersson spondylodiskitis is more rarely encountered (Fig. 34.12). It is characterized by inflammatory changes of two adjacent vertebral endplates, with or without inflammatory changes of the disk, but with frequent erosions of the endplates.

Inflammatory changes may also be identified involving the posterior structures of the spine and are highly specific (Hermann et al. 2012). Changes seen in the edges of the vertebral bodies typically reflect involvement of the costovertebral and costotransverse joints and rib heads and are better demonstrated on axial images. Transverse and spinous process edema, enthesitis of the interspinal, supraspinal and flaval ligaments, and facet joints arthritis may also be encountered. However, one should keep in mind that in the DESIR cohort (patients presenting with inflammatory back pain suggestive of axial SpA), only about 4% of patients with negative sacroiliac MRI findings were reclassified as SpA patients based on spinal MRI findings (Dougados et al. 2011).

34.3.2 Mimics and Pitfalls

34.3.2.1 Vertebral Corner Lesions

Although inflammatory vertebral corners represent the classical sign suggesting the diagnosis of SpA of the spine, these lesions have also been reported in asymptomatic volunteers, with one study giving a figure as high as 26% (Weber et al. 2009). Some of these pseudo-inflammatory vertebral corners are related to microtrauma of Sharpey fibers (the most peripheral fibers of the annulus fibrosus), which may be isolated or associated with disk degeneration (spondylosis deformans). These lesions are well known and demonstrated on radiographs or CT when the cleft representing the Sharpey fibers avulsion is filled with gas opposite a vertebral corner, frequently at L3 or L4 vertebral level (Fig. 34.13). The resulting local micro-mobility is thought to explain some traction exerted on the deep fibers of the longitudinal ligament and, as a consequence, osseous metaplasia with enthesophyte formation, typically located several millimeters below the corner (Yu et al. 1989). On MRI, such microtrauma may explain mildly increased signal intensity on T2-weighted images of one, sometimes two, and exceptionally three vertebral corners (Figs. 34.14 and 34.15). A cleft of the disk is sometimes observed opposite it, filled with fluid or enhancing after contrast agent administration, which confirm the diagnosis (Fig. 34.14). T1-weighted images are also particularly helpful when they may depict the traction enthesophyte at a distance from the vertebral corner (Fig. 34.14).

Other disorders potentially associated with pseudo-inflammatory corners include degenerative disks, because radial tears extend to the insertion of Sharpey fibers or because the bulging of the disk results in stretching of the insertion of the anterior longitudinal ligament (Fig. 34.16). Modic type 1 changes may also involve the

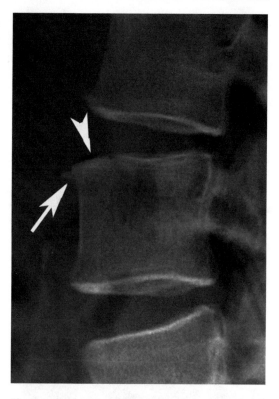

Fig. 34.13 Lateral radiograph shows gas (*arrowhead*) filling a Sharpey fibers avulsion of the anterosuperior corner of L4 vertebral body, associated with an enthesophyte (*arrow*)

vertebral corner, but BME is frequently more extensive along the vertebral endplate. Finally, vertebral collapse, whatever its cause, may be associated with adjacent shiny corners, possibly due to traction on the anterior longitudinal ligament (Fig. 34.17). Fatty vertebral corners are even more common in asymptomatic volunteers. Demonstration of these lesions mainly or solely involving the lumbar spine should be considered cautiously, particularly when seen in isolation (Fig. 34.18).

34.3.2.2 Infection

Infection may represent a tough differential diagnosis when SpA is revealed by Andersson spondylodiskitis or facet joints arthritis. Besides the different clinical and biological features, infectious spondylodiskitis and facet joint arthritis are rarely multifocal, and they are not associated with MRI signs of chronicity. The latter features include fat or sclerosis of the subchondral bone

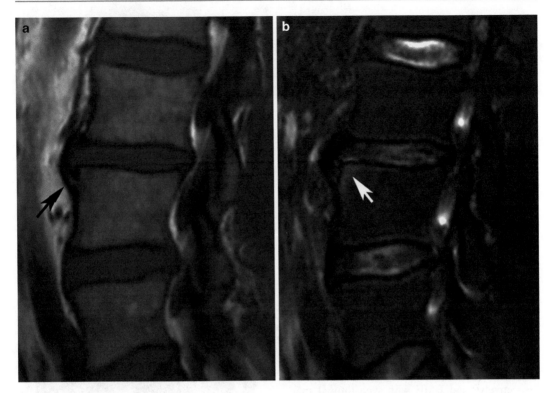

Fig. 34.14 Traction enthesophyte (*black arrow*) is well seen on (**a**) sagittal T1-W MR image. (**b**) Sagittal fat-suppressed T2-W MR image shows a cleft of the disk filled with fluid with adjacent BME (*white arrow*)

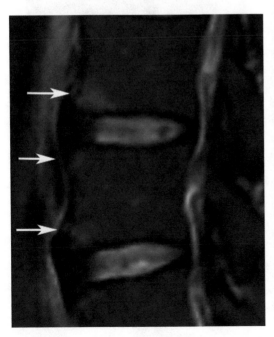

Fig. 34.15 Sagittal fat-suppressed T2-W MR image shows three vertebral corners affected by Sharpey fiber avulsion (*arrows*)

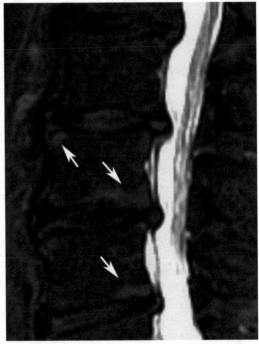

Fig. 34.16 Sagittal fat-suppressed T2-W MR image shows edema of vertebral body corners (*arrows*) associated with several degenerative disks

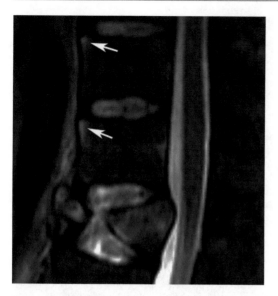

Fig. 34.17 Sagittal fat-suppressed T2-W MR image shows vertebral collapse associated with "shiny corners" of adjacent vertebral bodies (*arrows*)

(T1-hyperintense or T2-hypointense band, respectively) and BME with well-limited margins predominating at a distance from the subchondral bone (Fig. 34.12).

34.4 Peripheral Spondyloarthritis

34.4.1 Diagnosis

This disorder is notably characterized by the presence of peripheral arthritis, enthesitis, and/or dactylitis plus additional features, including psoriasis or inflammatory bowel disease (Rudwaleit et al. 2011). Peripheral arthritis may involve one or several joints. The hand and foot are most frequently involved, particularly at an early stage. Enthesitis is a key pathological lesion in peripheral SpA. It is defined by inflammation of the entheses, the sites where tendons, ligaments, fascias, or capsules insert into the bone. It frequently involves the heel, either at the Achilles tendon insertion or plantar aponeurosis, but any entheses can be affected (Fig. 34.19). Both ultrasound (US) imaging and MRI can demonstrate inflammatory features involving these entheses, but MRI may show the associated BME when present. Dactylitis,

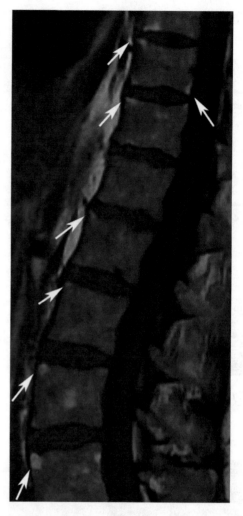

Fig. 34.18 Sagittal T1-W MR image shows nonspecific fatty vertebral corners (*arrows*)

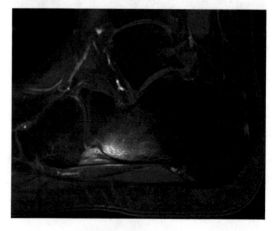

Fig. 34.19 Sagittal fat-suppressed T2-W MR image shows inflammatory changes of the calcaneocuboid ligament and of the adjacent calcaneus

or the "sausage digit," is defined as a diffuse swelling of a digit. It has long been recognized as one of the cardinal features of psoriatic arthritis. US imaging and MRI studies demonstrate that dactylitis is not only related to inflammation of the digital flexor tendon sheaths but also of the adjacent joints, periosteum, entheses, or soft tissue (Healy et al. 2008; Bakewell et al. 2013).

34.4.2 Mimics and Pitfalls

34.4.2.1 Other Joint Disorders

Septic arthritis is, of course, the main differential diagnosis when only one joint is affected. Imaging is neither sensitive nor specific for this diagnosis at an early stage, and its recognition relies on the identification of the organism (Mathews et al. 2007). The frequent involvement of the distal interphalangeal (DIP) joints and/or of the entire digit allows differentiation from rheumatoid arthritis and calcium pyrophosphate crystal deposition disease. In contrast, differentiation between osteoarthritis (OA) and psoriatic arthritis (psoA) can be difficult, as

both of these diseases can be associated with DIP joint space narrowing, chronic bony proliferation, and no periarticular osteoporosis on radiographs. However, when present, erosive changes are typically marginal in psoriatic arthritis and central in OA; bony proliferations are more fluffy, spiculated, and located at a distance from the joint space in psoA in contrast to the well-defined osteophytes in OA (Fig. 34.20). When MRI is performed, inflammatory changes can sometimes be depicted in the enthesis of the DIP joints affected by osteoarthritis, but they are much less marked than in psoriatic arthritis (Tan et al. 2006). Other joints such as the metacarpophalangeal (MCP) joints or the carpal joints can also be affected in psoA, with such distribution being more unusual in OA.

34.4.2.2 Complex Regional Pain Syndrome

Radiographic patchy osteopenia and/or patchy BME areas on MRI (Darbois et al. 1999) can be seen in complex regional pain syndrome (CRPS) and may be confusing, particularly when the foot is involved. Erosions and joint space narrowing are however absent. Moreover, BME typically

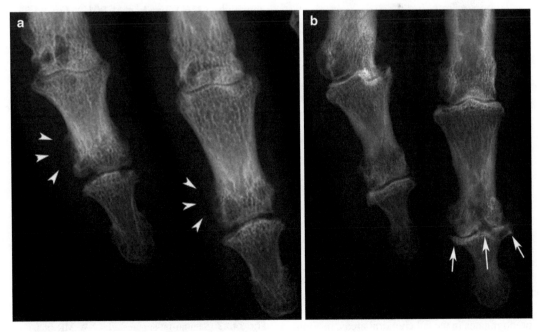

Fig. 34.20 Frontal radiographs of the DIP joints affected by (**a**) psoriatic arthritis and (**b**) osteoarthritis. Note the marginal erosions and irregular bony proliferations (*arrowheads*) at distance from the joint in psoA and the central erosions (*arrows*) and the osteophytes in OA

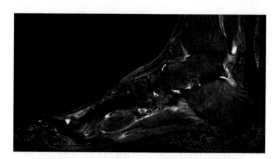

Fig. 34.21 Sagittal fat-suppressed T2-W MR image shows CRPS with BME affecting several bones

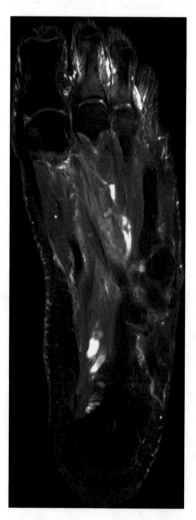

Fig. 34.22 Axial fat-suppressed T2-W MR image of the foot shows dactylitis of the second and third digits which was misdiagnosed as fat-suppression heterogeneity

predominates in the subchondral areas, in contrast to the BME seen in SpA which frequently predominates in the marginal areas or in front/opposite of entheses (Fig. 34.21). BME in CRPS is

also transient and sometimes migratory between two examinations (Malghem et al. 2003).

34.4.2.3 Dactylitis

Although dactylitis can be seen in other disorders (e.g., gout, sarcoidosis, hemolytic anemia), SpA is the main diagnosis in frequency, either at the hand or at the forefoot (Rothschild et al. 1998; Healy and Helliwell 2006). The presence of extensive osteitis and periostitis is highly suggestive of SpA, when present. This requires a good quality fat suppression of these anatomical areas when a large field of view is used (Fig. 34.22).

34.4.2.4 Mechanical Enthesopathy

Imaging performance for the differentiation between enthesitis and mechanical enthesopathy is still debated in the literature. Increased vascularization at the junction between the bone and the enthesis on power Doppler US imaging has been reported to be highly specific for enthesitis (D'Agostino et al. 2011). However, this feature and other ones were not found to be able to discriminate between these two disorders in the study of the foot (Feydy et al. 2012). Bone marrow edema on MRI was the only abnormality specific for SpA (94%), but it is associated with a poor sensitivity (22%) (Feydy et al. 2012) (Fig. 34.23).

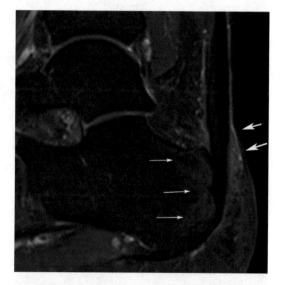

Fig. 34.23 Sagittal fat-suppressed T2-W MR image of the hindfoot shows mechanical Achilles enthesopathy. Note the inflammatory changes of the calcaneus (*thin arrows*) and adjacent soft tissue (*larger arrows*) that may be misleading on imaging

34.5 Rheumatoid Arthritis

34.5.1 Diagnosis

Rheumatoid arthritis (RA) is characterized by proliferative hypervascularized synovitis, which is secondarily responsible for bone erosions and cartilage damage. This disorder typically starts at the forefoot, wrist, and hand. Although radiography can provide only indirect information on synovitis and is insensitive to early bone damage, it is still widely used for bone erosion detection and remains the gold standard for evaluating structural damage. The lateral aspect of the fifth metatarsal bone; the radial aspect of the second and third metacarpal bones; the capitate, triquetrum, and lunate bones; and the ulnar styloid process are more frequently involved with bone erosions (Boutry et al. 2007). MRI and US imaging can detect pre-erosive synovitis. They can also identify early erosions before they become apparent on radiography. MRI also demonstrates BME, which may precede the development of bone erosions.

34.5.2 Mimics and Pitfalls

34.5.2.1 Synovitis

Frequent enhancement of the synovial tissue has been reported in the region of the peri-styloid process in a cohort of healthy subjects (Partik et al. 2002). However, rheumatoid synovitis is typically thick and extensive, with intense enhancement after gadolinium administration. Synovitis can also be found in many other disorders and is not specific to the disease (Boutry et al. 2005; Stomp et al. 2014). The profile of synovitis enhancement after gadolinium administration has also been studied in the literature, and although debated (Cimmino et al. 2012), rheumatoid and psoriatic arthritis do not seem to be differentiable based on this sole feature (Cimmino et al. 2005).

34.5.2.2 Pseudo-erosions

Because of the frequent involvement of the forefoot, wrist, and hand, analysis of these anatomical regions on radiography is commonly used for diagnosis, staging, and follow-up in RA. Analysis

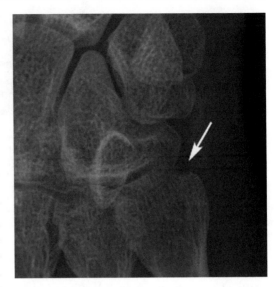

Fig. 34.24 Radiograph shows pseudo-erosion of the base of the fifth metacarpal bone (*arrow*)

of these images relies heavily on the detection of bone erosions. However, pseudo-erosions are frequently observed in these anatomical regions, particularly at the wrist. They can most often be explained by the presence of ligament insertions, which are associated with bone remodeling and a thinner bone lamina (McQueen et al. 2005; Wawer et al. 2014). Other causes include absence of radiographic tangency, presence of osteophytes, arterial foramen, and mucoid cyst (McQueen et al. 2005). Wawer et al. (2014) found that pseudo-erosions were mostly seen in the distal ulnar portion of the capitate, the distal radial portion of the hamate, the proximal ulnar portion of the base of the third metacarpal, the proximal radial portion of the base of the fourth metacarpal, the distal ulnar portion of the hamate, and the proximal portion of the base of the fifth metacarpal (Wawer et al. 2014) (Fig. 34.24).

On MRI, the definition of erosions requires their visualization in two planes according to the OMERACT (outcome measures in rheumatology) RA MRI scoring system (Østergaard et al. 2003). Slice thickness and field of view should be optimized to limit misdiagnosis of true erosions due to partial volume averaging. Mucoid cysts and arterial foramen may be misleading, but analysis of their bases (larger in erosions) and absence of significant associated synovitis may be used for this differentiation (Fig. 34.25).

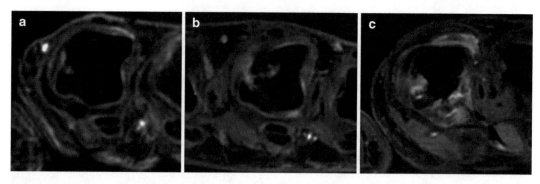

Fig. 34.25 Axial contrast-enhanced fat-suppressed T1-W MR images of the metacarpal base show (**a**) mucoid cyst and (**b**) vascular foramen – which are distinguishable from (**c**) erosion by their thinner bases and lack of synovitis

However, rare examples of pseudo-erosion and BME have been reported at the MCP joints and wrists of subjects free from RA (Ejbjerg et al. 2004). They might be related to synovial and bony hyperemia due to increased mechanical activity.

Conclusion

In conclusion, a good knowledge of the imaging features of the inflammatory arthritides, particularly at an early stage, is fundamental for accurate diagnosis of patients. Moreover, a good knowledge of the main imaging diagnostic pitfalls is mandatory to avoid inappropriate therapeutic management.

References

Ahovuo JA, Kiuru MJ, Visuri T (2004) Fatigue stress fractures of the sacrum: diagnosis with MR imaging. Eur Radiol 14:500–505

Bakewell CJ, Olivieri I, Aydin SZ et al (2013) Ultrasound and magnetic resonance imaging in the evaluation of psoriatic dactylitis: status and perspectives. J Rheumatol 40:1951–1957

Bennett AN, McGonagle D, O'Connor P et al (2008) Severity of baseline magnetic resonance imaging-evident sacroiliitis and HLA-B27 status in early inflammatory back pain predict radiographically evident ankylosing spondylitis at eight years. Arthritis Rheum 58:3413–3418

Bereau M, Prati C, Wendling D (2011) Sacroiliac edema by MRI does not always indicate spondylarthritis. Joint Bone Spine 78:646

Bollow M, Braun J, Kannenberg J et al (1997) Normal morphology of sacroiliac joints in children: magnetic resonance studies related to age and sex. Skeletal Radiol 26:697–704

Boutry N, Hachulla E, Flipo RM et al (2005) MR imaging findings in hands in early rheumatoid arthritis: comparison with those in systemic lupus erythematosus and primary Sjögren syndrome. Radiology 236: 593–600

Boutry N, Morel M, Flipo RM et al (2007) Early rheumatoid arthritis: a review of MRI and sonographic findings. AJR Am J Roentgenol 189:1502–1509

Bywaters EGL, Dixon ASJ, Scott JT (1963) Joint lesions of hyperparathyroidism. Ann Rheum Dis 22:171–187

Cimmino MA, Parodi M, Innocenti S et al (2005) Dynamic magnetic resonance of the wrist in psoriatic arthritis reveals imaging patterns similar to those of rheumatoid arthritis. Arthritis Res Ther 7:R725–731

Cimmino MA, Barbieri F, Boesen M et al (2012) Dynamic contrast-enhanced magnetic resonance imaging of articular and extraarticular synovial structures of the hands in patients with psoriatic arthritis. J Rheumatol Suppl 89:44–48

D'Agostino MA, Aegerter P, Bechara K et al (2011) How to diagnose spondyloarthritis early? Accuracy of peripheral enthesitis detection by power Doppler ultrasonography. Ann Rheum Dis 70:1433–1440

Darbois H, Boyer B, Dubayle P et al (1999) MRI symptomology in reflex sympathetic dystrophy of the foot. J Radiol 80:849–854

Dougados M, D'Agostino MA, Benessiano J et al (2011) The DESIR cohort: a 10-year follow up of early inflammatory back pain in France: study design and baseline characteristics of the 708 recruited patients. Joint Bone Spine 78:598–603

Egund N, Jurik AG (2014) Anatomy and histology of the sacroiliac joints. Semin Musculoskelet Radiol 18:332–339

Ejbjerg B, Narvestad E, Rostrup E et al (2004) Magnetic resonance imaging of wrist and finger joints in healthy subjects occasionally shows changes resembling erosions and synovitis as seen in rheumatoid arthritis. Arthritis Rheum 50:1097–1106

Feydy A, Lavie-Brion MC, Gossec L et al (2012) Comparative study of MRI and power Doppler ultrasonography of the heel in patients with spondyloarthritis with and without heel pain and in controls. Ann Rheum Dis 71:498–503

Healy PJ, Helliwell PS (2006) Dactyitis: pathogenesis and clinical considerations. Curr Rheumatol Rep 8:338–341

Healy PJ, Groves C, Chandramohan M et al (2008) MRI changes in psoriatic dactylitis – extent of pathology, relationship to tenderness and correlation with clinical indices. Rheumatology 47:92–95

Hermann KG, Baraliakos X, Van der Heijde DM et al (2012) Assessment in SpondyloArthritis international Society (ASAS). Description of spinal MRI lesions and definition of a positive MRI of the spine in axial spondyloarthritis: a consensual approach by the ASAS/OMERACT MRI study group. Ann Rheum Dis 71:1278–1288

Llauger J, Palmer J, Amores S et al (2000) Primary tumors of the sacrum: diagnostic imaging. AJR Am J Roentgenol 174:417–424

Malghem J, Vande Berg B, Lecouvet F et al (2003) Algodystrophie du pied. In: Chevrit A (ed) Imagerie du pied et de la cheville. Sauramps, Montpellier

Mau W, Zeidler H, Mau R et al (1987) Outcome of possible ankylosing spondylitis in a 10 years' follow-up study. Clin Rheumatol 6(Suppl 2):60–66

Mathews CJ, Kingsley G, Field M et al (2007) Management of septic arthritis: a systematic review. Ann Rheum Dis 66:440–445

McQueen F, Østergaard M, Peterfy C et al (2005) Pitfalls in scoring MR images of rheumatoid arthritis wrist and metacarpophalangeal joints. Ann Rheum Dis 64(Supp I):i48–i55

Olivieri I, Ferri S, Barozzi L (1996) Osteitis condensans ilii. Br J Rheumatol 35:295–297

Østergaard M, Peterfy C, Conaghan P et al (2003) OMERACT rheumatoid arthritis magnetic resonance imaging studies. Core set of MRI acquisitions, joint pathology definitions and the OMERACT RA-MRI scoring system. J Rheumatol 30:1385–1386

Partik B, Rand T, Pretterklieber ML et al (2002) Patterns of Gadopentetate-enhanced MR imaging of radiocarpal joints of healthy subjects. AJR Am J Roentgenol 179:193–197

Peh WCG, Khong PL, Yin Y et al (1996) Imaging of pelvic insufficiency fractures. Radiographics 16:335–348

Rothschild BM, Pingitore C, Eaton M (1998) Dactylitis: implications for clinical practice. Semin Arthritis Rheum 28:41–47

Rudwaleit M, Landewé R, van der Heijde D et al (2009a) The development of assessment of Spondyloarthritis International Society classification criteria for axial spondyloarthritis (part I): classification of paper patients by expert opinion including uncertainty appraisal. Ann Rheum Dis 68:770–776

Rudwaleit M, van der Heijde D, Landewé R et al (2009b) The development of Assessment of Spondyloarthritis International Society (ASAS) classification criteria for axial spondyloarthritis (part II): validation and final selection. Ann Rheum Dis 68:777–783

Rudwaleit M, Jurik AG, Hermann KGA et al (2009c) Defining active sacroiliitis on magnetic resonance imaging (MRI) for classification of axial spondyloarthritis: a consensual approach by the ASAS/OMERACT MRI group. Ann Rheum Dis 68:1520–1527

Rudwaleit M, Van der Heijde D, Landewé R et al (2011) The Assessment of Spondyloarthritis International Society classification criteria for peripheral spondyloarthritis and for spondyloarthritis in general. Ann Rheum Dis 70:25–31

Sheybani EF, Khanna G, White AJ et al (2013) Imaging of juvenile idiopathic arthritis: a multimodality approach. Radiographics 33:1253–1273

Shibata Y, Shirai Y, Miyamoto M (2002) The aging process in the sacroiliac joint: helical computed tomography analysis. J Orthop Sci 7:12–18

Stomp W, Krabben A, Van der Heijde D et al (2014) Are rheumatoid arthritis patients discernible from other early arthritis patients using 1.5T extremity magnetic resonance imaging? A large cross-sectional study. J Rheumatol 41:1630–1637

Stürzenbecher A, Braun J, Paris S et al (2000) MR imaging of septic sacroiliitis. Skeletal Radiol 29:439–446

Tan AL, Grainger AJ, Tanner SF et al (2006) A high-resolution magnetic resonance imaging study of distal interphalangeal joint arthropathy in psoriatic arthritis and osteoarthritis: are they the same? Arthritis Rheum 54:1328–1333

Tuite MJ (2008) Sacroiliac joint imaging. Semin Musculoskelet Radiol 12:72–82

Wawer R, Budzik JF, Demondion X et al (2014) Carpal pseudoerosions: a plain X-ray interpretation pitfall. Skeletal Radiol 43:1377–1385

Weber U, Hodler J, Kubik RA et al (2009) Sensitivity and specificity of spinal inflammatory lesions assessed by whole-body magnetic resonance imaging in patients with ankylosing spondylitis or recent-onset inflammatory back pain. Arthritis Rheum 61:900–908

Weber U, Zubler V, Pedersen SJ et al (2013) Development and validation of a magnetic resonance imaging reference criterion for defining a positive sacroiliac joint magnetic resonance imaging finding in spondyloarthritis. Arthritis Care Res 65:977–985

Yu SW, Haughton VM, Lynch KL et al (1989) Fibrous structure in the intervertebral disk: correlation of MR appearance with anatomic sections. Am J Neuroradiol 10:1105–1110

Metabolic Bone Lesions: Imaging Pitfalls

35

Eric A. Walker, Jonelle M. Petscavage-Thomas, Agustinus Suhardja, and Mark D. Murphey

Contents

35.1 **Introduction** 714

35.2 **Osteoporosis** 714
35.2.1 Regional Osteoporosis 714
35.2.2 Multiple Myeloma 715

35.3 **Hyperparathyroidism** 715
35.3.1 Acro-osteolysis 716
35.3.2 Resorption of the Distal Clavicle 717
35.3.3 Sacroiliitis Mimic 718
35.3.4 Brown Tumor 718

35.4 **Tumoral Calcinosis-Like Entities** 720
35.4.1 Secondary Tumoral Calcinosis 720
35.4.2 Tumoral Calcinosis 720
35.4.3 Scleroderma 720
35.4.4 Sarcoidosis 722
35.4.5 Other Calcified Masses 722

35.5 **Rickets** 722
35.5.1 Non-accidental Injury 724
35.5.2 Scurvy 724

35.6 **Dense Osseous Sclerosis** 724
35.6.1 Renal Osteodystrophy 724

35.6.2 Myelofibrosis 726
35.6.3 Mastocytosis 726
35.6.4 Osteopetrosis 726
35.6.5 Pyknodysostosis 726
35.6.6 Paget Disease 726
35.6.7 Other Sclerotic Lesions 727

35.7 **Rugger Jersey Spine** 727

35.8 **Thyroid Acropachy** 728

35.9 **Hypophosphatasia** 728
35.9.1 Osteogenesis Imperfecta 729
35.9.2 Achondrogenesis 730
35.9.3 Thanatophoric Dysplasia 730

35.10 **Tophaceous Gout** 730

35.11 **Intraosseous Hydroxyapatite Crystal Deposition Disease (HADD)** 730

35.12 **Hemophilia** 734

35.13 **Extramedullary Hematopoiesis in Thalassemia** 734

35.14 **Amyloidosis** 736

E.A. Walker, MD (✉)
Department of Radiology, Milton S. Hershey Medical Center, Pennsylvania State University, 500 University Drive, Hershey, PA 17033, USA

Department of Radiology and Radiological Sciences, Uniformed Services University of the Health Sciences, 4301 Jones Bridge Road, Bethesda, MD 20814, USA
e-mail: ewalker@hmc.psu.edu

J.M. Petscavage-Thomas, MD
Department of Radiology, Milton S. Hershey Medical Center, Pennsylvania State University, 500 University Drive, Hershey, PA 17033, USA
e-mail: jthomas5@hmc.psu.edu

A. Suhardja, MD
Musculoskeletal Section, American Institute for Radiologic Pathology, 1010 Wayne Avenue #320, Silver Spring, MD 20910, USA
e-mail: a_suhardja@yahoo.com

M.D. Murphey, MD
Musculoskeletal Section, American Institute for Radiologic Pathology, 1010 Wayne Avenue #320, Silver Spring, MD 20910, USA

Department of Radiology and Radiological Sciences, Uniformed Services University of the Health Sciences, 4301 Jones Bridge Road, Bethesda, MD 20814, USA
e-mail: mmurphey@acr.org

© Springer International Publishing AG 2017
W.C.G. Peh (ed.), *Pitfalls in Musculoskeletal Radiology*, DOI 10.1007/978-3-319-53496-1_35

35.14.1   Mimic: Pigmented Villonodular
          Synovitis   737
35.14.2   Mimic: Spondylodiskitis   738

Conclusion   739

References   740

Abbreviations

CT   Computed tomography
ESRD   End-stage renal failure
HPT   Hyperparathyroidism
MRI   Magnetic resonance imaging
RA   Rheumatoid arthritis

35.1   Introduction

Metabolic conditions may result in a variety of osseous and soft tissue manifestations. It is important to recognize how these lesions may present and be able to distinguish them from a variety of similar-appearing mimics. Regional osteoporosis may demonstrate a permeative osteolytic appearance and cortical tunneling that may mimic an aggressive neoplasm or multiple myeloma. Hyperparathyroidism (HPT) classically demonstrates bone resorption, brown tumors, osteosclerosis or osteopenia, and chondrocalcinosis. Intracortical resorption of the distal tufts in HPT can mimic other causes of acro-osteolysis. Rheumatoid arthritis and post-traumatic osteolysis can result in resorption of the distal clavicle similar to HPT. The subchondral bone resorption of HPT in the sacroiliac joints may mimic a sacroiliitis due to seronegative spondyloarthropathy. Brown tumors can be monostotic or polystotic and may be mistaken for osteolytic bone lesions. Periarticular calcified masses often seen in secondary HPT are indistinguishable from tumoral calcinosis by imaging. Rickets with widened, irregular, and frayed appearance of the metaphysis and rachitic rosary at the costochondral junction may be mistaken for non-accidental trauma.

Chronic renal failure often results in renal osteodystrophy. Osteosclerosis of the axial skeleton in renal osteodystrophy must be distin-guished from other possible causes such as diffuse sclerotic metastatic disease, myelofibrosis, mastocytosis, osteopetrosis, pyknodysostosis, and Paget disease. Characteristic horizontal bands of sclerosis adjacent to the vertebral endplates, known as rugger jersey spine, could be mistaken for the sandwich vertebra of osteopetrosis. Amyloid deposition in the hips could result in an intra-articular process with similar imaging characteristics to pigmented villonodular synovitis, and spine involvement in amyloidosis may resemble spondylodiskitis. This chapter will discuss what clinical features and imaging characteristics can be useful to distinguish these entities from their mimics.

35.2   Osteoporosis

Osteoporosis is the most common metabolic bone disease. It is defined by the World Health Organization (WHO) as "a skeletal disease, characterized by low bone mass and micro-architectural deterioration of bone tissue, with a consequent increase in bone fragility and susceptibility to fracture" (World Health Organization 2003). Osteoporosis may be generalized, as is seen in postmenopausal women due to accelerated trabecular bone resorption related to estrogen deficiency, or regional, only affecting a part of the skeleton (Guglielmi et al. 2011). Causes of regional osteoporosis include prolonged therapeutic bed rest, immobilization due to motor paralysis from injury of the nerves, and application of cast to treat fractures (Guglielmi et al. 2008).

35.2.1   Regional Osteoporosis

In regional osteoporosis, there is active bone remodeling with increased osteoclastic activity. Thus, localized or regional forms of osteoporosis can appear aggressive on imaging. Radiographs show multiple lucencies of varying size, cortical tunneling, and endosteal scalloping (Jones 1969) (Fig. 35.1a). The pattern of cortical lamellation and scalloping is due to an increased size of resorption

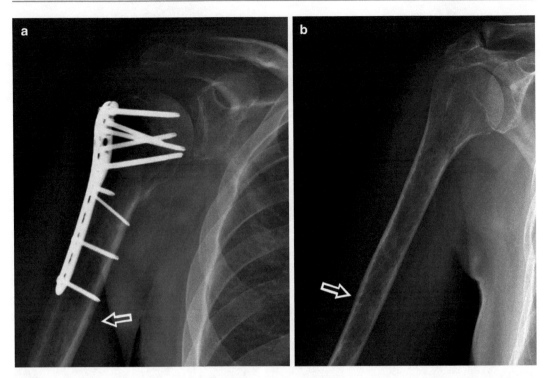

Fig. 35.1 Aggressive regional osteoporosis. (**a**) AP radiograph of the right humerus in a 56-year-old man shows plate and screw fixation of a healing surgical neck fracture. There is a permeative osteolytic pattern with cortical tunneling in the distal humerus (*arrow*) due to

aggressive regional osteoporosis. (**b**) AP radiograph of the right humerus in a 67-year-old man shows a similar permeative osteolytic appearance of the humeral diaphysis with endosteal scalloping (*arrow*). This patient had multiple myeloma

cavities along the endosteal or periosteal surface. Periostitis, bone expansion, and soft tissue masses are absent (Kattapuram et al. 1988). The humerus is a common bone associated with aggressive post-traumatic osteoporosis (Kattapuram et al. 1988).

35.2.2 Multiple Myeloma

The moth-eaten permeative pattern of regional osteoporosis may mimic that of aggressive rapidly progressing tumors such as multiple myeloma (Fig. 35.1b), metastatic disease, and lymphoma. However, with aggressive neoplasms, there is generally a central area of intense destruction, with diminished destruction at the margins rather than the uniform pattern with cortical tunneling and endosteal scalloping of aggressive osteoporosis (Kattapuram et al. 1988). Multiple myeloma may appear very similar to aggressive regional osteoporosis on imaging; however, focal

areas of endosteal scalloping associated with lucencies suggest mass replacement of the marrow by neoplasm, and clinical history may aid in the diagnosis.

35.3 Hyperparathyroidism

Hyperparathyroidism (HPT) is a metabolic disorder of excess parathyroid hormone production. The excess parathyroid hormone stimulates osteoclastic resorption of skeletal structures (Khan and Bilezikian 2000). The disorder can be primary or secondary in etiology. Primary disease is due to either diffuse parathyroid hyperplasia or an autonomously functioning parathyroid adenoma (McDonald et al. 2005). Secondary hyperparathyroidism is a response to sustained hypocalcemia, typically in patients with chronic renal failure or gastrointestinal malabsorption (Chew 2012).

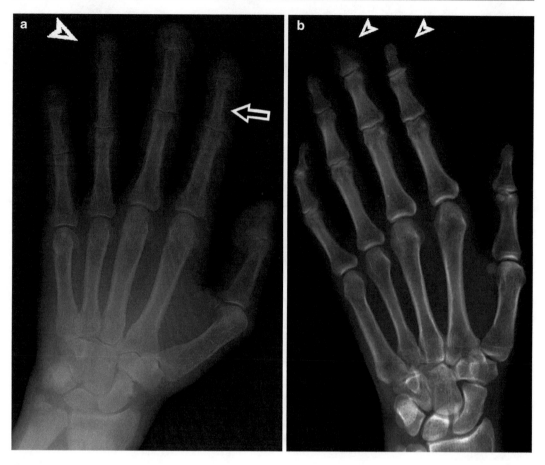

Fig. 35.2 Hyperparathyroid acro-osteolysis. (**a**) AP radiograph of the left hand in a patient with primary hyperparathyroidism shows distal tuft acro-osteolysis (*arrowhead*) and subperiosteal bone resorption (*arrow*) along the radial aspects of the middle and proximal pha-langes. (**b**) AP radiograph of the left hand in a 33-year-old woman with scleroderma shows soft tissue resorption and acro-osteolysis of the second and third distal phalanges (*arrowheads*)

Classical radiographic findings of hyperpara-thyroidism include bone resorption, brown tumors, osteosclerosis or osteopenia, and chondrocalcino-sis (more common in primary HPT) (McDonald et al. 2005; Chew 2012). Bone resorption can occur in subperiosteal, endosteal, intracortical, trabecu-lar, subligamentous, and subchondral locations. Subperiosteal resorption is virtually pathogno-monic for hyperparathyroidism and is most com-mon along the radial aspect of the middle phalanges of the index and middle fingers of the hands (Chew 2012) (Fig. 35.2a). Other common sites of subperi-osteal bone resorption include the proximal medial metaphyses of the humeri and tibia.

35.3.1 Acro-osteolysis

In the hands, intracortical resorption of the distal tufts can mimic other causes of acro-osteolysis, which refers to erosion of the terminal tufts of the distal phalanges (Fig. 35.2a). Other causes of acro-osteolysis include but are not limited to psoriatic arthritis, thermal injury, polyvinyl chlo-ride exposure, congenital insensitivity to pain, primary acro-osteolysis, Raynaud phenomena, scleroderma (Fig. 35.2b), and leprosy. Evaluation for subtle subperiosteal resorption should be performed to differentiate hyperparathyroidism from these other entities.

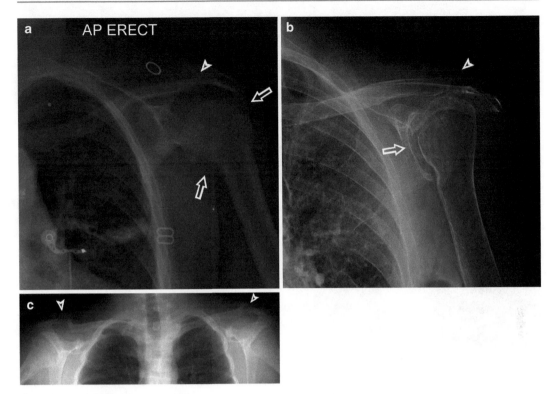

Fig. 35.3 Hyperparathyroidism – distal clavicle resorption. (**a**) Left shoulder radiograph of a 26-year-old woman on hemodialysis with secondary hyperparathyroidism shows resorption of the distal clavicle (*arrowhead*), subperiosteal bone resorption at the proximal medial metaphysis, and resorption at the rotator cuff insertion (*arrows*). (**b**) Left shoulder radiograph of a 60-year-old woman with rheumatoid arthritis shows resorption of the distal clavicle (*arrowhead*). There is severe secondary osteoarthritis from glenohumeral joint destruction (*arrow*) and loss of subacromial space secondary to rotator cuff tear. (**c**) AP radiograph of the clavicles shows cupping of the distal clavicles with resorption bilaterally (*arrowheads*) in an 18-year-old man who was a weight lifter. This appearance was due to distal clavicle osteolysis

35.3.2 Resorption of the Distal Clavicle

A frequently described site of bone resorption in hyperparathyroidism is the distal clavicle (Fig. 35.3a). The process is typically bilateral and involves primarily the clavicle rather than acromion. To distinguish clavicle resorption secondary to HPT from the other entities listed below, identification of additional areas of subperiosteal resorption at the medial proximal humeri and on the superior and inferior rib margins is helpful. Distal clavicle erosions may also be seen in rheumatoid arthritis (RA), scleroderma, and post-traumatic osteolysis. Both RA and HPT can have associated osteoporosis. In RA, the erosion usually occurs at the insertion of the coracoclavicular ligament, 2–4 cm from the distal end of the bone (Resnick and Niwayama 1976). Associated erosions are often seen in the coracoid process (Fig. 35.3b). In scleroderma, there is often associated soft tissue calcification. Distal clavicle osteolysis tends to be unilateral and related to a history of prior trauma from contact sports, falls, or weight lifting, usually in young men. Additionally, there may be acromial cupping, soft tissue swelling, and dystrophic calcification (Levine et al. 1976) (Fig. 35.3c). When the incident trauma stops, a reparative phase may occur, until the subchondral bone is reconstituted.

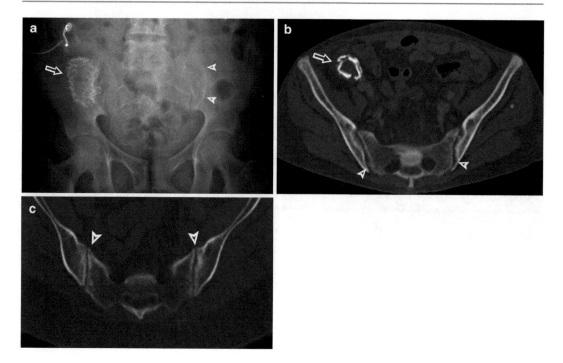

Fig. 35.4 Hyperparathyroidism with subchondral resorption simulating sacroiliitis. (**a**) AP pelvis radiograph and (**b**) axial CT image of a 26-year-old woman with secondary hyperparathyroidism and failed renal transplant. Note widening of the sacroiliac joints with subchondral iliac resorption (*arrowheads*) and coarse cal- cifications in the failed renal transplant graft within the right pelvis (*arrows*). (**c**) Axial CT image of the sacroiliac joints in a 53-year-old woman with ankylosing spondylitis shows sacroiliac joint space narrowing, subchondral scle- rosis, and erosions (*arrowheads*)

35.3.3 Sacroiliitis Mimic

At the sacroiliac joints, the subchondral bone resorption of HPT results in an articular disease that can masquerade as sacroiliitis due to sero- negative spondyloarthropathy. Similar to sacroili- itis, the findings are bilateral and affect the ilium more than the sacrum. There is an irregular articu- lar margin of the subchondral bone, similar to ero- sions (Prakash et al. 2014). In HPT, the joint is typically widened (Fig. 35.4a, b), while in sero- negative sacroiliac joint involvement, the joint space is narrowed with erosions and eburnation (Fig. 35.4c). Ankylosis may occur late in ankylos- ing spondylitis. Additionally, the presence of abnormal bone density, subperiosteal and subliga- mentous erosions, and involvement of other bones help in the differentiation of sacroiliac joint involvement in HPT from the seronegative spon- dyloarthropathies (Prakash et al. 2014).

35.3.4 Brown Tumor

Brown tumors, also known as osteitis fibrosa cys- tica, are a unique entity of hyperparathyroidism. They represent focal areas of bone resorption wherein the bone is replaced by fibrous tis- sue, hemorrhage, and osteoclasts. Hemosiderin imparts the brown color and name of the lesion. On radiographs, the lesions are round and osteo- lytic and can be central, eccentric, or cortical in location (Fig. 35.5a). Lesions can be single or multiple. The differential diagnosis for multiple brown tumors in the hands includes polyostotic acral metastatic lesions and multiple enchon- dromas in Ollier disease or Maffucci syndrome (Fig. 35.5b). In Ollier disease, the presence of chondroid matrix mineralization and the absence of other features of HPT should help in differ- entiation. Maffucci syndrome often has multiple phleboliths in the soft tissues.

Fig. 35.5 Brown tumors and mimics. (**a**) Oblique hand radiograph in a patient with primary hyperparathyroidism shows multiple expansile osteolytic lesions (*arrowheads*). (**b**) Hand radiograph of a 28-year-old woman with significant past medical history of Ollier disease also shows multiple expansile osteolytic lesions (*arrowhead*). Enchondromas of the hand frequently present without the characteristic chondroid matrix and can look similar to brown tumors. (**c**) Axial CT image of the pelvis in a 38-year-old woman with pain in the right anterior iliac crest shows multiple expansile osteolytic brown tumors (*arrowheads*) mimicking metastatic disease. Blood test showed dramatically elevated parathyroid hormone in this patient with left parathyroid adenoma

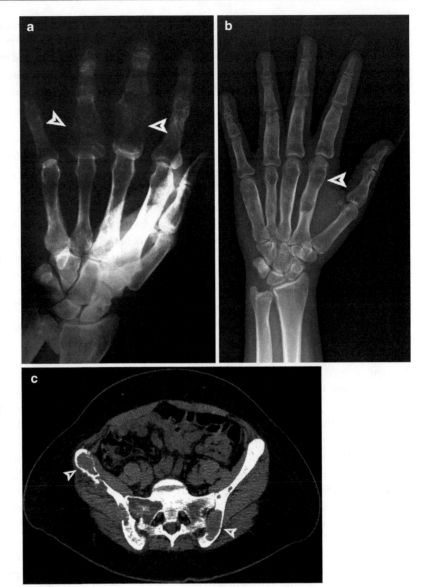

The differential diagnosis for a single brown tumor is extensive and includes the FEGNOMASHIC lesion differential of fibrous dysplasia, enchondroma, eosinophilic granuloma, giant cell tumor, non-ossifying fibroma, osteoblastoma, metastasis, myeloma, aneurysmal bone cyst, simple or unicameral bone cyst, HPT brown tumor, infection, and chondroblastoma or chondromyxoid fibroma. The differential diagnosis for multiple brown tumors (the polyostotic lesion differential) (Fig. 35.5c) includes the benign entities Langerhans cell histiocytosis, enchondromatosis, fibrous dysplasia, osteomyelitis, Paget disease, non-ossifying fibromas (in neurofibromatosis type 1 and Mazabraud syndrome), angiomatosis, and malignant lesions including polyostotic metastatic disease, multiple myeloma, and hemangioendothelioma.

On computed tomography (CT), brown tumor attenuation should be that of blood and fibrous tissue. On magnetic resonance imaging (MRI), the appearance can be solid, cystic, or mixed, depending on composition. Solid components are intermediate to hypointense on T1- and

T2-weighted MR images, while cystic components are hyperintense on T2-weighted MR images and may have fluid-fluid levels. The solid and septal components may enhance.

35.4 Tumoral Calcinosis-Like Entities

35.4.1 Secondary Tumoral Calcinosis

Chronic renal failure is the most frequent cause of periarticular calcified masses. This lesion is identified by many names in the literature, including secondary tumoral calcinosis, tumoral calcinosis-like lesion, uremic tumoral calcinosis, pseudotumor calcinosis, nonfamilial tumoral calcinosis, and tumoral calcification (Olsen and Chew 2006). These periarticular calcifications may be multifocal (Fig. 35.6a, b) and can extend into the adjacent joint. The most frequent sites affected include the phalanges, wrists, elbows, shoulders, hips, knees, and ankles. The presence of periarticular calcification is variable and increases with the duration of hemodialysis with 7% prevalence after 1 year, increasing to 55% after more than 4 years of hemodialysis (Massry et al. 1975). Factors contributing to soft tissue calcification include hypercalcemia, local tissue damage, alkalosis leading to the precipitation of calcium salts, and an increase in the calcium phosphorus product in extracellular fluids. Soft tissue calcifications are more common when the calcium-phosphorus product is greater than 75 mg/dL and generally uncommon when the product is under 70 mg/dL (Murphey et al. 1993).

35.4.2 Tumoral Calcinosis

Tumoral calcinosis, also known as Teutschlaender disease in the European literature, is a familial condition featuring solitary or multiple painless, periarticular masses. It has a familial tendency without gender predilection. There is a significantly higher incidence of this lesion in patients of African descent. Patients with tumoral calcinosis have a reduced fractional phosphate excretion, increased 1,25-dihydroxyvitamin D formation, and a normal dynamic response to parathyroid hormone in the proximal renal tubule (Olsen and Chew 2006). The term tumoral calcinosis is often incorrectly used to describe any periarticular calcified mass, such as the lesion associated with chronic renal failure. We refer to Teutschlaender disease as primary tumoral calcinosis and the lesion associated with chronic renal failure as secondary tumoral calcinosis. Primary tumoral calcinosis typically develops during the first two decades of life. The patient's serum calcium is typically normal. These lesions are usually at the extensor surface of a joint in the anatomical distribution of a bursa. The typical locations of primary tumoral calcinosis in descending order of frequency are the hip, elbow, shoulder, foot, and wrist (Olsen and Chew 2006).

There is no radiographic difference between primary and secondary tumoral calcinosis. The diagnosis must be made based on clinical history, serum chemistry, and glomerular filtration rate (Olsen and Chew 2006). The radiologic appearance is typically described as cloud-like or amorphous, cystic, and multilobular calcifications in a periarticular distribution. The chalky material can be seen as fluid levels on cross-sectional imaging (Murphey et al. 1993). CT may best demonstrate the mineral content. Two patterns have been described on T2-weighted MRI sequences. The lesion may be seen as a diffuse hypointense signal pattern or a hyperintense nodular pattern with alternating areas of signal hyperintensity and signal void. T1-weighted MRI sequences usually show heterogeneous lesions with signal hypointensity (Martinez et al. 1990). The differential diagnosis for calcified masses in the hands includes scleroderma, hyperparathyroidism, renal osteodystrophy, hypervitaminosis D, milk-alkali syndrome, dermatomyositis, polymyositis, and sarcoidosis.

35.4.3 Scleroderma

Scleroderma or progressive systemic sclerosis is a chronic autoimmune disease with thickening of the skin and connective tissues that can progress

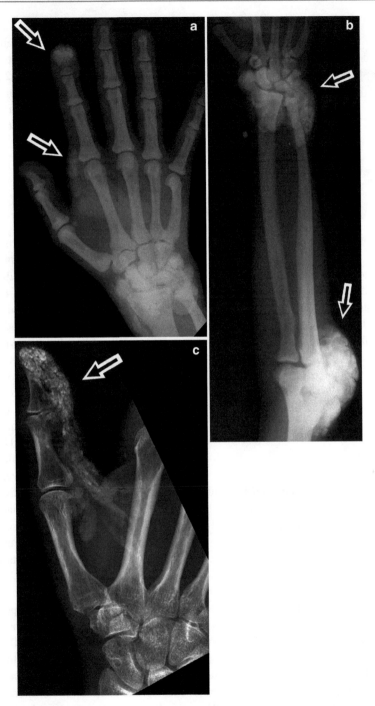

Fig. 35.6 Tumoral calcinosis-like lesions. Radiographs of the (**a**) hand and (**b**) forearm in a patient with secondary hyperparathyroidism show periarticular amorphous calcified masses (*arrows*) similar in appearance to tumoral calcinosis. (**c**) Lateral radiograph of the thumb in a 63-year-old woman with sarcoidosis shows a similar appearance of an amorphous calcified mass. The deposition is predominantly on the flexor surface of the thumb (*arrow*). Metastatic disease can mimic metabolic bone lesions and should be considered in most differential diagnoses. (**d**) Axial CT image shows an ovarian metastatic lesion (*arrow*) in the sternum of a 40-year-old woman after 20 years of remission. The lesion appears septated and amorphous and could easily be mistaken for primary or secondary tumoral calcinosis

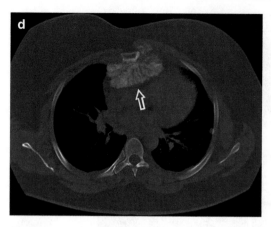

Fig.35.6 (continued)

to the internal organs. Radiographic findings in scleroderma include flexion contractures of the hands, soft tissue atrophy over the distal phalanges, and calcium hydroxyapatite deposits. Osseous resorption of the terminal tufts (acroosteolysis) is often noted, and occasionally, the fingertips are completely destroyed (acroscleroderma) (Bassett et al. 1981). Soft tissue atrophy results in cone-shaped fingertips.

35.4.4 Sarcoidosis

Sarcoidosis is a chronic granulomatous disorder of unknown etiology, which often involves multiple organ systems. Lung involvement is noted in approximately 95% of patients, and the skin, eye, and lymph nodes are also commonly involved. Hypercalcemia is a well-described complication of sarcoidosis, occurring in 4–11% of patients secondary to excess vitamin D (Demetriou et al. 2010). Sarcoidosis frequently demonstrates a lacelike pattern in the medullary cavity of the phalanges on radiographs. Several cases of tumoral calcinosis-like lesions (Fig. 35.6c) associated with sarcoidosis have been published in the literature (Wolpe et al. 1987; Carter and Warner 2003).

35.4.5 Other Calcified Masses

Hypervitaminosis D historically occurs in adults treated with excessive doses of vitamin D for conditions such as rheumatoid arthritis, gout,

and Paget disease, leading to generalized osteoporosis and metastatic calcifications in the periarticular soft tissues, joint capsules, and synovial bursa (Sidhu et al. 2012). The cause of milk-alkali syndrome is ingestion of an inappropriately high amount of calcium carbonate and milk or cream for the treatment of peptic ulcer disease (Resnick 2002).

35.5 Rickets

Rickets is a metabolic systemic disease seen in the pediatric population. In rickets, there is a lack of available calcium and/or phosphorous for osteoid mineralization of the growth plates (Chew 2012). Rickets typically results from pure vitamin D deficiency. In pure vitamin D deficiency, there is reduced calcium absorption by the gastrointestinal tract, resulting in hypocalcemia and secondary hyperparathyroidism. The systemic response is mobilization of calcium from the skeleton. This may occur in premature infants, maternal vitamin D deficiency, poor sun exposure, or unbalanced infant nutrition such as breastfeeding without vitamin D supplementation. Additional at-risk populations include immigrants, patients on total parenteral nutrition (TPN), and institutionalized individuals (Kumar et al. 2014). Other entities associated with a vitamin D deficiency include malabsorption, polyostotic fibrous dysplasia, neurofibromatosis, long-term use of anticonvulsants or aluminumcontaining antacids, and renal tubular absorptive defects (Chew 2012).

The characteristic radiographic finding of rickets is a widened, irregular, frayed appearance of the metaphysis (Donnelly 2001). The appearance results from cartilage growth in the absence of normal calcification and ossification. Weightbearing and stress on the thickened growth plate results in a more pronounced widening and cupping appearance of the metaphysis, coarsened trabeculae, and bowing deformities of the lower extremity bones (Chew 2012). Due to the poor osseous mineralization, there is increased risk of insufficiency fracture. Focal transverse zones of lucency on the concave side of long bones such as the femur and humerus are due to focal collections of non-mineralized osteoid. These are known as Milkman pseudofractures or Looser zones. Additional findings include delayed appearance of ossification centers, cortical spurs projecting at right angles to the metaphysis, and periosteal reaction (Swischuk and Hayden 1979).

Typical sites of involvement by rickets include the distal femur, tibia, distal radius and ulna, and proximal humerus. Another typical site of involvement is the rib, where there is expansion and nodularity of the anterior rib ends at the cos-tochondral junction (Fig. 35.7a), referred to as rachitic rosary. After treatment of rickets, there is calcification of the osteoid, resulting in a wide band of calcification and new periosteal bone for-mation. The rachitic rosary in rickets may simu-late multiple healing rib fractures in child abuse (Fig. 35.7b).

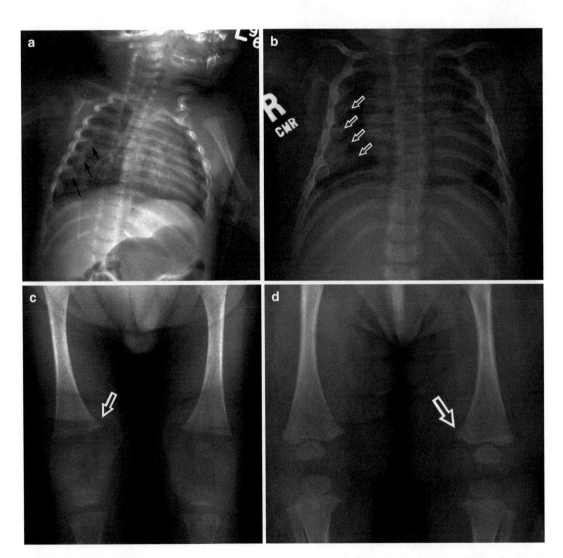

Fig. 35.7 Rickets versus non-accidental injury (NAI). (**a**) Oblique chest radiograph of a 1-year-old child with rick-ets shows expansion and nodularity of the anterior right ribs, known as rachitic rosary (*arrows*). (**b**) AP chest radiograph in a 2-month-old girl shows bilateral anterior and lateral rib nodularity (*arrows*), in this case due to the healing fractures of NAI. (**c**) AP radiograph of a 5-month- old boy with rickets shows the widened, irregular, frayed appearance of the femoral metaphyses (*arrow*). (**d**) Initial radiograph of a 2-month-old female victim of NAI who sustained subdural and subarachnoid hemorrhage and multiple fractures shows metaphyseal corner fractures (*arrow*) and (**e**) extensive periosteal reaction (*arrow*) on the 15-day follow-up radiograph

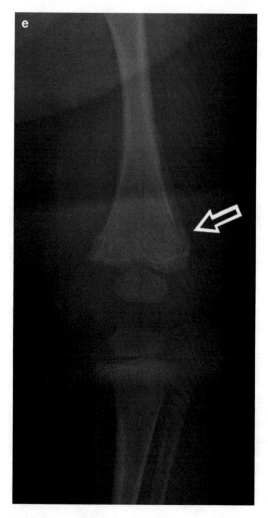

Leventhal et al. (2008) found that fractures in children younger than 36 months were attributed to abuse in 12% and to metabolic abnormalities such as rickets in only 0.12%. Thus, multiple fractures favor NAI, and a bone survey can help reveal more typical fractures of NAI, including those in the skull and sternum.

35.5.2 Scurvy

Another potential mimic of rickets is scurvy. Scurvy is a disorder of vitamin C deficiency with impaired collagen synthesis. Vitamin C deficiency can be related to inadequate food intake and imbalanced diet. Radiographic features include bone demineralization, periosteal reaction due to subperiosteal hemorrhage, metaphyseal spurs and cupped metaphyses (Pelkan spur), dense zones of provisional calcification, and Wimberger ring sign (a circular calcification surrounding the osteoporotic epiphyseal center of ossification in scurvy, which may occur secondary to bleeding) (Kirks and Griscom 1998; Weinstein et al. 2001; Fain 2005). Scurvy also affects the costochondral junction of the anterior ribs, mimicking rickets. In scurvy, the costochondral junction has a sharper step-off and is more angular. This appearance is known as scorbutic rosary.

Fig. 35.7 (continued)

35.5.1 Non-accidental Injury

In non-accidental injury (NAI), posteromedial rib involvement is a unique finding. These are caused when an adult grasps an infant around the chest causing compression (Lonergan et al. 2003). The flared widened metaphyses of rickets (Fig. 35.7c), with areas of cortical bone at right angles to the metaphysis with or without periostitis, may also resemble the healed metaphyseal corner fracture typical of NAI (Ebel and Benz-Bohm 1999) (Fig. 35.7d, e). Both entities are associated with other sites of osseous fracture, further complicating differentiation. The incidence of fractures in rickets has recently been shown to be low (Keller and Barnes 2008; Perez-Rossello et al. 2012).

35.6   Dense Osseous Sclerosis

35.6.1 Renal Osteodystrophy

Chronic renal failure induces low levels of vitamin D. These low vitamin D levels result in rickets in children or osteomalacia in adults. With chronic renal insufficiency, the kidneys are also unable to adequately excrete phosphate, leading to hyperphosphatemia. The parathyroid glands undergo hyperplasia of the chief cells secondary to phosphate retention and lowering of serum calcium, which leads to increased levels of parathyroid hormone. Excess production of parathyroid hormone affects the development of osteoclasts, osteoblasts, and osteocytes (Murphey et al. 1993). The most common cause of chronic renal insufficiency is diabetic end-stage renal disease (ESRD), followed by glomerulonephritis (Roderick 2002). ESRD is the irreversible loss of renal function to an extent that is incompatible with life without the use of dialysis or renal transplantation. The incidence of ESRD is increasing. The number of patients enrolled in the ESRD Medicare-funded program has increased from approximately 10,000 beneficiaries in 1973 to 615,899 as of December 31, 2011 (Obrador and Pereira 2014).

Renal osteodystrophy is a term describing a collection of musculoskeletal abnormalities that occur in the presence of chronic renal insufficiency, including secondary hyperparathyroidism, osteosclerosis, osteoporosis, osteomalacia, and soft tissue and vascular calcification.

Secondary hyperparathyroidism is a response to the sustained hypocalcemia typically caused by chronic renal failure or enteric malabsorption and may produce bone resorption, periosteal reaction, and brown tumors. Bone resorption is the most frequent alteration of chronic renal insufficiency and typically occurs in multiple locations, including subperiosteal, subchondral, trabecular, endosteal, and subligamentous. Brown tumors and periosteal reaction are much less common in chronic renal insufficiency. Osteosclerosis predominantly affects the axial skeleton (Fig. 35.8a) and may be the only radiographic indication of chronic renal insufficiency. The extent of soft tissue calcifications increases with the duration of hemodialysis (Murphey

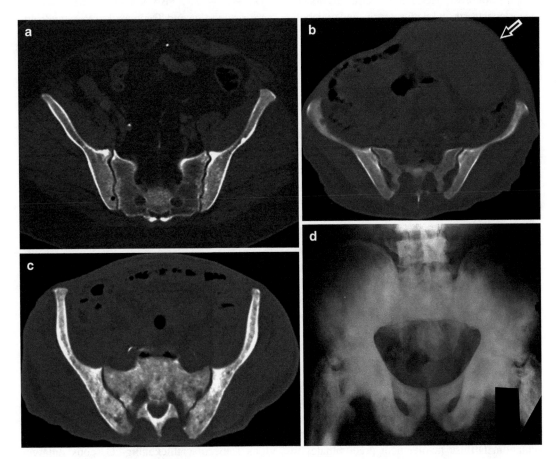

Fig. 35.8 Dense bones. (**a**) Axial CT image taken through the pelvis in a 59-year-old man with end-stage renal disease shows dense uniformly sclerotic bones in renal osteodystrophy. (**b**) Axial CT image taken through the pelvis in a 58-year-old woman with myelofibrosis shows sclerotic bones and massive splenomegaly (*arrow*). (**c**) Axial CT image taken through the pelvis in an 82-year-old man with mastocytosis shows mottled sclerotic bones. (**d**) AP radiograph of the pelvis in a patent with Paget disease shows the less frequently encountered osteoblastic phase. The sclerosis is less uniform and less symmetrical than the other entities shown in this figure

et al. 1993). Musculoskeletal manifestations of renal osteodystrophy are becoming increasingly common, owing to prolonged survival secondary to hemodialysis.

The cause of osteosclerosis in chronic renal insufficiency is not clearly understood. Parathyroid hormone is thought to be involved because of its stimulation of osteoblastic activity. Calcitonin may also play a role (Murphey et al. 1993). Increased bone density is well known in chronic renal insufficiency. It is reported as occurring in 9–34% of patients and may be the sole manifestation of renal osteodystrophy (Resnick et al. 1981). The differential diagnosis for diffuse osteosclerosis in the axial skeleton includes diffuse sclerotic metastatic disease (most often from prostate or breast cancer), myelofibrosis, sickle cell disease, mastocytosis, osteopetrosis, pyknodysostosis, and metabolic causes including fluorosis, hypervitaminosis A, Paget disease, and renal osteodystrophy.

35.6.2 Myelofibrosis

Myelofibrosis is a hematological disorder with replacement of bone marrow by collagenous connective tissue and progressive fibrosis. Osteosclerosis tends to be diffuse with a lack of architectural distortion (Fig. 35.8b). Sites of involvement include the axial skeleton, ribs, proximal humerus, and femur. Bone scintigraphy may give a "superscan" appearance. Non-osseous cross-sectional imaging findings include hepatomegaly and massive splenomegaly. Chest radiograph may reveal congestive heart failure from anemia (Resnick 2002).

35.6.3 Mastocytosis

Mastocytosis demonstrates skeletal involvement in 70% of cases. Bone involvement may be osteolytic or sclerotic (Fig. 35.8c) or have a mixed presentation. Diffuse involvement predominates in the axial skeleton and tends to be more common than a focal presentation. In the axial skeleton, there is loss of delineation of bone trabecula with a resulting radiodense appearance. Non-osseous imaging findings include thickened irregular

folds in the small bowel on fluoroscopy and hepatosplenomegaly on cross-sectional imaging (Resnick 2002).

35.6.4 Osteopetrosis

Osteopetrosis, also called Albers-Schönberg disease, is an uncommon hereditary bone dysplasia that results from dysfunctional osteoclasts. The bones become sclerotic and thick, but are weak and brittle (Kolawole et al. 1988)

35.6.5 Pyknodysostosis

Pyknodysostosis, also known as osteopetrosis acro-osteolytica and Toulouse-Lautrec syndrome (after the French painter), is a rare autosomal recessive bone dysplasia. It is characterized by osteosclerosis and short stature, particularly the limbs. Other imaging features include osteosclerosis with narrowed medullary cavities, delayed closure of cranial sutures, Wormian bones, frontal and occipital bossing, short broad hands with acro-osteolysis, hypoplasia of nails, obtuse angle of the mandible, and multiple long bone fractures following minimal trauma.

35.6.6 Paget Disease

Paget disease occurs in individuals older than 40 years of age. Three phases of Paget disease have been described: the osteolytic phase in which osteoclasts predominate, the mixed phase (most common), and the osteoblastic phase (Fig. 35.8d), in which osteoblasts predominate. Paget disease most commonly demonstrates bone expansion with cortical and trabecular thickening. In the long bones and pelvis, areas of sclerosis may develop and can be extensive in the osteoblastic phase, obliterating areas of previous trabecular thickening. Osseous enlargement is particularly common in the osteoblastic phase. There may be bowing of the long bones and insufficiency fractures on the convex side of bone, similar in appearance to Looser zones seen in osteomalacia, but which present on the concave side (Smith et al. 2002). Like diffuse metastatic disease, Paget disease is typically less symmetric than the entities described above.

35.6.7 Other Sclerotic Lesions

Fluorosis may also reveal spinal osteophytes, ligament calcification and ossification, and periostitis, in addition to osteosclerosis. The osteosclerosis observed in metastatic disease is usually less diffuse and less symmetrical than other enti-

ties featured in this section, and there are often associated osteolytic lesions.

35.7 Rugger Jersey Spine

When sclerosis of HPT involves the spine, it often presents with characteristic horizontal bands of sclerosis adjacent to the vertebral endplates. This is known as rugger jersey spine (McDonald et al. 2005; Chew 2012) (Fig. 35.9a). A mimic of the rugger jersey spine is the sandwich vertebra

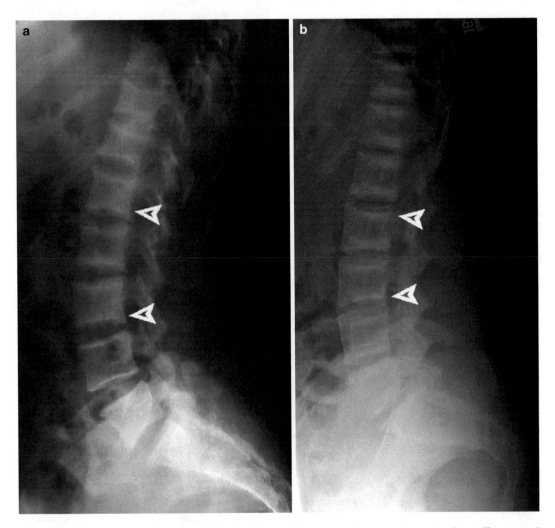

Fig. 35.9 Rugger jersey spine. (**a**) Lateral lumbar spine radiograph of a patient with parathyroid adenoma shows prominent sub-endplate density extending the length of the vertebral body giving the classic rugger jersey spine (*arrowheads*), simulating the transverse bands of a rugger jersey. (**b**) Lateral lumbar spine radiograph of a 37-year-old woman with recent diagnosis of type II autosomal dominant osteopetrosis shows the classic sandwich vertebra of osteopetrosis (*arrowheads*). The sclerotic endplates of osteopetrosis are often denser and more sharply defined than rugger jersey spine and do not extend to the anterior aspect of the vertebral body

(Fig. 35.9b) appearance of osteopetrosis, or Albers-Schönberg disease described above. The sandwich vertebral endplates of osteopetrosis are usually denser than those of rugger jersey spine and do not extend to the anterior vertebral body, helping in differentiation (Kolawole et al. 1988).

35.8   Thyroid Acropachy

Thyroid acropachy is an uncommon complication of autoimmune thyroid disease (Scanlon and Clemett 1964). It can occur in hypothyroid, euthyroid, or hyperthyroid conditions. The patient presents with an insidious onset of extremity swelling and clubbing, pretibial myxedema, and exophthalmos. On radiographs, there is periosteal new bone formation with either smooth flowing appearance or irregular, small, rounded radiolucent areas lending to a bubbled or lacy appearance (Rana et al. 2009) (Fig. 35.10a). The distribution of periostitis is typically along the midportion of the diaphysis of the bone, particularly the radial aspects of the bones of the hands and feet. In the hands, the first, second, and fifth metacarpals and proximal and middle phalanges are characteristically involved. Long bone involvement is rare, helping differentiate thyroid acropachy from secondary hypertrophic osteoarthropathy (Rana et al. 2009). Hypertrophic osteoarthropathy also tends to involve the entire diaphysis.

The primary mimic of thyroid acropachy is pachydermoperiostosis (Fig. 35.10b). This is a rare osteo-arthro-dermopathic syndrome, also known as primary hypertrophic osteoarthropathy (Rastogi et al. 2009). Pachydermoperiostosis is also more common in adolescent boys and in the African-American population. On imaging, the periosteal bone formation is symmetrical and shaggy and involves the metacarpals, metatarsals, and phalanges (Chew 2012) (Fig. 35.10b). Pachydermoperiostosis also involves the long bones, unlike thyroid acropachy. Additionally, in pachydermoperiostosis, there may be widening of the ends of bones, particularly at the wrist and knees.

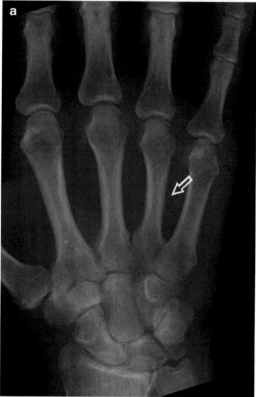

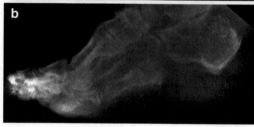

Fig. 35.10 Thyroid acropachy. (**a**) AP radiograph of the right wrist shows periosteal new bone formation along the fourth metacarpal bone (*arrow*) in a patient with underlying thyroid disease. (**b**) Lateral foot radiograph of a 25-year-old man with pachydermoperiostosis shows periosteal reaction that is most prominent along the calcaneus and fifth metatarsal base

35.9   Hypophosphatasia

Hypophosphatasia is an autosomal recessive disease with deficient activity of tissue-nonspecific isoenzyme of alkaline phosphatase, increased phosphoethanolamine and inorganic phosphate, and hypercalcemia when severe (Taybi and Lachman 1996). Serum calcium and phosphate levels are normal or high. The most

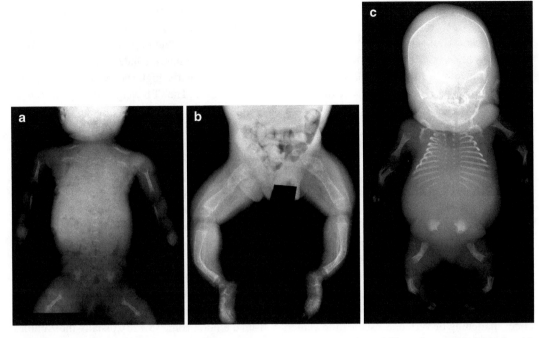

Fig. 35.11 Multiple fractures in a fetus suggest hypophosphatasia, osteogenesis imperfecta, or achondrogenesis. Radiographs of (**a**) stillborn term female with hypophosphatasia, (**b**) osteogenesis imperfecta, and (**c**) elective termination of 20-week gestational female with achondrogenesis. All show shortened extremities with severe osseous deformities and multiple fractures

severely affected infants die soon after birth, secondary to lack of bone support for the intracranial and thoracic structures (Resnick 2002). Fractures with deformity and shortening of the extremities may mimic dwarfism or osteogenesis imperfecta.

The infantile form of hypophosphatasia demonstrates marked delay of skeletal ossification, particularly in the growing ends of bones. Irregular prominent lucencies of uncalcified bone matrix extend from the growth plate into the metaphysis, sometimes resembling rickets. There is generalized de-ossification with coarse trabecular pattern, bowing deformities, and, often, healing fractures (Fig. 35.11a). There are short poorly ossified ribs. There may be craniosynostosis involving all the sutures and intersutural (Wormian) bones (Resnick 2002). Differential diagnosis for infantile hypophosphatasia with severe osseous deformities and shortening of the extremities includes achondrogenesis, rickets, thanatophoric dysplasia, and osteogenesis imperfecta. Bone fractures in a fetus suggest osteogenesis imperfecta, hypophosphatasia, or achondrogenesis.

35.9.1 Osteogenesis Imperfecta

The congenital forms of osteogenesis imperfecta (types 2 and 3) are severe and are characterized by osteopenia and multiple fractures at birth (Fig. 35.11b). Mutations cause structural defects in type 1 collagen. Extremities are shortened, broad, and crumpled, with bowing and angulation. There is demineralization and foci of localized bone thickening from callus formation. There are thin beaded ribs secondary to fractures, resulting in a bell-shaped chest. Skull findings include platybasia, basilar invagination, Wormian bones, enlarged sinuses, and abnormal teeth (Silence 1981). Other osseous findings include gracile bones, cortical thinning, popcorn calcification of the epiphyses, codfish vertebra, pectus excavatum, acetabular protrusion, and coxa vara (Goldman et al. 1980; Resnick 2002; Dighe et al. 2008).

35.9.2 Achondrogenesis

Achondrogenesis is an often-lethal autosomal recessive chondrodystrophy, with features of severe limb shortening (extreme micromelia), micrognathia, narrow fetal thorax, and disproportionately large head (Fig. 35.11c). Rib fractures can be present in the more severe type 1. There is poor mineralization of the skull and vertebra.

35.9.3 Thanatophoric Dysplasia

Thanatophoric dysplasia is the most common of the lethal skeletal dysplasias. Imaging features include a hypoplastic thorax with short horizontal ribs featuring cupped anterior ends, very short bowed (in type 1) extremities with metaphyseal flaring "telephone handle" appearance of long bones, flattening of vertebral ossification centers (platyspondyly), disproportionately large head with a prominent forehead (frontal bossing), and cloverleaf skull deformity (in type 2) (Dighe et al. 2008).

35.10 Tophaceous Gout

Gout is the most common form of crystal arthropathy in the United States, reportedly affecting 2% of the US population. The causes of hyperuricemia are often divided into primary (inborn defects of metabolism) and secondary. The secondary causes are more common and include disorders that lead to increased turnover of nucleic acids or impairment in renal excretion, as well as medication effects. Tophaceous gout results when there is localized precipitation of monosodium urate crystals in the soft tissues, with reactive inflammatory cells and foreign body giant cells. Tophaceous gout may occur in the tendons, ligaments, bursae, synovial spaces, cartilage, and bone. The most common locations include the pinna of the ear, olecranon bursa, and first metatarsophalangeal joints (Khoo and Tan 2011).

The MRI appearance of gouty tophi is variable. The appearance on T2-weighted sequences ranges from homogeneous hypointense to homogeneously hyperintense signal, depending on the extent of hydration and calcification. The most common T2-weighted appearance is a heterogeneous hypo- to intermediate signal intensity pattern. Tophi with high water content appear hyperintense. The T1-weighted appearance is more consistent, with homogeneously hypo- to intermediate signal intensity. Enhancement is also varied, but most commonly homogeneous and diffuse secondary to hypervascularity of the tophus (Khoo and Tan 2011). Dual-energy CT is an excellent problem-solving tool that can reliably diagnose the presence of gout in challenging clinical presentations (Nicolaou et al. 2010).

Several case reports in the literature discuss gouty tophi about the knee, mimicking a soft tissue tumor (Fig. 35.12a, b) on presentation (Amber 2012; Ozkan et al. 2013). Tendon xanthomas can present as a mass or masses arising from a tendon (Fig. 35.12c), usually the Achilles tendon. Clear cell sarcoma (Fig. 35.12d) often presents as a slowly enlarging mass intimately associated with or within a tendon, ligament, aponeurosis, or fascial structure and has a predilection for the lower extremity (Walker et al. 2011b). The differential diagnosis for soft tissue lesions with prominent areas of hypointense signal on T1- and T2-weighted sequences includes desmoid-type fibromatosis, densely calcified masses, pigmented villonodular synovitis (PVNS)/giant cell tumor of the tendon sheath (GCTTS), granular cell tumor, elastofibroma, desmoplastic fibroblastoma, and malignant fibrous histiocytoma/fibrosarcoma (Walker et al. 2010; Walker et al. 2011a; Walker et al. 2012).

35.11 Intraosseous Hydroxyapatite Crystal Deposition Disease (HADD)

Calcific tendinitis is a relatively common disorder (seen in about 3% of adults) that may be confused with osteoblastic metastasis or a bone island, when the hydroxyapatite crystal deposition extends into the adjacent bone. Pain is frequently the presenting symptom of calcific tendinitis, but patients may be asymptomatic.

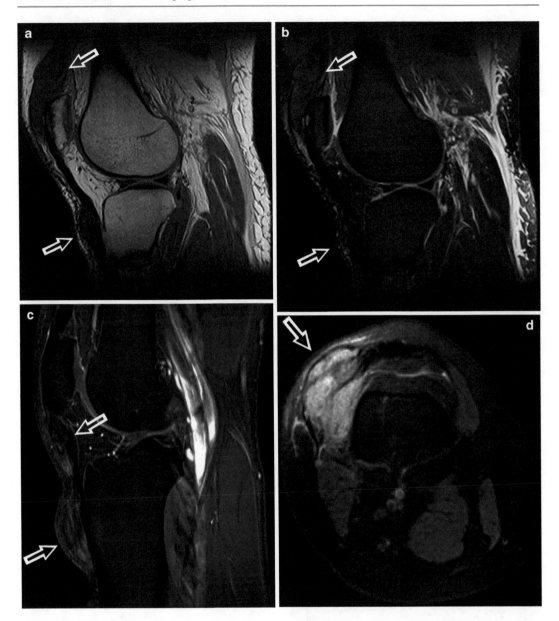

Fig. 35.12 Tophaceous gout and mimics. Sagittal (**a**) PD-W and (**b**) fat-suppressed T2-W MR images of a 45-year-old man with diabetes mellitus, hypertension, and gout who presented with knee masses show hypointense lesions extending from the quadriceps and patellar tendon insertions (*arrows*). These tophaceous gouty lesions arising from the tendon may be mistaken for tendon xanthomatosis or clear cell sarcoma arising from tendon. (**c**) Sagittal fat-suppressed T2-W MR image shows tendon xanthomas (*arrows*) with a similar imaging appearance at the knee in a 36-year-old man with familial hypercholesterolemia. (**d**) Axial contrast-enhanced fat-suppressed T1-W MR image shows clear cell sarcoma arising from the medial patellar tendon (*arrow*) in a 40-year-old woman

Radiographs classically show amorphous calcifications in variable amounts in the affected tendon or bursa. As the mineralized focus extends into the adjacent bone, there may be erosion of the underlying cortex or marrow change. Osseous involvement is most frequently noted at the proximal femur (gluteus maximus attachment) and at the proximal humerus (rotator cuff attachment).

Radiographs and CT most often reveal a solid sclerotic lesion representing intraosseous calcium deposition (Fig. 35.13a). The calcific concretions on MRI (Fig. 35.13b, c) are hypointense in signal on both T1- and T2-weighted images and are often discontinuous from the involved tendon. The majority of lesions demonstrate marked surrounding edema on fluid-sensitive MRI

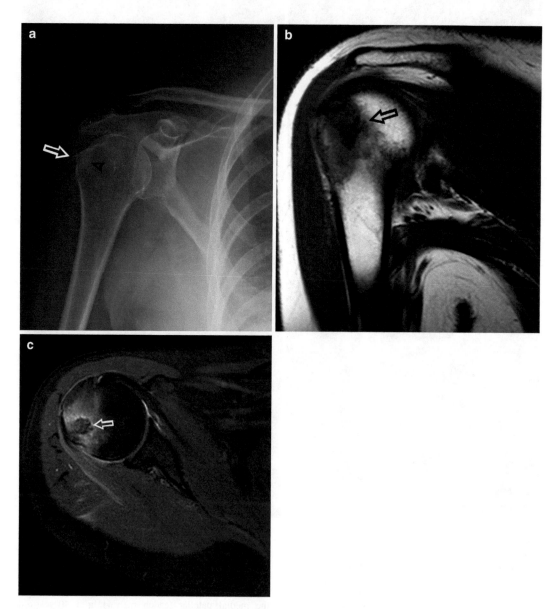

Fig. 35.13 Intraosseous hydroxyapatite crystal deposition disease and mimics. (**a**) Intraosseous hydroxyapatite crystal deposition manifesting as a sclerotic bone lesion in a 61-year-old woman with history of breast carcinoma and right shoulder pain with decreased range of motion for 10 days. AP radiograph shows a 1 cm sclerotic lesion at the greater tuberosity of the proximal humerus (*arrowhead*), which could easily be mistaken for a bone island or a small osteoblastic metastasis. Also note a small focus of crystal deposition in the adjacent supraspinatus tendon (*arrow*). (**b**) Coronal T1-W and (**c**) axial fat-suppressed T2-W MR images show a hypointense lesion (*arrows*) with marked surrounding bone marrow edema. The lesion (*arrow*) is "hot" on (**d**) Tc-99M bone scintiscans with greater uptake than the anterior iliac spines (*arrowhead*). (**e**) Sagittal fat-suppressed T2-W MR image in a 51-year-old woman with breast carcinoma and bone metastases shows the "halo sign" (*arrowhead*)

Fig. 35.13 (continued)

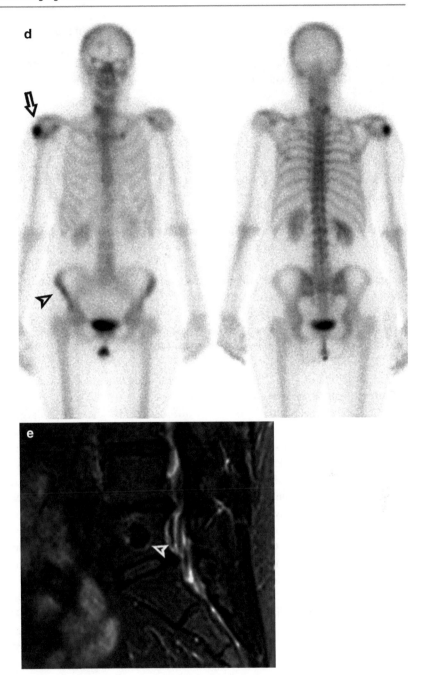

sequences. Delayed bone scintigraphy uptake (Fig. 35.13d) is marked in approximately 50% of cases (Flemming et al. 2003). Benign bone tumors commonly associated with bone marrow edema include osteoid osteoma, osteoblastoma, chondroblastoma, and Langerhans cell histiocytosis. The malignant primary bone tumors osteosarcoma, Ewing sarcoma, and chondrosarcoma may also be surrounded by bone marrow edema, although they are typically associated with a pathological fracture (James et al. 2008). Lymphoma may demonstrate edema without pathological fracture. A bone island typically shows spiculated margins on radiographs and CT and reveals no surrounding edema on MRI. Sclerotic metastatic lesions may occasionally have some intermediate T1- and hyperintense T2-weighted signal at the periphery. This signal hyperintensity surrounding the lesion has been termed the halo sign (Fig. 35.13e) (Schweitzer et al. 1993).

35.12 Hemophilia

Hemophilia is an X-linked recessive bleeding disorder occurring almost exclusively in males. Hemophilia A accounts for 80% of cases and is due to a deficiency of coagulation factor VIII. Hemophilia B and C account for the other 20% of cases and are deficiencies of factor IX and XI, respectively (Chew 2012). All types of hemophilia result in repetitive hemarthrosis and intraosseous bleeding. Typically, these first occur at 2–3 years of age and recur between 8 and 13 years. At least 50% of patients develop permanent osseous changes from hemorrhage (Brower and Flemming 2012).

Imaging findings of hemophilia include radiodense soft tissue swelling (due to hemorrhage or hemarthrosis), juxta-articular or diffuse osteoporosis related to hyperemia, subchondral cysts, and uniform joint space narrowing due to cartilage and synovial destruction (Brower and Flemming 2012). In the knee (Fig. 35.14a), there is characteristic ballooning or overgrowth of the femoral and tibial epiphyses, with widening of the intercondylar notch resulting from chronic hyperemia (Ng et al. 2005). The femoral condyles appear flattened, and the patella is ballooned and squared inferiorly. Knee findings are graded by the Arnold-Hilgartner classification system (Arnold and Hilgartner 1977):

Stage 0: normal joint
Stage I: no skeletal abnormalities, presence of soft tissue swelling
Stage II: osteoporosis and epiphysis overgrowth, no cysts, no narrowing of the cartilage space
Stage III: early subchondral bone cysts, squaring of the patella, widened notch of the distal femur or humerus, preservation of the cartilage space
Stage IV: findings of stage III, but more advanced; narrowed cartilage space

Stage V: fibrous joint contractures, loss of the joint cartilage space, extensive enlargement of the epiphyses with substantial disorganization of the joint

Juvenile idiopathic arthritis (JIA) may mimic the appearance of hemophilic arthritis at the knee (Fig. 35.14b). JIA is a disease of the pediatric population characterized by osteoporosis, soft tissue swelling, and joint effusions. At the ankle in hemophilic arthropathy, there is relative undergrowth of the lateral side of the tibial epiphysis, resulting in tibiotalar slanting, known as talar tilt (Brower and Flemming 2012). This talar tilt appearance is also seen in JIA. Findings suggesting JIA, as opposed to hemophilia, include ankylosis, erosions along areas of ligament insertion or thinner cartilage, and hand and wrist involvement (sites not typically involved in hemophilia) (Sheybani et al. 2013). In addition to the knee, other typical sites of involvement of hemophilia include the elbow, ankle, hip, and shoulder.

In chronic hemophilic arthropathy at the elbow, there are enlargement of the radial head, limited elbow motion, diffuse osteoporosis, uniform joint space narrowing, and secondary arthritis changes (Brower and Flemming 2012) (Fig. 35.14c). The findings are similar to those of rheumatoid arthritis (RA) (Fig. 35.14d). Findings suggesting RA include small joint involvement and more pronounced erosive changes. The late stages of elbow joint destruction can look very similar in hemophilia and RA.

35.13 Extramedullary Hematopoiesis in Thalassemia

Thalassemia is a group of biochemical disorders with splenomegaly and bone abnormalities seen in patients of Mediterranean decent. Alpha thalassemia is related to a deficiency of alpha globin chain synthesis. Beta thalassemia results from a deficiency of beta globin chain synthesis. Thalassemia major, also called Cooley anemia, is the homozygote type with two abnormal genes (Taybi and Lachman 1996; Resnick 2002).

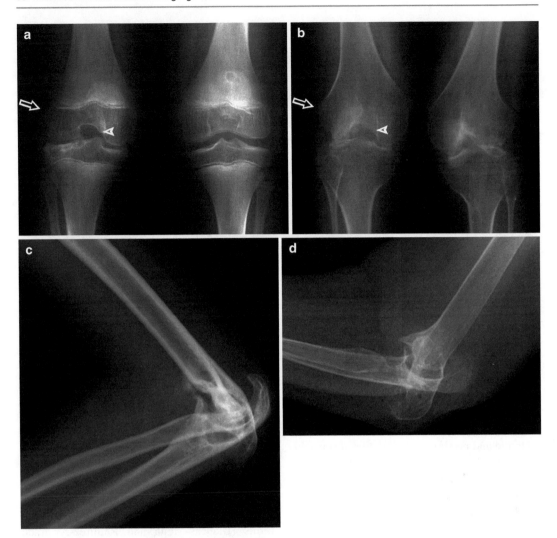

Fig. 35.14 Hemophilia and mimics. (**a**) AP radiograph of the knees in a 13-year-old boy with hemophilia shows osteopenia, joint space narrowing, condylar hypertrophy (*arrow*), and widening of the intercondylar notch (*arrowhead*) of the right knee secondary to chronic hyperemia. (**b**) AP radiograph of the knees in a 23-year-old woman with juvenile idiopathic arthritis shows diffuse osteopenia, joint space narrowing, symmetrical condylar hypertrophy (*arrow*), and widening of the intercondylar notch (*arrowhead*) in both knees secondary to chronic hyperemia. (**c**) Lateral radiograph of the right elbow in a 32-year-old hemophilic man shows erosions, subluxation, deformity, and osteopenia. The radial head is eroded and posteriorly dislocated. (**d**) Lateral radiograph of the right elbow in a 45-year-old woman with rheumatoid arthritis shows erosions, subluxation, deformity, and osteopenia. The radial head is eroded and posteriorly dislocated

Musculoskeletal imaging features of thalassemia are secondary to marrow hyperplasia and extramedullary hematopoiesis. The skull demonstrates widening of the diploic space and thinning of the outer table. Osseous production on the outer table leads to dense radial striations, giving the classic hair-on-end appearance most commonly demonstrated in thalassemia major.

Marrow hyperplasia in the nasal and temporal bones results in maxillary hypertrophy and forward displacement of the incisors, leading to the frequently described "rodent" facies. The proximal ribs may be expanded, with cortical thinning and osteoporosis (Resnick 2002). Extramedullary hematopoiesis is a compensatory mechanism due to chronic increased demand for erythrocytes.

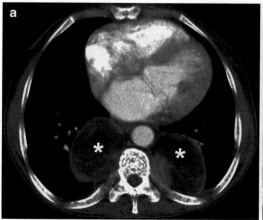

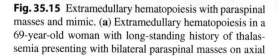

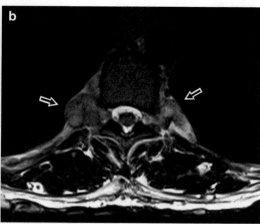

Fig. 35.15 Extramedullary hematopoiesis with paraspinal masses and mimic. (**a**) Extramedullary hematopoiesis in a 69-year-old woman with long-standing history of thalassemia presenting with bilateral paraspinal masses on axial CT. The significant fatty component (*asterisks*) suggests an inactive lesion. (**b**) Axial T2-W MR image shows bilateral neurofibromas (*arrows*) enlarging the neural foramen in this 31-year-old woman with neurofibromatosis type 1

The appearance is usually of a unilateral or bilateral paraspinal mass in the posterior mediastinum at the mid- and lower thorax. These masses are round or lobulated and do not contain calcifications. More active sites of paraspinal extramedullary hematopoiesis reveal immature and mature erythroid and myeloid cells and dilated sinusoids containing precursors of red cells. Inactive lesions may demonstrate elements of fatty tissue on cross-sectional imaging (Fig. 35.15a) and fibrosis or massive iron deposit (Tsitouridis et al. 1999).

The differential diagnosis of a paraspinal mass in the posterior mediastinum at the mid- and lower thorax includes other masses or mass-like processes of the posterior mediastinum, such as lipoma, liposarcoma, neural tumor, abscess, hematoma, and teratoma. Neural tumors (Fig. 35.15b), abscess, and hematoma would not have a significant lipid component. Bilaterality would only be expected in extramedullary hematopoiesis, neurofibroma (NF1), and lipomatosis syndrome. Neural tumors in this location often lead to widening of the neuroforamen and erosion of adjacent osseous structures (Walker et al. 2011a). The presence of osseous changes in the skull or face can confirm the diagnosis of extramedullary hematopoiesis.

35.14 Amyloidosis

Amyloidosis is a group of diseases characterized by tissue deposition of misfolded extracellular insoluble beta-pleated sheet proteins that demonstrate green birefringence under polarized microscopy when stained with Congo red (Blancas-Mejía and Ramirez-Alvarado 2013). Although there are at least 25 proteins capable of forming amyloid deposition, amyloidosis is mainly divided into primary and secondary forms (Blancas-Mejía and Ramirez-Alvarado 2013). While primary amyloidosis is hereditary, secondary amyloidosis can be due to a variety of chronic diseases including neoplastic process (antibody-producing plasma cell neoplasm such as multiple myeloma or lymphoma) or infectious/inflammatory processes such as tuberculosis, rheumatoid arthritis, or chronic renal failure on hemodialysis (Merlini et al. 2011). Since amyloid deposition could mimic both neoplastic and infectious or inflammatory process, distinction of this entity from the underlying chronic disease is essential.

In the musculoskeletal system, amyloid deposition mainly affects joints including the hip, shoulder, or wrist joints, often bilaterally, as well as the disk space. On radiographs, findings include well-defined osseous erosions with sclerotic margins and preservation of joint space, as well as juxta-articular soft tissue masses. CT (Fig. 35.16a) may be useful to further delineate bone erosions and periarticular soft tissue masses. Punctate calcifications may also be seen on CT and is much more common in primary disease (Georgiades et al. 2004). On MRI (Fig. 35.16b), amyloid proteins in the joint characteristically demonstrate hypointense signal on T1-weighted sequences and hypo-

to intermediate signal intensity on T2-weighted sequences (Otake et al. 1998).

35.14.1 Mimic: Pigmented Villonodular Synovitis

Pigmented villonodular synovitis (PVNS) is a neoplastic process of the synovium affecting

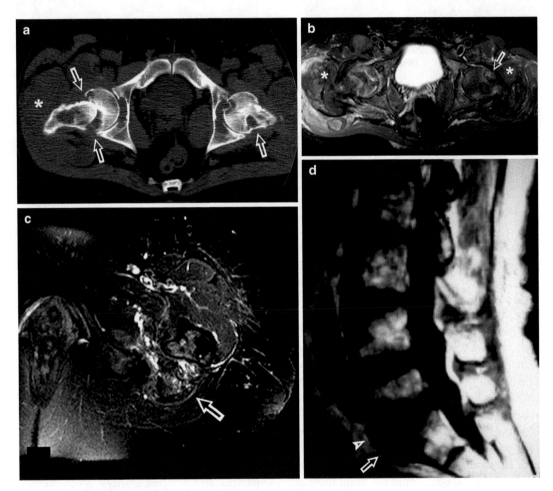

Fig. 35.16 Amyloidosis and mimics. (**a**) Amyloidosis of the hips in a patient with pathological fracture of the right hip secondary to extensive extrinsic bone erosion. CT of the pelvis shows multiple well-defined osteolytic lesions (*arrows*) and intra-articular soft tissue masses (*asterisk*). (**b**) Axial T2-W MR image shows multiple heterogeneous hypo- to intermediate signal intensity masses (*asterisks*) and erosions (*arrow*) involving both hip joints. (**c**) Axial fat-suppressed T2-W MR image in a 56-year-old woman with PVNS of the left hip shows a heterogeneously hypointense intraarticular mass (*arrow*). (**d, e**) Amyloid involve-ment in the spine may mimic infectious spondylodiskitis. Sagittal (**d**) T1-W and (**e**) T2-W MR images of the lumbar spine show endplate destruction (*arrowhead*) and signal hypointensity at the L5-S1 disk space (*arrow*). The fluid-sensitive sequence reveals predominantly hypointense tissue at L5-S1 disk space (*arrow*). (**f**) Sagittal fat-suppressed T2-W MR image in a 63-year-old woman with a history of multiple myeloma. She presented with gram-negative endocarditis, osteomyelitis/diskitis with fluid signal in the disk space and edema in the adjacent endplates (*arrow*), and an anterior epidural abscess (*arrowhead*)

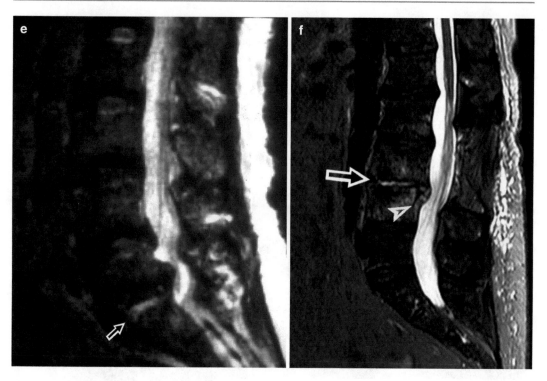

Fig. 35.16 (continued)

early- to middle-aged adults. It is characterized by benign synovial proliferation and hemosiderin deposition in a monoarticular distribution. On radiographs, PVNS of the hip may be seen as an articular or periarticular mass with osseous erosions affecting both sides of the joint. CT may better define osseous erosions. Calcification is rarely reported (Murphey et al. 2008). On MRI (Fig. 35.16c), PVNS reveals hypo- to intermediate signal intensity on both T1- and T2-weighted sequences and blooming artifacts on gradient-echo sequences (Murphey et al. 2008). Although both PVNS and amyloidosis can present as a lobulated mass within and adjacent to the joint, there are several features which can be helpful in distinguishing these two disorders. PVNS typically affects one joint, while amyloidosis related to systemic disease is usually polyarticular. In addition, blooming artifacts on gradient-echo sequences are typically only seen in PVNS (Murphey et al. 2008).

35.14.2 Mimic: Spondylodiskitis

Spondylodiskitis representing an infection of the vertebral body and intervertebral disk is usually due to hematogenous spread or direct inoculation following spinal procedures or surgery (Diehn 2012). It is characterized by disk space narrowing and vertebral endplate irregularities, which may be seen on radiographs but are better evaluated on CT. Contrast-enhanced CT can also be helpful in delineating paravertebral abscess. MRI is the best modality for evaluating spondylodiskitis due to its excellent soft tissue contrast resolution and its multiplanar capability. On fluid-sensitive sequences, signal hyperintensity can be observed in the disk space and adjacent endplates (Diehn 2012). On T1-weighted sequences, signal hypointensity is noted in the intervertebral disk and adjacent endplates, making them less distinct. There is usually disk enhancement following intravenous contrast administration (Ledermann et al. 2003). Following contrast agent injection, paraspinal soft tissue enhancement may represent phlegmon formation, while rim enhancement indicates paraspinal abscess (Ledermann et al. 2003).

When amyloid proteins are deposited in the intervertebral disk space, the spine may develop disk space collapse and endplate destruction on radiographs and CT, mimicking spondylodiskitis (Welk and Quint 1990). This is often designated as the destructive spondyloarthropathy associated with amyloid deposition. On MRI (Fig. 35.16d, e), amylod proteins in the disk space can show hypointense signal on T1-weighted sequences and hypo- to intermediate signal intensity on fluid-sensitive sequences (Marcelli et al. 1996). These imaging features, together with lack of surrounding paraspinal soft tissue edema, may allow distinction of infectious spondylodiskitis from amyloid. The presence of a paravertebral collection on contrast-enhanced CT or MRI indicates an infectious process, and it is not typically seen in amyloid spondylodiskitis.

Conclusion

Metabolic conditions may result in a variety of osseous manifestations. It is important to recognize how these lesions may present and be able to distinguish them from a variety of similar-appearing mimics. Regional osteoporosis may demonstrate a permeative osteolytic appearance and cortical tunneling that may mimic an aggressive neoplasm or multiple myeloma. With aggressive neoplasms, there is generally a central area of prominent osteolysis, with diminished destruction at the margins. Aggressive osteoporosis shows a uniform pattern of multiple lucencies and cortical tunneling, very similar to multiple myeloma. Intracortical resorption of the distal tufts in HPT can mimic other causes of acroosteolysis. Subperiosteal resorption along the radial aspect of the middle phalanges of the index and middle fingers is characteristic of HPT and can help make the diagnosis. Hyperparathyroidism, rheumatoid arthritis, and post-traumatic osteolysis can result in resorption of the distal clavicle. To distinguish

clavicle resorption secondary to HPT, look for subperiosteal resorption at the medial proximal humeri and on the superior and inferior rib margins. The subchondral bone resorption of HPT in the sacroiliac joints may mimic erosions due to seronegative spondyloarthropathy. In HPT, the sacroiliac joints are widened rather than narrowed as expected in the inflammatory arthropathies. Brown tumors can be singular or multiple and may be mistaken for lytic bone lesions. Brown tumor should be included in the differential for one or multiple osteolytic lesions in a patient with HPT. Periarticular calcified masses often seen in secondary HPT are indistinguishable from tumoral calcinosis by imaging and should be considered in the patient with chronic renal failure. Rickets with a widened, irregular, and frayed appearance of the metaphysis and rachitic rosary at the costochondral junction may be mistaken for non-accidental injury. Rickets is far less common than non-accidental injury, and a bone survey may reveal multiple healing fractures of various ages and characteristic locations of non-accidental trauma including the skull and sternum. Chronic renal failure often results in renal osteodystrophy, which is a combination of rickets or osteomalacia depending on patient age, secondary hyperparathyroidism, osteoporosis, and soft tissue and vascular calcifications increasing with the duration of hemodialysis.

Osteosclerosis may be noted in the axial skeleton in renal osteodystrophy and must be distinguished from other possible causes such as diffuse sclerotic metastatic disease, myelofibrosis, mastocytosis, osteopetrosis, pyknodysostosis, and Paget disease. Other musculoskeletal manifestations of renal osteodystrophy may aid in the diagnosis. Characteristic horizontal bands of sclerosis adjacent to the vertebral endplates known as rugger jersey spine could be mistaken for the sandwich vertebra of osteopetrosis, which are usually more dense and do not extend to the anterior vertebral body. The primary mimic of thyroid acropachy is pachydermoperiostosis (PDP), but PDP involves the long bones, unlike thyroid acropachy. Hemophilia and JIA demonstrate characteristic ballooning or overgrowth of the femoral condyles with widening of the intercondylar notch. Hemophilia may be distinguished if there is unilateral involvement or a dense effusion, unlike JIA. Amyloid deposition in the joints can result in an intraarticular process with similar imaging characteristics to PVNS. However, PVNS is monoarticular in distribution as opposed to polyarticular disease associated with amyloid. Spine involvement by amyloid may resemble infectious spondylodiscitis. Signal hyperintensity on fluid-sensitive MRI sequences in the disk or paraspinal abscess is much more indicative of infectious spondylodiscitis. Understanding the imaging characteristics of metabolic conditions and the most common mimics, along with obtaining adequate clinical history, can assist the radiologist to make the correct diagnosis or significantly narrow the differential diagnosis.

References

Amber H (2012) Gouty tophi mimicking synovial sarcoma of the knee joint. Turkish J Rheumatol 27:208–211

Arnold WD, Hilgartner MW (1977) Hemophilic arthropathy. Current concepts of pathogenesis and management. J Bone Joint Surg Am 59:287–305

Bassett LW, Blocka KL, Furst DE et al (1981) Skeletal findings in progressive systemic sclerosis (scleroderma). AJR Am J Roentgenol 136:1121–1126

Blancas-Mejía LM, Ramirez-Alvarado M (2013) Systemic amyloidoses. Annu Rev Biochem 82:745–774

Brower AC, Flemming DJ (2012) Arthritis in black and white, 5th edn. Saunders, Philadelphia

Carter JD, Warner E (2003) Clinical images: tumoral calcinosis associated with sarcoidosis. Arthritis Rheum 48:1770

Chew FS (2012) Skeletal radiology: the bare bones, 3rd edn. Lippincott Williams & Wilkins, Philadelphia

Demetriou ET, Pietras SM, Holick MF (2010) Hypercalcemia and soft tissue calcification owing to sarcoidosis: the sunlight-cola connection. J Bone Miner Res 25:1695–1699

Diehn FE (2012) Imaging of spine infection. Radiol Clin N Am 50:777–798

Dighe M, Fligner C, Cheng E et al (2008) Fetal skeletal dysplasia: an approach to diagnosis with illustrative cases 1. Radiographics 28:1061–1077

Donnelly LF (2001) Fundamentals of pediatric radiology. WB Saunders, Philadelphia

Ebel K-D, Benz-Bohm G (1999) Differential diagnosis in pediatric radiology. Thieme, New York

Fain O (2005) Musculoskeletal manifestations of scurvy. Joint Bone Spine 72:124–128

Flemming DJ, Murphey MD, Shekitka KM et al (2003) Osseous involvement in calcific tendinitis: a retrospective review of 50 cases. AJR Am J Roentgenol 181:965–972

Georgiades CS, Neyman EG, Barish MA, Fishman EK (2004) Amyloidosis: review and CT manifestations. Radiographics 24:405–416

Goldman AB, Davidson D, Pavlov H, Bullough PG (1980) "Popcorn" calcifications: a prognostic sign in osteogenesis imperfecta. Radiology 136:351–358

Guglielmi G, Muscarella S, Leone A, Peh WCG (2008) Imaging of metabolic bone diseases. Radiol Clin N Am 46:735–754

Guglielmi G, Muscarella S, Bazzocchi A (2011) Integrated imaging approach to osteoporosis: state-of-the-art review and update. Radiographics 31:1343–1364

James SLJ, Panicek DM, Davies AM (2008) Bone marrow oedema associated with benign and malignant bone tumours. Eur J Radiol 67:11–21

Jones G (1969) Radiological appearances of disuse osteoporosis. Clin Radiol 20:345–353

Kattapuram SV, Khurana JS, Ehara S, Ragozzino M (1988) Aggressive posttraumatic osteoporosis of the humerus simulating a malignant neoplasm. Cancer 62:2525–2527

Keller KA, Barnes PD (2008) Rickets vs. abuse: a national and international epidemic. Pediatr Radiol 38:1210–1216

Khan A, Bilezikian J (2000) Primary hyperparathyroidism: pathophysiology and impact on bone. Can Med Assoc J 163:184–187

Khoo JN, Tan SC (2011) MR imaging of tophaceous gout revisited. Singapore Med J 52:840–847

Kirks DR, Griscom NT (1998) Practical pediatric imaging. Lippincott Williams & Wilkins, Philadelphia

Kolawole TM, Hawass ND, Patel PJ, Mahdi AH (1988) Osteopetrosis: some unusual radiological features with a short review. Eur J Radiol 8:89–95

Kumar V, Abbas AK, Aster JC (2014) Robbins & Cotran pathologic basis of disease, 9th edn. Elsevier Health Sciences, Amsterdam

Ledermann HP, Schweitzer ME, Morrison WB, Carrino JA (2003) MR imaging findings in spinal infections: rules or myths? Radiology 228:506–514

Leventhal JM, Martin KD, Asnes AG (2008) Incidence of fractures attributable to abuse in young hospitalized children: results from analysis of a United States database. Pediatrics 122:599–604

Levine AH, Pais MJ, Schwartz EE (1976) Posttraumatic osteolysis of the distal clavicle with emphasis on early radiologic changes. AJR Am J Roentgenol 127:781–784

Lonergan GJ, Baker AM, Morey MK, Boos SC (2003) From the archives of the AFIP. Child abuse: radiologic-pathologic correlation. Radiographics 23:811–845

Marcelli C, Pérennou D, Cyteval C et al (1996) Amyloidosis-related cauda equina compression in long-term hemodialysis patients. Three case reports. Spine 21:381–385

Martinez S, Vogler JB, Harrelson JM, Lyles KW (1990) Imaging of tumoral calcinosis: new observations. Radiology 174:215–222

Massry SG, Bluestone R, Klinenberg JR, Coburn JW (1975) Abnormalities of the musculoskeletal system in hemodialysis patients. Semin Arthritis Rheum 4:321–349

McDonald DK, Parman L, Speights VO (2005) Best cases from the AFIP: primary hyperparathyroidism due to parathyroid adenoma. Radiographics 25:829–834

Merlini G, Seldin DC, Gertz MA (2011) Amyloidosis: pathogenesis and new therapeutic options. J Clin Oncol 29:1924–1933

Murphey MD, Sartoris DJ, Quale JL et al (1993) Musculoskeletal manifestations of chronic renal insufficiency. Radiographics 13:357–379

Murphey MD, Rhee JH, Lewis RB et al (2008) Pigmented villonodular synovitis: radiologic-pathologic correlation. Radiographics 28:1493–1518

Ng WH, Chu WCW, Shing MK et al (2005) Role of imaging in management of hemophilic patients. AJR Am J Roentgenol 184:1619–1623

Nicolaou S, Yong-Hing CJ, Galea-Soler S et al (2010) Dual-energy CT as a potential new diagnostic tool in the management of gout in the acute setting. AJR Am J Roentgenol 194:1072–1078

Obrador GT, Pereira B. Epidemiology of chronic kidney disease. 2014. https://www.uptodate.com/contents/epidemiology-of-chronic-kidney-disease.

Olsen KM, Chew FS (2006) Tumoral calcinosis: pearls, polemics, and alternative possibilities 1. Radiographics 26:871–885

Otake S, Tsuruta Y, Yamana D et al (1998) Amyloid arthropathy of the hip joint: MR demonstration of presumed amyloid lesions in 152 patients with long-term hemodialysis. Eur Radiol 8:1352–1356

Ozkan FU, Bilsel K, Turkmen I et al (2013) Tophi gout around the knee joint: an unusual presentation with a soft tissue mass. Int J Case Rep Images 4:593. http://doi.org/10.5348/ijcri-2013-11-388-CR-2.

Perez-Rossello JM, Feldman HA, Kleinman PK et al (2012) Rachitic changes, demineralization, and fracture risk in healthy infants and toddlers with vitamin D deficiency. Radiology 262:234–241

Prakash D, Prabhu SM, Irodi A (2014) Seronegative spondyloarthropathy-related sacroiliitis: CT, MRI features and differentials. Indian J Radiol Imaging 24:271–278

Rana RS, Wu JS, Eisenberg RL (2009) Periosteal reaction. AJR Am J Roentgenol 193:W259–W272

Rastogi R, Suma GN, Prakash R (2009) Pachydermoperiostosis or primary hypertrophic osteoarthropathy: a rare clinicoradiologic case. Indian J Radiol Imaging 19:123–126

Resnick D, Niwayama G (1976) Resorption of the under-surface of the distal clavicle in rheumatoid arthritis. Radiology 120:75–77

Resnick D, Deftos LJ, Parthemore JG (1981) Renal osteodystrophy: magnification radiography of target sites of absorption. AJR Am J Roentgenol 136:711–714

Resnick D (2002) Diagnosis of bone and joint disorders, 4th edn. WB Saunders, Philadelphia

Roderick P (2002) Epidemiology of end-stage renal disease. Clin Med (Lond) 2:200–204

Scanlon GT, Clemett AR (1964) Thyroid acropathy. Radiology 83:1039–1042

Schweitzer ME, Levine C, Mitchell DG et al (1993) Bull's-eyes and halos: useful MR discriminators of osseous metastases. Radiology 188:249–252

Sheybani EF, Khanna G, White AJ, Demertzis JL (2013) Imaging of juvenile idiopathic arthritis: a multimodality approach. Radiographics 33:1253–1273

Sidhu HS, Venkatanarasimha N, Bhatnagar G et al (2012) Imaging features of therapeutic drug–induced musculoskeletal abnormalities. Radiographics 32:105–127

Sillence D (1981) Osteogenesis imperfecta: an expanding panorama of variants. Clin Orthop Relat Res 159:11–25

Smith SE, Murphey MD, Motamedi K et al (2002) From the archives of the AFIP. Radiologic spectrum of Paget disease of bone and its complications with pathologic correlation. Radiographics 22:1191–1216

Swischuk LE, Hayden CK (1979) Rickets: a roentgenographic scheme for diagnosis. Pediatr Radiol 8:203–208

Taybi H, Lachman R (1996) Radiology of syndromes, metabolic disorders and skeletal dysplasias, 5th edn. Mosby, St Louis

Tsitouridis J, Stamos S, Hassapopoulou E et al (1999) Extramedullary paraspinal hematopoiesis in thalassemia: CT and MRI evaluation. Eur J Radiol 30:33–38

Walker EA, Song AJ, Murphey MD (2010) Magnetic resonance imaging of soft-tissue masses. Semin Roentgenol 45:277–297

Walker EA, Fenton ME, Salesky JS, Murphey MD (2011a) Magnetic resonance imaging of benign soft tissue neoplasms in adults. Radiol Clin N Am 49:1197–1217

Walker EA, Salesky JS, Fenton ME, Murphey MD (2011b) Magnetic resonance imaging of malignant soft tissue neoplasms in the adult. Radiol Clin N Am 49:1219–1234

Walker EA, Petscavage JM, Brian PL et al (2012) Imaging features of superficial and deep fibromatoses in the adult population. Sarcoma 2012(4):215810. http://doi.org/10.1155/2012/215810.

Weinstein M, Babyn P, Zlotkin S (2001) An orange a day keeps the doctor away: scurvy in the year 2000. Pediatrics 108:E55

Welk LA, Quint DJ (1990) Amyloidosis of the spine in a patient on long-term hemodialysis. Neuroradiology 32:334–336

Wolpe FM, Khedkar NY, Gordon D et al (1987) Tumoral calcinosis associated with sarcoidosis and positive bone and gallium imaging. Clin Nucl Med 12:529–532

World Health Organization (2003) Prevention and management of osteoporosis: report of a WHO scientific group. World Health Organization, Geneva

Multifocal and Multisystemic Bone Lesions: Imaging Pitfalls

36

Michael E. Mulligan

Contents

36.1	**Introduction**	743
36.2	**Imaging Modality Pitfalls**	744
36.3	**Normal Red Marrow and Marrow Reconversion**	749
36.4	**Mimics of Osteoblastic Metastases**	753
36.4.1	Bone Islands	753
36.4.2	Osteopoikilosis, Tuberous Sclerosis, and Mastocytosis	753
36.4.3	POEMS Syndrome	754
36.5	**Mimics of Osteolytic Metastases**	755
36.5.1	Osteoporosis	755
36.5.2	Polyostotic Fibrous Dysplasia	757
36.5.3	Langerhans Cell Histiocytosis	757
36.5.4	Infectious Conditions	758
36.5.5	Sarcoidosis	760
36.5.6	Brown Tumors	760
36.5.7	Paget Disease	761
36.6	**Treatment-/Medication-Related Lesions**	762
	Conclusion	764
	References	765

Abbreviations

CT	Computed tomography
MRI	Magnetic resonance imaging
PET	Positron emission tomography
PET/CT	Positron emission tomography/computed tomography
WBCT	Whole-body computed tomography
WBMRI	Whole-body magnetic resonance imaging

M.E. Mulligan, MD
Department of Diagnostic Radiology and Nuclear Medicine, University of Maryland School of Medicine, 22 South Greene Street, Baltimore, MD 21201, USA
e-mail: mmulligan@umm.edu

36.1 Introduction

Imaging studies that depict multifocal bone lesions in adults are most often regarded with much concern for the presence of metastatic disease or myeloma (Figs. 36.1 and 36.2). There is good reason for such concern. Approximately 30% of all patients with all forms of cancer develop metastatic disease, and 350,000 people die with bone metastases in the United States each year. The skeleton is the most common site of involvement and is the cause of the most morbidity for these patients (Coleman 2006). Myeloma is newly diagnosed in only 20,000 people in the United States each year, but more than 80% of the patients have focal osteolytic bone lesions discovered on staging imaging studies (Healy et al. 2011). In children with multifocal disease, one might prefer not to think of metastatic disease or other aggressive disease processes, but these are still possibilities. However,

© Springer International Publishing AG 2017
W.C.G. Peh (ed.), *Pitfalls in Musculoskeletal Radiology*, DOI 10.1007/978-3-319-53496-1_36

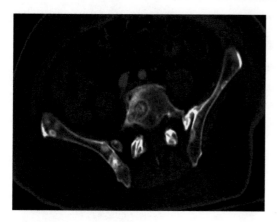

Fig. 36.1 A 72-year-old man with known prostate carcinoma. Axial CT imaging taken through the upper pelvis shows multiple osteoblastic lesions in the iliac wings and S1 vertebral body. These have a somewhat unusual ring-like appearance

Table 36.1 Some nonneoplastic causes of multifocal and multisystemic bone lesions

Langerhans cell histiocytosis

Leukemia and lymphoma

Polyostotic fibrous dysplasia

Multiple non-ossifying fibromas, Jaffe-Campanacci syndrome

Vascular lesions including focal hematopoietic hyperplasia, bone infarcts, hemangiomas, and angiosarcoma

Infectious diseases including tuberculosis, fungal infection, syphilis, yaws, cat scratch disease, and bacillary angiomatosis

Infectious-like conditions: chronic recurrent multifocal osteomyelitis and SAPHO syndrome

Sarcoidosis

Metabolic conditions that result in osteoporosis, brown tumors of hyperparathyroidism, amyloidosis, and red marrow reconversion

Developmental conditions including osteopoikilosis, osteopathia striata

Medication-related changes, e.g., those caused by voriconazole

Treatment-related changes, e.g., those caused by granulocyte colony stimulating factors

Miscellaneous conditions including Paget disease, mastocytosis, pyknodysostosis, and tuberous sclerosis

there are many other neoplastic conditions (both benign and malignant) and many nonneoplastic conditions that one should keep in mind, as alternative causes of multifocal lesions, in both children and adults (Table 36.1).

36.2 Imaging Modality Pitfalls

Selecting the most appropriate imaging modality will depend on the most likely etiology of the patient's condition and the type of equipment available at any given hospital. The limitations and pitfalls inherent in conventional radiography are well known, especially for lesions in the spine. Edelstyn et al. (1967) demonstrated experimentally that there must be 50–75% destruction in a

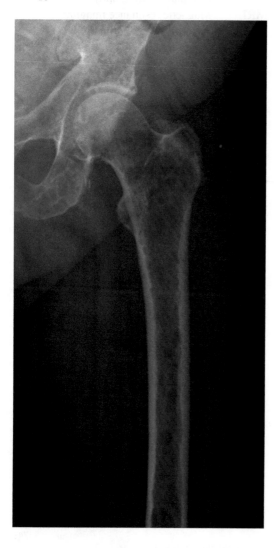

Fig. 36.2 A 77-year-old man with known multiple myeloma. AP radiograph of the proximal right femur shows multiple small osteolytic lesions consistent with extensive myelomatous involvement

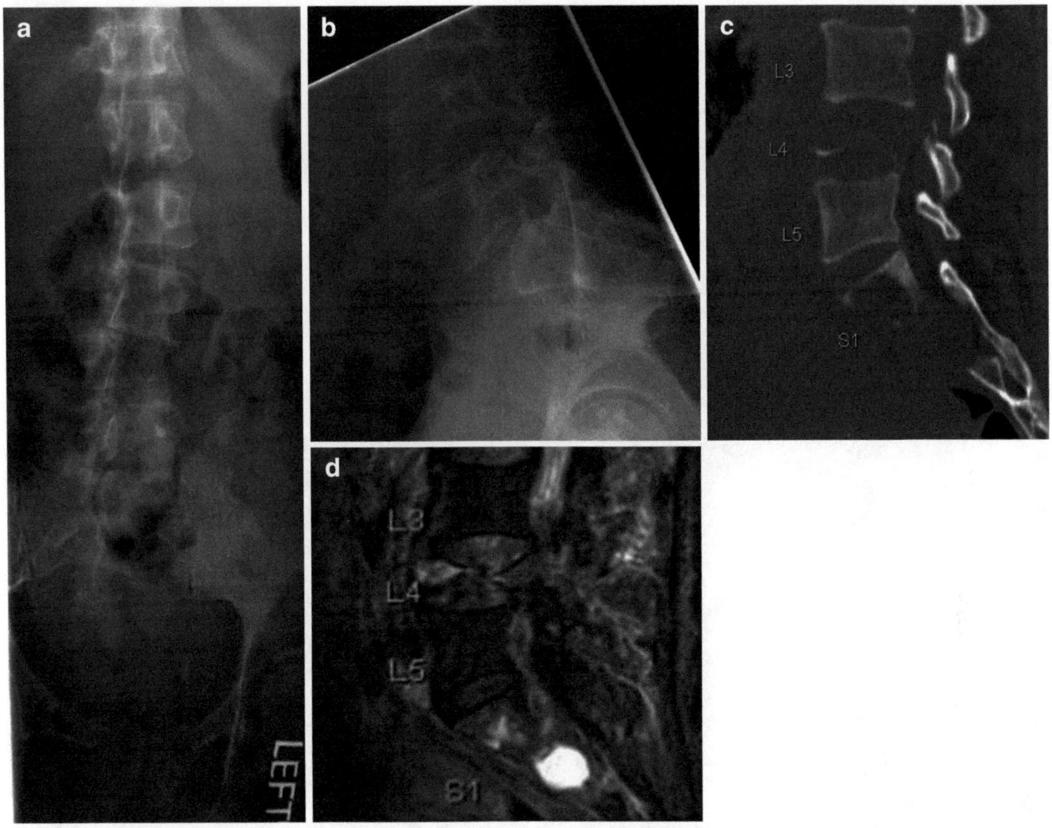

Fig. 36.3 A 46-year-old woman with history of HIV and metastatic cervical carcinoma. (**a**) AP and (**b**) lateral radiographs of the lumbar spine show pathological compression fracture of L4 vertebral body with no other obvious osteolytic lesions. However, sagittal lumbar spine (**c**) CT image and (**d**) STIR MR image show additional extensive involvement of S1 and S2 segments that is not evident, even in retrospect, on the radiographs, in addition to the L4 pathological compression fracture

vertebral body before a lesion will be evident on conventional radiographs (Fig. 36.3). This is also true in other areas of the skeleton, such as the pelvis and femoral necks, where there must be extensive cancellous bone destruction before a lesion becomes evident (Fig. 36.4). However, when cortical bone is directly involved, even lesions as small as 2–3 mm can be readily evident (Figs. 36.5 and 36.6). Although conventional radiographic skeletal surveys are a good initial screening study, when a more exact evaluation of extent of disease is needed, other whole-body techniques must be used. Whole-body imaging techniques that are currently available include nuclear scintigraphy (with a variety of different radionuclides); whole-body computed tomography (WBCT); positron emission tomography (PET), without or with concurrent computed tomography (PET/CT) or magnetic resonance imaging (PET/MRI); or stand-alone whole-body magnetic resonance imaging (WBMRI). Common pitfalls that are associated with these techniques are discussed in the following sections.

Standard technetium (Tc)-99m bone scintigraphy is useful for all multifocal conditions where lesions cause reactive bone formation (Fig. 36.7). A major pitfall arises when disease processes have limited reactive new bone formation or nonexistent reactive new bone formation, as is usually the case with multiple myeloma (Fig. 36.8). The explanation for this in myeloma patients is that they have osteoclast-activating factors and

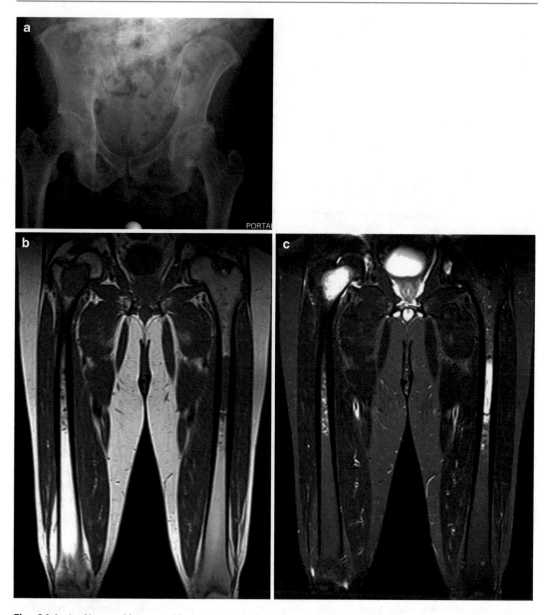

Fig. 36.4 A 61-year-old man with known multiple myeloma and report of worsening right hip pain. (**a**) AP radiograph of the pelvis shows a rounded lucency in the lateral aspect of the right femoral head that was stable when compared to prior studies dating back one full year. However, coronal (**b**) T1-W and (**c**) STIR MR images done later the same day show a 5 cm lesion involving the entirety of the right femoral neck with extension to the intertrochanteric region, as well as 8 cm lesion within the proximal left femoral shaft. The femoral neck lesion was at high risk for impending pathological fracture and was treated with internal fixation

osteoblast-suppressing factors that typically result in purely osteolytic lesions with no reactive bone formation (Delgado-Calle et al. 2014). This is true in most patients with myeloma even after successful treatment, although some newer treatment agents, such as Zometa, may allow reactive new bone formation in some patients (Fig. 36.9).

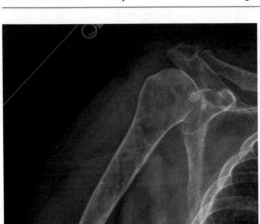

Fig. 36.5 A 77-year-old man with known multiple myeloma. AP radiograph of the right humerus from a skeletal survey shows multiple tiny punched-out osteolytic lesions throughout the entire shaft of the humerus. These are readily evident despite their small size, since they involve the adjacent endosteal cortical bone surface

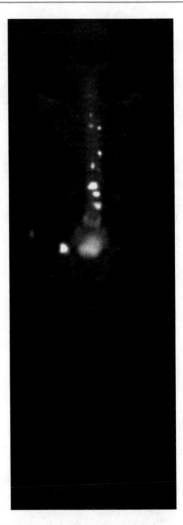

Fig. 36.7 A 64-year-old woman with known metastatic breast cancer. Tc-99m bone scintiscan shows multiple areas of abnormal uptake in a characteristic haphazard pattern throughout the spinal column and left acetabulum, typical of metastatic disease

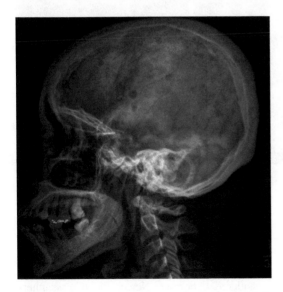

Fig. 36.6 A 55-year-old woman with known multiple myeloma. Lateral skull radiograph from a skeletal survey shows typical multiple small punched-out osteolytic lesions throughout the calvarium

CT and/or PET/CT with fluorodeoxyglucose (FDG) is commonly used to stage patients with various cancers and other conditions, including multiple myeloma, leukemia, and lymphoma. One pitfall is that mild diffuse infiltration in the spinal column and in the flat bones such as the scapula and pelvis may not show PET/CT abnormalities or elevated FDG uptake (Breyer et al. 2006). Another pitfall regarding PET/CT FDG uptake is false-negative problems with bone

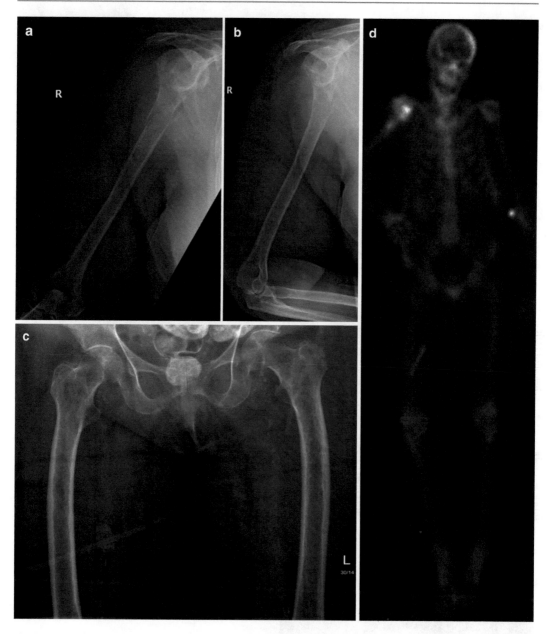

Fig. 36.8 An 87-year-old woman with known multiple myeloma and new right arm pain. (**a**) AP and (**b**) lateral radiographs of the humerus show a minimally displaced pathological fracture through the proximal humeral shaft, as well has multiple tiny osteolytic lesions throughout the entire shaft of the humerus. Patient had extensive myelomatous bone changes throughout the entire skeleton shown on the (**c**) AP radiograph of both proximal femurs and other images from skeletal survey. (**d**) Anterior image from Tc-99m bone scintiscan shows abnormal uptake only at the pathological fracture site in the proximal right humerus

lesions that are less than 5 mm in size. Any FDG uptake in small myeloma lesions, regardless of its standardized uptake value (SUV), should be considered abnormal. Newer PET/CT scanners are being developed that will allow for detection of lesions that are less than 5 mm in size. Another

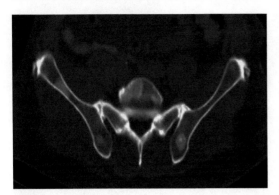

Fig. 36.9 A 60-year-old man with known myeloma undergoing routine restaging status posttransplant and Zometa therapy for 1 year prior to the current exam. Axial CT image of the pelvis shows multiple sclerotic bone lesions consistent with healing response

pitfall is that some malignancies and their bone marrow metastases are not very FDG-avid, including lobular breast cancer, hepatocellular carcinoma, and prostate carcinoma (Ulaner et al. 2013). One way to avoid these pitfalls is to consider using WBMRI as a complementary study, when there is a need to know the full extent of bone marrow involvement. This is especially true for staging patients who have multiple myeloma. The combination of PET/CT and WBMRI for initial diagnosis, staging, and follow-up of myeloma patients was recommended at a meeting of the International Myeloma Working Group that was held in Kyoto, Japan, in 2014 (Brioli et al. 2014).

Another pitfall is to fail to recognize that not all lesions detected on such screening studies represent areas of metastatic disease from the known primary disease process or are areas of metastatic disease or myelomatous involvement (Fig. 36.10). A study of 482 patients from Memorial Sloan-Kettering Cancer Center demonstrated a second cancer, when biopsy of a suspicious lesion was done, in 3% of the cases (Raphael et al. 2013). The US National Cancer Institute Surveillance, Epidemiology, and End Results (SEER) program data report a cumulative incidence of second primary malignancies in 14% of cancer patients after 25 years of follow-up (Yang et al. 2012). Likewise, myeloma patients are known to have an increased

risk for second malignancies such as acute myelogenous leukemia (AML), chronic myelogenous leukemia (CML), and Kaposi sarcoma. AML is the most common second malignancy in myeloma patients (Yang et al. 2012).

WBMRI is an evolving, excellent technique but is costly and time-consuming and may not be available worldwide. A pitfall with MRI is a lag in the change of appearance of successfully treated disease when one uses standard imaging sequences. One way to avoid this pitfall is to consider using additional MRI techniques, such as diffusion-weighted imaging and/or dynamic contrast enhancement, for better detection of lesion response (or lack of response) to treatment (Giles et al. 2014). Certain MRI techniques can be used to avoid the pitfall of misidentifying a lesion as a pathologic focus. One such technique is in-phase and out-of-phase imaging. This technique can be performed very quickly on most MRI systems. It allows one to determine if there are coexistent pixels of fat and water within a suspected bone marrow lesion (Figs. 36.11 and 36.12). The signal dropout one sees on the out-of-phase images allows one to confidently report that the lesion is not malignant (Disler et al. 1997). The change in signal intensity usually can be appreciated by simply visually comparing the two sequences without having to determine absolute values. However, if a number is needed, it has been reported that a 20% decrease in signal intensity is reliable for distinguishing benign from malignant foci in spinal bone marrow (Zajick et al. 2005).

36.3 Normal Red Marrow and Marrow Reconversion

Normal red marrow or areas of red marrow reconversion can mimic pathology (as can focal hematopoietic hyperplasia). Normal adult red marrow skeletal distribution pattern is established in most people by the age of 25 years. Therefore, it is normal to see patchy or focal areas of red marrow in the spinal column, shoulder girdle regions, pelvis/

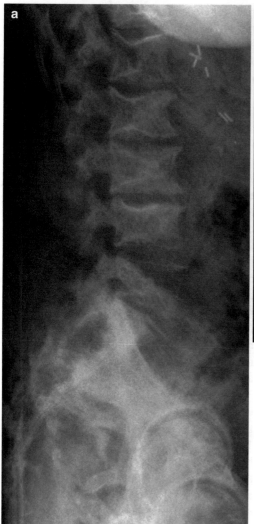

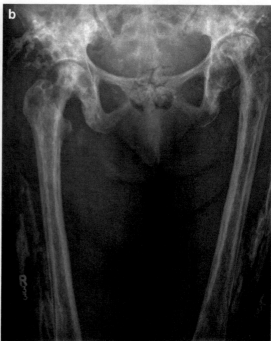

Fig. 36.10 A 66-year-old woman undergoing staging for new diagnosis of multiple myeloma. (**a**) Lateral radiograph of the lumbar spine and (**b**) AP radiograph of the lower pelvis and proximal femurs show multifocal osteosclerotic changes of sickle cell disease with "H"-shaped vertebral bodies and characteristic bone infarcts within the femoral shafts. There is unusual heterotopic ossification in the soft tissues of the pelvis and thighs. Patient also had known sickle cell trait and had chronic complaints of bone pain

hip regions, and proximal long bones (Fig. 36.13). Normal red marrow is distinguished from pathological processes in these areas on MRI by its signal intensity, distribution, and feathered edge appearance. T1-weighted signal intensity of normal red marrow should be more hyperintense than adjacent skeletal muscle, and hyperintensity of T2-weighted signal intensity is typically minimal.

Fig. 36.12 A 71-year-old man with new diagnosis of lung cancer and complaints of vague left hip pain. Initial coronal (**a**) T1-W and (**b**) STIR MR images show patchy areas of bone marrow change with more focal questionable abnormality in the left ischium. Axial (**c**) in-phase and (**d**) out-of-phase MR images show signal dropout, indicative of normal red marrow, not metastatic disease

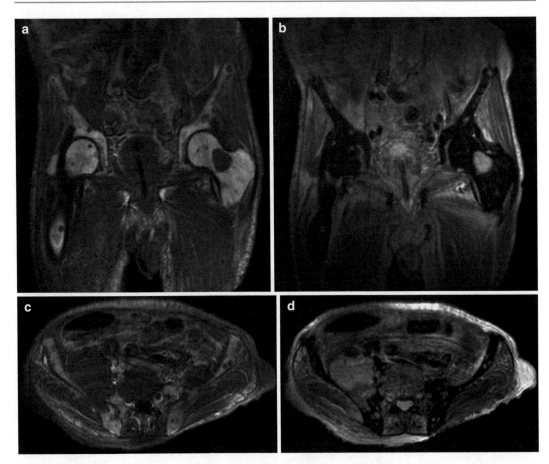

Fig. 36.11 An 85-year-old man with known prostate cancer and complaints of left hip pain. Initial coronal (**a**) T1-W and (**b**) STIR MR images show multiple focal areas of T1 signal hypointensity and STIR signal hyperintensity consistent with metastases. Axial (**c**) in-phase and (**d**) out-of-phase (**d**) images show no signal dropout, most readily evident in the lesions involving the left iliac wing, which also indicate pathologic marrow process consistent with metastatic disease

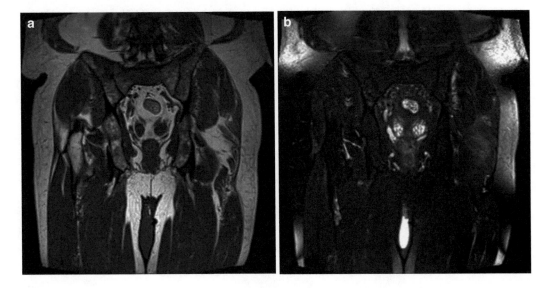

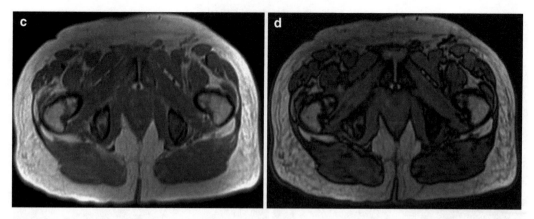

Fig. 36.12 (continued)

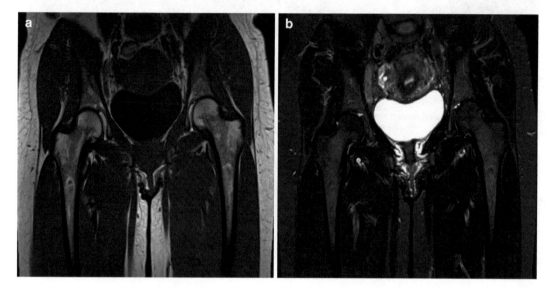

Fig. 36.13 A 46-year-old woman with history of lymphoma and new left groin pain after running. Coronal (**a**) T1-W and (**b**) STIR MR images show normal areas of red marrow within each acetabular roof and each proximal femur with feathery pattern and T1 signal intensity higher than adjacent skeletal muscle and no significant increase in signal intensity on STIR images. Findings are characteristic of normal red marrow

When there is red marrow reconversion of previous yellow marrow areas (especially in distal long bones), red marrow is usually confined to the metaphysis and usually does not extend into the epiphysis, although there are exceptions to this rule. Red marrow reconversion is reported to result from many different causes and conditions including obesity, smoking, heavy menses, high-altitude living, and increased demand in high-performance athletes (Wilson et al. 1996). However, when there is complete red marrow reconversion in the metaphysis of the distal femur, as might be seen on routine knee MRI (Fig. 36.14), correlation with laboratory studies is suggested, since a study by Gonzalez et al. (2016) indicated that half of the patients with such findings would demonstrate a

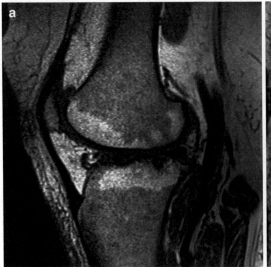
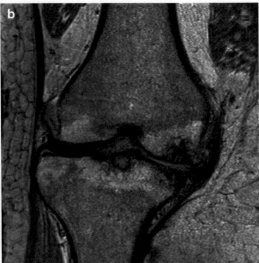

Fig. 36.14 A 47-year-old woman with persistent knee pain after a fall 1 month prior. Routine (**a**) sagittal T1-W and (**b**) coronal PD-W MR images of the knee show extensive red marrow reconversion throughout the entire metaphyses of the distal femur and proximal tibia. There is even extension into the epiphyses. Such extensive red marrow reconversion is concerning for anemia despite the

presence of other factors, including obesity and history of smoking. Knee pain is secondary to medial meniscus tear and associated degenerative changes in the medial compartment, with extensive articular cartilage loss and subchondral bone changes in the medial femoral condyle and medial tibial plateau

true anemia, whether the patient was obese or not. Please also refer to Chap. 37 on hematological and circulatory bone lesions: imaging pitfalls for further information on red marrow reconversion.

36.4   Mimics of Osteoblastic Metastases

36.4.1 Bone Islands

Bone islands (enostoses) are foci of normal cortical bone that are found in the cancellous bone or marrow compartment. They have a characteristic radiographic appearance of a feathered edge that blends into the adjacent bony trabeculae without any surrounding bone destruction (Fig. 36.15). Their appearance on CT is similar to osteoblastic metastases, but in addition, CT will show uniform dense mineralization with very high Hounsfield

units (HU), typically measuring >1000 HU. These findings should allow confident distinction of a bone island from an osteoblastic metastasis. Bone islands show uniform hypointense signal on all MRI pulse sequences. They do not typically have significant increased uptake on Tc-99m bone scintigraphy.

36.4.2 Osteopoikilosis, Tuberous Sclerosis, and Mastocytosis

These three conditions do not usually pose much of a diagnostic dilemma, since the patients have other characteristic clinical manifestations that allow for distinction from osteoblastic metastases. Patients with osteopoikilosis have multiple small osteoblastic foci in many areas of the skeleton that have been present from early in life. The long bone lesions are clustered proximally and

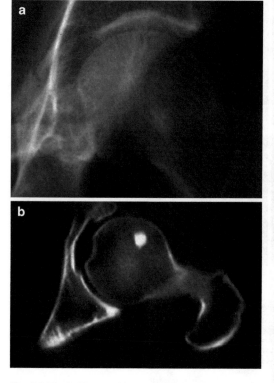

Fig. 36.15 A 59-year-old man with left hip pain. (**a**) AP radiograph shows a small focal osteoblastic lesion within the femoral neck that has characteristic feathered edges blending into the normal adjacent trabecular bone. (**b**) Axial CT image confirms a homogeneous densely osteoblastic lesion characteristic of a bone island

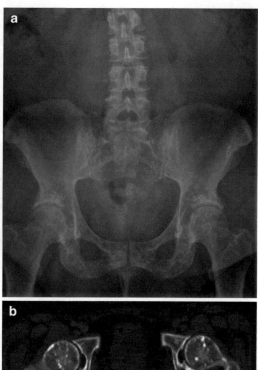

Fig. 36.16 A 38-year-old woman with complaints of abdominal pain. (**a**) Abdominal radiograph shows numerous tiny osteoblastic foci throughout the bones of the pelvis as well as within the femoral heads and necks. (**b**) Axial CT image from the abdominal/pelvic exam confirms multiple intramedullary osteoblastic foci characteristic of osteopoikilosis

involve the epiphyses (Fig. 36.16). Epiphyseal involvement is not a usual feature of metastatic disease. Patients with tuberous sclerosis, or tuberous sclerosis complex, are usually diagnosed in infancy or early childhood, based on the presence of typical calcified tubers in the brain, visceral organs, and other sites like the skin. Those with mastocytosis must have the systemic form to develop sclerotic changes of the bone. One pitfall, however, is that patients with mastocytosis may show abnormal areas of uptake on PET/CT (Djelbani-Ahmed et al. 2015).

36.4.3 POEMS Syndrome

POEMS syndrome is an unusual disorder with a classic description of five features: polyneuropathy, organomegaly, endocrine abnormalities, monoclonal gammopathy, and skin lesions. More recently, major and minor criteria have been established, since patients often present with more than the five classic features. The three major criteria that must be met are polyneuropathy, monoclonal gammopathy, and presence of bone lesions (Dispenzieri 2015). A review of imaging findings in 24 patients with POEMS syndrome by Glazebrook et al. (2015) indicated that 75% had at least five bone lesions. The most common pattern was multiple small lesions, usually less than 1 cm in size (Fig. 36.17). Larger lesions had central osteolytic areas that can help to distinguish them from other osteoblastic entities such as bone islands (Glazebrook et al. 2015).

36.5 Mimics of Osteolytic Metastases

36.5.1 Osteoporosis

Age-related decrease in bone mineral density is a global health problem that affects older women more than older men. The major health concern relates to fractures of vertebral bodies and hips with their attendant morbidity and mortality. As a result of their symptoms, these patients frequently have imaging studies of the spine (Fig. 36.18) and pelvis that can present a confusing picture. Focal areas of osteolysis can be mistaken for osteolytic metastases. One easy way to avoid this pitfall on CT is to measure the HU within the areas of osteolysis and to measure the overall value within the L1 vertebral body. Focal marrow-related changes of osteoporosis will have HU less than 20, whereas osteolytic destructive metastases will have HU typically greater than 40. Generalized L1 vertebral body measurements less than 110 HU correlate

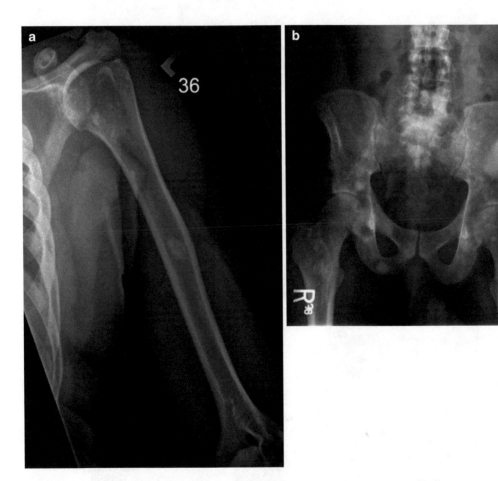

Fig. 36.17 A 51-year-old man with new clinical diagnosis of POEMS syndrome. Selected radiographs from a complete skeletal survey show multiple focal osteoblastic lesions throughout the (**a**) left humeral shaft, (**b**) pelvis, and (**c**) lumbar spine. Axial and sagittal CT images of the (**d**) lumbar spine, (**e**) upper chest, and (**f**) lower pelvis also show multiple densely osteoblastic intramedullary lesions, consistent with the clinical diagnosis

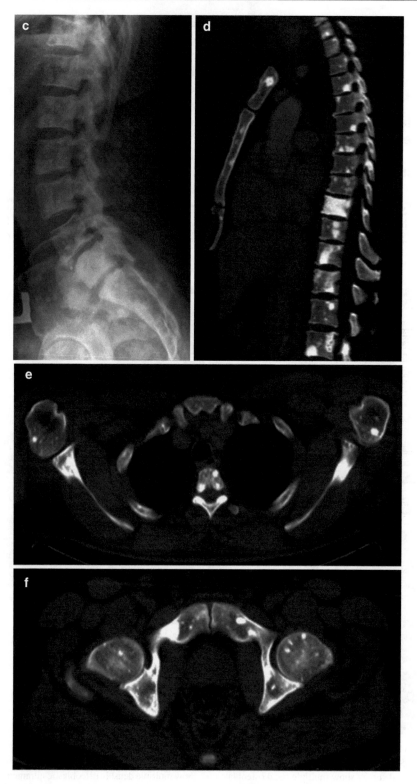

Fig. 36.17 (continued)

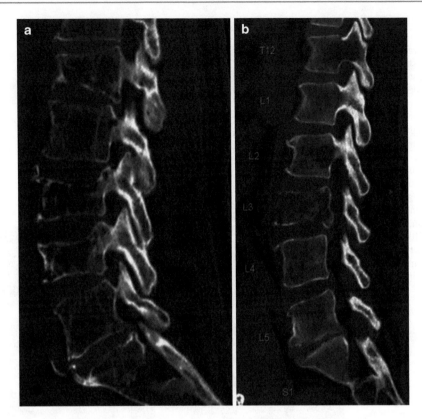

Fig. 36.18 An example of osteoporosis mimicking metastatic disease. (**a**) Sagittal CT image of the lumbar spine in a patient with osteoporosis shows compression fractures at *L1*, *L3*, and *L4* vertebral bodies with end plate deformities but no bone destruction. Compare this CT image to the CT of a 63-year-old woman with persistent back pain after a fall 1 month previously. (**b**) Sagittal CT image shows multiple osteolytic lesions, most predominantly involving *T12*, *L2*, and *L3* vertebrae. There is pathologic compression fracture of *L3* vertebra. Discrete focal pattern of osteolysis, especially with extension into the pedicles and posterior elements at *T12* level, indicates a pathological process and not simple osteoporosis. This lesion was subsequently proven to be from previously unknown breast cancer

well with diagnosis of decreased bone mineral density by dual energy X-ray absorptiometry (DXA) studies (Pickhardt et al. 2013; Lee et al. 2016).

36.5.2 Polyostotic Fibrous Dysplasia

Polyostotic fibrous dysplasia lesions typically have a characteristic radiographic appearance of focal osteolysis with expanded remodeling and cortical thinning. The classic "ground glass" matrix mineralization may not be detectable with conventional radiographs (Fig. 36.19). On CT, the "ground glass" matrix mineralization can be detected more readily, especially if one measures the HU of the lesion. This usually will be in the range of 70–130 HU. Unusual cases have been reported that mimic metastatic disease (Lee et al. 2014).

36.5.3 Langerhans Cell Histiocytosis

Langerhans cell histiocytosis usually affects children and has three major presentations, namely, a

Fig. 36.19 A 45-year-old man with right hip pain. (**a**) AP radiograph of the pelvis shows large osteolytic lesions with sclerotic borders involving the right ilium and intertrochanteric area of the right femur. These are benign-appearing but nonspecific. (**b, c**) Axial CT images show more characteristic ground glass appearance with Hounsfield units averaging 110 in the (**c**) intertrochanteric area of the femur, confirming diagnosis of fibrous dysplasia

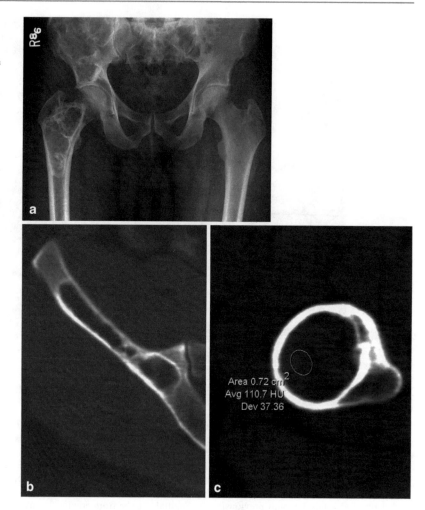

solitary form also known as eosinophilic granuloma, a multifocal form with the designation Hand-Schüller-Christian disease, and a severe systemic form known as Letterer-Siwe disease. Even the usual solitary form may present with more than one skeletal lesion and can cause concern for more aggressive processes, including metastatic disease (Nguyen et al. 2010). Early in their course, the lesions can have an aggressive appearance, with focal osteolysis and periosteal reaction (Fig. 36.20). A common differential diagnostic consideration is osteomyelitis. When there is involvement of the skull, recognition of the classic beveled edge sign and the presence of a sequestrum can help to make the correct diagnosis (Fig. 36.21). Sequestra are not common in metastatic lesions.

36.5.4 Infectious Conditions

Many infectious agents are endemic around the globe and cause tremendous pain and suffering. Single focal areas of skeletal involvement (osteomyelitis) are not usually confusing to the trained clinician or radiologist. However, patients with multifocal disease can have a confusing presentation. Infectious conditions that may have multiple areas of skeletal involvement include tuberculosis,

Fig. 36.20 A 14-month-old boy with arm swelling. (**a**) AP and (**b**) lateral radiographs show an osteolytic lesion within the proximal ulna with extensive surrounding sclerosis and periosteal reaction, suggestive of osteomyelitis. Subsequently proven to represent eosinophilic granuloma

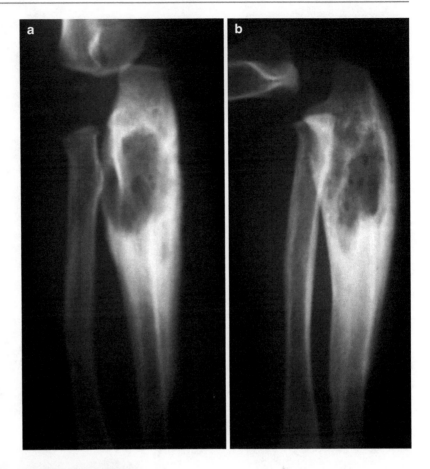

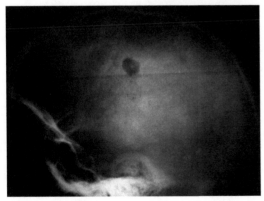

Fig. 36.21 Lateral radiograph of a 3-year-old child shows a focal osteolytic lesion in the skull, which demonstrates the characteristic central sequestrum of eosinophilic granuloma

syphilis, yaws, and many others. Noninfectious syndromes, including chronic recurrent multifocal osteomyelitis (CRMO) and SAPHO syndrome

(acronym for synovitis, acne, pustulosis, hyperostosis, and osteitis), may be similarly confusing. For these latter two, characteristic distribution of areas of involvement and other nonskeletal findings will help to make the diagnosis. Another unique patient group includes those with human immunodeficiency virus (HIV)/acquired immunodeficiency syndrome (AIDS). This is another worldwide problem. Patients frequently have imaging of the chest and abdomen for nonskeletal reasons but may demonstrate areas of skeletal abnormality. In this patient group, one entity to be aware of is bacillary angiomatosis. This process is caused by *Bartonella henselae* or *quintana* and can result in a multifocal osteomyelitis (Frean et al. 2002). Lesions usually are reported to appear as focal areas of osteolysis, but osteoblastic foci also may be seen.

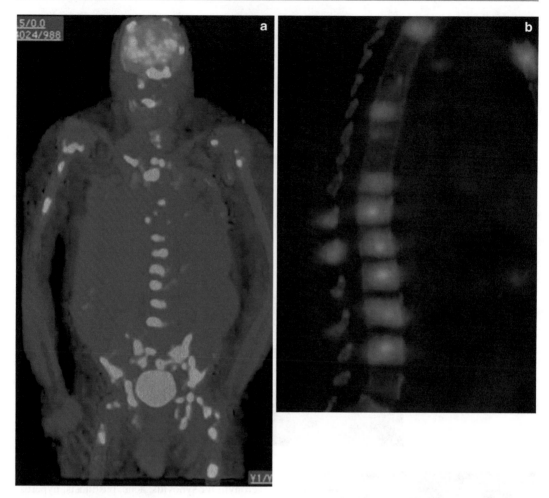

Fig. 36.22 Example of sarcoid mimicking metastatic disease. 47-year-old Caucasian man who presented to local emergency department with complaint of flank pain. He was found to have incidental osteolytic lesions on CT done to evaluate for renal calculi. Subsequent bone survey showed multiple lesions throughout the axial skeleton and long bones thought to be due to metastatic disease. (**a**) AP and (**b**) lateral PET/CT images also show multiple focal areas of abnormal uptake throughout the skeleton including the skull, proximal humeri, spine, pelvis, and proximal femurs. Patient had open biopsy of humeral lesion with pathologic diagnosis of sarcoidosis

36.5.5 Sarcoidosis

Sarcoidosis is a non-caseating granulomatous disease that is common in people of African descent. When typical pulmonary findings are present on chest radiographs, the diagnosis is not difficult. Multifocal osseous involvement is most common in the small bones of the hands, where it is also not usually a diagnostic puzzle when the characteristic lacelike pattern is present in the phalanges. However, some cases of multifocal axial skeletal involvement (Fig. 36.22), with or without other more typical findings, have been reported (Talmi et al. 2008) In these cases, biopsy of individual lesions may be needed to exclude unknown metastatic disease.

36.5.6 Brown Tumors

Brown tumors may be encountered in patients with various forms of hyperparathyroidism. They

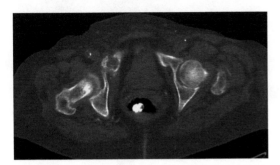

Fig. 36.23 A 64-year-old patient with end-stage renal disease, diabetes mellitus, and groin pain. Axial CT image taken through the lower pelvis shows a focal osteolytic lesion in the right superior pubic ramus that was biopsy-proven to represent a brown tumor

may be solitary or multifocal. The usual imaging appearance is an osteolytic lesion with expansile remodeling (Fig. 36.23). They can mimic metastases from primary tumors that are prone to have the osteolytic/blowout pattern, as is common in patients with primary renal or thyroid cancers (Fig. 36.24).

36.5.7 Paget Disease

Paget disease has several different phases including osteolytic, mixed, sclerotic, and sarcomatous (Figs. 36.25 and 36.26). Osteolytic phase lesions,

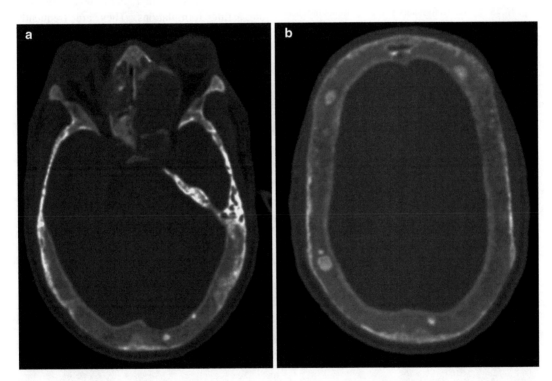

Fig. 36.24 A 35-year-old man with chronic hypertension, end-stage renal disease, and tertiary hyperparathyroidism. Axial CT images taken through the (**a**) face and (**b**) upper skull show an expanded blowout-type osteolytic lesion in the left ethmoid sinus that was biopsy-proven to represent a brown tumor. There is generalized abnormality of the calvarium secondary to osteitis fibrosa cystica

especially osteoporosis circumscripta of the skull, can be mistaken for metastases. Skeletal involvement can be unifocal or multifocal.

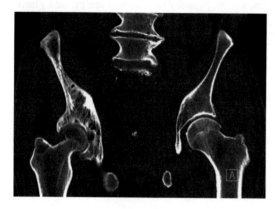

Fig. 36.25 Coronal reformatted CT image shows the characteristic changes of Paget disease involving the right hemipelvis with cortical thickening and trabecular coarsening, which is obvious when compared to the normal *left side*

36.6 Treatment-/Medication-Related Lesions

Voriconazole is a medication that is often given to patients after organ transplant (especially lung transplant) for prophylaxis against the development of aspergillosis. This agent is a trifluoro compound that can give rise to a painful, reactive periostitis within a matter of days of its administration (Fig. 36.27). The reactive periostitis is commonly seen along the clavicles, proximal long bones, ribs, and pelvic bones and can be mistaken for more aggressive processes including metastatic disease (Chen and Mulligan 2011).

Granulocyte colony-stimulating factors (GCSF) are medications found in both short- and long-acting formulations. They are frequently used in cancer patients, in addition to chemotherapy agents, to counter the effect of chemotherapy

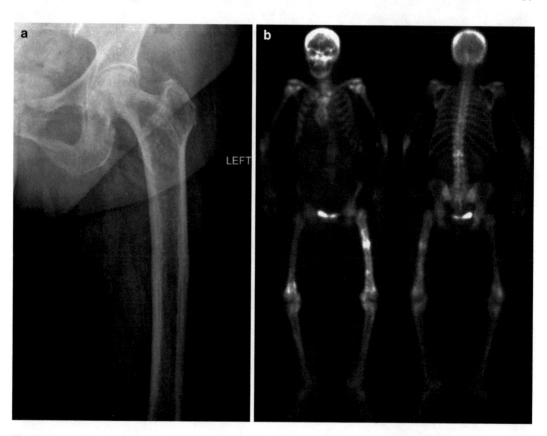

Fig. 36.26 A 73-year-old woman with left thigh pain. (**a**) Radiograph of the left femur shows cortical thickening and trabecular coarsening typical of Paget disease. (**b**) Tc-99m bone scintiscan shows focal areas of abnormal uptake at two separate locations within the femoral shaft, most intense in the subtrochanteric region. (**c**) FDG PET/CT image shows extensive increased uptake throughout the entire shaft of the femur. Coronal (**d**) T1-W and (**e**) STIR MR images show abnormal bone marrow replacement throughout the entire shaft of the femur that raised concerns for sarcomatous degeneration or other neoplastic involvement. Open biopsy revealed metastasis from newly diagnosed lung carcinoma

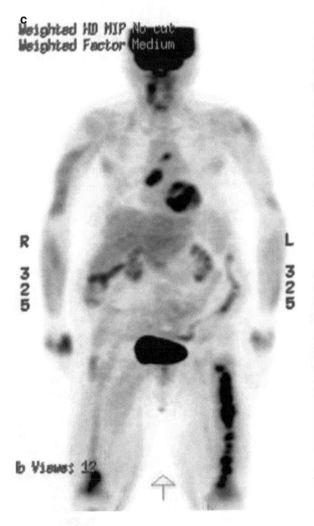

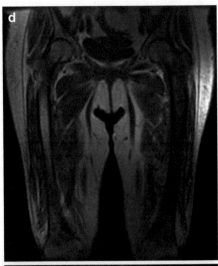

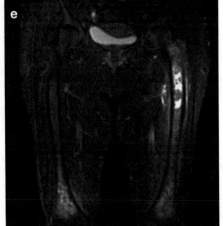

Fig. 36.26 (continued)

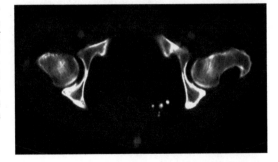

Fig. 36.27 A 37-year-old woman with known acute myelogenous leukemia in remission who complained of abdominal pain. CT of the abdomen/pelvis shows several areas of proliferative new bone formation along the anterior margins of the pubic rami and proximal femoral shafts, atypical for osseous involvement by leukemia. The patient's medications included voriconazole which is known to be associated with periosteal new bone formation

on bone marrow suppression. The bone marrow stimulation effects of GCSF agents can mimic persistent or progressive disease because they can cause multiple focal areas of red marrow to appear or to be more prominent. Follow-up imaging in patients receiving such agents should be scheduled to avoid the time frame when there would be an expected bone marrow response. One must also consider the patient's overall response to their treatment. If their primary tumor and any other known areas of metastatic disease are responding to treatment, then it would not be likely that new areas of "disease" would be appearing.

Diffusion-weighted imaging, with b values of 50 s/mm^2 and 800 or 900 s/mm^2 with an apparent diffusion coefficient (ADC) value cutoff of 774 μm^2/s, has been reported as one way to make the distinction between normal and abnormal bone marrow foci, thereby avoiding this pitfall (Padhani et al. 2013). Bone marrow response can be generalized or focal. Focal hematopoietic hyperplasia also can mimic pathological conditions. However, if there is a correlating CT study, one can evaluate the focus of abnormality by CT

for the presence of bone osteolysis or osteosclerosis. Focal hematopoietic hyperplasia does not demonstrate areas of osteosclerosis or osteolytic destruction (Biffar et al. 2010).

Conclusion

Remember that individual cases do not always follow the standard or usual path. Do not always expect "classic" imaging features, for example, do not exclude prostate cancer metastases from your differential diagnosis of multiple osteolytic lesions in older men (Fig. 36.28). A final pitfall when evaluating imaging studies is to ignore the

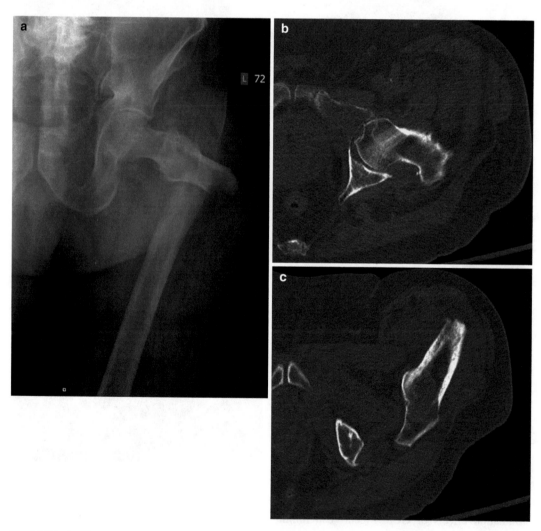

Fig. 36.28 An 87-year-old man presenting with left thigh pain. Patient had no known history of malignancy. (**a**) Initial AP radiograph of the left hip shows a pathological subtrochanteric fracture. Note osteolytic destruction of the left superior pubic ramus at the acetabular junction. (**b**,

c) Axial CT images confirm osteolytic destruction of the left superior pubic ramus and permeative destruction at the subtrochanteric fracture site. Patient was subsequently proven to have metastatic prostate carcinoma with unusual osteolytic lesions

information from other recent imaging examinations. For example, it has been shown that combining the information from spine MRI and PET/CT studies in myeloma patients can be helpful for predicting impending pathological fractures (Mulligan et al. 2011).

References

Biffar A, Baur-Melnyk A, Schmidt GP et al (2010) MRI assessment of normal-appearing and diseased vertebral bone marrow. Eur Radiol 20:2679–2689

Breyer RJ 3rd, Mulligan ME, Smith SE et al (2006) Comparison of imaging with FDG PET/CT with other imaging modalities in myeloma. Skeletal Radiol 35: 632–640

Brioli A, Morgan GJ, Durie B et al (2014) The utility of newer imaging techniques as predictors of clinical outcomes in multiple myeloma. Expert Rev Hematol 7:13–16

Chen L, Mulligan M (2011) Voriconazole medication-induced periostitis in lung transplant patients: periostitis deformans revisited. Skeletal Radiol 40:143–148

Coleman R (2006) Clinical features of metastatic bone disease and risk of skeletal morbidity. Clin Cancer Res 12:6243s–6249s

Delgado-Calle J, Bellido T, Roodman GD (2014) Role of osteocytes in multiple myeloma bone disease. Curr Opin Support Palliat Care 8:407–413

Disler D, McCauley T, Ratner L et al (1997) In-phase and out-of-phase MR imaging of bone marrow: prediction of neoplasia based on the detection of coexistent fat and water. AJR Am J Roentgenol 169:1439–1447

Dispenzieri A (2015) POEMS syndrome: update on diagnosis, risk-stratification, and management. Am J Hematol 90:951–962

Djelbani-Ahmed S, Chandesris MO, Mekinian A et al (2015) FDG-PET/CT findings in systemic mastocytosis: a French multicentre study. Eur J Nucl Med Mol Imaging 42:2013–2020

Edelstyn GA, Gillespie PJ, Grebbell FS (1967) The radiological demonstration of osseous metastases. Experimental observations. Clin Radiol 18:158–162

Frean J, Arndt S, Spencer D (2002) High rate of Bartonella henselae infection in HIV-positive outpatients in Johannesburg, South Africa. Trans R Soc Trop Med Hyg 96:549–550

Giles SL, Messiou C, Collins DJ et al (2014) Whole-body diffusion-weighted MR imaging for assessment of treatment response in myeloma. Radiology 271:785–794

Glazebrook K, Bonilla F, Johnson A et al (2015) Computed tomography assessment of bone lesions in patients with POEMS syndrome. Eur Radiol 25:497–504

Gonzalez F, Mitchell J, Monfred E et al (2016) Knee MRI patterns of bone marrow reconversion and relationship to anemia. Acta Radiol 57:964–970

Healy CF, Murray JG, Eustace SJ, et al. Multiple myeloma: a review of imaging features and radiological techniques. Bone Marrow Res. 2011;2011:article ID 583439.

Lee JH, Kim SY, Lee JE et al (2014) Polyostotic fibrous dysplasia mimicking multiple bone metastases in a patient with ductal carcinoma in situ. J Breast Cancer 17:83–87

Lee SJ, Binkley N, Lubner MG et al (2016) Opportunistic screening for osteoporosis using the sagittal reconstruction from routine abdominal CT for combined assessment of vertebral fractures and density. Osteoporos Int 27:1131–1136

Mulligan M, Chirindel A, Karchevsky M (2011) Characterizing and predicting pathologic spine fractures in myeloma patients with FDG PET/CT and MR imaging. Cancer Invest 29:370–376

Nguyen BD, Roarke MC, Chivers SF (2010) Multifocal Langerhans cell histiocytosis with infiltrative pelvic lesions: PET/CT imaging. Clin Nucl Med 35:824–826

Padhani A, van Ree K, Collins D et al (2013) Assessing the relationship between bone marrow signal intensity and apparent diffusion coefficient in diffusion-weighted MRI. AJR Am J Roentgenol 200: 163–170

Pickhardt PJ, Pooler BD, Lauder T et al (2013) Opportunistic screening for osteoporosis using abdominal computed tomography scans obtained for other indications. Ann Intern Med 158:588–595

Raphael B, Hwang S, Lefkowitz RA et al (2013) Biopsy of suspicious bone lesions in patients with a single known malignancy: prevalence of a second malignancy. AJR Am J Roentgenol 20:1309–1314

Talmi D, Smith S, Mulligan ME (2008) Central skeletal sarcoidosis mimicking metastatic disease. Skeletal Radiol 37:757–761

Ulaner G, Hwang S, Landa J et al (2013) Musculoskeletal tumours and tumour-like conditions: common and avoidable pitfalls at imaging in patients with known or suspected cancer. Part B: malignant mimics of benign tumours. Int Orthop 37:877–882

Wilson AJ, Hodge JC, Pilgram TK et al (1996) Prevalence of red marrow around the knee joint in adults as demonstrated on magnetic resonance imaging. Acad Radiol 3:550–555

Yang J, Terebelo H, Zonder J. Secondary primary malignancies in multiple myeloma: an old nemesis revisited. Adv Hematol. 2012;2012:article ID 801495.

Zajick D, Morrison W, Schweitzer M et al (2005) Benign and malignant processes: normal values and differentiation with chemical shift MR imaging in vertebral marrow. Radiology 237:590–596

Hematological and Circulatory Bone Lesions: Imaging Pitfalls

37

Suphaneewan Jaovisidha, Khalid Al-Ismail, Niyata Chitrapazt, and Praman Fuengfa

Contents

37.1 **Introduction** 767

37.2 **Bone Marrow: Normal and Variants** 768
37.2.1 MRI of Normal Bone Marrow 768
37.2.2 Normal Marrow Conversion 768
37.2.3 Reconversion of Bone Marrow 771

37.3 **Osteonecrosis** 772
37.3.1 Introduction and Pathophysiology 772
37.3.2 Treatment Decision-Making 772
37.3.3 Imaging Diagnosis 773
37.3.4 Femoral Head Osteonecrosis:
       Imaging Pitfalls 782
37.3.5 Osteonecrosis at the Other Sites: Imaging
       Pitfalls 786
37.3.6 Malignant Transformation of
       Osteonecrosis 789

37.4 **Thalassemia** 789
37.4.1 Introduction and Pathophysiology 789
37.4.2 Imaging Bone Changes 792
37.4.3 Pitfalls, Mimics, and Differentials 801

37.5 **Sickle Cell Disease** 803
37.5.1 Introduction and Pathophysiology 803
37.5.2 Imaging Bone Changes 804
37.5.3 Pitfalls and Mimics of Bone Changes 809

Conclusion 814

References 814

Abbreviations

CT   Computed tomography
EMH   Extramedullary hematopoiesis
MRI   Magnetic resonance imaging
SCD   Sickle cell disease

S. Jaovisidha, MD (✉) • N. Chitrapazt, MD
P. Fuengfa, MD
Department of Diagnostic and Therapeutic
Radiology, Faculty of Medicine, Mahidol University,
Ramathibodi Hospital, 270 Rama VI Road,
Ratchatewi, Bangkok 10400, Thailand
e-mail: rasjv@yahoo.com; mail_nit@yahoo.com;
time_today@hotmail.com

K. Al-Ismail, MD
Department of Radiology, King Faisal Specialist
Hospital & Research Centre, Zahrawi Street, Al
Maather, Riyadh 12713, Kingdom of Saudi Arabia
e-mail: kalismail@yahoo.com

37.1 Introduction

In this chapter, hematological and circulatory bone diseases refer to two types of benign hematological conditions: abnormal red blood cell production (hemoglobinopathy) and decreased blood flow, including their subsequent complications. Magnetic resonance imaging (MRI) features of normal bone marrow from birth to elderly, along with the normal variants that may be diagnostic pitfalls, are addressed. Since this chapter has been written by authors located in the endemic areas of thalassemia and sickle cell disease (SCD), these two entities ideally illustrate abnormal red blood cell production. Both thalassemia and SCD are hemoglobinopathies that produce a large variety of imaging findings. Some

© Springer International Publishing AG 2017
W.C.G. Peh (ed.), *Pitfalls in Musculoskeletal Radiology*, DOI 10.1007/978-3-319-53496-1_37

imaging features are similar, while some may overlap with each other and with other diseases. Decreased blood flow or ischemic change of bone can occur from many causes and may result in osteonecrosis, with resultant characteristic imaging findings. Imaging pitfalls and mimics can be encountered in every disease. There are many normal variants that radiologists should know and not misinterpret as disease. Some of the pathological processes may be misinterpreted as being normal structures. This chapter will review characteristic imaging findings of each entity, addressing the imaging pitfalls including how to avoid them.

37.2 Bone Marrow: Normal and Variants

37.2.1 MRI of Normal Bone Marrow

There are two types of bone marrow, namely, red and yellow marrow, which are defined by their physiology. Red marrow is active hematopoietic marrow. The chemical compositions of red marrow are 40% water, 40% fat, and 20% protein, whereas the cellular compositions are 60% hematopoietic cells and 40% fat cells. Yellow marrow is inactive hematopoietic marrow. The chemical compositions of yellow marrow are 80% fat, 15% water, and 5% protein, and the cellular compositions are 95% fat cells and 5% nonfat cells (Vogler and Murphy 1988; Malkiewicz and Dziedzic 2012). The different cellularity and fat in bone marrow are indicated by the different signal intensities on the various MRI sequences.

In the spine, red marrow shows intermediate or slight signal hypointensity on T1-weighted MR images as compared to skeletal muscle, but signal intensity is higher than the intervertebral disk. Red marrow signal hyperintensity seen on T2-weighted images is slightly lower than that of yellow marrow. Because signal intensities of water and fat on T2-weighted image are closer, detection of a pathological lesion on T2-weighted images may be limited. T2-weighted images with addition of fat suppression may be more helpful since the hyperintense signal is clearly observed (Shah and Hanrahan 2011; Bracken et al. 2013) (Fig. 37.1). Due to high fat component of the yellow marrow, signal intensity of the yellow marrow is high on T1-weighted images, similar to the subcutaneous fat. On T2-weighted images, yellow marrow shows signal hyperintensity compared to muscle and intermediate to slightly hypointense signal compared to subcutaneous fat. On fat-suppressed T2-weighted images, yellow marrow shows signal hypointensity (Shah and Hanrahan 2011; Bracken et al. 2013).

37.2.2 Normal Marrow Conversion

In the neonate, the bone marrow is hematopoietic and gradually converts to fatty marrow with age. Conversion of bone marrow begins in the first year of life. Complete marrow conversion in the appendicular skeleton parallels skeletal maturation, whereas marrow conversion in the axial skeleton is observed throughout life. In general, the adult pattern of bone marrow is achieved at the age of 25 years (Volger and Murphy 1988). The proportion of red marrow slowly decreases with age. Marrow conversion has a predictable pattern. It begins in the periphery and gradually extends to the central part of the appendicular skeleton. Fatty marrow occurs at the epiphysis and then diaphysis and lastly at the metaphysis (Fig. 37.2). The metaphysis of the proximal humeri and femurs is the last area of fatty transformation. However, red marrow in these areas may persist in normal adult (Volger and Murphy 1988; Malkiewicz and Dziedzic 2012) and is generally confined within the metaphysis.

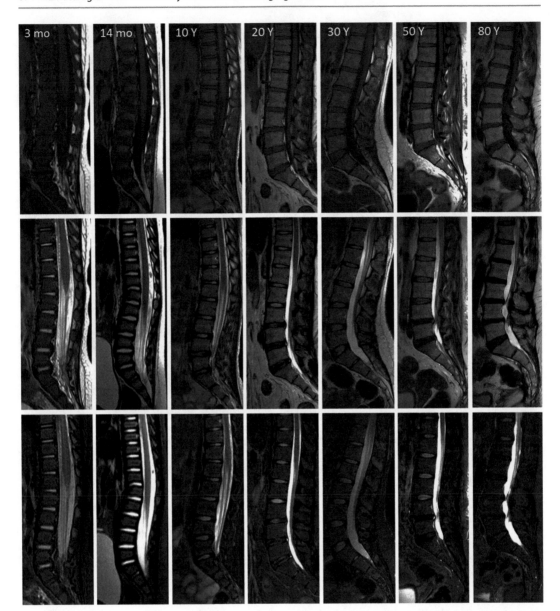

Fig. 37.1 Normal marrow conversion in the spine. Sagittal T1-W (*upper row*), T2-W (*middle row*), and STIR (*bottom row*) MR images of different patients with different ages (*mo: month; Y: year*). In children, most of bone marrow at the spine is red marrow so the signal intensity on the T1-W images is intermediate and on T2-W images is slightly hyperintense compared to skeletal muscle. Slightly progressively increased signal intensity of the bone marrow on the T1- and T2-W images is observed when the age increases and the red marrow converts to yellow marrow. Slightly hyperintense signal of the bone marrow on STIR images in children is due to red marrow, and the signal decreases with age as the proportion of the fat component increases in yellow marrow

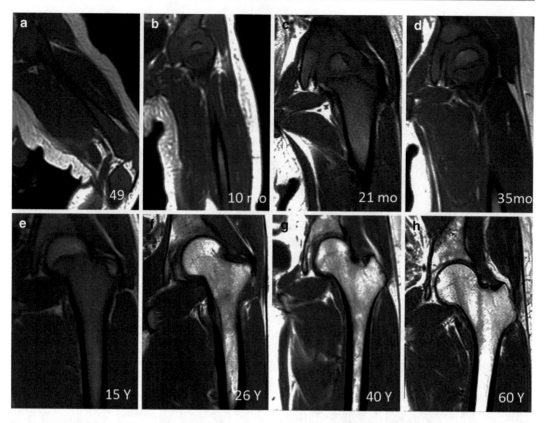

Fig. 37.2 Normal marrow conversion in the long bone. Coronal T1-W MR images of the bone marrow of the proximal femurs in different patients with varying ages: (**a**) 49 days, (**b**) 10 months, (**c**) 21 months, (**d**) 35 months, (**e**) 15 years, (**f**) 26 years, (**g**) 40 years, and (**h**) 60 years (*d: day; mo: month; Y: year*). Red marrow in early childhood is seen as intermediate signal intensity of the bone marrow at the femur. When the epiphysis begins to ossify, the ossified portion appears T1-hyperintense at the epiphysis. There is slow progression of increased T1 signal intensity from intermediate to high which corresponds to decreased proportion of red marrow and increased amount of yellow marrow, according to normal marrow conversion. When the bone is mature, the marrow pattern becomes an adult pattern so that T1 signal hyperintensity is seen in most of the femoral bone marrow, and small areas of intermediate signal red marrow are present at the metaphysis

On T1-weighted MR images, the signal intensity of "residual" red marrow is lower than that of fat, but generally higher than that of skeletal muscle due to an admixture of fatty elements with hematopoietic elements. On fat-suppressed T2-weighted MR images, the signal intensity is higher than that of yellow marrow and often is similar to or slightly higher than that of skeletal muscle. Residual red marrow is symmetrical in distribution, and hence its observation in both proximal femurs on pelvic MRI does not usually cause any diagnostic confusion (Stacy and Dixon 2007). Residual red marrow is often seen in the distal femur on MRI of the knee as well, particularly in adolescents, women of menstruating age, and obese subjects. They appear in a focal, streaky, patchy, or geographic pattern that mimics an infiltrative intramedullary lesion or neoplasm (Fig. 37.3). In females, hematopoietic marrow in the femur may occupy up to one-half or two-thirds of the shaft, without evidence of anemia or excessive blood loss (Shillingford 1950) (Fig. 37.3). The epiphysis always contains fatty marrow in adults, so any extension of red marrow into the epiphysis should raise the suspicion of abnormality (Shillingford 1950; Volger and Murphy 1988; Poulton et al. 1993; Stacy and Dixon 2007; Malkiewicz and Dziedzic 2012) (Fig. 37.4).

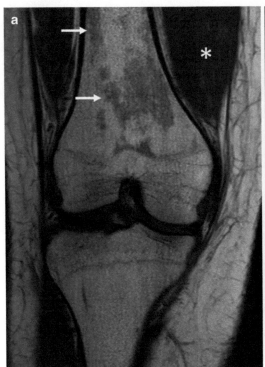
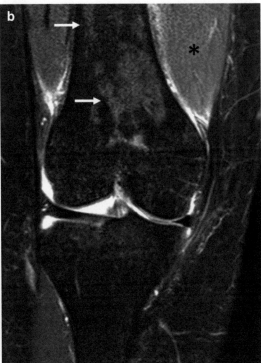

Fig. 37.3 Residual hematopoietic (or red) marrow. (**a**) Coronal T1-W MR image of a 33-year-old woman shows patchy regions of intermediate signal intensity (*arrows*) in the distal femur. These regions have signal intensity higher than that of the nearby skeletal muscle (*) and do not extend

into the epiphysis. (**b**) Sagittal fat-suppressed PD-W MR image shows a patchy area (*arrow*) with signal intensity similar to that of skeletal muscle (*). These characteristics are suggestive of residual red marrow. MRI findings of these features may be misinterpreted as potential malignancy

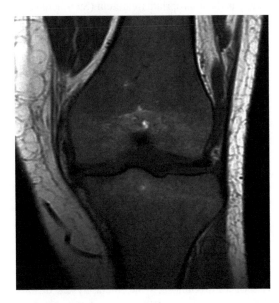

Fig. 37.4 Thalassemia. Coronal T1-W MR image shows hematopoietic marrow completely occupying the medullary cavity of the femur and tibia. The epiphyses are involved. This finding suggests disease process rather than residual marrow which is a normal variation

37.2.3 Reconversion of Bone Marrow

When the demand of hematopoietic cell is increased, yellow marrow can reconvert to red marrow in the reverse pattern of marrow conversion. Marrow reconversion starts from the proximal to peripheral regions, i.e., the process begins at the axial skeleton and progresses to the long bones. In long bones, marrow reconversion begins in the proximal metaphysis, followed by distal metaphysis and diaphysis, respectively. The causes of bone marrow reconversion are chronic anemia (i.e., thalassemia and sickle cell anemia) (Fig. 37.4), increased oxygen consumption (i.e., living at high altitude and athletes), hematopoietic growth factor (Volger and Murphy 1988; Laor and Jaramillo 2009; Malkiewicz and Dziedzic 2012), heart failure (Shillingford 1950), and smoking (Poulton et al. 1993). A pathological study regarding hematopoietic marrow in the femur in relation to cardiovascular diseases showed that essential hypertension alone has no effect on the hematopoietic marrow, but when cardiac failure has been present, there is a marked increase in the red marrow. This increase of red marrow, although present, does not occur to such an extent in heart failure associated with emphysema or mitral stenosis (Shillingford 1950). In smokers, it is not known whether marrow reconversion occurs as a result of tissue hypoxia from increased carboxyhemoglobin and resultant stimulation of red blood cell production or from other factors (Poulton et al. 1993).

37.3 Osteonecrosis

37.3.1 Introduction and Pathophysiology

Osteonecrosis, like infarction in other organs, results from significant reduction or obliteration of blood supply to the affected area of bone. Pathogenic mechanisms of osteonecrosis consist of ischemic changes, direct cellular toxicity, and altered differentiation of mesenchymal stem cells. The ischemic change may result from vascular disruption (i.e., trauma or surgery), vascular compression or constriction, and intravascular occlusion (i.e., thrombosis of any cause). Direct cellular toxicity can occur after irradiation, pharmacologic agents (i.e., chemotherapy), and oxidative stress. Osteonecrosis has been linked to human immunodeficiency virus (HIV); perhaps these patients have more risk factors (e.g., corticosteroid, alcohol, and antiviral therapy). Altered differentiation of mesenchymal stem cells, i.e., decreased osteogenesis and increased adipogenesis, as in patients with corticosteroid usage or alcohol consumption, may result in osteonecrosis of the bone by extrinsic compression to the vessels by the increased adipose cells (Resnick et al. 2002; Zalavras and Lieberman 2014; Mont et al. 2015).

Multiple risk factors have been described in osteonecrosis, which relate to the pathogenic mechanisms, including trauma, excessive alcohol consumption, corticosteroid, hemoglobinopathies, coagulation disorders, dysbaric phenomena, autoimmune diseases (generally cause vasculitis with resultant thickening of the vascular wall and, hence, varying degree of decreased blood flow), smoking, and hyperlipidemia (Resnick et al. 2002). Any patient exposed to more than one risk factors, i.e., connective tissue disease treated with corticosteroids, will increase the risk of osteonecrosis (Resnick et al. 2002; Zalavras and Lieberman 2014; Mont et al. 2015).

37.3.2 Treatment Decision-Making

Regarding the recent treatment options of osteonecrosis of the femoral head, which is the most well-recognized location involved by osteonecrosis, small medially located asymptomatic lesions may be treated with observation alone (Mont et al. 2015). For the symptomatic pre-collapse lesion, the treatment options are decompression (Marker et al. 2008; Rajagopal et al. 2012), osteotomy (Seki et al. 2008; Hamanishi et al. 2014), and non-vascularized or vascularized bone grafting (Mont et al. 2007; Zhang et al. 2013). When the patients reach the post-collapse stage, satisfactory results can be achieved with total hip arthroplasty or bone grafting (Amstutz and Le Duff 2010; Wang et al. 2013). When the signs of degenerative acetabular changes appear on radiographs, total hip arthroplasty is the appropriate treatment (Steinberg et al. 2008; Johannson et al. 2011). It is clear that imaging findings affect the treatment decision.

Imaging should provide adequate information for the physicians. Such information consists of (1) lesion size and location, (2) the presence or absence of head collapse, (3) degree of head depression, and (4) acetabular involvement (Schmitt-Sody et al. 2008; Mont et al. 2010; Lee and Steinberg 2012). Although a number of staging systems have been proposed, unfortunately, no validated classification system has received universal acceptance (Zibis et al. 2007; Schmitt-Sody et al. 2008; Lee and Steinberg 2012). The extent (size) of involvement is important for management (Mont et al. 2015). Subchondral lesions are also of concern because of the high risk of joint collapse, while metaphyseal lesions are less ominous. MRI is considered the gold standard for detecting the pre-collapse lesion of osteonecrosis or avascular necrosis (AVN) when without subchondral bone fracture (Zibis et al.

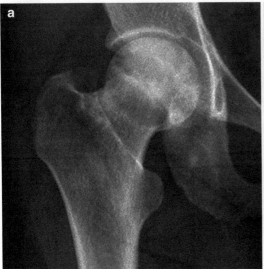
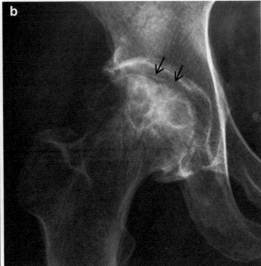

Fig. 37.5 Osteonecrosis of epiphysis on radiographs. (**a**) Frontal radiograph of a 36-year-old woman with history of using steroids shows ill-defined patchy radiolucent areas and sclerosis involving the femoral head. (**b**) Frontal radiograph of the right hip in a 74-year-old man shows arc-like subchondral bone collapse (*black arrows*) and subjacent multiple cystic changes. The joint space is preserved

2007; Lee et al. 2014; Zalavras and Lieberman 2014) or when osteonecrosis is considered clinically but radiographs look normal. When subchondral fracture is suspected but is not clearly delineated on radiographs, further investigation, i.e., computed tomography (CT) or MRI, should be performed with CT considered as the best modality in this clinical situation (Yeh et al. 2009). Once collapse or acetabular involvement is present on radiographs, no further imaging is needed for treatment decision-making.

37.3.3 Imaging Diagnosis

37.3.3.1 Radiography

Imaging evaluation of osteonecrosis should begin with radiography, as it is the least expensive and most widely available method of radiological assessment (Murphey et al. 2014). The radiographical findings of osteonecrosis at the epiphysis, metaphysis, or diaphysis of long bones or flat or irregular bones are so characteristic that additional diagnostic methods are frequently not required. Arc-like subchondral radiolucent lesions, patchy lucent areas and sclerosis, osseous collapse, and preserved joint space in the epiphyseal region are typical signs of osteonecrosis (Fig. 37.5). However, these abnormalities do not appear for several months after clinical onset in many patients, and, therefore, radiographs are not a sensitive indication for early disease (Strecker et al. 1988; Munk et al. 1989).

37.3.3.2 Bone Scintigraphy

Since radiography is relatively insensitive and establishing early diagnosis will help improve efficacy of treatment, this led to the use of other imaging techniques. Scintigraphy with bone-seeking radiopharmaceutical agents may be useful to evaluate clinically suspected femoral head osteonecrosis when the radiograph is still normal, or to study the contralateral "silent" hip in cases with unilateral osteonecrosis of the femoral head (Conklin et al. 1983; Kulkarni et al. 1987; Steinberg et al. 2008). Immediately after interruption of the osseous blood supply, bone scintigraphy can reveal an area of decreased or absent blood supply or a "cold" lesion and may require pinhole collimation (Fig. 37.6). This latter finding has been reported to appear earlier than MRI, when the MR images are still normal (Gohel et al. 1973; Conklin et al. 1983; Kulkarni et al. 1987; Murphey et al. 2014). The possible diseases

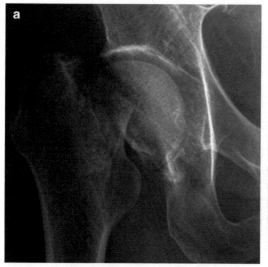

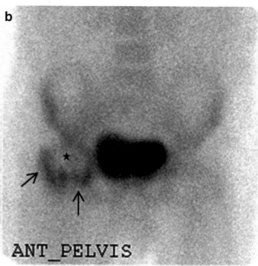

Fig. 37.6 Osteonecrosis of epiphysis seen as a cold lesion on bone scintigraphy. (**a**) Frontal radiograph of a 56-year-old man shows fracture of the femoral neck. The femoral head looks normal. (**b**) Tc-99 m bone scintiscan taken 2 days after the radiograph shows an area of increased uptake across the right femoral neck due to fracture (*black arrows*) and a large photopenic area in the right femoral head due to osteonecrosis (*black star*)

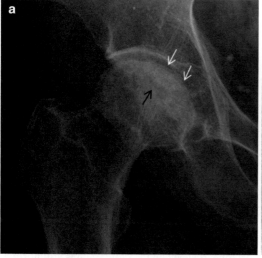

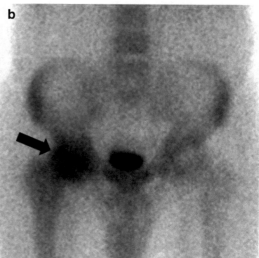

Fig. 37.7 Osteonecrosis of epiphysis seen as a hot lesion on bone scintigraphy. (**a**) Frontal radiograph of a 69-year-old man shows patchy sclerosis with fracture line (*black arrow*) and flattening of the right femoral head suggesting subchondral bone collapse (*white arrows*). These are late findings of osteonecrosis. (**b**) Tc-99 m bone scintiscan taken 13 days after the radiograph shows prominent increased uptake at the femoral head (*thick black arrow*) due to osteonecrosis

that can cause this cold area include infection, skeletal metastasis, hemangioma, plasma cell myeloma, and irradiation. Knowing the clinical history and correlation with radiographs is necessary to achieve the correct diagnosis.

After weeks or months, reparative process and revascularization in the surrounding bones lead to accumulation of the radioisotope, or a "hot" lesion (Alavi et al. 1977; D'Ambrosia et al. 1978) (Fig. 37.7). Even when abnormal, the result is not specific and should be interpreted together with the clinical and radiographical findings (D'Ambrosia et al. 1978). In between these two stages, the bone scintigraphic examination can be normal. The addition of single photon emission computed tomography (SPECT) may improve the accuracy of radionuclide imaging for diagnosis of osteonecrosis. SPECT has been found to be more sensitive than MRI (100% versus 66%) in detecting early osteonecrosis in renal transplant patients (Ryu et al. 2002; Luk et al. 2010).

37.3.3.3   Computed Tomography

Multidetector CT has not been extensively studied in evaluation of osteonecrosis. CT assessment of early (non-collapsed) osteonecrosis, particularly of the femoral head, needs knowledge of the normal cross-sectional pattern of the trabeculae and CT reconstructed images (Resnick et al. 2002). Within the femoral head, the primary compressive trabeculae and medial portion of the primary tensile trabeculae combine to form an area of apparent condensation of the bone, which appear as a radiating pattern on axial images, the "asterisk" or "star" sign (Fig. 37.8a). Alteration of this pattern is considered evidence of early osteonecrosis (Dihlmann 1982) (Fig. 37.8b). However, CT is not recommended in early detection of osteonecrosis and is less sensitive than bone scintigraphy or MRI (Hauzeur et al. 1987). In later stages, the osteonecrosis is well detected by CT, showing a serpentine sclerotic margin, similar to that seen on radiography. Reformation of CT data in the coronal or sagittal plane is useful because it can delineate areas of subchondral bone fracture and buckling or collapse of the articular surface. The articular surface collapse typically occurs at the junction of the serpentine sclerotic rim and the articular surface, where stress is maximally exerted (Fig. 37.8c). These findings of the post-collapse stage are indications for surgery, with total hip arthroplasty or bone grafting providing satisfactory results. In addition, three-dimensional (3D) reformatted CT can help assess the degree of osseous involvement.

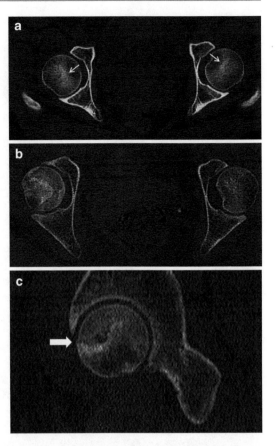

Fig. 37.8 Asterisk sign of osteonecrosis on CT. (**a**) Axial CT image of an intact femoral head shows the characteristics of a normal asterisk sign (*white arrows*). This pattern represents an area of condensation of the bone formed by the primary compressive group and the medial portion of the primary tensile group. (**b**) Axial CT image in a 41-year-old woman with osteonecrosis shows loss of normal asterisk sign (compared to **a**). (**c**) Sagittal reformatted CT image shows buckling of articular surface, or step sign (*thick white arrow*), at the junction of serpentine sclerotic rim and the articular surface

37.3.3.4   Magnetic Resonance Imaging

MRI is considered the imaging gold standard for osteonecrosis, particularly in the pre-collapse stage, although a negative MRI examination does not exclude osteonecrosis histologically (Koo et al. 1994). The accuracy of MRI is 97–100% (Glickstein et al. 1988; Bradbury et al. 1994; Resnick et al. 2002; Kamata et al. 2008; Piyakunmala et al. 2009; Sen et al. 2012). Two

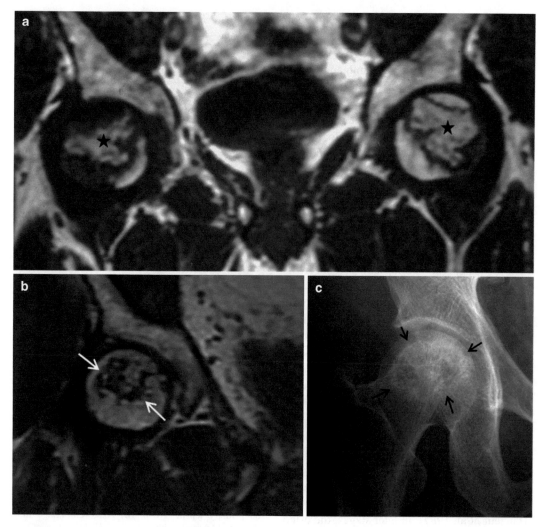

Fig. 37.9 MRI appearances of osteonecrosis. (**a**) Coronal T1-W MR image of both hips shows a geographic sclerotic rim of hypointense signal surrounding a central region whose signal characteristics are identical to those of fat (*black stars*). (**b**) Coronal T1-W MR image shows a ringlike sclerotic rim in the right femoral head (*white arrows*) corresponding to the (**c**) radiographical appearance (*black arrows*). Note the preserved joint space

MRI features that indicate an increased risk of development of femoral head osteonecrosis are (a) a thick physeal scar and (b) early conversion to yellow marrow (Jiang and Shih 1994). Variations are encountered in the pattern of MRI abnormalities and are due to individual differences in distribution, extent, and host responses. The regions of involvement may be homogeneous or heterogeneous. The most common MRI pattern is an area of yellow marrow surrounded by a hypointense rim on all pulse sequences, corresponding to the pathology that is walled-off by sclerosis. Since the viable and devitalized adipose tissues show identical signal intensity on MRI, the signal intensity of yellow marrow is maintained. The sclerotic rim may appear as geographic, crescentric, ringlike, wedge shaped, or band-like in epiphyseal osteonecrosis (Fig. 37.9).

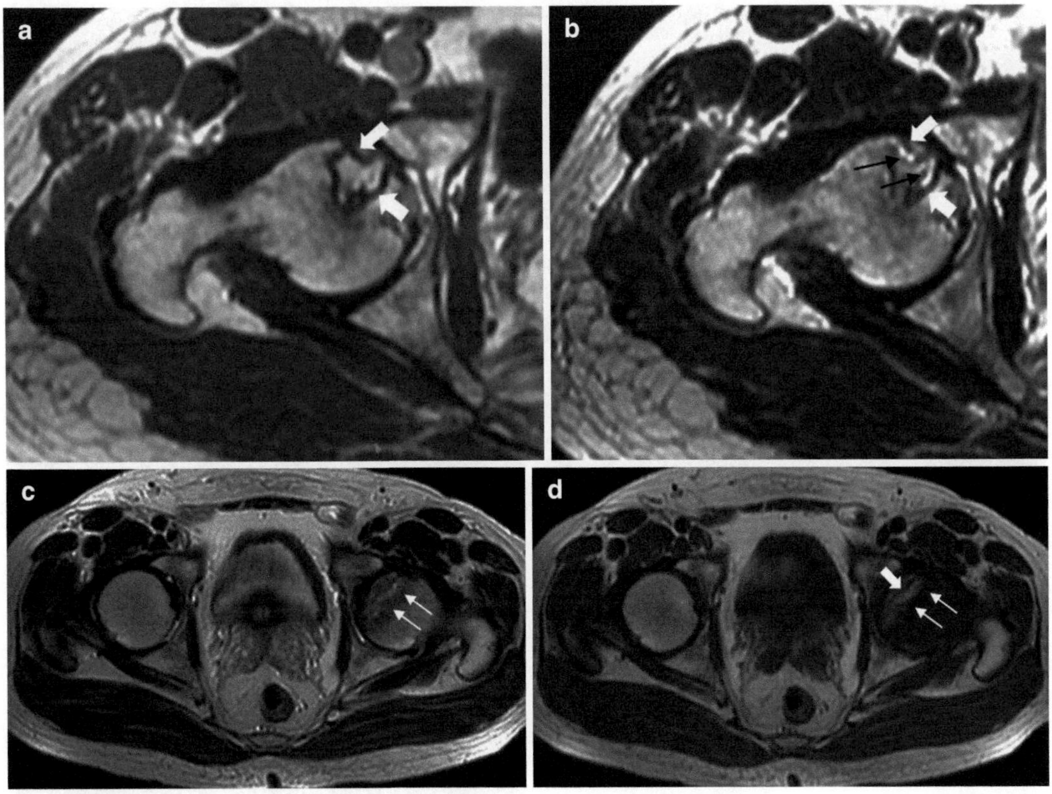

Fig. 37.10 Double-line sign of osteonecrosis on MRI. (**a**) Axial T1-W SE MR image shows a geographic sclerotic rim at the right femoral head (*thick white arrows*). (**b**) Corresponding T2-W SE MR image shows a hyperintense inner rim representing reactive interface (*small black arrows*). (**c**) Axial T2-W SE MR image of another patient, a 46-year-old man, shows what appears to be the double-line sign (*thin white arrows*). (**d**) Corresponding T1-W SE MR image shows signal intensity of fat at the area of signal hyperintensity on the T2-W image (*thick white arrow*). This patient did not have osteonecrosis

The most characteristic pattern, the "double-line sign," has been described in 65–85% of cases of osteonecrosis (Mitchell et al. 1987; Vande Berg et al. 1993b) and is best evaluated on T2-weighted spin echo (SE) MR images at the interface between ischemic and nonischemic bone (Mitchell and Kressel 1988; Zurlo 1999). On T1-weighted SE MR images, this interface is identified as a hypointense line, reflecting granulation tissue and, to a lesser extent, sclerotic bone. On T2-weighted SE images, a narrow outer zone of hypointense signal reflecting bone sclerosis and inner zone of hyperintense signal indicating reparative granulation tissue of the reactive inter-face are apparent. This combination of findings is designated as the double-line sign (Fig. 37.10a, b). Since the signal intensity of fat is bright on T2-weighted images and resembles the signal intensity of fluid, it is mandatory to obtain the T1-weighted images to obviate pitfalls in diagnosing the double-line sign (Fig. 37.10c, d). However, if the patients came in the late stage of disease, with or without articular surface collapse, the double-line sign may not be identified. This double-line sign may also partially result from chemical shift misregistration artifact (Duda et al. 1993). Because a focal lesion predominates in osteonecrosis of the femoral head, such lesions

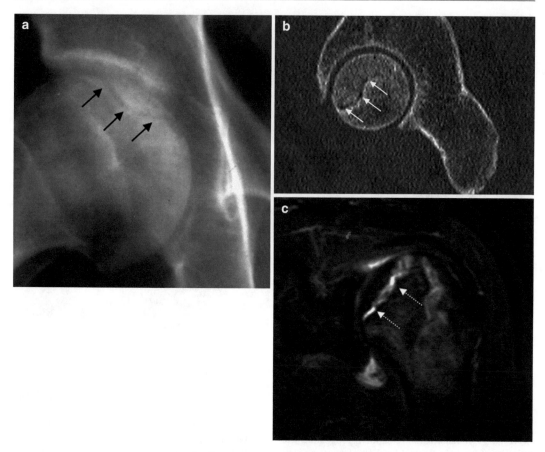

Fig. 37.11 Crescent sign of osteonecrosis. (**a**) Frontal radiograph shows a curvilinear lucency within an area of patchy sclerosis at the femoral head, due to fracture of the necrotic portion (*black arrows*). (**b**) Coronal CT image of another patient shows the curvilinear collection of gas in a fracture of a necrotic femoral head (*white arrows*). (**c**) Coronal fat-suppressed T2-W MR image shows the fracture, or crescent, containing fluid (*dotted white arrows*)

without the double-line sign may simulate a number of normal variations such as normal hematopoietic (red) marrow, fovea centralis, synovial herniation pit, and other disease entities such as subchondral bone cyst, osteochondral lesion, subchondral insufficiency fracture in osteoporosis, and tumor (Jackson and Major 2004).

The "crescent sign" is a thin curvilinear lucency occurring in the subchondral bone and is located at the weight-bearing portion. It is related to fracture of the necrotic portion of the femoral head or other epiphyseal osteonecrosis and is frequently visible with routine radiography. Its appearance on CT or MRI is variable because the fracture gap may be filled with fluid or gas (Pappas 2000) (Fig. 37.11). Further collapse may result in a "step sign," in which cortical offset is noted (Fig. 37.8c). The "snowcap

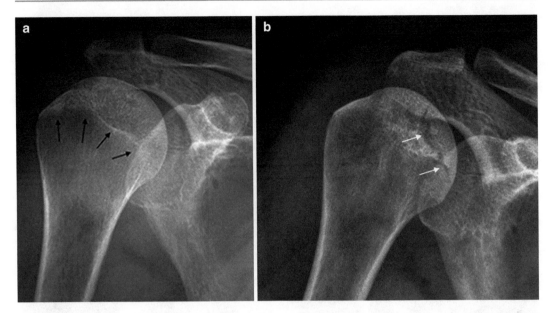

Fig. 37.12 Snowcap sign of osteonecrosis. (**a**) Frontal radiograph shows diffuse sclerosis involving the right humeral head, resembling a snowcapped mountain (*black arrows*), in this female patient who had underlying sys-temic lupus erythematosus (SLE). (**b**) Frontal radiograph of the right humeral head shows a crescent sign within a snowcap appearance (*white arrows*), designating fracture of the necrotic portion

sign" refers to diffuse sclerosis of the femoral head or humeral head on radiographs which resembles a snowcapped mountain and is seen only if the repair process is sufficient in the revascularization phase (Fridinger et al. 2001; Weerakkody et al. 2016) (Fig. 37.12). The associated findings commonly encountered with epiphyseal osteonecrosis are joint effusion and marrow edema; the latter may, but not certainly, precede osteonecrosis for 6–8 weeks. Diffuse marrow edema has been reported as either an early or late finding of osteonecrosis and has to be distinguished from transient osteoporosis of the hip, infection, or tumor (Mitchell 1989; Hayes et al. 1993; Vande Berg et al. 1993a). It may be associated with pain and tendency for bone collapse (Kenan et al. 1998; Koo et al.

1999; Iida et al. 2000). If the marrow edema occurs following subchondral bone collapse, it indicates a poor prognosis, with a tendency for progression of disease (Fig. 37.13).

No uniform agreement exists regarding the imaging plane or specific sequence to evaluate osteonecrosis. Because the reparative process and the presence of granulation tissue make a substantial contribution to the MR signal changes, imaging sequences to detect water content in such tissue, i.e., STIR, heavily T2-weighted fast SE, and fat-suppressed T2-weighted sequences, may be beneficial in assessment of the presence and extent of osteonecrosis (Mirowitz et al. 1994). The use of contrast-enhanced MRI in osteonecrosis is not necessary for diagnosis or assessment in the vast majority of cases. The

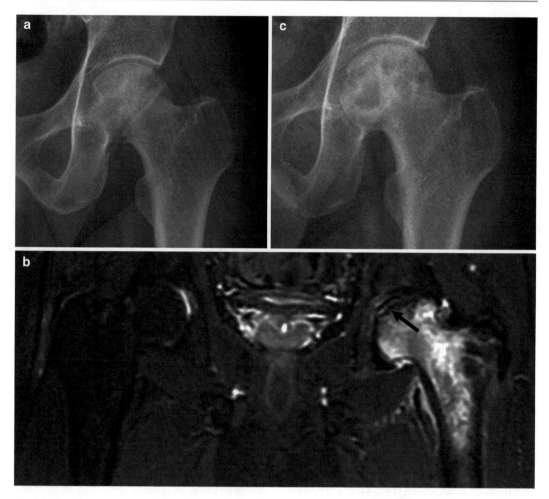

Fig. 37.13 Marrow edema in osteonecrosis. (**a**) Frontal radiograph shows patchy lucency and sclerosis of the left femoral head. (**b**) Coronal fat-suppressed T2-W MR image shows subchondral bone collapse (*black arrow*) with extensive marrow edema extending down to the proximal femoral shaft, suggesting increased intramedullary pressure that can cause worse progression of the disease. (**c**) Radiograph taken 8 months later shows progression of the disease although the collapse of the femoral head still cannot be well appreciated

appearance on contrast-enhanced MRI is lack of enhancement of the devitalized tissue, with a peripheral rim of enhancement corresponding to the granulation tissue (Fig. 37.14). These may help discriminate osteonecrosis from other disease processes. Variable patterns of enhancement, perhaps due to mixtures of ischemia and fibrosis, have also been reported (Hauzeur et al. 1992; Li and Hiette 1992). MRI with T2 mapping, diffusion sequences, and apparent diffusion coefficient (ADC) mapping techniques to evaluate osteonecrosis remains under investigation (Camporesi et al. 2010; Oner et al. 2011; Mackenzie et al. 2012).

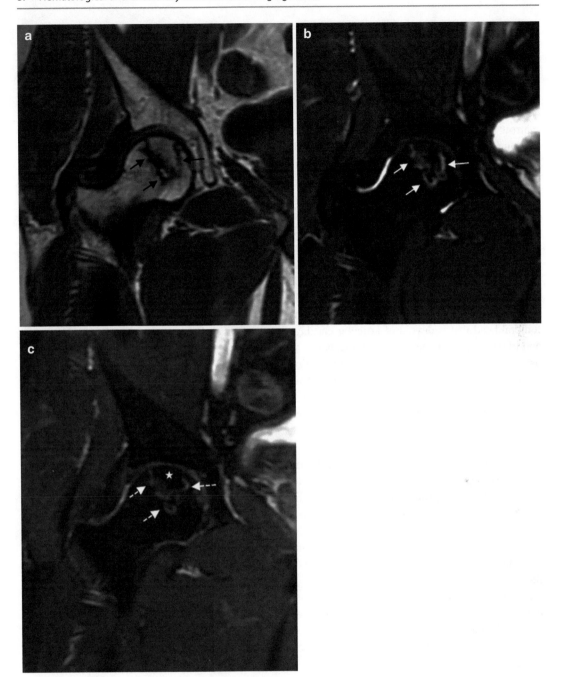

Fig. 37.14 Contrast enhancement in osteonecrosis. (**a**) Coronal T1-W MR image shows a geographic hypointense rim (*black arrows*) in the right femoral head. (**b**) Coronal fat-suppressed T2-W MR image shows signal hyperintensity along the hypointense lines on T1-W image due to reactive interface or granulation tissue (*white arrows*). (**c**) Coronal contrast-enhanced fat-suppressed T1-W image shows lack of enhancement in the devitalized tissue (*white star*) with peripheral rim of enhancement (*dotted white arrows*)

37.3.4 Femoral Head Osteonecrosis: Imaging Pitfalls

Persistent normal hematopoietic marrow can potentially be misinterpreted as osteonecrosis on MRI. In some individuals, residual islands of red marrow can persist in a subchondral location of the humerus and femoral head and are typically found in women. The reliable means to distinguish normal red marrow from a pathological process is to compare its signal intensity with adjacent muscle on T1-weighted MR images. The signal intensity of normal red marrow is higher than that of adjacent muscle, whereas the signal intensity of pathological processes, including osteonecrosis, is lower than that of the adjacent muscle (Jackson and Major 2004) (Fig. 37.15). The fovea centralis is a normal anatomical component of the femoral head that is devoid of articular cartilage and to which the ligamentum teres attaches. It is usually seen as a medially located indentation with a rim of hypointense signal on T1-weighted images. Recognition of this normal structure is important because it is frequently misinterpreted as osteonecrosis with subchondral bone collapse (Fig. 37.16).

Synovial herniation pit is a benign lesion caused by ingrowth of fluid, fibrous, and cartilaginous elements through a perforation in the femoral cortex. Its appearance is similar to subchondral bone cyst, with the difference that the herniation pit does not involve the articular surface but is located at the superolateral quadrant of the femoral neck (in the coronal plane), or femoral head-neck junction, with anterior cortical extension (Nokes et al. 1989). Although an osteonecrotic lesion tends to be in the anterior location, it typically occurs at the 10 o'clock to 2 o'clock position. This will help differentiate a herniation pit from osteonecrosis (Fig. 37.17). Subchondral bone cyst associated with degenerative disease may appear similar to osteonecrosis on radiographs and MRI. The important distinguishing features are: (1) Subchondral bone cyst has a

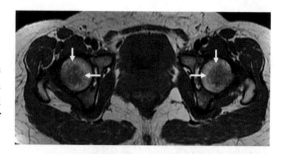

Fig. 37.15 Persistent red marrow. Axial T1-W MR image shows intermediate signal intensity within the femoral heads (*white arrows*). Note that the red marrow signal is brighter than the skeletal muscle

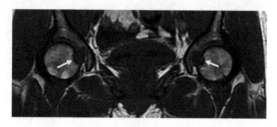

Fig. 37.16 Fovea centralis. Coronal T1-W MR image shows an area of decreased signal at the medial aspect of the femoral heads with hypointense rim (*white arrows*). This is different from osteonecrosis which frequently affects the weight-bearing area

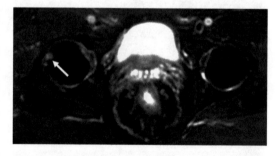

Fig. 37.17 Synovial herniation pit. Axial fat-suppressed T2-W MR image shows small cystic lesions at the right femoral head-neck junction with extension to the cortex (*arrow*). This is at about the 10 o'clock position along the cortical surface

relatively smooth and regular margin which is different from serpiginous margin of osteonecrosis. (2) Simultaneous findings of joint space narrowing and osteophytes, when present, favor

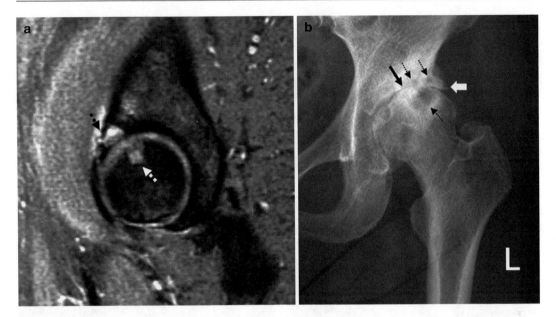

Fig. 37.18 Subchondral bone cysts – degenerative changes. (**a**) Sagittal GRE T2*-W MR image shows subchondral bone cysts at both the femoral head (*white dotted arrow*) and acetabular sides (*black dotted arrow*). (**b**) Frontal radiograph of the left hip clearly shows multiple bone cysts (*dotted black arrows*), eccentric joint space narrowing (*black arrow*), and marginal osteophyte (*thick white arrow*)

degenerative process. (3) Subchondral cysts are present on both sides of the joint (Fig. 37.18). However, degenerative changes and osteonecrosis can coexist in the advanced stage.

Osteochondral lesions are traumatic injuries that tend to occur in young adults and elite athletes who use a wide range of motion of the hips (Weaver et al. 2002). Typically, lesions occur at the medial or inner aspect of the femoral head and extend to the chondral surface. The lesions do not involve the lateral aspect of the femoral head, in contrast to osteonecrosis. The lesion appears as a focal wedge-shaped area of hypointense signal on T1-weighted MR images, with surrounding edema on T2-weighted images. Characteristic imaging findings combined with the clinical history should allow differentiation of osteochondral injury from osteonecrosis. Subchondral insufficiency fractures are nontraumatic flattened lesions located at the superolateral aspect of the femoral head. It occurs in

healthy older adults (more than 60 years of age). Radiographs may be normal in the early stage. On MRI, the fracture line is detected with surrounding reactive marrow edema (Dubost et al. 1996; Raffi et al. 1997). In cases with equivocal findings, the clinical history (patient's age, evidence of osteoporosis, history of radiation therapy) can help distinguish subchondral insufficiency fractures from osteonecrosis (Fig. 37.19).

Transient osteoporosis of the hip is an entity of painful hip occurring in young and middle-aged adults, with a male-to-female ratio of approximately 3:1. In women, the left hip is involved much more frequently and has been associated with the third trimester of pregnancy. It presents with a spontaneous and insidious onset of pain and resolves spontaneously within 3–12 months after symptomatic support. Radiographs may demonstrate osteopenia of the affected hip; however, this finding can be difficult

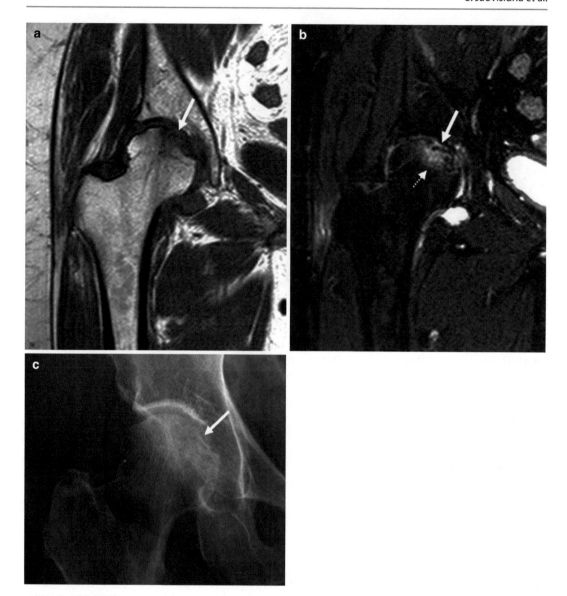

Fig. 37.19 Subchondral insufficiency fracture in a 63-year-old woman. Coronal (**a**) T1-W and (**b**) fat-suppressed T2-W MR images and (**c**) frontal radiograph show a fracture line (*white arrow*) at the subchondral region of the right femoral head with surrounding marrow edema (*dotted white arrow* in **b**). Note that there is no lesion with a hypointense rim on the (**a**) T1-W MR image. This case was histologically proved to be insufficiency fracture of the femoral head

to appreciate. MRI shows hypointense signal on T1-weighted images and hyperintense signal on T2-weighted images, extending from the femoral head to the intertrochanteric region. Patients often have large joint effusions. Signal intensity of the acetabulum is normal (Hayes et al. 1993; Vande Berg et al. 1993b) (Fig. 37.20, Table 37.1).

Metastasis or primary bone tumor is uncommon in the femoral head but, when present, can be mistaken for osteonecrosis. The clinical history of known malignancy, presence of multiple lesions elsewhere, and absence of serpiginous appearance will help exclude osteonecrosis (Fig. 37.21).

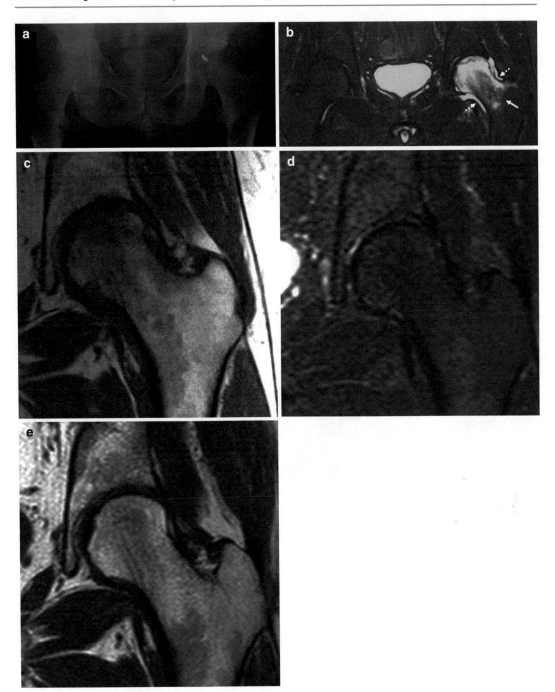

Fig. 37.20 Transient osteoporosis of the hip. (**a**) Frontal radiograph of the pelvis shows osteopenia of the left proximal femur. Coronal (**b**) fat-suppressed T2-W and (**c**) T1-W MR images show extensive marrow edema affecting the femoral head and neck and down to intertrochanteric region (*white arrow*). Small effusion is also observed (*dotted white arrow*). Follow-up coronal (**d**) fat-suppressed T2-W and (**e**) corresponding T1-W MR images taken at 12 months later show that the marrow signal has returned to normal

Table 37.1 Differentiation between osteonecrosis and transient osteoporosis of the hip

	Osteonecrosis	Transient osteoporosis of the hip
Border	True segmental, focal lesion (low signal intensity rim)	Non-segmental (diffuse)
Marrow edema	Nonhomogeneous Involves the femoral head and neck	Homogeneous Involves the femoral head and neck and may go down to intertrochanteric region
Clinical setting	Middle-aged adult Usually associated with risk factors of osteonecrosis May progress	Middle-aged men or women in the third trimester of pregnancy Do not have risk factors of osteonecrosis Spontaneous onset of pain, usually progressive over several weeks Return to normal in 3–12 months Radiographical features lagging behind clinical improvement 4–8 weeks

Compiled from Hayes et al. (1993), Vande Berg et al. (1993b)

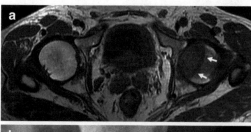

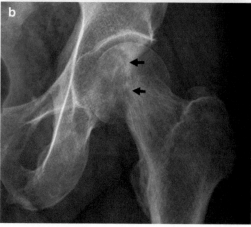

Fig. 37.21 Malignant round cell tumor in a 63-year-old man who presented with left hip pain. (**a**) Axial T1-W MR image shows a hypointense lesion involving the medial half of the left femoral head (*white arrows*). No hypointense rim is detected. (**b**) Frontal radiograph shows a well-defined geographic area of bone destruction without sclerotic border (*black arrows*). With this appearance, malignancy cannot be excluded

37.3.5 Osteonecrosis at the Other Sites: Imaging Pitfalls

Ischemic changes at other skeletal sites, i.e., the humeral head, around the knees, talus and other tarsal bones, carpus, and diametaphyseal regions of tubular bones, although appearing with less frequency, can be assessed with radiography. Lucent shadows with a peripheral rim of sclerosis and periostitis in the diametaphyseal regions (Figs. 37.22a–b) and patchy lucent areas and sclerosis with bony collapse in a flat or irregular bone (Fig. 37.22c) are typical signs of osteonecrosis (Strecker et al. 1988; Munk et al. 1989). The basic MRI characteristics are similar to those seen in osteonecrosis of the femoral head (Fig. 37.23), specific for the diagnosis of osteonecrosis, and explain the radiographical changes (Munk et al. 1989). The MRI changes in the diametaphyseal regions of long bones may vary according to the stage of process. Early infarcts may have intermediate signal intensity on T1-weighted sequences and hyperintense signal on T2-weighted sequences. Chronic infarcts are typically of hypointense signal on both T1- and T2-weighted images (Munk et al. 1989; Rajah et al. 1995). In both

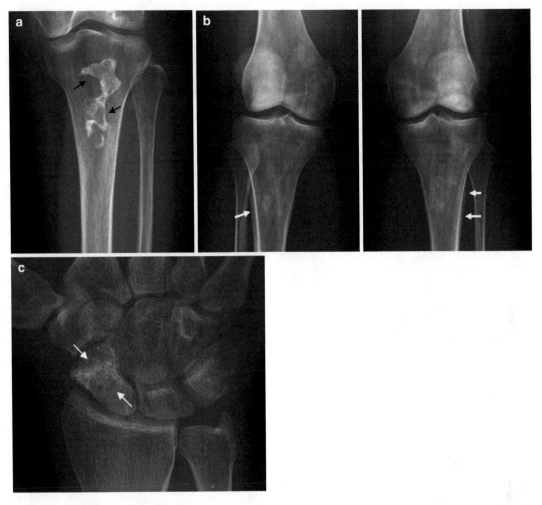

Fig. 37.22 Osteonecrosis at other sites. (**a**) Frontal radiograph of the proximal tibia shows a geographic lesion with a serpentine rim of sclerosis (*black arrows*). (**b**) Frontal radiograph of both knees in a patient with overlapping syndrome (SLE and scleroderma) shows patchy lucent areas and sclerosis in the distal femurs and proximal tibias with periostitis (*white arrows*). (**c**) Radiograph shows a patchy lucent and sclerotic area with bony collapse in the scaphoid (*white arrows*). Example of osteonecrosis in a flat bone

instances, a serpentine zone of hypointense signal, reflecting bone sclerosis or fibrosis, may surround the necrotic region.

Difficulty in diagnosis and pitfalls may be encountered in cases of acute bone infarction and in detection of infarction in hyperplastic marrow or infiltrative intramedullary conditions. In such cases, the island of trapped fat within the lesion may help differentiate osteonecrosis from surrounding diseased marrow.

The T2-weighted sequence and the use of intravenous contrast administration may also be helpful (Vande Berg et al. 1993a) (Fig. 37.24). Another pitfall is enchondroma in the long bone, a benign cartilaginous tumor in which the presence of the internal chondroid matrix may assist to achieve the correct diagnosis (Fig. 37.25). In some instances, the radiographical findings may be subtle, mottled, or poorly defined, so as to simulate aggressive

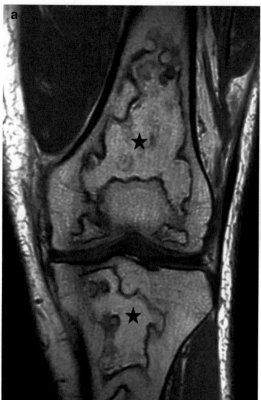
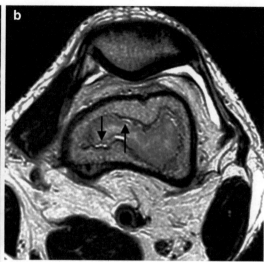

Fig. 37.23 MRI of metadiaphyseal osteonecrosis. (**a**) Coronal T1-W and (**b**) axial T2-W MR images show area of osteonecrosis in the distal femur and proximal tibia with maintained central fat signal intensity (*black stars*) and the double-line sign (*black arrows* in **b**)

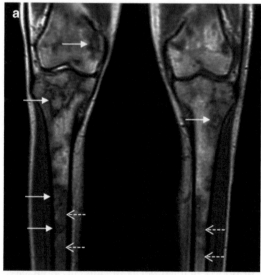
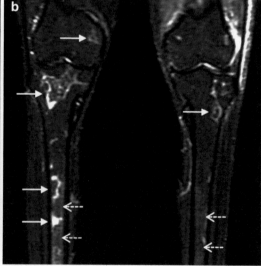

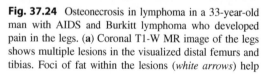

Fig. 37.24 Osteonecrosis in lymphoma in a 33-year-old man with AIDS and Burkitt lymphoma who developed pain in the legs. (**a**) Coronal T1-W MR image of the legs shows multiple lesions in the visualized distal femurs and tibias. Foci of fat within the lesions (*white arrows*) help discriminate osteonecrosis from hyperplastic marrow (*thin dotted white arrows*). Corresponding coronal (**b**) fat-suppressed T2-W image and (**c**) contrast-enhanced fat-suppressed T1-W MR images show the differences more clearly

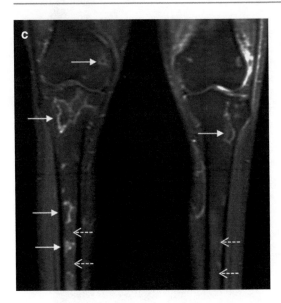

Fig. 37.24 (continued)

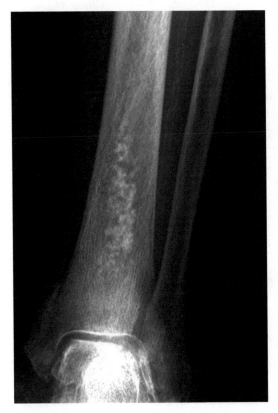

Fig. 37.25 Enchondroma. Frontal radiograph shows an intramedullary lesion in the distal tibia. The ring and arc pattern of calcification designates a cartilaginous lesion

lesion, e.g., osteomyelitis or even bone sarcoma (Fig. 37.26).

37.3.6 Malignant Transformation of Osteonecrosis

Sarcoma associated with osteonecrosis is almost exclusively seen in metadiaphyseal lesions and requires a long latent period (Domson et al. 2009; Dua et al. 2011; Murphey et al. 2014). It was presumed that osteonecrotic lesions turn to be malignant at the reactive interface where there is a high degree of reparative change, followed by the possible excessive proliferation (Dorfman 1972). The most common sarcoma is malignant fibrous histiocytoma (69%), followed by osteosarcoma (17%) and angiosarcoma (9%), with these three lesions accounting for 95% of reported cases (Domson et al. 2009). The majority of lesions (60%) arise around the knee, and 75% of osteonecrosis-associated sarcomas have multiple areas of bone infarctions. Prognosis of patients with osteonecrosis-associated sarcomas is poor. This condition leads to patient demise in 60% of cases, and the disease-free survival is less than 33% at 2 years following the diagnosis. The poor prognosis is related to the high-grade poorly differentiated histology and metastasis to the lungs. The diagnosis can be appreciated on radiographs. MRI will help depict a mass-like replacement of the bone marrow around the areas of osteonecrosis, associated cortical destruction, and probable soft tissue mass (Fig. 37.27).

37.4 Thalassemia

37.4.1 Introduction and Pathophysiology

In 1925, Cooley and Lee described a form of severe anemia associated with bone abnormalities and splenomegaly which they designated thalassemia, from the Greek word for "the sea" since the patients were of Mediterranean origin (Resnick 1995). It is now known that thalassemia is a group of genetic blood disorders passed down

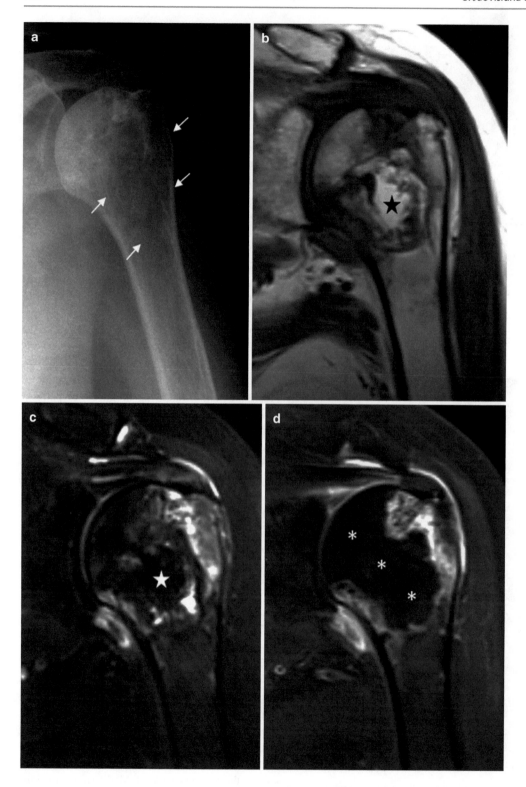

Fig. 37.27 Malignancy superimposed on osteonecrosis. (**a**) Lateral radiograph of the left knee of a 40-year-old man with acute lymphoblastic leukemia in complete remission. There is an area of intramedullary osteonecrosis (*black arrows*). The patient developed spastic knee pain 8 months later. (**b**) Repeat lateral radiograph shows a new soft tissue mass displacing the pre-femoral fat pad (*white arrows*). (**c**) Sagittal T1-W MR image confirmed the soft tissue mass (*dotted white arrows*). The preexisting osteonecrotic lesion in the distal femur was infiltrated by the new lesion (*white asterisk*), while the ones in the proximal tibia were not (*black asterisk*). The new lesion was histologically proved to be lymphoma

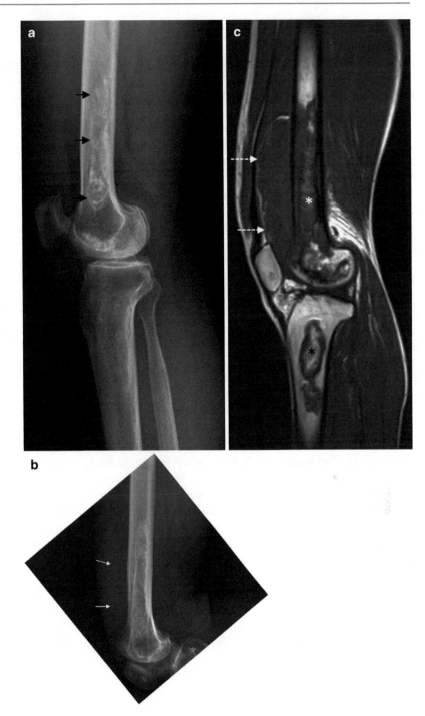

Fig. 37.26 Osteonecrosis simulating an aggressive lesion. (**a**) Frontal radiograph shows a geographic osteolytic lesion with an ill-defined border at the proximal humerus (*arrows*). A malignant process cannot be excluded. Coronal (**b**) T1-W and (**c**) fat-suppressed T2-MR images show a fat-containing lesion with internal inhomogeneity (*star*). (**d**) Coronal contrast-enhanced fat-suppressed T1-W MR image shows a non-enhancing area continuing from the subchondral area down to the level of the surgical neck (*white asterisks*). MRI finding was first interpreted as intraosseous lipoma. Histology revealed osteonecrosis, and no malignancy was found

through families (i.e., inherited) in which the body produces an abnormal form of hemoglobin. Hemoglobin is the oxygen-carrying component of the red blood cell and consists of two different proteins: the alpha globin and beta globin. Thalassemia occurs when there is a defect in the gene that controls production of these globin proteins (Spritz and Forget 1983). This contributes to imbalanced globin-chain production, leading to ineffective erythropoiesis and hemolysis. The result is chronic anemia that lasts throughout life (Spritz and Forget 1983; Forget 1993).

There are two main groups of thalassemia, alpha thalassemia and beta thalassemia, and several distinct disorders exist in these groups. Thalassemia minor refers to a heterozygous form in which the patients have mild anemia. Physicians often mistake the small red blood cells of the patients with thalassemia minor as iron deficiency anemia. Thalassemia intermedia represents a poorly defined intermediate variety of the disease. However, the lack of globin protein is great enough to cause a moderately severe anemia, bone deformities, and splenomegaly. The borderline between thalassemia intermedia and, the most severe form, thalassemia major can be confusing. The more dependent the patient is on blood transfusion, the more likely he or she is to be classified as thalassemia major. In general, the patients with thalassemia intermedia need blood transfusion to improve their quality of life rather than to survive. Thalassemia major is a homozygous form of disease in which the lack of globin protein is complete. Most individuals with alpha thalassemia major die before or shortly after birth. Patients with beta thalassemia major, or Cooley anemia, are normal at birth and develop severe anemia during the first year of life (Resnick 1995; Gersten et al. 2014).

37.4.2 Imaging Bone Changes

37.4.2.1 Marrow Hyperplasia

The skeletal changes in thalassemia are secondary to hematopoietic or red marrow proliferation. This results in widening of the marrow cavity, a coarse trabeculated appearance, with cortical thinning of the skeleton (Fernbach 1984). The changes in thalassemia major are much more severe than those in thalassemia minor. Initially, both the axial and appendicular skeleton is altered. As the patients reach puberty, the appendicular skeletal changes decrease, due to normal regression of hematopoietic marrow from the peripheral skeleton. In the skull, the frontal bones reveal the earliest and most severe changes, whereas the inferior part of occiput is believed to be unaffected. The findings range from granular osteoporosis, widening of the diploic space, and thinning of the outer table. Bone proliferation of the outer table creates the "hair-on-end" appearance (Hamperl and Weiss 1955) (Fig. 37.28). Computed tomography (CT) reveals the coarse trabeculation more clearly than radiographs. MRI is considered a very accurate method for detecting iron deposition in various tissues, due to the strong paramagnetic properties of intracellular ferritin and hemosiderin that cause T2 relaxation time shortening and signal intensity (SI) reduction in SE and gradient-echo (GRE) sequences (Levin et al. 1995).

In thalassemia, the signal intensity of the bone marrow is related not only to the red marrow hyperplasia but also the treatment received. The untreated patients demonstrate signal consistent with red marrow throughout the central and peripheral skeleton. Although thalassemic patients are treated by transfusion and chelation, iron deposition can occur at the sites of

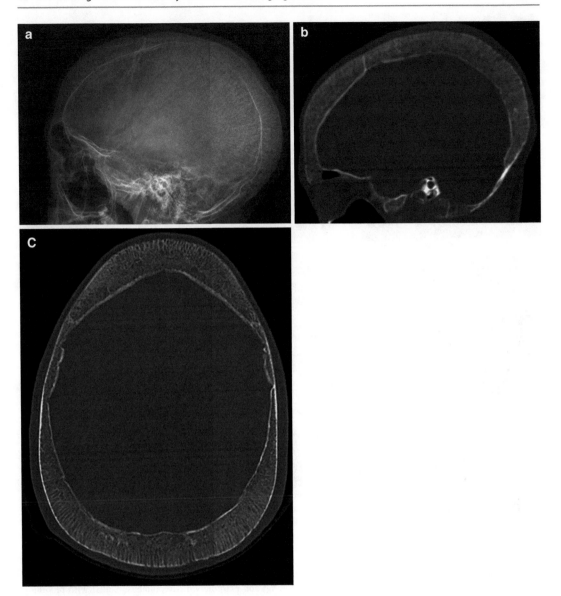

Fig. 37.28 Thalassemia major with marrow hyperplasia. (a) Lateral radiograph of the skull shows bony proliferation in the outer table of cranial vault creating a "hair-on-end" appearance, with dense striations traversing the thickened calvarium. The inferior part of the occipital bone is preserved. These bony changes are more obvious when viewing the bone windows of the (b) sagittal and (c) axial CT images

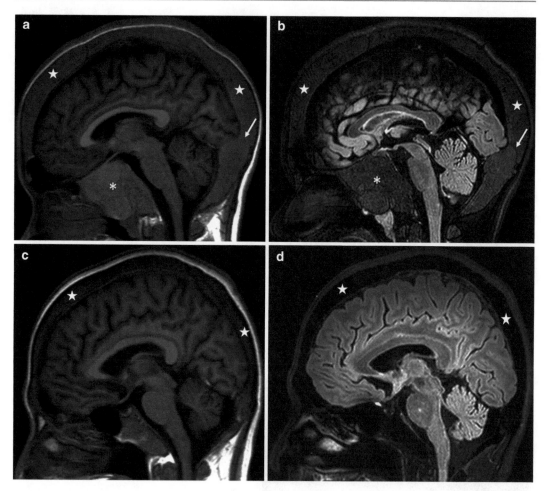

Fig. 37.29 Thalassemia major with marrow hyperplasia. Sagittal (**a**) T1-W and (**b**) fat-suppressed T2-W MR images of the skull in a 18-year-old man show widening of the diploic space (*white stars*), with a greater degree at the clivus (*white asterisk*). It contains proliferated red marrow which appears slightly hyperintense on the T1-W image, with signal reduction on the T2-W image due to prominent trabeculation, intracellular ferritin, and hemo-siderin deposition. The occipital bone has a mass-like area at its superior portion (*arrow*) which represents pronounced hematopoiesis. Sagittal (**c**) T1-W and (**d**) fat-suppressed T2-W MR images in a 55-year-old thalassemic patient with longtime blood transfusion show the visualized marrow space exhibiting slightly T1-hypointense signal and extremely T2-hypointense signal with blooming (*white stars*) due to hemosiderin deposition

active red marrow, despite chelation therapy. As red marrow retreats centrally with age, so does the pattern of iron deposition (Drakonaki et al. 2007) (Fig. 37.29). Besides the skull, marrow hyperplasia extends to involve the facial bones. The expansion of the temporal and nasal bones causes obliteration of the maxillary sinuses, resulting in lateral displacement of the orbits, malocclusion of the jaws, and displacement of dental structures, giving rise to the "rodent facies" (Fernbach 1984) (Fig. 37.30). In the spine, osteoporosis is evident. This is due to reduction in number of trabeculae, thinning of subchondral bone plate, accentuation of the

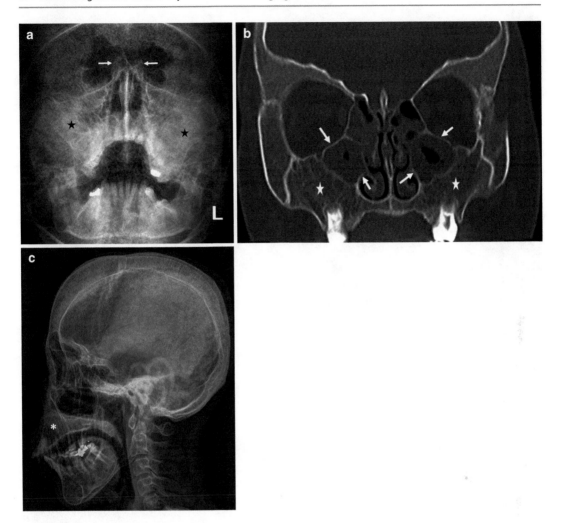

Fig. 37.30 Facial bones in thalassemia major. (**a**) Waters view radiograph of a 43-year-old man shows overgrowth of the facial bones (*black stars*) causing almost total obliteration of both maxillary sinuses. Expansion of the nasal bone is also observed (*white arrows*) which produces lateral displacement of the orbits leading to hypertelorism. (**b**) Coronal CT image of the sinus in another patient shows small size of both maxillary sinuses with sinusitis (*white arrows*). The expanded sinus walls show coarse trabeculation (*white stars*). (**c**) Lateral radiograph of the skull in another 48-year-old man shows the "hair-on-end" appearance of the skull and expansion of the maxilla bone (*white asterisk*) which resulted in malocclusion of the jaws and displacement of the teeth

vertical trabeculation, and biconcave deformities (fish vertebra).

Medullary hyperplasia also appears in other bones of axial skeleton, including the clavicle, ribs, and pelvis (Fig. 37.31) along with the bones of appendicular skeleton. Posterior aspects of multiple ribs frequently reveal significant expansion (Fig. 37.32). Additional rib changes are subcortical radiolucent lesions and localized radiolucency which is called the "rib-within-a-rib" appearance. Long bones are similarly involved, revealing widened marrow space, coarse and trabeculated

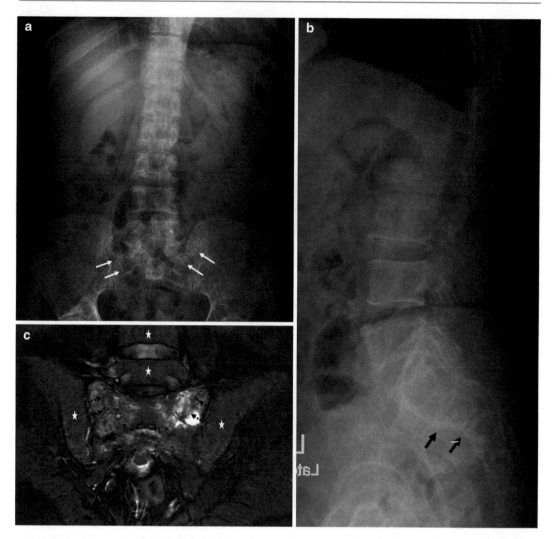

Fig. 37.31 Axial skeleton in thalassemia major. (**a**) Anteroposterior and (**b**) lateral radiographs of the lumbar spine in a 44-year-old woman show generalized osteoporosis with diffusely coarse and trabeculated appearance. Thinning of subchondral endplates and vertical trabeculation is detected. The sclerotic bands in both sacral wings (*white arrows*) and deformed S2 segment (*black arrows*) are evidence of insufficiency fractures. (**c**) Oblique coronal fat-suppressed T2-W MR image shows the fracture lines (*dotted black arrows*) parallel to the sacroiliac joints with nearby marrow edema. The visualized marrow space shows signal intensity of red marrow (*white stars*)

appearance, and cortical thinning. These findings are more severe if the hemoglobin level cannot be maintained by transfusion (Lawson et al. 1981a, b). A recent study has reported the correlation of trabeculation with nucleated red blood cell count in patients with thalassemia intermedia. This is due to longtime treatment of thalassemia major patients with blood transfusion and the efficacy of this type of treatment to lower marrow hyperplasia (Foroughi et al. 2015), resulting in diminished red blood cell production and decreased trabeculation. The contour of long bones may be altered, with the normal concavity lost and becoming straight or convex; this is called "undertubulation." The widening of metaphysis resembles an "Erlenmeyer flask" (Fig. 37.33).

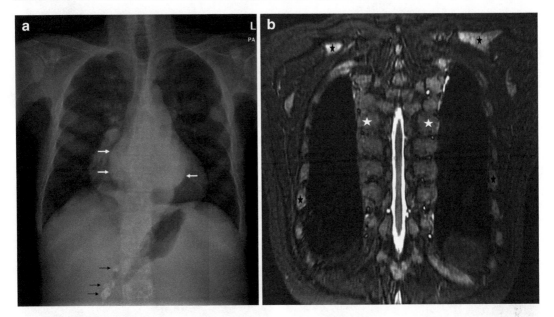

Fig. 37.32 Thalassemia major with marrow hyperplasia of the ribs. (**a**) Posteroanterior chest radiograph shows generalized osteopenia with multifocal bone expansion, particularly at the posterior portion of the ribs. Retrocardiac lobulated shadows represent extramedullary hematopoiesis (*white arrows*). Gallstones are also detected (*black arrows*) along with hepatosplenomegaly. (**b**) Coronal fat-suppressed T2-W MR image of the thorax in another patient shows marrow reconversion and symmetrical marrow space expansion at posterior ribs (*white stars*). Other portions of ribs and scapulas are also involved (*black stars*)

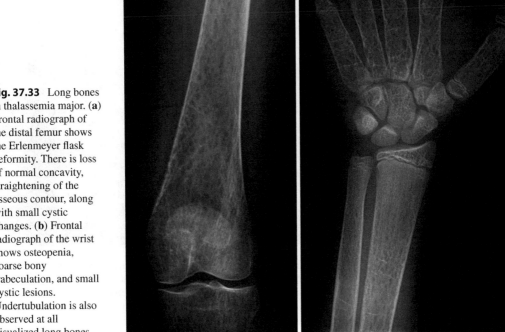

Fig. 37.33 Long bones in thalassemia major. (**a**) Frontal radiograph of the distal femur shows the Erlenmeyer flask deformity. There is loss of normal concavity, straightening of the osseous contour, along with small cystic changes. (**b**) Frontal radiograph of the wrist shows osteopenia, coarse bony trabeculation, and small cystic lesions. Undertubulation is also observed at all visualized long bones

37.4.2.2 Growth Disturbances

The Erlenmeyer flask deformity of long bones is only one of the growth disturbances that can be encountered in patients with thalassemia. Additional findings that reflect growth disturbances are the irregular transverse radiodense lines near the ends of long bones, which represent growth recovery lines (Fig. 37.34). Premature fusion of the physis (growth plate) has been noted in 10–15% of patients, particularly in children, with thalassemia major, and usually occurs after the age of 10 years (Currarino and Erlandson 1964; Dines et al. 1976).

37.4.2.3 Fractures

Spontaneous fracture is not uncommon in patients with thalassemia, with one or more fractures occurring in about one-third of the patients (Dines et al. 1976). The most frequent locations are long bones of lower extremities, particularly the femur, bones of forearms, and the vertebrae (Finsterbush et al. 1985) (Fig. 37.35).

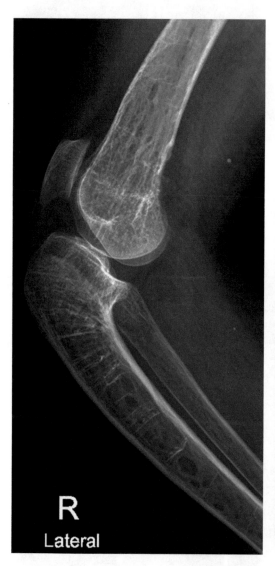

Fig. 37.34 Thalassemia major with growth disturbance. Lateral radiograph shows multiple growth recovery lines, along with coarse trabeculation, multiple cystic lesions, and a deformed knee joint

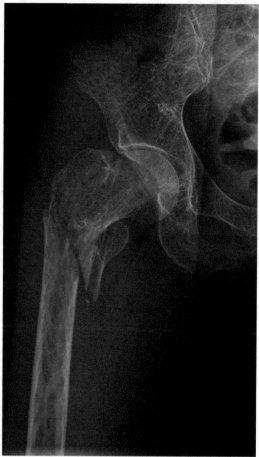

Fig. 37.35 Thalassemia major with fracture. Frontal radiograph of the right femur shows extreme osteoporosis in the pelvis and lower extremity, with an oblique fracture traversing the subtrochanteric region of the right femur

37.4.2.4 Arthropathy

Multiple types of arthropathy can be encountered during the clinical course of thalassemia, i.e., secondary hemochromatosis due to repeated blood transfusion, and hyperuricemia, including gouty arthritis. Some forms of thalassemia, particularly thalassemia minor, have been reported to have a relationship with several articular abnormalities such as osteomyelitis, septic arthritis, rheumatoid arthritis, chronic seronegative arthritis, and osteonecrosis (Dorwart and Schumacher 1981; Gerster et al. 1984; Orzincolo et al. 1986; Resnick 1995).

37.4.2.5 Extramedullary Hematopoiesis

Extramedullary hematopoiesis (EMH) refers to hematopoiesis occurring outside the medulla of the bone. It may be physiological process, i.e., during fetal development in the liver and spleen (Ginzel et al. 2012; Hashmi et al. 2014). However, it is more frequently associated with pathological processes which include various chronic hematological disorders that lead to ineffective hematopoiesis or inadequate bone marrow function (i.e., hemolytic anemia, hemoglobinopathies such as thalassemias, polycythemia rubra vera, myelofibrosis of many causes, leukemia, and lymphoma) (Haidar et al. 2010; Orphanidou-Vlachou et al. 2014). Hematological disorders associated with poor blood cell formation will first lead to conversion of yellow marrow to red marrow throughout the skeleton (Sauer et al. 2007; Ginzel et al. 2012). There are two sources of EMH. The first source is normal hematopoietic tissue that expands outside the medullary cavity through permeative erosion of the bony cortex. This causes expansion of the marrow space, thinning of the cortical bone, resorption of the medullary bone, and resultant coarse trabeculation, leading to osteoporosis. Bone expansion can be observed at the ribs, vertebral column including the sacrum, skull, long bones, and facial bones. The second source is the previous hematopoietic tissue that becomes reactivated, i.e., the liver, spleen, lymph nodes, and, most commonly, the

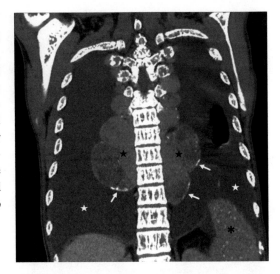

Fig. 37.36 Thalassemia major with extramedullary hematopoiesis in a 48-year-old man. Coronal contrast-enhanced CT image of the thorax shows multiple posterior mediastinal paraspinal masses simulating a tumorous process (*black stars*). The rim calcification is due to post-treatment change (*white arrows*). Coarse bony trabeculation is present, as well as bilateral pleural effusion (*white stars*). The visualized portion of the spleen has numerous tiny calcifications (*black asterisk*). This is the same patient as in Fig. 37.32 whose chest radiograph shows multiple lobulated retrocardiac masses and CT was requested to exclude lung cancer

paravertebral regions. The thymus, pleura, heart, breasts, kidneys, adrenal glands, retroperitoneal tissue, broad ligaments, prostate, skin, spinal canal, and peripheral and cranial nerves may also be involved (Sohawon et al. 2012; Hashmi et al. 2014). These sites are thought to have active hematopoietic tissue in the fetus, which ceased activity at birth. However, the extramedullary hematopoietic vascular connective tissues still retain the ability to produce red cells, particularly when there is ineffective hematopoiesis (Haidar et al. 2010; Orphanidou-Vlachou et al. 2014).

EMH may appear as large masses and mimic malignancies (Sohawon et al. 2012; Zhu et al. 2012) (Figs. 37.36 and 37.37). A recent study has reported the correlation of patients' age and paravertebral mass in the thalassemia intermedia group, suggesting that the older age the patients are, the more tolerance they have to

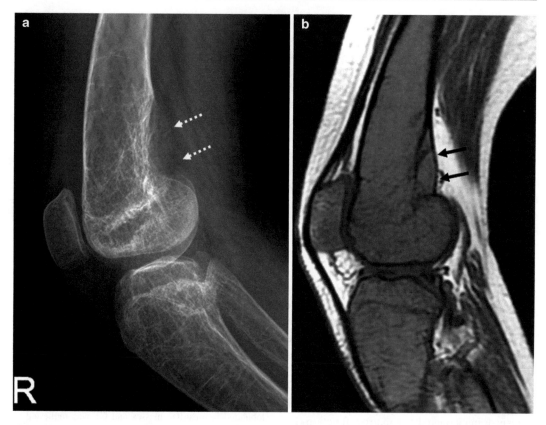

Fig. 37.37 Thalassemia major with extramedullary hematopoiesis in the peripheral skeleton of a 23-year-old woman. (**a**) Lateral radiograph of the knee shows an area of bone destruction at the posterior cortex of the distal femur (*dotted white arrows*). Malignancy cannot be excluded. Extreme osteoporosis, coarse trabeculation, and multiple growth recovery lines in the tibia represent thalassemic bone changes. (**b**) Sagittal T1-W MR image shows generalized red marrow hyperplasia breaking through the posterior femoral cortex and forming a mass-like lesion (*black arrows*)

the anemia (Foroughi et al. 2015). Tsitouridis et al. (1999) divided the CT and MRI pattern of paraspinal EMH into four groups. The first group with massive iron deposition has high CT density and signal hypointensity in both T1- and T2-weighted MR images without enhancement. This pattern occurs when patients are treated with blood transfusion, even with chelation (Figs. 37.29c, d). The second group refers to active EMH. The CT density is similar to that of soft tissue, with intermediate signal intensity in both T1- and T2-weighted MR images with some enhancement (Tsitouridis et al. 1999; Orphanidou-Vlachou et al. 2014). The third group exhibits fat replacement, revealing negative CT density and signal hyperintensity on both T1- and T2-weighted MRI, representing fatty tissue. Fat replacement related to oxidative stress, which leads to lipid peroxidation of the cell membrane, is encountered in non-transfused, non-chelated patients. The fourth group is a mixed type, with foci of fat and different foci of some activity (Tsitouridis et al. 1999). Ginzel et al. (2012), in an attempt to diagnose EMH accurately, reported that 90% of axial EMH had multiple masses with 70% containing fat, while those in non-axial locations did not have internal fat. When such imaging features

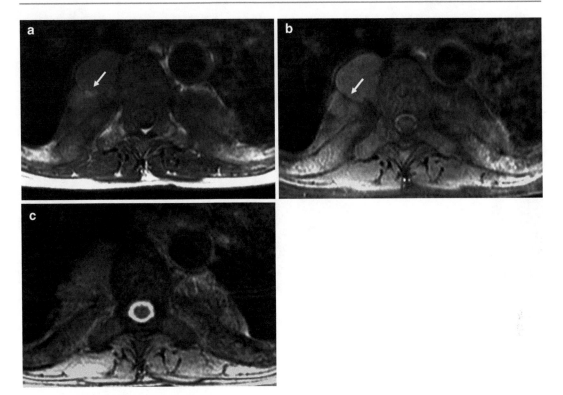

Fig. 37.38 Extramedullary hematopoiesis in a 44-year-old woman. Axial (**a**) T1-W and (**b**) fat-suppressed T1-W MR images show paraspinal extramedullary hematopoiesis in which a T1-hyperintense focus (*white arrow*) was completely suppressed in the fat-suppressed T1-W sequence, suggestive of fat. Other portions of the lesion show intermediate signal intensity on the T1-W (**a**) and T2-FFE (**c**) sequences

are localized to the axial skeleton, EMH should be considered, particularly when occurring in the setting of predisposing medical conditions (Ginzel et al. 2012) (Fig. 37.38).

37.4.3 Pitfalls, Mimics, and Differentials

37.4.3.1 Differentiation from Anemia
Thickening of the cranial vault and the "hair-on-end" appearance is most characteristic of thalassemia, occurring in sickle cell disease in only 5% of cases. Marrow hyperplasia in the peripheral skeleton is most common and marked in thalassemia, while bone infarction is common in sickle cell disease (Resnick 1995).

37.4.3.2 Differentiation from Other Conditions
Fibrous dysplasia (leontiasis ossea) can lead to hyperostosis of the skull but usually predominates in the frontal region. When involving facial bones, it will cause a ground-glass appearance, which is different from the coarse and trabeculated appearance in thalassemia (Fig. 37.39). Hyperostosis frontalis interna is confined to anterior aspect of the cranial vault. Paget disease, acromegaly, and hypoparathyroidism may produce diffuse calvarial thickening (Fig. 37.40). Bone infarction, particularly in the femoral head, is observed in exogenous and endogenous steroid excess, Legg-Calve-Perthes disease, Gaucher disease, alcoholism with pancreatitis, connective tissue disease,

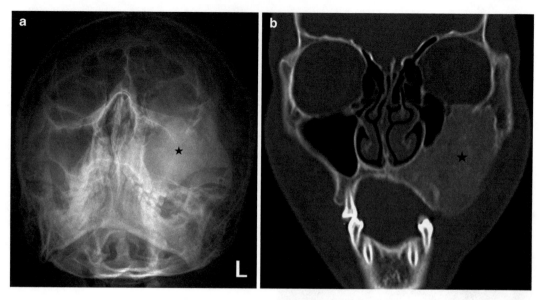

Fig. 37.39 Fibrous dysplasia in facial bones. (**a**) Waters view radiograph of a male patient with fibrous dysplasia of the left maxilla shows maxillary wall thickening with ground-glass appearance, more apparent on the (**b**) coro- nal CT image (*black star*). The density and architecture of the bone are different from the osteopenia and coarse tra- beculated appearance in thalassemia (compared to Fig. 37.30)

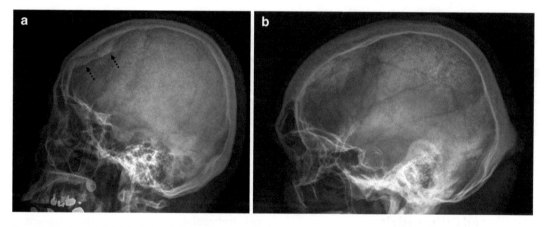

Fig. 37.40 Potential pitfalls in the skull. (**a**) Hyperostosis frontalis interna where the lesion is confined to anterior aspect of the cranial vault (*dotted black arrows*). (**b**) Acromegaly generally produces diffuse calvarial thickening

radiation therapy, as well as following trauma (Resnick 1995).

Fish vertebrae may be observed in anemia but are not specific, as they appear in all forms of osteoporosis and conditions that cause dif- fuse weakening of the bone (Fig. 37.41). EMH leading to enlargement of ribs simulates fibrous dysplasia, and lobulated posterior mediastinal masses or expansion of bones may resemble tumors (Ginzel et al. 2012; Sohawon et al. 2012). However, the ribs involved by fibrous dysplasia usually show varying degree of sclerosis due

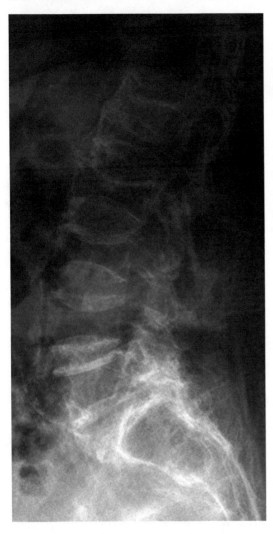

Fig. 37.41 Potential pitfalls on lateral radiograph of the spine. Fish vertebrae are observed at multiple lumbar vertebral bodies in this 93-year-old woman with osteoporosis. They may be observed in all forms of osteoporosis, many types of anemia, and the conditions that cause diffuse weakening of the bone

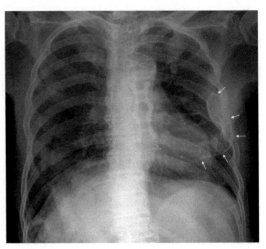

Fig. 37.42 Potential pitfalls – rib. Posteroanterior chest radiograph shows expansion of a single left lower rib from its posterior to anterior portion with sclerotic change (*white arrows*), consistent with fibrous dysplasia. The bony structure is otherwise unremarkable

37.5 Sickle Cell Disease

37.5.1 Introduction and Pathophysiology

Sickle cell anemia or sickle cell disease (SCD) is an autosomal recessive disorder resulting from gene mutation of the beta globin, characterized by production of abnormal hemoglobin S (HbS) that is associated with different risks of morbidity and mortality. Many genotypes and phenotypes of SCD have been discussed in the literature. Each has its own musculoskeletal and systemic manifestations, according to the severity of the disease and the associated environmental factors (Jastaniah 2011). The disease manifestations on musculoskeletal system are multifactorial, depending on the age, site affected, and associated complications. It has been agreed in many reports that the etiology of the musculoskeletal and systemic clinical disease manifestations is related to three mechanisms: (1) vaso-occlusive crisis, (2) chronic anemia, and (3) infections (Saito et al. 2010).

to calcification within the fibrous matrix in the marrow compartment. Although fibrous dysplasia may involve multiple ribs, the nearby ribs usually appear normal in size and bony architecture (Fig. 37.42). The known presence of anemia will help differentiate EMH from other disease entities (Figs. 37.32, 37.36, 37.37, and 37.38).

The most common clinical presentation of the patients in most research studies is bone pain involving one or multiple sites. MRI is the most sensitive noninvasive tool to diagnose various musculoskeletal abnormalities in SCD which may help in early initiation of therapy. MRI is very sensitive in detecting early stages of osteonecrosis, red marrow persistence, EMH, changes of arthritis, infections, and joint effusion (Sachan et al. 2015). The acute, painful vaso-occlusive crises are the most common and the earliest clinical manifestations of SCD. More than 50% of all patients with SCD experience a painful crisis by 5 years of age. The pain is usually described as bone pain, although crises may involve virtually any organ. They are presumed to be caused by microvascular occlusion with subsequent tissue ischemia.

37.5.2 Imaging Bone Changes

37.5.2.1 Vaso-occlusive Crisis (Infarction)

Infants younger than 6 months are usually at low risk of having sickling due to the presence of fetal hemoglobin. In infants between 6 months and 2 years of age, the vaso-occlusive crises most commonly manifest as dactylitis, a painful swelling of the hands, fingers, feet, and toes (Ejindu et al. 2007) (Fig. 37.43). In older children and adults, bone infarction is common. Acute infarcts cause osteolytic changes that become heterogeneous with time and end as a coarse trabeculation pattern in the chronic phase, with the thickening and lamination of the cortex resulting in a "bone-within-bone appearance" (Fig. 37.44).

In the spine, infarction may appear as a central, square-shaped endplate depression, resulting from endplate microvascular occlusion and subsequent overgrowth of the surrounding portions of the endplate. This appearance is seen in approximately 10% of patients, but it is essentially pathognomonic for SCD and has been called the "Lincoln log" or "H-shaped vertebra" deformity (Lonergan et al. 2001) (Fig. 37.45). Epiphyseal

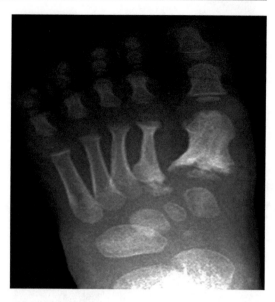

Fig. 37.43 Dactylitis in SCD. Anteroposterior radiograph of the right foot shows squaring and increased sclerosis of the first and second metatarsal bones secondary to the vaso-occlusive insult of the SCD

osteonecrosis is commonly encountered, with the proximal femurs and humeri being most commonly affected. It appears as a subchondral crescent-shaped lucency with surrounding sclerosis on radiographs, giving the classical double-line sign on T2-weighted MRI (Fig. 37.46).

37.5.2.2 Chronic Hemolytic Anemia (Extramedullary Hematopoiesis)

Over time, the disease produces various musculoskeletal abnormalities as a result of chronic anemia. These include marrow hyperplasia, reversion of yellow marrow to red marrow, and, occasionally, extramedullary hematopoiesis (EMH) that is more common in sickle cell thalassemia (HbS-Thal) and in thalassemic patients once compared to patients with HbS (Fig. 37.47). Thinning of the bones and eventually pathological fractures might occur in rare cases, especially

Fig. 37.44 Septic arthritis in SCD. (**a**) Anteroposterior and (**b**) lateral radiographs of the right knee in a patient with SCD show heterogeneous mixed osteolytic and sclerotic bone lesions, along with coarse trabeculation of the right femur and the right tibia due to SCD bone changes. Small amount of joint effusion is detected (*white star*) and was proved to be septic arthritis by ultrasound-guided aspiration and culture

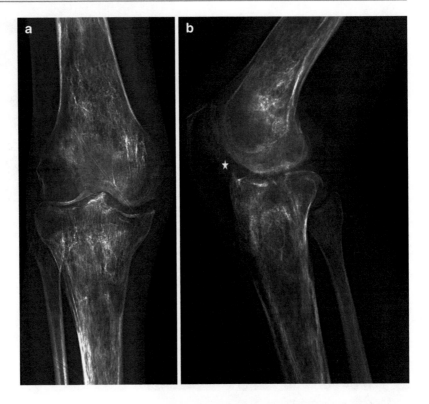

when osteoporosis is present (Martinoli et al. 2011; Sheehan et al. 2015).

37.5.2.3 Infection

With disease development, the spleen will be involved by veno-occlusive infarctions, leading to splenic dysfunction. This increases the susceptibility to infection, which includes septic arthritis, osteomyelitis, and subperiosteal hemorrhage. Septic arthritis and osteomyelitis most commonly occur at the diaphysis of the femur, tibia, and humerus. The vertebrae may also be involved. The most commonly encountered organisms are *Salmonella* and *Staphylococcus aureus*. Septic arthritis is less common than osteomyelitis and often arises in conjunction with bone infarction (Bahebeck et al. 2004) (Fig. 37.48). The diagnosis of osteomyelitis in SCD patients is somewhat challenging,

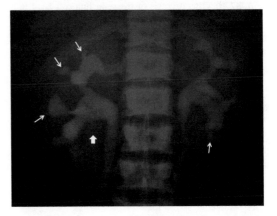

Fig. 37.45 H-shaped vertebrae in SCD. Intravenous urogram image shows evidence of papillary necrosis (*white arrows*). There is also generalized bone sclerosis and H-shaped vertebrae resulting from secondary changes of SCD. Note multiple gallstones projected over the right renal shadow (*thick white arrow*). As in other hemolytic anemias, these gallstones are bilirubinated stone secondary to hemolysis

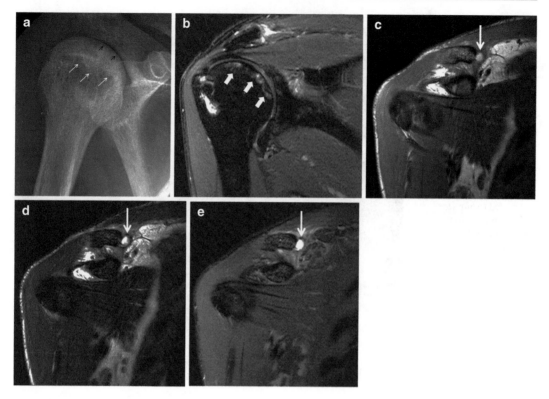

Fig. 37.46 Osteonecrosis of the right humeral head in a patient with known SCD who complained of right shoulder pain. (**a**) Anteroposterior radiograph of the right shoulder shows coarse trabeculation of the humeral head with patchy sclerosis involving the epiphyseal region (snowcap sign – *white arrows*) along with thin curvilinear radiolucent line at the subchondral region (crescent sign – *small black arrows*). (**b**) Coronal STIR MR image shows osteonecrosis of the humeral epiphysis (*thick white arrows*). Coronal (**c**) T1-W, (**d**) T2-W, and (**e**) fat-suppressed T2-weighted MR images show a hyperintense spot at the conoid tubercle of the right clavicle, due to focal bleeding

especially differentiating it from acute vaso-occlusive crisis (Madani et al. 2007). Several diagnostic tools have been tried to solve this dilemma, and MRI has the highest sensitivity in this aspect (Delgado et al. 2015). Some of MRI findings are more helpful in the diagnosis of infection rather than infarction. Cortical irregularity/destruction, fluid collections in the adjacent soft tissue, bone marrow enhancement, and intraosseous abscess (irregular bone marrow enhancement around a non-enhanced center) are suggestive of infection (Ejindu et al. 2007). MRI may also act as a guide to intervention by identifying focal bone marrow or soft tissue fluid collection that can be aspirated for further evaluation (Rifai and Nyman 1997). Ultrasound imaging is also one of the best tools for aspiration-guided procedures. Scintigraphic studies carry a high specific rate for infection and inflammation detection in conjunction with other modalities such as MRI and ultrasound imaging (Ahmad et al. 2010).

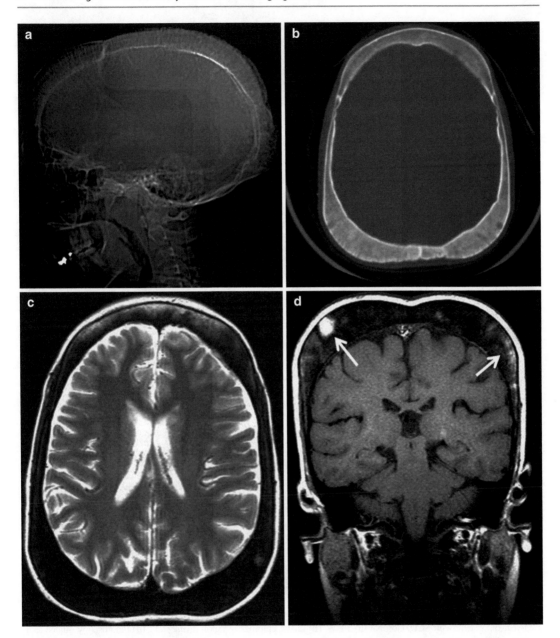

Fig. 37.47 Extramedullary hematopoiesis of the skull in SCD. (**a**) Lateral scout CT image shows widening of the diploic space with the "hair-on-end" appearance, confirmed on (**b**) axial CT images obtained with bone window. (**c**) Axial T2-W MR image shows hyperplasia of bone marrow with areas of active red marrow in the frontal region. (**d**) Coronal contrast-enhanced T1-W MR image shows enhancing foci of active red marrow (*white arrows*)

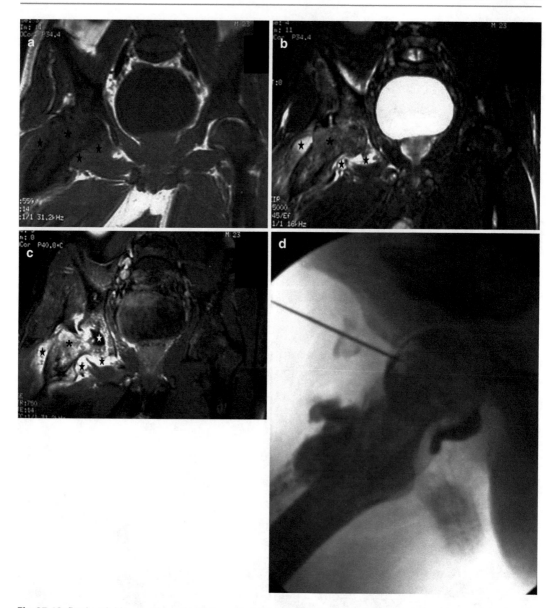

Fig. 37.48 Septic arthritis superimposed on osteonecrosis in a 23-year-old patient with SCD. Coronal (**a**) T1-W, (**b**) fat-suppressed T2-W, and (**c**) contrast-enhanced fat-suppressed T1-W MR images show enhancing thickened synovium (*black stars*), enhancing marrow edema (*black asterisks*), and non-enhancing osteonecrotic change at the femoral epiphyseal region (*white star*). (**d**) Fluoroscopy-guided aspiration confirmed the diagnosis of *Staphylococcus aureus* septic arthritis and osteomyelitis. Note the vertebral body and bone marrow which show bone changes due to SCD

37.5.3 Pitfalls and Mimics of Bone Changes

37.5.3.1 Subchondral Insufficiency Fracture

Subchondral insufficiency fractures in SCD occur secondary to osteoporosis. They are seen as a hypointense band-like region in the superolateral femoral head which is convex toward the articular surface (as opposed to concave in osteonecrosis). Contrast enhancement is frequently apparent proximal to this region, being found in 90% of cases (Ikemura et al. 2010) (Fig. 37.49), different from osteonecrosis in which there is lack of enhancement proximal to such a fracture line.

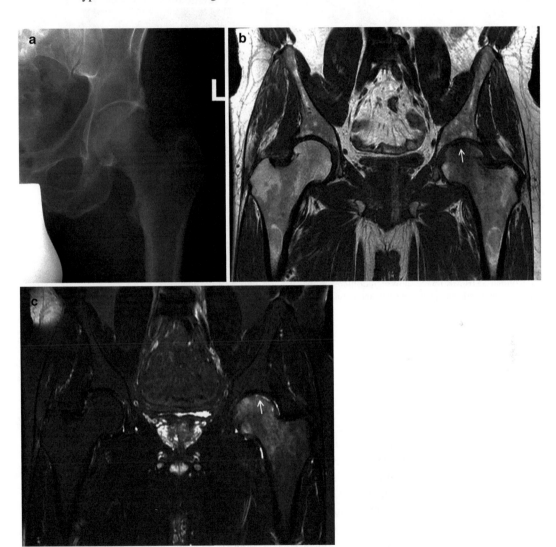

Fig. 37.49 Subchondral insufficiency fracture. (**a**) Anteroposterior radiograph of the left hip shows osteopenia of the left proximal femur. (**b**) Coronal T1-W MR image shows a thin convex-shaped hypointense line at the subchondral area of the left femoral head (*white arrow*) with surrounding marrow edema seen as signal hypoin- tensity. (**c**) Coronal STIR image shows hyperintense signal involving the femoral head and neck, which continues to the intertrochanteric region. This corresponds to the area of signal hypointensity on the T1-W image, confirming extensive marrow edema. Subchondral insufficiency fracture is *arrowed*

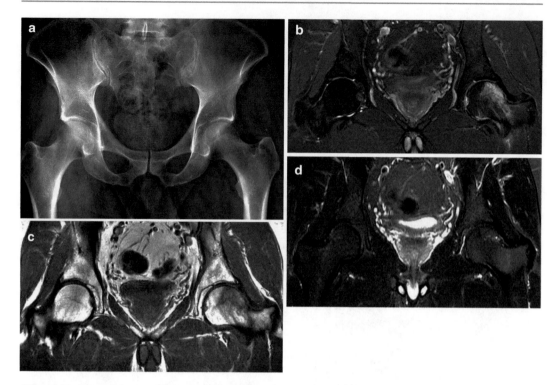

Fig. 37.50 Transient osteoporosis of the hip. (**a**) Anteroposterior radiograph of the pelvis shows osteopenia of the left proximal femur, compared to the right side. (**b**) Coronal STIR MR image shows hyperintense signal at the femoral head and neck regions, indicating marrow edema. (**c**) Coronal T1-W MR image shows no fracture line or evidence of osteonecrosis. (**d**) Follow-up coronal STIR MR image taken 2 months later shows complete resolution of the edema

37.5.3.2 Transient Osteoporosis of the Hip

Transient osteoporosis of the hip is seen as femoral head osteopenia at radiography and markedly increased radionuclide uptake in the femoral head (without central photopenia as in osteonecrosis). On MRI, there is markedly increased signal intensity on long repetition time images in the femoral head marrow, which shows diffuse enhancement after contrast agent administration (without signal variation or non-enhancement in the superolateral femoral head as in osteonecrosis) (Murphey et al. 2014) (Fig. 37.50).

37.5.3.3 Intramedullary Sclerosis

The imaging findings of osteonecrosis itself, particularly the epiphyseal region, may mimic septic arthritis since the joint effusion and thickened synovium (synovitis) can similarly occur (Fig.37.51). On the other hand, intramedullary bone infarction causes the usual serpentine sclerotic-line appearance on radiographs or CT (Fig. 37.52) which may mimic other disease entities such as enchondroma. Enchondroma may be differentiated from bone infarct by the typical ring and arc pattern of calcification, the MRI signal of the bone marrow and chondroid matrix, as well as the pattern of enhancement (Fig. 37.53).

Other pitfalls are calcified or ossified simple bone cyst/fibrous dysplasia (Fig. 37.54). The differentiation is more easily done finding a cystic component and expansion, if present. Wang et al. (2015) described intramedullary calcifications mimicking the bone infarction secondary to intraosseous arteriovenous malformation of the tibia. Osteonecrosis can be caused by certain disease entities other than SCD; one example is systemic lupus erythematosus (SLE) with typical bilateral osteonecrotic features of the femoral

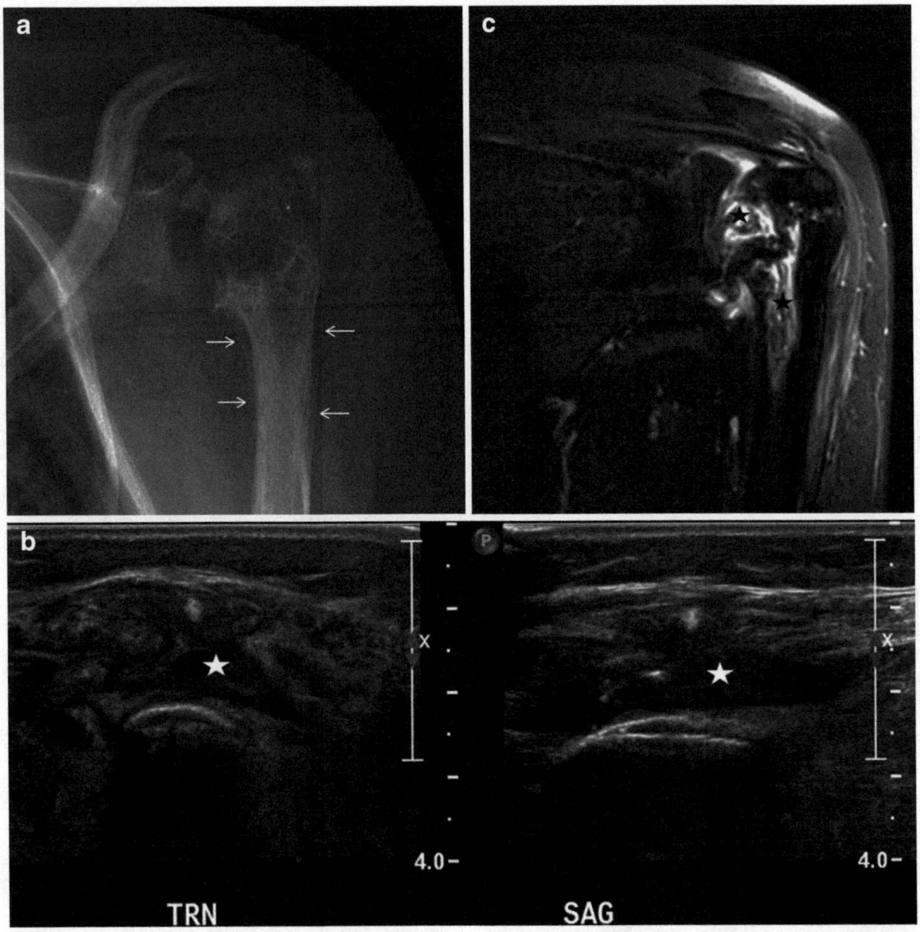

Fig. 37.51 Osteonecrosis and SCD bone changes simulating infection. (**a**) Anteroposterior radiograph of the left shoulder shows coarse trabeculation of bony structure, deformity of the humeral head with bone destruction, and periosteal reaction (*white arrows*). (**b**) Transverse (*left*) and sagittal (*right*) ultrasound images of the left shoulder show turbid effusion (*white stars*). (**c**) Coronal STIR MR image shows bone destruction and turbid joint fluid (*black stars*) simulating infection. No marrow edema is observed in this patient, which may help differentiate osteonecrosis from infection. Ultrasound-guided aspiration was negative for infection

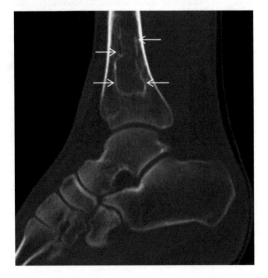

Fig. 37.52 Medullary bone infarction. Sagittal CT image shows calcification in distal tibia which has a serpentine outline and ground-glass to lucent center (*white arrows*), representing intramedullary bone infarction

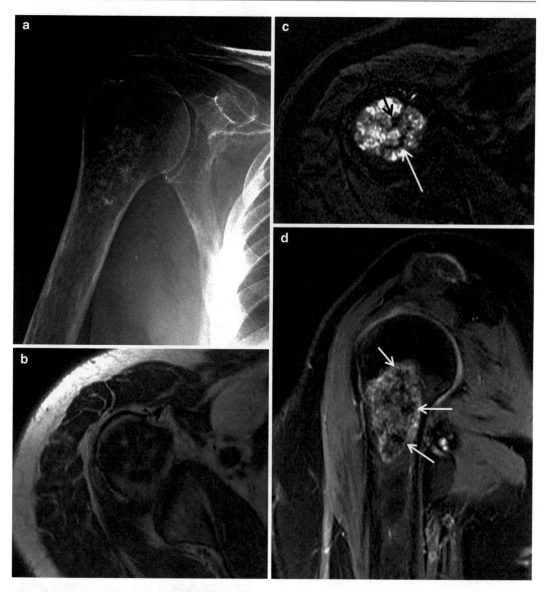

Fig. 37.53 Enchondroma. (**a**) Anteroposterior radiograph of the right shoulder shows intramedullary calcifications with a ring and arc appearance at the right proximal humerus. (**b**) Axial T1-W MR image shows signal hypointensity at the area of calcification. (**c**) Axial fat-suppressed T2-W MR image shows hyperintense signal of the hyaline cartilage with very hypointense dots inside, representing foci of calcification (*arrows*). (**d**) Sagittal contrast-enhanced fat-suppressed T1-W MR image shows faint enhancement of the lesion, but the calcific foci are still obvious (*white arrows*). Lack of serpentine appearance, the ring and arc calcification distribution within the lesion, and pattern of enhancement can help differentiate enchondroma from medullary bone infarct

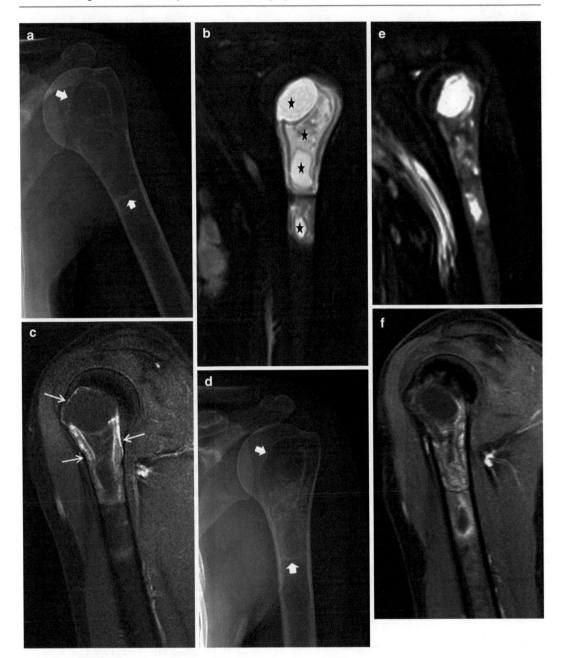

Fig. 37.54 Unicameral (simple) bone cyst. (**a**) Anteroposterior radiograph of the left shoulder shows an intramedullary elongated osteolytic lesion with calcified margins and mild endosteal scalloping (between *thick white arrows*). (**b**) Coronal fat-suppressed T2-W and (**c**) sagittal contrast-enhanced fat-suppressed T1-W MR images show a cystic component (*black stars*) with peripheral enhancement (*thin white arrows*). Follow-up imaging obtained 3 years later consisting of corresponding (**d**) radiograph and (**e**) coronal fat-suppressed T2-W and (**f**) sagittal contrast-enhanced fat-suppressed T1-W MR images shows a decreased cystic component and increased calcification suggesting a healing process and benignity of the lesion. The lack of serpentine appearance, osteolytic bone destruction, cystic component, and pattern of enhancement can help differentiate unicameral bone cyst from medullary bone infarct

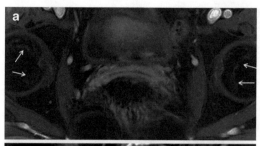

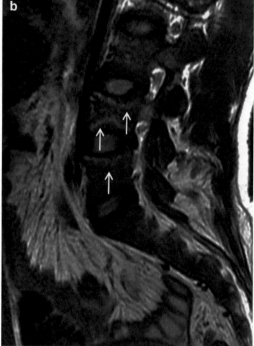

Fig. 37.55 Osteonecrosis in SLE. (**a**) Axial fat-suppressed T1-W MR image of a patient with SLE on steroid therapy shows the typical geographic lesion of osteonecrotic changes at the femoral heads (*white arrows*). (**b**) Sagittal T2-W MR image shows the codfish appearance of the vertebral bodies with endplate edema due to osteoporosis (*arrows*)

heads. Generalized bone softening of the vertebrae causing "codfish" appearance and subchondral endplate edema changes (Fig. 37.55) help discriminate SLE from the pathognomonic "H-shaped vertebra" deformity seen in SCD.

Conclusion

In this chapter, pitfalls in hematological and circulatory bone diseases represent only certain pitfalls that may possibly occur. To achieve the best result in imaging

interpretation, radiologists may need to understand the pathophysiology of each disease that can explain what appears in the images. Differential diagnoses should be offered, when appropriate. Awareness of normal variants and potential pitfalls, good clinical information about the patient, and clear understanding of the modality limitations can help radiologists to avoid misinterpretation in their clinical practice.

References

Ahmad S, Khan ZA, Rehmani R et al (2010) Diagnostic dilemma in sicklers with acute bone crisis: role of subperiosteal fluid collection on MRI in resolving this issue. J Pak Med Assoc 60:819–822

Alavi A, McCloskey JR, Steinberg ME (1977) Early detection of avascular necrosis of the femoral head by 99m technetium diphosphonate bone scan: a preliminary report. Clin Orthop Relat Res 127:137–141

Amstutz HC, Le Duff MJ (2010) Hip resurfacing results for osteonecrosis are as good as for other etiologies at 2 to 12 years. Clin Orthop Relat Res 468:375–381

Bahebeck J, Atangana R, Techa A et al (2004) Relative rates and features of musculoskeletal complications in adult sicklers. Acta Orthop Belg 70:107–111

Bracken J, Nandurkar D, Radhakrishnan K et al (2013) Normal paediatric bone marrow: magnetic resonance imaging appearances from birth to 5 years. J Med Imaging Radiat Oncol 57:283–291

Bradbury G, Benjamin J, Thompson J et al (1994) Avascular necrosis of bone after cardiac transplantation: prevalence and relationship to administration and dosage of steroids. J Bone Joint Surg Am 76:1385–1388

Camporesi EM, Vezzani G, Bosco G et al (2010) Hyperbaric oxygen therapy in femoral head necrosis. J Arthroplast 25:118–123

Conklin JJ, Alderson PO, Zizic TM et al (1983) Comparison of bone scan and radiography sensitivity in the detection of steroid induced ischemic necrosis of bone. Radiology 147:221–226

Currarino G, Erlandson ME (1964) Premature fusion of epiphyses in Cooley's anemia. Radiology 83:656–664

D'Ambrosia RD, Shoji H, Riggins RS et al (1978) Scintigraphy in the diagnosis of osteonecrosis. Clin Orthop Relat Res 130:139–143

Delgado J, Bedoya MA, Green AM et al (2015) Utility of unenhanced fat-suppressed T1-weighted MRI in children with sickle cell disease – can it differentiate bone infarcts from acute osteomyelitis? Pediatr Radiol 45:1981–1987

Dihlmann W (1982) CT analysis of the upper end of the femur: the asterisk sign and ischemic bone necrosis of the femoral head. Skeletal Radiol 8:251–258

Dines DM, Canale VC, Arnold WD (1976) Fractures in thalassemia. J Bone Joint Surg Am 58:662–666

Domson GF, Shahlaee A, Reith JD et al (2009) Infarct-associated bone sarcomas. Clin Orthop Relat Res 467:1820–1825

Dorfman HD (1972) Proceedings: malignant transformation of benign bone lesions. Proc Natl Cancer Conf 7:901–913

Dorwart BB, Schumacher HR (1981) Arthritis in beta thalassaemia trait: clinical and pathological features. Ann Rheum Dis 40:185–189

Drakonaki EE, Maris TG, Papadakis A et al (2007) Bone marrow changes in beta-thalassemia major: quantitative MR imaging findings and correlation with iron stores. Eur Radiol 17:2079–2087

Dua SG, Purandare N, Shah S et al (2011) Bone infarct-associated sarcoma detected on FDG PET/CT. Clin Nucl Med 36:218–220

Dubost JJ, Rami S, Carcanagues Y et al (1996) Subchondral insufficiency fracture of the femoral head. Rev Rheum Engl Ed 63:859–861

Duda SH, Laniado M, Schick F et al (1993) The double-line sign of osteonecrosis: evaluation on chemical shift MR images. Eur J Radiol 16:233–238

Ejindu VC, Hine AL, Mashayekhi M et al (2007) Musculoskeletal manifestations of sickle cell disease. Radiographics 27:1005–1021

Fernbach SK (1984) Case report 274. Beta thalassemia affecting the facial bones and skull (intermediate form). Skeletal Radiol 11:307–309

Finsterbush A, Farber I, Mogle P et al (1985) Fracture patterns in thalassemia. Clin Orthop Relat Res 192:132–136

Forget BG (1993) The pathophysiology and molecular genetics of beta thalassemia. Mt Sinai J Med 60:95–103

Foroughi AB, Ghaffari H, Haghpanah S et al (2015) Comparative study of radiographic and laboratory findings between beta thalassemia major and beta thalassemia intermedia patients with and without treatment by hydroxyurea. Iran Red Crescent Med J 17:e23607. doi:10.5812/ircmj.23607

Fridinger S, Mick TJ, Rich J (2001) Avascular necrosis and related disorders. https://www.nwhealth.edu

Gersten T, Zieve D, Ogilvie I (2014) Thalassemia. https://www.nlm.nih.gov

Gerster JC, Dardel R, Guggi S (1984) Recurrent episodes of arthritis in thalassemia minor. J Rheumatol 11:352–354

Ginzel AW, Kransdorf MJ, Peterson JJ et al (2012) Mass-like extramedullary hematopoiesis: imaging features. Skeletal Radiol 41:911–916

Glickstein MF, Burk DL Jr, Schiebler ML et al (1988) Avascular necrosis versus other diseases of the hip: sensitivity of MR imaging. Radiology 169:213–215

Gohel VK, Dalinka MK, Edeiken J (1973) Ischemic necrosis of the femoral head simulating chondroblastoma. Radiology 107:545–546

Haidar R, Mhaidli H, Taher AT (2010) Paraspinal extramedullary hematopoiesis in patients with thalassemia intermedia. Eur Spine J 19:871–878

Hamanishi M, Yasunaga Y, Yamasaki T et al (2014) The clinical and radiographic results of intertrochanteric curved varus osteotomy for idiopathic osteonecrosis of the femoral head. Arch Orthop Trauma Surg 134:305–310

Hamperl H, Weiss P (1955) Spongius hyperostosis of skulls in old-Peru. Virchows Arch 327:629–642

Hashmi MA, Guha S, Sengupta P et al (2014) Thoracic cord compression by extramedullary hematopoiesis in thalassemia. Asian J Neurosurg 9:102–104

Hauzeur JP, Pasteels JL, Orloff S (1987) Bilateral non-traumatic aseptic osteonecrosis in the femoral head: an experimental study of incidence. J Bone Joint Surg Am 69:1221–1225

Hauzeur JP, Sintzoff S Jr, Appelboom T et al (1992) Relationship between magnetic resonance imaging and histologic findings by bone biopsy in nontraumatic osteonecrosis of the femoral head. J Rheumatol 19:385–392

Hayes CW, Conway WF, Daniel WW (1993) MR imaging of bone marrow edema pattern: transient osteoporosis, transient bone marrow edema syndrome, or osteonecrosis. Radiographics 13:1001–1011

Iida S, Harada Y, Shimizu K et al (2000) Correlation between bone marrow edema and collapse of the femoral head in steroid-induced osteonecrosis. AJR Am J Roentgenol 174:735–743

Ikemura S, Yamamoto T, Motomura G et al (2010) MRI evaluation of collapsed femoral heads in patients 60 years old or older: differentiation of subchondral insufficiency fracture from osteonecrosis of the femoral head. AJR Am J Roentgenol 195:W63–W68

Jackson SM, Major NM (2004) Pathologic conditions mimicking osteonecrosis. Orthop Clin N Am 35:315–320

Jastaniah W (2011) Epidemiology of sickle cell disease in Saudi Arabia. Ann Saudi Med 31:289–293

Jiang CC, Shih TT (1994) Epiphyseal scar of the femoral head: risk factor of osteonecrosis. Radiology 191:409–412

Johannson HR, Zywiel MG, Marker DR et al (2011) Osteonecrosis is not a predictor of poor outcomes in primary total hip arthroplasty: a systematic literature review. Int Orthop 35:465–473

Kamata N, Oshitani N, Sogawa M et al (2008) Usefulness of magnetic resonance imaging for detection of asymptomatic osteonecrosis of the femoral head in patients with inflammatory bowel disease on long-term corticosteroid treatment. Scand J Gastroenterol 43:308–313

Kenan S, Abdelwahab IF, Hermann G et al (1998) Malignant fibrous histiocytoma associated with a bone infarct in a patient with hereditary bone dysplasia. Skeletal Radiol 27:463–467

Koo KH, Kim R, Cho SH et al (1994) Angiography, scintigraphy, intraosseous pressure, and histologic findings in high-risk osteonecrotic femoral heads with negative magnetic resonance images. Clin Orthop Relat Res 308:127–138

Koo KH, Ahn IO, Kim R et al (1999) Bone marrow edema and associated pain in early stage osteonecrosis of the femoral head: prospective study with serial MR images. Radiology 213:715–722

Kulkarni MV, Tarr RR, Kim EE et al (1987) Potential pitfalls of magnetic resonance imaging in the diagnosis of avascular necrosis. J Nucl Med 28:1052–1054

Laor T, Jaramillo D (2009) MR imaging insights into skeletal maturation: what is normal? Radiology 250:28–38

Lawson JP, Ablow RC, Pearson HA (1981a) The ribs in thalassemia I. The relationship to therapy. Radiology 140:663–672

Lawson JP, Ablow RC, Pearson HA (1981b) The ribs in thalassemia II. The pathogenesis of the changes. Radiology 140:673–679

Lee GC, Steinberg ME (2012) Are we evaluating osteonecrosis adequately? Int Orthop 36:2433–2439

Lee GC, Khoury V, Steinberg D et al (2014) How do radiologists evaluate osteonecrosis? Skeletal Radiol 43:607–614

Levin TL, Sheth SS, Ruzai-Shapiro C et al (1995) MRI marrow observations in thalassemia: the effects of the primary disease, transfusional therapy, and chelation. Pediatr Radiol 25:607–613

Li KC, Hiette P (1992) Contrast-enhanced fat saturation magnetic resonance imaging for studying the pathophysiology of osteonecrosis of the hips. Skeletal Radiol 21:375–379

Lonergan GJ, Cline DB, Abbondanzo SL (2001) Sickle cell anemia. Radiographics 21:971–974

Luk WH, Au-Yeung AW, Yang MK (2010) Diagnostic value of SPECT versus SPECT/CT in femoral avascular necrosis: preliminary results. Nucl Med Commun 31:958–961

Mackenzie JD, Hernandez A, Pena A et al (2012) Magnetic resonance imaging in children with sickle cell disease: detecting alterations in the apparent diffusion coefficient in hips with avascular necrosis. Pediatr Radiol 42:706–713

Madani G, Papadopoulou AM, Holloway B et al (2007) The radiological manifestations of sickle cell disease. Clin Radiol 62:528–538

Małkiewicz A, Dziedzic M (2012) Bone marrow reconversion – imaging of physiological changes in bone marrow. Pol J Radiol 77:45–50

Marker DR, Seyler TM, Ulrich SD et al (2008) Do modern techniques improve core decompression outcomes for hip osteonecrosis? Clin Orthop Relat Res 466:1093–1103

Martinoli C, Bacigalupo L, Forni GL et al (2011) Musculoskeletal manifestations of chronic anemias. Semin Musculoskelet Radiol 15:269–280

Mirowitz SA, Apicella P, Reinus WR et al (1994) MR imaging of bone marrow lesions: relative conspicuousness on T1-weighted, fat-suppressed T2-weighted, and STIR images. AJR Am J Roentgenol 162:215–221

Mitchell DG, Joseph PM, Fallon M et al (1987) Chemical shift MR imaging of the femoral head: an in vitro study of normal hips and hips with avascular necrosis. AJR Am J Roentgenol 148:1159–1164

Mitchell DG, Kressel HY (1988) MR imaging of early avascular necrosis. Radiology 169:281–282

Mitchell DG (1989) Using MR imaging to probe the pathophysiology of osteonecrosis. Radiology 171:25–26

Mont MA, Marulanda GA, Seyler TM et al (2007) Core decompression and nonvascularized bone grafting for the treatment of early stage osteonecrosis of the femoral head. Instr Course Lect 56:213–220

Mont MA, Zywiel MG, Marker DR et al (2010) The natural history of untreated asymptomatic osteonecrosis of the femoral head: a systematic literature review. J Bone Joint Surg Am 15:2165–2170

Mont MA, Cherian JJ, Sierra RJ et al (2015) Nontraumatic osteonecrosis of the femoral head: where do we stand today? J Bone Joint Surg Am 97:1604–1627

Munk PL, Helms CA, Holt RG (1989) Immature bone infarct: findings on radiographs and MR scans. AJR Am J Roentgenol 152:547–549

Murphey MD, Foreman KL, Klassen-Fischer MK et al (2014) From the radiologic pathology archives. Imaging of osteonecrosis: radiologic-pathologic correlation. Radiographics 34:1003–1028

Nokes SR, Vogler JB III, Spritzer CE et al (1989) Herniation pits of the femoral neck: appearance at MR imaging. Radiology 172:231–234

Öner AY, Aggunlu L, Akpek S et al (2011) Staging of hip avascular necrosis: is there a need for DWI? Acta Radiol 52:111–114

Orphanidou-Vlachou E, Tziakouri-Shiakalli C, Georgiades CS (2014) Extramedullary hemotopoiesis. Semin Ultrasound CT MRI 35:255–262

Orzincolo C, Castaldi G, Scutellari PN et al (1986) Aseptic necrosis of femoral head complicating thalassemia. Skeletal Radiol 15:541–544

Pappas JN (2000) The musculoskeletal crescent sign. Radiology 217:213–214

Piyakunmala K, Sangkomkamhang T, Chareonchonvanitch K (2009) Is magnetic resonance imaging necessary for normal plain radiography evaluation of contralateral non-traumatic asymptomatic femoral head in high osteonecrosis risk patient. J Med Assoc Thai 92:S147–S151

Poulton TB, Murphy WD, Duerk JL et al (1993) Bone marrow reconversion in adults who are smokers: MR imaging findings. AJR Am J Roentgenol 161:1217–1221

Rafii M, Mitnick H, Klug J et al (1997) Insufficiency fracture of the femoral head: MR imaging in three patients. AJR Am J Roentgenol 168:159–163

Rajagopal M, Balch Samora J et al (2012) Efficacy of core decompression as treatment for osteonecrosis of the hip: a systematic review. Hip Int 22:489–493

Rajah R, Young J, Conway WF (1995) Acute hemorrhagic infarct with edema. Skeletal Radiol 24:158–159

Resnick D (1995) Hemoglobinopathies and other anemias. In: Resnick D (ed) Diagnosis of bone and joint disorders, 3rd edn. WB Saunders, Philadelphia

Resnick D, Sweet DE, Madewell JE (2002) Osteonecrosis: diagnostic techniques, specific strategies, and complications. In: Resnick D (ed)

Diagnosis of bone and joint disorders, 4th edn. WB Saunders, Philadelphia

Rifai A, Nyman R (1997) Scintigraphy and ultrasonography in differentiating osteomyelitis from bone infarction in sickle cell disease. Acta Radiol 38:139–143

Ryu JS, Kim JS, Moon DH et al (2002) Bone SPECT is more sensitive than MRI in the detection of early osteonecrosis of the femoral head after renal transplantation. J Nucl Med 43:1006–1011

Sachan AA, Lakhkar BN, Lakhkar BB et al (2015) Is MRI necessary for skeletal evaluation in sickle cell disease. J Clin Diagn Res 9:TC08–TC12

Saito N, Nadgir RN, Flower EN et al (2010) Clinical and radiologic manifestations of sickle cell disease in the head and neck. Radiographics 30:1021–1034

Sauer B, Buy X, Gangi A et al (2007) Exceptional localization of extramedullary hematopoiesis: presacral and periureteral masses. Acta Radiol 48:246–248

Schmitt-Sody M, Kirchhoff C, Mayer W et al (2008) Avascular necrosis of the femoral head: inter- and intraobserver variations of Ficat and ARCO classifications. Int Orthop 32:283–287

Seki T, Hasegawa Y, Masui T et al (2008) Quality of life following femoral osteotomy and total hip arthroplasty for nontraumatic osteonecrosis of the femoral head. J Orthop Sci 13:116–121

Sen RK, Tripathy SK, Aggarwal S et al (2012) Early results of core decompression and autologous bone marrow mononuclear cells instillation in femoral head osteonecrosis: a randomized control study. J Arthroplast 27:679–686

Shah LM, Hanrahan CJ (2011) MRI of spinal bone marrow: part I, techniques and normal age-related appearances. AJR Am J Roentgenol 197:1298–1308

Sheehan SE, Shyu JY, Weaver MJ et al (2015) Proximal femoral fractures: what the orthopedic surgeon wants to know. Radiographics 35:1563–1584

Shillingford JP (1950) The red bone marrow in heart failure. J Clin Pathol 3:24–39

Sohawon D, Lau KK, Lau T et al (2012) Extra-medullary haematopoiesis: a pictorial review of its typical and atypical locations. J Med Imaging Radiat Oncol 56:538–544

Spritz RA, Forget BG (1983) The thalassemias: molecular mechanisms of human genetic disease. Am J Hum Genet 35:333–361

Stacy GS, Dixon LB (2007) Pitfalls in MR image interpretation prompting referrals to an orthopedic oncology clinic. Radiographics 27:805–828

Steinberg ME, Lai M, Garino JP et al (2008) A comparison between total hip replacement for osteonecrosis and degenerative joint disease. Orthopedics 31:360

Strecker W, Gilula LA, Kyriakos M (1988) Case report 479: idiopathic healing infarct of bone simulating osteosarcoma. Skeletal Radiol 17:220–225

Tsitouridis J, Stamos S, Hassapopoulou E et al (1999) Extramedullary paraspinal hematopoiesis in thalassemia: CT and MRI evaluation. Eur J Radiol 30:33–38

Vande Berg B, Malghem J, Labaisse MA et al (1993a) Apparent focal bone marrow ischemia in patients with marrow disorders: MR studies. J Comput Assist Tomogr 17:792–797

Vande Berg BE, Malghem JJ, Labaisse MA et al (1993b) MR imaging of avascular necrosis and transient marrow edema of the femoral head. Radiographics 13:501–520

Vogler JB 3rd, Murphy WA (1988) Bone marrow imaging. Radiology 168:679–693

Wang B, Zhao D, Liu B et al (2013) Treatment of osteonecrosis of the femoral head by using the greater trochanteric bone flap with double vascular pedicles. Microsurgery 33:593–599

Wang HH, Yeh TT, Lin YC et al (2015) Imaging features of an intraosseous arteriovenous malformation in the tibia. Singapore Med J 56:e21–e25

Weaver CJ, Major NM, Garrett WE et al (2002) Femoral head osteochondral lesions in painful hips of athletes: MR imaging findings. AJR Am J Roentgenol 178:973–977

Weerakkody Y, Goel A (2016) Snowcap sign. http://www.radiopaedia.org/articles/snowcap-sign

Yeh LR, Chen CK, Huang YL et al (2009) Diagnostic performance of MR imaging in the assessment of subchondral fractures in avascular necrosis of the femoral head. Skeletal Radiol 38:559–564

Zalavras CG, Lieberman JR (2014) Osteonecrosis of the femoral head: evaluation and treatment. J Am Acad Orthop Surg 22:455–464

Zhang HJ, Liu YW, Du ZQ et al (2013) Therapeutic effect of minimally invasive decompression combined with impaction bone grafting on osteonecrosis of the femoral head. Eur J Orthop Surg Traumatol 23:913–919

Zhu G, Wu X, Zhang X et al (2012) Clinical and imaging findings in thalassemia patients with extramedullary hematopoiesis. Clin Imaging 36:475–482

Zibis AH, Karantanas AH, Roidis NT et al (2007) The role of MR imaging in staging femoral head osteonecrosis. Eur J Radiol 63:3–9

Zurlo JV (1999) The double-line sign. Radiology 212:541–542

Pediatric Nontraumatic Musculoskeletal Lesions: Imaging Pitfalls

38

Eu Leong Harvey James Teo

Contents

38.1	**Introduction**	819
38.2	**Pitfalls in Normal Development and Variants**	820
38.2.1	Diaphysis	820
38.2.2	Epiphysis	822
38.2.3	Metaphysis	826
38.2.4	Apophysis	830
38.2.5	Spine	830
38.2.6	Individual Bones and Joints	833
38.3	**Bone Age Assessment**	836
38.4	**Bone Marrow**	836
38.5	**Bone Lesions**	837
38.5.1	"Don't Touch" Lesions	837
38.5.2	Osteofibrous Dysplasia and Adamantinoma	838
38.5.3	Osteochondral Lesions	838
38.5.4	Cystic or Cystic-Appearing Bone Lesions	839
38.5.5	Legg-Calve-Perthes Disease and Differential Diagnosis	841
38.6	**Infection**	841
38.6.1	Septic Arthritis of the Hip	841
38.6.2	Osteomyelitis	842
38.7	**Inflammation**	844
38.7.1	Chronic Recurrent Multifocal Osteomyelitis	844
38.7.2	Juvenile Idiopathic Arthritis	845
38.8	**Soft Tissue Masses**	845
	Conclusion	849
	References	849

Abbreviations

CT Computed tomography
MRI Magnetic resonance imaging
US Ultrasound

38.1 Introduction

Nontraumatic pitfalls in the pediatric musculoskeletal system occur frequently, and it is important to recognize these pitfalls in order to avoid unnecessary further imaging, intervention, and treatment. These nontraumatic pitfalls may arise due to unfamiliarity with the appearance of normal development or variants in the growing child. They may also arise because of overlap in the imaging features between benign and malignant lesions in children. Pitfalls occurring in the long bones and the axial skeleton, as well as some individual bones, along with the problems related to the assessment of bone age, bone marrow development, cystic-appearing bone lesions, infection, juvenile inflammatory arthritis, and soft tissue masses, will be discussed.

E.L.H.J. Teo
Department of Diagnostic Imaging and Intervention, KK Women's and Children's Hospital, 100 Bukit Timah Road, Singapore 229899, Republic of Singapore
e-mail: Harvey.teo.el@kkh.com.sg

© Springer International Publishing AG 2017
W.C.G. Peh (ed.), *Pitfalls in Musculoskeletal Radiology*, DOI 10.1007/978-3-319-53496-1_38

38.2 Pitfalls in Normal Development and Variants

38.2.1 Diaphysis

38.2.1.1 Physiological Periosteal New Bone

Bones develop through membranous or endo-chondral ossification. Membranous ossification is the process where mesenchymal cells transform directly into cortical bone without an intervening cartilaginous matrix. Secondary membranous ossification occurs in the periosteum of growing long bones. This is seen as periosteal new bone formation in an infant between 1 and 5 months of age, due to rapid bone growth at this age. It commonly occurs in the tibia, femur, and humerus and, less frequently, in the other long bones. It is bilateral and is usually symmetrical (Kwon et al. 2002) (Fig. 38.1). Other conditions associated with periosteal new bone formation include metabolic disorders such as scurvy, rickets, hypervitaminoses A and D, prostaglandin administration, congenital syphilis, or malignancies such as neuroblastoma, leukemia, and trauma. The periosteal new bone formation seen in these conditions is not as symmetrical as the physiological form and will have other distinguishing radiological features present. Physiological periosteal new bone

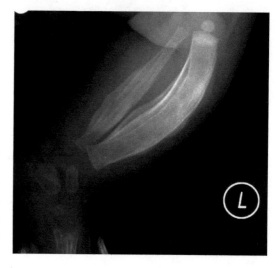

Fig. 38.2 A 4-month-old child with infantile cortical hyperostosis. Radiograph shows thick lamellated periosteal reactions over the shafts of the left tibia and fibula. These resolved and the bones returned to normal when the child developed further

formation should also not be confused with infantile cortical hyperostosis (Caffey disease) which is a self-limiting disorder occurring in infants up to 6 months of age due to a recurrent arginine-to-cysteine substitution (R836C) in the $\alpha 1$(I) chain of type I collagen (Nistala et al. 2014). It is characterized by thick lamellated periosteal reactions classically involving the ulna, clavicle, and mandible. The bones remodel over time and return to normal as the child develops (Fig. 38.2). Also see Sect. 38.2.3.4.

38.2.1.2 Vascular Nutrient Channels

Bones are penetrated by nutrient vessels. These are commonly seen in the diaphysis of long bones and appear as lucent lines on radiographs (Fig. 38.3). They occur bilaterally and symmetrically and traverse the bone obliquely. They may have a sclerotic edge and are not associated with soft tissue swelling or bony malalignment that may be seen in fractures.

38.2.1.3 Diaphyseal Sclerosis in the Newborn

The bones in newborns may appear more sclerotic than the bones in the older child because of the relatively thicker cortex of the bone relative to the medullary cavity. This usually resolves

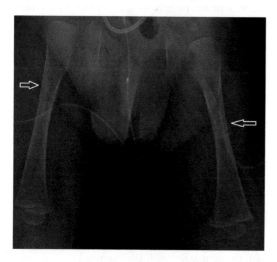

Fig. 38.1 Normal periosteal reaction in an infant. Frontal radiograph shows normal periosteal new bone formation in the diaphyseal regions of both femurs (*arrows*) in this ex-premature infant

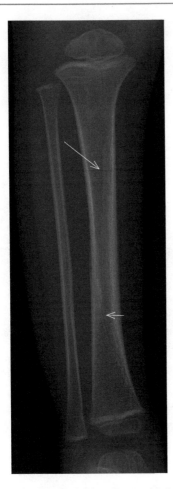

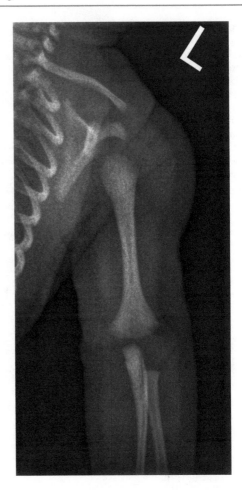

Fig. 38.3 Vascular channel in a 2-year-old child with a toddler fracture of the distal tibia (*short arrow*). Frontal radiograph shows a linear lucency in the upper tibia (*long arrow*) which should not be confused with a fracture

Fig. 38.4 Normal diaphyseal sclerosis in the newborn. Frontal radiograph of the left upper limb shows the visualized bones to be sclerotic because of the relative thicker cortex of the bone relative to the medullary cavity

spontaneously in 2–3 months. Differential diagnoses that may give rise to a similar appearance include osteosclerotic bony dysplasias such as osteopetrosis and pyknodysostosis, idiopathic hypercalcemia (William syndrome), neonatal infections, erythroblastosis fetalis, and the battered baby syndrome (Nadvi et al. 1999) (Fig. 38.4). These conditions will usually have systemic signs and symptoms such as anemia, motor development, or neurological deficits that are not present in newborns with diaphyseal sclerosis.

38.2.1.4 Bowing

Genu varus angulation is normally seen in neonates, and this is usually corrected within 6 months of walking or between 18 and 24 months of age. Thereafter, genu valgus is normally seen and this reverts to the normal adult pattern at 6–7 years of age. Physiological bowing of the tibia is said to occur when there is an exaggerated varus angulation centered at the knee during the second year of life (Cheema et al. 2003) (Fig. 38.5). It occurs in a posteromedial direction, and radiographs show mild enlargement and depression of the proximal tibial metaphyses posteromedially, without fragmentation or beaking. The medial tibial cortices are thickened and the ankle joints are tilted, with the medial side higher. The metaphyseal-diaphyseal angle is the angle between a parallel line drawn along the top of the metaphysis and a line drawn perpendicular to the long

Fig. 38.5 Tibial bowing in a 3-year-old girl. (**a**) Radiograph of both lower limbs show bilateral genu varum. (**b**) Radiograph of both lower limbs obtained 18 months later in the same patient shows the left genu varum to be resolving, but Blount disease has developed in the right lower limb

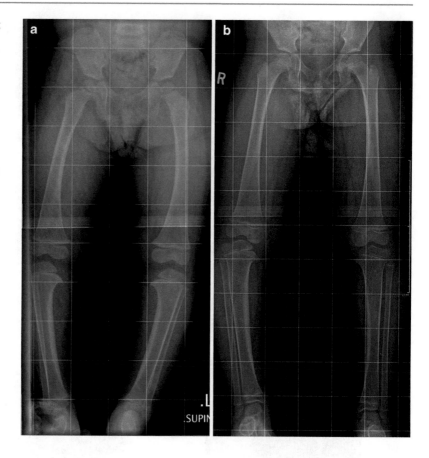

axis of the tibia, tangential to the cortex (Fig. 38.6). This angle is 5° ±2.8 in physiological bowing.

Physiological bowing should be differentiated from Blount disease which is a growth disorder of the medial aspect of the proximal tibial physis, resulting in progressive lower limb deformity. The cause of Blount disease is unknown but is thought to be the effects of weight on the growth plate. Children with indeterminate angles between 8° and 11° should be followed up. Other radiographic findings of Blount disease include genu varum, depression and irregularity, fragmentation of the tibial metaphysis posteromedially, and deficiency of the epiphysis medially. Lateral subluxation of the tibia and genu recurvatum may occur in late cases.

38.2.2 Epiphysis

38.2.2.1 Epiphyseal Irregularity

Endochondral ossification is the process of bone development where cartilage cells transform into bone. This occurs in the physeal plates and in the secondary ossification centers of long bones. Nonuniform ossification of the epiphysis may result in a fragmented appearance of the epiphysis. This is frequently seen in the lateral femoral condyle and is due to rapid growth in the width of the epiphysis between 2 and 6 years of age (Caffey et al. 1958) (Fig. 38.7). Independent ossification centers may appear separate from the main secondary ossification center and, on radiographs, appear as separate bony fragments. These should not be interpreted as loose bony fragments such as

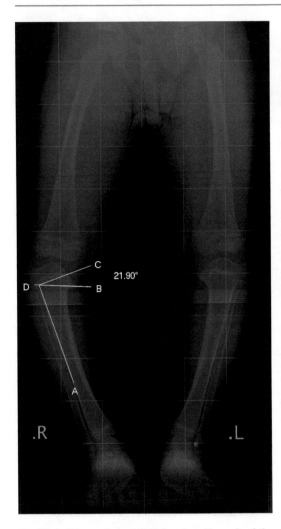

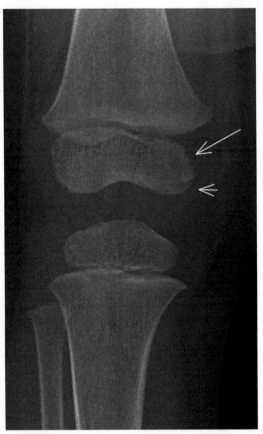

Fig. 38.7 Epiphyseal irregularity. Radiograph of the knee in a 1-year 5-month-old child shows normal irregularity of the medial aspect of the ossifying epiphysis (*long arrow*). A fragment can be seen separate from the main epiphysis (*short arrow*) but is still within the unossified cartilaginous part of the epiphysis and should not be interpreted as a loose body

Fig. 38.6 Blount disease. Full-length radiograph of the lower limbs in a 3-year-old girl shows bilateral genu varum. There is bilateral depression, irregularity, and fragmentation of the tibial metaphyses. The metaphyseal-diaphyseal angle is 21.9°. This is the angle created between lines DC, which is perpendicular to a line drawn along the long axis of the tibia (DA) and DB which is a line drawn parallel to the top of the proximal tibial metaphysis. In Blount disease, the metaphyseal-diaphyseal angle is greater than 11 degrees

those that may occur in osteochondritis dissecans. Further investigation is unnecessary, but should magnetic resonance imaging (MRI) be performed, an intact overlying articular cartilage, the presence of an accessory ossification center corresponding to the bony fragment seen on the radiograph, and

lack of bone marrow edema distinguish this normal developmental finding from an osteochondral lesion (OCL) (Gebarski and Hernandez 2005). Similar epiphyseal irregularities also occur frequently in many other bones, and differentiating normal irregularity from genuine pathology may be difficult. For example, tibial tuberosity irregularity may be a normal finding in some children but may also be seen in patients with Osgood-Schlatter disease (Fig. 38.8). Clinical correlation is needed to diagnose Osgood-Schlatter disease.

Enchondral ossification irregularity may also be seen in the carpal and tarsal bones of the hands

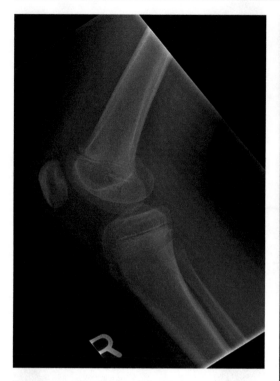

Fig. 38.8 Tibial tuberosity irregularity in a 9-year-old boy. Lateral radiograph shows a bony fragment at the tibial tuberosity. This is a normal developmental finding. This patient's symptoms were unrelated to the tibial tuberosity

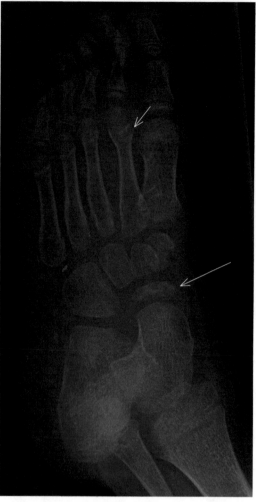

Fig. 38.9 Navicular irregularity in an 8-year-old girl. AP radiograph shows flattening, sclerosis, and fragmentation of the navicular bone identical to what would be seen in Kohler disease (*long arrow*). The patient's symptoms were unrelated, and she presented with a fracture of the head of the second metatarsal (*short arrow*). Subsequent follow-up radiographs showed normal development of the navicular bone

and feet, respectively. An example of this is navicular irregularity which is frequently seen in young children (Fig. 38.9). The navicular is the last of the tarsal bones to ossify and does not develop symmetrically and bilaterally. Differentiation from Kohler disease may be difficult on a single examination, although extreme flattening and sclerosis of the navicular are usually seen only in Kohler disease and not in enchondral ossification irregularity. However, in many symptomatic cases, an identical appearance is also seen in the opposite asymptomatic foot. The diagnosis of Kohler disease can be made definitively, only if the changes occur in a previously normal navicular bone. If necessary, bone scintigraphy may be diagnostic, by showing decreased tracer uptake in the early phase with increased uptake during the revascularization phase (Ozonoff 1992a).

The appearance of hyaline cartilage on ultrasound (US) imaging and MRI should be recognized. On US imaging, the hyaline cartilage is seen as a well-defined hypoechoic layer surrounding the ossification center of the epiphysis (Fig. 38.10). It should be distinguished from a joint effusion. On MRI, the signal intensity of the hyaline articular cartilage and the signal intensity of the physis are intermediate, when compared with that of the bony epiphysis. As the child grows, areas within the epiphyseal cartilage about to form bone appear as foci of hyperintense T2 signal and should not be interpreted as intra-epiphyseal abscesses (Thapa et al. 2012b; Zember et al. 2015). After intravenous contrast agent administration, the cartilage will enhance and show linear and punctate areas of signal hyperintensity, corresponding to vascular channels (Fig. 38.11). Some of these extend from the metaphysis to the epiphysis in younger infants and children up to approximately 18 months of age, after which they regress, leaving behind metaphyseal hairpin channels that are limited by the physis. Epiphyseal vascular canals increase in diameter with increasing maturity. These vascular channels may become more prominent during osteomyelitis.

38.2.2.2 Cone-Shaped Epiphyses

Cone-shaped epiphyses are epiphyses that invaginate into cup-shaped metaphyses (Fig. 38.12). Cone-shaped epiphyses occurring in the first distal and the fifth middle phalanges are normal and unassociated with syndromes in most cases but are abnormal when they are seen in the middle phalanx of the third and fourth digits and in the first proximal and fifth distal phalanges (Scanderbeg and Dallapicolla 2001). Some con-

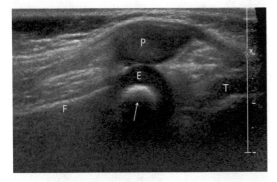

Fig. 38.10 Sagittal US image of the distal femur and knee joint in a 2-year-old boy shows the normal hypoechoic epiphyseal cartilage (*E*) surrounding the ossification center of the distal femur (*arrow*). The epiphyseal cartilage of the proximal tibia can also be partially seen (*T*). The patella has yet to ossify (*P*). It should not be interpreted as a knee joint effusion. [*F = femur*]

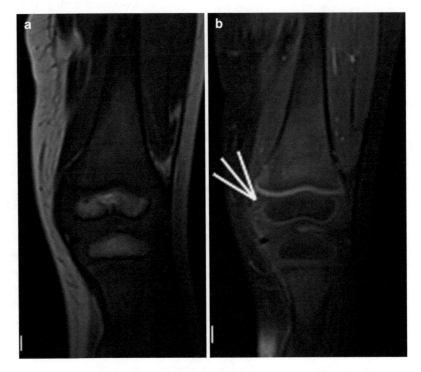

Fig. 38.11 MRI of epiphyseal vessels and cartilage in the knee of a 2-year-old boy.
(**a**) Coronal T1-W MR image shows the cartilage surrounding the ossification centers in the epiphyses of the distal femur and proximal tibia to be isointense to muscle.
(**b**) Coronal contrast-enhanced T1-W MR image shows the vessels within the epiphyseal cartilage as areas of punctate and linear areas of enhancement (*arrow*)

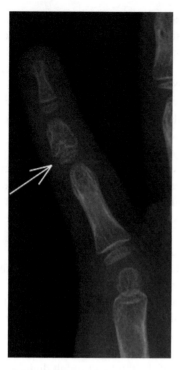

Fig. 38.12 Cone-shaped epiphysis in a 4-year-old girl. Radiograph shows a cone-shaped epiphysis of the middle phalanx of the little finger invaginating into the proximal metaphysis (*arrow*). This is a normal variant

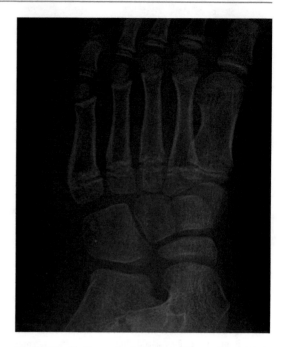

Fig. 38.13 Radiograph of a 6-year-old boy with multiple pseudoepiphysis in the proximal metatarsals of the foot. The pseudoepiphyses in the proximal second to fifth metatarsals are normal variants, and the epiphysis in the proximal first metatarsal is a normal occurrence

ditions associated with bony dysplasias are achondroplasia, acrodysostosis, chondrodysplasia punctata, cleidocranial dysplasia, and multiple epiphyseal dysplasia.

38.2.2.3 Pseudoepiphyses

The epiphyses of the metacarpals and metatarsals occur proximally in the first digit and distally in the second to fifth digits of the hands and feet, respectively. Pseudoepiphyses are notches or clefts that occur on the opposite ends of these bones and are common incidental findings (Limb and Loughenbury 2012) (Fig. 38.13). They do not contribute to bone growth and may occasionally be seen in hypothyroidism and cleidocranial dysplasia.

38.2.2.4 Ivory Epiphyses

Ivory epiphyses may be seen in up to 8% of boys and 4% of girls and refer to the dense appearance of the epiphyses, usually in the distal and middle phalanges of the small finger. It is usually a normal variant, although it has been supported to be

associated with growth retardation, renal osteodystrophy, Cockaynes syndrome, rhino-trichophalangeal syndrome, and various types of multiple epiphyseal dysplasia (Kuhns et al. 1973) (Fig. 38.14). Clinical correlation should distinguish normal from syndromic cases.

38.2.3 Metaphysis

38.2.3.1 Metaphyseal Irregularity

Metaphyseal irregularity may also be seen in the growing child (Fig. 38.15) and should not be interpreted as being indicative of an erosive process. It is due to uneven ossification in the adjacent physeal plate during growth. These findings disappear as the child matures. Metaphyseal step-offs are perpendicular projections adjacent to the physeal plate seen in young children, usually in the bones around the wrist and knee. Metaphyseal beaks or spurs are similar findings and should not be mistaken for the corner fractures of child abuse (Kleinman et al. 1991) (Fig. 38.16).

Fig. 38.14 Ivory epiphysis.
(**a**) Radiograph of a 7-year-old boy shows ivory epiphysis of the distal phalanx of the little finger (*arrow*).
(**b**) Radiograph of a 5-year-old boy shows ivory epiphyses of the distal phalanges of the big toes of both feet (*arrows*)

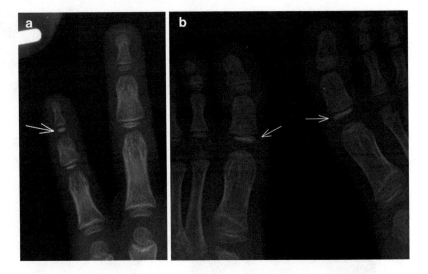

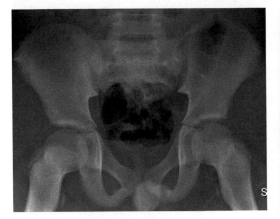

Fig. 38.15 Metaphyseal irregularity in a 12-year-old boy. Frontal pelvic radiograph shows irregularity of both iliac crests. This is a normal finding and should not be interpreted as erosions

38.2.3.2   Fibrous Cortical Defects and Avulsive Cortical Irregularity

These lesions are both situated in the posteromedial aspect of the distal femoral metaphyses. Fibrous cortical defects occur in the latter half of the first decade up to the early part of the second decade. They are present in up to 40% of children and appear radiographically as well-defined lucencies when seen in the frontal projection and cortical irregularities when seen in the lateral projection. As the patient grows, they migrate

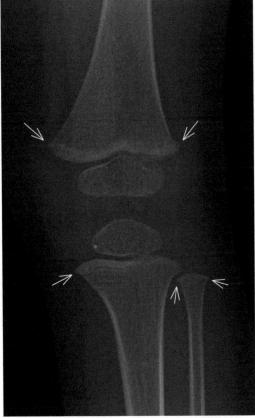

Fig. 38.16 Metaphyseal spurs in a 2-year-old boy. Radiograph of the knee shows subtle metaphyseal spurs in the distal femur, proximal tibia, and fibula (*arrows*). These are normal findings and should not be mistaken for the corner fractures of child abuse

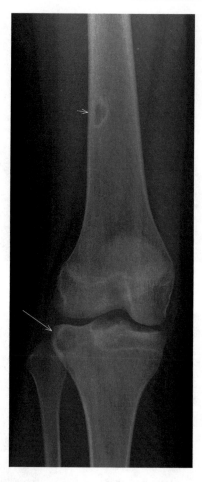

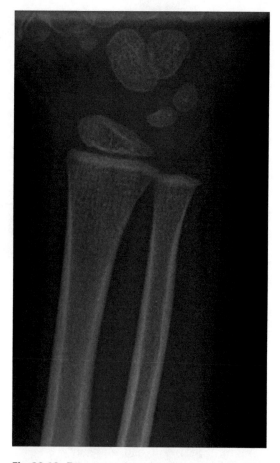

Fig. 38.17 Fibrous cortical defect in a 13-year-old girl. Frontal radiograph shows a fibrous cortical defect in the medial diaphysis of the femur (*short arrow*). Fibrous cortical defects grow away from the physis as the patient grows. The patient presented with knee pain due to the chondroblastoma of the proximal tibial metaphysis (*long arrow*)

Fig. 38.18 Dense metaphyseal lines in a 5-year-old boy. Radiograph of the distal radius and ulna shows dense metaphyseal lines adjacent to the physis in the distal radius and ulna

away from the growth plate (Fig. 38.17). Avulsive cortical irregularity or cortical desmoids occur in older children between the ages of 10 and 15 years. They are avulsive lesions occurring at the posteromedial aspect of the distal femoral metaphyses due to repetitive vigorous activity involving the adductor magnus muscle. They may be bilateral. On radiographs, CT, and MRI, they appear as areas of cortical irregularity and sclerosis. Histologically, periosteal thickening embedded in the cortex with proliferating fibrous tissue has been described (Pai and Strouse 2011).

Fibrous cortical defects and avulsive cortical irregularity should not be mistaken for malignant neoplasms.

38.2.3.3 Metaphyseal Lines

Dense metaphyseal lines may be seen on radiographs in the metaphysis of children between the ages of 2 and 5 years. This is due to increased bone density within the zone of provisional calcification (Fig. 38.18). This finding is normal, but it may simulate the dense metaphyseal lines seen in renal osteodystrophy, healing rickets, and lead and other heavy metal poisoning (Raber 1999). Correlation with clinical findings is needed to distinguish

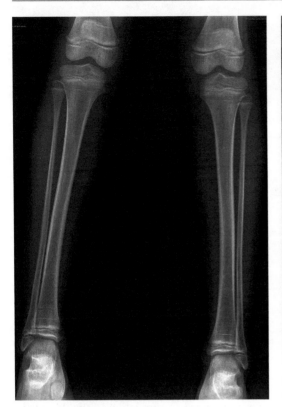

Fig. 38.19 Metaphyseal growth lines in a 6-year-old child with past history of clear cell sarcoma of the kidney currently in remission. Radiograph of the knees and lower legs shows multiple, bilateral symmetrical growth arrest lines in the metaphyseal regions of the distal femurs and the proximal and distal metaphyses of the tibiae and fibulae

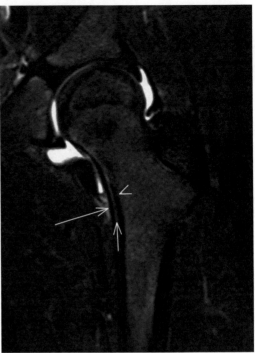

Fig. 38.20 Metaphyseal stripe in a 5-year-old boy with transient synovitis of the left hip. Coronal fat-suppressed T2-W MR image shows the cambium layer of the periosteum as a hyperintense metaphyseal stripe (*short arrow*) between the hypointense cortex (*arrowhead*) and the outer fibrous layer of the periosteum (*long arrow*)

normal from abnormal causes of these dense metaphyseal lines. Metaphyseal Harris growth lines (or lines of Park) appear as thin white lines perpendicular to the long axis of the bone and are most marked in the rapidly growing end of bones such as the distal femur and proximal tibia (Fig. 38.19). They appear when normal growth resumes after a period of nutritional deprivation, generalized illness, or prolonged immobilization.

38.2.3.4 Metaphyseal Stripe on MRI

The periosteum comprises of an inner cambium layer and an outer fibrous layer. The cambium layer of the periosteum is situated just adjacent to the cortex of the bone. The cambium layer is highly vascularized in the young infant and has been shown to play a role in intramembranous bone growth. On MRI, this layer is seen as a smooth, circumferential area with signal hyperintensity on T2-weighted and contrast-enhanced T1-weighted images, measuring 1–2 mm in width and separating the hypointense cortex from the hypointense fibrous periosteum (Fig. 38.20). It should not be mistaken for subperiosteal disease caused by tumor, fracture, or osteomyelitis. In these conditions, the subperiosteal disease typically appears as uneven and irregular stripping of the fibrous periosteum away from the cortex. The presence of other signs on MRI such as surrounding edema and bone destruction helps to distinguish these entities from the normal metaphyseal stripe (Zember et al. 2015) (Fig. 38.21).

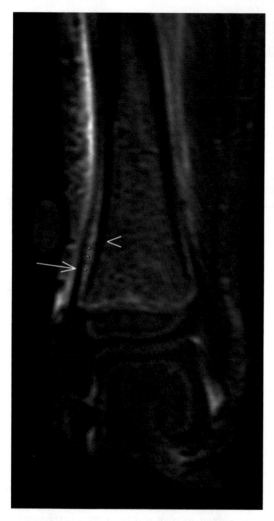

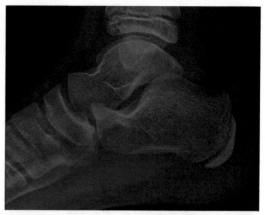

Fig. 38.22 Dense calcaneal apophysis in a 9-year-old girl. Lateral foot radiograph shows the calcaneal apophysis to be denser than the body of the calcaneus. This is a normal finding

Fig. 38.21 A 4-year-old boy with osteomyelitis of the distal tibia. Coronal fat-suppressed T2-W MR image shows a subperiosteal abscess (***) causing undulating elevation of the fibrous layer of the periosteum (*arrow*) away from the cortex of the bone (*arrowhead*). There is overlying soft tissue swelling and heterogeneous signal intensity in the metaphyseal region of the tibia due to inflammation

38.2.4 Apophysis

Apophyses are normal developmental outgrowths from bones which arise from separate ossification centers. They do not contribute to bone length growth, and they will eventually fuse to the bone when they completely ossify. They may serve as attachments for tendons or

ligaments. The calcaneal apophysis may appear normally extremely sclerotic and fragmented, as it ossifies (Fig. 38.22). Calcaneal apophysitis (Sever disease) is a cause of heel pain in children and may have similar radiographic findings. Clinical correlation should help differentiate the normal heel from apophysitis. Despite the nonspecific findings, a routine lateral radiograph is still advised because lesions requiring more aggressive treatment may be missed, e.g., calcaneal stress fractures and bone cysts (Rachel et al. 2011).

38.2.5 Spine

38.2.5.1 Bone-In-Bone Appearance

A bone-in-bone appearance of the vertebral bodies is a normal radiographic finding during infancy. This is usually seen in the thoracic and lumbar vertebrae in the first few months of life and is due to rapid growth of the vertebral body and where the fetal spine contour has not been remodeled (Ozonoff 1992c). An abnormal bone-in-bone appearance may occur in pathological conditions such as sickle cell disease, thalassemia, heavy metal ingestion, hypervitaminosis A, renal osteodystrophy, osteopetrosis, and other rarer conditions, but in these conditions, the

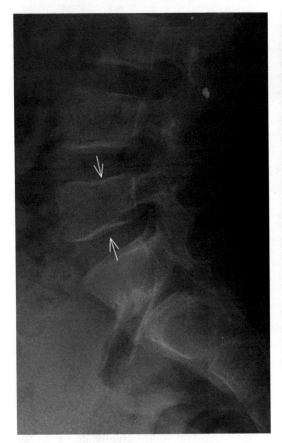

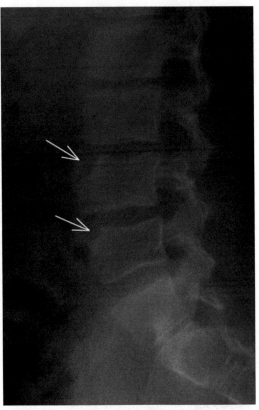

Fig. 38.23 Schmorl nodes in a 10-year-old boy. Lateral spine radiograph shows mild indentations on the superior and inferior endplates of the L5 vertebral body (*arrows*) due to Schmorl nodes

Fig. 38.24 Lateral spine radiograph shows limbus vertebrae (*arrows*) at the anterosuperior aspects of L4 and L5 vertebral bodies in a 14-year-old boy. The patient was followed up for 2 years and the findings remained stable

bone-in-bone appearance usually occurs at a later age. Correlation with the clinical history should help provide the correct diagnosis.

38.2.5.2   Schmorl Nodes and Limbus Vertebra

Schmorl nodes are protrusions of disk material (nucleus pulposus) into the surface of the endplates of the adjacent vertebral bodies (Fig. 38.23). They are commonly seen in the thoracic spine in adolescents and may or may not be symptomatic. Limbus vertebra is a closely related developmental anomaly where the nucleus pulposus herniates through the vertebral body endplate through the ring apophyses (Fig. 38.24). These lesions should not be confused with limbus fractures or infection (Ghelman and Freiberger 1976).

38.2.5.3   Interpedicular Widening and Vertebral Body Scalloping

The interpedicular distance in the frontal projection of the spine radiograph may appear relatively widened in children, compared to adults. This is normal and is frequently seen in the cervical and lumbar regions (Fig. 38.25). A minor degree of concavity of the posterior vertebrae is commonly seen in up to 50% of cases and should not be interpreted as being diagnostic of a space-occupying lesion in the spinal canal (Wakely 2006). This finding can also be seen on CT and MRI. Pronounced posterior scalloping of the vertebral bodies occurs in bony dysplasias such as achondroplasia, the mucopolysaccharidoses, and dural ectasia. These diagnoses should be clinically apparent.

Fig. 38.25 Widening of the interpedicular distance in two different patients. (**a**) Frontal radiograph of the cervical spine in a 5-year-old boy shows normal widening of the cervical interpedicular distance at C5 level compared to the thoracic spine at T1 level. (**b**) Frontal radiograph of the cervical spine in a 3-year-old child shows normal widening of the interpedicular distance of the lumbar and sacral vertebrae from L1 to S1 levels

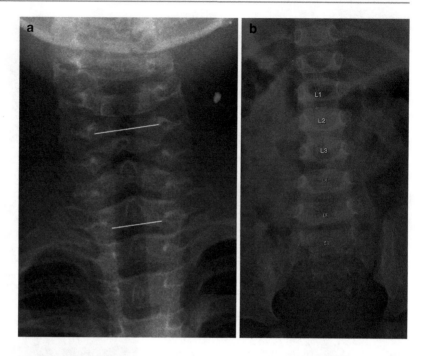

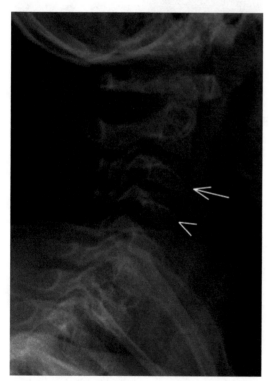

Fig. 38.26 Wedge-shaped cervical vertebrae in a 6-year-old girl. Lateral cervical spine radiograph shows wedge-shaped C3 (*arrow*) and C4 (*arrowhead*) vertebral bodies. These are normal variants

38.2.5.4 Wedge-Shaped Cervical Vertebrae

The third through seventh ossified parts of the cervical vertebral bodies usually appear wedge shaped on the lateral cervical radiograph. The vertebral body becomes squared off when the child reaches 7 to 8 years old. This is a normal variant and should not be misinterpreted as being part of a syndrome or due to compression fractures (Swischuk et al. 1993) (Fig. 38.26).

38.2.5.5 Fusion of the Posterior Neural Arches

Each vertebra has two separate ossification centers in the posterior neural arches that begin to fuse in the lumbar region, beginning in the first year of life. The fusion progresses cephalad to the cervical region, and fusion is complete in the third year of life (Prenger and Ball 1991). The separation between the posterior neural arches can be visualized on the anterior cervical spine or chest radiographs and should not be interpreted as being due to spina bifida (Fig. 38.27).

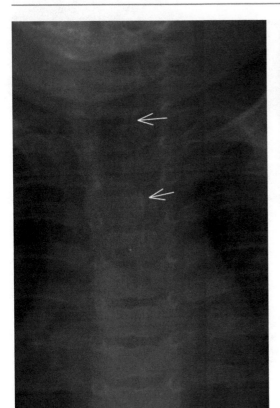

Fig. 38.27 Frontal radiograph coned down to the cervicothoracic spine of an 8-month-old girl shows unfused posterior neural arches at several levels in the thoracic vertebrae. These are normal findings and they fuse by the age of 3 years. They should not be interpreted as spina bifida

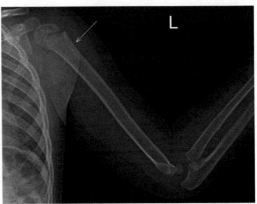

Fig. 38.28 Radiograph of the humerus taken in external rotation in a 3-year-old boy shows the presence of the bicipital groove (*arrow*) projected laterally, appearing as a pseudo-lesion of the metaphysis of the humerus

38.2.6   Individual Bones and Joints

Some individual bones and joints have their own unique pitfalls related to normal growth or radiographic technique. A few of the more common pitfalls within these individual bones will be discussed.

38.2.6.1   Humerus

The proximal humeral epiphysis consists of two or sometimes three ossification centers which appear at different times. The first to appear is situated in the medial aspect of the epiphysis, and this may appear laterally displaced and dislocated if the radiograph is taken with the humerus in internal rotation. The bicipital groove may appear to be a cortical-based pseudo-lesion, if the radiograph is taken with the humerus in external rotation (Keats and Strouse 2008) (Fig. 38.28). The greater tuberosity of the humerus frequently appears lucent on radiographs. This is a normal phenomenon and should not be interpreted as a destructive lesion. The supracondylar process is a normal bony projection on the anterior surface of the humeral shaft and occurs in about 1% of the population. This should not be interpreted as an exostosis.

38.2.6.2   Clavicle

The clavicle may appear distorted due to shoulder positioning or rotation of the patient during chest radiography (Fig. 38.29). Familiarity with this finding should prevent misdiagnosis.

38.2.6.3   Sternum

The sternum ossifies from five separate centers, and these may be misinterpreted as pulmonary nodules if a chest radiograph is obtained with the patient rotated. On a rotated radiograph, the manubrium sterni may be projected over the mediastinum, mimicking a mediastinal mass (Fig. 38.30).

38.2.6.4   Ribs

The anterior aspects of the ribs may normally appear bulbous and cupped in infants (Fig. 38.31).

Fig. 38.29 Clavicle distortion. (**a**) Coned-down view of a chest radiograph in a 10-month-old child shows the left clavicle to appear distorted due to patient rotation. The child was clinically well. (**b**) Dedicated radiograph of the left clavicle shows it to be normal without evidence of a fracture. It appears almost identical to the right side on the chest radiograph

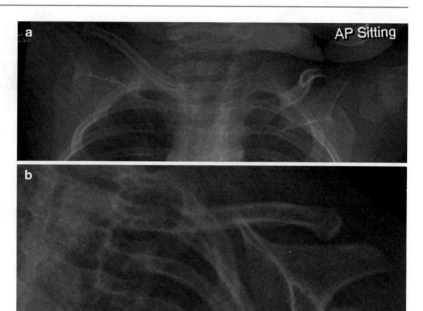

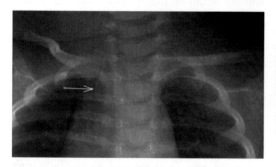

Fig. 38.30 Coned-down view of a rotated chest radiograph shows the manubrium sterni projected over the right superior mediastinum (*arrow*). This should not be mistaken for an abnormal mediastinal lesion

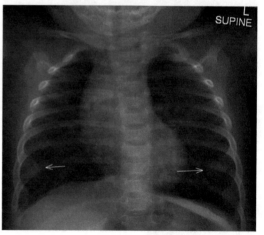

Fig. 38.31 Chest radiograph in a 3-year-old child shows the anterior aspects of the ribs to be cupped (*arrows*). This is a normal finding and should not be interpreted as that seen in healing rickets or bony dysplasias

A similar appearance may be seen in treated rickets, clinically known as the "rachitic rosary" sign. However, the bulbous appearance of the costochondral junction is usually more severe in rickets, and other bones will also be involved.

38.2.6.5   Joints

The vacuum phenomenon is the transient presence of gas in the joint space caused by the spontaneous extraction of gas from joint fluid (Sakamoto et al. 2011). This finding has been

seen in many joints in the body and in diarthrodial joints and is considered to be a normal phenomenon.

38.2.6.6   Patella

A dorsal defect of the patella is an area of fibrosis, with or without bone necrosis, situated in the

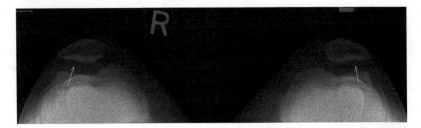

Fig. 38.32 Dorsal patella defect in a 10-year-old child who presented with left patella dislocation. Bilateral skyline radiographs of the knee shows bilateral subtle patella defects seen in the dorsal-lateral aspects of both patellae (*arrows*). These are normal variants. The right knee was asymptomatic

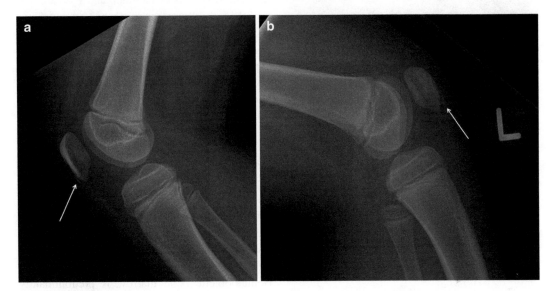

Fig. 38.33 Patella ossification. Lateral radiographs of the (**a**) right and (**b**) left knees show a linear ossification center in the inferior aspects of both patellae that have yet to fuse with the main body of the patella (*arrows*). These are normal variants and should not be interpreted as avulsion injuries

superolateral aspect of the articular surface of the patella (Fig. 38.32). It is a normal variant due to irregular ossification and is present in 0.3–1% of the population. On radiographs, it appears as a rounded lucency, frequently with a sclerotic border, measuring 4–26 mm in diameter. The cartilage over the defect is usually, but not always, intact. On T1-weighted MR images, the signal of a dorsal defect is heterogeneous, and on gradient-echo images, the signal is equal to or greater than that of the cartilage. The lesion disappears spontaneously as the child grows (Ho et al. 1991).

The patella ossifies from several different foci. These may occur irregularly and are normal findings (Fig. 38.33). A bipartite patella develops when a secondary ossification center fails to fuse

to the main part of the patella. It is usually asymptomatic but may cause anterior knee pain if chronic, or direct trauma involves the synchondrosis between the ossification centers (Thapa et al. 2012a). In symptomatic cases, MRI may show abnormal signal within the synchondrosis, edema in the bipartite fragment, and cartilage discontinuity.

38.2.6.7 Calcaneus

The unique trabecular architecture of the calcaneus can give rise to a cyst-like lesion in the mid-portion of the bone (Fig. 38.34). This is recognized as a normal variant, but other lesions may also involve this region, making diagnosis challenging. Another view of the calcaneus can

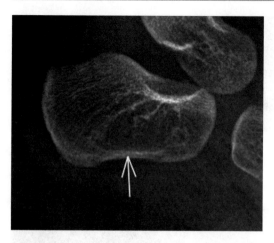

Fig. 38.34 Calcaneal pseudocyst in a 2-year-old boy. Lateral radiograph of the calcaneus shows a pseudocyst in the midportion of the bone (*arrow*) caused by unique trabecular pattern of the bone in this region of the calcaneus

usually confirm the absence of a true lesion. Differential diagnosis includes simple bone cyst and lipoma. These lesions will usually still be visible on the second view (Weger et al. 2013). Symptoms lasting more than 10 days are also suspicious for a true lesion, and if necessary, contrast-enhanced MRI is advised for further evaluation.

38.3 Bone Age Assessment

Bone age assessment is important in the treatment of limb length discrepancies and endocrine and metabolic disorders where children may have accelerated or delayed bone ages. Radiographic evaluation of bone age is most frequently performed using the standards of Greulich and Pyle. These standards were published in 1959 and with data collected between 1931 and 1942 in a Caucasian middle class population in the United States of America (Greulich and Pyle 1959). These standards may not be applicable in all populations due to differences in ethnicity and socioeconomic factors (Calfee et al. 2010). However, they are still useful in following-up of the growth and maturity in an individual patient.

Bone age evaluation is subjective and proper technique must be judiciously adhered to in order to avoid interpretation errors. Evaluation is performed by comparing the radiograph of the left hand of the subject to the standards of Greulich and Pyle. The appearance, size, and fusion of the epiphyses of the metacarpals and phalanges are matched with these standards which are grouped by gender and age. The carpal bones are also assessed but are more variable than the epiphyses. The standards of Greulich and Pyle are less useful in children younger than 2 years of age because the carpal bones are largely unossified and the epiphyses show little change in the appearance of the ossification centers. In these cases, standards of the knee (Pyle and Hoerr 1969) and the foot and ankle (Hoerr et al. 1962) should be referred to.

38.4 Bone Marrow

The marrow of the skeleton contains both fat and hematopoietic cells. Hematopoietic marrow is predominantly present in the pediatric age group and converts in an orderly but variable manner to fatty yellow marrow as the child grows. Hematopoietic bone marrow is predominantly seen in neonates. Conversion of red marrow to yellow fatty marrow begins at 1 year of age in the appendicular skeleton and progresses until early adulthood. Conversion begins in the distal parts of the long bone followed by the proximal bones. In any given long bone, conversion begins in the epiphysis and apophysis, followed by the diaphysis, and gradually progresses to the distal and proximal metaphysis (Vande Berg et al. 1998).

On MRI, hematopoietic marrow is lower in signal intensity than fatty marrow and equal to or slightly higher in signal intensity than skeletal muscle on T1-weighed sequences. It is of intermediate signal on fluid-sensitive sequences. Fatty marrow is hyperintense on T1-weighed and hypointense on fat-saturated T2-weighted and STIR sequences. Remnant red marrow can appear as scattered, flamed-shaped, geographic, ill-defined areas of T2-hyperintense signal in the

Fig. 38.35 Bone marrow pitfall in a 15-year-old boy. (**a**) Coronal T1-W MR image of the knee shows remnant red marrow around the knee (*arrows*) appearing as areas of hypointense signal, compared to fatty marrow. (**b**) Corresponding coronal STIR MR image shows these areas to be hyperintense compared to fatty marrow which is hypointense due to fat saturation (*arrows*)

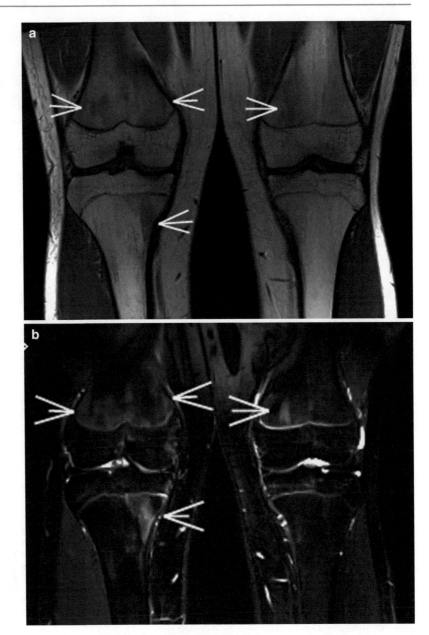

knee, foot, and ankle and should not be mistaken for pathological edema or neoplasm (Shabshin et al. 2006) (Fig. 38.35). Occasionally, red marrow may be focal, geographic, or patchy, mimicking an intramedullary lesion. Marrow reconversion may occur if there is increased hematopoietic demand. This commonly occurs in a patient with a known malignancy where mixed marrow signals may be seen and should not be mistaken for pathology.

38.5 Bone Lesions

38.5.1 "Don't Touch" Lesions

It is important for the radiologist to recognize characteristic benign lesions on radiographs for which further imaging workup or biopsy is unnecessary. Some examples of these lesions include the fibrous cortical defect, heterotopic

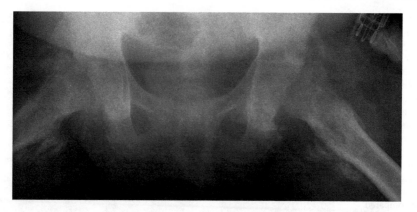

Fig. 38.36 Heterotopic ossification in a 17-year-old boy who had brain injury and neurological delay. Frontal pelvic radiograph shows patchy and flocculent soft tissue ossification around the upper aspects of both femurs typical for heterotopic ossification. These findings are diagnostic and no further workup is necessary

ossification, bone island, pseudotumor of the calcaneum, osteopoikilosis, geode, cortical desmoid, and avulsive cortical irregularity (Helms 2014) (Figs. 38.17 and 38.36).

38.5.2 Osteofibrous Dysplasia and Adamantinoma

These lesions are most often found in the tibia, and histopathological, immunohistochemistry, ultrastructure, and cytogenetic studies indicate that these lesions are closely related. Only adamantinoma has malignant potential. Osteofibrous dysplasia may cause limb bowing, leading to fractures and even pseudoarthrosis formation (Teo et al. 2007) (Fig. 38.37). These lesions have very similar radiographic appearances, although the diagnosis of classical adamantinoma is suggested by an extensive lesion with moth-eaten margins and complete involvement of the medullary cavity. Misdiagnosis on needle biopsy may occur in up to one-fifth of cases, and radiological features can assist in making the correct diagnosis (Khanna et al. 2008).

38.5.3 Osteochondral Lesions

Osteochondral lesions (OCLs) involve osteochondral fractures in an area of avascular necrosis in subchondral bone and overlying cartilage.

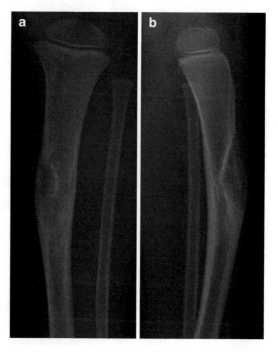

Fig. 38.37 Osteofibrous dysplasia in a 2-year-old boy. (**a**) Frontal and (**b**) lateral radiographs show a well-defined anterior cortical-based lesion typical for an osteofibrous dysplasia. It should not be confused with a fibrous dysplasia which is medullary based and has typical ground-glass opacification. There are overlapping features between osteofibrous dysplasia and adamantinoma and it is often difficult to distinguish these two lesions

Repetitive trauma is believed to be the primary cause in most cases (Grimm et al. 2014). Juvenile OCL usually occurs in the older child or adolescent more than 13 years old. Initial radiographs

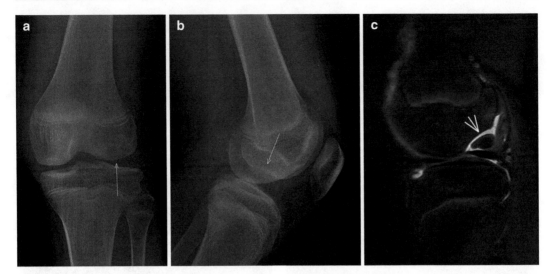

Fig. 38.38 Subtle osteochondral lesion of the left knee in a 13-year-old boy. (**a**) Frontal and (**b**) lateral radiographs show a subtle lucency in the lateral femoral condyle (*arrows*) suspicious for an osteochondral lesion. (**c**) Sagittal STIR MR image shows fluid separating the osteochondral fragment within the cavity in the lateral femoral condyle from the underlying bone, indicating an unstable lesion (*arrow*)

may show an area of rarefaction in the epiphysis which may be subtle (Fig. 38.38). Further progression to a bone fragment within a defect may occur. Later, this lesion may heal or progress further to flattening, further fragmentation, and cystic change in the epiphysis. MRI is performed to detect separation of the osteochondral fragment. The detection of a hyperintense line demarcating the fragment from the underlying bone on fluid-sensitive sequences indicates an unstable lesion.

OCL should be differentiated from bone bruising on MRI, osteochondral cyst, stress fracture, and Panner disease of the elbow. The latter condition is an osteochondrosis of the capitellum occurring in the dominant elbow in boys aged 5–12 years (Kobayashi et al. 2004). It occurs in a younger age group than OCL. On radiographs, an initial area of lucency is noted adjacent to the articular cartilage with some degree of sclerosis. In 1–2 years, the epiphysis returns to normal, without loose body formation. On MRI, an area of signal hyperintensity is seen in the affected area of the capitellum without overlying articular cartilage irregularity. The prognosis is excellent. Panner disease and OCL may be a continuum of a similar disorder but with different clinical outcomes (Kobayashi et al. 2004).

38.5.4 Cystic or Cystic-Appearing Bone Lesions

Cystic or cystic-appearing bone lesions commonly occur in children and are often a diagnostic dilemma. They are well-defined osteolytic lesions which may have a sclerotic margin. Frequently encountered lesions in children are the unicameral bone cyst, aneurysmal bone cyst, fibrous dysplasia, and Langerhans cell histiocytosis. Tuberculosis or a Brodie abscess may give similar appearances on radiographs but are far less common. Although these lesions have overlapping imaging appearances, close correlation to the clinical history and some imaging clues can point us to the correct diagnosis in many cases, obviating the need for further imaging and biopsy.

Unicameral (or simple) bone cyst usually occurs in the medullary region of the metaphysis in long bones, most commonly in the proximal humerus. As the bone grows, the lesion appears to migrate away from the growth plate toward the diaphysis. In actual fact, the physeal plate grows away from the lesion. It is generally unilocular but may occasionally contain fine septations. It is prone to fracture which is a common mode of

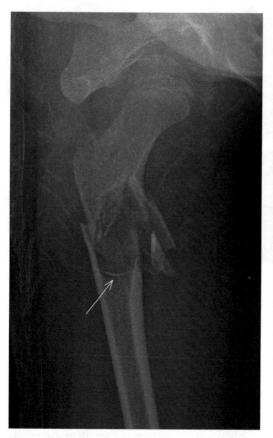

Fig. 38.39 Fallen fragment sign in a 7-year-old boy with a pathological fracture through a unicameral (simple) bone cyst. Frontal radiograph shows a fragment of the bone in the dependent portion of the cyst (*arrow*). This is pathognomonic of a unicameral bone cyst and further imaging is unnecessary

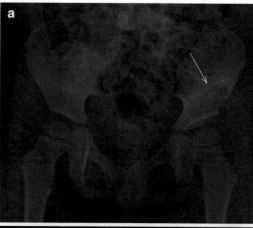

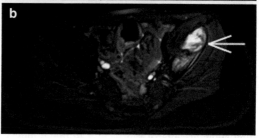

Fig. 38.40 Fluid-fluid level within Langerhans cell histiocytosis in a 3-year-old boy. (**a**) Radiograph of the pelvis shows a nonspecific lucent bone lesion in the left iliac bone (*arrow*). (**b**) Axial T2-W MR image shows a fluid-fluid level within the lesion (*arrow*). At biopsy, 6 ml of fluid was withdrawn. Langerhans cell histiocytosis was diagnosed histologically

presentation. The "fallen fragment sign," where a fragment of the bone is situated in the dependent portion of the cyst, is pathognomonic of this entity (Struhl et al. 1989) (Fig. 38.39). Cross-sectional imaging is unnecessary for diagnosis.

Aneurysmal bone cysts are lesions that occur secondary to hemorrhage in a preexisting lesion, such as a unicameral bone cyst or even a malignant tumor. It usually has a well-defined, thin, expansile, multiloculated "soap-bubble" appearance and frequently occurs in the metaphysis of long bones and in the posterior elements of the spine. Cross-sectional imaging characteristically shows the presence of fluid-fluid levels. However, fluid-fluid levels may also occur in numerous other lesions (O'Donnell and Saifuddin 2004)

(Fig. 38.40). The presence of a solid component suggests the coexistence of another lesion which should be investigated further.

Langerhans cell histiocytosis (LCH) presenting as a solitary bone lesion, commonly referred to as an eosinophilic granuloma, typically occurs in children between 5 and 10 years of age. They are usually found in the skull, mandible, spine, and long bones, commonly the femur and tibia. In long bones, lesions usually arise in the diaphysis or metaphysis. Radiographically, these appear as osteolytic lesions with variably defined margins with or without sclerosis, endosteal scalloping, and cortical thinning. Associated lamellated or solid periosteal reaction may occur. MRI is used for local staging of the lesion but is limited in diagnosis. Lesions have hyperintense signal on T2-weighted images and are isointense to muscle on T1-weighted images. After contrast agent administration, there is diffuse enhancement of lesion as well as surrounding reactive changes. LCH should be considered in the differential diagnosis of many osteolytic lesions in children, given the variable clinical and radiological features it may portray. In most cases biopsy is necessary for diagnosis (Azouz et al. 2005).

Fibrous dysplasia is a lesion in which fibroosseous tissue replaces the normal medullary space. It is usually monostotic, with polyostotic disease occurring in about 30% of cases. The ribs, long bones, and base of the skull are commonly affected. Polyostotic disease predominates on one side of the body and may be part of the McCune-Albright syndrome which consists of at least two of three features, namely, (1) polyostotic fibrous dysplasia, (2) café-au-lait skin pigmentation, and (3) autonomous endocrine hyperfunction. Radiographically, fibrous dysplasia has a characteristic "ground-glass" density. It frequently occurs in the medullary cavity of the diaphysis of long bones, causing endosteal scalloping. Bowing deformity of the bones may occur. Fibrous dysplasia may cause marked cranial deformity and cranial nerve palsies, when it occurs in the base of the skull. MRI is seldom useful in establishing the diagnosis, with the lesions typically appearing iso- to hypointense to skeletal muscle on T1-weighted imaging and intermediate to hyperintense on T2-weighted imaging, with variable contrast enhancement (Jee et al. 1996; Shah et al. 2005). Occasionally, fibrous dysplasia can be confused with osteofibrous dysplasia because both lesions have similar radiographic appearances (Fig. 38.37). However, osteofibrous dysplasias tend to occur in the cortex of bone, with a predilection for the anterior tibial cortex, whereas fibrous dysplasias occur in the medullary cavity.

38.5.5 Legg-Calve-Perthes Disease and Differential Diagnosis

Legg-Calve-Perthes (LCP) disease is an idiopathic necrosis of the proximal femoral epiphysis in children. Radiographically, LCP goes through several phases, beginning with the ossific nucleus of the affected hip appearing smaller than its normal counterpart. This is the stage of avascularity and the ossific nucleus also becomes increasingly dense. MRI performed at this stage shows no enhancement of the epiphysis. In the next stage of revascularization, the epiphysis becomes denser than before, and a subchondral fracture or "crescent sign" may be seen. With increased disease progression, the epiphysis becomes increasingly fragmented and flattened, with cystic changes appearing in the metaphysis and associated widening. MRI at this stage shows synovial proliferation and enhancement. During the healing phase, the epiphysis regains its height. The degree of rejuvenation depends on the amount of coverage by the acetabulum. The greater the epiphysis is covered by the acetabulum, the greater the remodeling occurs. Residual deformity such as coxa magna, coxa breva or short femoral neck, coxa vara, or valgus may occur (Smith and Jaramillo 2008).

Osteonecrosis related to other causes such as sickle cell anemia, steroids, and Gaucher disease has identical radiological findings and should be excluded before a diagnosis of LCP is made. Meyer dysplasia is a rare developmental condition that is characterized by irregular ossification of the proximal femoral epiphysis. It occurs in a younger age group (less than 4 years) than LCP and has a good prognosis with no significant long-term complications. Radiographs obtained 2–4 years after the initial presentation show a near-normal appearance of the femoral head. In contrast to LCP, the signal intensity of the femoral epiphysis is normal on MRI (Harel et al. 1999). Multiple epiphyseal dysplasia is an autosomal dominant short-limbed skeletal dysplasia that is also characterized by irregular ossification of the femoral head. It can be distinguished from the other conditions by detecting involvement of the epiphyses of other bones and genetic studies (Lachman et al. 2005).

38.6 Infection

38.6.1 Septic Arthritis of the Hip

Hip pain is a common clinical problem in children with an extensive differential diagnosis. Septic arthritis is a medical emergency and should be diagnosed early because it may give rise to significant morbidity and mortality. Diagnosis may be difficult in the early stage because the signs and symptoms may be subtle and overlap with other causes. Radiographs are usually normal. Early changes may manifest as osteopenia of the femoral head and surrounding soft tissue swelling. A frequently mentioned sign on the radiograph is effacement or outward bulging of the fat line adjacent to the hip joint which is indicative of a joint effusion. This has been shown through anatomical studies to be false, and that the radiographic sign of "capsular swelling" is due to lateral rotation and abduction of the hip (Brown 1975).

CT and MRI have also shown that there is little contact between the fat planes and the joint capsule. Evaluation for the presence or absence of hip effusion on radiographs has largely been rendered irrelevant because US imaging is now performed to detect the presence or absence of an effusion (Fig. 38.41). The echogenicity of the joint fluid cannot distinguish septic and non-septic etiologies. Comparison with the opposite side is important because a small amount of fluid may be seen in a normal joint, and joint effusions are only considered significant if they measure more than 5 mm or are more than 2 mm when compared to the asymptomatic contralateral hip (Tsung and Blaivas 2008). Positioning the probe perpendicular to the skin is also important in preventing the anisotropic effect which is an artifact that can falsely diagnose joint fluid when none is present.

Clinical parameters have been found to be valuable in distinguishing septic arthritis from other causes. Caird et al. (2006) did a prospective study of children who presented with findings that were highly suspicious for septic arthritis of the hip and found that fever (oral temperature > 38.5 °C) was the best predictor of septic arthritis, followed by elevated C-reactive protein level, elevated erythrocyte sedimentation rate (ESR), refusal to bear weight, and elevated serum white blood cell count. In their study group, C-reactive protein level of >2.0 mg/dL (>20 mg/L) was a strong independent risk factor and a valuable tool for assessing and diagnosing children suspected of having septic arthritis of the hip (Caird et al. 2006). While US imaging is

useful in determining the presence or absence of an effusion, it has a limited field of view, and MRI is more useful in evaluating the extent of disease (Fig. 38.41). MRI also provides better contrast resolution than US. On imaging, if gross displacement of the femoral head is seen, it is most likely due to septic arthritis and this sign is rare in non-septic causes (Ozonoff 1992b).

38.6.2 Osteomyelitis

Osteomyelitis may occur from hematogenous spread, spread from adjacent infected soft tissue or joint or direct implantation from a foreign body or surgery. The earliest change that is seen on radiographs is deep soft tissue edema. Bony changes occur late, and a normal radiograph does not exclude osteomyelitis and should not be relied upon to make the diagnosis. Three-phase bone scintigraphy may be used for the diagnosis of osteomyelitis, and the affected area appears as an area of increased tracer activity in all three phases of the bone scintiscans. A possible pitfall is the difficulty in diagnosing areas of involvement within the metaphysis, close to the physeal plate, because the increased tracer uptake in the physeal plate may mask pathological uptake in the metaphysis. Other pathologies such as fractures, sickle cell disease, and tumors may mimic osteomyelitis on three-phase bone scintigraphy because they also demonstrate uptake on all three phases (Love et al. 2003). In these instances, correlation with the clinical findings and blood investigations should be useful in distinguishing among the differential diagnoses in most cases.

Subperiosteal abscesses can be seen on US imaging, CT, or MRI before bony changes are detectable on radiographs, and in the appropriate clinical setting, the detection of a subperiosteal abscess is diagnostic of osteomyelitis unless proven otherwise. US imaging may be performed to distinguish cellulitis from osteomyelitis by detecting the presence of a subperiosteal abscess underlying the area of pain and erythema. However, the finding of a subperiosteal abscess is a late change. Furthermore, US imaging cannot diagnose the extent of marrow involvement, and MRI may be indicated for early evaluation in some

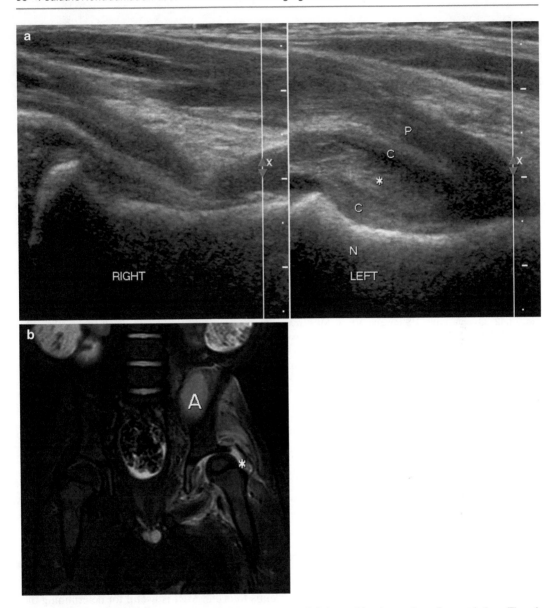

Fig. 38.41 Septic arthritis in a 1-year-old boy. (**a**) Sagittal US images of the right and left hips show an echogenic effusion in the left hip joint (*) within the joint capsule (*C*). No effusion is seen in the right hip [*N*, femoral neck; *P*, iliopsoas muscle]. (**b**) Coronal STIR MR image shows the left hip effusion (*) with lateral displacement of the left femoral head away from the acetabulum. There is marked surrounding soft tissue inflammation and an abscess within the iliacus muscle (*A*). MRI provides a more panoramic view of the surrounding structures and better contrast resolution

cases (Fig. 38.42). MRI is the modality of choice in many institutions because of its excellent sensitivity and ability to provide excellent anatomical information. The ability to provide panoramic anatomical images in multiple planes is useful for surgical planning and follow-up. Disadvantages include increased cost and the necessity for sedation or general anesthesia in some cases.

While the diagnosis of osteomyelitis should be clinically obvious in most cases, Ewing sarcoma may present with nearly identical clinical features, anemia, leukocytosis, and elevated ESR. The imaging findings on MRI may also be similar to osteomyelitis. Henninger et al. (2013) showed that the most clear-cut pattern for determining the correct diagnosis was the presence of a sharp and

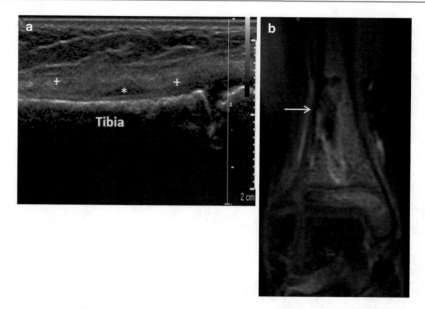

Fig. 38.42 Osteomyelitis: US imaging versus MRI in a 6-year-old boy presenting with swelling, pain, and edema over the shin. (**a**) Sagittal US image of the distal tibia shows increased echogenicity of the soft tissue overlying the distal tibia, consistent with soft tissue edema (+). A small subperiosteal collection is seen (*). These findings are consistent with underlying tibial osteomyelitis. (**b**) Coronal contrast-enhanced fat-suppressed T1-W MR image shows enhancement within the bone marrow of the tibia with a rim-enhancing collection within the medullary cavity *(arrow)* – these findings cannot be seen on US

defined margin of the bone lesion and the presence of an enhancing soft tissue mass which is seen in Ewing sarcoma and not in osteomyelitis.

38.7 Inflammation

38.7.1 Chronic Recurrent Multifocal Osteomyelitis

Chronic recurrent multifocal osteomyelitis (CRMO) is a rare autoinflammatory disease that presents with recurrent bone pain, with or without a fever. The pain is due to the presence of one or more foci of nonbacterial osteomyelitis. CRMO is now considered the pediatric equivalent of synovitis, acne, pustulosis, hyperostosis, and osteitis (SAPHO) syndrome in adults (Wipff et al. 2011). Diagnosis of this condition is difficult because it has nonspecific symptoms and imaging features. It is often not considered in the diagnosis because of its rarity, and is a diagnosis of exclusion. Early in the disease, radiographs may show a lucent lesion in the metaphysis adjacent to the physis. Progressive sclerosis then occurs around the lytic lesion, so that chronic lesions may be predominantly sclerotic with associated hyperostosis. The lesions have a nonspecific appearance.

The tibia is the commonest bone to be involved. The clavicle is also frequently involved. This, in fact, is a clue to the diagnosis because the clavicle is an unusual site for bacterial osteomyelitis to occur. MRI is useful for determining the extent of disease and for follow-up. In the early active phase of the disease, MRI shows marrow edema. Periostitis, soft tissue inflammation, and transphyseal disease may be seen as the disease progresses (Khanna et al. 2009). Bone biopsy is required in nearly all patients with a unifocal lesion to distinguish this disease from tumor or infection. Biopsies usually show a nonspecific inflammation, with numerous plasma cells. Cultures are negative. Radiologists can play a role in diagnosis by suggesting the diagnosis in patients with the abovementioned clinical history and radiological findings.

38.7.2 Juvenile Idiopathic Arthritis

Juvenile idiopathic arthritis (JIA) is a diagnosis of exclusion and is defined as an arthritis that develops in a patient before the age of 16 years, persists for at least 6 weeks, and has no identifiable cause. Although it is classified into several subtypes, chronic inflammation of the synovium is common to all subtypes. With disease progression, the proliferative synovium erodes into the underlying articular cartilage and bone, with progressive deformity and ankylosis. Historically, radiographs have been used to image the disease. However, radiographs are insensitive in detecting early articular damage because the pediatric epiphysis is mostly cartilaginous and early erosions may not be visualized. Furthermore, the development of new disease-modifying antirheumatic drugs (DMARDs) that are able to suppress the inflammatory changes in the joints has increased the demand for more sensitive imaging modalities that are able to detect active disease before irreversible structural change occurs.

Thus, modalities such as US imaging and MRI are increasingly being used to detect the early signs of JIA. They are also being used to assess the adequacy of DMARD therapy in patients. This has highlighted the need to establish norms and standard references in healthy children regarding the imaging anatomy of joints in healthy children, including growth changes over time. Several studies have evaluated MRI-based semiquantitative scoring systems for assessment of synovitis in JIA with varying results (Damasio et al. 2012). Bony depressions occur normally in the wrists of healthy children, and it may be difficult to distinguish these from bony erosions caused by JIA (Fig. 38.43). The temporomandibular joint (TMJ) is frequently involved in JIA and is thus frequently imaged. Age-related changes are seen in the mandibular condyle that may be misinterpreted for joint erosion. The variable enhancement pattern of the synovium of the TMJ also makes evaluation for disease activity difficult (Karlo et al. 2010; von Kalle et al. 2015).

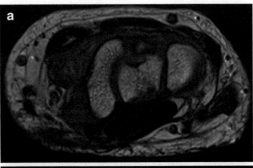

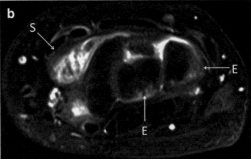

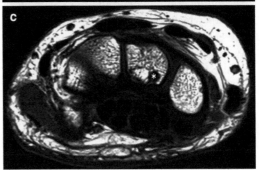

Fig. 38.43 Carpal erosions due to juvenile idiopathic arthritis (JIA). Axial (**a**) T1-W and (**b**) contrast-enhanced fat-suppressed T1-W MR images of the wrist in an 11-year-old boy show synovial enhancement (*S*) surrounding the carpal bones with erosions (*E*). (**c**) Axial T1-W MR image of the wrist in a 13-year-old boy who presented with injury while playing rugby shows a depression in the capitate bone (*asterisk*). These are commonly seen in children and it may be difficult to distinguish these from bony erosions caused by JIA. The presence of these findings makes the establishment of accurate scoring systems challenging

38.8   Soft Tissue Masses

US imaging and MRI are the modalities most often used to evaluate soft tissue masses in children. US imaging is initially used if the lesion is superficial and small in size. The presence or absence of a mass can be confirmed. Occasionally, there is no focal lesion present and the "mass" noted clinically is due to asymmetrically distributed soft tissue. This negates the necessity for further workup. The next step is to determine if the mass is cystic or solid in nature. Ganglion cysts, synovial cysts, bursae, and lymphatic malformations are common cystic lesions seen in children. If necessary, MRI may be performed if the lesion is large or infiltrative. It is important to ensure that the entire lesion is covered but using as small a coil as possible to ensure good quality images. The lesion should be imaged in at least two orthogonal planes using both T1- and T2-weighted images. Contrast-enhanced fat-suppressed images should also be obtained if a lesion is present. The latter sequence may give information regarding the degree of vascularity within the lesion. MR angiographic images may give information regarding the blood supply to the lesion which is useful for surgical planning.

A broad array of solid benign masses (e.g., myxomas, peripheral nerve sheath tumors, certain vascular lesions, glomus tumors, and malignant solid masses, including undifferentiated pleomorphic sarcomas, myxofibrosarcomas, myxoid liposarcomas, synovial sarcomas, extraskeletal myxoid chondrosarcomas, and, less frequently, soft tissue metastases) may exhibit hyperintense T2 signal on MRI, thereby simulating a cyst. On the other hand, fluid-filled lesions with associated complications (e.g., bleeding or inflammatory changes) may have a more complex appearance (Bermejo et al. 2013). Imaging is limited in its ability to distinguish benign from malignant soft tissue lesions, and in many cases, the role of the radiologist is to confirm the presence of a lesion and to determine its extent. With knowledge of the clinical history, lesion location, and imaging characteristics, some lesions may be specifically diagnosed or the differential diagnosis narrowed. Indeterminate lesions may need to be biopsied.

Soft tissue masses in children are most often benign and vascular in origin. Radiologists should be familiar with the International Society for the Study of Vascular Anomalies classification of vascular anomalies. This classification divides vascular anomalies into two distinct groups, namely, vascular tumors and vascular malformations (www.issva.org). Vascular tumors are due to endothelial proliferation. The commonest example is the infantile hemangioma which has a typical growth cycle and usually regresses completely during childhood. Vascular malformations are due to dysplastic vessels that do not proliferate or regress. They can be divided into fast or slow flow lesions The imaging features of vascular anomalies are diagnostic in many cases, and it is important for the radiologist to correctly classify these lesions because the management is different for each type (Mulligan et al. 2014) (Fig. 38.44).

Lipomas are tumors composed of mature fat cells. Lipoblastoma and lipoblastomatosis are terms applied to discrete and diffuse forms, respectively, of a lipoma variant that is named for its resemblance to fetal adipose tissue (Bancroft et al. 2006). Lipomas and lipoblastomas are well-defined focal lesions that have echogenicity or signal intensities similar to subcutaneous adipose tissue. Additionally, lipoblastomas have areas of non-lipomatous tissue corresponding to immature adipocytes with a richly vascular myxoid matrix. These have a nonspecific imaging appearance and are T1 hypointense and T2 hyperintense on MRI. These areas also enhance after the contrast agent administration. The appearance of lipoblastoma is identical to liposarcoma but is exceedingly rare in children. Diagnosis of lipomas and lipoblastomas are usually straightforward, given the predominance of adipose tissue within these lesions. However, in some cases, the myxoid components predominate with only small elements of fat, making diagnosis difficult (Murphey et al. 2004) (Fig. 38.45).

Benign peripheral nerve sheath tumors are schwannomas and neurofibromas; the latter may occur sporadically or be associated with neurofibromatosis type 1. On imaging, these lesions are well-defined fusiform lesions that are aligned along the course of a nerve. On MRI, they are T1-hypointense but T2-hyperintense and have avid contrast enhancement. In some lesions, a

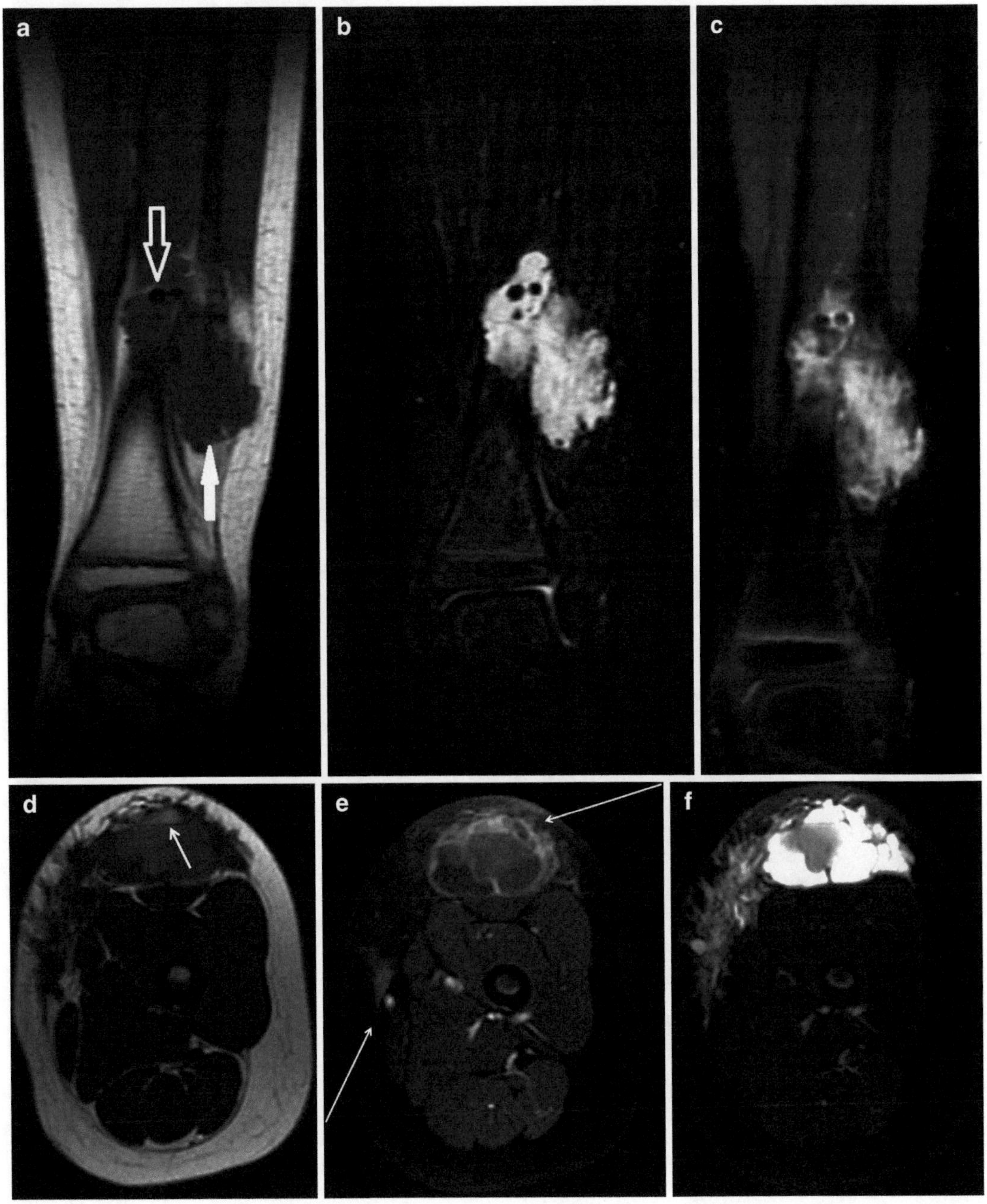

Fig. 38.44 Two types of vascular malformations. (**a**–**c**) Venous malformation. Coronal (**a**) T1-W, (**b**) STIR, and (**c**) contrast-enhanced fat-suppressed T1-W MR images show a venous malformation over the distal tibia (*solid arrow*). A phlebolith (*open arrow*) is seen, typical for a venous malformation. (**d**–**f**) Mixed lymphatic and venous malformation. Axial (**d**) T1-W, (**e**) contrast-enhanced fat-suppressed T1-W, and (**f**) fat-suppressed T2-W MR images show a soft tissue lesion with cystic and solid components. The cystic component contains fluid-fluid levels which may be due to hemorrhage within the lymphatic malformation (*short arrow*). The solid part of the lesion enhances slightly (*long arrows*) but is quite prominent on the T2-W image. The appearance of this lesion is consistent with a predominantly lymphatic malformation with a smaller component of venous malformation

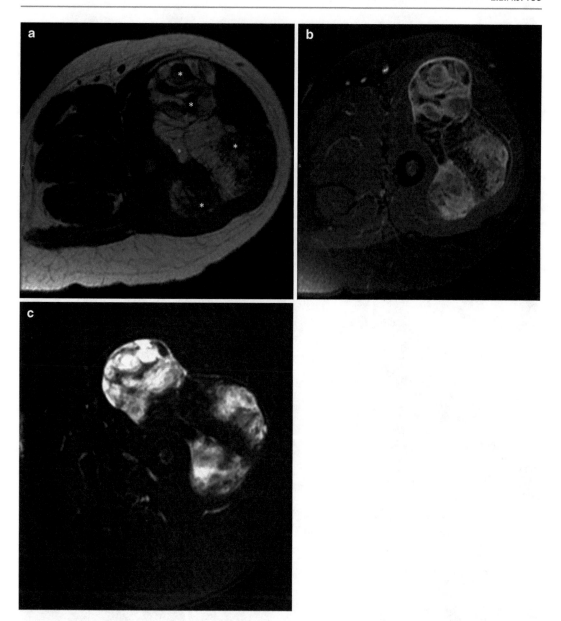

Fig. 38.45 Lipoblastoma in a 4-year-old boy. (**a**) Axial T1-W MR image shows a large soft tissue lesion in the anterolateral aspect of the left thigh. The lesion is predominantly fatty in signal intensity with several areas of signal hypointensity within it (*). These corresponded to richly vascular myxoid areas in the tumor on the histopathological specimen. (**b**) Axial contrast-enhanced fat-suppressed T1-W MR image shows the fatty areas within the lesion to be identical in signal intensity to the subcuta-neous adipose tissue. The previously noted areas of signal hypointensity enhance markedly, reflecting the rich vascularity seen in the myxoid areas. (**c**) Axial fat-suppressed T2-W MR image again shows the fatty areas within the lesion to be identical in signal intensity to the subcutaneous adipose tissue. The previously noted areas of signal hypointensity on the T1-W image which enhanced markedly is hyperintense on this T2-W image, reflecting the high water content

characteristic "target sign" can be seen (Fig. 38.46). Another common group of benign soft tissue masses is the fibromatous tumors, of which there is a wide spectrum. Infantile myofibromatosis is the commonest type. Most of these lesions are benign and slow growing, but some may be aggressive and infiltrative. Imaging features of fibrous tumors are nonspecific. The commonest malignant lesion is rhabdomyosarcoma. Non-rhabdomyosarcoma soft tissue tumors

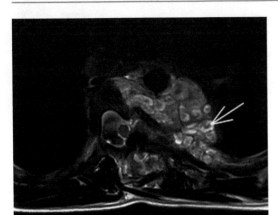

Fig. 38.46 Neurofibroma in a 14-year-old boy with scoliosis. Axial T2-W MR image shows a large paraspinal neurofibroma with both intra- and extra-thoracic components. The characteristic "target sign" is seen (*arrow*)

include but are not limited to fibrosarcoma, pleomorphic sarcoma, synovial sarcoma, and peripheral primitive neuroectodermal tumors. The imaging features of these lesions overlap and are again nonspecific. The role of the radiologist is to determine the extent of the lesion and to guide biopsy (Wu and Hochman 2009).

Conclusion

Nontraumatic pitfalls in imaging the pediatric musculoskeletal system may arise due to unfamiliarity with normal development or normal variants and overlapping imaging features between benign and malignant lesions. Pitfalls may occur anywhere within the musculoskeletal system and across a wide range of pathological conditions. It is necessary to be familiar with these in order to avoid unnecessary investigation, biopsy, and treatment.

References

Azouz EM, Saigal G, Rodriguez MM, Podda A (2005) Langerhans' cell histiocytosis: pathology, imaging and treatment of skeletal involvement. Pediatr Radiol 35:103–115

Bancroft LW, Kransdorf MJ, Peterson JJ, O'Connor MI (2006) Benign fatty tumors: classification, clinical course, imaging appearance, and treatment. Skeletal Radiol 35:719–733

Bermejo A, De Bustamante TD, Martinez A et al (2013) MR imaging in the evaluation of cystic-appearing soft-tissue masses of the extremities. Radiographics 33:833–855

Brown I (1975) A study of the "capsular" shadow in disorders of the hip in children. J Bone Joint Surg Br 57:175–179

Caffey J, Madell SH, Royer C, Morales P (1958) Ossification of the distal femoral epiphysis. J Bone Joint Surg Am 40-A:647–654

Caird MS, Flynn JM, Leung YL et al (2006) Factors distinguishing septic arthritis from transient synovitis of the hip in children. A prospective study. J Bone Joint Surg Am 88:1251–1257

Calfee RP, Sutter M, Steffen JA, Goldfarb CA (2010) Skeletal and chronological ages in american adolescents: current findings in skeletal maturation. J Child Orthop 4:467–470

Cheema JI, Grissom LE, Harcke HT (2003) Radiographic characteristics of lower-extremity bowing in children. Radiographics 23:871–880

Damasio MB, Malattia C, Tanturri de Horatio L et al (2012) MRI of the wrist in juvenile idiopathic arthritis: proposal of a paediatric synovitis score by a consensus of an international working group. Results of a multicentre reliability study. Pediatr Radiol 42:1047–1055

Gebarski K, Hernandez RJ (2005) Stage-I osteochondritis dissecans versus normal variants of ossification in the knee in children. Pediatr Radiol 35:880–886

Ghelman B, Freiberger RH (1976) The limbus vertebra: an anterior disc herniation demonstrated by discography. AJR Am J Roentgenol 127:854–855

Greulich WW, Pyle SI (1959) Radiographic atlas of skeletal development of the hand and wrist, 2nd edn. Stanford University Press, Stanford

Grimm NL, Weiss JM, Kessler JI, Aoki SK (2014) Osteochondritis dissecans of the knee: pathoanatomy, epidemiology, and diagnosis. Clin Sports Med 33:181–188

Harel L, Kornreich L, Ashkenazi S et al (1999) Meyer dysplasia in the differential diagnosis of hip disease in young children. Arch Pediatr Adolesc Med 153:942–945

Helms CA (2014) "Don't touch" lesions. In: Helms CA (ed) Fundamentals of skeletal radiology, 4th edn. Elsevier, Philadelphia

Henninger B, Glodny B, Rudisch A et al (2013) Ewing sarcoma versus osteomyelitis: differential diagnosis with magnetic resonance imaging. Skeletal Radiol 42:1097–1104

Ho VB, Kransdorf MJ, Jelinek JS, Kim CK (1991) Dorsal defect of the patella: MR features. J Comput Assist Tomogr 15:474

Hoerr NL, Pyle SI, Francis CC (1962) Radiographic atlas of skeletal development of the foot and ankle. Charles C Thomas, Springfield

Jee WH, Choi KH, Choe BY et al (1996) Fibrous dysplasia: MR imaging characteristics with radiopathologic correlation. AJR Am J Roentgenol 167:1523–1527

von Kalle T, Stuber T, Winkler P et al (2015) Early detection of temporomandibular joint arthritis in children with juvenile idiopathic arthritis - the role of contrast-enhanced MRI. Pediatr Radiol 45:402–410

Karlo CA, Stolzmann P, Habernig S et al (2010) Size, shape and age-related changes of the mandibular condyle during childhood. Eur Radiol 20:2512–2517

Keats EK, Strouse PJ (2008) Anatomic variants. In: Slovis TL (ed) Caffey's pediatric diagnostic imaging, 11th edn. Mosby, Philadelphia

Khanna M, Delaney D, Tirabosco R, Saifuddin A (2008) Osteofibrous dysplasia, osteofibrous dysplasia-like adamantinoma and adamantinoma: correlation of radiological imaging features with surgical histology and assessment of the use of radiology in contributing to needle biopsy diagnosis. Skeletal Radiol 37: 1077–1084

Khanna G, Sato TS, Ferguson P (2009) Imaging of chronic recurrent multifocal osteomyelitis. Radiographics 29:1159–1177

Kleinman PK, Belanger PL, Karellas A, Spevak MR (1991) Normal metaphyseal radiologic variants not to be confused with findings of infant abuse. AJR Am J Roentgenol 156:781–783

Kobayashi K, Burton KJ, Rodner C et al (2004) Lateral compression injuries in the pediatric elbow: Panner's disease and osteochondritis dissecans of the capitellum. J Am Acad Orthop Surg 12:246–254

Kuhns LR, Poznanski AK, Harper HA, Garn SM (1973) Ivory epiphyses of the hands. Radiology 109: 643–648

Kwon DS, Spevak MR, Fletcher K, Kleinman PK (2002) Physiologic subperiosteal new bone formation: prevalence, distribution, and thickness in neonates and infants. AJR Am J Roentgenol 179:985–988

Lachman RS, Krakow D, Cohn D et al (2005) MED, COMP, multilayered and NEIN: an overview of multiple epiphyseal dysplasia. Pediatr Radiol 35:116–123

Limb D, Loughenbury PR (2012) The prevalence of pseudoepiphyses in the metacarpals of the growing hand. J Hand Surg Eur 37:678–681

Love C, Din AS, Tomas MB et al (2003) Radionuclide bone imaging: an illustrative review. Radiographics 23:341–358

Mulligan PR, Prajapati HJ, Martin LG, Patel TH (2014) Vascular anomalies: classification, imaging characteristics and implications for interventional radiology treatment approaches. Br J Radiol 87:20130392

Murphey MD, Carroll JF, Flemming DJ et al (2004) From the archives of the AFIP: benign musculoskeletal lipomatous lesions. Radiographics 24:1433–1466

Nadvi SZ, Kottamasu SR, Bawle E, Abella E (1999) Physiologic osteosclerosis versus osteopetrosis of the newborn. Clin Pediatr (Phila) 38:235–238

Nistala H, Mäkitie O, Jüppner H (2014) Caffey disease: new perspectives on old questions. Bone 60:246–251

O'Donnell P, Saifuddin A (2004) The prevalence and diagnostic significance of fluid-fluid levels in focal lesions of bone. Skeletal Radiol 33:330–336

Ording Muller LS, Boavida P, Avenarius D et al (2013) MRI of the wrist in juvenile idiopathic arthritis: erosions or normal variants? A prospective case-control study. Pediatr Radiol 43:785–795

Ozonoff MB (1992a) The foot. In: Ozonoff MB (ed) Pediatric orthopedic radiology, 2nd edn. WB Saunders, Philadelphia

Ozonoff MB (1992b) The hip. In: Ozonoff MB (ed) Pediatric orthopedic radiology, 2nd edn. WB Saunders, Philadelphia

Ozonoff MB (1992c) The spine. In: Ozonoff MB (ed) Pediatric orthopedic radiology, 2nd edn. WB Saunders, Philadelphia

Pai DR, Strouse PJ (2011) MRI of the pediatric knee. AJR Am J Roentgenol 196:1019–1027

Prenger EC, Ball WS (1991) Spine and contents. In: Kirks DR (ed) Practical pediatric imaging: diagnostic radiology of infants and children. Little Brown and Co, Boston

Pyle SI, Hoerr NL (1969) A radiographic standard of reference for the growing knee. Charles C Thomas, Springfield

Raber SA (1999) The dense metaphyseal band sign. Radiology 211:773–774

Rachel JN, Williams JB, Sawyer JR et al (2011) Is radiographic evaluation necessary in children with a clinical diagnosis of calcaneal apophysitis (Sever's disease)? J Pediatr Orthop 31:548–550

Sakamoto FA, Winalski CS, Schils JP et al (2011) Vacuum phenomenon: prevalence and appearance in the knee with 3T magnetic resonance imaging. Skeletal Radiol 40:1275–1285

Scanderbeg AC, Dallapicolla B (2001) Congenital defects, malformation syndromes and skeletal dysplasias. In: Guglielmi G, Van Kuijik C, Genant HK (eds) Fundamentals of hand and wrist imaging. Springer, Berlin

Shabshin N, Schweitzer ME, Morrison WB et al (2006) High-signal T2 changes of the bone marrow of the foot and ankle in children: red marrow or traumatic changes? Pediatr Radiol 36:670–676

Shah ZK, Peh WCG, Koh WL, Shek TWH (2005) Magnetic resonance imaging appearances of fibrous dysplasia. Br J Radiol 78:1104–1115

Smith JD, Jaramillo D (2008) Osteochondroses. In: Slovis TL (ed) Caffey's pediatric diagnostic imaging, 11th edn. Mosby, Philadelphia

Struhl S, Edelson C, Pritzker H et al (1989) Solitary (unicameral) bone cyst. The fallen fragment sign revisited. Skeletal Radiol 18:261–265

Swischuk LE, Swischuk PN, John SD (1993) Wedging of C-3 in infants and children: usually a normal finding and not a fracture. Radiology 188:523–526

Teo HEL, Peh WCG, Akhilesh M, Tan SB, Ishida T (2007) Congenital osteofibrous dysplasia associated with pseudoarthrosis of the tibia and fibula. Skeletal Radiol 36(Suppl 1):S7–14

Thapa MM, Chaturvedi A, Iyer RS et al (2012a) MRI of pediatric patients: part 2, normal variants and abnormalities of the knee. AJR Am J Roentgenol 198:W456–W465

Thapa MM, Iyer RS, Khanna PC, Chew FS (2012b) MRI of pediatric patients: part 1, normal and abnormal cartilage. AJR Am J Roentgenol 198:W450–W455

Tsung JW, Blaivas M (2008) Emergency department diagnosis of pediatric hip effusion and guided arthrocentesis using point-of-care ultrasound. J Emerg Med 35:393–399

Vande Berg BC, Malghem J, Lecouvet FE et al (1998) Magnetic resonance imaging of the normal bone marrow. Skeletal Radiol 27:471–483

Wakely SL (2006) The posterior vertebral scalloping sign. Radiology 239:607–609

Weger C, Frings A, Friesenbichler J et al (2013) Osteolytic lesions of the calcaneus: results from a multicentre study. Int Orthop 37:1851–1856

Wipff J, Adamsbaum C, Kahan A, Job-Deslandre C (2011) Chronic recurrent multifocal osteomyelitis. Joint Bone Spine 78:555–560

Wu JS, Hochman MG (2009) Soft-tissue tumors and tumorlike lesions: a systematic imaging approach. Radiology 253:297–316

Zember JS, Rosenberg ZS, Kwong S et al (2015) Normal skeletal maturation and imaging pitfalls in the pediatric shoulder. Radiographics 35:1108–1122

Shigeru Ehara

Contents

39.1	**Introduction**	853
39.2	**Assessment of the Whole Spine**	854
39.2.1	Numbering of Vertebral Bodies	854
39.2.2	Correlation of Vertebral Segments and Spinal Nerve Territories	855
39.3	**Articulation Between the Skull Base and Atlas/Axis**	855
39.4	**Vertebral Bodies**	858
39.4.1	Atlas/Axis	858
39.4.2	Other Vertebrae	859
39.4.3	Reactive Changes at the Vertebral Body Corners	860
39.4.4	Transitional Vertebrae	860
39.4.5	Thoracic Vertebrae: Relationship with the Ribs	861
39.4.6	Lumbar Vertebra	862
39.5	**Intervertebral Disks**	862
39.5.1	Anatomy	862
39.5.2	Normal MRI Findings	864
39.5.3	Degenerative Process	864
39.5.4	Disk Calcification	867
39.5.5	Traumatic Change at Endplates in Adolescents	868
39.5.6	Degenerative Change at Vertebral Endplates (Modic Classification)	870
39.5.7	Joint of Luschka	870
39.6	**Facet (Zygapophyseal) Joint**	872
39.7	**Posterior Elements**	872
39.8	**Ligaments Around the Vertebral Bodies and Laminae**	873
39.8.1	Anterior Longitudinal Ligament	873
39.8.2	Posterior Longitudinal Ligament	875
39.8.3	Ligamentum Flavum	876
39.8.4	Interspinous and Supraspinous Ligaments	876
39.8.5	Iliolumbar Ligament	878
39.9	**Vascular Anatomy**	878
39.10	**Spinal Cord, Cauda Equina, and Nerve Roots**	878
39.11	**Extradural Space of the Spinal Canal**	879
Conclusion		880
References		880

Abbreviations

CT   Computed tomography
MRI   Magnetic resonance imaging

39.1 Introduction

In imaging of the spine, errors in numbering of the vertebrae may result in inaccurate diagnosis and even wrong site surgery. There are numerous congenital anomalies such as the skull base-upper cervical articulation and atlas/axis and transitional vertebra that may result in diagnostic pitfalls. Degenerated intervertebral disks, traumatic vertebral endplate changes in adolescents, degenerative vertebral endplate changes, and variants in the

S. Ehara, MD
Department of Radiology, Iwate Medical University,
19-1 Uchimaru, Morioka 020-8505, Japan
e-mail: ehara@iwate-med.ac.jp

© Springer International Publishing AG 2017
W.C.G. Peh (ed.), *Pitfalls in Musculoskeletal Radiology*, DOI 10.1007/978-3-319-53496-1_39

joints and ligaments around the vertebrae, as well as the blood vessels and nerve roots, may contribute to imaging misinterpretation. This chapter aims to highlight some anatomical variants and degenerative findings in the spine which may pose diagnostic problems in clinical imaging.

39.2 Assessment of the Whole Spine

39.2.1 Numbering of Vertebral Bodies

Errors in the numbering of vertebral segments are one of the typical causes of wrong site surgery. The typical number of vertebral bodies, i.e., 7 cervical vertebrae, 12 thoracic vertebrae, and 5 lumbar vertebrae, does not apply in all the subjects. Exceptions are not rare (more than 10%), particularly in the thoracic and lumbar vertebrae (Standring 2005). In order to avoid inaccuracy by counting at each segment, counting of vertebrae should start from C2 level (Peh et al. 1999) (Fig. 39.1). The C1 vertebra (atlas) is often hypoplastic or a part of the vertebra may be deficient, particularly in the lamina. Scout images on computed tomography (CT) or magnetic resonance imaging (MRI) need to include C2 vertebra and below. Counting from the sacrum upward to the upper vertebrae may cause an error due to variations in the number of

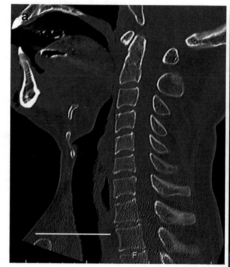

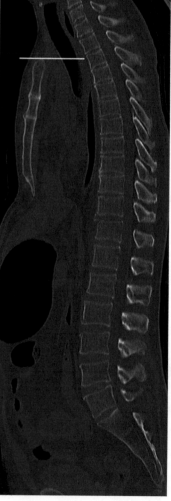

Fig. 39.1 The whole spine is used for counting vertebral levels in a 44-year-old man. Sagittal reformatted CT image of the (**a**) cervical vertebrae and (**b**) thoracolumbar vertebrae. High-quality sagittal images can be readily used for assessing the level of the vertebral column. The superior margin of the manubrium of the sternum (*white line*) is a relatively stable marker, corresponding to T2 or T3 level

the lumbar and thoracic vertebrae and lumbosacral transitional vertebra. Variations in the number of the cervical vertebrae are relatively uncommon, and cervical rib may be a cause of error.

There are several markers to count the vertebrae, as described below.

(a) The first thoracic vertebra connects to the first rib, whose anterior aspect connects to the manubrium of the sternum, just below the clavicle (different from cervical rib).

(b) The upper edge of the sternal notch is often located at T2 or T3 level on the sagittal localization images (Standring 2005) (Fig. 39.1).

(c) Aortic bifurcation is most often located at L4 level although variations exist (Standring 2005).

(d) Tracheal bifurcation is most commonly located at the upper border of T5 vertebra (Standring 2005), but it is not so reliable because of the difficulty in determining bifurcation on sagittal image.

(e) Posterior tubercle is a characteristic finding at the lowest thoracic vertebra, i.e., T12 (Ehara et al. 1990).

(f) The iliolumbar ligament, connecting the transverse process and the iliac crest, is a specific structure of the lowest lumbar vertebra, connecting the transverse process of the fifth lumbar vertebra and the iliac crest (Hughes and Saiffudin 2006) (Fig. 39.2).

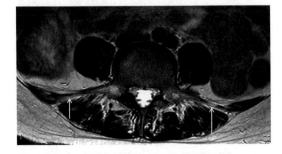

Fig. 39.2 Iliolumbar ligament in a 48-year-old woman. Axial T1-W MR image shows the iliolumbar ligament (*arrows*) which connects the transverse process of the lowest (fifth) lumbar vertebrae and iliac crests

39.2.2 Correlation of Vertebral Segments and Spinal Nerve Territories

Typical focal neurological signs may explain where the lesion is. At the level of cervical vertebrae, vertebral segments correspond to the spinal cord segments. At the upper thoracic spine, cord segments are two levels more cranial than the vertebral segments. At the lower thoracic vertebrae, cord segments are more than three levels more cranial. Levels of clinical signs and symptoms need to be correlated with lesions on imaging studies.

39.3 Articulation Between the Skull Base and Atlas/Axis

Assimilation of atlas is an uncommon anomaly of the craniovertebral junction and is classified into complete and partial (Fig. 39.3). It may be associated with basilar invagination, block vertebrae, and other dysplasia of the occiput and is a rare cause of atlantoaxial subluxation. Atlantoaxial fusion is a rare anomaly. The atlas-dens interval (ADI) is a gap between the anterior arch of the atlas and the dens. Normally it is less than 2 mm in width and considered widened if more than 4 mm. It is normally wider in children, with the normal range being less than 5 mm. There are also several variations in this C1–2 articulation. A V-shaped ADI is considered normal (Bohrer et al. 1985) (Fig. 39.4).

Soft tissue masses may be seen on the posterior aspect of the dens, particularly in patients with atlantoaxial instability, such as in rheumatoid arthritis (RA). These soft tissue masses may be due to the pannus of RA or non-specific inflammatory reaction, "pseudotumor." Retrodental pseudotumor is an inflammatory pseudotumor with non-specific reactive change histologically, and it is often associated with instability (Yonezawa et al. 2013) (Fig. 39.5). The cruciate ligament of the atlas consists of the transverse ligament, accessory atlantoaxial ligament (between the base of the lateral mass and the dens), and the alar ligament. The small apical ligament is located at the tip of the dens. The transverse ligament is

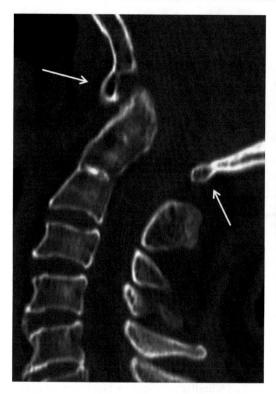

Fig. 39.3 Occiput–C1 vertebral assimilation in a 78-year-old woman. Sagittal reformatted CT image shows that the anterior and the posterior arches of C1 are united to the skull base (*arrows*)

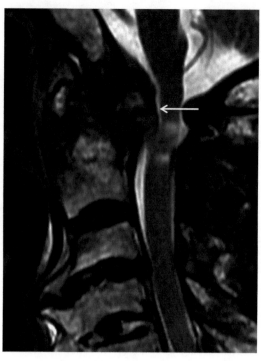

Fig. 39.5 Retrodental pseudotumor in a 83-year-old man with DISH. Sagittal T2-W MR image shows a hypointense mass lesion at the posterior aspect of the dens (*arrow*). The signal intensity of the spinal cord is increased at this level

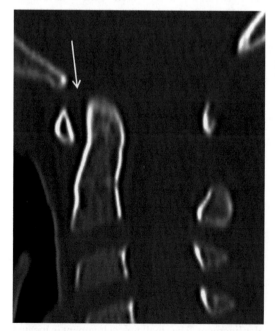

Fig. 39.4 V-shaped atlas-dens interval in a 7-year-old boy. Sagittal reformatted CT image shows superior widening of ADI (*arrow*). This is a frequent finding with no clinical significance

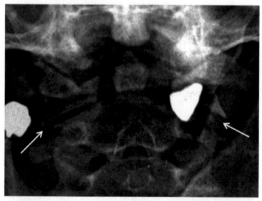

Fig. 39.6 C1–2 vertebral offset in a 58-year-old woman. Frontal open-mouth view radiograph shows C1–2 offset (*arrows*) which is a sign of burst fracture of the atlas (Jefferson fracture), but it may also be seen in normal subjects

considered to be disrupted when the combined lateral displacement of the lateral mass is 6.9 mm or more (rule of Spence) (Perez-Orribo et al. 2016). The lateral margin of the atlas and axis should be well aligned, but occasionally bilateral offset is noted with no fractures ("pseudo-spread") (Suss et al. 1983) (Fig. 39.6).

Posterior tilt of the dens is a common normal configuration (Swischuck et al. 1979) (Fig. 39.7). On the other hand, anterior tilt of the dens is a sign of malunion of dens fracture. Accessory ossification may be seen at the tip of the dens. There are two types:

(a) Os terminale is a secondary ossification at the tip of the dens (Fig. 39.8). It appears by 3 years of age and unites with the dens by 12 years of age.

(b) Os odontoideum is a larger ossification at the superior aspect of the dens (Fig. 39.9). It is considered to be a non-united ossification after fracture and is often symptomatic.

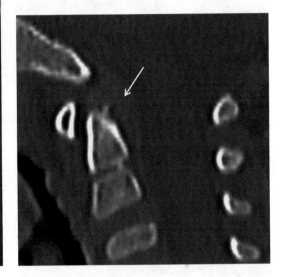

Fig. 39.7 Posteriorly tilted dens in a 14-year-old girl. Sagittal reformatted CT image shows posterior tilt of the dens. This is a normal finding

Fig. 39.8 Os terminale in a 29-month-old boy. Sagittal reformatted CT image shows a small ossification center (*arrow*) at the tip of the dens

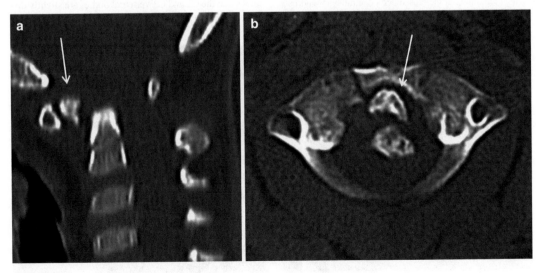

Fig. 39.9 Os odontoideum in a 4-year-old girl. (**a**) Sagittal reformatted and (**b**) axial CT images show an extra ossification (*arrow*) between the anterior arch of the atlas and the dens. It is relatively small. Spinal canal is narrowed at this level

39.4 Vertebral Bodies

39.4.1 Atlas/Axis

Specific shapes are noted in the upper two cervical vertebrae, i.e., the atlas and axis. No vertebral body exists in the atlas. The dens and vertebral body of the axis are united at the age of 5–8 years.

Scar of the dentocentral synchondrosis varies on MRI (Fig. 39.10). Open synchondroses may simulate a fracture (Smith et al. 1993) (Fig. 39.11). The Mach effect at the base of the dens may also simulate a fracture (Daffner 1977). In the upper cervical vertebrae in young children, apparent anterior displacement may occur in otherwise normal children, the so-called pseudosubluxation (Swischuck 1977) (Fig. 39.12).

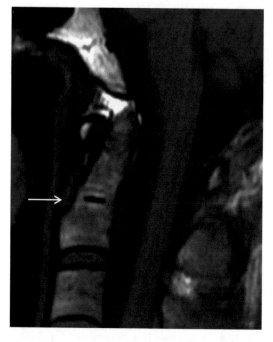

Fig. 39.10 Scar of dentocentral synchondrosis in a 28-year-old man. Sagittal T1-W MR image shows hypointense signal change remaining at the closed dentocentral synchondrosis. Most common feature is linear sclerosis (*arrow*)

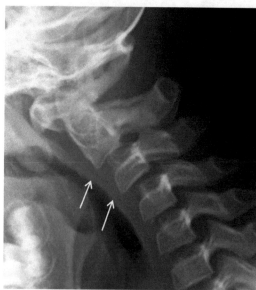

Fig. 39.12 Pseudosubluxation in a 6-year-old boy. Lateral radiograph of the cervical vertebra taken in flexion shows that the C2 and C3 vertebral bodies are slightly displaced anteriorly (*arrows*)

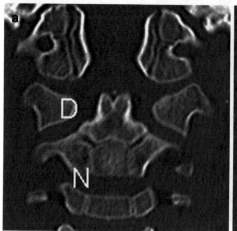
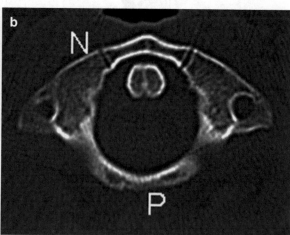

Fig. 39.11 Open synchondroses in a 3-year-old boy. (**a**) Coronal reformatted CT image shows open dentocentral (*D*) and neurocentral (*N*) synchondroses. (**b**) Axial CT image shows open neurocentral (*N*) and closed posterior (*P*) synchondroses

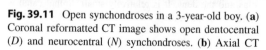

39.4.2 Other Vertebrae

Variations in the number of vertebral segments are common in the lumbar vertebrae. They may be four or six in approximately 10% of cases (Fig. 39.13). The next common variation is the thoracic vertebrae, in which 11 or 13 segments may be accompanied by ribs (Fig. 39.13). The anterior and the posterior edges of the vertebral bodies should be well aligned. However, exceptions in the alignment of the anterior and the posterior margin of the vertebral bodies exist: one at the C1 posterior arch that may be located anteriorly because of relative hypoplasia of the atlas (Fig. 39.14), and the other at T1 vertebral body, whose posterior margin of the vertebral body exists posteriorly because of relatively large T1 body compared with C7 vertebral body (Fig. 39.15). At the lumbosacral junction, significance of the apparent posterior displacement of L5 vertebra on the lateral view is controversial, and it is often believed to be due to rotation, and

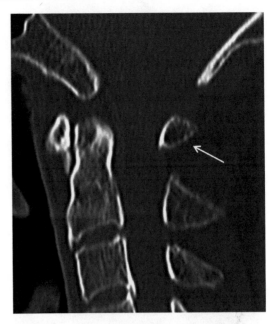

Fig. 39.14 Anteriorly displaced posterior arch of C1 vertebra in a 58-year-old man. Sagittal reformatted CT image shows anterior displacement of the posterior C1 arch (*arrow*), because of a small C1 ring. This is a normal finding

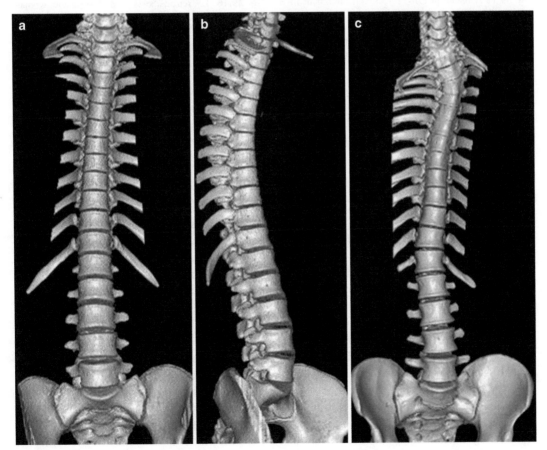

Fig. 39.13 3D whole spine reformatted CT images in two different patients with scoliosis. (**a, b**) 12 thoracic and 5 lumbar vertebrae are present in this 12-year-old girl. (**c**) 13 thoracic and 4 lumbar vertebrae are seen in this 17-year-old man

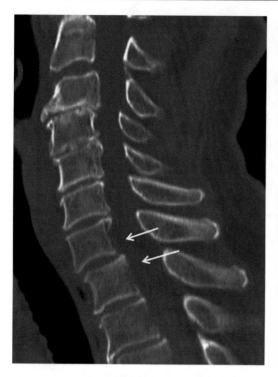

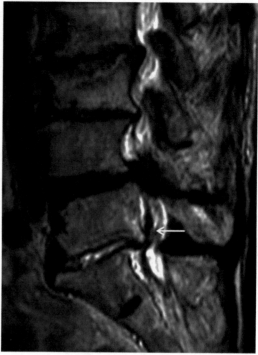

Fig. 39.15 Change in C7–T1 vertebral alignment in a 73-year-old woman. Sagittal reformatted CT image shows posterior location of the T1 vertebral body (*arrows*), because of relatively small size of C7 vertebral body compared to T1 body. The anterior margins of C7 and T1 vertebral bodies are well aligned

Fig. 39.16 L5 retrolisthesis in a 71-year-old woman. Sagittal T2-W MR image shows that L5 vertebral body is located posteriorly compared to S1 body (*arrow*)

not real retrolisthesis. However, in the author's experience, real retrolisthesis may be seen, particularly with multilevel instability (Fig. 39.16).

39.4.3 Reactive Changes at the Vertebral Body Corners

The anterosuperior and anteroinferior edges of the vertebral bodies are the attachment sites of the anterior longitudinal ligament and annulus of the intervertebral disks, and they constitute the entheses. Bone overgrowth may occur at the attachment of these ligamentous fibers due to chronic traction, forming osteophytes of the vertebral bodies. "Traction spur" and "claw spur" may be due to the difference in the direction of stress (MacNab 1971) (Fig. 39.17). Enthesis is also a known site of inflammatory change, i.e., spondyloarthropathy. Enthesitis or enthesopathy, representing mineralization and reactive marrow change at the edge of vertebral bodies, is a known

as "shiny corner sign" that is also seen on MRI in a relatively early disease phase (Fig. 39.18).

39.4.4 Transitional Vertebrae

Transitional vertebrae are the vertebrae associated with characteristic features of both upper and lower segments. Thoracolumbar transitional vertebrae are characterized by the following three features: (1) unilateral rib; (2) lumbar rib articulation with the tip of the transverse process; and (3) variation in the shape of the transverse process, with characteristic posterior tubercle of T12 vertebral body (Fig. 39.19). Lumbosacral transitional vertebrae are characterized by the following two features: (1) partially sacralized lateral mass (Fig. 39.20) and (2) hypoplastic disk (Fig. 39.21). Lumbosacral transitional vertebra is often a cause of mechanical load imbalance, if the osseous connection is rigid. Bertolotti syndrome refers to low back pain related to an asymmetric lateral mass of the sacrum.

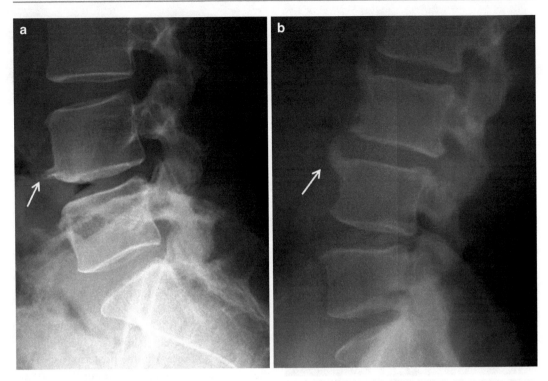

Fig. 39.17 Osteophytes in two different patients. (**a**) Lateral lumbar spine radiograph shows traction osteophytes in a 44-year-old woman, seen as small linear ossifications parallel to the endplates (*arrow*). (**b**) Lateral lumbar spine radiograph shows claw osteophytes in a 50-year-old man, seen as claw-shaped ossification at L3 and L4 vertebral bodies (*arrow*)

39.4.5 Thoracic Vertebrae: Relationship with the Ribs

The relationship with the ribs is important for assessing the level of thoracic vertebrae. The anterior aspect of the first rib is always located just caudal to the medial aspect of the clavicle, and it is used to exclude a cervical rib. The number of the ribs is used to decide the level of thoracic spine, but the knowledge of the costovertebral joint is important to avoid errors. Typical vertebrae have two articulations with the rib, namely, articular facets at the lateral aspect of vertebral body and at the lateral aspect of transverse process.

The articular facet of the costovertebral joint on the lateral aspect of the vertebral bodies is

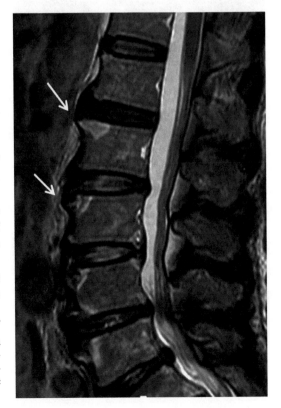

Fig. 39.18 Shiny corners of the vertebral bodies in a 75-year-old man. Sagittal T2-W MR image shows deposition of bone marrow fat at the anterior corners of the vertebral bodies of the lumbar vertebrae representing chronic reactive change in spondyloarthropathy (*arrows*)

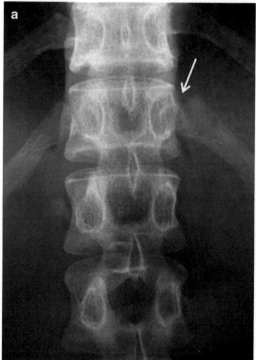

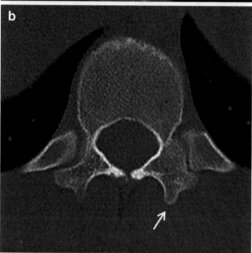

Fig. 39.19 Target pedicle of T12 vertebra in a 22-year-old man. (**a**) AP radiograph of the lumbar spine shows a double ring at T12 pedicles (*arrow*). (**b**) Axial CT image shows the posterior tubercle at T12 vertebra (*arrow*)

often located at the superior aspect and articulates with the one vertebra above (Fig. 39.22). At the first thoracic vertebra, the articular facet of the first costovertebral joint is incomplete at the

superior aspect of the vertebral body, and the first rib articulates also with the seventh cervical vertebra. The 10th–12th ribs are floating ribs, with no connection at the anterior aspect. As they are mechanically weak, this is a cause of high frequency of compression fractures at the lower thoracic and upper lumbar vertebrae.

39.4.6 Lumbar Vertebra

The lumbar vertebral bodies are larger than thoracic and cervical vertebrae. Their trabeculae consist of three components: cortical framework, vertical trabeculae, and horizontal trabeculae (Fig. 39.23). Y-shaped basivertebral veins exist in the center of the vertebral body (Fig. 39.24). Interosseous arteries are complex and different in the center and metaphyseal region of the vertebral bodies. Overall, more blood flow is present in the posterior aspect of the vertebral bodies (Ratcliffe 1980) (Fig. 39.25). Fatty conversion of the bone marrow occurs in the older age group. Such fatty marrow conversion typically starts from the region adjacent to the basivertebral veins. It is often heterogeneous, and it may mimic neoplastic lesions (Fig. 39.26), and it can be differentiated by chemical shift or contrast enhancement (Montazel et al. 2003; Zajick et al. 2005). On the other hand, bone marrow (red marrow) conversion may be caused by hemolysis or destruction of hematopoietic tissue.

39.5 Intervertebral Disks

39.5.1 Anatomy

39.5.1.1 Endplates
The cartilaginous endplate consists of hyaline cartilage cranial and caudal to the vertebral bodies. However, differentiation between nucleus pulposus and osseous endplate may not be easy by the current contrast and spatial resolution of MRI.

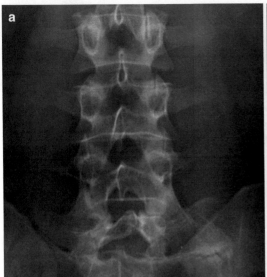

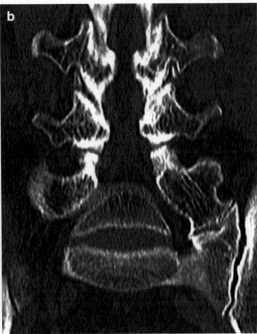

Fig. 39.20 Partially sacralized lateral mass in two different patients. (**a**) AP radiograph of the lumbar spine shows an enlarged left lateral mass at L5 vertebra of a 20-year-old woman. (**b**) Coronal reformatted CT image also shows an enlarged left lateral mass of L5 vertebra of a 52-year-old man

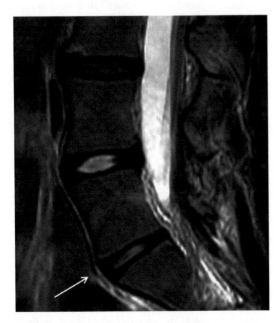

Fig. 39.21 Hypoplastic intervertebral disk in a 16-year-old girl. Sagittal T2-W MR image shows a small intervertebral L5–S1 disk (*arrow*), compared to the complete L4–5 disk. The signal intensity is higher than the degenerated L3–4 disk

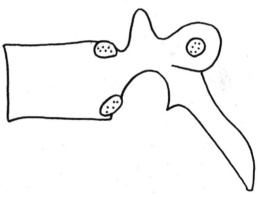

Fig. 39.22 Diagram shows the costovertebral joints. Except for the upper and lower thoracic levels, articular facets are located at the superior aspect of the vertebral body and transverse process for the same level, and the lower aspect of the vertebral body for one lower level

39.5.1.2 Annulus Fibrosus

The annulus fibrosus is the outer layer of the disk consisting of thin collagen fibers which are short and taut and are tightly attached to the anterior

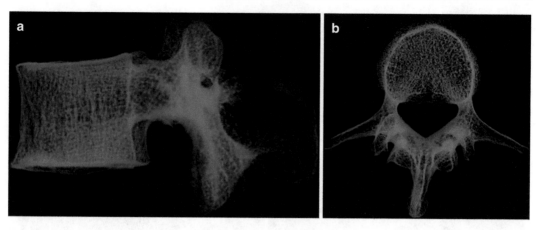

Fig. 39.23 Trabecular pattern of the 3rd lumbar vertebra. (**a**) Lateral and (**b**) axial images show typical trabeculae of the vertebra that become more evident during the process of osteoporosis

and posterior aspects of the disk. Such fibers are ring shaped, attached to the epiphyseal ring, and merge with the fibers of the anterior and posterior longitudinal ligaments. These structures constitute the protective mechanism for compressive forces. Blood flow only exists in the posterior and outer aspect of the annulus, mainly supplied by small vessels. Transverse or concentric tears of the annulus are often present incidentally, with no clinical symptoms.

39.5.1.3   Nucleus Pulposus

Nucleus pulposus is the soft component consisting of mucoid elements, and it is remnant of notochord. Its water content is high (80–90%), and proteoglycan is rich. The margin with the annulus fibrosus is not clear, and no significant blood flow is present. Decrease in height is often seen due to ageing.

39.5.2 Normal MRI Findings

Differentiation between the annulus fibrosus and the nucleus pulposus is often difficult. There is least thickness at the upper thoracic spine, and an increase in thickness toward the lumbosacral junction is the rule. The intranuclear cleft is seen in the normal disk, mainly in subjects of 30 years and older (Aguila et al. 1985) (Fig. 39.27). It may not be seen in the diseased disk with inflammation.

39.5.3 Degenerative Process

Degeneration of the disk related to ageing is represented by signal hypointensity on T2-weighted MR images. Such changes are present in 85–95% of cases at autopsy. Tear, regeneration of chondrocytes, and granulation occur in cartilaginous endplates. At the annulus fibrosus, degeneration is the cause of decreased type 2 collagen, decreased water content (70%), and decreased aggregated proteoglycan. Radial tears appear at the inner and middle layer of the annulus fibrosus. The disk volume decreases from 15 to 1 ml.

39.5.3.1   Morphologic Changes of Degenerated Intervertebral Disk

Bulging   Annular bulging is the result of degeneration. There is no tear of the annulus fibrosus, but the annular fibers are loosened. The outer margin of the disk projects externally (Fig. 39.28). Large "bulging" is usually associated with a radial tear of the annulus fibrosus, and it should be called protrusion, not bulging. Annular tears are classified into concentric type (fluid collec-

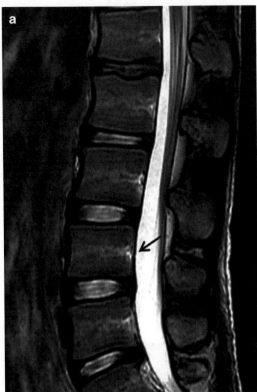

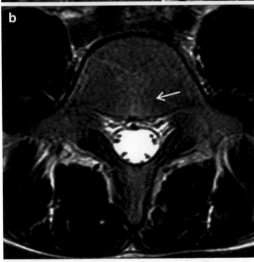

Fig. 39.24 Basivertebral veins in a 22-year-old man. (**a**) Sagittal and (**b**) axial T2-W MR images show basivertebral veins in the center of the vertebral bodies and in the midline posteriorly. Signal hyperintensity on T2-weighted image represents venous blood. In addition, increased bone marrow fat around the vein contributes to the high signal intensity (*arrow*)

tion among fibrous layers), radial type (disruption of the whole layer of the annulus), and transverse type (disruption of Sharpey fibers at the margin of the annulus or apophysis).

Protrusion Protrusion is the extension of the nucleus pulposus through the annular defect. The disk margin projects outward, but it is still contained in the normal annulus fibrosus or the posterior longitudinal ligament (PLL) fibers ("contained disk") (Fig. 39.29). Signal intensity of the nucleus pulposus decreases on T2-weighted images. The protruded disk may erode the cortical margin of the lateral recess or neural foramen.

Extrusion The extruded disk herniates through the annular defect, constituting a free extradural mass (Fig. 39.30). Extrusion is classified into the subligamentous type (contained within PLL) and transligamentous type (extending outside through PLL). Since fibers of PLL and dura mater merge in the midline, transligamentous extrusion may result in an intradural lesion. Because of taut midline septum (merged fibers from annulus and PLL) in the lumbar vertebrae, the herniated disk material tends to be present off midline.

Sequestration When extruded disk material loses continuation from the disk, it exists as a free fragment in extradural space. This is called a sequestered disk and may be mistaken for a intraspinal tumor (Fig. 39.31). The sequestered disk tends to decrease in size or may even disappear in relatively short period of time.

39.5.3.2 Diagnosis of Intervertebral Disk Herniation

The above 2–4 categories are defined as disk herniation. It is clinically significant, mainly in the lower lumbar vertebrae, but it may occur anywhere, and lesions at any levels can be clinically significant. Herniation of the thoracic disk is commonly seen at T11–12 level. Disk herniation at the cervical spine level most often occurs at C5–6 and C6–7 levels. Symptomatic cases are more common in younger age group (30s and 40s). Spontaneous regression is known to occur in 30–100%. Larger herniation tends to regress

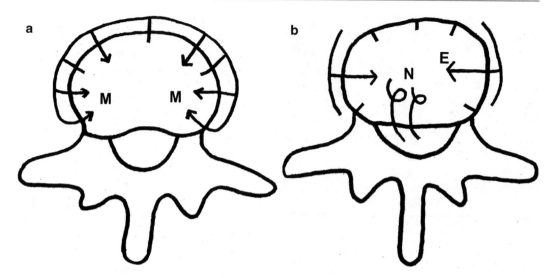

Fig. 39.25 Diagrams show arteries of the lumbar vertebrae. (**a**) Metaphyseal network with prominent metaphyseal arteries (*M*). (**b**) Anterolateral equatorial artery (*E*) arising from lumbar artery and nutrient arteries (*N*) entering the vertebral body from the posterior aspect (based on Ratcliffe JF 1980)

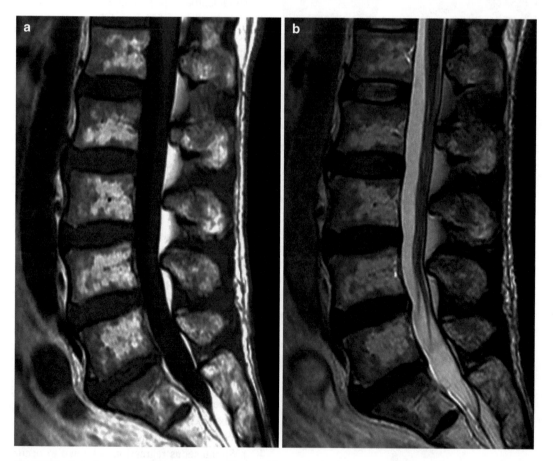

Fig. 39.26 Fatty bone marrow conversion in a 62-year-old man. Sagittal (**a**) T1-W and (**b**) T2-W MR images of the lumbar spine show areas of signal hyperintensity in the bone marrow representing fatty bone marrow conversion

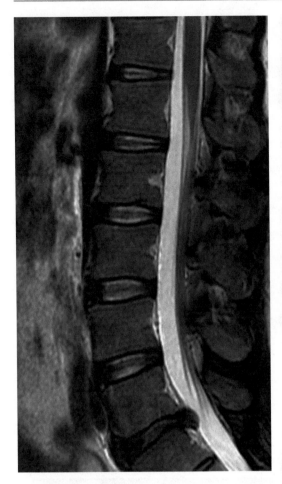

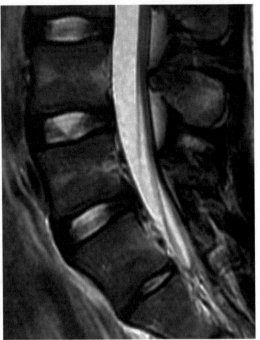

Fig. 39.28 Disk bulging in a 16-year-old boy. Sagittal T2-W MR image of the lumbar spine shows that the L5 segment is partially sacralized with a hypoplastic L5–S1 disk. Mild disk bulging with normal hyperintense signal is noted at L4–5 level

Fig. 39.27 Intranuclear cleft in a 37-year-old man. Sagittal T2-W MR image shows linear bands of hypointense signal in the center of the intervertebral disks, except for the degenerated and protruded L5–S1 disk

more frequently. Poor correlation exists between the type and size of the herniation and clinical features. At the lumbar vertebral levels, symptoms tend to occur at a more cranial level because the lower nerve roots tend to be compressed because of their descending course. Contrast-enhanced MRI is often useful because granulation around the nerve roots may be enhanced.

39.5.4 Disk Calcification

Disk calcification may be caused by trauma, infection, metabolic abnormalities, and degeneration. The most common cause is degeneration. MRI signal usually decreases, but occasionally

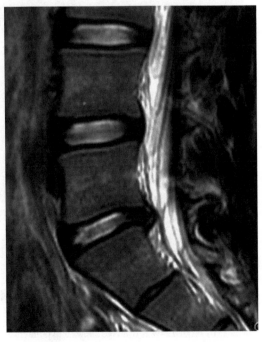

Fig. 39.29 Disk protrusion in a 22-year-old man. Sagittal T2-W MR image shows central posterior disk protrusion at L5–S1 level

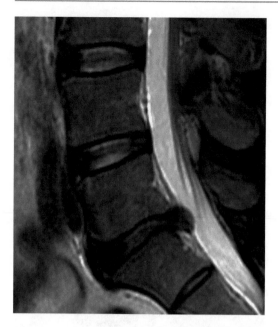

Fig. 39.30 Disk extrusion in a 37-year-old man. Sagittal T2-W MR image shows posteriorly displaced disk material beyond the confines of the annulus and PLL

the signal intensity on T1-weighted images is increased (Major et al. 1993) (Fig. 39.32). This is caused by T1 shortening due to surface relaxation mechanism by calcium particles. At 1.5 T, calcium particles increase T1 signal with 30 weight% and decrease T1 signal above 30 weight%.

39.5.5 Traumatic Change at Endplates in Adolescents

Persistent ring apophyses at the anterosuperior aspect of the vertebral bodies are typical traumatic change in adolescents, and ossification in the vertebral endplates becomes irregular. If irregularities occur in the center of the vertebral endplates, the osseous excavation due to the herniated disk material is called Schmorl nodes (Fig. 39.33). If herniation occurs at the margin of ring apophysis, the persistent ossification of the ring apophysis is

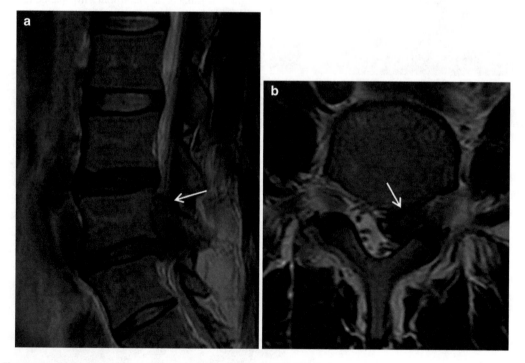

Fig. 39.31 Sequestered disk in a 31-year-old man. (**a**) Sagittal T2-W MR image shows a hypointense mass at L4 level (*arrow*). (**b**) Axial T2-W MR image shows a hypointense disk fragment at the left lateral recess (*arrow*)

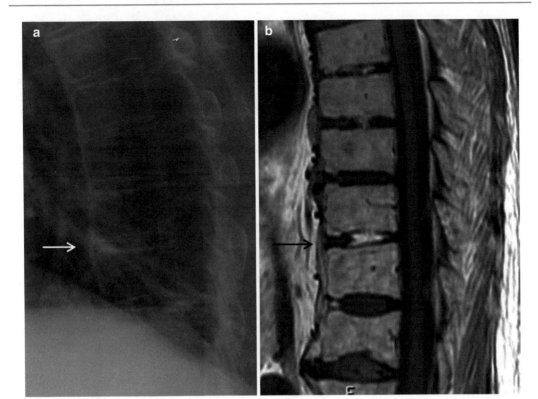

Fig. 39.32 Calcified disk in a 78-year-old man. (**a**) Lateral radiograph shows a calcified disk at the lower thoracic level (*arrow*). (**b**) Sagittal T1-W MR imaging shows a hyperintense disk at the lower thoracic level (*arrow*)

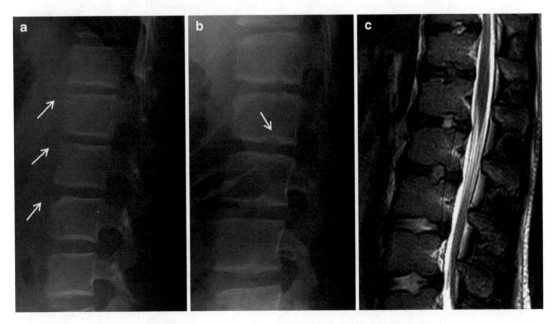

Fig. 39.33 Traumatic changes in the vertebral endplates of two different patients. (**a**) Lateral radiograph shows lumbar Scheuermann disease in a 13-year-old girl. Persistent ring apophysis (*upper two arrows*) and limbus vertebra (*lowest arrow*) secondary to disk herniation through the margin of the ossification center are present. (**b**) Lateral radiograph and (**c**) sagittal T2-W MR image show lumbar Scheuermann disease in a 12-year-old boy. Multiple excavations of the endplate represent Schmorl nodes (*arrow*). Disk degeneration is noted on MR imaging

called limbus vertebra. Low back pain syndrome with such irregular endplates in the thoracolumbar spine is called lumbar or atypical Scheuermann disease, and it is a cause of low back pain in adolescents (Blumenthal et al. 1987).

39.5.6 Degenerative Change at Vertebral Endplates (Modic Classification)

Various MRI signal intensity changes may be seen in the vertebral endplates due to degeneration. Type I disk is associated with endplates that have hypointense signal on T1-weighted images and hyperintense signal on T2-weighted images and are slightly contrast enhanced (Fig. 39.34). It represents the signal intensity of vascularized fibrous tissue, similar to osteomyelitis. The lack of abnormal signal extending into the disk may help differentiate it from infection. Type I disk tends to change into type

II (Modic et al. 1988). Type II disk is associated with endplates with hyperintense signal on T1-weighted images and slightly hyperintense signal intensity on T2-weighted images, representing fatty bone marrow (Fig. 39.35). This disk type is stable with no further signal change. Type III disk is associated with endplates with hypointense signal both on T1- and T2-weighted MR images, corresponding to sclerosis subjacent to the endplate (Fig. 39.36).

39.5.7 Joint of Luschka

Joint of Luschka (uncovertebral joint) is located in the cervical vertebra with an oblique notch at the side of the disk, contributing to stability to the lateral translation. It constitutes the anteromedial wall of the neural foramen. The uncinate process exists at the superolateral aspect of the vertebral body (Fig. 39.37). It is a common site of degenerative change with osteophytes.

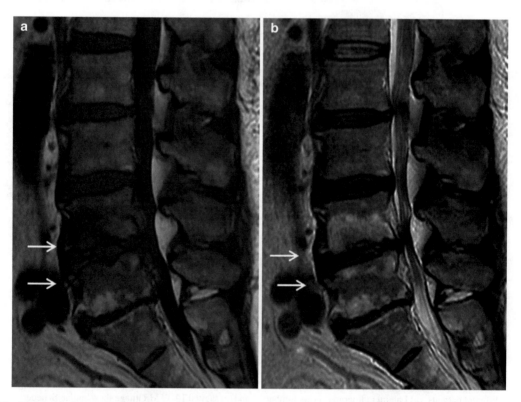

Fig. 39.34 Modic type I disk degeneration in a 57-year-old man. Sagittal (**a**) T1-W and (**b**) T2-W MR images show areas of T1 hypointensity and T2 hyperintensity in the vertebral bodies adjacent to the L4–5 disk (*arrows*). This represents the reactive changes to disk degeneration

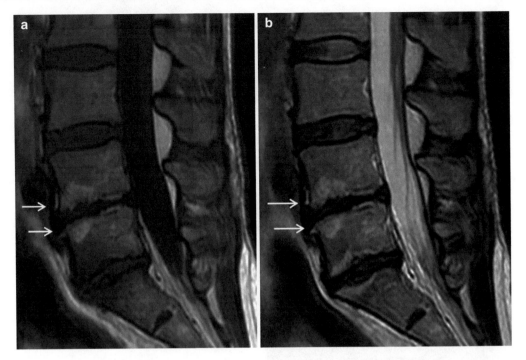

Fig. 39.35 Modic type II disk degeneration in a 47-year-old woman. Sagittal (**a**) T1-W and (**b**) T2-W MR images show signal intensity of fat at the endplates of vertebral bodies adjacent to the L4–5 disk (*arrows*)

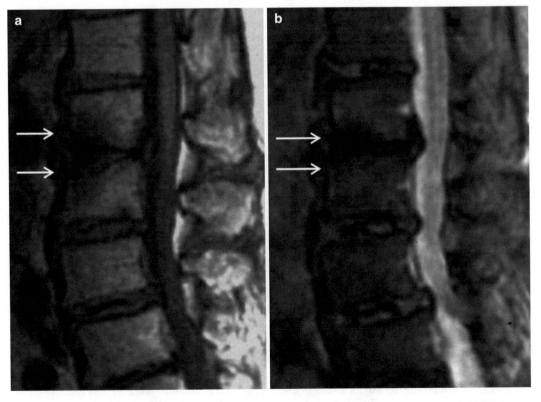

Fig. 39.36 Modic type III disk degeneration in a 64-year-old woman. Sagittal (**a**) T1-W and (**b**) T2-W MR images show signal hypointensity in the endplates adjacent to the L2–3 disk (*arrows*). This represents sclerotic change

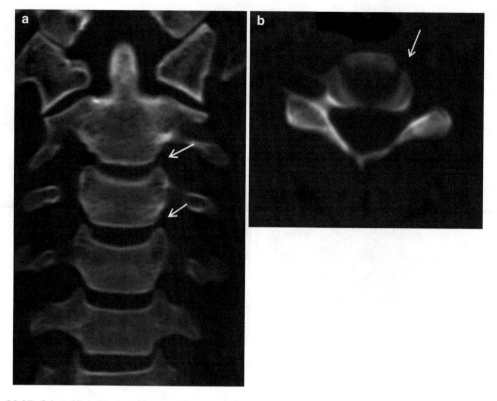

Fig. 39.37 Joint of Luschka in a 38-year-old man. (**a**) Coronal reformatted and (**b**) axial CT images show a notch on the lateral aspect of the vertebral bodies of the cervical vertebrae which represents the joint of Luschka (*arrows*)

39.6 Facet (Zygapophyseal) Joint

The facet (or zygapophyseal) joint consists of an articular process covered by a 2–4 mm thick hyaline cartilage and joint space extending below ligamentum flavum along the superior and inferior articular surfaces. The synovial joint space is small and may extend into the ligaments. Relationship between the articular cartilage and axis of the joint may change by the level (Fig. 39.38). At most levels, these joints are best viewed on sagittal images.

Degeneration of the joint may occur early, even in the young subjects. Dislocation or subluxation usually occurs in significant trauma. "Naked facet," the lack of opposing facet, is the sign of dislocation of facet joint (Fig. 39.39). The retrodural space of Okada is the potential space between the right and left facet joints and the posterior epidural space (Murthy et al. 2011) (Fig. 39.40). A lesion in one side of the facet joint may extend through the posterior aspect of the dura and involves the other side of the facet joint. This can be a route of spread of the infection or hemorrhage.

39.7 Posterior Elements

The posterior elements of the vertebra consist of the lamina, the articular process, and the spinous process. The seventh cervical vertebra is known to have a long spinous process, but it is usually not readily identified on the sagittal images. A characteristic feature of the 12th thoracic vertebra is the posterior tubercle (also called superior tubercle), a cause of "target pedicle" on anteroposterior (AP) radiographs (Fig. 39.19). It constitutes the posterior element of the transverse process.

The shape of the posterior element of the lumbar vertebra may be complex, including the mammary process (osseous projection from the posterior edge of the articular process) and accessory process (osseous projection from the posterior aspect of the base of the transverse process) (Fig. 39.41).

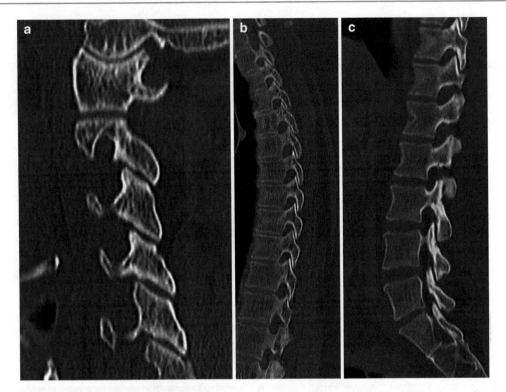

Fig. 39.38 Sagittal reformatted CT images of the zygapophyseal joints in a (**a**) 44-year-old man, (**b**) 58-year-old woman, and (**c**) 40-year-old man. The orientation of zygapophyseal joint is more horizontal at the cervical level and more vertical at the thoracolumbar level. In the lower lumbar level, it becomes slightly horizontal

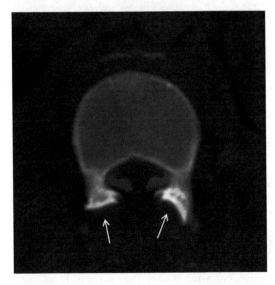

Fig. 39.39 Naked facet in a 26-year-old man with T12–L1 dislocation. Axial CT image shows no articular facet opposing the superior articular process of the lower vertebra (*arrows*)

Osseous clefts in the lamina, pedicle, and articular process are considered to be congenital or traumatic. They are classified as retrosomatic cleft, isthmic cleft (pars interarticularis defect), retroisthmic cleft, and median cleft (Nakayama and Ehara 2015) (Fig. 39.42). No clinical significance is attached to the median cleft, while the other clefts may be traumatic (fatigue fracture) and are associated with spondylolisthesis.

39.8 Ligaments Around the Vertebral Bodies and Laminae

39.8.1 Anterior Longitudinal Ligament

The anterior longitudinal ligament (ALL) is the ligament that extends over the anterior aspect of

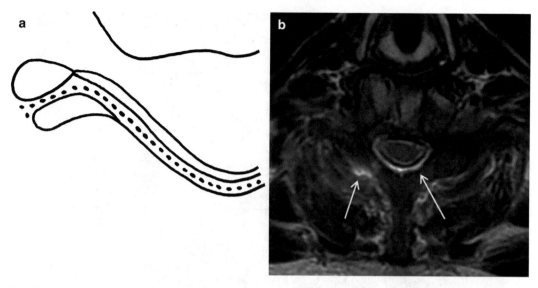

Fig. 39.40 Retrodural space of Okada. (**a**) Diagram shows that the joint space of the zygapophyseal joint is connected to an extradural space at the posterior aspect of the spinal canal. (**b**) Axial T2-W MR image of the cervical spine in a 56-year-old man with septic arthritis of the zygapophyseal joint and epidural space. Fluid is seen at the right zygapophyseal joint and the posterior extradural space (*arrows*)

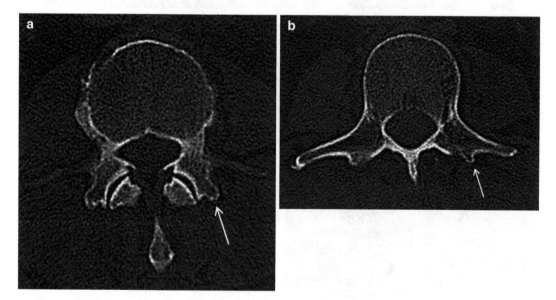

Fig. 39.41 Mammillary and accessory processes in a 50-year-old woman. Axial CT images show the (**a**) mammillary process (*arrow*) and (**b**) accessory process (*arrow*)

the vertebral body from the upper to the lower vertebrae (Fig. 39.43). At thoracic level, it is narrow and thick. Longitudinal fibers connect the intervertebral disks and cartilaginous endplates. It consists of three components, namely, deep layer (localized to one level), intermediate layer (connecting several levels), and superficial layer (connecting 4–5 levels). They are loosely attached to the fibrous annulus, but it firmly connects to the vertebral bodies at the upper and lower edges

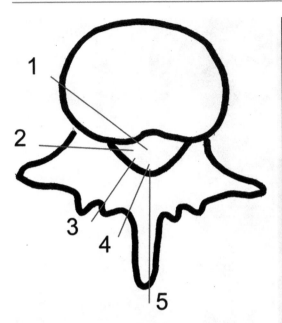

Fig. 39.42 Diagram shows classification of spondylolysis. *1*, neurocentral synchondrosis; *2*, pedicular (retrosomatic) cleft; *3*, pars interarticularis (isthmic) cleft; *4*, retroisthmic cleft; *5*, spinous cleft (spina bifida)

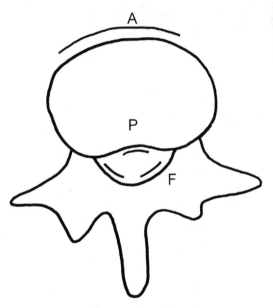

Fig. 39.43 Diagram shows vertebral ligaments. Anterior longitudinal ligament (*A*), posterior longitudinal ligament (*P*), ligamentum flavum (*F*)

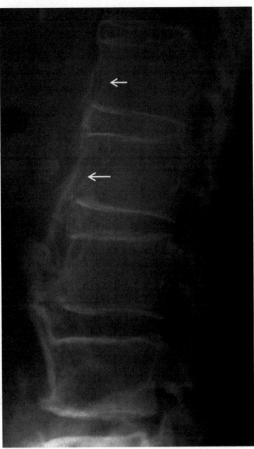

Fig. 39.44 Ossified ALL in a 71-year-old man with DISH. Lateral radiograph of the lumbar spine shows ossification of the anterior aspect of the vertebral bodies, which are separated from the anterior margin of the vertebral bodies (*arrows*)

contiguous levels and is typically separated from the vertebral body (Fig. 39.44).

39.8.2 Posterior Longitudinal Ligament

The posterior longitudinal ligament (PLL) is the ligament connecting the posterior aspect of the C2 (axis) vertebral body and the sacrum (Fig. 39.43). It attaches to the tectorial membrane superiorly. Fibrous connection exists between the vertebral endplate and the edge of the vertebral body, with communicating fibers at the outer layer of the intervertebral disk. These fibers extend transver-

of the vertebral bodies. Ossified PLL, a feature of diffuse idiopathic skeletal hyperostosis (DISH), is characterized by ossification of more than four

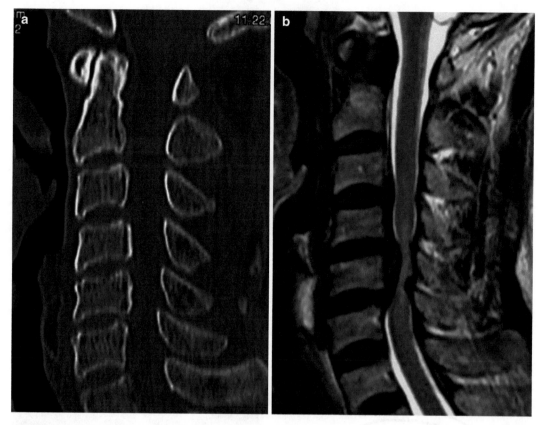

Fig. 39.45 Thick PLL in a 70-year-old woman. (**a**) Sagittal reformatted CT image shows no ossification of PLL. (**b**) Sagittal T2-W MR image shows significant thickening of PLL at C4–6 levels. Flattening and signal hyperintensity are noted at the spinal cord

sally and connect with the fibers of the annulus fibrosus. It is very thin in the lumbar vertebrae. Ligament fibers are separated from the cortices of the lumbar vertebral bodies but attached to the annulus fibrosus. However, it cannot be separated from the vertebral body cortex on MRI. It may be thickened, resulting in spinal canal stenosis, and may be finally ossified. Thickening is considered to be a predisposing condition of ossification (Fig. 39.45). It connects with the periosteum at the midline via the plica mediana dorsalis and constitutes a T-shaped fibrous structure on the posterior surface of the vertebral bodies.

39.8.3 Ligamentum Flavum

The ligamentum flavum (or yellow ligament) connects the right and left and upper and lower laminae (Fig. 39.43). The right and left components of the ligament are incompletely connected at the midline, and they are penetrated by veins. Its MRI signal is slightly hyperintense, due to high elastin content (80%) and low type I collagen content (20%). Its thickness is 3–5 mm, reinforcing medial aspect of the facet joint. Thickening and ossification can cause spinal canal stenosis (Fig. 39.46).

39.8.4 Interspinous and Supraspinous Ligaments

The interspinous ligaments consist of three layers. The ventral portion of the ligamentum flavum extends to the inferior aspect of the anterior half of the upper spinous process. The central portion extends from the anterior half of the inferior spinous process to the posterior half of the upper spinous process. The dorsal portion connects from

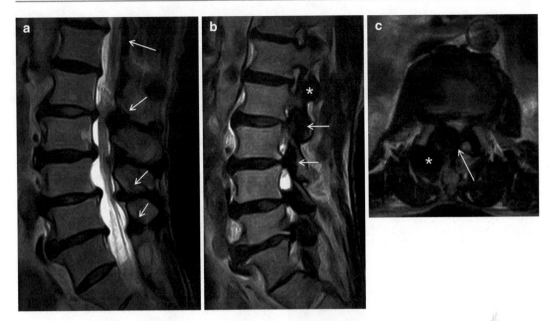

Fig. 39.46 Thick ligamentum flavum in an 81-year-old man. (**a**) Midsagittal, (**b**) parasagittal, and (**c**) axial T2-W MR image shows that the ligamentum flavum is exten- sively thickened (*arrows*). Capsule of zygapophyseal joint is also thickened (*)

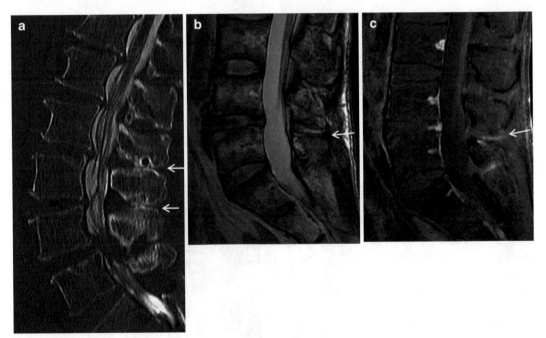

Fig. 39.47 Baastrup disease in different patients. (**a**) Baastrup disease in a 60-year-old woman. Sagittal reformat- ted CT myelogram image of the thoracolumbar spine shows sclerosis and erosions of the lower spinous processes which abut each other. Sagittal (**b**) T2-W and (**c**) contrast-enhanced fat-suppressed T1-W MR images of a 48-year-old man with Baastrup disease show degenerated interspinous ligament with enhancement in the wall of the bursa-like lesion (*arrow*)

the posterior half of the inferior spinous process to the supraspinous ligament. Degeneration of the ligament due to the direct contact of the spinous processes is common, and it may be a cause of low back pain (Baastrup disease) (Kwong et al. 2011) (Fig. 39.47).

39.8.5 Iliolumbar Ligament

The iliolumbar ligament of the lowest lumbar vertebra connects the transverse process of L5 body and the iliac crest (Hughes and Saiffudin 2006) (Fig. 39.2).

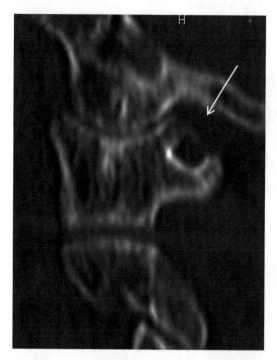

Fig. 39.48 Ponticulus posticus in a 71-year-old woman. Sagittal reformatted CT image shows an osseous arch formed at the superior aspect of the lamina that covers the vertebral artery (*arrow*)

39.9 Vascular Anatomy

The vertebral artery enters into the transverse foramen at C7 level, extending up to C3 level. It changes the course from vertical to horizontal at the C2 articular process, courses upward to C1 level, and penetrates the dura mater just above C1 level. An osseous arch is formed at the superior aspect of C1 arch, forming ponticulus posticus, or arcuate foramen. It covers the retrocondylar vertebral artery (Fig. 39.48). The segmental radiculomedullary branch of segmental lumbar artery distributes the dura mater. The most important artery is the artery of Adamkiewicz arising at T9–12 levels in slightly more than 60 % of cases (Fig. 39.49). Hairpin curve configuration on the anterior aspect of the spinal cord is characteristic. Spinal radicular veins (intervertebral veins) connect anterior internal vertebral vein and ascending lumbar vein. The posterior inferior venous plexus connects the intervertebral veins.

39.10 Spinal Cord, Cauda Equina, and Nerve Roots

A small fissure, the anterior median fissure, exists at the midline of the ventral aspect of conus medullaris and is located at T12–L1 levels. It may contain terminal ventricle, a cystic dilatation of the spinal cord canal. The cauda equina consists

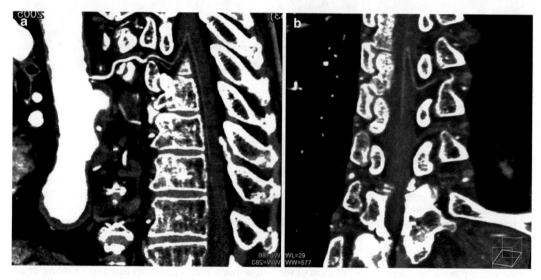

Fig. 39.49 Artery of Adamkiewicz. (**a**) Sagittal and (**b**) oblique coronal reformatted CT images show the artery of Adamkiewicz. Hairpin curve configuration is typical on the anterior aspect of the spinal cord

Fig. 39.50 Fibrolipoma of the filum terminale in a 50-year-old man. (**a**) Sagittal T1-W and (**b**) axial T2-W MR images show hyperintense fat in the filum terminale (*arrow*)

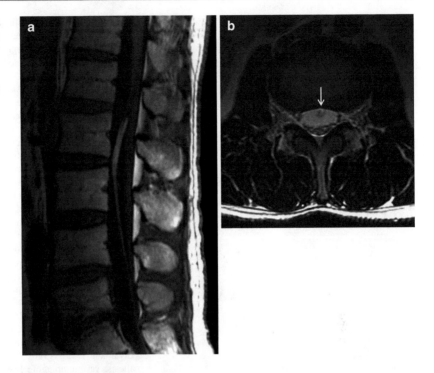

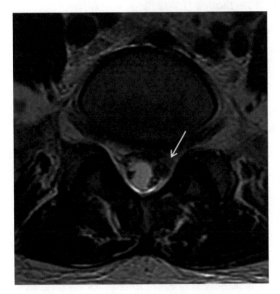

Fig. 39.51 Conjoint nerve root in a 41-year-old woman. Axial T2-W MR image shows a relatively large left nerve root at the left neural foramen which represents a conjoint nerve root, containing two nerve roots (*arrow*)

of the nerves arising from the spinal cord, constituting nerve roots in the neural foramina. Fat signal is seen in the film terminale in 5% of cases on T1-weighted images, named "fibrolipoma of filum terminale," which usually has no clinical significance (Fig. 39.50).

The neural foramen is formed by the pedicles (upper and lower walls), posterolateral aspect of the vertebral bodies (lateral wall), disk (anterior and medial walls), and articular process (lateral wall). The nerve root can be classified into entrance zone, midzone (running laterally at the inferior aspect of the pedicle, entering into neural foramen, up to root ganglion), and exit zone (lateral to the root ganglion). Conjoint nerve root is one of the causes of an enlarged nerve root, containing two nerve root segments in one nerve sleeve (Fig. 39.51).

39.11 Extradural Space of the Spinal Canal

The space between the vertebra and thecal sac is occupied by fat, but it does not usually exist at the posterior aspect at L5–S1 level. It is sometimes thick with small thecal sac (epidural lipomatosis) (Fig. 39.52). Epidural lipomatosis is known to be caused by Cushing syndrome, but its clinical significance in most cases is questionable. The venous network around the thecal sac is prominent, particularly anteriorly, adjacent to vertebral bodies.

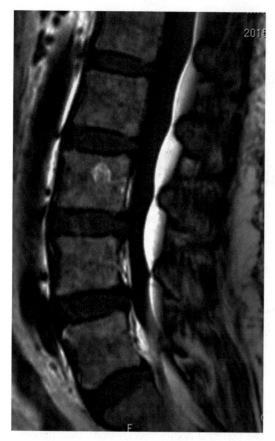

Fig. 39.52 Epidural lipomatosis in a 52-year-old woman. Sagittal T1-W MR image shows increased epidural fat and a small thecal sac

Conclusion

In imaging of the spine, there are numerous congenital, developmental, and degenerative anomalies that may lead to inaccuracies in interpretation. Familiarity with the imaging features of these anomalies as well as anatomical variants is essential to avoid diagnostic pitfalls.

References

Aguila LA, Piriano DW, Modic MT et al (1985) The intranuclear cleft of the intervertebral disk: magnetic resonance imaging. Radiology 155:155–158

Blumenthal SL, Roach J, Herring JA (1987) Lumbar Scheuermann's disease: a clinical series and classification. Spine 12:929–932

Bohrer SP, Klein A, Martin W III (1985) "V" shaped predens space. Skeletal Radiol 14:111–116

Daffner RH (1977) Pseudofracture of the dens: mach bands. AJR Am J Roentgenol 128:607–612

Ehara S, El-Khoury GY, Bergman RA (1990) The target pedicle of T-12: radiologic-anatomic correlation. Radiology 174:871–872

Hughes RJ, Saiffudin A (2006) Numbering of lumbosacral transitional vertebrae on MRI: role of iliolumbar ligaments. AJR Am J Roentgenol 187:W59–W65

Kwong Y, Rao N, Latif K (2011) MDCT findings in Baastrup disease: diseases or normal feature of the aging spine? AJR Am J Roentgenol 196:1156–1159

MacNab I (1971) The traction spur: an indicator of segmental instability. J Bone Joint Surg Am 53:663–670

Major NM, Helms CA, Genant HK (1993) Calcification demonstrated as high signal on T1-weighted MR images of the disks of the lumbar spine. Radiology 189:494–496

Modic MT, Steinberg PM, Ross JS et al (1988) Degenerative disk disease: assessment of changes in vertebral bone marrow with MR imaging. Radiology 166:193–199

Montazel JL, Divine M, Lapage E et al (2003) Normal spinal bone marrow in adults: dynamic gadolinium-enhanced MR imaging. Radiology 229:703–709

Murthy NS, Maus TP, Aprill C (2011) The retrodural space of Okada. AJR Am J Roentgenol 196:W784–W789

Nakayama T, Ehara S (2015) Spondylolytic spondylolisthesis: various imaging features and natural courses. Jpn J Radiol 33:3–12

Peh WCG, Siu TH, Chan JHM (1999) Determining the lumbar vertebral segments on magnetic resonance imaging. Spine 24:1852–1855

Perez-Orribo L, Kalb S, Snyder LA et al (2016) Comparison of CT versus MRI measurements of transverse atlantal ligament integrity in craniovertebral junction injuries. Part 2: a new CT-based alternative for assessing transverse ligament integrity. J Neurosurg Spine 26:1–7

Ratcliffe JF (1980) The arterial anatomy of the adult human lumbar vertebral body: a microangiographic study. J Anat 131:57–79

Smith JT, Skinner SP, Shonnard NH (1993) Persistent synchondrosis of the second cervical vertebra simulating Hangman's fracture in a child. J Bone Joint Surg Am 75:1228–1230

Standring S (ed) (2005) Gray's anatomy: the anatomical basis of clinical practice, 39th edn. Elsevier/Churchill-Livingstone, Edinburgh

Suss RA, Zimmerman RD, Leeds NE (1983) Pseudospread of the atlas: false sign of Jefferson fracture in children. AJR Am J Roentgenol 140:1079–1082

Swischuck LE (1977) Anterior displacement of C2 in children: physiologic or pathologic. Radiology 122:759–763

Swischuck LE, Hayden CK Jr, Sarwar M (1979) The posterior tilted dens: normal variation simulating fracture. Pediatr Radiol 8:27–28

Yonezawa I, Okuda T, Won J et al (2013) Retrodental mass in rheumatoid arthritis. J Spinal Disord Tech 26:E65–E69

Zajick DC Jr, Morrison WB, Schweizer ME et al (2005) Benign and malignant processes: normal values and differentiation with chemical shift MR imaging in vertebral marrow. Radiology 237:590–596

Cartilage Imaging Pitfalls

40

Klaus Bohndorf

Contents

40.1 **Introduction** 881

40.2 **MRI Inherent Artifacts Applicable to Cartilage Imaging** 882
40.2.1 Chemical Shift Artifact 882
40.2.2 Susceptibility Artifact 883
40.2.3 Truncation Artifact 884
40.2.4 Magic Angle Artifact 885
40.2.5 Partial Volume Averaging Artifact 886

40.3 **Sequence-Related Pitfalls in Cartilage Imaging** 886
40.3.1 Ambiguity of Cartilage Surface in the Posterior Femoral Condyle 886
40.3.2 Linear Area of Signal Intensity in Cartilage Deep Zone 886

40.4 **Potential Pitfalls Related to Anatomy and Composition of Cartilage** 887
40.4.1 Cartilage Thinning Adjacent to Anterior Horn of Lateral Meniscus 887
40.4.2 Decreased Signal Intensity in the Distal Part of the Trochlear Cartilage 887

40.5 **Developmental Pitfalls of Cartilage Imaging** 887
40.5.1 Shoulder Joint 887
40.5.2 Elbow Joint 887
40.5.3 Hip Joint 889

Conclusion 891

References 891

K. Bohndorf, MD
The High Field MR Center, Department of
Biomedical Imaging and Image-guided Therapy,
Medical University of Vienna,
Währinger Gürtel 18-20, 1090 Wien, Austria
e-mail: klaus@bohndorf-radiologie.de

Abbreviations

CT   Computed tomography
FSE   Fast spin-echo
GRE   Gradient-echo
MRI   Magnetic resonance imaging
SE   Spin-echo

40.1 Introduction

Hyaline cartilage and its pathology can only be delineated using radiography or computed tomography (CT) when cartilage is calcified or when fluid or air is applied intra-articularly. Today, magnetic resonance imaging (MRI) is the modality of choice to assess cartilage noninvasively. Rheumatoid diseases and trauma-induced cartilage injury are relevant disorders for individual patients and for society as well, bearing in mind the socioeconomic impact. New therapeutic drugs and surgical techniques are being developed for their treatment, including autografting and autologous chondrocyte implantation. These new therapeutic entities will substantially enhance the importance of MRI for diagnosis, patient care, and follow-up. The relative signal intensity of normal articular cartilage is dependent on the pulse sequences that are used. Fluid-sensitive MR images in two to three orthogonal planes are best suited for assessing focal cartilage defects. Fat-suppressed or water excitation T1-weighted gradient-echo or double-echo steady-state (DESS)

© Springer International Publishing AG 2017
W.C.G. Peh (ed.), *Pitfalls in Musculoskeletal Radiology*, DOI 10.1007/978-3-319-53496-1_40

images with a maximum of 1.5 mm slice thickness and a < 0.35 mm in-plane resolution are suited for cartilage thickness analysis (Eckstein et al. 2014). MRI of cartilage is however subject to a variety of MRI inherent artifacts (Waldschmidt et al. 1997; Yoshioka et al. 2004), which will be discussed in this chapter. In addition, several normal variants can be seen in MRI of the cartilage.

40.2   MRI Inherent Artifacts Applicable to Cartilage Imaging

MRI is prone to several artifacts which may lead to an incorrect diagnosis. Motion artifacts and flow artifacts have to be considered but are beyond the scope of this chapter. For further information, please see Chap. 4 on MRI artifacts. Protocol-error artifacts include saturation, wraparound, radiofrequency interference, and shading, and partial volume averaging artifacts are generally due to improper parameter selection or poor protocol planning (Peh and Chan 2001). However, these operator-dependent artifacts are preventable with adequate training and experience. In contrast, several MRI artifacts are inherent to the technique and may substantially degrade cartilage imaging. They have to be addressed including the strategy to reduce or even avoid them.

40.2.1 Chemical Shift Artifact

Because 1H protons of fat are better shielded by electron clouds compared to 1H protons of water, the effects of an externally applied magnetic field to these protons are different. A fat proton experiences a slightly weaker local magnetic field and will resonate at a slightly lower frequency than a nearby water proton. In routine MRI, spatial position is assigned along the frequency-encoding direction on the basis of the resonant frequency. If both water and lipid protons coexist in a voxel, the signal emitted by the lipid proton will have a lower frequency than that of the water proton.

The computer assumes all protons to precess at the same frequency, and the signal from fat is

mapped to a different location corresponding to the frequency at which it is precessing. This artifact appears as areas or lines of hyperintense signal where signals of fat and water overlap or hypointense signal areas where their signals spread apart. The interface between cartilage (water containing) and the bone marrow (fat containing) is especially prone to chemical shift artifacts. To reduce the artifact, an increased bandwidth and switching of the phase- and frequency-encoding direction are helpful (Fig. 40.1). To avoid the artifact, fat-suppression

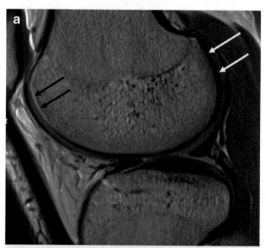

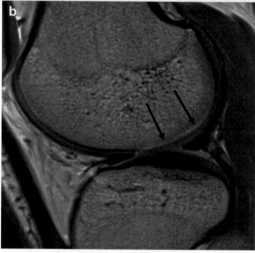

Fig. 40.1 Chemical shift artifact (*arrows*) on sagittal proton density MR images of the knee joint. Dependency on frequency-encoding direction. (**a**) Frequency-encoding direction is anteroposterior. (**b**) Frequency-encoding direction is cranio-caudal. Both images were obtained with the same MRI parameters [TR 3750, TE 24, SL 2.5; FOV 160 × 160, matrix 384 × 384, pixel bandwidth 240]

techniques should be carried out. Fat-suppression techniques that are based on chemical shift fat selection tend to work better at higher magnetic field strengths (Del Grande et al. 2014).

40.2.2 Susceptibility Artifact

Magnetic susceptibility is variable for different tissues and directly proportional to the magnetic field strength. Artifacts occur at the interfaces between substances of different susceptibilities. Cartilage imaging can be degraded by the susceptibility artifact in case of air/gas, intra-articular hemosiderin deposition, and metal located near to cartilage (Fig. 40.2). The magnetic field distortions created by susceptibility effects vary the precessional frequency across the patient and even within individual voxels. These frequency changes, in turn, produce signal loss from T2* dephasing and spatial mismapping of the MR signal. The MRI characteristics reflect both of these physical mechanisms: geometric distortion with focal areas of signal void and regions of very bright signal resulting from "piling up" signal assigned to the wrong areas. In general, susceptibility artifacts may occur in all pulse sequences.

They are minimal in spin-echo (SE) sequences because the 180° refocusing radiofrequency (RF) pulse corrects for T2* effects. However, these artifacts are strong in gradient-echo (GRE) sequences (Elster 2015a) (Fig. 40.2).

The effects of magnetic susceptibility can be reduced by using fast SE (FSE) sequences with short echo times or by increasing the receiver bandwidth. Use of small field of view (FOV), high-resolution matrix, and high gradient strength has also been found to reduce susceptibility artifacts (Lee et al. 2007). The more severe metal artifacts may be reduced by specific metal artifact reduction pulse sequences and, to some extent, may overcome the inherent limitation of MRI in the presence of metal (Singh et al. 2014). Gas may be extracted from intra-articular fluid due to negative pressure. This "vacuum phenomenon" is well known on radiographs and CT. On MRI, gas leads to intra-articular susceptibility artifacts, seen as signal voids. This phenomenon is more pronounced at higher fields and has been reported with a prevalence of 1.3% in a large series of knee MRI at 3.0 T (Sakamoto et al. 2011). Although important for meniscal imaging, no relevant problems concerning cartilage imaging have been reported.

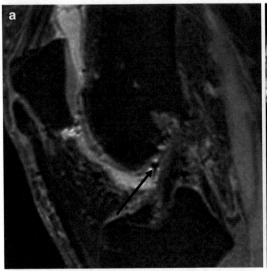 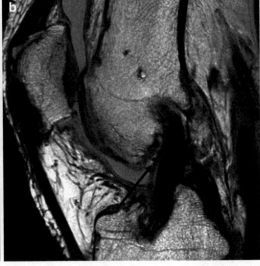

Fig. 40.2 Susceptibility artifacts due to metal debris (*arrow*) in the knee joint. Dependency on sequence selection with increased effect on the gradient-echo sequence. (**a**) GRE (fat-suppressed 3D-FFE) compared to (**b**) intermediate-weighted FSE sagittal MR images of the knee

40.2.3 Truncation Artifact

In the early days of clinical MRI, it was already suggested that the laminar appearance within the articular cartilage on gradient-echo images is predominantly attributable to truncation artifacts (also known as Gibbs ringing artifacts) rather than to histologic zonal anatomy (Erickson et al. 1996; Frank et al. 1997). It does not indicate degenerative change of the articular cartilage (Yoshioka et al. 2004). The artifact is a consequence of using Fourier transformations to reconstruct MR signals into images. In theory, any signal can be represented as an infinite summation of sine waves of different amplitudes, phases, and frequencies. In MRI, however, only a finite number of frequencies can be sampled, and therefore, the image has to be approximated by using only a relatively few harmonics in its Fourier representation. The Fourier series, then, is cut short or "truncated," hence the name for this artifact (Elster 2015b).

Truncation artifacts in principle appear as alternating dark and bright lines that run parallel to a sharp change in signal intensity. Classical examples are truncation artifacts at the boundary between layers of subchondral bone and hyaline cartilage, especially the cartilage of both the patellofemoral compartments and the posterior region of the femoral condyles. The artifact is prominent in fat-suppressed three-dimensional (3D)-spoiled gradient-echo (SPGR), but also seen in fast low-angle shot (FLASH) sequences (Takahashi et al. 2014) (Fig. 40.3). Interestingly, FSE images sometimes show a truncation artifact in the patellofemoral compartment that appears as a linear area of high signal intensity in the cartilage (Yoshioka et al. 2004). Because truncation artifacts arise as a fundamental consequence of the Fourier representation of an image, they occur in both the phase- and frequency-encoding directions. However, because fewer samples are usually taken in the phase-encoding direction, the artifact is usually most prominent in the phase-encoding direction. Truncation errors can be minimized by increasing the matrix in both phase- and frequency-encoding direction or by reducing the FOV (Fig. 40.4).

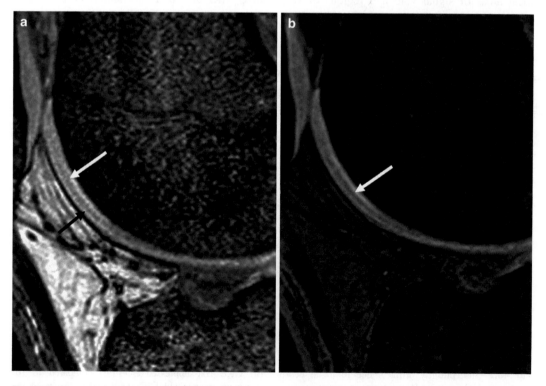

Fig. 40.3 Demonstration of similar truncation artifacts (*arrows*) on 3D-GRE sequences with different sequence parameters but same in-plane resolution (0.5 × 0, 5 × 1.5).

Sagittal MR images of the knee with parameters: (**a**) 3D FLASH, 20/8 12°, compared to (**b**) fat-suppressed 3D FLASH 40/7 45°

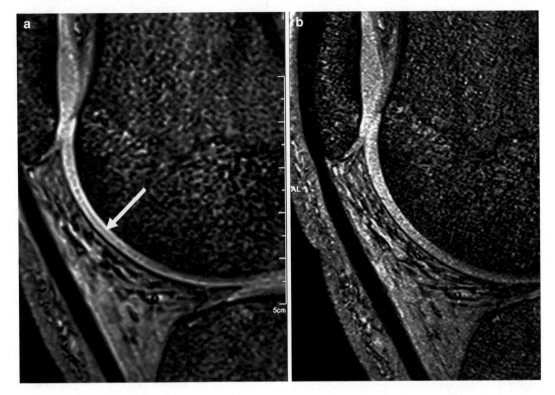

Fig. 40.4 Truncation artifact in GRE sequence (3D FLASH, 20/8 12°, SL 1.5 mm) (*arrow* in (**a**). Dependency of appearance on spatial resolution. Sagittal MR images of the knee with parameters: (**a**) matrix 256 × 320, compared to (**b**) matrix 410 × 512

40.2.4 Magic Angle Artifact

On T2-weighted imaging, the signal strength and contrast within cartilage is dependent on the direction of parallel-oriented substructures within the cartilage with reference to the direction of the external static magnetic field (B0). This angle dependence is called the "magic angle effect." Substructures such as collagen within the cartilage are oriented parallel but not randomly in space. Packed collagen fibers exhibit a maximum in signal intensity when the main direction of their orientation is parallel to the magic angle of 54.7° (or 125.3°) with reference to the external magnetic field B0. At other orientations, the signal is decreased. This leads to an inhomogeneous appearance of signal within the cartilage ("magic angle artifact"). This artifact should not be confused with degenerative changes in the cartilage substance (Fig. 40.5).

The cartilage signal change produced by the magic angle effect can be greatly reduced by increasing the echo time (TE). At TE values of 70 ms in

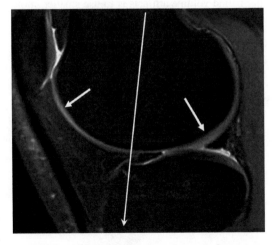

Fig. 40.5 Sagittal fat-suppressed proton density (TR 3750, TE 24) MR image of the knee shows the magic angle artifact (*arrows*) at approximately 55° to the *z*-axis (*line*) of the static magnetic field. The line representing the *z*-axis is tilted to compensate oblique positioning of acquired data volume

FSE imaging and 30 ms in GRE imaging, no artifacts will be produced (Li and Mirowitz 2003). Although the critical TE is lower in GRE compared to FSE, in clinical practice, TEs of 30 ms are rarely applied; which makes the artifact a phenomenon to be considered in most of the GRE sequences. In routine clinical intermediate FSE MRI, the artifact can be ignored at a value of around 40 ms and above. A detailed explanation of the physical principles of the angle dependence of cartilage and the "magic angle effect" is beyond the scope of this chapter. The reader is referred to the excellent review article by Xia (2000).

40.2.5 Partial Volume Averaging Artifact

Partial volume artifacts occur when signals of different objects are encompassed in one slice. For example, if two slices contain only fat or water signal, and a larger slice might contain a combination of the two, the large slice possesses a signal intensity equal to the weighted average of the quantity of water and fat present in the slice. This results in impaired resolution and erroneous intensity. Volume averaging can also decrease the visualization of low-contrast abnormalities and blur or distort affected structures. The main strategy for decreasing partial volume artifacts is to use smaller, more sharply defined voxels. This means thinner sections, smaller FOV, and/or higher imaging matrix sizes. In high-end cartilage imaging, acquisition of 3D data sets is particularly useful, because it provides thin sections with no intervening gaps (Fig. 40.4).

40.3 Sequence-Related Pitfalls in Cartilage Imaging

40.3.1 Ambiguity of Cartilage Surface in the Posterior Femoral Condyle

On fat-suppressed 3D-SPGR images, the surface contour of the cartilage cannot be delineated well in the majority of cases. This finding appears to be due to low contrast between cartilage and meniscus or adjacent structures such as the joint capsule, synovial fluid, and muscle. This finding was also observed in FLASH imaging (Takahashi et al. 2014) (Fig. 40.6).

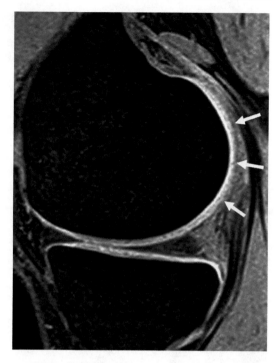

Fig. 40.6 Sagittal GRE (fat-suppressed 3D FLASH 40/7 45°) MR image of the knee shows ambiguity of cartilage surface at the posterior femoral condyle (*arrows*)

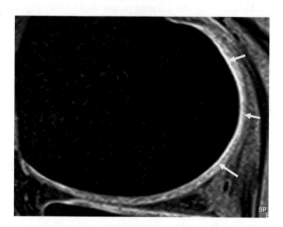

Fig. 40.7 Sagittal GRE (fat-suppressed 3D FLASH 40/7 45°) MR image of the knee shows a linear area of high signal in the deep zone (*arrows*)

40.3.2 Linear Area of Signal Intensity in Cartilage Deep Zone

This artifact is frequently seen in cartilage imaging with fat-suppressed 3D-GRE imaging (Fig. 40.7). The origin of this linear area of hyperintense signal in fat-suppressed 3D-SPGR is uncertain (Yoshioka et al. 2004). The finding described represents a major pitfall in the segmentation of cartilage for generation of 3D thickness maps (Steines et al. 2000).

40.4 Potential Pitfalls Related to Anatomy and Composition of Cartilage

40.4.1 Cartilage Thinning Adjacent to Anterior Horn of Lateral Meniscus

This finding is independent of the sequences applied. It is important to recognize this normal variant to distinguish it from true thinning resulting from degenerative change or trauma in this region. Smooth transition of the cartilage thickness is one of the characteristics that differentiate healthy cartilage from true cartilage defects (Fig. 40.8).

40.4.2 Decreased Signal Intensity in the Distal Part of the Trochlear Cartilage

This phenomenon is a normal signal pattern. In the study of Yoshioka et al. (2004), it was

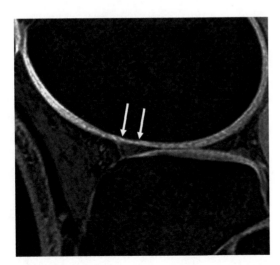

Fig. 40.8 Sagittal GRE (fat-suppressed 3D FLASH 40/7 45°, SL 1.5 mm) MR image of the knee shows cartilage thinning adjacent to anterior horn of the lateral meniscus (*arrows*)

observed in all volunteers and in all sequences (Fig. 40.9). The cause of the very low signal intensity in this region is not clear, but is presumably related to the anisotropic arrangement of collagen fibers.

40.5 Developmental Pitfalls of Cartilage Imaging

40.5.1 Shoulder Joint

A smooth benign-appearing full-thickness cartilage defect ("bare spot") without thickened underlying bone can be seen as a normal variant, not to be mistaken for chondromalacia (Figs. 40.10 and 40.11). This so-called bare spot has been described as a normal variant in adults and occasionally in children, adolescents, and young adults in the range between 10 and 20 years of age (Ly et al. 2004; Kim et al. 2010).

40.5.2 Elbow Joint

40.5.2.1 Transverse Trochlear Ridge
In most persons, the trochlear groove is traversed by a cartilage-free bony ridge at the junction of the olecranon and the coronoid process, either along the full transverse extension or partially in the radial or ulnar sides of the trochlear groove. Rosenberg et al. (1994) were the first to demonstrate in detail this transverse ridge on sagittal MR images as a central elevation of the articular surface of the trochlear groove in 70–80% of the MRI studies. The height of the ridge varied from a minimal wrinkle of the surface of the groove to a distinct central elevation which could be mistaken for an osteophyte.

40.5.2.2 Pseudo-Defect of the Trochlear Groove
Located peripheral to the bony ridge traversing the trochlear groove, there is an inward tapering of the trochlear groove of the ulna at the junction of the coronoid process and the olecranon. This tapering results in a gentle ulnar waist and small cartilage-free areas at the medial and lateral edges of this waist (Fig. 40.12).

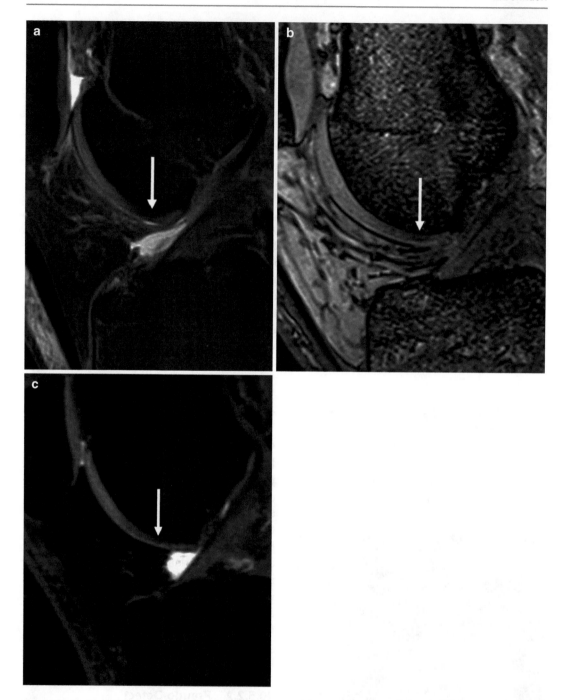

Fig. 40.9 Sagittal MR images obtained with a variety of sequences in different patients and volunteers all show decreased signal intensity in the distal part of the trochlear cartilage (*arrows*). (**a**) IM FS (TR 3500, TE 37 ms, SL 2.5 mm), (**b**) 3D FLASH (20/8–12°, SL 1.5 mm), (**c**) 3D DESS water excitation (40/5 40°, SL 1 mm)

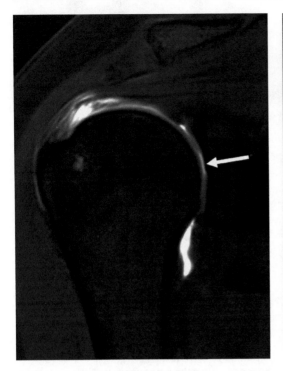

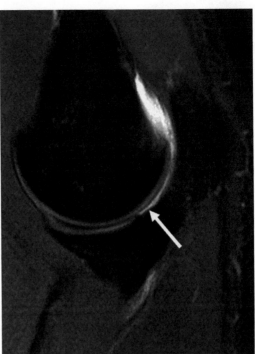

Fig. 40.10 Coronal MR arthrographic image shows the "bare spot" variant in the center of the glenoid labral cartilage of the shoulder joint (*arrow*) (Courtesy of Karl-Friedrich Kreitner, Mainz, Germany)

Fig. 40.12 Sagittal MR image of the elbow shows the pseudo-defect of the trochlear groove (*arrow*). Inward tapering of the trochlear groove of the ulna at the junction of the coronoid process and the olecranon may result in a small cartilage-free area at the medial and lateral edges

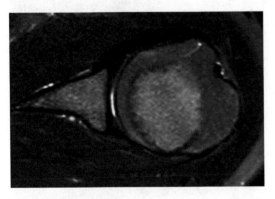

Fig. 40.11 Axial FSE T2-W MR image shows the "bare spot" variant in the center of the glenoid labral cartilage of the shoulder joint (Courtesy of Peter Bureik, Germany)

40.5.2.3   Pseudo-Defect of the Capitellum

This pseudo-defect is another anatomical variation frequently seen in the elbow. It occurs posterolaterally where the normal cartilage-covered surface of the capitellum ends abruptly, resulting in a step-off at the border with the non-articular portion of the distal humerus. The posterior part of the radius lies opposite to this non-articular cartilage-deprived portion of the lateral condyle. This is identified in the MRI as a notch, easily identified in sagittal images but also seen in the coronal plane (Fig. 40.13). It can be more subtle or more conspicuous and can simulate an osteochondral lesion of the capitellum. In case of osteochondral fractures, these traumatic lesions are regularly accompanied by bone bruises.

40.5.3   Hip Joint

40.5.3.1   Supra-Acetabular Fossa

The supra-acetabular fossa (SAF) can be identified on MRI in the coronal and sagittal planes at the superior weight-bearing region of the acetabulum seen at the 12 o'clock position. It may mimic an acetabular cartilage defect but is usually easily distinguishable from an osteochondral lesion because

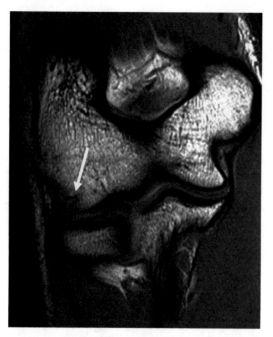

Fig. 40.13 Coronal MR image shows the pseudo-defect of the capitellum posterolaterally where the normal cartilage-covered surface of the capitellum ends abruptly, resulting in a step-off at the border with the non-articular portion of the distal humerus (*arrow*)

it has relatively smooth margins and there is normal underlying marrow signal (DuBois and Omar 2010) (Fig. 40.14). In the study of Dietrich et al. (2012), the SAF was a common finding at MR arthrography of the hip in their patient population, with a frequency of 1.6% for SAF type 1 filled with contrast material and 8.9% for SAF type 2 with a bony fossa filled with cartilage. SAF type 1 was more common in younger patients. Thus, the authors assume that SAF type 1 may undergo some remodeling with time and appear later as SAF type 2. Their correlation with arthroscopic findings underlines the theory that the SAF represents a variant because no distinct cartilage defect was seen at arthroscopy at this location. However, the cause of the SAF is not known.

40.5.3.2 Stellate Crease

This represents a bare area deficient of hyaline cartilage within the lunate surface of the acetabulum. At arthroscopy, this lesion is frequently seen near and above the anterior apex of the acetabular fossa. It has the appearance of an indentation that the untrained eye may confuse for early

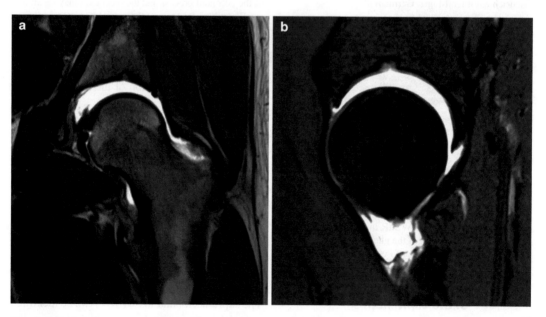

Fig. 40.14 (**a**) Coronal and (**b**) sagittal MR arthrographic images of the hip show a supra-acetabular fossa at the 12 o'clock position (Courtesy of Christian Pfirrmann, Zurich, Switzerland)

degenerative change (Keene and Villar 1994). On MRI, it is rarely detectable (Christian Pfirrmann, personal communication).

Conclusion

Several pitfalls may affect the assessment of cartilage on MRI. These include MRI inherent artifacts, sequence-related pitfalls such as the ambiguity of the cartilage surface in the posterior femoral condyle and the linear area of signal intensity in cartilage deep zone on 3D gradient-echo sequences, potential pitfalls related to anatomy and composition of cartilage, and developmental pitfalls at the shoulder, elbow, and hip joints.

Acknowledgment The author would like to thank Andreas Berg, Vienna, for reviewing and improving the contents of the chapter and Vladimir Mlynarik, Vienna, for fruitful discussions.

References

Del Grande F, Santini F, Herzka DA et al (2014) Fat-suppression techniques for 3-T MR imaging of the musculoskeletal system. Radiographics 34:217–233

Dietrich TJ, Suter A, Pfirrmann CW et al (2012) Supraacetabular fossa (pseudodefect of acetabular cartilage): frequency at MT arthrography and comparison with findings at MR arthrography and arthroscopy. Radiology 263:484–491

DuBois DF, Omar IM (2010) MR imaging of the hip: normal anatomic variants and imaging pitfalls. Magn Reson Imaging Clin N Am 18:663–674

Eckstein F, Guermazi A, Gold G et al (2014) Imaging of cartilage and bone: promises and pitfalls in clinical trials of osteoarthritis. Osteoarthr Cartil 22:1516–1532

Elster AD (2015a) Susceptibility artifacts. Questions and answers in MRI. https://www.mriquestions.com. Accessed 12 Dec 2015

Elster AD (2015b) Truncation artifacts. Questions and answers in MRI. https://www.mriquestions.com. Accessed 15 Dec 2015

Erickson SJ, Waldschmidt JG, Czervionke LE, Prost RW (1996) Hyaline cartilage: truncation artifact as a cause of trilaminar appearance with fat-suppressed three-dimensional spoiled gradient-recalled sequences. Radiology 201:260–264

Frank LR, Brossmann JB, Buxton RB, Resnick D (1997) MR imaging truncation artifacts can create a false laminar appearance in cartilage. AJR Am J Roentgenol 168:547–554

Keene GS, Villar RN (1994) Arthroscopic anatomy of the hip: an in vivo study. Arthroscopy 10:392–399

Kim HK, Emery KH, Salisbury SR (2010) Bare spot of the glenoid fossa in children: incidence and MRI features. Pediatr Radiol 40:1190–1196

Lee MJ, Kim S, Lee SA et al (2007) Overcoming artifacts from metallic orthopedic implants at high field strength MR imaging and multi-detector CT. Radiographics 27:791–803

Li T, Mirowitz SA (2003) Manifestation of magic angle phenomenon: comparative study on effects of varying echo time and tendon orientation among various MR sequences. Magn Reson Imaging 21:741–744

Ly JQ, Bui-Mansfield LT, Kline MJ (2004) Bare area of the glenoid: magnetic resonance appearance with arthroscopic correlation. J Comput Assist Tomogr 28:229–232

Peh WCG, Chan JHM (2001) Artifacts in musculoskeletal magnetic resonance imaging: identification and correction. Skeletal Radiol 30:179–191

Rosenberg ZS, Beltran J, Cheung YY (1994) Pseudodefect of the capitellum: potential MR imaging pitfall. Radiology 191:821–823

Sakamoto FA, Winalski CS, Schils JP et al (2011) Vacuum phenomenon: prevalence and appearance in the knee with 3T magnetic resonance imaging. Skeletal Radiol 40:1275–1285

Singh DR, Chin MSM, Peh WCG (2014) Artifacts in musculoskeletal MR imaging. Semin Musculoskelet Radiol 18:12–22

Steines D, Berger F, Cheng C, Napel S, Lang P (2000) 3D thickness maps of articular cartilage for quantitative assessment of osteoarthritis (abstr). In: Proceedings of the 64th meeting of the American College of Rheumatology, Philadelphia, p 1717

Takahashi M, Fujinaga Y, Fukamatsu F et al (2014) MR findings that mimic disease of knee cartilage in osteoarthritis patients: comparison between SPGR at 1.5T and FLASH at 3T. ECR Poster 2014/C-0835. http://posterng.netkey.at

Waldschmidt JG, Rilling RJ, Kajdacsy-Balla AA et al (1997) In vitro and in vivo MR imaging of hyaline cartilage: zonal anatomy, imaging pitfalls, and pathologic conditions. Radiographics 17:1387–1402

Xia Y (2000) Magic-angle effect in magnetic resonance imaging in articular cartilage. A review. Invest Radiol 35:602–621

Yoshioka H, Stevens K, Genovese M et al (2004) Articular cartilage of knee: normal patterns at MR imaging that mimic disease in healthy subjects and patients with osteoarthritis. Radiology 231:31–39

Giuseppe Guglielmi, Federico Ponti, Sara Guerri, and Alberto Bazzocchi

Contents

41.1	**Introduction**	893
41.2	**Epidemiology**	894
41.3	**Physical Concepts and Technological Advances**	894
41.4	**Role of DXA Scan in Clinical Practice**	896
41.5	**Pitfalls in Bone Mineral Densitometry**	898
41.5.1	Wrong Demographic Information	898
41.5.2	Improper Patient Preparation and Positioning	899
41.5.3	Data Analysis Errors	900
41.5.4	Mistakes in Interpretation	905
41.5.5	Serial BMD Measurements and Pitfalls in Follow-Up	908
Conclusion		921
References		921

G. Guglielmi (✉)
Department of Radiology, University of Foggia,
Viale Luigi Pinto 1, 71100 Foggia, Italy

Department of Radiology, Scientific Institute "Casa Sollievo della Sofferenza" Hospital,
Viale Cappuccini 1, 71013 San Giovanni Rotondo, Italy
e-mail: giuseppe.guglielmi@unifg.it

F. Ponti
Department of Specialized, Diagnostic and Experimental Medicine, University of Bologna,
Sant'Orsola – Malpighi Hospital,
Via G. Massarenti 9, 40138 Bologna, Italy

The "Rizzoli" Orthopaedic Institute,
Via G. C. Pupilli 1, 40136 Bologna, Italy

S. Guerri
Department of Specialized, Diagnostic and Experimental Medicine, University of Bologna,
Sant'Orsola – Malpighi Hospital,
Via G. Massarenti 9, 40138 Bologna, Italy

A. Bazzocchi
The "Rizzoli" Orthopaedic Institute,
Via G. C. Pupilli 1, 40136 Bologna, Italy

Abbreviations

BMD	Bone mineral density
DXA	Dual-energy X-ray absorptiometry
QCT	Quantitative computed tomography
ROI	Region of interest
WHO	World Health Organization

41.1 Introduction

Dual-energy X-ray absorptiometry (DXA) was introduced in late 1980s to assess bone mineral density (BMD). Nowadays, thanks to several technological advances, it represents the gold standard for diagnosis and monitoring osteoporosis and low bone mass conditions. DXA also represents an innovative technique for fracture risk assessment and to study body composition, in terms of fat mass and non-bone lean mass, both at a regional and whole-body level (Toombs et al. 2012). Despite all of this, DXA is often little understood among radiologists who lack confidence in the operation of the machines and in the technique of acquisition, analysis and interpretation of the

W.C.G. Peh (ed.), *Pitfalls in Musculoskeletal Radiology*, DOI 10.1007/978-3-319-53496-1_41

results, thus incurring into frequent mistakes that could easily be avoided (Lorente Ramos et al. 2012). The pitfalls can be divided into: (1) technical ones, taking place during the examination, and (2) interpretative ones that, when often unnoticed, can lead to mistakes in the management of the patient. Contrary to widely held assumptions, DXA, like other diagnostic tools, is not an automatic technique. To achieve the best results, each step of the diagnostic process (from appropriate clinical indications to correct acquisition and data interpretation) should be validated and fully understood. Moreover, a periodic quality control (QC) program and precision assessment of the facilities are vital to obtain reliable and reproducible results, as well as constant training of technologists (Lorente Ramos et al. 2012; Kim and Yang 2014).

41.2 Epidemiology

According to National Institutes of Health (NIH) Consensus Statement (March 27–29, 2000), osteoporosis is "a skeletal disorder characterized by compromised bone strength predisposing to an increased risk of fracture." Bone strength is determined by two different parameters, namely, (1) bone density, the amount of mineral per unit area or unit volume in bones (expressed as g/cm^2 or g/cm^3), reflecting the integration between the peak bone mass and the amount of bone loss, and (2) bone quality, which refers to the micro-architecture of the tissue and to aspects of its composition (NIH Consensus Development Panel 2001). Osteoporosis is a steadily rising disease, due to aging of the population and the widespread long-term glucocorticoid administration in rheumatologic diseases, chronic obstructive pulmonary disease, and post-organ transplant. About 27.6 million of adults in Europe (22.0 million of women and 5.6 million of men) were estimated to have osteoporosis in the year 2010 (Hernlund et al. 2013).

Recently the National Osteoporosis Foundation estimated that in the United States of America (USA), by the year 2010, osteoporosis and low bone mass conditions affect a total of 53.6 million adults aged 50 years and older. This is currently approximately one-half of the total adult population in the USA that is affected by these pathological conditions, especially non-Hispanic white women (Wright et al. 2014). The prevalence of osteoporosis in the Asian continent is largely unknown, but it will be an issue in the very near future, due to the rapidly increasing age of its population (Mithal and Kaur 2012). The burden of osteoporosis is extremely high in term of morbidity and socioeconomic costs associated with the disease and its complications. In the year 2000, approximately nine million osteoporotic fractures occur worldwide; the total disability-adjusted life years (DALYs) lost was 5.8 million, of which 51% were accounted for by fractures that occurred in America and Europe (Johnell and Kanis 2006). It is therefore very important to evaluate patients at risk for osteoporosis to correctly diagnose this pathological condition, to assess the fracture risk, and to monitor the effects of treatment.

41.3 Physical Concepts and Technological Advances

Since the World Health Organization (WHO) set threshold levels for the diagnosis of osteoporosis and osteopenia in 1994, DXA became the technique of reference to establish BMD *in vivo* (Guglielmi et al. 2011). Before reporting on the pitfalls of DXA, it is useful to have a brief overview of technical aspects and correct execution of this exam. A DXA scanner consists essentially of three components, namely, (1) a mobile X-ray source, (2) a detector array on the opposite side, and (3) a patient table. Dedicated software to process and analyze the acquired images is provided by the manufacturers, with the three major manufacturers of DXA instruments being Hologic Inc. (Bedford, MA, USA), GE Lunar Inc. (Madison, WI, USA), and Cooper Surgical (Norland; Trumbull, CT, USA). The X-ray source is placed under the patient table, and during scanning, it moves coupled with the detector array located at the opposite site of patient's body. The operating principle of DXA lies in differential attenuation of the X-ray beam, depending on energy of the X-ray beam itself and density and thickness of tissue it runs through. Attenuation is less with high photon energy, whereas it is greater when the X-ray beam passes through high-density material such as bone.

In order to determine BMD and body composition, DXA scanners use two X-ray beams: a high energy one (140 kV) and a low energy one (70–100 kV). While the patient is being scanned, the computer constructs the image of the examined section pixel by pixel. To each pixel corresponds a specific degree of attenuation of the two beams. The ratio between the degree of attenuation of the lower energy and the higher energy beam is the "R" value. The threshold value to discriminate between the pixels that contain bone and those that cover only soft tissue is obtained by manufacturers using complex, multifactorial algorithms. From the R value, it is possible, using other specific formulas, to assess the percentage and the amount of bone mineral content (BMC) and soft tissue in pixels containing bone. In pixels without bone, soft tissue can be further characterized as fat mass and non-bone lean mass. By subtracting the pixels with soft tissue attenuation values from the acquired image, a computer algorithm determines bone edge profiles and then calculates the area of the pixels that correspond to bone tissue. The BMD (expressed in g/cm^2) is finally calculated as the ratio BMC/area (Pietrobelli et al. 1996; Toombs et al. 2012).

Since the introduction of DXA in 1987, many technical developments have taken place. First-generation DXA scanners use a pencil-width X-ray beam, tightly collimated and rigidly coupled with a single detector, that moves in tandem in a rectilinear manner across the anatomical site of interest. The disadvantage of this technology is the relatively long scanning time (about 5–10 min per site and 10–20 min for the whole body). Fan-beam densitometers were introduced in 1993 and use a wider beam of photons and multiple detectors. Images are obtained in a single sweep, scanning in a longitudinal fashion across the anatomical site, allowing a faster scan speed (about 1 min per site and 5 min for the whole body) and a better resolution (0.8–2 mm for fan-beam densitometers versus 1.5–2.5 mm for pencil-beam densitometers). Disadvantages of this technology include a higher radiation dose

(even though it is still very small) and the magnification of scanned structures because of the shorter distance from the X-ray source. In practice, magnification is responsible for mistakes in measurement of BMC and of bone area. To overcome this limitation, some important advances have been introduced recently: narrow fan-beam scans come with a beam wider than first-generation machines, but still narrower than the previous-generation fan-beam densitometers. This type of DXA scan works in a rectilinear manner, with each individual sweep overlapping the previous one. Although scanning time is slightly longer, narrow fan-beam densitometers allow estimation of the real depth and size of bone more accurately (Toombs et al. 2012).

One of the latest generation of scanners is represented by the iDXA, a system with a larger number of detectors and a narrow-angle fan-beam that provides images of enhanced resolution (1.05 mm longitudinally and 0.6 mm laterally) (Toombs et al. 2012). Moreover, current fan-beam systems have a rotating C-arm able to perform lateral scanning with the patient in the supine position. By rotating this C-arm 90°, the X-ray tube provides lateral projections without the superimposition of vascular calcifications, posterior vertebral elements, and marginal osteophytes, thus giving a more accurate picture of bone density (Guglielmi et al. 1994).

Over the past few years, there has been an impressive increase in the use of bone densitometry. In the USA, the number of DXA examinations performed has grown from 501,105 in 1996 to 2,195,548 in 2002, and this trend is expected to continue over the next few years. Accordingly, topics concerning dose justification and dose optimization have indeed become extremely important (Intenzo et al. 2005; Damilakis et al. 2010). One of the leading advantages of DXA is the low radiation dose received by patients. Patient dose from X-ray exams can be expressed by effective dose (in Sv) which allows an estimation of the radiogenic risk of selective body exposure that typically occurs when different organs are exposed to different doses. Moreover, effective dose allows comparison of radiogenic risk from different X-ray examinations and natural background radiation. For a DXA examination, the radiation dose depends on various parameters like the length of the exam itself, patient size, scan model, beam filtration, tube current (mA), and tube potential (kVp) (Damilakis et al. 2010). For current systems, the effective dose to an adult from a spine and hip examination is approximately between 1 and 10 μSv; this dose is even smaller than one incurred in obtaining a chest radiograph (Kalender 1992; Wall and Hart 1997; Hawkinson et al. 2007).

To compare radiogenic risk of different X-ray examinations, we can also refer to the time of exposure to natural background radiation. The worldwide average ionizing radiation dose is 2.4 mSv/year, equivalent to 6.7 μSv a day. While examinations such as chest CT correspond to several years of exposure to natural background radiation, a whole-body or regional DXA scan corresponds approximately to 1 day of exposure, or even less. The latest narrow fan-beam DXAs allow adapting the scanning surface to underline the skeletal structure of every individual and, thus, achieve an important reduction in time of scanning and radiation dose received both by patients and operators (Hawkinson et al. 2007).

41.4 Role of DXA Scan in Clinical Practice

Currently, DXA scan has a key role in the diagnosis and follow-up of osteoporosis and low bone density conditions. The International Society of Clinical Densitometry (ISCD) recently revised the correct indications for performing a DXA scan (Schousboe et al. 2013) (Table 41.1). DXA examination has three main roles, namely, the diagnosis of osteoporosis, fracture risk assessment, and monitoring treatment response (Blake and Fogelman 2010). In a central DXA scan, two skeletal sites are commonly analyzed: BMD results at the lumbar spine (L1 through L4) and at the proximal femur (i.e., hip). These are, by consensus, interpreted using the WHO T-score definitions of osteoporosis and osteopenia: a T-score of −2.5 or lower is defined as osteoporosis (WHO 1994) (Table 41.2).

Table 41.1 Current indications for BMD testing

| Women aged 65 years and older |
| Postmenopausal women under age 65 years and women during the menopausal transition with one or more of the following risk factors: |
| Low body weight |
| Prior fracture |
| High-risk medication use |
| Disease or condition associated with bone loss |
| Men aged 70 years and older |
| Men under age 70 years with one or more of the following risk factors: |
| Low body weight |
| Prior fracture |
| High-risk medication use |
| Disease or condition associated with bone loss |
| Adults with a fragility fracture |
| Adults with a disease or condition associated with low bone mass or bone loss |
| Adults taking medication associated with low bone mass or bone loss |
| Anyone being considered for pharmacological therapy |
| Anyone being treated, to monitor treatment effect |
| Anyone not receiving therapy in whom evidence of bone loss would lead to treatment |

Table 41.2 The World Health Organization definitions of osteoporosis and osteopenia

Normal	$T \geq -1.0$
Low bone mass (osteopenia)	$-2.5 < T < -1.0$
Osteoporosis	$T \leq -2.5$
Established osteoporosis	$T \leq -2.5$ in the presence of one or more fragility fractures

The WHO definition of osteoporosis applies to postmenopausal women and to men older than 50 years old. According to the ISCD guidelines, in premenopausal women, in men younger than 50 years old, and in children, the Z-score is used, comparing individual BMD measurement to the mean BMD of an age-matched population of the same gender and ethnic group. A Z-score value lower than −2 is defined as "below the expected range for age," although it is very important to underscore that osteoporosis cannot be defined just on the basis of the DXA BMD alone in these populations (Link 2012). Since osteoporosis is a systemic disease, similar trends in T-score values may be expected at the spine and at the hip; but in reality, osteoporosis affects the different skeletal sites differently, and a discordant T-score at hip and spine is commonly encountered. A large discordance with differences in T-score greater of 1.5 may indicate an underlying disease, and in this case, other examinations should be requested (Lenchik et al. 1998).

Even if DXA represents the most available and used technique to assess BMD, other advanced radiological modalities aim to study the geometry of the bone and to better understand the metabolic status of bone and its strength. While DXA is able to provide areal bone mineral density (BMDa, g/m^2), quantitative computed tomography (QCT) estimates volumetric bone mineral density (BMDv, mg/cm^3) and is extremely useful for early diagnosis of osteoporosis and to monitor the response to consequent treatment. QCT has the ability to assess BMD in cortical and trabecular bone, which are affected differently by this disease, separately. This technique and some of its improvements such as peripheral QCT (pQCT) and high-resolution pQCT (HR-pQCT), that provide BMD in the appendicular skeleton to more accurately evaluate bone density and microarchitecture, are however more commonly used as second-level methods or only in field of research (Guglielmi et al. 2011). Another innovative technology of growing use among different centers and that does not involve ionizing radiations exposure is quantitative ultrasound (QUS). While DXA represents the gold standard to diagnose osteoporosis, QUS allows estimation of the bone strength and to classify patients according to their risk of experiencing a fracture (Guglielmi et al. 2009).

In a clinical setting, an individualized approach is recommended for the evaluation of osteoporotic patients, and three major imaging modalities are commonly used to assess bone strength, namely, DXA, QCT, and calcaneal ultrasonography. The choice of which of these examinations to use depends on many factors, including patient age and the presence of risk factors for osteoporotic fractures. In patients without osteoporotic risk factors, calcaneal ultrasonography represents the screening modality of choice. When multiple risk factors are present, a DXA scan or a QCT should be performed on the skeletal area at greater

risk of fracture. In women younger than 65 years old, vertebral fractures are of greater concern than hip fractures, so DXA or QCT should be performed on the spine. In women older than 65 years old, osteoporotic fractures are more prevalent at the hip, and aortic calcification and degenerative spinal changes could overestimate the BMD at lumbar spine. Thus, in this population, posteroanterior spinal DXA should be avoided in favor of a DXA scan of the hip or of the lateral spine and QCT of the spine (Brunader and Shelton 2002). In addition, several studies suggest that hip BMD represents the most reliable measurement to estimate hip fractures risk, whereas spine BMD represents the most reliable one for monitoring treatment (Marshall et al. 1996; Stone et al. 2003; Johnell et al. 2005). According to the ISCD, if DXA and QCT are both available and if they provide comparable information, then DXA should be preferred to limit radiation dose received by patients (Shepherd et al. 2015).

The second main role of DXA examination is fracture risk assessment. Vertebral compression fractures (VCFs) represent an ever-increasing problem among elderly, with prevalence among women and men older than 50 years old being approximately 10–26%. About 75% of all VCFs, however, are not clinically apparent at the time of their occurrence. DXA lateral spine, also known as vertebral fracture assessment (VFA), is typically performed at the same time as a bone density test. It allows the identification of clinically unrecognized or undocumented vertebral fractures, improves fracture prediction, and evaluates the need for prevention therapy (Rosen et al. 2013). VCFs represent an independent risk factor for future VCFs and for fragility fractures at other skeletal sites; in presence of a VCF, the relative risk of future VCFs increases more than four times (Klotzbuecher et al. 2000).

According to ISCD, lateral spine imaging (with standard radiography or densitometric VFA) is indicated when the T-score is less than −1.0, and one or more of the following applies: (1) women aged >70 years or men aged >80 years, (2) height loss >4 cm, (3) prior vertebral fracture (self-reported but undocumented), and (4) glucocorticoid therapy (>5 mg of prednisone or equivalent per day for >3 months) (Rosen et al. 2013). In VFA, the patient lies on the scanning table in a lateral decubitus or in supine lateral position, if DXA has a rotary C-arm. Dedicated post-processing-specific tools allow the manipulation of acquired images and the placing of point markers at the anterior, middle, and posterior margins of the vertebral endplates so that vertebral heights can be measured. According to ISCD, the Genant visual semiquantitative method (combination of morphometric and visual assessment) is the technique of choice for diagnosing vertebral fractures with VFA (Lewiecki and Laster 2006). In clinical practice, during the initial evaluation of a back pain of suspected skeletal etiology, the first examination performed is generally a spine radiograph. This examination has good spatial resolution and low cost and is widely available. Even if the spatial resolution is not as good as in a standard radiography, VFA has important advantages: it can be performed concurrently with BMD measurement and patient radiation dose is very low, as discussed above. Once a fracture is detected, CT or magnetic resonance imaging (MRI) may be done to better define the anatomy or when an underlying disease (e.g., malignancy) is suspected (Lewiecki and Laster 2006).

Recently, there has been great interest concerning the possible relation between the prolonged bisphosphonate (BP) therapy and femoral subtrochanteric and shaft fractures. These fractures are classified as "atypical," as opposed to "typical fractures" occurring at the femoral neck and trochanteric area, and are typically stress- or low-trauma-related fractures (Shane et al. 2014; Im and Jeong 2015). As suggested by recent studies, in patients with chronic BP therapy who undergo DXA exam, it is useful to extend the length of the femur image, as only in this way is it possible to diagnose unrecognized atypical femoral fractures (McKenna et al. 2013). Localized periosteal reaction with focal lateral cortical thickening and transverse fracture are reliable signs for diagnosis (Rosenberg et al. 2011).

Even if the subject falls outside the field of interest of this chapter, it is interesting to note that DXA can be used to determine body composition (lean, fat, and mineral mass) in various body compartments (Bazzocchi et al. 2016). This type of examination offers new diagnostic insights for a large variety of diseases and can be used to monitor treatment response (Guglielmi et al. 2016). According to ISCD, DXA total body composition with regional analysis is validated in three main situations: (1) to assess fat distribution in HIV patients treated with anti-retroviral agents associated with a risk of lipoatrophy, (2) in obese patients undergoing bariatric surgery when weight loss exceeds approximately 10%, and (3) in patients with muscle weakness or poor physical functioning. In the two last situations, DXA helps to assess fat and lean mass changes, but the impact on clinical outcomes is uncertain (Hangartner et al. 2013; Shepherd et al. 2013).

41.5 Pitfalls in Bone Mineral Densitometry

Performing a DXA study correctly is very important in order to make correct diagnosis and clinical decisions (Watts 2004). According to Watts (2004) and Garg and Kharb (2013), pitfalls in DXA can be divided in four main categories, namely, wrong demographic information, improper patient positioning, data analysis errors, and mistakes in interpretation (Messina et al. 2015).

41.5.1 Wrong Demographic Information

The first step in performing a correct DXA study is ensuring the correct identification of the patient: it is very important to enter the patient's biographical information with utmost care because mistakes in gender assignment, patient's race, and weight can affect both the T-score and Z-score (Khan et al. 2007). Date of birth, gender, and ethnicity are all used to calculate the Z-score. In calculating the T-score, the gender of the patient is used as well by all manufacturers, while there is inconsistency over the use of patient race. The ISCD recommends calculating the T-scores regardless of the race of the subject in North America because using race-adjusted T-scores results in a similar prevalence of osteoporosis among different racial groups; thus, it does not reflect the true situation faithfully (Watts 2004).

41.5.2 Improper Patient Preparation and Positioning

Patient preparation is important. Information such as height and weight must be carefully obtained before performing the scan, because changes in this data can affect DXA results. If possible, stadiometric measurements should be used because of height reduction is an indicator of spinal compression fracture (Lenchik et al. 1998; Khan et al. 2007). The technologists should always ask female patients if there is a chance of pregnancy, and if pregnancy cannot be excluded, the scan must be delayed. Having recently given birth and breastfeeding are not contraindications, but since they produce transient and reversible changes in bone mass, BMD testing should be delayed for 6 months postpartum. DXA also needs to be postponed if the patient has received calcium supplements within 2 h, a previous radioactive isotope administration within 72 h, or if a radiographic procedure involving contrast material has been performed within the last 14 days (Khan et al. 2007). Patients should list accurately all previous fractures. The results may not be valid if a fracture lies within the regions of interest (ROIs) of the scan; for example, a spurious increase in BMD can result when a vertebral body becomes compressed in a smaller volume after a fracture. Even if it lies outside the ROIs of the scan, a previous fracture is an independent risk factor for future fractures (Lenchik et al. 1998).

Prior to getting onto the scanning table, the patient must be asked to remove any footwear and all metal items overlying the scan area, such as buttons, buckles, zippers, jewelry, keys, and coins, since all of these can cause artifacts (Khan et al. 2007). Incorrect positioning of the patient is one of the most common mistakes in DXA examinations (Messina et al. 2015). Before performing the examination, technologists should ensure that the patient is correctly positioned on the scanning table; and positioning should be double-checked by the reporting physician before the patient leaves (Watts 2004). If, during the initial scanning, there is evidence of suboptimal positioning, the technologists should stop the scanning, reposition the patient correctly, and start the scan again (Messina et al. 2015).

For DXA lumbar spine scan, the patient should be lying straight on his back on the scanning table. It is extremely important that the spine is centered on the table, ideally with the same amount of soft tissue on both sides of the spinal column. The right and left anterior superior iliac spines (ASIS) must be at the same distance from the tabletop. The arms should be placed on each side of the body, and knees must be flexed over a 90° support pad in order to straighten the lumbar spine, to partially flatten its lordosis, and to facilitate segmentation of lumbar levels. In patients with scoliosis, who cannot lie straight and centered on the scanning table, measurement of BMD by DXA lumbar spine is not always valid (Watts 2004; Khan et al. 2007).

For assessing BMD at the hip, the patient should lie supine on the table with arms on the chest. For proper positioning, the femoral shaft should be aligned straight to the long axis of the scanning table (so that it will appear parallel to the edge of the picture) with 15–25° of internal rotation. To help the patient rest in this position, a specific foot support is used. This degree of internal rotation guarantees that the long axis of the femoral neck is perpendicular to the X-ray beam, in order to scan the greatest area and the lowest BMC (and BMD). In patients with severe hip arthritis, achieving the adequate degree of internal rotation can be difficult; in this case, an easy reproducible position should be preferred (Watts 2004; Khan et al. 2007). Since a "dominant" hip that could affect BMD measurement does not appear to exist, the scan can be performed on both sides in absence of a focal lesion or prior surgery (Fig. 41.1). If the exam has to be performed again sometime after, it is necessary to choose the same side (Hamdy et al. 2002).

The third site that can be used to measure BMD is the forearm. The 33% radius, also called one-third radius, of the non-dominant forearm is used for diagnosis; the other forearm is not recommended. This scan is performed when spine or hip BMD cannot be assessed (e.g., patients with severe scoliosis or degenerative changes, multiple compression fractures, spine surgical devices or bilateral hip prosthesis, severe obesity) and in case of primary hyperparathyroidism, because this pathological condition affects more

Fig. 41.1 Proximal femoral DXA scans can be performed indiscriminately on both sides in absence of focal lesion or prior surgery. (**a**) In the case of unilateral metallic instrumentations (e.g., metal pins, rods or plates, and screws placed into the bone), the opposite side should be selected. (**b**) In the case of bilateral hip prosthesis, another skeletal site to scan should be selected

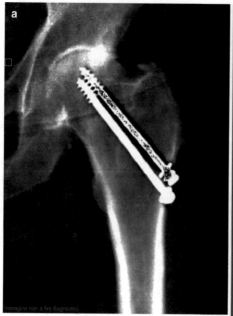
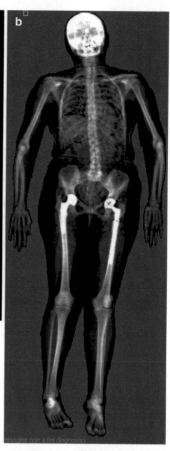

directly cortical bone than trabecular bone, thus affecting the forearm before the axial skeleton (Hamdy et al. 2002). The non-dominant forearm is expected to have a lower BMD than the dominant one. The forearm should not be scanned in case of internal hardware or previous wrist fractures. The patient is seated, side against the table, in a standard height chair with the forearm lying in a special support. The elbow is flexed between 90° and 105°, and forearm length is measured (Khan et al. 2007).

41.5.3 Data Analysis Errors

During scanning, densitometers produce a bone map using an algorithm that distinguishes different density gradients between bone and soft tissue and then automatically marks the ROIs both at the spine and hip. Inaccuracies occurring in any of the steps of this procedure are known as "data analysis errors." They include incorrect bone mapping

and misplacement of analysis boxes that can lead to mistakes in BMD measurement. Analysis represents a key step between the acquisition of the image and data interpretation. The operator should check each time for these types of mistakes, correct them manually, and make adjustments if necessary (Messina et al. 2015). It is also the reason why the scan should be analyzed before the patient leaves the testing unit, in case repeat scanning is necessary (Watts 2004).

41.5.3.1 Pitfalls in Lumbar Spine Data Analysis

Spine ROIs consist of vertebrae from L1 to L4 levels. Scan acquisition should extend from a point 2.5–5 cm below the anterior margin of iliac crest, to include the middle of L5 vertebra and all of L4 vertebra, up to about 4 cm above the tip of the sternum until the middle of T12 vertebra appears (Fig. 41.2). Scan acquisition should be interrupted and restarted if anatomical landmarks are not correctly displayed or if the spine is not centered (the spine must be

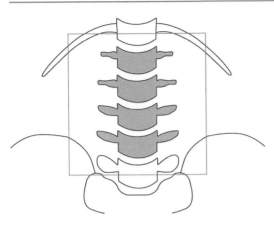

Fig. 41.2 Graphic illustration of a correctly acquired DXA spine scan

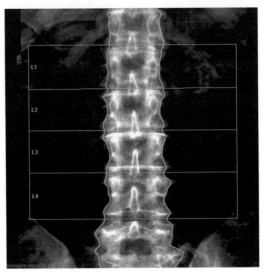

Fig. 41.3 Spine lumbar DXA and spine ROIs

centered in the scan field with the same amount of soft tissue on both sides). Previous DXA scans should be reviewed, if available, to ensure identical ROIs placement (Hamdy et al. 2002; Theodorou and Theodorou 2002). Once the image is acquired, auto-analysis software identifies the bone edges and places the global ROI and the intervertebral lines. The spine global ROI represents the anatomical area included in the analysis. It has a defined and not-modifiable pixel width (the box can just be moved to the left or to the right to be centered around the vertebral column) and adjustable length. The superior border of the spine global ROI should be positioned at the level of the T12–L1 intervertebral space and the inferior border at the level of the L4–L5 intervertebral space. Three more intervertebral lines are positioned between L1–L2, L2–L3, and L3–L4 levels. For the correct positioning of the intervertebral lines, the analysis software identifies the point of lower mineral density between two adjacent vertebrae; all these horizontal lines can be slightly angled in case of scoliosis. Then the system automatically labels the vertebral bodies from L1 to L4 vertebrae, defining the bone map for the lumbar spine (Fig. 41.3).

The global ROI box, the intervertebral markers, and the bone edges are usually appropriately positioned by the latest generation of DXA scanners that, thanks to good contrast resolution, automatically remove all recognizable artifacts. Even so, technologists are asked to check each time for possible mistakes, confirming or modifying the global ROI, the intervertebral lines, and the bone map. Changes should be done only if

absolutely necessary and should be performed in an easily reproducible way to facilitate follow-up scanning and monitoring of the patient. Finally, the results are generated: the estimated area (in cm²) and the estimated BMC (in grams) are measured and the BMD (g/cm²) is calculated separately for each vertebra. Even if the latest scanners allow the performing of lateral projections, thanks to a rotating C-arm, lateral scanning has, at the moment, just a role in monitoring and should not be used for diagnosis (Hamdy et al. 2002; Schousboe et al. 2013).

Mistakes in determination of spinal levels and in ROIs placement may invalidate BMD measurement. Correct positioning of the analysis box is critical because among lumbar vertebrae, BMD increases from L1 to L4 vertebrae. About 15% of population has an anatomical variation, such as four or six lumbar vertebrae or the last set of ribs on T11 or L1, that can lead to errors in the numbering of vertebrae and, thus, to over- or underestimations of BMD at the spine (Watts 2004). To avoid mistakes (e.g., including a T12 vertebra without ribs that would significantly lower the BMD), numbering should start from bottom up, and if in doubt, morphology can help to correctly identify vertebrae (Garg and Kharb 2013). The vertebrae can be correctly labeled by identifying L4 and L5 vertebrae by their characteristic shape: L4 has an H-shaped appearance, while L5 is looks like a capital I lying on its side (Bonnick

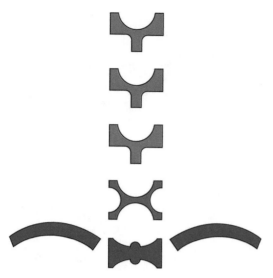

Fig. 41.4 Schematic rappresentation of vertebral morphology (from L1 to L5) at lumbar DXA scan

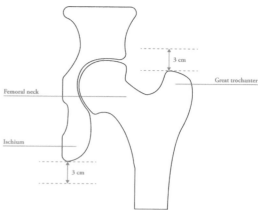

Fig. 41.5 Correct scan acquisition in proximal femur DXA. The scan includes all of the greater trochanter, the femoral neck, and the ischium, with a minimum of 3 cm of soft tissue proximal to the great trochanter and distal to the ischium

2010). Another clue is that the L3 vertebra commonly has the widest transverse processes among lumbar vertebrae (Peel et al. 1993) (Fig. 41.4).

41.5.3.2 Pitfalls in Proximal Femur Data Analysis

Femoral analysis can be challenging. Conventionally, the laser is positioned on the midline of the thigh, 4 cm distal to the greater trochanter or 1 cm distal to the pubic symphysis (Khan et al. 2007). The acquired image should include the great trochanter, the femoral neck, and the ischium, with a minimum of 3 cm of soft tissue proximal to the great trochanter and distal to the ischium. The acquisition of the scan should be stopped and then restarted, if anatomical landmarks are not correctly displayed or if femoral shaft is not aligned to the center of the image (Fig. 41.5). Once the scan is acquired, the analysis software applies the ROIs that, like those in lumbar spine, should be each time confirmed and/or corrected by the technologists. The global ROI box for the hip (i.e., the anatomical area to be evaluated) should include the great trochanter, femoral neck, and part of the ischium and appears like a rectangular box with four adjustable borders. The lesser trochanter is not included in this image if the legs are internally rotated correctly (Watts 2004; Khan et al. 2007). The upper border is typically positioned at the superomedial border of the acetabular rim, about 5 pixels (pixel size, approximately 1 × 1 mm) above

the femoral head. The upper left corner is positioned in the soft tissue region of the pelvic cavity. The lateral border is positioned in the soft tissue approximately 5 pixels outside the great trochanter (the great trochanter should be included in its entirety). To include all of the femoral head, the medial border of the box is typically placed about 5 pixels medially on the outer rim of the acetabulum. The lower border of the box is conventionally placed along femoral long axis at a point twice the length of the greater trochanter (or 10 pixels below the lesser trochanter).

The system then automatically labels the bone edges, defining the bone map for the proximal femur, places the ROIs, and draws the midline of the narrowest part of the femoral neck. The midline should be centered adequately for correct placement of the ROIs. The standard ROIs for the proximal femur are the (1) femoral neck, (2) Ward triangle (or Ward area), (3) trochanteric region, (4) intertrochanteric region (or shaft region), and (5) total femur. To place these ROIs, the software automatically defines the origin of a coordinate system (about 7 pixels distal to the point of minimal width along the symmetry axis of the femoral neck). A line is drawn from the origin of the coordinate system to the base of the great trochanter to delineate the trochanteric region. The intertrochanteric region extends, within the box, distally from the femoral neck and trochanteric region (Steiger et al. 1992). The total hip is defined as the sum of the neck, the trochanteric, and the shaft/intertrochanteric region (Watts 2004):

(BMC femoral neck + BMC trochanter + BMC shaft)/(femoral neck area + trochanter area + shaft area)

Femoral neck ROI is automatically positioned perpendicular to the midline. Therefore, technologists must ensure that the midline is angled in the same way in each scan and reposition it, if required (Steiger et al. 1992). Placement of the rectangular femoral neck ROI differs among different manufacturers. For Hologic, the infero-lateral corner of the box should touch the notch of

junction between the trochanter and femoral neck (Fig. 41.6a). For GE Lunar, the box should be placed at the narrowest and lowest density section of the neck, i.e., about halfway between the trochanter and femoral head (Fig. 41.6b, c). For Norland Cooper Surgical, a box 1.5 cm long is automatically centered in the narrowest area of the femoral neck. For all manufactures, the ROI should include only the femoral neck (with soft tissue on both sides), and the rectangular box should not extend to include part of the ischium or the trochanter. Since having part of the ischium in the neck ROI would falsely elevate the BMD,

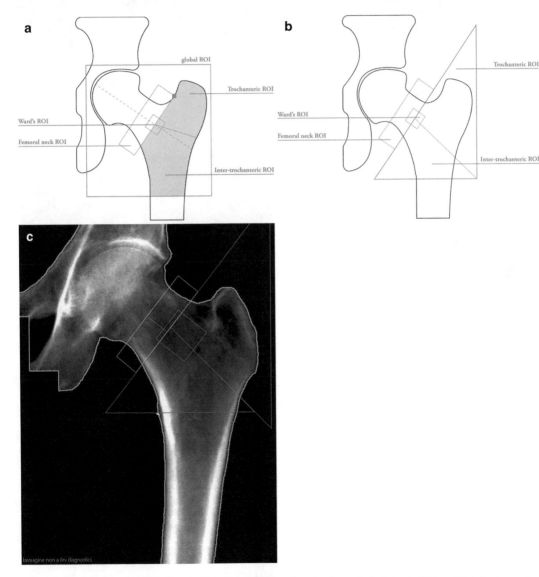

Fig. 41.6 (a) Correct hip ROIs for the Hologic scanner. (b) Correct hip ROIs for the GE Lunar scanner. (c) DXA exam of the left hip acquired on a GE Lunar scanner. Note that the femoral shaft is straight and that the lesser trochanter is not seen on the scan, indicating a proper internal rotation of the femur

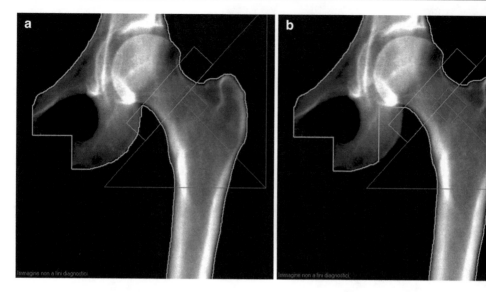

Fig. 41.7 Typical example of data analysis pitfall. Femoral neck ROI must include only the femoral neck (with soft tissue on both sides), and the rectangular box should not extend to include part of the ischium or the trochanter. (**a**) In this case, the ROI includes part of the ischium, affecting the BMD measurement. (**b**) In postprocessing the lateral part of the ischium was excluded from the ROI

newer machines exclude the ischium automatically; otherwise, it should be painted out manually (Watts 2004) (Fig. 41.7). For the evaluation of status of the bone, the femoral neck is used as the reference ROI, or the total proximal femur is preferred, whichever is lowest (Schousboe et al. 2013). Other hip ROIs, including Ward area and the greater trochanter, should not be used for diagnosis; as BMD and T-score at Ward area result in an overdiagnosis of osteoporosis and in fracture risk overestimation. The mean hip BMD can be used for monitoring, with the total hip being preferred (Hamdy et al. 2002; Schousboe et al. 2013).

41.5.3.3   Pitfalls in Forearm Data Analysis

Forearm scanning has distinct manufacturer's recommendations. During the scan, the forearm must be centered and placed straight in the scan field, with an adequate amount of air on the ulnar side. To scan the 33% of the radius, the laser is positioned at the level of the first row of carpal bones; and the distal end of the ulna should be included in the image (Khan et al. 2007) (Fig. 41.8). According to manufacturer's instructions, the forearm length should be measured and the distal

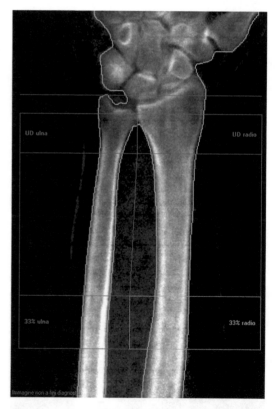

Fig. 41.8 DXA exam of the left forearm acquired on a GE Lunar scanner

one-third of its length should then be used to place the distal radius ROI at the first DXA examination and follow-up scans.

41.5.4 Mistakes in Interpretation

This last group includes errors related to the presence of artifacts. The latest generations of DXA scanners allow positioning of bone map and placement of ROIs, but are not able to differentiate between bone and other calcified structures or high-attenuation material included in the ROIs that can falsely elevate the BMD value (Theodorou and Theodorou 2002). Metallic items and/or local structural changes represent typical artifacts that can invalidate scan results; as already mentioned, all metal items (e.g., surgical clips, buckles, zippers, navel rings) must be removed before performing the scan. Scoliosis and other degenerative diseases and focal structural changes should also be noted, and the ROI should be repositioned to exclude the abnormal area. If this is not possible, an alternate skeletal site should be selected for the examination (Fig. 41.9). A different skeletal site should also be picked if orthopedic hardware precludes the accurate assessment of the BMD (e.g., spinal instrumentation or total hip replacement) (Theodorou and Theodorou 2002).

Regarding the lumbar spine, degenerative changes (e.g., intervertebral disk space narrowing, subchondral bone sclerosis, facet osteoarthritis, osteophytes, and soft tissue calcifications) can falsely elevate BMD by 2, 3, or more T-score units (Figs. 41.10 and 41.11); if available, correlation with prior radiographs is helpful (Bazzocchi et al. 2012a) (Fig. 41.12). Absent bone or conditions like spina bifida falsely lowers BMD (Watts 2004). Compression fractures or degenerative changes may be identified on DXA scan, even if not immediately visible, due to the nonuniform BMD trend among adjacent vertebrae affected. Lumbar vertebrae are larger and have greater BMC from L1 to L4 levels. Normally, the BMD value increases from L1 to L4 levels, but not uncommonly, it could be similar in L3 and L4 or greater in L3 vertebrae (Watts 2004). T-scores

among adjacent vertebrae should be within one standard deviation (SD) of each other. A compression fracture manifests as a reduction in vertebral body height and in a spurious elevation of BMD, which typically increases by about 0.07 g/cm^2; this can lead to a variation of the Z-score (age-matched reference population) from -2.3 to -1.6 (Theodorou and Theodorou 2002; Bazzocchi et al. 2012b). These statements do not apply to the hip, where differences bigger than one SD between various hip sites can occur because of different rate of loss of trabecular and cortical bone (Watts 2004).

According to ISCD, all evaluable vertebrae from L1 to L4 levels should be included in BMD measurement for more accuracy. At least two evaluable vertebrae are required to assess spine BMD. If only one vertebra remains, after excluding all the others, then the diagnosis of osteoporosis should be based on another valid skeletal site. Only vertebrae affected by local structural changes (e.g., fractures, vertebral compression or collapse, focal lesion) or artifacts (such as metal devices or surgical changes) should be excluded. In these cases, a spine radiograph or additional imaging can help to determine the cause of the local structural changes (Hamdy et al. 2002) (Fig. 41.13). Specific criteria are used to decide if one or more vertebra should be excluded, namely, (1) evidence of focal abnormalities affecting some but not all vertebrae in the scan range on DXA or X-ray image and (2) unusual discrepancy in BMC between adjacent vertebrae in the scan range and/or unusual discrepancy in T-score between adjacent vertebrae in the scan range (difference in individual T-scores higher than one SD among adjacent vertebrae) (Schousboe et al. 2013) (Figs. 41.14 and 41.15).

In the hip, some of the most common abnormalities that can affect the BMD value are osteoarthritis, calcific tendinitis, enostosis, fractures, vascular calcifications, and Paget disease. All these conditions can increase the BMD measurement, if included in the ROIs. ROI repositioning is required or, if not possible, another skeletal site to scan should be selected. On the contrary, avascular necrosis of the femoral head and dysplasia of the hip do not affect BMD value, because

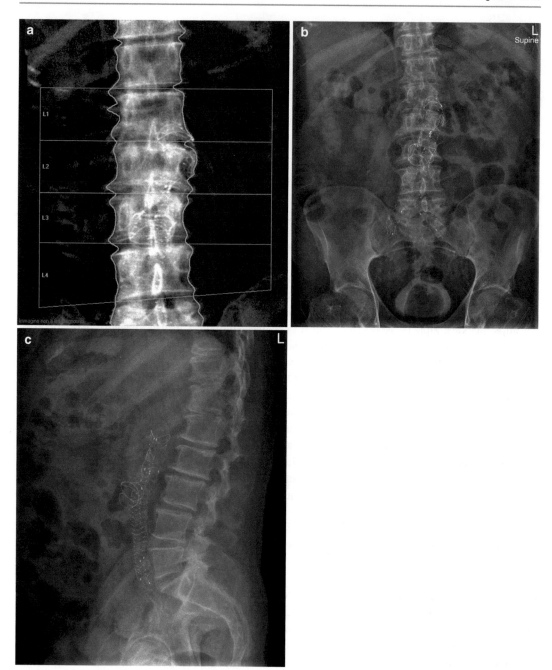

Fig. 41.9 76-year-old man had a central DXA scan. (**a**) Lumbar spine scan shows an aortoiliac endoprosthesis superimposed on the vertebral body in the lumbar spine projection leading to a misleading increase in bone mineral density from L1 to L4 levels. (**b**, **c**) On subsequent inspection, the metallic prosthesis is also evident in previous abdomen radiographs. In these circumstances, lumbar spine DXA cannot be used, and the diagnosis of osteoporosis should be done just on the basis of a proximal femoral scan

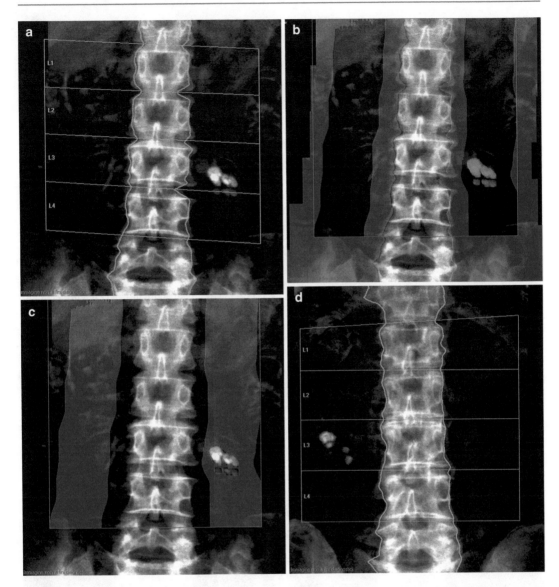

Fig. 41.10 Artifacts in soft tissues commonly influence BMD measurement if included in soft tissue typing. Even if they are localized outside the edge of the spine field, these artifacts affect the soft tissue contribution to X-ray attenuation (and thus the bone density of the spine). The latest software automatically identifies and eliminates soft tissue artifacts. With older versions, it is up to the technologists to manually neutralize them from the soft tissue baseline calculations, by typing them as "neutral" or "artifact" with the aid of specific post-processing tools. (**a**) Initial DXA scan shows some high-density artifacts on the left of the lumbar spine which were incorrectly typed as soft tissue. (**b**, **c**) Manual adjustment was made to type them as "neutral." In these cases, further examinations can help in determining their nature. (**d**, **e**) Another similar case of artifacts in the soft tissues

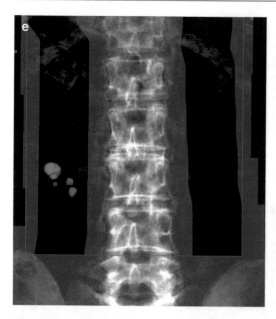

Fig. 41.10 (continued)

usually they do not extend to the femoral neck ROI (Theodorou and Theodorou 2002). The forearm site is relatively free of artifacts compared to the lumbar spine and hip. Nevertheless, it is important to note that prior unrecognized fractures included in the ROI can spuriously elevate BMD by 20% (Garg and Kharb 2013).

41.5.5 Serial BMD Measurements and Pitfalls in Follow-Up

Patients with diagnosis of osteoporosis or with several risk factors frequently undergo repeated DXA examinations to monitor relevant changes in BMD over time or to evaluate response to treatment. The interval between subsequent BMD testing is determined considering the clinical status of each patient. Under most circumstances, the DXA scan

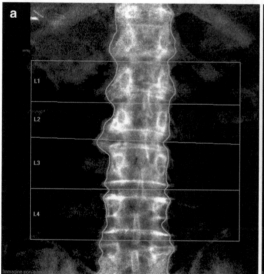

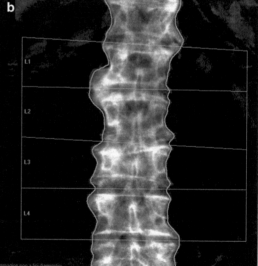

Fig. 41.11 In elderly patients, the presence of exuberant anterior and marginal osteophytes is a common cause of spurious BMD elevation. Images should always be reviewed to determine if any artifacts in the soft tissue or bone affect the BMD measurement. (**a**, **b**) Lumbar DXA images show two different examples of exuberant marginal osteophytes. (**c**, **d**) Once identified, these artifacts are removed from the soft tissue baseline calculations by typing them as "neutral" or "artifact." (**e**) At a previous radiograph performed on the first patient (**a**), an exuberant osteophyte is noted at the L2–L3 level. Some vascular calcifications are also visible

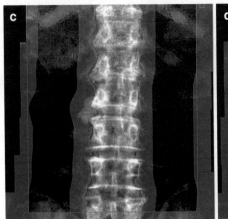 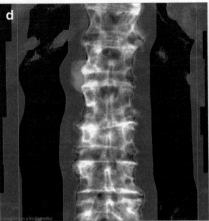 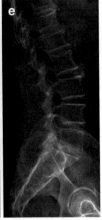

Fig. 41.11 (continued)

is repeated 1 year after a therapy is started or changed. Once the therapeutic effect is established by finding stability or an increase in BMD, intervals can be longer. In case of glucocorticoid therapy or other conditions associated to high rates of bone turnover, DXA scan should be repeated at briefer intervals. If in serial BMD testing, a loss of bone density is found, a reevaluation of the therapy is needed, and a secondary cause of osteoporosis should be suspected (Schousboe et al. 2013). In women 65 years or older who undergo BMD examination to screen for osteoporosis, the interval between the following BMD test can be planned depending on the *T*-score value: (1) 15 years for women with normal BMD (*T*-score, −1.00 or higher) and for women with a *T*-score between −1.01 and −1.49, (2) 5 years if the *T*-score is between −1.50 and −1.99, and (3) 1 year if the *T*-score is below −2.0 (Gourlay et al. 2012).

Since bone turnover in normal conditions is relatively slow, changes in BMD value are usually small. To ensure that a change in BMD value on repeated measurement is significant, each DXA center should perform a quality assurance (QA) program to determine the normal variance of the test (Guglielmi et al. 2012). Otherwise, compari-

son of serial measurement would be potentially misleading. QA is mandatory to ensure that DXA facility is working within acceptable range, monitoring both operator and machine variability. It consists of two distinct parts: instrument quality control and technologist quality control (Khan et al. 2007). Firstly, at least once a week, a scan of a phantom of known density should be performed to assess system calibration and thus the accuracy of results. The scanner must be recalibrated if results are not within a range of 1%. Phantom scanning and calibration should be repeated after any service is performed on the densitometer (Schousboe et al. 2013).

The second part of the quality assessment consists in determination of the precision error (PE) and least significant change (LSC). Precision refers to the degree of obtaining consistent BMD from the same patient via repeated measurement in a short time, and it is essential to ensure that the measured value is related to an actual biological change and not just caused by an error (Kim and Yang 2014). The PE results from the summation of inherent machine fluctuation and inaccuracies of the technologists who carry out the examination (e.g., imperfections in patient positioning, in

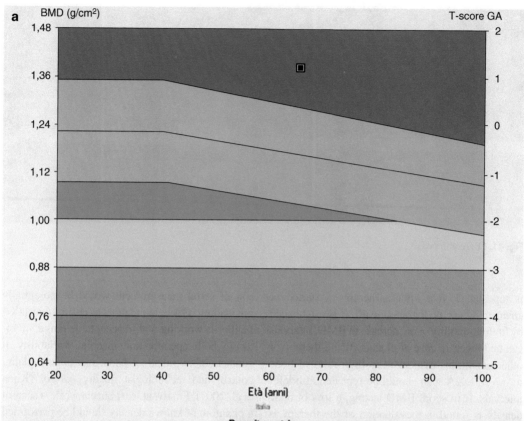

Densitometria

	Regione	BMD (g/cm²)	GA T-score	PE Z-score
■	L1	1,071	-0,7	0,0
□	L2	1,026	-1,8	-1,1
■	L3	1,383	1,2	1,9
■	L4	1,390	1,2	1,9
■	L1-L2	1,050	-1,2	-0,5
■	L1-L3	1,165	-0,4	0,3
■	L1-L4	1,228	0,1	0,8
■	L2-L3	1,215	-0,2	0,5
■	L2-L4	1,281	0,3	1,0
■	L3-L4	1,386	1,2	1,9

Fig. 41.12 A 69-year-old white man had (**a**) DXA scan that shows a L1–L4 *T*-score value of 0.1 and a femoral neck *T*-score of −2.8 with a comment of "osteoporosis." (**b, c**) On a closer inspection, the L2–L3 vertebral endplate is not clearly detectable, making it difficult to place the intervertebral markers even with the aid of the AP spine histogram. In addition, the shapes of the L2 and L3 vertebrae appear unusual. (**d**) Previous lumbar spine radiograph shows that the L2–L3 vertebral body were fused with the formation of an acquired block vertebra. Technologists should always review previous examinations to recognize abnormal vertebral anatomy in order to avoid this kind of mistakes. To correctly evaluate this test, L2 and L3 vertebral bodies should be excluded from examination. L4 vertebra should also be eliminated because of the unusual increase in *T*-score value based on osteoarthritis. In cases like this one, the diagnosis should be based on the *T*-score at the hip and at the forearm

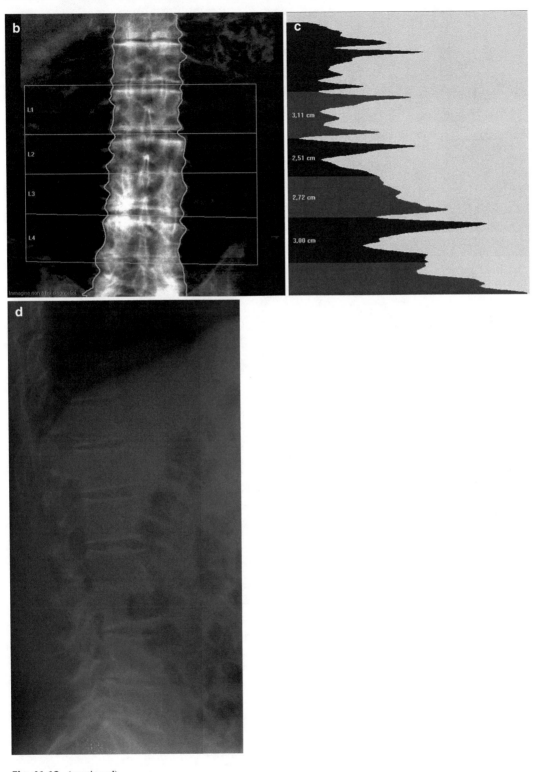

Fig. 41.12 (continued)

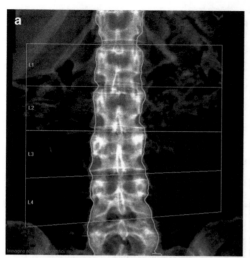

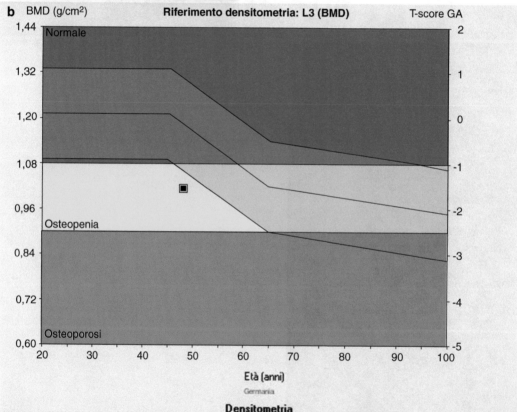

b BMD (g/cm²)   **Riferimento densitometria: L3 (BMD)**   T-score GA

Età (anni)

Germania

	Regione	BMD (g/cm²)	GA T-score	PE Z-score
	L1	0,893	-2,0	-1,7
	L2	0,931	-2,2	-2,0
	L3	1,015	-1,5	-1,3
	L4	0,882	-2,6	-2,4
	L1-L2	0,913	-2,1	-1,9
	L1-L3	0,950	-1,8	-1,6
	L1-L4	0,931	-2,1	-1,8
	L2-L3	0,975	-1,9	-1,6
	L2-L4	0,941	-2,2	-1,9
	L3-L4	0,945	-2,1	-1,9

Densitometria

ROIs selection, device manipulation). According to the ISCD, the minimum acceptable precision is 1.9% at the lumbar spine, 2.5% at the femoral neck, and 1.8% at the total hip. If a technologist's precision error exceeds these values, retraining is required. Each DXA facility should determine its precision error (the precision error supplied by the manufacturer should not be used). If two or more technologists work on the same DXA scan, an average precision error that combines data from all technologists is used. The precision assessment should be repeated after a new DXA system is installed and if the skills of the technologist change (Schousboe et al. 2013).

Once the PE for each DXA skeletal site is known, the next step of QA consists in determin-ing the LSC. The LSC is needed to ensure that change in two BMD values separated by time reflects biological significance. The LSC is cal-culated by multiplying PE × 2.77, where 2.77 is the multiplication factor required to enclose a confidence interval of 95%. For follow-up, the value to study is the BMD and not the T-score. If the degree of change in BMD value is above the LSC, change is considered to be significant (Kim and Yang 2014). Since there is a slight variance in how BMD is measured among different facili-ties, ideally the follow-up examinations should be performed on the same machine by the same technologist. Results obtained from different DXA scanners should not be compared (Garg and Kharb 2013).

Fig. 41.13 Postmenopausal woman had (**a, b**) DXA scan that shows a L1–L4 T-score value of −2.1 and (**c, d**) femo-ral neck T-score of −2.5 with a comment "osteoporosis" based on this last result. More thorough examination of lumbar spine DXA shows an unusual discrepancy in T-score value between L3 and L4 (the difference in indi-vidual T-scores was higher than 1 SD among adjacent ver-tebrae). (**e**) VFA was then performed, leading to the identification of a clinically unrecognized compression fracture with moderate deformity of the L3 body (grade 2, according to Genant classification). (**f**) After the exclusion of L3 vertebra from the study, the L1–L4 (L3) T-score value turned out to be −2.2. MRI exam was then per-formed to better define the fracture and to exclude an underlying disease. Sagittal (**g**) T1-W and (**h**) T2-W MR images show an endplate defect and edema-like altera-tions in marrow signal intensity in the L3 vertebral body. Bilateral radicular cysts were also reported

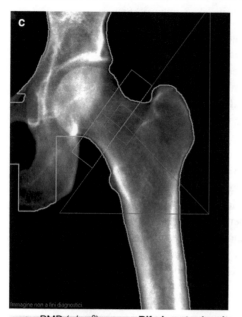

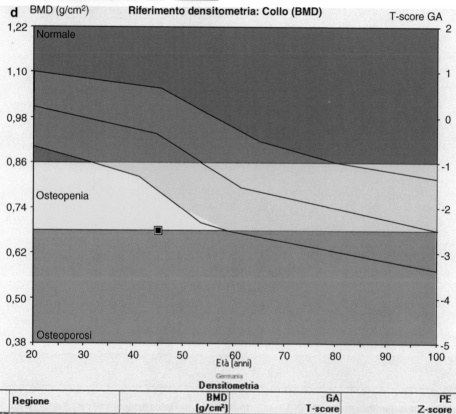

Fig. 41.13 (continued)

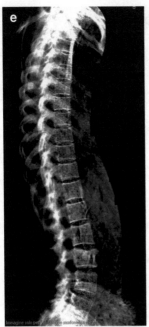

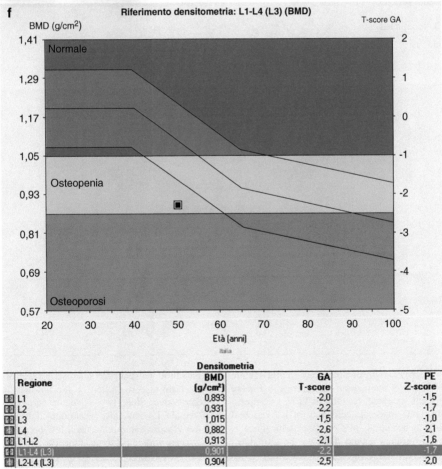

Fig. 41.13 (continued)

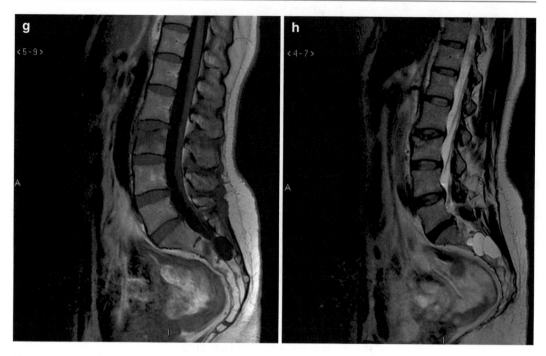

Fig. 41.13 (continued)

Fig. 41.14 (**a, b**) Example of unknown vertebral fracture suspected because of the unusual discrepancy in T-score among adjacent vertebrae. (**c**) On the VFA, a compression fracture with moderate deformity of L1 vertebral body (grade 2, according to Genant classification) is identified; L1 vertebra should therefore be eliminated from the analysis. Note that typical features of disk degeneration with endplate sclerosis are seen at L4 vertebra and are also suggested by the unusual increase in T-score value. Since two evaluable vertebrae (L2–L3) still remain, L4 could also be eliminated; in so doing, the L2–L3 T-score value indicates a low bone condition in accordance with the T-score at the hip

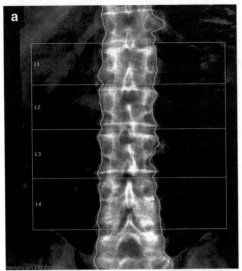

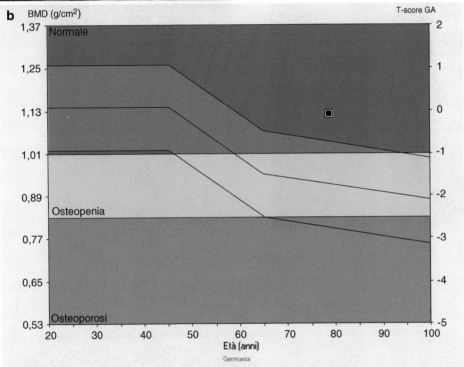

Densitometria

Regione	BMD (g/cm²)	GA T-score	PE Z-score
L1	1,118	-0,1	1,6
L2	1,051	-1,2	0,5
L3	1,051	-1,2	0,5
L4	1,158	-0,4	1,3
L1-L2	1,083	-0,7	1,0
L1-L3	1,072	-0,8	0,9
L1-L4	1,097	-0,7	1,0
L2-L3	1,051	-1,2	0,5
L2-L4	1,091	-0,9	0,8
L3-L4	1,108	-0,8	0,9

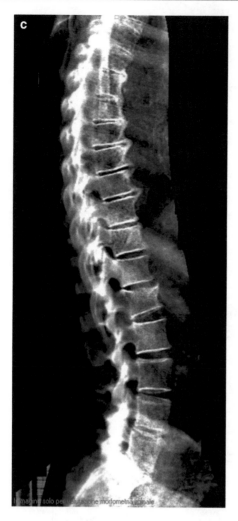

Fig. 41.14 (continued)

Fig. 41.15 Postmenopausal woman had a central DXA scan. (**a**, **b**) Proximal femoral DXA shows a total hip T-score value of −2.3. (**c**, **d**) The lumbar spine DXA shows a L1–L3 T-score value of −3.7 with a comment of "osteoporosis." L4 was excluded because of the unusual discrepancy in T-score value between L3 and L4 vertebra, due to severe osteoarthritis that was confirmed by VFA performed at the same time. (**e**) Note that aortic calcifications can be detected by VFA. Vascular calcifications are often invisible in PA projections and can falsely elevate the BMD at the spine. In this specific case, the T-score value at lumbar spine was diagnostic for osteoporosis despite this superimposed artifact, with no need to invalidate the lumbar spine scan

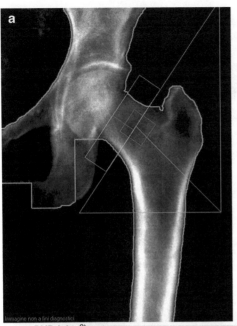

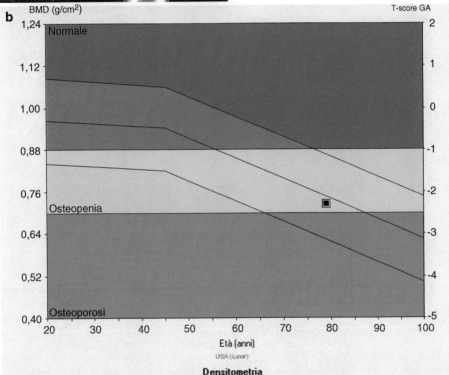

Densitometria			
Regione	**BMD** (g/cm²)	**GA** T-score	**PE** Z-score
Collo	0,721	-2,2	0,1
Collo superiore	0,588	-1,9	0,3
Collo inferiore	0,854	.	.
Ward	0,552	-2,8	0,0
Trocantere	0,513	-2,5	-0,9
Diafisi	0,921	.	.
Intero	0,724	-2,3	-0,1

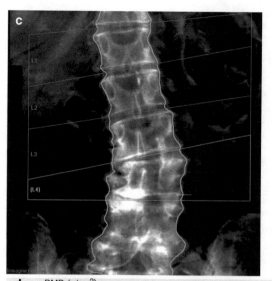

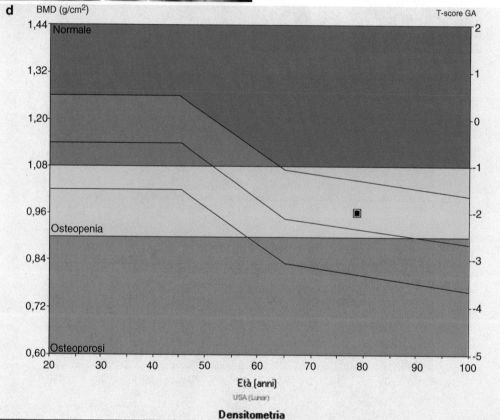

Densitometria			
Regione	**BMD** **(g/cm²)**	**GA** **T-score**	**PE** **Z-score**
L1	0,725	-3,4	-1,1
L2	0,661	-4,5	-2,2
L3	0,785	-3,5	-1,1
L4	0,963	-2,0	0,3
L1-L2	0,692	-3,9	-1,6
L1-L3	0,726	-3,7	-1,4
L2-L3	0,726	-3,9	-1,6

Fig. 41.15 (continued)

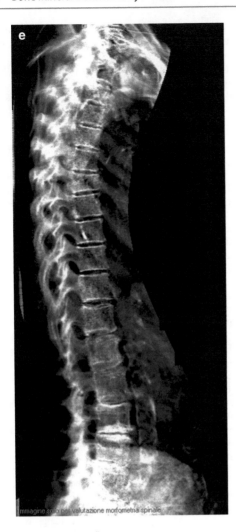

Fig. 41.15 (continued)

Conclusion

DXA represents the technique of choice for diagnosis of osteoporosis and low bone mass conditions and for monitoring the response to treatment. An in-depth knowledge of the technical aspects and pitfalls of this exam is required for proper interpretation and for clinically useful data analysis. The technologists performing bone densitometry, as well as the physicians interpreting and reporting a DXA scan, must have sufficient expertise in identifying the source of mistakes commonly encountered in scan acquisition and analysis that frequently lead to detecting spurious BMD alterations.

Acknowledgment The authors thank Duccio Fattori of Prato, Italy, for drawing Figs. 41.2, 41.4, 41.5, and 41.6.

References

Bazzocchi A, Ferrari F, Diano D et al (2012a) Incidental findings with dual-energy X-ray absorptiometry: spectrum of possible diagnoses. Calcif Tissue Int 91:149–156

Bazzocchi A, Spinnato P, Fuzzi F et al (2012b) Vertebral fracture assessment by new dual-energy X-ray absorptiometry. Bone 50:836–841

Bazzocchi A, Ponti F, Albisinni U et al (2016) DXA: Technical aspects and application. Eur J Radiol 85:1481–1492

Blake GM, Fogelman I (2010) An update on dual-energy x-ray absorptiometry. Semin Nucl Med 40:62–73

Bonnick SL (2010) Bone Densitometry in Clinical Practice. Humana Press, New York

Brunader R, Shelton DK (2002) Radiologic bone assessment in the evaluation of osteoporosis. Am Fam Physician 65:1357–1364

Damilakis J, Adams JE, Guglielmi G, Link TM (2010) Radiation exposure in X-ray-based imaging techniques used in osteoporosis. Eur Radiol 20:2707–2714

Garg MK, Kharb S (2013) Dual energy X-ray absorptiometry: pitfalls in measurement and interpretation of bone mineral density. Indian J Endocrinol Metabol 17:203–210

Gourlay ML, Fine JP, Preisser JS et al (2012) Bone-density testing interval and transition to osteoporosis in older women. N Engl J Med 366:225–233

Guglielmi G, Grimston SK, Fischer KC, Pacifici R (1994) Osteoporosis: diagnosis with lateral and posteroanterior dual x-ray absorptiometry compared with quantitative CT. Radiology 192:845–850

Guglielmi G, Adams J, Link TM (2009) Quantitative ultrasound in the assessment of skeletal status. Eur Radiol 19:1837–1848

Guglielmi G, Muscarella S, Bazzocchi A (2011) Integrated imaging approach to osteoporosis: state-of-the-art review and update. Radiographics 31:1343–1364

Guglielmi G, Damilakis J, Solomou G, Bazzocchi A (2012) Quality assurance of imaging techniques used in the clinical management of osteoporosis. Radiol Med 117:1347–1354

Guglielmi G, Ponti F, Agostini M et al (2016) The role of DXA in sarcopenia. Aging Clin Exp Res 28:1047–1060

Hamdy RC, Petak SM, Lenchik L (2002) Which central dual X-ray absorptiometry skeletal sites and regions of interest should be used to determine the diagnosis of osteoporosis? J Clin Densitom 5(Suppl):S11–S18

Hangartner TN, Warner S, Braillon P et al (2013) The official positions of the International Society for Clinical Densitometry: acquisition of dual-energy X-ray absorptiometry body composition and considerations regarding analysis and repeatability of measures. J Clin Densitom 16:520–536

Hawkinson J, Timins J, Angelo D et al (2007) Technical white paper: bone densitometry. J Am Coll Radiol 4:320–327

Hernlund E, Svedbom A, Ivergard M et al (2013) Osteoporosis in the European Union: medical management, epidemiology and economic burden. A report prepared in collaboration with the International Osteoporosis Foundation (IOF) and the European Federation of Pharmaceutical Industry Associations (EFPIA). Arch Osteoporos 8:136. doi:10.1007/s11657-013-0136-1

Im GI, Jeong SH (2015) Pathogenesis, management and prevention of atypical femoral fractures. J Bone Metabol 22:1–8

Intenzo CM, Parker L, Rao VM, Levin DC (2005) Changes in procedure volume and service provider distribution among radiologists and nonradiologists in dual-energy x-ray absorptiometry between 1996 and 2002. J Am Coll Radiol 2:662–664

Johnell O, Kanis JA, Oden A et al (2005) Predictive value of BMD for hip and other fractures. J Bone Mineral Res 20:1185–1194

Johnell O, Kanis JA (2006) An estimate of the worldwide prevalence and disability associated with osteoporotic fractures. Osteoporos Int 17:1726–1733

Kalender WA (1992) Effective dose values in bone mineral measurements by photon absorptiometry and computed tomography. Osteoporos Int 2:82–87

Khan AA, Colquhoun A, Hanley DA et al (2007) Standards and guidelines for technologists performing central dual-energy X-ray absorptiometry. J Clin Densitom 10:189–195

Kim HS, Yang SO (2014) Quality control of DXA system and precision test of radio-technologists. J Bone Metabol 21:2–7

Klotzbuecher CM, Ross PD, Landsman PB et al (2000) Patients with prior fractures have an increased risk of future fractures: a summary of the literature and statistical synthesis. J Bone Mineral Res 15:721–739

Lenchik L, Rochmis P, Sartoris DJ (1998) Optimized interpretation and reporting of dual X-ray absorptiometry (DXA) scans. AJR Am J Roentgenol 171:1509–1520

Lewiecki EM, Laster AJ (2006) Clinical applications of vertebral fracture assessment by dual-energy x-ray absorptiometry. J Clin Endocrinol Metab 91:4215–4222

Link TM (2012) Osteoporosis imaging: state of the art and advanced imaging. Radiology 263:3–17

Lorente Ramos RM, Azpeitia Arman J, Arevalo Galeano N et al (2012) Dual energy X-ray absorptimetry: fundamentals, methodology, and clinical applications. Radiologia 54:410–423

Marshall D, Johnell O, Wedel H (1996) Meta-analysis of how well measures of bone mineral density predict occurrence of osteoporotic fractures. BMJ (Clin Res ed) 312:1254–1259

McKenna MJ, van der Kamp S, Heffernan E, Hurson C (2013) Incomplete atypical femoral fractures: assessing the diagnostic utility of DXA by extending femur length. J Clin Densitom 16:579–783

Messina C, Bandirali M, Sconfienza LM et al (2015) Prevalence and type of errors in dual-energy x-ray absorptiometry. Eur Radiol 25:1504–1511

Mithal A, Kaur P (2012) Osteoporosis in Asia: a call to action. Curr Osteoporos Rep 10:245–247

NIH Consensus Development Panel (2001) NIH consensus development panel on osteoporosis prevention, diagnosis, and therapy. JAMA 285:785–795

Peel NF, Johnson A, Barrington NA et al (1993) Impact of anomalous vertebral segmentation on measurements of bone mineral density. J Bone Mineral Res 8:719–723

Pietrobelli A, Formica C, Wang Z, Heymsfield SB (1996) Dual-energy X-ray absorptiometry body composition model: review of physical concepts. Am J Phys 271:E941–E951

Rosen HN, Vokes TJ, Malabanan AO et al (2013) The official positions of the International Society for Clinical Densitometry: vertebral fracture assessment. J Clin Densitom 16:482–488

Rosenberg ZS, La Rocca VR, Chan SS et al (2011) Bisphosphonate-related complete atypical subtrochanteric femoral fractures: diagnostic utility of radiography. AJR Am J Roentgenol 197:954–960

Schousboe JT, Shepherd JA, Bilezikian JP, Baim S (2013) Executive summary of the 2013 International Society for Clinical Densitometry Position Development Conference on bone densitometry. J Clin Densitom 16:455–466

Shane E, Burr D, Abrahamsen B et al (2014) Atypical subtrochanteric and diaphyseal femoral fractures: second report of a task force of the American Society for Bone and Mineral Research. J Bone Mineral Res 29:1–23

Shepherd JA, Baim S, Bilezikian JP et al (2013) Executive summary of the 2013 International Society for Clinical Densitometry Position Development Conference on Body Composition. J Clin Densitom 16:489–495

Shepherd JA, Schousboe JT, Broy SB et al (2015) Executive Summary of the 2015 ISCD Position Development Conference on Advanced Measures From DXA and QCT: Fracture Prediction Beyond BMD. J Clin Densitom 18:274–286

Steiger P, Cummings SR, Black DM et al (1992) Age-related decrements in bone mineral density in women over 65. J Bone Mineral Res 7:625–632

Stone KL, Seeley DG, Lui LY et al (2003) BMD at multiple sites and risk of fracture of multiple types: long-term results from the study of osteoporotic fractures. J Bone Mineral Res 18:1947–1954

Theodorou DJ, Theodorou SJ (2002) Dual-energy X-ray absorptiometry in clinical practice: application and interpretation of scans beyond the numbers. Clin Imaging 26:43–49

Toombs RJ, Ducher G, Shepherd JA, De Souza MJ (2012) The impact of recent technological advances on the trueness and precision of DXA to assess body composition. Obesity 20:30–39

Wall BF, Hart D (1997) Revised radiation doses for typical X-ray examinations. Report on a recent review of doses to patients from medical X-ray examinations in the UK by NRPB. National Radiological Protection Board. Br J Radiol 70:437–439

Watts NB (2004) Fundamentals and pitfalls of bone densitometry using dual-energy X-ray absorptiometry (DXA). Osteoporos Int 15:847–854

WHO Study Group (1994) Assessment of fracture risk and its application to screening for postmenopausal osteoporosis. Report of a WHO Study Group. World Health Organ Tech Rep Ser 843:1–129

Wright NC, Looker AC, Saag KG et al (2014) The recent prevalence of osteoporosis and low bone mass in the United States based on bone mineral density at the femoral neck or lumbar spine. J Bone Mineral Res 29:2520–2526

Congenital Skeletal Dysplasias: Imaging Pitfalls

42

Richa Arora and Kakarla Subbarao

Contents

42.1	Introduction	925
42.2	Thanatophoric Dysplasia and Achondrogenesis	926
42.3	Chondroectodermal Dysplasia and Jeune Syndrome	927
42.4	Osteogenesis Imperfecta, Non-accidental Injury, Rickets, Hypophosphatasia, and Juvenile Idiopathic Osteoporosis	929
42.5	Osteopetrosis, Pyknodysostosis, and Cleidocranial Dysostosis	931
42.6	Morquio and Hurler Syndromes and Spondyloepiphyseal Dysplasia Tarda	935
42.7	Achondroplasia and Pseudoachondroplasia	939
42.8	Chondrodysplasia Punctata, Multiple Epiphyseal Dysplasia, Meyer Dysplasia, Perthes Disease, and Cretinism	941
42.9	Metaphyseal Chondrodysplasia (Schmid Type) and Rickets	943
42.10	Camurati-Engelmann Disease, Ghosal-Type Hemato-Diaphyseal Dysplasia, Ribbing Disease, Caffey Disease, Intramedullary Osteosclerosis, and Erdheim-Chester Disease	944
42.11	Osteopoikilosis and Sclerotic Metastases	946
Conclusion		948
References		948

R. Arora, MD, MMed, FRCR (✉) • K. Subbarao, FRCR, FACR, FICP, FCCP, FICR
Department of Radiology & Imageology, Nizam's Institute of Medical Sciences,
Punjagutta, Hyderabad, Telangana 500082, India
e-mail: dr.richaarora@gmail.com;
subbaraokakarla25@gmail.com

42.1 Introduction

Skeletal dysplasias (or osteochondrodysplasias) comprise of a large heterogeneous group of disorders of the bone or cartilage growth, which continue to evolve throughout life and are due to genetic mutations. Thus, they differ from dysostosis which can be defined as malformation of single or multiple bones occurring due to abnormal blastogenesis *in utero* and which remain phenotypically static throughout life (Resnick 1994; Yochum and Rowe 2005). There are 450 different dysplasias mentioned in the literature (Warman et al. 2011), and various epidemiologic studies have reported their overall prevalence of 2.3–7.6 per 10,000 births (Rasmussen et al. 1996). Majority of these disorders are confusing and have overlapping features with the other entities. It is important to be familiar with their imaging features and those of various other radiologically similar dysplasias and non-dysplastic pathologies, to aid in their accurate diagnosis and for early institution of the appropriate therapy, prognostication, and counseling of the family regarding inheritance pattern and risk of recurrence. This would also prevent serious sequelae or complications associated with some of these dyspla-sias. This chapter focuses on the imaging mimics found in commonly encountered skeletal dysplasias.

42.2 Thanatophoric Dysplasia and Achondrogenesis

Thanatophoric dysplasia is the second most common lethal dysplasia (the most common is osteogenesis imperfecta type 2). It is character-ized by marked short-limbed dwarfism with bow-ing of tubular bones, macrocephaly with frontal bossing, small thoracic cage, and severe platyspondyly (Yochum and Rowe 2005). The vast majority of cases are due to sporadic muta-tions coding for the fibroblast growth receptor 3 (FGFR3) located in chromosome 4p16.3. Patients often die within the first 48 h of birth, either from pulmonary hypoplasia caused by a narrow thorax or brain stem and cervical cord compression from foramen magnum stenosis. It has two subtypes (Miller et al. 2009). The typical radiographic fea-tures (Fig. 42.1) include macrocephaly with fron-tal bossing (with cloverleaf skull appearance in type II), narrow chest with short horizontal ribs, small scapulae, marked platyspondyly with flat-tening of the vertebral bodies and widened disk spaces against a backdrop of well-formed neural arches giving the "H" or "inverted U" appearance (on frontal radiograph of the spine), relatively normal trunk length, small squared iliac wings with horizontal acetabular roofs and small sacro-sciatic notches, shortening of proximal portions of long limbs (rhizomelia), and bowing of long tubular bones (commonly humeri and femurs) giving the "telephone handle" appearance with metaphyseal flaring (in type I). Clinically, these fetuses have flat facies with a depressed nasal bridge and proptosis (Keats et al. 1970; Kozlowski et al. 1970; Miller et al. 2009).

Achondrogenesis is another lethal type of osteochondrodysplasia characterized by poor or deficient ossification of the vertebral column, sacrum, and pelvic bones and shortening of tubu-lar bones (but this is quite rare). It is divided into

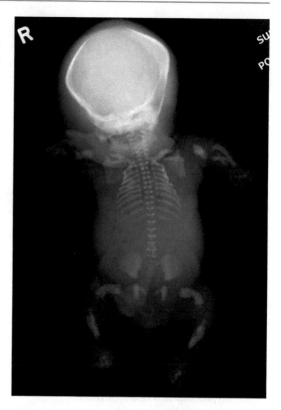

Fig. 42.1 Babygram of a fetus with thanatophoric dys-plasia shows severe platyspondyly with well-formed neu-ral arches (giving a "H"-shaped appearance), narrow and elongated chest (normal trunk length), small squared iliac bones, shortening of tubular bones with bowing deformity (telephone handle deformity, particularly in bilateral femurs and humeri), and relatively large skull (Courtesy of Dr. Hani Al Salam with permission from Radiopaedia. org)

two types, and type I (which is more severe and is associated with multiple rib fractures and involve-ment of the hands) has further two subtypes. Type I is caused by recessive mutation in the DTDST gene (responsible for encoding the dia-strophic dysplasia sulfate transporter), and type II is caused by the dominant mutation in the COL2A1 gene. Although all types are lethal, type II has fewer stillbirths, longer survival, and rela-tively larger baby with longer limbs (Kapur 2007). The characteristic imaging features (Fig. 42.2) include short tubular bones (more pro-nounced in type I) with metaphyseal flaring and spurring (resembling thorn apples), poor or absent ossification of carpals and phalanges, poor

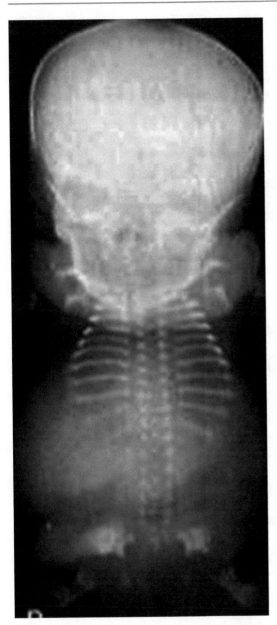

Fig. 42.2 Babygram of a fetus with achondrogenesis shows poor ossification of the vertebral column (with ossified pedicles) and pelvis, narrow chest with short horizontal ribs, small scapulae, markedly shortened bilateral femurs with metaphyseal flaring and spurring, and relatively large skull (Reproduced with permission from: Subbarao (2014))

or deficient ossification of the vertebral column with pedicles generally ossified, narrow thorax with short ribs (ribs are thin and show multiple

fractures in type IA), pulmonary hypoplasia, small iliac bones (with only upper portion ossified in type IA) with poor ossification of the ischium, normal-sized skull (which appears relatively large compared to hypoplastic skeleton and with poor ossification in type I), and micrognathia. Antenatal ultrasound (US) imaging may show polyhydramnios and hydrops fetalis (Kapur 2007).

Both these entities have common features of poorly ossified spine (with posterior elements generally well formed), narrow thorax, shortened tubular bones, and small pelvis. However, the presence of short trunk with narrow thorax (in contrast to narrow and elongated thorax in thanatophoric dysplasia), marked shortening of tubular bones without bowing deformity, rib fractures, micrognathia, and polyhydramnios and hydrops fetalis favor achondrogenesis. Cloverleaf skull, if present, suggests thanatophoric dysplasia (Keats et al. 1970; Kozlowski et al. 1970; Kapur 2007; Miller et al. 2009).

42.3   Chondroectodermal Dysplasia and Jeune Syndrome

Chondroectodermal dysplasia (also known as Ellis-van Creveld syndrome) is a rare autosomal recessive skeletal dysplasia, which belongs to the short-rib dysplasia group of osteochondrodysplasias and is due to mutation affecting the EVC gene on locus 4p160 (Baujat and Le Merrer 2007). It is characterized by the involvement of ectoderm along with the skeleton and was first described by Richard WB Ellis and Simon van Creveld in 1940 (Chauss 1955). This condition manifests at birth with characteristic features of disproportionate short-limb dwarfism; dysplastic nails, teeth, and hair; postaxial polydactyly (hexadactyly); multiple labiogingival frenula; congenital cardiac defects (most common being single atrium and atrioventricular cushion defects); cryptorchidism; and epispadias. The imaging features (Fig. 42.3) include narrowing of the thorax with short ribs, progressive acromeso-

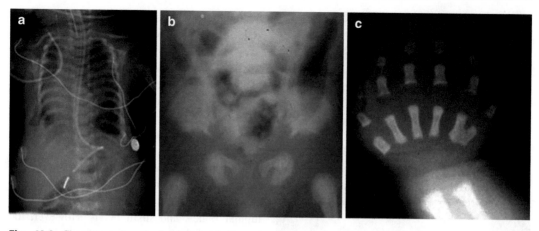

Fig. 42.3 Chondroectodermal dysplasia. (**a**) Frontal chest radiograph shows narrowing of the thorax with short horizontal ribs. (**b**) Frontal radiograph of the pelvis shows short flared iliac wings with trident acetabula. (**c**) Frontal radiograph of the hands shows postaxial polydactyly with fusion of the fifth and sixth metacarpals and disproportionate shortening of middle and distal phalanges (Courtesy of Dr. Radswiki with permission from Radiopaedia.org)

Fig. 42.4 Jeune syndrome. (**a**) Frontal chest radiograph shows short horizontal ribs with a narrow thorax. (**b**) Radiograph of the pelvis shows small flared iliac bones with trident acetabula (same as in chondroectodermal dysplasia) (Courtesy of Dr. Radswiki with permission from radiopaedia.org)

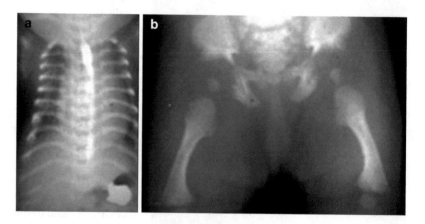

melia (shortening of distal and middle segments as opposed to proximal segments – involving forearms and lower legs – and disproportionate shortening of distal and middle phalanges in the hands), postaxial hexadactyly in the hands and sometimes in the toes, carpal fusion involving the capitate and hamate, cone-shaped epiphysis of phalanges of the hands, premature ossification of femoral capital epiphysis, hypoplastic lateral proximal tibial epiphysis, genu valgum, short pelvis with flared iliac wings and narrow base, and trident acetabula (horizontal acetabular roof with three downward-projecting spikes). The differential diagnosis includes asphyxiating thoracic dysplasia and other short-rib syndromes (with or without polydactyly) (Chauss 1955; Baujat and Le Merrer 2007; Weiner et al. 2013).

Jeune syndrome (or asphyxiating thoracic dystrophy) is another autosomal recessive short-rib dysplasia with a severely narrow thorax. The imaging features are almost same (Fig. 42.4) as those seen in chondroectodermal dysplasia except that it can be differentiated by the absence of involvement of ectodermal structures (such as the hair, nail, and teeth), lack of cardiac anomalies, absence of both carpal fusion, and hypoplastic lateral proximal tibial epiphysis. Unlike chondroectodermal dysplasia, polydactyly is seen rarely in Jeune syndrome, and involvement of the thorax is more severe (Chauss 1955; Baujat and Le Merrer 2007; de Vries et al. 2009; Tüysüz et al. 2009; Thakkar et al. 2012; Weiner et al. 2013). Additional manifestations, including liver fibrosis, cystic renal dysplasia, cystic pancreatic disease, and retinal pigmentary degeneration, have also been described in some cases of Jeune syndrome (de Vries et al. 2009; Tüysüz et al. 2009; Thakkar et al. 2012).

42.4 Osteogenesis Imperfecta, Non-accidental Injury, Rickets, Hypophosphatasia, and Juvenile Idiopathic Osteoporosis

Osteogenesis imperfecta (OI) (also known as brittle bone disease) is a genetic disorder of collagen type I production (involving connective tissues and bones) due to mutations in either the COL1A1 or the COL1A2 gene. The clinical features are variable – based on its subtype – and include osteoporosis, increased bone fragility, blue sclera, dental fragility, and hearing loss

(Renaud et al. 2013; Greenspan 2015). The hallmarks on imaging (Fig. 42.5) include osteopenia, bone fractures, and bone deformities. Osteopenia occurs due to cortical bone thinning and trabecular bone rarefaction. Bone densitometry by dual-energy X-ray absorptiometry (DXA) is the appropriate method to detect decreased bone mineral density. However, it is important to exclude other entities such as rickets, hypophosphatasia, and juvenile idiopathic osteoporosis (and rarely prematurity, leukemia, hypogonadism, growth hormone deficiency, hyperthyroidism, juvenile diabetes mellitus) causing reduced bone mineral density. Fractures can involve the axial and appendicular skeleton and often involve diaphysis of long bones with exuberant callus formation. Vertebral compression fractures and spondylolysis of L5 vertebra are also seen. Bone deformities occur due to excessive bone malleability and plasticity and include deformed gracile over-tubulated bones with diaphyseal bowing and angulation, basilar invagination, codfish vertebrae, platyspondyly, kyphoscoliosis, pectus carinatum or excavatum, protrusio acetabuli, and

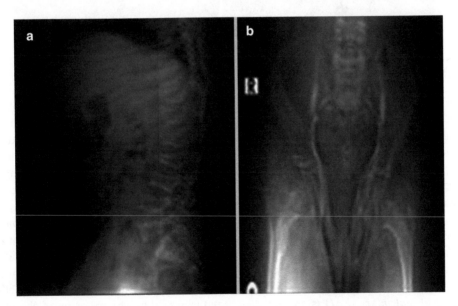

Fig. 42.5 Osteogenesis imperfecta. (**a**) Lateral radiograph of the thoracolumbar spine shows osteopenia with thin cortices, codfish vertebrae in the lumbar spine, and compression fractures with anterior wedging involving the L1 and L2 vertebrae. (**b**) Frontal radiograph of the pelvis shows osteopenia and triangular pelvis with bilateral protrusio acetabuli. (**c**, **d**) Frontal radiographs of both femurs show osteopenia with bowing deformities

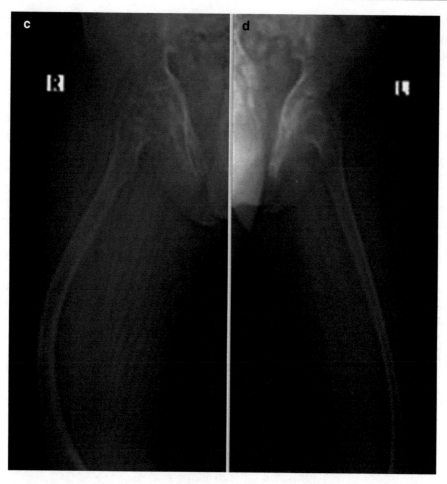

Fig. 42.5 (continued)

coxa vara. Other features include wormian bones, popcorn calcification in the metaphyses and epiphyses (especially in the knee) due to micro-traumatic fragmentation and disordered maturation of the growth plate, ossification of the interosseous membrane, and dense metaphyseal bands leading to the zebra stripe sign (in children receiving bisphosphonates) (Renaud et al. 2013; Greenspan 2015). It is difficult to diagnose milder forms of OI (types I and IV) especially in cases with negative family history and with no obvious extraskeletal manifestations.

Non-accidental injury (NAI) is an important differential in young children. Nevertheless, certain features, namely, fractures of varying ages, no evidence of osteopenia, peculiar fractures (such as metaphyseal corner fractures (Fig. 42.6), posterior rib fractures, and complex skull fractures), subdural hematomas, retinal hemorrhage, absence of wormian bones, and modeling deformities, favor NAI (Ablin et al. 1990). *Rickets* and *hypophosphatasia* are other differentials as they show defective skeletal mineralization, bone fractures, and deformities. Hypophosphatasia is a rare autosomal recessive metabolic disorder characterized by a reduced tissue-nonspecific isoenzyme of alkaline phosphatase (TNSALP) and increased urinary excretion of phosphoethanolamine. However, the presence of metaphyseal changes (cupping, fraying, and splaying with

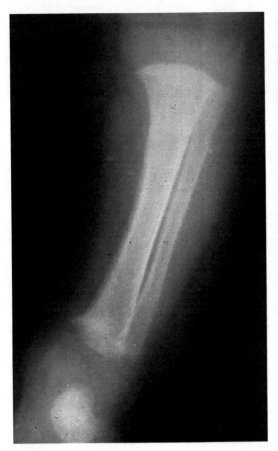

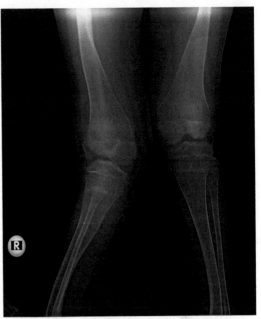

Fig. 42.7 Rickets. Frontal radiograph of both knees shows osteopenia with bowing deformity resulting in knock-knees. Additionally, metaphyseal changes in the form of splaying, fraying, cupping, and widened growth plates are also seen

Fig. 42.6 Non-accidental injury. Frontal radiograph of the tibia and fibula shows a distal metaphyseal corner fracture in the tibia along with the periosteal reaction. Bone density is normal

Fractures often involve vertebrae and metaphysis of long bones (Imerci et al. 2015).

42.5 Osteopetrosis, Pyknodysostosis, and Cleidocranial Dysostosis

widened growth plate) (Fig. 42.7) and presence of biochemical changes help in differentiating both these entities from OI (Grover et al. 2003). *Idiopathic juvenile osteoporosis* is a rare sporadic disorder which manifests with pain in bones, osteoporosis, fractures, and deformity of the axial and appendicular skeleton (Fig. 42.8), often between 2 and 14 years of age. Diagnosis is established by excluding other causes of osteoporosis (normal biochemical findings and negative findings on hormone assays), negative family history, and in an appropriate clinical setting, with no features of hearing loss or blue sclera.

Osteopetrosis (also known as marble bones or Albers-Schonberg disease) is a rare hereditary disorder which occurs due to defective osteoclasts, resulting in lack of resorption of primitive osteochondrous tissue, leading to diffusely sclerotic and brittle bones. It has three subtypes: benign autosomal dominant form, severely malignant autosomal recessive form, and an intermediate recessive type with renal tubular acidosis (Machado et al. 2015). Radiographic features (Fig. 42.9) include diffuse increase in bone density without trabeculation

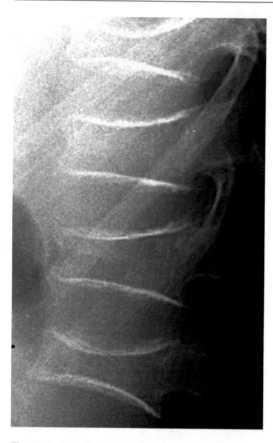

Fig. 42.8 Juvenile idiopathic osteoporosis. Lateral radiograph of the thoracolumbar shows osteopenia with thin cortices and multiple compression fractures (Courtesy of Dr. Anwar Adil, Karachi X-rays CT and Ultrasound Centre, Pakistan)

and with loss of cortical and medullary differentiation; bone-within-a-bone appearance (also known as endobones that represent fetal vestiges which are normally removed) particularly involving innominate bones, calcaneum, and ribs; multiple transverse fractures (banana fractures) with abundant callus formation; failure of metaphyseal remodeling resulting in "Erlenmeyer flask" deformity (see Table 42.1 for list of differentials); uniformly sclerotic vertebrae or dense bands adjacent to vertebral end plates giving the appearance of "sandwich vertebrae;" sclerosis of calvarial vault and base of the

skull; and poor pneumatization of the paranasal sinuses. In type III osteopetrosis (associated with tubular acidosis), rachitic changes are an additional finding (Resnick 1994; Machado et al. 2015). Complications include pathological fractures, hydrocephalus, cranial nerve palsies, optic atrophy, deafness, dental caries secondary to faulty dentition, anemia, infections, leukemia, and sarcoma (Resnick 1994; Yochum and Rowe 2005; Machado et al. 2015).

Pyknodysostosis is also known as *Toulouse-Lautrec syndrome*, named after the French painter who was affected with this disease. It is a rare autosomal recessive, lysosomal disorder with abnormal osteoclast function due to genetic deficiency in cathepsin K which has been mapped to chromosome 1q21, leading to increase in bone density. It is a hybrid between osteopetrosis and cleidocranial dysostosis and shares its imaging features with both. It presents in early childhood with short stature (Resnick 1994; Bathi and Masur 2000). The main radiological abnormality (Figs. 42.10 and 42.11) is generalized osteosclerosis with preservation of medullary canal (unlike osteopetrosis, in which medullary canal is encroached upon, resulting in anemia and extramedullary hematopoiesis). The osteosclerosis is most pronounced in the limbs, followed by the clavicles, mandible, skull, and spine. Another major feature mimicking osteopetrosis is the presence of transverse fractures in the long bones. However, metaphyseal remodeling is normal. Other features which are exclusively seen in pyknodysostosis and differentiate it from osteopetrosis (Table 42.2) include marked delay in sutural closure, persistent fontanelles, wormian bones, frontoparietal bossing, nasal beaking, obtuse mandibular gonial angle often with relative prognathism, persistence of deciduous teeth, clavicular hypoplasia, and, lastly, aplasia of terminal phalanges simulating acro-osteolysis. Platybasia and vertebral segmentation anomalies (spool-shaped vertebrae) are also common, particularly at the craniovertebral and lumbosacral regions. Osteomyelitis of the jaw is a frequent complica-

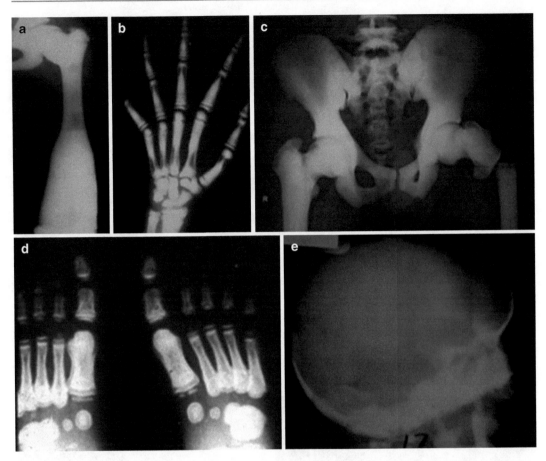

Fig. 42.9 Osteopetrosis. (**a**) Frontal radiograph of the femur shows osteosclerosis with abnormal distal metaphyseal remodeling resulting in the "Erlenmeyer flask" deformity. (**b**) Frontal hand radiograph shows the "bone-within-a-bone" appearance (endobones) along with increased bone density. (**c**) Frontal radiograph of the pelvis shows osteosclerosis with obliteration of the trabeculae along with "banana" type of fracture in the left proximal femur. (**d**) Frontal radiograph of both feet shows generalized increased bone density. (**e**) Lateral skull radiograph shows sclerosis of the base of the skull with no evidence of widened sutures/fontanelles or wormian bones (Reproduced with permission from: Subbarao (2013))

Table 42.1 Erlenmeyer flask deformity: causes and differentiating features

Etiology	Other characteristic features
Osteopetrosis	Diffuse osteosclerosis, transverse fractures with abundant callus, bone-within-a-bone appearance, sandwich vertebrae, other manifestations
Pyle disease	Lucent and flask-shaped metaphysis with narrow and sclerotic shafts
Thalassemia	Coarsened trabeculations producing a "cobweb" appearance
Niemann-Pick and Gaucher disease	Osteopenia with thin cortices, avascular necrosis of bones, hepatosplenomegaly
Lead poisoning	Dense metaphyseal bands

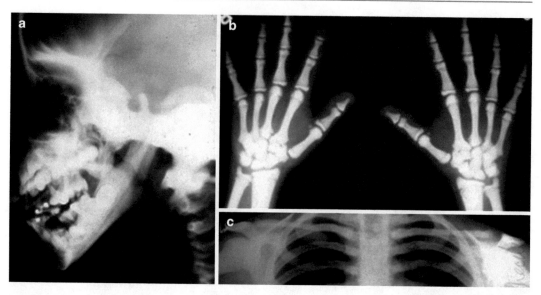

Fig. 42.10 Skeletal survey in a patient with pyknodysostosis. (a) Oblique radiograph of the mandible shows osteosclerosis with obtuse angle of the mandible. (b) Frontal radiograph of both hands shows terminal phalangeal hypoplasia mimicking acro-osteolysis (apart from osteosclerosis). (c) Frontal radiograph of both clavicles shows hypoplasia of the lateral aspect of the left clavicle and the junction of medial one-third and lateral two-thirds of the right clavicle (Reproduced with permission from: Subbarao (2013))

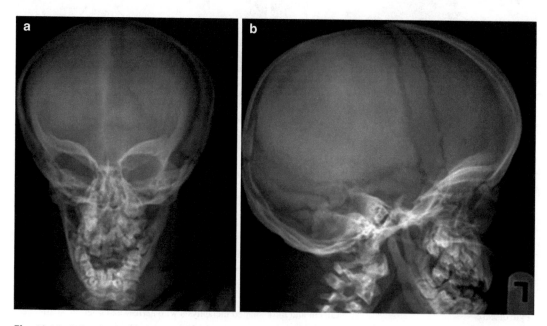

Fig. 42.11 Pyknodysostosis. (a) Frontal and (b) lateral skull radiographs show widened sutures and wormian bones, apart from osteosclerosis (Courtesy of Dr. Mark Holland with permission from Radiopaedia.org)

Table 42.2 Imaging pitfalls and differentiating features between osteopetrosis and pyknodysostosis

Imaging pitfalls	Osteopetrosis (exclusive features)	Pyknodysostosis (exclusive features)
Generalized osteosclerosis and transverse fractures in the bones	Obliteration of trabeculae and involvement of medullary canal leading to anemia and extramedullary hematopoiesis	Medullary canal is spared
	Erlenmeyer flask deformity in the long bones Bone-within-a-bone appearance Sandwich vertebrae	Delay in suture closure and persistent fontanelles Wormian bones Obtuse angle of the mandible Clavicle hypoplasia Terminal phalangeal aplasia mimicking acro-osteolysis

tion (Resnick 1994; Bathi and Masur 2000; Yochum and Rowe 2005).

Cleidocranial dysostosis is a rare non-sclerosing, autosomal dominant skeletal dysplasia predominantly affecting development of intramembranous and enchondral bones. It is caused by mutation in CBFA1 gene on chromosome 6. Skull and clavicular anomalies and incomplete ossification of midline skeletal structures are classic hallmarks of this entity. The typical clinical features are large head, small face, and excessively mobile drooping shoulders. Dwarfism is not present though height is slightly reduced in the affected patients (Shen et al. 2009). The radiographic features (Fig. 42.12) include delayed ossification of the calvaria, widening of skull sutures (sagittal and coronal) and persistent fontanelles, wormian bones, persistent metopic suture, frontoparietal bossing/brachycephaly, underdeveloped facial bones including nasal bone and the maxilla with hypoplastic paranasal sinuses, large mandible, delayed and defective dentition, hypoplasia/aplasia of lateral clavicle, small and elevated scapulae, narrow and bell-shaped chest, pseudo-widening of the symphysis pubis (due to absent/delayed ossification of the pubic bones), delayed mineralization of the vertebrae along with segmentation anomalies in the spine, and hypoplastic radius and fibula (Shen et al. 2009). The pitfalls and the differentiating features from pyknodysostosis are tabulated in Table 42.3.

42.6 Morquio and Hurler Syndromes and Spondyloepiphyseal Dysplasia Tarda

Morquio syndrome is an autosomal recessive type IV mucopolysaccharidosis (MPS), which occurs due to deficiency of N-acetyl galactosamine-6-sulfatase resulting in excess accumulation of the keratan sulfate in the various tissues, particularly the cartilage, nucleus pulposus of intervertebral disks, and cornea. Diagnosis is established by keratosulphaturia, which differentiates it from Hurler syndrome. Patients present in the early childhood with features of short-trunk dwarfism, thoracolumbar kyphosis, protuberant sternum, and deafness. The mental capacity in the affected patients is normal, unlike Hurler syndrome (Langer and Carey 1966; Mikles and Stanton 1997; Di Cesare et al. 2012). Radiological features (Fig. 42.13) include universal platyspondyly with anterior central vertebral beaking and posterior scalloping, round vertebra, posteriorly displaced and hypoplastic L1 or L2 vertebra, normal or increased disk heights, odontoid hypoplasia, atlantoaxial subluxation, goblet-shaped flared iliac wings, hypoplastic acetabuli, flattened capital femoral epiphysis, unstable hip, coxa vara or valga, short and wide tubular bones with or without metaphyseal flaring, proximal metacarpal tapering, hand and foot deformities, pectus carinatum,

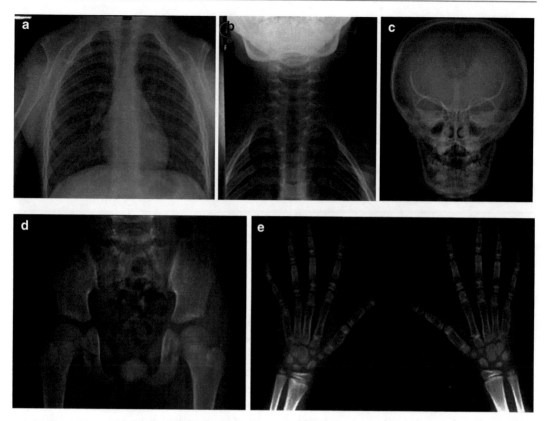

Fig. 42.12 Cleidocranial dysplasia. (**a**) Frontal chest radiograph shows the absence of both clavicles with omovertebral bones articulating with the T3 transverse processes on both sides, bell-shaped chest, small and high scapulae, and non-visualization of both glenoid fossa with inferiorly located humeral heads. (**b**) Frontal radiograph of the cervicothoracic spine shows bifid C7 to T2 vertebrae. (**c**) Frontal skull radiograph shows widened anterior and posterior fontanelles, wormian bones, and a large mandible. (**d**) Frontal radiograph of the pelvis shows diastasis of the pubic symphysis, hypoplastic iliac bones, and bilateral short femoral necks causing coxa vara deformity. (**e**) Frontal radiograph of both hands shows an elongated second metacarpal bone and hypoplastic distal phalanges of both hands with pointed terminal tufts. Note that the bone density is normal in all the visualized bones (Courtesy of Dr. Sharifah Intan with permission from Radiopaedia.org)

Table 42.3 Imaging pitfalls and differentiating features between pyknodysostosis and cleidocranial dysostosis

Imaging pitfalls	Pyknodysostosis (exclusive features)	Cleidocranial dysostosis (exclusive features)
Widened skull sutures with persistent fontanelles, wormian bones, frontoparietal bossing, platybasia	Short stature	Small and elevated scapulae
	Obtuse angle of the mandible	Narrow bell-shaped chest
Defective dentition sometimes causing dental caries and osteomyelitis of the jaw	Diffuse osteosclerosis with transverse fractures particularly in the limbs	Pseudo-widening of the pubic symphysis
Hypoplastic clavicles and terminal phalanges		

and late-onset aortic regurgitation (Langer and Carey 1966; Resnick 1994; Mikles and Stanton 1997; Rasalkar et al. 2011; Di Cesare et al. 2012).

Hurler syndrome is a rare autosomal recessive disorder of mucopolysaccharide metabolism (MPS type 1), which is characterized clinically

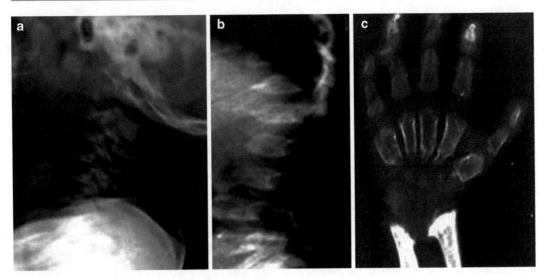

Fig. 42.13 Morquio syndrome. (**a**) Lateral radiograph of the cervical spine shows universal platyspondyly. Hypoplasia of the odontoid process is also noted. Intervertebral disk spaces are normal. (**b**) Lateral thoracolumbar spine radiograph shows platyspondyly with cen- tral beaking and posterior scalloping. (**c**) Frontal hand radiograph shows pointed proximal metacarpals with irregular articular ends of the radius and ulna (Reproduced with permission from: Subbarao (2014))

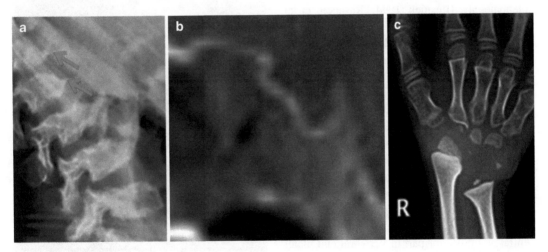

Fig. 42.14 Hurler syndrome. (**a**) Lateral thoracolumbar spine radiograph shows platyspondyly with anteroinferior beaking (*arrows*). (**b**) Sagittal-reconstructed CT image of the sella (bone window) shows a "J"-shaped sella. (**c**) Frontal radiograph of the wrist shows tilting of the ulna toward the radius and bullet-shaped proximal ends of the metacarpals (Reproduced with permission from: Subbarao (2014))

by mental retardation, corneal clouding, deaf- ness, and cardiac disease. Dermatan sulfate and heparin sulfate are the mucopolysaccharides excreted excessively in the urine. The prognosis is poor in most patients, with death in the first decade due to cardiac disease (Rasalkar et al. 2011). The radiographic findings (Fig. 42.14) in the spine consist of hypoplastic vertebra at the thoracolumbar junction, mainly at the anterosu- perior aspect with anterior inferior vertebral beaking causing thoracolumbar kyphosis. Atlantoaxial subluxation, proximal metacarpal tapering, short and wide tubular bones, flaring of iliac bones, and coxa vara or valga are also seen

Table 42.4 Imaging pitfalls and differentiating features between Morquio syndrome and Hurler syndrome

Imaging pitfalls	Morquio syndrome (exclusive features)	Hurler syndrome (exclusive features)
Anterior vertebral beaking and posterior vertebral scalloping Hypoplastic vertebra at thoracolumbar junction with thoracolumbar kyphosis Atlantoaxial subluxation Small flared iliac bones Coxa vara or valga Short and wide tubular bones Proximal metacarpal tapering	Universal platyspondyly with anterior central vertebral beaking Pectus carinatum Cardiac abnormalities Normal intelligence	Anterior inferior vertebral beaking Skull changes – macrocephaly, frontal bossing, large J-shaped sella, calvarial thickening, craniosynostosis, hydrocephalus Short thick clavicles Oar-shaped ribs Osteoporosis Hepatosplenomegaly Mental retardation

in the affected patients. However, the differentiating features (Table 42.4) include the presence of macrocephaly, frontal bossing, calvarial thickening, craniosynostosis involving sagittal and lambdoid sutures, hydrocephalus, enlarged J-shaped sella, widening of anterior ribs (oar-shaped/paddle ribs), osteoporosis, and hepatosplenomegaly (Resnick 1994; Rasalkar et al. 2011; Greenspan 2015).

Spondyloepiphyseal dysplasia (SED) refers to hereditary chondrodysplasia characterized by predominant involvement of the spine and epiphysis of the long bones, leading to disproportionate dwarfism. The inheritance is X-linked recessive, autosomal dominant, and autosomal recessive. It has two subtypes, namely, SED congenita and SED tarda. SED tarda is the milder form, which manifests in late childhood or adolescence (Lakhar and Raphael 2003). The cardinal imaging features (Fig. 42.15) include platyspondyly with mounds of dense bone over central and posterior part of vertebral end plates causing hump-shaped vertebra or absence of ossification in the anterior parts of vertebral end plates giving the appearance of anterior vertebral beaking. Thin intervertebral disk spaces, odontoid hypoplasia (seen in SED congenita), flattened and dysplastic epiphysis of long bones (particularly proximal femoral epiphysis), small iliac wings, and kyphoscoliosis are the other important radiographic features (Lakhar and Raphael 2003; Greenspan 2015). Complications include premature osteoarthritis and atlantoaxial subluxation. Morquio syndrome is a close differential due to the presence of diffuse platyspondyly

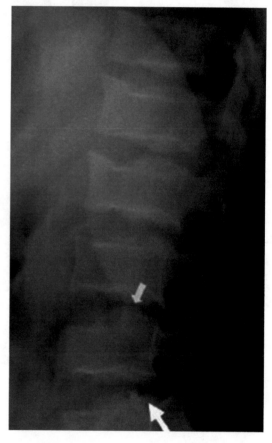

Fig. 42.15 Spondyloepiphyseal dysplasia tarda. Lateral thoracolumbar spine radiograph shows hyperostotic bone deposited at the posterior two-thirds of the vertebral end plates causing a "hump-shaped" or "heaping up" vertebra (*arrows*) along with the thin disk spaces (Reproduced with permission from: Subbarao (2014))

with hump-shaped vertebra (mimicking anterior vertebral beaking) and presence of dysplastic epiphysis. However, the absence of imaging features, namely, anterior central vertebral beaking and posterior scalloping, normal disk height, proximal metacarpal tapering, and systemic manifestations (cardiac and visceral involvement, corneal clouding, and metabolic abnormality), point toward SED (Resnick 1994; Lakhar and Raphael 2003; Greenspan 2015).

42.7 Achondroplasia and Pseudoachondroplasia

Achondroplasia is a short-limb dwarfing dysplasia characterized by abnormal epiphyseal chondroblastic growth and maturation. It occurs due to sporadic mutation in about 80% of the cases, and autosomal dominant transmission occurs in the remaining ones. The enchondral ossification centers (particularly at the base of the skull and ends of long bones) are involved more than others, and the periosteal and membranous ossification are normal. The disease presents at birth and commonly involves the skull, spine, pelvis, and limbs (Resnick 1994; Subbarao 2014).

The pathognomonic radiographic features (Fig. 42.16) include:

► *Limbs*: Symmetrical rhizomelic limb shortening, widening of the shafts (due to normal periosteal ossification), splaying and cupping of the metaphysis with V-shaped growth plates (chevron sign), short and thick tubular bones of the hands and feet, trident hand (separation of the middle and ring fingers with all fingers of the same length), and delayed appearance of the carpal bones

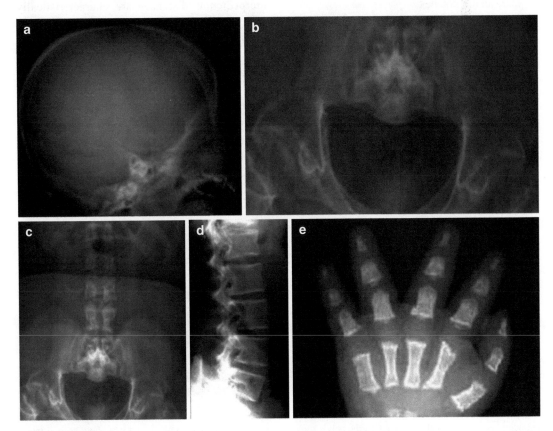

Fig. 42.16 Skeletal survey in a patient with achondroplasia. (**a**) Lateral skull radiograph shows a large skull with a narrow base. (**b**) Frontal radiograph of the pelvis shows a champagne glass appearance of the pelvic inlet with horizontal acetabular roofs. (**c**) Frontal and (**d**) lateral radiographs of the lumbosacral spine show short thick pedicles with progressive caudal narrowing of the interpedicular distance and lumbar canal stenosis, along with posterior scalloping of vertebrae. The sacrum is oriented horizontally. (**e**) Frontal hand radiograph shows a trident hand with short and stubby phalanges (Reproduced with permission from: Subbarao (2014))

► *Skull*: Large cranium (with short anteroposterior dimension – brachycephaly), small base of the skull often with stenotic foramen magnum (causing cervicomedullary kink), basilar impression, and prominent frontal and small nasal bones

► *Spine*: Posterior vertebral scalloping, bullet-shaped vertebrae, widened intervertebral disk height (due to increased amount of cartilage), progressive caudal narrowing of interpedicular distance in the lumbar spine, short and thick pedicles (causing spinal stenosis), and exaggerated lumbar lordosis with increased angle between the sacrum and lumbar spine (horizontally oriented sacrum)

► *Pelvis*: Small pelvis with champagne glass pelvic inlet, horizontal acetabular roofs, squared (tombstone) iliac wings, and narrow sacrosciatic notches

► *Chest*: Anteroposterior shortening of the ribs with anterior flaring

► Neurological complications are seen in many cases and vary from cervicomedullary compression and hydrocephalus due to small foramen magnum and cord compression due to lumbar canal stenosis (Resnick 1994; Yochum and Rowe 2005; Subbarao 2014).

Pseudoachondroplasia is a rarer and similar skeletal dysplasia which features the rhizomelic type of dwarfism. The inheritance is autosomal dominant in majority of the cases. In contrast to achondroplasia, most patients are normal at birth and present around 2–3 years of age with delay in walking/abnormal waddling gait or lower limb deformity. The most obvious discriminating feature is the presence of normal skull and facial bones and normal facies (Tandon et al. 2008; Radlović et al. 2013; Subbarao 2014). The radiographic changes (Fig. 42.17) are quite similar to achondroplasia, especially in the pelvis and limbs, except that the epiphyses are also involved in limbs, which are small and fragmented with a delayed appearance. Proximal femoral and humeral epiphyses are affected in most cases, with medial beaking of the femoral neck. Spinal features also resemble achondroplasia, but the interpedicular distances are characteristically normal. Therefore, stenosis of the foramen magnum and lumbar canal is not seen. In addition, marked platyspondyly and odontoid dysplasia are the other spinal abnormalities often seen in patients with pseudoachondroplasia exclusively. However, the skull is normal, unlike achondroplasia (Yochum and Rowe 2005; Tandon et al. 2008; Radlović et al. 2013; Subbarao 2014). The pitfalls and differences between achondroplasia and pseudoachondroplasia are summarized in Table 42.5.

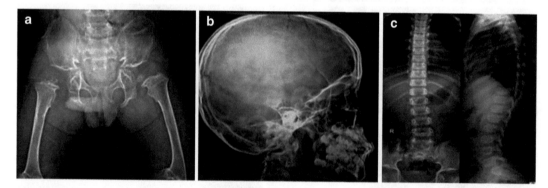

Fig. 42.17 Skeletal survey in a patient with pseudoachondroplasia. (**a**) Frontal radiograph of the pelvis shows a champagne glass pelvic inlet (same as achondroplasia) along with delayed appearance of bilateral proximal femoral epiphysis which are flattened and fragmented. (**b**) Lateral skull radiograph is normal. (**c**) Frontal and (**d**) lateral thoracolumbar spine radiographs show normal interpedicular distances (Reproduced with permission from: Subbarao (2014))

Table 42.5 Imaging pitfalls and differentiating features between achondroplasia and pseudoachondroplasia

Anatomical region	Imaging pitfalls/mimics	Achondroplasia (exclusive features)	Pseudoachondroplasia (exclusive features)
Limbs	Rhizomelic dwarfism with flaring and cupping of the metaphysis	None	Additional involvement of epiphysis (small, fragmented, and delayed appearance)
Spine	Bullet-nose vertebrae, widened disk spaces, posterior vertebral scalloping	Short and thick pedicles, caudal narrowing of interpedicular distance, lumbar canal stenosis	Platyspondyly
Pelvis	Small squared pelvis with champagne glass pelvic inlet and horizontal acetabular roofs	None	None
Skull and facial bones	None	Large cranium with small base of the skull	Normal (Fig. 42.17b)

42.8 Chondrodysplasia Punctata, Multiple Epiphyseal Dysplasia, Meyer Dysplasia, Perthes Disease, and Cretinism

Chondrodysplasia punctata (also known as dysplasia epiphysealis punctata) is a genetically heterogeneous epiphyseal dysplasia characterized by punctate or stippled calcification of multiple epiphyseal centers. It can be classified into several subtypes: the autosomal recessive (rhizomelic type associated with peroxisomal enzyme disorder and death often in the first few years of life) and the X-linked dominant (CDPX2 or Conradi-Hünermann-Happle syndrome). A third rare subtype is the brachytelephalangic type with X-linked recessive inheritance. In addition to genetically inherited forms, chondrodysplasia punctata may also be seen with embryotoxicity due to maternal use of coumarin-like compounds or phenytoin during gestation, or babies born to mothers with autoimmune diseases like systemic lupus erythematosus. It is important to identify the radiological type in order to prognosticate the patient. Punctate calcifications tend to disappear after the first year of life, thus necessitating early diagnosis (Morthy et al. 2002; Figueirêdo et al. 2007; Irving et al. 2008). Radiological features of the rhizomelic and Conradi-Hünermann subtypes

(Fig. 42.18) of chondrodysplasia punctata are tabulated in Table 42.6.

Multiple epiphyseal dysplasia (also known as *dysplasia epiphysealis multiplex or Fairbank-Ribbing disease*) is a genetically heterogeneous skeletal dysplasia caused by mutations in at least six genes, characterized by flattening and fragmentation of epiphyses. The transmission is autosomal dominant in most of the cases (Unger et al. 2008; Panda et al. 2014). Unlike chondrodysplasia punctata, multiple epiphyseal dysplasia presents in older children (after 2–4 years of age, when the child begins to walk) with complaints of waddling gait and difficulty in running. Short stature is not a feature. The radiographic features (Fig. 42.19) include bilateral symmetrical involvement of epiphysis of the hips, knees, ankles and, less commonly, the shoulders, wrists, hands, and feet which are flattened and fragmented (with hypoplastic femoral and tibial condyles with shallow intercondylar notch). In contrast, the stippling in chondrodysplasia punctata is finer than the fragmentation seen in multiple epiphyseal dysplasia. The lateral tibiotalar slant (due to thinning of lateral tibial epiphysis) and double-layered patella are the other differentiating features. The involvement of the spine is uncommon and, if it occurs, is mild with features including mild endplate irregularity, anterior wedging, multiple Schmorl nodes (like

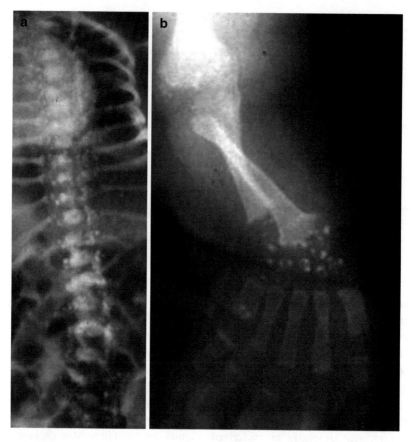

Fig. 42.18 Chondrodysplasia punctata (Conradi-Hünermann subtype). (**a**) Frontal radiograph of the thoracolumbar spine shows punctate calcifications adjacent to vertebrae with vertebral deformities. (**b**) Radiograph of the forearm shows stippling of the wrist (Reproduced with permission from: Subbarao (2014))

Table 42.6 Imaging features of the rhizomelic and Conradi-Hünermann subtypes of chondrodysplasia punctata

Rhizomelic type (lethal+ mental retardation +)	Conradi-Hünermann type (normal intelligence and life span)
Epiphyseal stippling noted mainly in large joints, such as the hips, shoulders, knee, and wrists	Stippling at ends of long bones as well as short tubular bones in the hands and feet
Short tubular bones in the hands and foot spared	Metaphyses and diaphyses are normal
Metaphyses are often flared	Occasional asymmetric limb shortening
Symmetrical rhizomelic limb shortening	Stippling in the spine present
Stippling in the spine absent (coronal clefts in vertebrae are present)	Stippling may also involve ends of ribs, hyoid bone, thyroid cartilage, larynx and trachea, and base of the skull

in Scheuermann disease), and scoliosis with absent platyspondyly. Dens agenesis is also seen in some cases causing atlantoaxial subluxation. Complications include premature degenerative changes, slipped capital femoral epiphysis, and osteochondritis dissecans (Unger et al. 2008; Panda et al. 2014).

Legg-Calve-Perthes disease, Meyer dysplasia, and *cretinism* can have similar radiographic features as multiple epiphyseal dysplasia. However, the symmetrical nature, involvement of characteristic joints, and absence of other systemic features are helpful in differentiating points that favor multiple epiphyseal dysplasia. Legg-Calve-Perthes disease (osteonecrosis of proximal femoral epiphysis) can be bilateral in 10–15% of cases; however, it is more often sequential rather than simultaneous. Bilateral symmetrical involvement favors epiphyseal dysplasia. Meyer dysplasia is a subtype

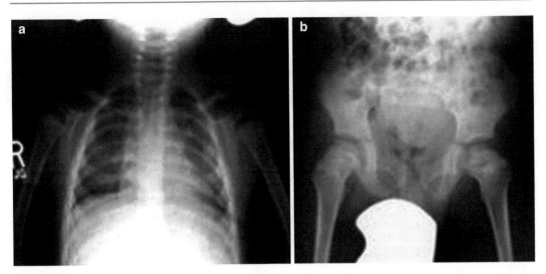

Fig. 42.19 Multiple epiphyseal dysplasia. (**a**) Frontal chest radiograph shows the absence of proximal humeral ossification centers. (**b**) Frontal radiograph of the pelvis shows symmetrical flattening of bilateral proximal femo- ral epiphysis (Courtesy of Professor L Das Narla, Virginia Commonwealth University Medical Center, Richmond, USA)

of epiphyseal dysplasia confined to the hips, which is often asymptomatic or has milder symptoms, unlike Legg-Calve-Perthes disease. The absence of involvement of other epiphysis differentiates Meyer dysplasia from multiple epiphyseal dysplasia. Cretinism (congenital hypothyroidism) shows fragmented and dysplastic epiphysis, with delayed bone age. The spine is also involved in some cases, causing anterior vertebral beaking. Therefore, delayed skeletal maturation, the presence of other systemic features and proper clinical history, along with hormonal assays, distinguish it from multiple epiphyseal dysplasia (Yochum and Rowe 2005; Panda et al. 2014).

42.9 Metaphyseal Chondrodysplasia (Schmid Type) and Rickets

Schmid-type metaphyseal chondrodysplasia is a rare autosomal dominant disorder characterized by moderately short stature with short limbs, bowing of long bones, waddling gait, and coxa vara. It is caused by mutations in the COL10A1 (6q21-q22) gene encoding the collagen alpha-1(X) chain. *Spahr-type metaphyseal chondrodysplasia* is a similar condition which is autosomal

recessive and presents with moderate short stature. It is due to MMP 13 mutations which cause disruption of a crucial hydrogen bond in the calcium-binding region of the catalytic domain of the matrix metalloproteinase. Molecular confirmation is required for distinction of both the conditions. Patients often present in second to third year of life (Lachman et al. 1988; Elliott et al. 2005; Mäkitie et al. 2005). The radiographic changes (Fig. 42.20) are similar to those of *rickets* (particularly *nutritional rickets*) (Fig. 42.21) and consist of cupping, flaring, and fraying of the metaphysis with widening of the growth plate (most pronounced at the knees); coxa vara; bowing of long bones (commonly femur); enlarged capital femoral epiphysis in early childhood; cupping, splaying, and sclerosis of the anterior aspect of the ribs; and a normal spine. Positive family history and no abnormality in biochemical analysis (serum calcium, phosphate, parathyroid hormone, and alkaline phosphatase levels) help in differentiating metaphyseal chondrodysplasias from rickets. Rickets is a metabolic bone disease which is due to deficiency in one or more of calcium, phosphorus, and 1,25 di-hydroxy vitamin D (Lachman et al. 1988; Dahl and Birkebaek 1996; Elliott et al. 2005; Mäkitie et al. 2005; Bonafé et al. 2014).

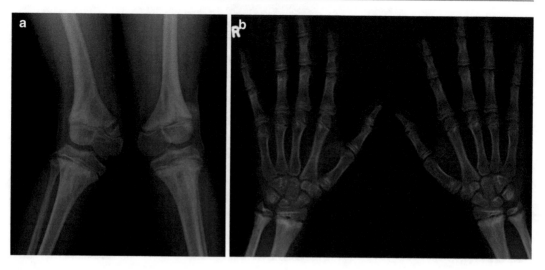

Fig. 42.20 Metaphyseal dysplasia (Schmid type). Frontal radiographs of (**a**) both knees and (**b**) both wrists show expansion, sclerosis, and irregularity of the metaphyses of the femurs, tibiae, radii, and ulnae bilaterally, with widened growth plates

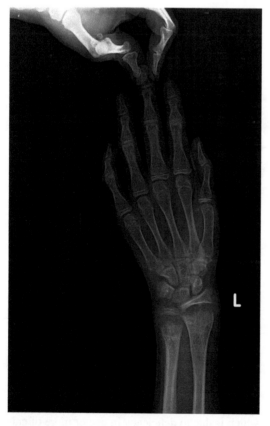

Fig. 42.21 Frontal radiograph of the left wrist in a patient with rickets shows cupping, splaying, and fraying of the distal metaphysis of the left radius and ulna, with widened growth plates

42.10 Camurati-Engelmann Disease, Ghosal-Type Hemato-Diaphyseal Dysplasia, Ribbing Disease, Caffey Disease, Intramedullary Osteosclerosis, and Erdheim-Chester Disease

Camurati-Engelmann disease (also known as *Engelmann disease* or *progressive diaphyseal dysplasia*) is a rare autosomal dominant sclerosing bony dysplasia characterized by bilateral, symmetrical, fusiform thickening of the cortical bone in the diaphysis of long tubular bones (Fig. 42.22). Engelmann disease affects long bones and bones formed by intramembranous ossification; therefore, calvarial hyperostosis is also as frequently seen as the involvement of long bones. The disorder manifests in the first decade of life with symptoms of bone and muscle pain, weakness and atrophy, waddling and broad-based gait, and delayed puberty. It is more common in boys (Vanhoenacker et al. 2003; Bartuseviciene et al. 2009; Damiá Ade et al. 2010).

Ghosal hemato-diaphyseal dysplasia is a similar autosomal recessive disorder which features metadiaphyseal dysplasia of long bones and

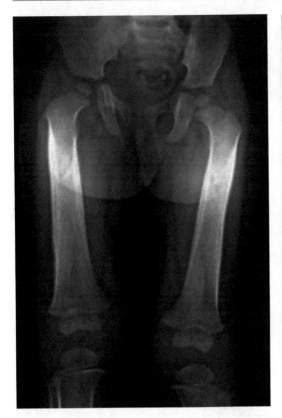

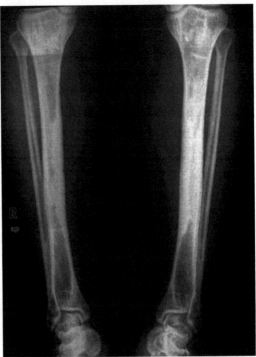

Fig. 42.23 Ribbing disease. Frontal radiograph of both legs shows asymmetrical cortical thickening of the diaphysis of both tibiae (left > right) (Reproduced with permission from: Damle et al. (2011))

Fig. 42.22 Engelmann disease. Frontal radiograph of the pelvis and both femurs shows symmetrical cortical thickening involving the diaphysis of both femurs (Reproduced with permission from: Subbarao (2013))

hematologic abnormalities due to fibrosis or sclerosis of the bone marrow. The differentiating features from Engelmann disease include involvement of both metaphysis and diaphysis of long bones (unlike only diaphyseal involvement in Engelmann disease), presence of defective hematopoiesis, absence of gait abnormalities, elevated levels of immunoglobulins, and autosomal recessive mode of inheritance (in contrast to autosomal dominant in Engelmann disease) (Arora et al. 2015).

Ribbing disease (also known as *hereditary multiple diaphyseal sclerosis*) is another rare sclerosing dysplasia which closely resembles Engelmann disease and is characterized by benign endosteal and periosteal new bone formation confined to the diaphysis of the long bones of the lower extremities (Fig. 42.23). However, unlike Engelmann disease, it is of autosomal

recessive inheritance (with no gender predominance) and presents later in life (after puberty) with just pain in the involved extremity. It is either unilateral or asymmetrically and asynchronously bilateral (unlike bilateral symmetrical involvement of the former two disorders). There is no involvement of the skull and hematological abnormalities are not seen. Histologically, Ribbing disease shows isolated osteoblastic activity with progressive obstruction of the haversian systems, whereas Engelmann disease features both osteoblastic and osteoclastic activity, implying bone formation and resorption with trabecular thickening and normal or enlarged haversian systems. Some authors have proposed that both entities represent phenotypic variations of the same disorder (Seeger et al. 1996; Damle et al. 2011; Oztürkmen and Karamehmetoğlu 2011).

Caffey disease (also known as *infantile cortical hyperostosis*) is a largely self-limiting inherited disorder with both autosomal dominant and recessive inheritances (sporadic cases also seen infrequently). It is characterized by a clinical triad of (1) presentation within first 6 months of life; (2) hyperirritability, bony lesions, and soft tissue swelling; and (3) mandibular involvement. Other sites of involvement include the ulna, clavicle, and, less commonly, other long bones, scapula, ribs, and skull. Radiological findings (Fig. 42.24) include lamellated periosteal reactions with cortical thickening and soft tissue swelling involving the diaphysis. It often resolves spontaneously within 6 months to 1 year (Kutty et al. 2010; Panda et al. 2014).

Intramedullary osteosclerosis is a non-hereditary condition that mimics Ribbing disease and is characterized by unilateral or asymmetrical, intramedullary diaphyseal osteosclerosis of one or more long bones of one or both lower extremities. There is no periosteal new bone formation and soft tissue involvement, with onset in adulthood. However, female predominance, lack of family history, and medullary sclerosis as the dominant imaging findings differentiate between the two disorders (Chanchairujira et al. 2001).

Erdheim-Chester disease is a rare nonfamilial, non-Langerhans cell lipogranulomatous disorder with infiltration by lipid-laden histiocytes, Touton giant cells, and variable amount of fibrosis. It often presents in middle age, with a slight male predominance. It is a multisystem disorder, and its manifestations include musculoskeletal involvement (most common), diabetes insipidus, exophthalmos (due to retro-orbital involvement), and involvement of the lungs and kidneys. Like Engelmann disease, it shows bilateral symmetrical metadiaphyseal osteosclerosis with cortical thickening (Fig. 42.25). However, onset in adulthood with absent family history, multisystem involvement, moderate anemia, elevated erythrocyte sedimentation rate and C-reactive protein, abnormal lipid metabolism, sparing of axial skeleton, and partial epiphyseal involvement with bone infarcts (in some cases) are the contrasting points (Dion et al. 2006).

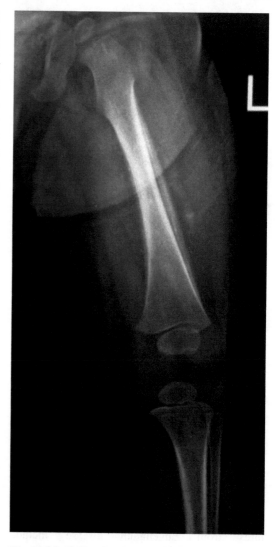

Fig. 42.24 Caffey disease. Frontal radiograph of the left femur and knee in an 8-month-old boy shows lamellated periosteal reaction involving the diaphysis of the femur with soft tissue swelling

42.11 Osteopoikilosis and Sclerotic Metastases

Osteopoikilosis is a rare autosomal dominant sclerosing dysplasia characterized by multiple small (1–10 mm), symmetrical, uniform, sclerotic, ovoid opacities (bone islands) parallel to surrounding trabeculae and clustered around joints (Fig. 42.26). The common sites of

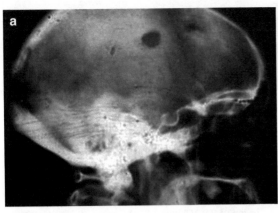

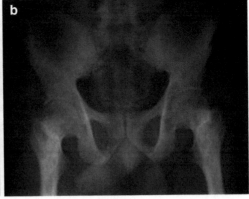

Fig. 42.25 Erdheim-Chester disease. (**a**) Lateral radiograph of the skull shows a well-defined rounded radiolucent lesion with beveled edges in the parietal bone, with another similar lesion also noted in the frontal bone. (**b**)

Frontal radiograph of the pelvis and hips shows symmetrical metadiaphyseal sclerosis involving both proximal femurs. Patchy areas of sclerosis and radiolucency are also seen involving both pelvic bones

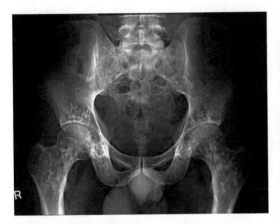

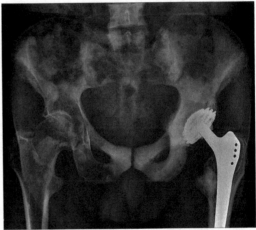

Fig. 42.26 Osteopoikilosis. Frontal radiograph of the pelvis shows multiple, bilateral symmetrical, sclerotic lesions of uniform size around both hip joints (Reproduced with permission from: Subbarao (2013))

Fig. 42.27 Frontal radiograph of the pelvis shows multiple sclerotic foci of variable sizes involving the pelvic bones and proximal femurs bilaterally, with variable distribution in a patient with osteoblastic metastasis from prostate carcinoma. Left hip implant is noted (Courtesy of Dr. Stefan Ludwig with permission from Radiopaedia. org)

involvement include ends of long bones, carpals, tarsals, and peri-acetabular and subglenoid areas. The spine, skull, and ribs are involved rarely. They often develop in childhood and do not regress (so are seen in all age groups). It often coexists with osteopathia striata and melorheostosis. They do not demonstrate increased uptake on bone scintigraphy and have no malignant potential (Benli et al. 1992; Stacy et al. 2002; Karwar et al. 2005).

Sclerotic metastases are an important differential and can be differentiated by the variable size and distribution of the lesions (Fig. 42.27). Additionally, they show increased uptake on bone scintigraphy (Stacy et al. 2002; Karwar et al. 2005; Panda et al. 2014).

Conclusion

Imaging enables the correct diagnosis of skeletal dysplasias and their distinction from other dysplastic and non-dysplastic conditions. This would help in targeted workup and prevent unnecessary investigations. An accurate diagnosis of these complex abnormalities is also essential for their early management, assessment of prognosis, and genetic counseling.

References

Ablin D, Greenspan A, Reinhart M, Grix A (1990) Differentiation of child abuse from osteogenesis imperfecta. AJR Am J Roentgenol 154:1035–1046

Arora R, Aggarwal S, Deme S (2015) Ghosal hematodiaphyseal dysplasia – a concise review including an illustrative patient. Skeletal Radiol 44:447–450

Bartuseviciene A, Samuilis A, Skucas J (2009) Camurati-Engelmann disease imaging: clinical features and differential diagnosis. Skeletal Radiol 38:1037–1043

Bathi RJ, Masur VN (2000) Pyknodysostosis – a report of two cases with a brief review of the literature. Int J Oral Maxillofac Surg 29:439–442

Baujat G, Le Merrer M (2007) Ellis-van Creveld syndrome. Orphanet J Rare Dis 2:27

Benli IT, Akalin S, Boysan E et al (1992) Epidemiological, clinical and radiological aspects of osteopoikilosis. J Bone Joint Surg Br 74:504–506

Bonafé L, Liang J, Gorna MW et al (2014) MMP13 mutations are the cause of recessive metaphyseal dysplasia, Spahr type. Am J Med Genet A 164:1175–1179

Chanchairujira K, Chung CB, Lai YM et al (2001) Intramedullary osteosclerosis: imaging features in nine patients. Radiology 220:225–230

Chauss J (1955) Chondroectodermal dysplasia (Ellis van Creveld disease) 1. Radiology 65:213–217

Dahl M, Birkebaek NH (1996) Metaphyseal chondrodysplasia as differential diagnosis to rickets. Ugeskr Laeger 158:1683–1684

Damiá Ade B, Morón CC, Pérez PA et al (2010) Bone scintigraphy in Engelmann-Camurati disease. Clin Nucl Med 35:559–560

Damle NA, Patnecha M, Kumar P et al (2011) Ribbing disease: uncommon cause of a common symptom. Indian J Nucl Med 26:36–39

De Vries J, Yntema J, van Die C et al (2009) Jeune syndrome: description of 13 cases and a proposal for follow-up protocol. Eur J Pediatr 169:77–88

Di Cesare A, Di Cagno A, Moffa S et al (2012) A description of skeletal manifestation in adult case of Morquio syndrome: radiographic and MRI appearance. Case Rep Med 2012:1–6

Dion E, Graef C, Miquel A et al (2006) Bone involvement in Erdheim-Chester disease: imaging findings including periostitis and partial epiphyseal involvement. Radiology 238:632–639

Elliott AM, Field FM, Rimoin DL et al (2005) Hand involvement in Schmid metaphyseal chondrodysplasia. Am J Med Genet A 132:191–193

Figueirêdo SDS, Araújo JS, Kozan JEM et al (2007) Rhizomelic chondrodysplasia punctata: a case report and brief literature review. Radiol Bras 40:69–72

Greenspan A (2015) Orthopedic imaging: a practical approach, 6th edn. Lippincott Williams & Wilkins, Philadelphia

Grover SB, Kumar S, Taneja DK (2003) Radiological quiz- skeletal radiology. Indian J Radiol Imaging 13:335–338

Imerci A, Canbek U, Haghari S, Sürer L, Kocak M (2015) Idiopathic juvenile osteoporosis: a case report and review of the literature. Int J Surg Case Rep 9:127–129

Irving MD, Chitty LS, Mansour S et al (2008) Chondrodysplasia punctata: a clinical diagnostic and radiological review. Clin Dysmorphol 17:229–241

Kapur R (2007) Achondrogenesis. Pediatr Dev Pathol 10:253–255

Karwar J, Gupta R, Sharma G (2005) Osteopoikilosis: a case report. Indian J Radiol Imaging 15:453–454

Keats T, Riddervold H, Michaelis L (1970) Thanatophoric dwarfism. AJR Am J Roentgenol 108:473–480

Kozlowski K, Prokop E, Zybaczynski J (1970) Thanatophoric dwarfism. Br J Radiol 43:565–568

Kutty N, Thomas D, George L et al (2010) Caffey disease or infantile cortical hyperostosis: a case report. Oman Med J 25:134–136

Lachman RS, Rimoin DL, Spranger J (1988) Metaphyseal chondrodysplasia, Schmid type. Clinical and radiographic delineation with a review of the literature. Pediatr Radiol 18:93–102

Lakhar BN, Raphael R (2003) Spondyloepiphyseal dysplasia: an evaluation of six cases. Indian J Radiol Imaging 13:199–203

Langer LO, Carey LS (1966) The roentgenographic features of the Ks mucopolysaccharidosis of Morquio (Morquio-Brailsford's disease). AJR Am J Roentgenol 97:1–20

Machado CDV, Siquara Da Rocha MCB, Telles PDDS et al (2015) Infantile osteopetrosis associated with osteomyelitis. BMJ Case Rep pii: bcr2014208085

Mäkitie O, Susic M, Ward L et al (2005) Schmid type of metaphyseal chondrodysplasia and COL10A1 mutations-findings in 10 patients. Am J Med Genet A 137:241–248

Mikles M, Stanton RP (1997) A review of Morquio syndrome. Am J Orthop 26:533–540

Miller E, Blaser S, Shannon P, Widjaja E (2009) Brain and bone abnormalities of thanatophoric dwarfism. AJR Am J Roentgenol 192:48–51

Morthy NL, Venkataratnam I, Rao RP et al (2002) Images: chondrodysplasia punctata. Indian J Radiol Imaging 12:397–398

Oztürkmen Y, Karamehmetoğlu M (2011) Ribbing disease: a case report and literature review. Acta Orthop Traumatol Turc 45:58–65

Panda A, Gamanagatti S, Jana M et al (2014) Skeletal dysplasias: a radiographic approach and review of common non-lethal skeletal dysplasias. World J Radiol 6:808–825

Radlović V, Smoljanić Z, Radlović N et al (2013) Pseudoachondroplasia: a case report. Srp Arh Celok Lek 141:676–679

Rasalkar DD, Chu WCW, Hui J et al (2011) Pictorial review of mucopolysaccharidosis with emphasis on MRI features of brain and spine. Br J Radiol 84:469–477

Rasmussen S, Bieber F, Benacerraf B et al (1996) Epidemiology of osteochondrodysplasias: changing trends due to advances in prenatal diagnosis. Am J Med Genet 61:49–58

Renaud A, Aucourt J, Weill J et al (2013) Radiographic features of osteogenesis imperfecta. Insights Imaging 4:417–429

Resnick D (1994) Diagnosis of bone and joint disorders, 4th edn. Saunders, Philadelphia

Seeger LL, Hewel KC, Yao L et al (1996) Ribbing disease (multiple diaphyseal sclerosis): imaging and differential diagnosis. AJR Am J Roentgenol 167:689–694

Shen Z, Zou CC, Yang RW, Zhao ZY (2009) Cleidocranial dysplasia: report of 3 cases and literature review. Clin Pediatr 48:194–198

Stacy GS, Heck RK, Peabody TD et al (2002) Neoplastic and tumor like lesions detected on MR imaging of the knee in patients with suspected internal derangement: part I, intraosseous entities. AJR Am J Roentgenol 178:589–594

Subbarao K (2013) Skeletal dysplasia (sclerosing dysplasias) Part I. NJR 3:1–10

Subbarao K (2014) Non-sclerosing skeletal dysplasias. NJR 4:1–11

Tandon A, Bhargava SK, Goel S et al (2008) Pseudoachondroplasia: a rare cause of rhizomelic dwarfism. Indian J Orthop 42:477–479

Thakkar P, Aiyer S, Shah B (2012) Asphyxiating thoracic dystrophy (Jeune syndrome). JCR 2012:15–17

Tüysüz B, Barış S, Aksoy F, Madazlı R, Üngür S, Sever L (2009) Clinical variability of asphyxiating thoracic dystrophy (Jeune) syndrome: evaluation and classification of 13 patients. Am J Med Genet A 149:1727–1733

Unger S, Bonafé L, Superti-Furga A (2008) Multiple epiphyseal dysplasia: clinical and radiographic features, differential diagnosis and molecular basis. Best Pract Res Clin Rheumatol 22:19–32

Vanhoenacker FM, Janssens K, Van Hul W et al (2003) Camurati-Engelmann disease. Review of radioclinical features. Acta Radiol 44:430–434

Warman M, Cormier Daire V, Hall C et al (2011) Nosology and classification of genetic skeletal disorders 2010 revision. Am J Med Genet A 155:943–968

Weiner D, Jonah D, Leighley B et al (2013) Orthopaedic manifestations of chondroectodermal dysplasia the Ellis–van Creveld syndrome. J Child Orthop 7:465–476

Yochum TR, Rowe LJ (2005) Yochum and Rowe's essentials of skeletal radiology, 3rd edn. Lippincott Williams & Wilkins, Baltimore

Yun Young Choi, Jae Sung Lee,
and Seoung-Oh Yang

Contents

43.1 **Introduction** 951

43.2 **Basic Principles** 952
43.2.1 Planar Scintigraphy and SPECT
Radioisotopes 952
43.2.2 PET Radioisotopes 952
43.2.3 SPECT/CT and PET/CT 953
43.2.4 PET/MRI 953

43.3 **Pitfalls in Interpretation** 954
43.3.1 Instrument-Related Pitfalls: Improper
Photopeak Window Setting 954
43.3.2 Technique-Related Pitfalls: Injection
Pitfalls 954
43.3.3 Patient-Related Pitfalls 957

Conclusion 975

References 975

Y.Y. Choi, MD
Department of Nuclear Medicine, Hanyang
University Medical Center, Seoul, South Korea
e-mail: yychoi@hanyang.ac.kr

J.S. Lee, PhD
Departments of Nuclear Medicine and Biomedical
Sciences, Seoul National University,
Seoul, South Korea
e-mail: jaes@snu.ac.kr

S.-O. Yang, MD (✉)
Department of Nuclear Medicine, Dongnam Institute
of Radiological and Medical Science,
267-2, Jwadong-ri Jangan-eup, Gijang-gun,
Busan 619-953, South Korea
e-mail: sosoyangmd@gmail.com

Abbreviations

CT   Computed tomography
MRI   Magnetic resonance imaging
PET   Positron-emission tomography
SPECT   Single photon emission computed
        tomography
TOF   Time-of-flight

43.1 Introduction

Nuclear medicine departments have to comply with and maintain a strict state policy to process radionuclides, radiopharmaceuticals, and body fluids along with an up-to-date inventory log. In general, the most frequent unexpected or nondiagnostic but preventable events are injecting wrong dosage of radionuclides or radiopharmaceuticals intravenously, applying incorrect peak or window setting on patients who were given other treatment of examination using radiopharmaceuticals with long half-life, or increased background radiation due to careless management of radiopharmaceuticals. Pitfalls in nuclear medicine imaging can be categorized into radionuclide production and detection, human error, and patient-related factors. Unlike anatomical imaging, knowing the proper half-life of isotopes is important for effective scanning, which is critical for optimal investigation and treatment planning.

© Springer International Publishing AG 2017
W.C.G. Peh (ed.), *Pitfalls in Musculoskeletal Radiology*, DOI 10.1007/978-3-319-53496-1_43

The two main imaging systems used in nuclear medicine for visualizing the *in vivo* distribution of radioisotope-emitting radiation (mostly gamma rays) and radiopharmaceuticals labeled with those radioisotopes are the gamma camera and positron-emission tomography (PET) scanner. Single photon emission computed tomography (SPECT) is a tomographic technique performed using rotating gamma cameras. Additionally, insufficient morphological information in PET and SPECT images are compensated for by combining them with morphological imaging devices, such as computed tomography (CT) and magnetic resonance imaging (MRI) (Seo et al. 2008; Townsend 2008 Lee and Kim 2014; Vandenberghe and Marsden 2015).

Whole-body bone scintigraphy has been widely used for evaluation of benign and malignant bone diseases for decades, and until recently, no other single study could replace this role. Many sources of diagnostic errors, including factors related to history and physical examination, the patient's condition, radiopharmaceuticals, technique, and factors associated with interpretation, are well known. Recently, the introduction of SPECT/CT and the additional role of SPECT/CT have enabled more accurate diagnosis through enhanced sensitivity of SPECT and additional anatomical information from CT.

43.2 Basic Principles

43.2.1 Planar Scintigraphy and SPECT Radioisotopes

The radioisotopes typically used in planar scintigraphy and SPECT using gamma cameras are technetium (Tc)-99m, iodine (I)-123, I-131, and thallium (Tl)-201. These radioisotopes emit gamma rays with different energies (e.g., Tc-99m, 140 keV; I-123, 159 keV). Most gamma cameras comprise a mechanical collimator, a single large-area NaI (Tl) scintillation crystal and an array of photomultiplier tubes (PMTs) optically coupled to the back face of the crystal. The collimator is used to collect only the gamma rays moving in certain directions (e.g., perpendicular direction to

the crystal surface with parallel-hole collimator). The NaI (Tl) crystal detects gamma rays and emits scintillation light photons, and PMTs convert the scintillation light to electrical current. The amount of scintillation light photons and the amplitude of PMT output signal are proportional to the energy of detected gamma rays, enabling the measurement of gamma ray energy and rejection of scattered gamma events based on this energy information.

The scattered events that degrade image contrast are primarily rejected by applying energy windows centered on the photopeak positions, and dual- or triple-energy window-based or convolution-subtraction-based scatter correction algorithms are applied to enhance the image contrast if necessary. Because each radioisotope used in single photon imaging has a different gamma ray energy, wrong energy window settings cause the blurring of images and visualization of PMT array patterns. Nonuniform light output from scintillation crystal and position-dependent response and light correction efficiency of PMTs cause image nonuniformity and nonlinearity, which lead to the distortion in count and shape, if they are not properly corrected for. Selection of the proper collimator type is important because each isotope and examination have different requirements of collimator design. For example, the use of medium-energy collimator in I-131 scan causes the higher fraction of unwanted collimator scatter and septal penetration events (Dewaraja et al. 2013).

43.2.2 PET Radioisotopes

In PET, unstable neutron-poor radioisotopes undergo decay and emit a positron. The positron then combines with an electron in the surrounding tissue, and their masses are converted into photon energy, resulting in the annihilation of two 511 keV photons in nearly exact opposite directions. The PET scanner collects the coincidence events in which the annihilated photons are detected in a coincidence time window. Currently, cerium-doped LSO and LYSO scintillation crystal arrays coupled with the arrays of PMT, avalanche photodiode, or silicon photomultiplier are used in most state-of-the-art clinical whole-body PET, PET/CT, and PET/MRI scanners. The most advanced PET and hybrid systems provide time-of-flight (TOF) information that allows more accurate localization of annihilation points during the PET image reconstruction, leading to image quality enhancement (Karp et al. 2008; Conti 2011).

Random coincidence events occur when two unrelated photons that originate from different annihilation positions are detected accidentally within the coincidence window. The ratio between random and true coincidences increases as the total radioactivity increases. Another unwanted event in PET is scatter coincidence that occurs when one of the annihilated photons undergoes Compton scattering. Both random and scatter events cause the loss of image contrast and quantitative accuracy. The most significant physical artifact in PET is photon attenuation that is caused by both absorption and scattering of the primary photons. Because the attenuation correction factor in PET is huge (approximately 20), quantification is impossible without the proper attenuation compensation (Bailey 1998; Zaidi and Hasegawa 2003). Normalization in PET is a procedure to correct for nonuniformity of PET detector elements, and the failure of accurate normalization leads to rings or other artifacts and nonuniform activity distribution in reconstructed images (Badawi and Marsden 1999).

43.2.3 SPECT/CT and PET/CT

In PET/CT and SPECT/CT, attenuation maps required for attenuation and scatter corrections are derived from the CT Hounsfield units using their piecewise linear relationship. The CT-based attenuation correction has considerably reduced whole-body PET scan time relative to the use of external rotating radioisotope (Ga-68/Ge-68 or Cs-137) for attenuation correction. In addition, the CT-based attenuation correction provides essentially noiseless attenuation correction factor (Kinahan et al. 1998). However, artifacts (e.g., metal artifacts) shown on CT images are propagated into the reconstructed PET images (Barrett and Keat 2004). CT streak artifacts around the metallic implants cause over- or underestimation of PET activity around the implants (Goerres et al. 2003; Kamel et al. 2003). The different breathing patterns in CT and PET/SPECT scans cause anatomical mismatch between transmission CT and emission PET data, leading to artifacts in attenuation-corrected PET images. The anatomical regions most affected by the patient respiration include bases of the lung and upper pole of the liver (Beyer et al. 2003; Osman et al. 2003). Other motions arising between CT and PET/SPECT scans are also the source of error in PET/SPECT quantification.

43.2.4 PET/MRI

PET attenuation correction in PET/MRI is not straightforward because MRI intensity is largely determined by tissue hydrogen density, and relaxation properties which are not directly related to photon attenuation. Thus, in PET/MRI, PET attenuation correction methods based on the segmentation of individual MR images or transformation of template or atlas data into individual space are used (Yoo et al. 2015; Mehranian et al. 2016). However, three (soft tissues, lung, and air) or four (water, fat, lung, and air) tissue segments used in current whole-body or torso PET/MRI studies do not account for bone tissues. Ignoring the bone tissues results in considerable PET quantification errors in bone and neighboring lesions (Eiber et al. 2011, 2014; Kim et al. 2012). Although the MRI segmentation-based PET attenuation correction can account for the large variation in the shapes and positions of various organs in the body (Vandenberghe and Marsden 2015), inaccurate segmentation of MRI leads to PET quantification errors. It is also difficult to account for subject-specific and local variations in attenuation coefficients (Kim et al. 2012; Marshall et al. 2012). In addition, the smaller field of view of MRI compared to PET sometimes causes the truncation of arms of patients in the attenuation map and associated PET quantification error (Delso et al. 2010; Schramm et al. 2013).

TOF information in PET allows more accurate localization of the annihilation positions of gamma ray photons along the line of response. Thus, better image quality is yielded by the fine timing resolution of TOF PET. The TOF information is also useful for the mitigation of artifacts due to inaccurate physical corrections (e.g., mismatch between emission and transmission images, wrong normalization and scatter corrections, artifacts in transmission images) because TOF image reconstruction is more robust to the inconsistent or missing data in PET measurements (Conti 2011). In addition, the TOF information improves the performance of joint estimation of radioactivity and attenuation factors from only the emission PET data without attenuation information (Defrise et al. 2012; Rezaei et al. 2012). Accordingly, the joint estimation of emission and transmission enhanced by the fine TOF information is expected to remove the PET artifacts due to the inaccurate and inconsistent attenuation information.

43.3 Pitfalls in Interpretation

Many sources of diagnostic errors may occur during whole-body bone scintigraphy, including factors related to history and physical examination (e.g., prior history of trauma or recent radionuclide studies), factors related to patient's condition (e.g., age, body habitus, underlying diseases, medications, hydration status, lack of cooperation during scanning), factors related to radiopharmaceuticals (e.g., radiochemical impurities, introduction of air into vial during preparation), factors related to technique (e.g., intra-arterial injection, extravasation, suboptimal image due to inadequate count collection, full bladder), and factors associated with interpretation (e.g., normal and abnormal pattern recognition).

In this section, clinical case reviews of some classical pitfalls associated with technical and patient-related factors, and clinical cases of whole-body bone scintigraphy with equivocal diagnosis at presentation, which were correctly diagnosed with additional SPECT/CT or PET/

CT, are presented. Each case provides learning points, specifically aimed at avoidance of technical pitfalls and patient-related factors during the imaging process. The factors for best possible quality and interpretation include: (1) obtaining the relevant clinical information, (2) proper preparation of patients, (3) meticulous positioning of patients and adequate acquisition, (3) familiarity of the normal imaging appearances at different age groups and of normal variants, (4) awareness of technical pitfalls, and (5) knowledge of strengths and limitations of each modality.

43.3.1 Instrument-Related Pitfalls: Improper Photopeak Window Setting

Gamma cameras are equipped with pulse height analyzers which allow the operator to select an optimal range of energies for accepting photons for the bone scintiscan images, which is centered at the photopeak energy of Tc-99m. The typical energy window for Tc-99m bone scan agents is the 10–20% window centered at 140 keV (Naddaf et al. 2004). Co-57 flood sources are used for daily quality control (QC) of field homogeneity, which has an energy peak (122 keV) similar to that of Tc-99m. The energy peak of the gamma camera should be reset after the daily QC and before imaging commences. If this is not done, subsequent scanning using Tc-99m bone scan agents will produce low-resolution images, resulting from loss of photopeak count and increased lower-energy scatter counts (Sokole et al. 2010; Wyngaert et al. 2016) (Fig. 43.1).

43.3.2 Technique-Related Pitfalls: Injection Pitfalls

43.3.2.1 Intra-arterial Injection

The uptake mechanism of bone-seeking agents is influenced not only by osteoblastic activity but also by other factors including blood flow, sympathetic tone, and bone surface area. Intra-arterial

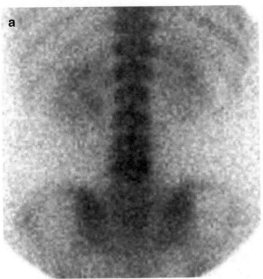

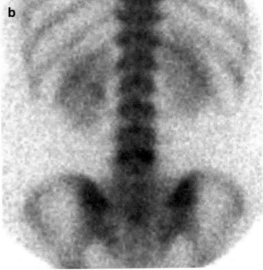

Fig. 43.1 Off-photopeak energy window. (**a**) Initial bone scintiscan image shows diffusely increased soft tissue activity with poor visualization of the bones. The photopeak energy window was found to be centered errone- ously lower at 122 keV, the energy of Co-57. This was corrected. (**b**) Repeat bone scintiscan image taken 10 min later shows marked improvement in image quality

injection may cause increased delivery of bone-seeking agent to the area distal to injection site and results in increased bone uptake. The "glove" phenomenon was previously described in cases with increased uptake in distal forearm bone and soft tissues after intra-arterial injection in the antecubital region. The "sock" pattern was also introduced as an intra-arterial injection artifact of the lower limb (Giammarile et al. 2014). The explanation for hyperfixation mechanism could be secondary to the increased arterial blood flow at the first step of the radiotracer binding mechanism. Intra-arterial injection should be considered when exaggerated diffuse increased bone uptake is seen in an extremity distal to the injection site, especially with no demonstrable history and radiographic findings (Fig. 43.2). Differential diagnosis includes reflex sympathetic dystrophy (Bozkurt and Uğur 2001), frostbite injury, and tourniquet effect (Gunay and Erdogan 2011).

43.3.2.2   Tourniquet Effect

Release of a tourniquet results in increase of blood flow and radiotracer uptake distal to the injection site. This phenomenon is associated with reactive hyperemia induced by transient ischemia during perfusion and blood pool phases of three-phase bone scintigraphy, due to prolonged compression (Kirsh and Tepperman 1985; Lecklitner and Douglas 1987). On delayed bone scans, diffusely increased uptake in the extremity distal to the injection site can be seen in cases where the tourniquet is maintained in place during injection (Weiss and Conway 1984; Orzel et al. 1989; Sohn et al. 2010) (Fig. 43.3). The opposite finding of decreased localization of radionuclide in an extremity can also occur due to tight elastic stockings or elastic bandage wrappings, representing an ischemic condition (Weiss and Conway 1984) (Fig. 43.4).

43.3.2.3   Radiopharmaceutical Extravasation

Extravasation and subcutaneous infiltration of radiopharmaceutical into surrounding soft tissues induce increased activity at the site of injection, which can create a star artifact on bone scintigraphy, if a large amount has leaked (Andrich and Chen 1996). Incidental visualization of the ipsilateral

Fig. 43.2 Intra-arterial injection in a 75-year-old man who had bone scintigraphy performed for evaluation of back pain. (**a**) Whole-body images show intense uptake in the left hand distal to radioisotope injection site in the left wrist. (**b**) On regional images of the hand, increased uptake of the radiopharmaceutical is more prominent on the radial side of the left hand, where the radial artery supplies dominantly. This finding is due to injection of bone-seeking agent into the left radial artery, instead of the vein

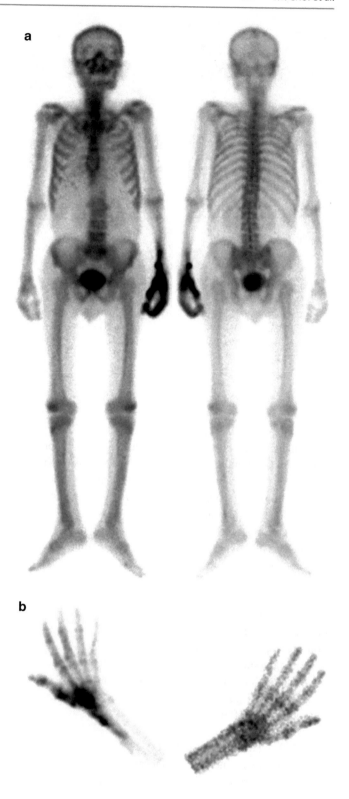

Fig. 43.3 Tourniquet effect in an 82-year-old woman who complained of pain in the chest wall and upper back after several sittings on a massage machine. She was injected in her right antecubital vein after tight binding with a rubber tourniquet. Whole-body bone scintigraphy shows focal uptake lesions in the right and left anterior thoracic cage which were confirmed as acute fractures and another focal uptake at T5–6 level that was revealed as an acute compression fracture. There is incidentally detected diffusely increased uptake in the right arm distal to the right elbow injection site, due to tight binding of the tourniquet

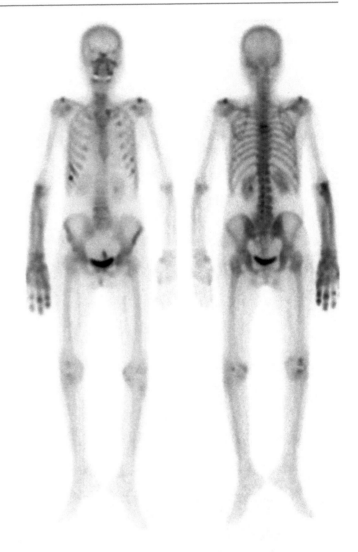

axillary or elbow lymph node has been reported (Ongseng et al. 1995; Shih et al. 2001). The lymphatic system is an accessory route for drainage of interstitial fluid. Large molecular weight substances, which cannot be directly absorbed into capillaries, are readily accommodated by lymphatics and incorporated into the chylous network draining into regional nodes. Tc-99m methylene diphosphonate (MDP) is a large molecular weight substance and therefore is preferentially captured by the lymphatic system. Axillary lymph node uptake should be differentiated from superimposed bony structures by

adding oblique spot views and not be misinterpreted as a pathological focus (Wallis et al. 1987; Ongseng et al. 1995) (Fig. 43.5).

43.3.3 Patient-Related Pitfalls

43.3.3.1 Influence of Recent Nuclear Medicine Study

Unexpected abnormal uptake lesion can occur due to the influence of a recent nuclear medicine study. Prior administration of a higher-energy

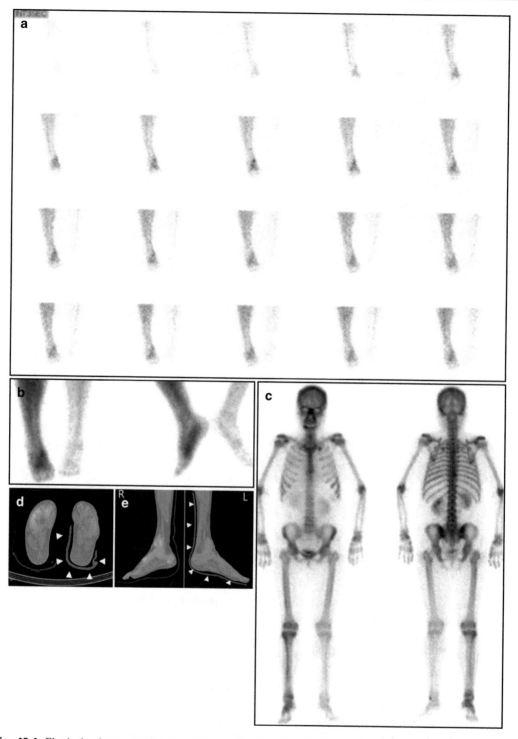

Fig. 43.4 Elastic bandage wrapping in a 52-year-old woman who had pain and tenderness in the lateral malleolar area of the left ankle after a slip and fall. She underwent three-phase bone scintigraphy 11 days after trauma which shows asymmetrical diffusely decreased (**a**) perfusion, (**b**) blood pool activity, and (**c**) bone uptake in the left lower leg. These findings could be present in the chronic phase of complex regional pain syndrome. But the patient's secret was revealed on (**d**, **e**) SPECT/CT images. She was wearing an elastic bandage and short leg cast (*arrowheads*) during three-phase bone scan, with the latter well seen on the (**d**) axial and (**e**) sagittal SPECT/CT images

a

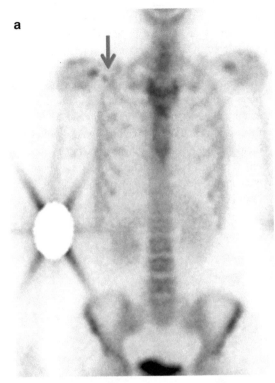

b

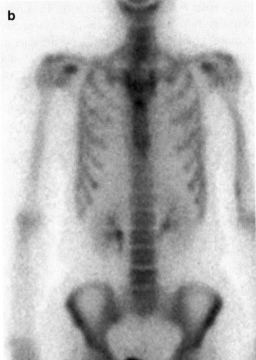

Fig. 43.5 Axillary lymph node uptake of extravasated radiopharmaceutical in a 36-year-old woman who complained of polyarthralgia. (**a**) The star artifact in the right elbow, which resulted from leakage of radiopharmaceutical at the injection site, is masked. There is a focal uptake lesion in right axillary area (*arrow*), indicating axillary lymph node activity, which was newly visualized compared to the (**b**) prior bone scintiscan taken 3 months before. The venous route in the left upper arm can just be traced

radionuclide or of a preceding examination with another Tc-99m radiopharmaceutical that accumulates in an organ could obscure or confound skeletal activity (Wyngaert et al. 2016). Therefore, relevant information that may assist in interpretation of imaging findings, including history of recent nuclear medicine studies, should be checked with the patient before injection of radiopharmaceutical (Donohoe et al. 1996; Wyngaert et al. 2016). In lymphoscintigraphy, which uses very small doses compared to bone scintigraphy, most of the injected colloid material remains at the intradermal or subdermal injection site and could be seen as focal uptake even 48 h after injection. It is postulated that intradermal injection of a small dose of Tc-99m colloid has not been cleared via the kidney or liver within this time period (Fig. 43.6).

43.3.3.2 Attenuation Artifacts

Photon-deficient areas detected on the bone scintigraphy are commonly encountered attenuation artifacts caused by metallic objects external to the patients, such as jewelry, pacemakers, coins in pockets, metallic belt buckles, snaps, zippers, and external breast prosthesis. Therefore, patients should be asked to remove metallic objects, wherever possible before performing the scan (Gnanasegaran et al. 2009) (Fig. 43.7). Photon-deficient areas due to avascular change may be differentiated in some cases (Fig. 43.8).

43.3.3.3 Optimum Timing of Bone Scintiscan After Trauma

Whole-body bone scintigraphy is a highly sensitive modality in the evaluation of fractures, and the majority of fractures will manifest a positive three-phase bone scan immediately. However, potential false-negative results are a concern, because it may take up to a week for the scan to become positive in a small percentage of the elderly patients (Martin 1979; Taylor et al. 2000) (Fig. 43.9).

43.3.3.4 Abnormal Non-osseous Uptake Lesions

Incidentally detected abnormal non-osseous uptake is often noted on whole-body bone scintiscans. True non-osseous findings are usually related to the uri-

nary system (Figs. 43.10 and 43.11). Visualization of other organs can be expected to be associated with dystrophic or metastatic microcalcification (Fig. 43.12), resolving hematoma (Fig. 43.13), rhabdomyolysis, and effusion. Appropriate assessment of the patient's condition and obtaining a relevant medical history, including a review of medications and other imaging studies, will clarify incidental soft tissue findings on the bone scintigraphy (Fig. 43.14) and will be helpful for diagnosis of incidentally detected diseases (Weiner et al. 2001; Loutfi et al. 2003).

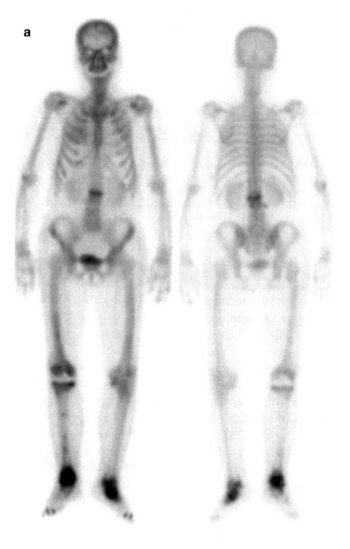

a

Fig. 43.6 Influence of recent nuclear medicine study in a 65-year-old woman who complained of bilateral leg swelling for 3 weeks. She had a 4-year history of rheumatoid arthritis and underwent right total knee replacement 3 months before. (**a**) Whole-body bone scintigraphy and (**b**) regional images show increased uptake lesions in both ankles and left hindfoot. Unexpectedly, focal spotty uptake lesions are noted in 2nd and 3rd MTP joint areas of both feet (**a, b**). There is no demonstrable bone or joint lesion on (**c**) radiographs of both feet. On regional blood pool and bone images (**b**), the definition of lesions is too clear; therefore, artifacts could be considered. The recent past history of the patient was reviewed, and it was found that she underwent (**d**) lymphoscintigraphy 2 days before the whole-body bone scintiscan. (**d, e**) Tc-99m phytate (1 mCi syringe was prepared for each site, residual activity in each syringe was about 0.25 mCi, so nett injected dose was 0.75 mCi) was given. Intradermal injection of such a small dose of Tc-99m colloid could remain after 2 days, because it has not been excreted via the kidney or liver

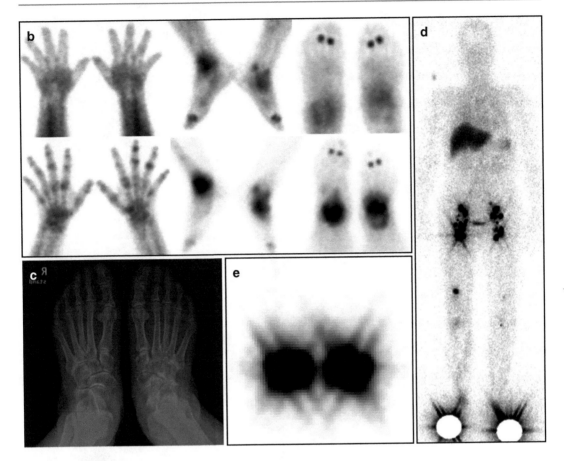

Fig. 43.6 (continued)

Fig. 43.7 Examples of attenuation artifacts. Focal or diffusely decreased uptake associated with attenuation artifact due to (**a**) metallic button (*arrow*), (**b**) coin (*arrow*), and (**c**) sandbag. (**c**) The posterior view (*right image*) of the whole-body bone scintigraphic image of an 18-year-old girl with intestinal lymphoma shows diffusely decreased uptake at L3–L5 vertebral levels, which proved on (**d**, **e**) CT images to be attenuation artifact due to sandbag applied after bone marrow aspiration biopsy

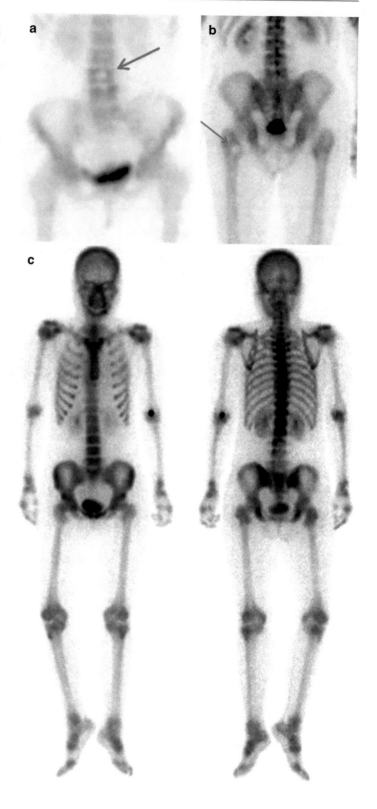

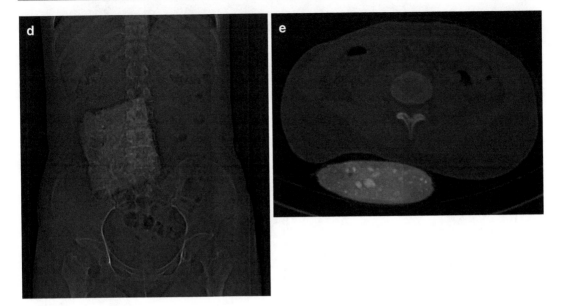

Fig. 43.7 (continued)

Fig. 43.8 Differential diagnosis of photon-deficient lesions in two different patients with similar whole-body bone scintigraphic anterior view images, with each showing a cold defect in the femur. (**a**) 75-year-old man with lung cancer has a focal defect in the left proximal femoral shaft (*arrow*). (**b**) 16-year-old boy has a cold defect in the mid-shaft of the right femur (*arrow*). To distinguish an attenuation artifact from a true lesion, the key is looking carefully at the posterior view images. (**c**) There is no defect in the left proximal femur on the posterior view image of the 75-year-old man, indicating an attenuation artifact (*arrow*), while (**d**) there still a cold defect in the mid-shaft of the femur of the 16-year-old boy (*arrow*) on both anterior and posterior views. (**e**) Radiographs of the 16-year-old boy showed a badly overlapped left femoral shaft fracture; therefore, the (**f**) scintigraphic cold defect (*arrow*) was thought to represent avascular change. (**g**) On follow-up bone scintiscans and radiographs of the 16-year-old boy, cortical bone uptake is seen in the medial femur (*arrows* at POD 2 weeks), matched with periosteal bone formation (*arrow* POD 1.5 months), but there was still a cold defect in the lateral cortex (*arrow* POD 1 week), suggestive of avascular state. After 1.5 years, healed fracture with minimal lateral angulation is noted

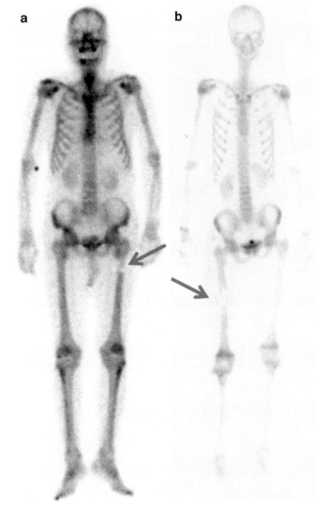

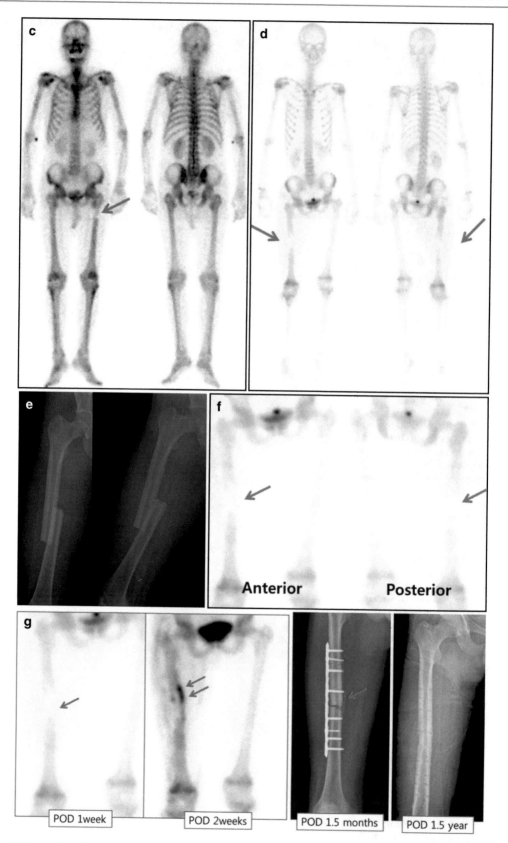

Fig. 43.8 (continued)

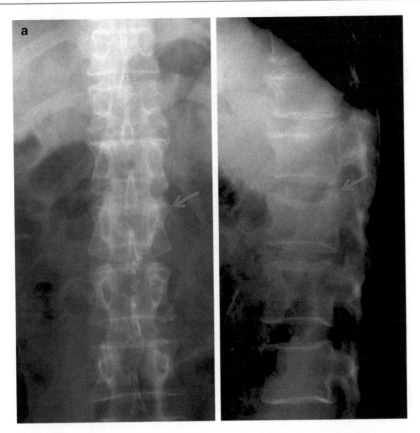

Fig. 43.9 Optimum time of bone scintiscan after trauma was not achieved in a 58-year-old man who had back pain after a slip and fall. (**a**) Radiographs show multiple compression fractures in the lower thoracic and upper lumbar vertebral bodies. L1 vertebra is arrowed. (**b**) Bone scinti-scans obtained after 2 days show subtle uptake at T11-L1 vertebral level (*arrows*). As the patient was concerned about an acute compression fracture, the bone scintiscan was repeated after 1 week. (**c**) Repeat bone scintiscan showed intense uptake at L1 vertebral level (*arrow*), while T11 and T12 vertebrae did not show increased activity compared to initial study. Those findings are suggestive of an acute compression fracture of L1 vertebra and old T11 and T12 compression fractures

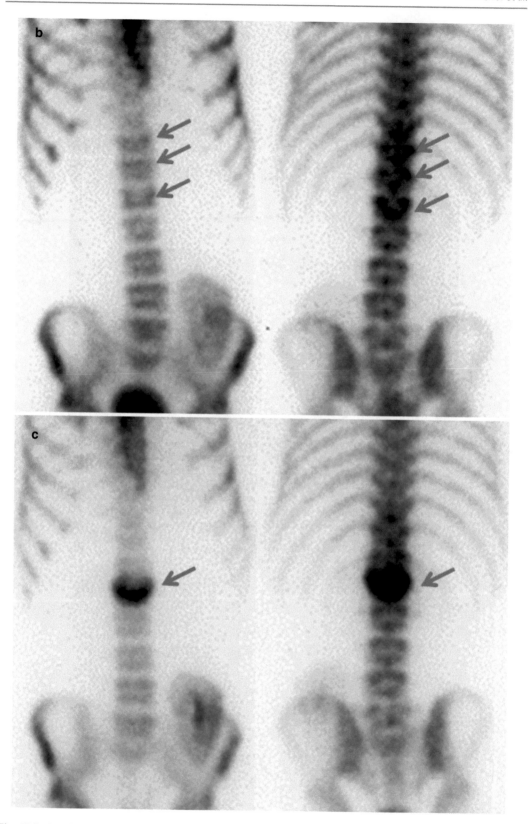

Fig. 43.9 (continued)

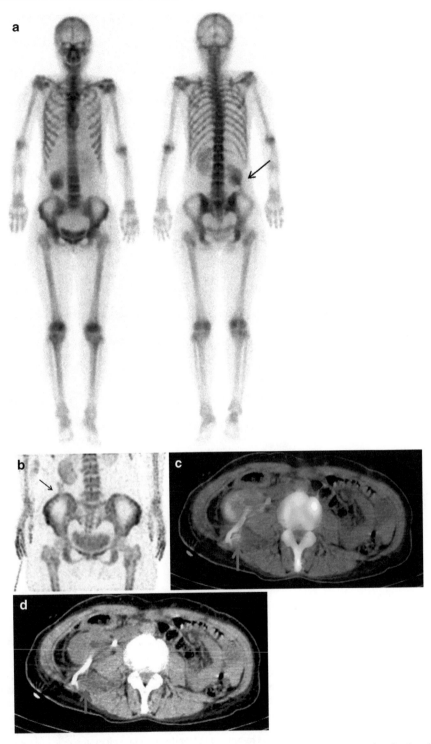

Fig. 43.10 Urinoma due to urine leakage from percutaneous nephrectomy (PCN) catheter in a 50-year-old woman who complained of right pelvic pain for 1 week. She had total gastrectomy due to stomach cancer 8 years previously. Right PCN catheter was inserted 3 weeks before because of right hydronephrosis resulting from periureteral metastasis. (**a**) Whole-body and (**b**) regional bone scintigraphy shows asymmetrical radioactivity retention in the right kidney, with linear increased uptake in the soft tissues (*arrow*), which was suspected to be due to PCN catheter activity. (**c**, **d**) Pelvic SPECT/CT image, taken for evaluation of pelvic pain, show focal radioactivity retention in right back muscle adjacent to the catheter route, which is swollen compared to the contralateral side, due to intramuscular urinoma (*arrow*)

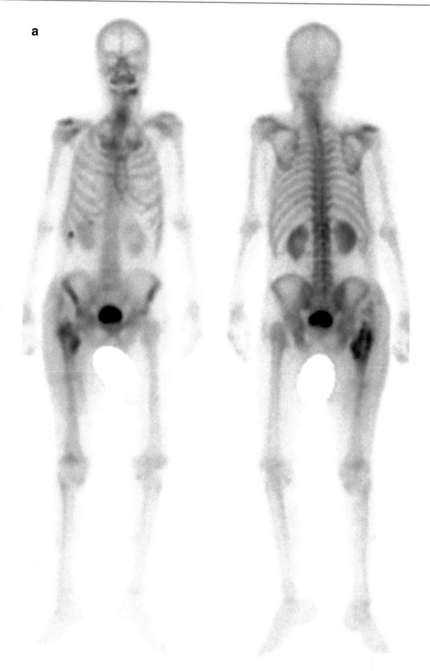

Fig. 43.11 Focal uptake in bladder diverticula of a 79-year-old man who had an operation for right femoral neck fracture. (**a–d**) SPECT/CT was taken for evaluation of vascularity of the right femoral head. There are three incidentally detected hot spots (*arrows*) in the posterior wall of bladder on MIP images (**b, c**), which were not clearly defined on whole-body image (**a**). Tiny calcific densities (*arrow in right CT image*) are scattered in the dependent portion of bladder, and focal radioactivity retention is seen between the calcifications (*arrow in left SPECT/CT image*) (**d**). The lesions were proven to be bladder diverticulum on cystoscopic examination

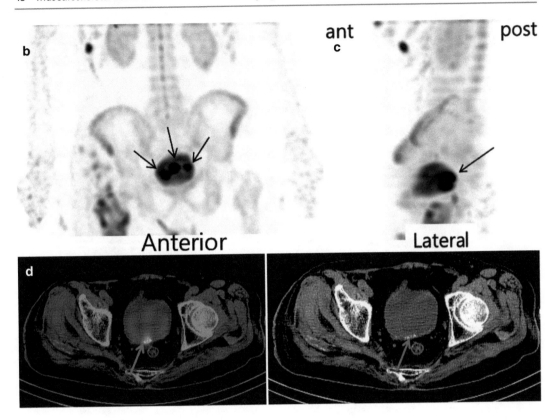

Fig. 43.11 (continued)

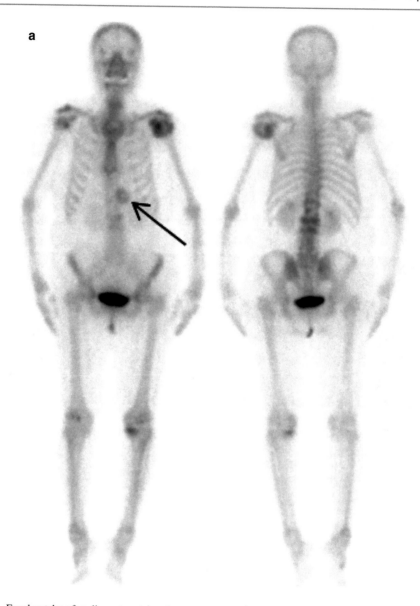

Fig. 43.12 Focal uptake of malignant gastric submucosal tumor incidentally detected on bone scintigraphy in a 73-year-old woman who had left shoulder pain. (**a**) Curvilinear soft tissue uptake (*arrow*) is incidentally noted in the left upper abdomen on the whole-body bone scintiscan. (**b**) Additional SPECT/CT images show uptake in the calcific density of exophytic gastric submucosal mass (*arrows*), suggestive of a gastrointestinal stromal tumor (GIST). (**c**, **d**) Enhanced abdominal CT images, performed for further evaluation, better show details of the calcified mass. Subsequent excision revealed malignant GIST. Careful evaluation of soft tissue uptake enabled early diagnosis of malignant tumor

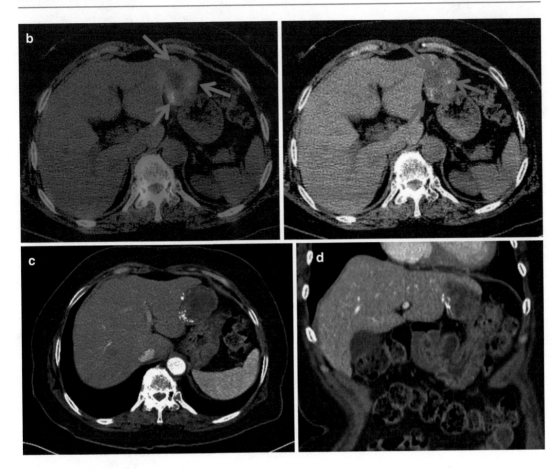

Fig. 43.12 (continued)

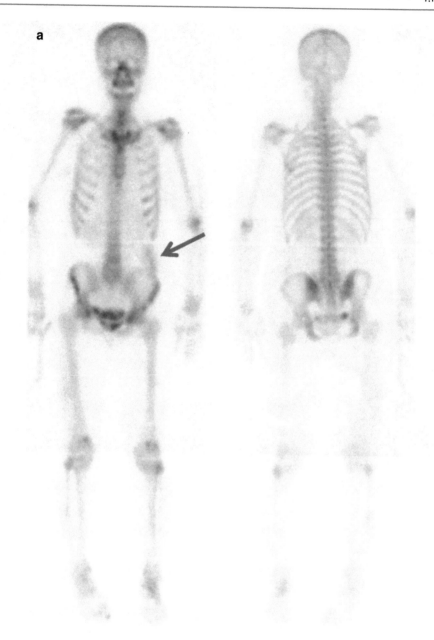

Fig. 43.13 Diffuse uptake in a resolving hematoma due to abdominal wall contusion in a 57-year-old woman. She was hit by a motorcycle the day before and presented with complaints of left hip and elbow pain. Linear increased soft tissue uptake (*arrows*) is noted along the left lower anterior abdominal wall on (**a**) whole-body and (**b**) regional bone scintigraphic images, which was proven to be a resolving hematoma (*arrow*) on (**c**) coronal reformatted CT image of the abdomen

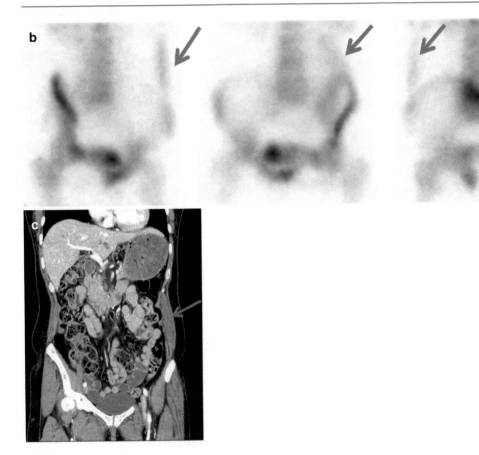

Fig. 43.13 (continued)

Fig. 43.14 Hepatic cyst manifesting as a cold defect in a 66-year-old woman who had intramedullary nailing of both femurs, due to a displaced fracture on the right and atypical fracture on the left. (**a**) Whole-body bone scintiscan taken 10 days after surgery shows a huge cold defect in right upper abdomen seen only on the anterior view image (*arrows*). (**b**) This was shown to be due to a large cyst in right hepatic lobe on CT images. No definite attenuation in the overlying ribs suggests that the cold defect may not be an attenuation artifact but a space-occupying lesion of liver

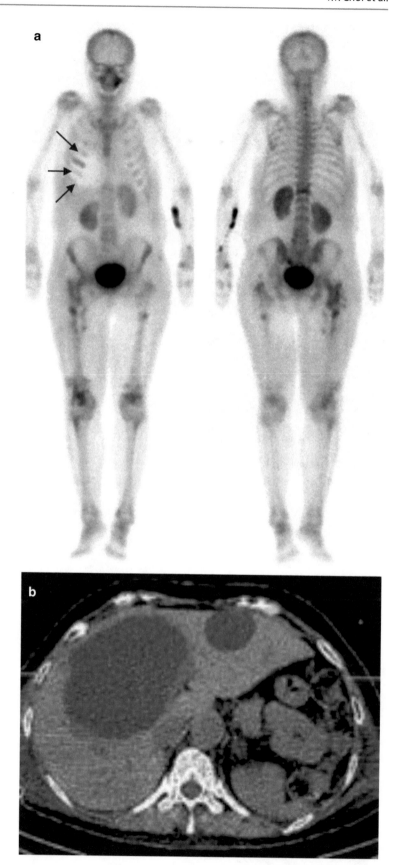

Conclusion

In musculoskeletal nuclear medicine imaging, unexpected results are rare and may occur from many factors. Generally, these unexpected outcomes are not life-threatening, but they cause time delay from repeated examinations, additional cost, and unnecessary radiation exposure to the patient. Other technical errors in radionuclide processing are relatively frequent, along with cross-contamination of different radionuclide vials. In the nuclear medicine department, standard protocols for technician education and awareness, well-maintained devices, and proper easy access to the patient information can reduce many problems. In case of unexpected situations, prepared guidelines may be helpful in explaining errors. Knowledge and recognition of errors, additional safety precautions, and solutions are necessary to prevent same mistakes from occurring again and promote further improvement. In this chapter, many illustrative cases may be useful as a ready reference guide when unexpected scan findings are encountered, and knowledge and awareness can result in the prompt institution of corrective solutions. To achieve high-quality diagnostic nuclear medicine images, details of the patient's history, appropriate management of radionuclides, proper maintenance of imaging device, equipment calibration, correct patient records, and physician's expertise are essential.

References

Andrich MP, Chen CC (1996) Bone scan injection artifacts. Clin Nucl Med 21:260–262

Badawi RD, Marsden PK (1999) Developments in component-based normalization for 3D PET. Phys Med Biol 44:571–594

Bailey DL (1998) Transmission scanning in emission tomography. Eur J Nucl Med 25:774–787

Barrett JF, Keat N (2004) Artifacts in CT: recognition and avoidance. Radiographics 24:1679–1691

Beyer T, Antoch G, Blodgett T et al (2003) Dual-modality PET/CT imaging: the effect of respiratory motion on combined image quality in clinical oncology. Eur J Nucl Med Mol Imaging 30:588–596

Bozkurt MF, Uğur O (2001) Intra-arterial Tc-99m MDP injection mimicking reflex sympathetic dystrophy. Clin Nucl Med 26:154–156

Conti M (2011) Focus on time-of-flight PET: the benefits of improved time resolution. Eur J Nucl Med Mol Imaging 38:1147–1157

Defrise M, Rezaei A, Nuyts J (2012) Time-of-flight PET data determine the attenuation sinogram up to a constant. Phys Med Biol 57:885–899

Delso G, Martinez-Möller A, Bundschuh RA, Nekolla SG, Ziegler SI (2010) The effect of limited MR field of view in MR/PET attenuation correction. Med Phys 37:2804–2812

Dewaraja YK, Ljungberg M, Green AJ et al (2013) MIRD pamphlet No. 24: Guidelines for quantitative 131I SPECT in dosimetry applications. J Nucl Med 54: 2182–2188

Donohoe KJ, Henkin RE, Royal HD et al (1996) Procedure guideline for bone scintigraphy: 1.0. J Nucl Med 37:1903–1906

Eiber M, Martinez-Mo̎ller A, Souvatzoglou M et al (2011) Value of a Dixon-based MR/PET attenuation correction sequence for the localization and evaluation of PET-positive lesions. Eur J Nucl Med Mol Imaging 38:1691–1701

Eiber M, Takei T, Souvatzoglou M et al (2014) Performance of whole body integrated 18F-FDG PET/MR in comparison to PET/CT for evaluation of malignant bone lesions. J Nucl Med 55:191–197

Giammarile F, Mognetti T, Paycha F (2014) Injection artefact displaying "sock" pattern on bone scan: "glove" sign equivalent resulting from bisphosphonate-(99mTc) injection in foot venous system. Eur J Nucl Med Mol Imaging 41:1644–1645

Gnanasegaran G, Cook G, Adamson K, Fogelman I (2009) Patterns, variants, artifacts, and pitfalls in conventional radionuclide bone imaging and SPECT/CT. Semin Nucl Med 39:380–395

Goerres GW, Ziegler SI, Burger C et al (2003) Artifacts at PET and PET/CT caused by metallic hip prosthetic material. Radiology 226:577–584

Gunay EC, Erdogan A (2011) Asymmetrically increased uptake in upper extremities on 99mTc-MDP bone scintigraphy caused by intra-arterial injection: different uptake patterns in three cases. Rev Esp Med Nucl 30:372–375

Kamel EM, Burger C, Buck A, von Schulthess GK, Goerres GW (2003) Impact of metallic dental implants on CT-based attenuation correction in a combined PET/CT scanner. Eur Radiol 13:724–728

Karp JS, Surti S, Daube-Witherspoon ME, Muehllehner G (2008) Benefit of time-of-flight in PET: experimental and clinical results. J Nucl Med 49:462–470

Kim JH, Lee JS, Song IC, Lee DS (2012) Comparison of segmentation-based attenuation correction methods for PET/MRI: evaluation of bone and liver standardized uptake value with oncologic PET/CT data. J Nucl Med 53:1878–1882

Kinahan PE, Townsend DW, Beyer T, Sashin D (1998) Attenuation correction for a combined 3D PET/CT scanner. Med Phys 25:2046–2053

Kirsh JC, Tepperman PS (1985) Assessment of hand blood flow: a modified technique. AJR Am J Roentgenol 144:781–783

Lecklitner ML, Douglas KP (1987) Increased extremity uptake on three-phase bone scans caused by peripherally induced ischemia prior to injection. J Nucl Med 28:108–111

Lee JS, Kim JH (2014) Recent advances in hybrid molecular imaging systems. Semin Musculoskelet Radiol 18:103–122

Loutfi I, Collier BD, Mohammed A (2003) Nonosseous abnormalities on bone scans. J Nucl Med Technol 31:149–153

Marshall HR, Prato FS, Deans L et al (2012) Variable lung density consideration in attenuation correction of whole-body PET/MRI. J Nucl Med 53:977–984

Martin P (1979) The appearance of bone scans following fractures, including immediate and long-term studies. J Nucl Med 20:1227–1231

Mehranian A, Arabi H, Zaidi H (2016) Magnetic resonance imaging-guided attenuation correction in PET/MRI: challenges, solutions, and opportunities. Med Phys 43:1130–1155

Naddaf SY, Collier BD, Elgazzar AH, Magdy MK (2004) Technical errors in planar bone scanning. J Nucl Med Technol 32:148–153

Ongseng F, Goldfarb R, Finestone H (1995) Axillary lymph node uptake of technetium-99m-MDP. J Nucl Med 36:1797–1799

Orzel JA, Rosenbaum DM, Weinberger E (1989) "tourniquet effect" can alter delayed static bone scan. AJR Am J Roentgenol 152:896

Osman MM, Cohade C, Nakamoto Y, Wahl RL (2003) Respiratory motion artifacts on PET emission images obtained using CT attenuation correction on PET-CT. Eur J Nucl Med Mol Imaging 30:603–606

Rezaei A, Defrise M, Bal G et al (2012) Simultaneous reconstruction of activity and attenuation in time-of-flight PET. IEEE Trans Med Imaging 31:2224–2233

Schramm G, Langner J, Hofheinz F et al (2013) Influence and compensation of truncation artifacts in MR-based attenuation correction in PET/MR. IEEE Trans Med Imaging 32:2056–2063

Seo Y, Mari C, Hasegawa BH (2008) Technological development and advances in single-photon emission computed tomography/computed tomography. Semin Nucl Med 38:177–198

Shih WJ, Collins J, Kiefer V (2001) Visualization in the ipsilateral lymph nodes secondary to extravasation of a bone-imaging agent in the left hand: a case report. J Nucl Med Technol 29:154–155

Sohn MH, Lim ST, Jeong YJ et al (2010) Abnormally increased uptake on bone scintigraphy in the long bone proximal to a tourniquet: an injection artifact. Clin Nucl Med 35:349–350

Sokole EB, Plachcinska A, Britten A et al (2010) Routine quality control recommendations for nuclear medicine instrumentation. Eur J Nucl Med Mol Imaging 37:662–671

Taylor A, Schuster DM, Alazraki N (2000) The skeletal system. In: A clinician's guide to nuclear medicine, 2nd edn. Society of Nuclear Medicine, Reston, pp 209–229

Townsend DW (2008) Dual-modality imaging: combining anatomy and function. J Nucl Med 49:938–955

Vandenberghe S, Marsden PK (2015) PET-MRI: a review of challenges and solutions in the development of integrated multimodality imaging. Phys Med Biol 60:R115–R154

Wallis JW, Fisher S, Wahl RL (1987) 99mTc-MDP uptake by lymph nodes following tracer infiltration: clinical and laboratory evaluation. Nucl Med Commun 8:357–363

Weiner GM, Jenicke L, Muller V, Bohuslavizki KH (2001) Artifacts and non-osseous uptake in bone scintigraphy. Imaging reports of 20 cases. Radiol Oncol 35:185–191

Weiss SC, Conway JJ (1984) An injection technique artifact. J Nucl Med Technol 12:10–12

Wyngaert T, Strobel K, Kampen W et al (2016) The EANM practice guidelines for bone scintigraphy. Eur J Nucl Med Mol Imaging 43:1723–1738

Yoo HJ, Lee JS, Lee JM (2015) Integrated whole body MR/PET: where are we? Korean J Radiol 16:32–49

Zaidi H, Hasegawa B (2003) Determination of the attenuation map in emission tomography. J Nucl Med 44:291–315